UNDERSTANDING ANESTHESIA EQUIPMENT

Construction, Care and Complications

THIRD EDITION

UNDERSTANDING ANESTHESIA EQUIPMENT

Construction, Care and Complications

THIRD EDITION

Jerry A. Dorsch, M.D.

*Mayo Clinic
Jacksonville, Florida*

Susan E. Dorsch, M.D.

*St. Vincent's Medical Center
Jacksonville, Florida*

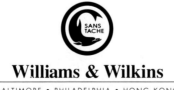

Williams & Wilkins

BALTIMORE • PHILADELPHIA • HONG KONG
LONDON • MUNICH • SYDNEY • TOKYO

A WAVERLY COMPANY

Editor: David C. Retford
Project Managers: Marjorie Kidd Keating, Kathleen Courtney Millet
Copy Editor: Candace B. Levy
Designer: Norman W. Och
Illustration Planner: Wayne Hubbel

Copyright © 1994
Williams & Wilkins
428 East Preston Street
Baltimore, Maryland 21202, USA

Accurate indications, adverse reactions, and dosage schedules for drugs are provided in this book, but it is possible that they may change. The reader is urged to review the package information data of the manufacturers of the medications mentioned.

Printed in the United States of America

First Edition 1975
Second Edition 1984

Library of Congress Cataloging in Publication Data

Dorsch, Jerry A., 1941–
    Understanding anesthesia equipment : construction, care and complications / Jerry
A. Dorsch, Susan E. Dorsch. — 3rd ed.
      p.   cm.
    Includes bibliographical references and index.
    ISBN 0-683-02616-X
    1. Anesthesiology—Apparatus and instruments.   I. Dorsch, Susan E., 1942–
II. Title.
    [DNLM: 1. Anesthesiology—instrumentation. WO 240 D717u 1994]
RD78.8.D67 1994
617.9′6′028—dc20
DNLM/DLC
for Library of Congress
                                         93-28417
                                           CIP

93 94 95 96 97
1 2 3 4 5 6 7 8 9 10

This book is dedicated to all our fellow anesthesia personnel who are

GAINING understanding
SHARPENING their skill
IMPROVING patient care
VOLUNTEERING their services
STRIVING to improve patient care in developing countries
PRESERVING our heritage
CONDUCTING research
INVENTING new devices
ORGANIZING meetings
SERVING on committees
ALERTING us to dangers
EDITING journals
CLEANING equipment
UPDATING their knowledge
LEARNING from mistakes
MAINTAINING their idealism
TRAINING other personnel
PROTECTING the environment
MAKING more efficient use of resources
PROMOTING disease prevention
DEVELOPING new concepts
GIVING lectures
PARTICIPATING in politics
LEADING societies
WRITING books and articles
REVIEWING articles
MAINTAINING apparatus

and CELEBRATING more than 150 years of providing relief from pain
for patients all over the planet.

Preface to the Third Edition

When updating a textbook, it is always exciting to discover just how much a subject has advanced. Since the second edition was published in 1984, there have been many changes in anesthesia equipment and much new information has become available. Our goals in writing this edition were to update information on the subjects discussed in previous editions and to cover new and important subjects.

Subjects covered in previous editions, including cylinders, hospital pipelines, anesthesia machines, breathing systems, control of trace gas airways, laryngoscopes, tracheal tubes, equipment checking and maintenance, and cleaning and sterilization have been updated and enlarged. Sections on oxygen concentrators, the laryngeal mask, and double-lumen and endobronchial tubes have been added.

Nonrebreathing valves are seldom used for anesthesia at present but are used frequently in resuscitation devices. Accordingly, we eliminated the chapter on nonrebreathing valves and replaced it with one on manual resuscitators.

Humidification has taken on more importance as longer general anesthetics are being undertaken. We have chosen to underscore the importance of various means of providing humidification by discussing the subject in a separate chapter.

The most dramatic changes in anesthesia equipment since the second edition have been the introduction of new vigilance aids and improvement in existing ones. Two chapters have been devoted to these. Vigilence aids have been judged so important that the specialty has established practice guidelines that indicate what parameters need to be measured and the technologies to be used to accomplish this end. Never before has a specialty been so specific about the standard of care.

Another new chapter in this edition is anesthesia ventilators. There has been a transformation in ventilators in recent years with increased complexity and integration into the anesthesia machine.

Our aim in writing the third edition of *Understanding Anesthesia Equipment* was to bring together knowledge of commonly used anesthesia equipment and the problems associated with their use. It should be especially helpful to anesthesia residents and student CRNAs, but it is our hope that even the most experienced anesthesiologist and CRNAs will find some pearls. One only needs to look at the present-day anesthesia machine to be impressed by complexity never dreamed of in past versions. While new equipment seems unduly complex, with proper understanding it can be very friendly.

A trend that has been especially gratifying to us is the increased interest in equipment as a subject. This is evident in the formation of the Society for Technology in Anesthesia and the number of papers on equipment presented at anesthesia meetings. The *Journal of Clinical Monitoring* is in large part concerned with anesthesia equipment. Equipment has become a basic science in the study of anesthesia. We hope this book will stir up further interest.

Preface to the First Edition

As in most areas of medicine the anesthesiologist and nurse anesthetist are finding it necessary to rely more and more upon increasingly sophisticated equipment. While this increased reliability allows the practitioner more flexibility in technique and more accuracy, it also requires a thorough understanding of the equipment. The responsibility of the practitioner for the safe and efficient performance of his equipment should be a fundamental consideration in his care for patients.

Most anesthesia equipment does not come with an instruction manual, or if it does, it is soon lost in a busy department. Most general anesthesia textbooks cover some pieces of equipment, often in a fair degree of detail. However, components are often treated individually with no attempt to bring them together into a comprehensive whole. A working knowledge of one's equipment, therefore, must usually come from practice or be imparted by those with experience in its use. Unfortunately, this experience is usually incomplete and lacking in true understanding.

This book has been written to fulfill a need to inform practitioners in anesthesia about their equipment. The authors feel that an understanding of commonly used equipment is not prevalent and this lack causes incorrect selection and use. Accordingly, we have selected for discussion the equipment about which the least information is readily available in the literature. Equipment which has been covered well in other books, e.g., ventilators, monitors, etc., has not been included. While we feel that all practitioners of anesthesia will be benefited by it, it should be especially useful to the resident anesthesiologist or student nurse anesthetist who is faced with a bewildering assortment of strange gadgets.

A final word of caution should be issued to the readers. Proper use of equipment is but one facet in the safe administration of anesthesia. There is always a danger that attention to the equipment may replace attention to the patient. Even with the finest equipment, vigilance is still necessary to prevent accidents that result in patient mortality and morbidity. Horton summed it up very well: "The value of an adequate physical environment is not that it makes vigilance unnecessary, but that it makes it effective."*

---

*National Fire Protection Association: Recommended safe practice for hospital operating rooms. Bulletin No. 56, July, 1956.

Acknowledgments

The authors wish to express their sincere thanks to the many people whose help made this text possible. We have had a great deal of assistance from the equipment manufacturers who have supplied pictures and information on their products. Credits have been included with their pictures.

Although it is impossible to list all the individuals who have helped us, we would like to recognize David Tufenkjian, Mark Peterson, Joseph Condurso, William Stewart, James Willick, Renee Johnson, CRNA, and Paul Baumgart who have been especially helpful in providing needed information.

Special thanks is due to Dr. Neil Feinglass and Dr. A. I. J. Brain for reviewing manuscripts.

Our most profound gratitude is extended to Billy Atkins who serviced our computers. Day or night, he was always prompt.

Special thanks to Barbara Murphy who provided a place to work during the storm of the century in March 1993.

Literature searches and reprints were furnished by the Borland Medical Library of Jacksonville.

Finally, we could never have produced this book without the superb talent and professional expertise of Duncan Sawyer, who was never too busy to help and did such a great job taking photographs.

Contents

Chapter 1

Medical Gas Cylinders and Containers

Definitions

PSIA, PSIG, PSI

Psi stands for pounds per square inch. *Psig* stands for pounds per square inch gauge, which is the difference between the measured pressure and surrounding atmospheric pressure. Most gauges are constructed to read 0 at atmospheric pressure. *Psia* stands for pounds per square inch absolute. Absolute pressure is based on a 0 reference point, the perfect vacuum. Psia is psig plus the local atmospheric pressure. For example, at sea level we are at 0 psig, but we are at 14.7 psia.

COMPRESSED GAS

A compressed gas is defined as "any material or mixture having in the container an absolute pressure exceeding 40 psi at 70°F or, regardless of the pressure at 70°F, having an absolute pressure exceeding 104 psi at 130°F or any liquid having a vapor pressure exceeding 40 psia at 100°F" (1).

NONLIQUEFIED COMPRESSED GAS

A nonliquefied compressed gas is a gas that does not liquefy at ordinary terrestrial temperatures and under pressures that range up to 2000 to 2500 psig (13,789 to 17,237 kPa) (1). Examples include oxygen, nitrogen, air, and helium. These gases do become liquids at very low temperatures, when they are generally referred to as cryogenic liquids (1).

LIQUEFIED COMPRESSED GAS

A liquefied compressed gas is a gas that becomes liquid to a very large extent in containers at ordinary temperatures and at pressures from 25 to 2500 psig (172.4 to 17,237 kPa) (1). Examples include nitrous oxide and carbon dioxide.

MEDICAL GAS CYLINDER (2)

A medical gas cylinder is a tank containing a high-pressure gas or gas mixture at a pressure that may be in excess of 2000 psig.

MEDICAL GAS CONTAINER (2)

A medical gas container is a low-pressure, vacuum-insulated vessel containing gas(es) in liquid form.

INTERNATIONAL SYSTEM OF UNITS (SI UNITS)

The SI system of metric units is an attempt to standardize systems of measurement used by different countries throughout the world. Table 1.1 gives some SI units, their equivalent U.S. units, and conversion factors.

Regulatory Agencies and Industry Standards

All those who produce, supply, transport or use, medical gases must comply with a variety of safety regulations promulgated and enforced by agencies at the federal, state, provincial, and local levels of government.

Medical gases must meet the purity specifications described in the *Pharmacopoeia of the United States* or *National Formulary.* They are also subject to regulation by the Food and Drug Administration.

The Department of Transportation (DOT) and Transport Canada (TC) have published requirements for the manufacturing, marking, labeling, filling, qualification, transportation, storage, handling, maintenance, requalification, and disposition of medical gas cylinders and containers. U.S. states and Canadian provinces vary widely in their regulations for compressed gases (1). In addition, many local governments have regulations that apply to compressed gases.

The U.S. government regulates matters affecting the safety and health of employees in all industries through the Department of Labor and the Occupational Safety and Health Act (OSHA). The National Fire Protection Association (NFPA), the Compressed Gas Association (CGA), and the Canadian Standards Association (CSA) have published a number of standards for safe practices. Although termed *voluntary,* many regulatory agencies have made adherence to these mandatory.

Table 1.1. U.S. and SI Units

Category	U.S. Unit	Multiplied by	SI Metric Unit
Pressure	lb/in.^{2}(psi)	6.894757	kPa
Pressure	kg/cm^2	98.06650	kPa
Pressure	atm	101.325	kPa
Temperature	F	(F − 32)/1.8	C^a
Density	lb/cu ft	16.01846	kg/m^3
Volume	cu ft	0.02831685	m^3
Specific volume	cu ft/lb	0.06242796	m^3/kg
Heat	Btu/lb	2.326	kJ/kg
Heat	Btu/cu ft	37.25895	kJ/m^3
Heat	Btu/gal	278.7163	kJ/m^3
Specific heat	Btu/(lb)(F)	4.1868	kJ/(kg)(C)
Mass	lb	0.4535924	kg
Length	inch	0.0254	m
Length	foot	0.3048	m
Length	mile	1.609344	km

^{a}The recommended SI unit of temperature is the degree Kelvin (K), but degree Celsius (C) values are acceptable for commonly used temperature measurements. A degree difference on the Celsius scale is the same as a degree difference on the Kelvin scale. 0 K equals −273.15 C.

Medical Gas Cylinders

COMPONENTS

Body (3,4)

Most medical gas cylinders (tanks) are constructed of steel, with various alloys added for strength. In recent years cylinders made from aluminum have become available. These are especially useful when anesthesia is administered in a magnetic resonance imaging (MRI) environment. Cylinders have flat bottoms so that they may stand on end. The other end tapers into a neck that is fitted with screw threads for attachment of the cylinder valve.

Valve (Spindle Valve)

Cylinders are filled and discharged through a valve that is attached to the neck by means of a tapered thread. The valve, which is made of bronze or brass, is an integral part of the cylinder and should be removed only during testing or maintenance of the cylinder.

Port

The port is the point of exit for the gas. It should be protected in transit by a covering. When installing a small cylinder on an anesthesia machine, it is important not to mistake the port for the conical depression on the opposite side of the valve, which is designed to receive the retaining screw on the yoke. Screwing the retaining screw into the port may damage the port and/or the index pins. Damage to the port may prevent a tight seal.

Stem

Each valve contains a stem, or shaft, that closes the valve by sealing against the seat. When the valve is opened the stem is moved upward, allowing gas to flow to the port.

Packed Valve. Most cylinder valves are of the packed type (Fig. 1.1). In these, the stem is sealed by a resilient packing such as Teflon, which prevents leakage around the threads. This type of valve is also called direct acting, because turning the stem causes the seat to turn. In the large cylinder valve, the force is transmitted by means of a driver

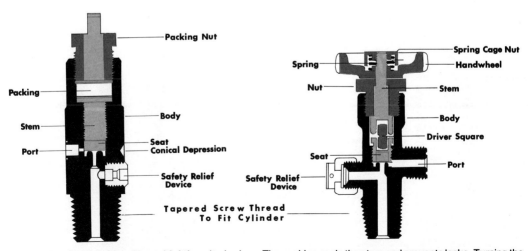

Figure 1.1. Small **(left)** and large **(right)** packed valves. The packing seals the stem and prevents leaks. Turning the stem on the large cylinder valve counterclockwise causes the seat to turn in its thread, opening the valve. From drawings furnished by Puritan-Bennett Corp.

square (Fig. 1.1, *right*). This type of valve is capable of withstanding high pressures.

Diaphragm Valve. In the diaphragm valve (Fig. 1.2), the stem is separated from the seat. A flexible diaphragm seals the opening to the internal parts. Turning the stem raises or lowers the diaphragm.The downward force of the stem is opposed by a spring acting on the seat. Turning the stem clockwise lowers the diaphragm, which, in turn, lowers the seat and closes the valve. When the stem is turned counterclockwise, the diaphragm is raised and the force of the spring raises the seat, opening the valve. This type of valve has the following advantages (5):

1. It can be opened fully using a one-half to three-quarters turn, whereas the packed valve requires two or three full turns.
2. The seat does not turn and is therefore less likely to leak.
3. No stem leakage can occur because of the diaphragm.

For these reasons, the diaphragm type is generally preferable when the pressures are relatively low and when no leaks can be allowed, such as with flammable gases. It is somewhat more expensive than the packed type.

Handle or Handwheel

A handle or handwheel must be used to open or close a cylinder valve. It is turned counterclockwise to open the valve and clockwise to close it. This causes the stem to turn. The large cylinder valve has a permanently attached handwheel that uses a spring and nut to hold it firmly in place (see Figs. 1.1 and 1.2).

A handle is used to open a small cylinder valve. These come in a variety of shapes (Fig. 1.3). Some handles, such as the one in the middle of Figure 1.3, have a hexagonal opening that fits the packing (gland) nut of the valve (see Fig. 1.1). This handle may be used to tighten the nut should it become loose. A hazard associated with this handle is that a person unacquainted with cylinders could loosen the packing nut under the mistaken impression that he or she was opening the valve. This could cause the valve stem and retaining nut to shoot off the cylinder with great force (6).

A ratchet-type handle is supplied with certain anesthesia machines (see Fig. 1.3). After the cylinder is opened, the handle must be removed, inverted, and reapplied to close the cylinder. A burn from freezing nitrous oxide during these maneuvers has been reported (7).

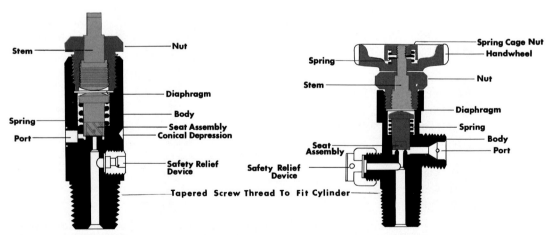

Figure 1.2. Small **(left)** and large **(right)** diaphragm valves. Turning the handle clockwise forces the diaphragm downward and closes the seat. Upon opening the valve, the upward force of the spring opens the seat. From drawings furnished by Puritan-Bennett Corp.

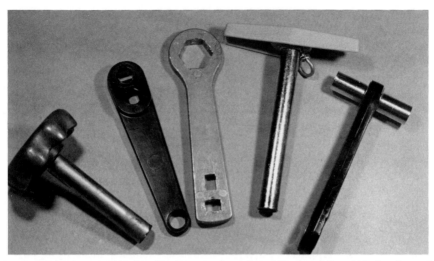

Figure 1.3. Small cylinder valve handles. The hexagonal opening at the top of the middle handle can be used to tighten the packing nut on the cylinder valve. A ratchet handle is at the right. After a cylinder has been opened, this handle must be removed, inverted and reapplied to close the cylinder valve.

A good practice is to chain a handle to each anesthesia machine or other apparatus for which it may be needed.

Pressure Relief Device (1)

The pressure relief device is also called the safety relief device and safety device. Every cylinder is fitted with a device that lets gas escape if the pressure of the enclosed gas increases to a dangerous level.

Rupture Disc

The rupture disc (frangible disc or burst disc) is a nonreclosing device with a disc held against an orifice (Fig. 1.4). When the predetermined pressure is reached, the disc ruptures and allows the cylinder contents to be discharged. The pressure opening is the orifice against which the disc functions. The rated burst pressure is the pressure at which the disc is designed to burst. It is determined by the material, thickness and shape of the disc, and the diameter of the pressure opening. This device is used on some air, carbon dioxide, carbon dioxide–oxygen, helium, nitrous oxide, helium-oxygen, nitrogen, and oxygen cylinders. It protects against excess pressure as a result of high temperatures or overfilling.

Fusible Plug

The fusible plug is a thermally operated, nonreclosing pressure-relief device with the plug held against the discharge channel. It offers protection from excessive pressure caused by a high temperature but not from improper charging practices. The yield temperature is the temperature at which the fusible material becomes sufficiently soft to extrude from its holder so that cylinder contents are discharged. A fusible plug with

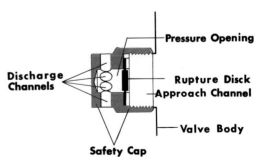

Figure 1.4. Rupture disc device. When the rated burst pressure is exceeded, the disc ruptures and gas flows from the approach channel into the pressure opening and to atmosphere through the discharge channels. From Anonymous. Frangible disc safety device assembly. Pamphlet S-3. New York: Compressed Gas Society, p. 4.

a yield temperature of 212°F is sometimes used on certain nitrogen and air cylinders.

Combination Rupture Disc/Fusible Plug

A combination rupture disc/fusible plug can be used to prevent bursting at a predetermined pressure unless the temperature is high enough to cause yielding of the fusible material. Such a device with a yield temperature of 165°F may be found on cylinders of air, oxygen, nitrogen, nitrous oxide, helium, helium-oxygen mixtures, carbon dioxide, and carbon dioxide–oxygen mixtures. Because it functions only in the presence of both excessive heat and excessive pressure, it does not offer protection against overpressure from improper filling.

Pressure Relief Valve

The pressure relief valve (Fig. 1.5) is a spring-loaded device designed to reclose and prevent discharge of cylinder contents after normal conditions have been restored. The set pressure, at which it will start to discharge, is marked on the valve. A pressure relief valve may be found on air, helium, oxygen, nitrogen, helium-oxygen mixture, carbon dioxide, and carbon dioxide–oxygen mixture cylinders with up to 500 psig charging pressure. Pressure relief valves are generally more susceptible to leakage than rupture discs or fusible plugs (1).

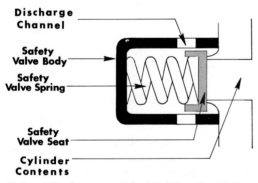

Figure 1.5. Pressure relief valve. When the set pressure is exceeded, the pressure in the cylinder forces the spring to the left and gas flows around the safety valve seat to the discharge channel. From a drawing furnished by Ohmeda, a division of the BOC Group, Inc.

Conical Depression

Above the safety relief device on small cylinders is the conical depression that receives the retaining screw of the yoke (Fig. 1.6; see also Figs 1.1 and 1.2). It must be distinguished from the safety relief device. If the retaining screw is tightened into the safety relief device, the device may be damaged and the cylinder contents may escape (8,9).

Noninterchangeable Safety Systems (1)

With widespread use of cylinders containing different gases, a potential hazard is connection of a cylinder to equipment intended for a different gas. To help solve this problem, color coding was developed; however this did not give complete protection against human error. Through the cooperation of the CGA and others, two noninterchangeable systems were developed. Both of these systems are located between the cylinder valve and the regulator and should not be confused with the Diameter Index Safety System which is on the low pressure side of the regulator and will be discussed in Chapter 2.

Pin Index Safety System

The Pin Index Safety System is used on size E and smaller cylinders. It consists of two pins projecting from the inner surface of the yoke and so positioned as to fit into two corresponding holes in the cylinder valve (Fig. 1.7; see also Fig. 1.6). Combinations of pins assigned to gases or gas mixtures in anesthesia are shown in Table 1.2. Unless the pins and holes are aligned, the port will not seat against the washer of the yoke. It is possible for a yoke without pins to receive any cylinder valve, but ordinarily it is not possible for an undrilled cylinder valve to be placed in a yoke containing pins.

Valve Outlet Connections for Large Cylinders

Size M and larger cylinders are equipped with valves that have threaded outlet connections. The essential components are shown

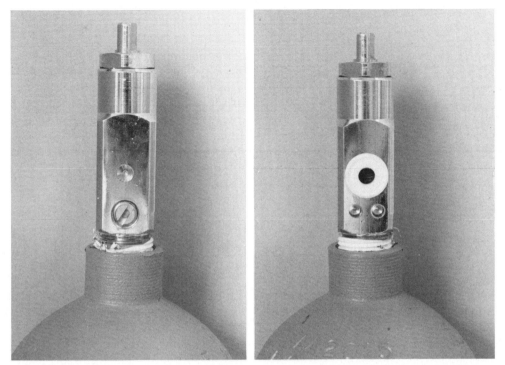

Figure 1.6. Small cylinder valves. **Left,** the conical depression is above the pressure relief device. **Right,** the port is above the Pin Index Safety System holes. A washer is over the port.

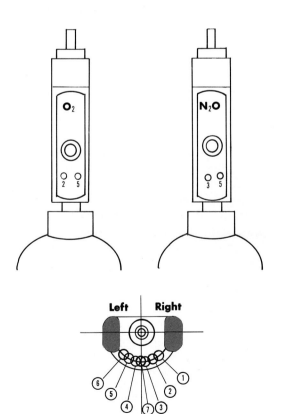

Figure 1.7. Pin Index Safety System. The **bottom** figure shows the six index positions as seen on the yoke. The pins are 4 mm in diameter and 6 mm long, except for pin 7, which is slightly thicker. The seven hole positions are on the circumference of a circle of $^9/_{16}$ inch radius centered on the port.

Table 1.2. Pin Index System

Gas	Index Pins
Oxygen	2, 5
Nitrous oxide	3, 5
Cyclopropane	3, 6
O_2-CO_2 (CO_2 < 7.5%)	2, 6
O_2-CO_2 (CO_2 > 7.5%)	1, 6
O_2-He (He > 80.5%)	4, 6
O_2-He (He < 80.5%)	2, 4
Air	1, 5
Nitrogen	1, 4
N_2O-O (N_2O 47.5–52.5%)	7

in Figure 1.8. The cylinder valve has a threaded outlet. When the threads of this outlet mesh with those of the nut, the nut may be tightened by turning it clockwise, causing the nipple to seat against the valve outlet. In this way the gas channel of the valve is aligned with the channel of the nipple. The outlets and connections are indexed by diameter, thread size, right- or left-handed threading, external or internal threading, and the nipple-seat design.

SIZES

Historically, gas suppliers have classified cylinders using a letter code, with A being the smallest. Table 1.3 gives the approximate di-

mensions and capacities for some commonly used cylinders. Cylinder sizes and letter designations have varied over the years and between suppliers (2). Size E is the cylinder most commonly used on anesthesia machines and for patient transport and resuscitation. Aluminum cylinders are shorter and have a larger diameter than steel cylinders (3).

CONTENTS AND PRESSURE

As illustrated in Figure 1.9, in a cylinder containing a nonliquefied gas, the pressure declines steadily as the contents are withdrawn. Therefore, the pressure can be used to measure the cylinder contents. The weight of the cylinder can also be used to estimate contents.

In a cylinder containing a liquefied gas, the pressure depends on the vapor pressure of the liquid and is not an indication of the amount of gas remaining in the cylinder as long as the contents are partly in the liquid phase. The pressure remains nearly constant (if the temperature remains constant) until all the liquid has evaporated, after which the pressure declines until the cylinder is exhausted. Weight can be used to determine

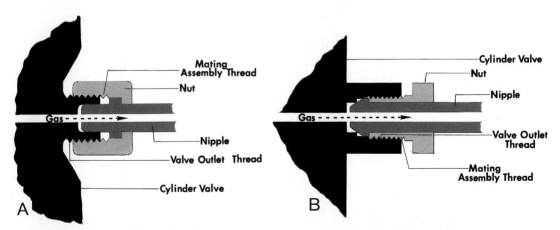

Figure 1.8. Valve outlet connections for large cylinders. **Left,** the valve outlet thread is external, i.e., the threads are on the outside of the cylinder valve outlet and the nut screws over the valve outlet. **Right,** the valve outlet thread is internal, so that the nut screws into the outlet. The specification for cylinder connections are often shown as in the following example for oxygen: 0.903-14-RH EXT. The first number is the diameter in inches of the cylinder outlet. The next number gives the number of threads per inch. The letters following this indicate whether the threads are right hand or left hand and external or internal. Redrawn courtesy of the Compressed Gas Association.

Table 1.3.   Typical Medical Gas Cylinders, Volumes, Weights, and Pressures

Cylinder Size	Cylinder Dimensions (O.D. × Length in inches)	Empty Cylinder Weight (lb)	Capacities and Pressures (at 70°F)	Air	Carbon Dioxide	Helium	Nitrous Oxide	Oxygen	Nitrogen	Helium-Oxygen Mixtures[a]	Carbon Dioxide–Oxygen Mixtures[a]
B	3½ × 13	5	liters		370			200			
			psig		838			1,900			
D	4½ × 17	11	liters	375	940	300	940	400	370	300	400
			psig	1,900	838	1,600	745	1,900	1,900	+	+
E	4¼ × 26	14	liters	625	1,590	500	1,590	660	610	500	660
			psig	1,900	838	1,600	745	1,900	1,900	+	+
M	7 × 43	63	liters	2,850	7,570	2,260	7,570	3,450	3,200	2,260	3,000
			psig	1,900	838	1,600	745	2,200	2,200	+	+
G	8½ × 51	97	liters	5,050	12,300	4,000	13,800			4,000	5,300
			psig	1,900	838	1,600	745			+	+
H	9¼ × 51	119	liters	6,550		6,000	15,800	6,900[b]	6,400		
			psig	2,200		2,200	745	2,200[b]	2,200		

[a]The + indicates that the pressures of these mixed gases will vary according to the composition of the mixture.
[b]7,800-liter cylinders at 2,490 psig are available.

cylinder contents regardless of the state of gas in the cylinder.

During common use, the temperature is not likely to remain constant. Evaporation of the liquid requires energy in the form of heat, which is supplied mainly by the liquid in the cylinder. This results in cooling. As the temperature falls, the vapor pressure of the liquid also falls, so that a progressive fall in pressure accompanies the release of gas from the cylinder at a constant flow (10). If the outer surface of a cylinder that contains liquefied gas becomes cold as gas is discharged, this is an indication there is residual liquid left in the cylinder (10). If liquid remains when withdrawal stops, cylinder pressure will slowly increase to its original level as the temperature rises.

TESTING (1)

A cylinder must be inspected and subjected to internal hydrostatic pressure testing at least every 5 years or, with a special permit, up to every 10 years. The test date (month and year) must be permanently stamped on the cylinder.

Each cylinder must pass an internal and external visual check. Doubtful containers must be returned to the supplier. Cylinders are checked for leaks and retention of structural strength by testing to a minimum of 1.66 (1.5 in Canada) times their service pressures. The service pressure is the maximum pressure to which the cylinder may be filled at 70°F. Table 1.4 gives the service pressures for gases commonly used in anesthesia. A cylinder that leaks or expands more than the allowable limit must be rejected.

FILLING (1)

If a cylinder containing gas under a safe pressure at normal temperatures is subjected to higher temperatures, the pressure may increase to a dangerous level. To prevent this, the DOT has drawn up regulations limiting the amount of gas a cylinder may contain.

1. The pressure in a filled cylinder at 70°F may not exceed the service pressure marked on the cylinder except for some nonliquefied, nonflammable gases such as oxygen, helium, carbon dioxide–oxygen mixtures and helium-oxygen mixtures, which may be allowed an additional 10%.

2. For gases other than nitrous oxide and

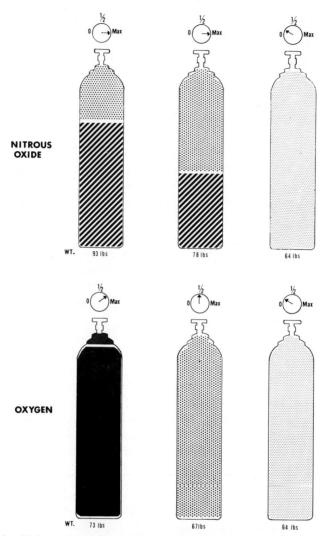

Figure 1.9. The relationship between cylinder weight, pressure, and contents. A gas stored partially in liquid form, such as nitrous oxide, will show a constant pressure (assuming constant temperature) until all the liquid has evaporated, at which time the pressure will drop in direct proportion to the rate at which gas is withdrawn. A nonliquefied gas such as oxygen will show a steady decline in pressure until the cylinder is evacuated. Each cylinder, however, will show a steady decline in weight as gas is discharged.

carbon dioxide, the pressure in the cylinder at 130°F may not exceed 1.25 times the maximum permitted filling pressure at 70°F.

3. As illustrated in Figure 1.9, in a cylinder containing a liquefied gas, the pressure will remain nearly constant as long as there is liquid in the cylinder. Thus, if only the pressure was limited, these cylinders could be filled with any amount of liquid. To prevent a cyl-

inder containing a liquefied gas from being overfilled, the maximum amount of gas allowed is defined by a filling density (filling ratio) for each gas. The filling density is defined as "the percent ratio of the weight of gas in a container to the weight of water that the container would hold at 60°F" (1). The filling densities of gases commonly used in anesthesia are shown in Table 1.4.

Table 1.4. Medical Gases

Gas	Formula	United States	International	State in Cylinder	Filling Density
Oxygen	O_2	Green	White	Nonliquefied[a]	
Carbon dioxide	CO_2	Gray[b]	Gray	Liquefied (below 88°F)	68%
Nitrous oxide	N_2O	Blue	Blue	Liquefied (below 98°F)	68%
Helium	He	Brown[c]	Brown	Nonliquefied	
Nitrogen	N_2	Black	Black	Nonliquefied	
Air		Yellow[d]	White & black	Nonliquefied	

[a] Special containers for liquid oxygen are discussed in Chapter 2.
[b] In carbon dioxide–oxygen mixtures in which the CO_2 is greater than 7%, the cylinder is predominately gray and the balance is green. If the CO_2 is less than 7%, the predominant color is green.
[c] If helium is greater than 80% in a helium-oxygen mixture, the predominant color is brown and the balance is green.
[d] Air, including oxygen-nitrogen mixtures containing 19.5–23.5% oxygen, is color coded yellow. Cylinders with nitrogen-oxygen mixtures other than those containing 19.5–23.5% oxygen are colored black and green.

The filling density is not the same as the volume of the full cylinder occupied by the liquid phase. For example, in a full nitrous oxide cylinder, the liquid phase occupies about 90% to 95% of total cylinder volume, whereas the filling density is 68%.

COLOR (1)

Accidental confusion of cylinders has been a significant cause of mortality in the past. Color can be used as a means to aid in identifying gases in use. The color code used in the United States is shown in Table 1.4. The top and shoulder (the part sloping up to the neck) of each cylinder are painted the color assigned to the gas it contains or the entire cylinder may be covered using a nonfading, durable, water-insoluble paint. In the case of a container containing more than one gas, the colors must be applied in a way that will permit each color to be seen when viewed from the top.

An international color code (see Table 1.4) has been adopted by several countries, including Canada. This system differs from the one used in the United States in that oxygen's color is white and air is black and white rather than yellow. A number of countries other than the United States use a color code that differs from the international code (11). When people trained in one country

work in another country that has a different code, confusion frequently results.

Because of variations in color tones, chemical changes in paint pigments, lighting effects and differences in color perception by personnel, color should be not be used as the primary means for identification of cylinder contents. However, it does provide a useful check on labeling accuracy.

PERMANENT MARKINGS (1)

DOT and TC regulations require specific markings on each cylinder. These are usually stamped into the shoulder. Representative markings are shown in Figure 1.10. The first number is the DOT or TC specification number. This indicates the type of material used in construction. This is followed by the service pressure for the cylinder in pounds per square inch. Next is a serial number and the identifying symbol of the purchaser, user, or manufacturer.

The initial qualifying test date with the inspector's mark between the month and year of the test date may appear last or may be on the opposite side of the shoulder. If a cylinder has been retested, the retest date and testing facility must appear after the original qualifying test date. A five-pointed star stamped after the most recent test date indicates that the cylinder may be retested every 10 instead

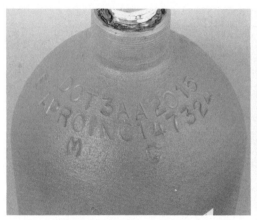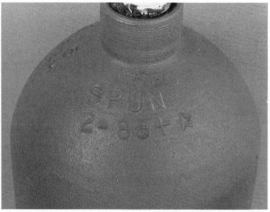

Figure 1.10. Cylinder markings. **Left,** "DOT3AA" is the DOT specification number; "2015" is the service pressure in psig. The next line shows the identifying symbol of the manufacturer and the serial number of the cylinder. **Right,** "SPUN" indicates that the end of the cylinder was closed by a spinning process. The initial qualifying date is shown with the inspector's mark between the month and year. The plus sign indicates that the cylinder is authorized for charging up to 10% in excess of the marked service pressure. The star indicates that the cylinder may be retested every 10 instead of every 5 years.

of every 5 years. If a plus (+) sign appears immediately after the test date marking on a cylinder, it means that the cylinder is authorized to be charged up to 10% in excess of the marked service pressure. The word *spun* or *plug* must be stamped where an end closure has been made by spinning or by spinning, drilling, and plugging.

LABELING (1)

Each cylinder must bear a label or decal that may, when space permits, be on the shoulder of the cylinder (but may not cover any permanent markings) or on the side of the cylinder, approximately two-thirds of the distance from the cylinder bottom to the top of the valve or cap.

Figure 1.11 shows a typical cylinder label that uses a diamond-shaped figure denoting the hazard class of the contained gas and a white panel with the name of the contained gas to the left. The diamond indicates whether the contents contain an oxidizer (yellow), a nonflammable gas (green), or a flammable gas (red). A signal word (*DANGER, WARNING,* or *CAUTION,* depending on whether the release of gas would create an immediate, less than immediate, or no immediate hazard to health or property) is present. Following the signal word is the statement of hazard, which gives the dangers present in connection with the customary or reasonably anticipated handling or use of the gas. A brief precautionary statement that gives measures to be taken to avoid injury or damage is usually present.

The label should contain the name and address of the cylinder manufacturer or distributor and a statement as to its content, usually the volume in liters at 70°F. Other information such as the cylinder weight when empty and full may also be present.

DOT regulations permit the use of a combination label-tag, one side of which contains the prescribed wording of the DOT label, while the other side is used as a shipping tag with space for the names and addresses of the shipper and consignee. Medical gas manufacturers in general use these on large cylinders, attached to the cylinder cap. The tag is perforated so that when the cylinder is empty part of the tag may be torn off at the perforation, obliterating the label wording. The part of the tag that remains attached to the cylinder contains the return address of the supplier.

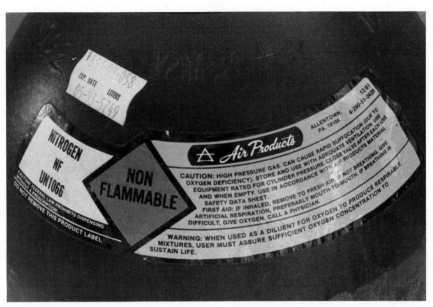

Figure 1.11. Cylinder label, showing the basic CGA marking system. The diamond-shaped figure denotes the hazard class of the contained gas (NONFLAMMABLE). To the left is a white panel with the name of contained gas (NITROGEN). The signal word (CAUTION) is to the right, following by a statement of hazards and measures to be taken to avoid injury.

TAGS

Tags normally bear the same color as the cylinder. The tag is primarily a means of denoting cylinder contents and not an identification device. A typical tag is shown in Figure 1.12. It has three sections labeled FULL, IN USE, and EMPTY connected by perforations. When a cylinder is first opened the FULL portion of the tag should be detached. When the cylinder is empty, the IN USE portion should be removed. The tag sometimes contains a washer to fit between the small cylinder valve and the yoke or regulator.

RULES FOR SAFE USE OF CYLINDERS (1,15)

General Rules

1. Cylinders should be handled only by personnel well trained in safe procedures. Frequently personnel involved in the transport, storage, and use of cylinders do not receive adequate instructions regarding their safe handling (12). Even those that do receive adequate training may become complacent in regard to safe practices.

2. Valves, regulators, gauges, and fittings should never be permitted to come into contact with oils, greases, organic lubricants, rubber, or any other combustible substance. Oil plus oxygen or nitrous oxide under pressure can cause an explosion. Cylinders or valves should not be handled with hands, rags, or gloves contaminated with oil or grease. Polishing or cleaning agents should not be applied to the valve, because they may contain combustible chemicals.

3. No part of any cylinder should ever be subjected to a temperature above 130°F (54°C). A flame, torch, or sparks from any source should never be permitted to come in contact with any part of a cylinder. A cylinder should not be supported by or placed in proximity to a radiator, steam pipe or heat duct. If a cylinder is exposed to a high temperature, it should be returned to the manufacturer for testing. Exposure to extremes of cold should also be avoided. Should ice or

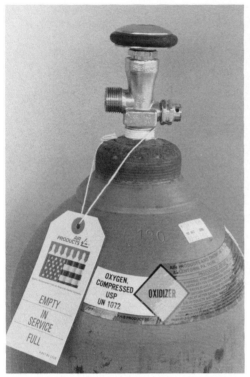

Figure 1.12. Cylinder tag. When the cylinder is first opened, the FULL portion of the tag should be removed. When the cylinder is empty, the IN SERVICE portion should be removed. On this cylinder label, the hazard class is OXIDIZER, the contained gas is OXYGEN, and the signal word is WARNING.

snow accumulate on a cylinder, it should be thawed at room temperature or with water at a temperature not exceeding 130°F.

4. Connections to piping, regulators, and other appliances should always be kept tight to prevent leakage. If a hose is used, it should be kept in good condition.

5. The discharge port of a pressure relief device or the valve outlet must not be obstructed.

6. Regulators, gauges, or other appliances designed for use with one gas should never be used with cylinders containing other gases.

7. Adapters to change the outlet size of a cylinder valve should not be used, because this defeats the whole purpose of standardizing valve outlets.

8. The cylinder valve should be kept closed except when the gas is in use. It should be turned off with no more force than is necessary, or damage to the seating may result.

9. The valve is the most easily damaged part of the cylinder. Valve protection caps—metal caps that screw over the valve on large cylinders (Fig. 1.13)—are available and should be kept securely in place, except when the cylinder is connected for use.

10. No part of the cylinder or its valve should be tampered with, painted, altered, repaired or modified by the user. Any cylinder whose proper functioning is in doubt for any reason should be returned to the supplier. Cylinders should be repainted only by the supplier.

11. Markings, labels, decals, or tags applied by the supplier must not be defaced, altered, or removed.

12. A cylinder should not be used for a

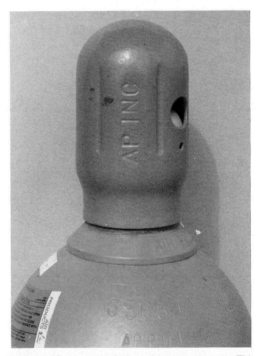

Figure 1.13. Large cylinder valve protection cap. This cap should be kept in place at all times, except when the cylinder is connected for use.

roller, support, or any other purpose other than that for which it was intended, even if the cylinder is believed to be empty.

13. A cylinder should not be placed where it might come into contact with electrical apparatus or circuits.

14. Cylinders should not be dragged, slid, or rolled, even for short distances. Cylinders should be transported on a cart or carrier made especially for that purpose and secured by a chain, strap, or other suitable device.

15. Cylinders should be properly secured at all times to prevent them from falling or being knocked over. They should not be dropped or permitted to strike each other or other surfaces violently. They must not be chained to portable or movable apparatus such as beds.

16. Cylinders should never be used where they could become contaminated by other gases or foreign material.

17. The owner of the cylinder should be notified if any damage that might impair its safety has been noticed or if any condition has occurred that might permit a foreign substance to enter the cylinder or valve.

18. Disposition of unserviceable cylinders is potentially dangerous and should be done only by qualified personnel (1).

19. Wrappings should be removed and cylinders should be cleaned before being taken into a clean area such as an operating room suite.

Storage

1. A definite area should be designated for storage of cylinders.

2. The storage area should be in a cool, dry, clean, well-ventilated room that is constructed of fire-resistant materials. Conductive flooring must be present where flammable gases are stored but is not required where only nonflammable gases are stored. Adequate ventilation should be provided so that if there is a leak in a cylinder gas will not accumulate in the room. Easily visible signs with texts such as "GAS CYLINDERS. RE-

MOVE TO A SAFE PLACE IN THE EVENT OF FIRE" and "OFF LIMITS TO UNAUTHORIZED PERSONNEL" should be hung outside the storage area. Signs reading "NO SMOKING," "NO OPEN FLAMES OR SPARKS," "NO OIL OR GREASE," and "NO COMBUSTIBLE MATERIALS" should be posted inside the room and on the door. Cylinders should not be stored in an operating room.

3. Cylinders may be stored in the open but should be protected against extremes of weather and from the ground beneath. During winter, stored cylinders must be protected against accumulations of ice and snow. In summer, cylinders must be protected from continuous exposure to direct rays of the sun in localities where high temperatures prevail. Smoking or open flames should be prohibited in oxygen or flammable gas cylinder storage areas.

4. Cylinders should be stored in a secure area, subject to removal only by authorized personnel. Cylinders in public areas should be protected from tampering.

5. Cylinders of nitrous oxide should be stored where the opportunity for theft and/or indiscriminate use is minimized. There should be a system for detecting unusually heavy use or loss of nitrous oxide (1). Any theft should be reported promptly to the police and the supplier.

6. Cylinders containing flammable gases should not be stored in an enclosure containing oxidizing gases (nitrous oxide, oxygen, or compressed air). Other nonflammable (inert) medical gases may be stored in the same enclosure as oxidizing gases.

7. Combustible materials should not be kept near cylinders containing oxygen or nitrous oxide. An exception to this may be made in the case of cylinder shipping cartons or crates (2). Cylinder storage racks may be made of wood.

8. Sources of heat in storage locations must be protected or located so that cylinders are not heated to the point of activation of in-

tegral safety devices. In no case shall the temperature of the cylinder exceed 130°F.

9. Cylinders should not be exposed to continuous dampness, corrosive chemicals, or fumes, because these may damage the cylinders and/or cause valve protection caps to stick.

10. Cylinders should be protected from abnormal mechanical shock. They should not be stored where heavy moving objects may strike them or fall on them.

11. Small cylinders are best stored upright or horizontally in bins or racks constructed of a nonflammable material that will not damage the cylinder surface when it is moved. Large cylinders should be stored upright against a wall and chained in place.

12. Wrappers should be removed from cylinders before storage. Their presence in the storage area is undesirable because they are frequently dirty, provide a combustible medium, and conceal the cylinder labels.

13. A cylinder should not be draped with any material. A combustible mixture may accumulate under the drape and its removal could provide a spark.

14. When different types of gases are stored in the same location, containers should be grouped by contents and by sizes (if different sizes are present). Full cylinders should be stored so that they are used in the order they were received from the supplier. Empty cylinders should be marked as such and segregated from full cylinders to avoid confusion and delay if a full cylinder is needed in a hurry.

15. There should be a system of inventory for both empty and full cylinders.

Use

1. Before use, the contents of the cylinder should be identified by reading the label. The color of a cylinder should not be relied on for identification of its contents. If the label is missing, illegible, or altered or if the cylinder color and label do not correspond, the cylinder should be returned to the manufacturer unused. The user should also read the pre-

cautionary information on the label and follow the recommendations.

2. The cylinder should be inspected before use. Only cylinders with the letters *DOT* or *ICC* (for Interstate Commerce Commission) should be used. In Canada equivalent cylinders are marked *BTC* (Board of Transport Commissioners) or *CTC* (Canadian Transport Commission). A cylinder that does not show evidence of inspection within the required period should not be used. The cylinder valve, especially the pressure relief device, outlet, and pin index holes, should be checked for defects. The valve outlet should be checked to see that it is pin indexed or has a proper large valve outlet connection and that it is clean. Any defective cylinder should be clearly marked as such and returned to the vendor.

3. A pressure-reducing regulator should always be used. For small cylinders attached to an anesthesia machine, the regulator inside the machine performs this function. Needle valves or similar devices without pressure-regulating mechanisms should not be used because excessive pressures may develop downstream of such devices and result in damage to equipment or injury to personnel.

4. Full small cylinders are usually supplied with a protective cover over the outlet to prevent contamination (Fig. 1.14). This should be removed immediately before fitting the cylinder to the dispensing equipment.

5. On large cylinders, the valve protection cap should be removed just before connecting the cylinder for use. If the cap is extremely difficult to remove, excessive force should not be applied nor should the cap be pried loose with a bar inserted into the ventilation openings. A label or tag identifying the problem should be attached to the cylinder and the cylinder should be returned to the supplier.

6. Before a regulator is connected to a cylinder it should be inspected for signs of damage and to make certain it is free of foreign materials. Regulators should be kept in good

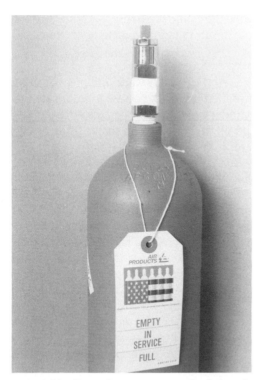

Figure 1.14. Protective cover over small cylinder valve outlet.

condition and stored in plastic bags to avoid contamination.

7. Before any fitting is applied to the cylinder valve particles of dust, metal shavings, and other foreign matter should be cleared from the outlet by momentarily opening ("cracking") the valve with the port pointed away from the user and any other persons. This reduces the possibility of a flash fire or explosion when the valve is later opened with the fittings in place; also the dust will not be blown into the anesthesia machine or other equipment where it could clog filters or interfere with the internal workings.

8. A sealing washer (gasket) in good condition should always be used with a small cylinder valve. It fits over the port (see Fig. 1.6). Only one washer should be used. If more than one is used, the pins on the yoke or regulator may not extrude out far enough to engage the mating holes, and the safety of the

Pin Index Safety System will be negated or a leak may occur (13).

9. The threads on the regulator-to-cylinder valve connection or the pin indexing devices on the yoke-to-cylinder valve connections should mate properly. Connections that do not fit should never be forced.

10. Outlets and connections should be tightened only with wrenches or other tools provided or recommended by the manufacturer. Wrenches with malaligned jaws should not be used because they may damage the equipment or slip and injure personnel. Excessive force should not be used as it may cause damage. The handwheel should never be hammered in an attempt to open or close the valve.

11. If a Bourdon gauge-type regulator is being used, the adjusting knob should be turned counterclockwise until it turns freely before the cylinder valve is opened. If the cylinder is attached to the yoke of an anesthesia machine or a regulator/flowmeter, the flow control valve should be closed before the cylinder valve is opened.

12. The person opening a cylinder valve should position himself or herself and the apparatus so that the valve outlet and/or the face of the regulator gauge points away from all persons.

13. A cylinder valve should always be opened SLOWLY (12). If gas passes quickly into the space between the valve and the yoke or regulator, the rapid recompression in this space will generate large amounts of heat. Because there is little time for dissipation of this heat, this constitutes an adiabatic process (one in which heat is neither lost nor gained from the environment). Particles of dust, grease, etc. present in this space may be ignited by the heat, causing a flash fire or explosion (14). Opening the valve slowly prolongs the time of recompression and permits some of the heat to dissipate. The cylinder valve should continue to be opened slowly until the pressure on the gauge stabilizes, then it can be opened to the full limit of its travel.

14. After the cylinder valve is opened the pressure should be checked. A cylinder with a pressure substantially greater than the service pressure should not be used, but marked and returned to the supplier. A cylinder arriving with a pressure substantially below the service pressure should be checked for leaks.

15. If a cylinder valve is open but no pressure is registered on the gauge or no gas flows, the cylinder valve should be closed and the cylinder should be disconnected from the dispensing apparatus, marked defective, and returned to the supplier with a note indicating the problem.

16. If a hissing sound is heard when the valve is opened, a large leak exists and the connection should be tightened. If the sound does not disappear, the sealing washer should be replaced (in the case of a small cylinder valve). However, under no circumstances should more than one washer be used. If the hissing sound persists, soapy water, a commercial leak detection fluid or other suitable solution should be applied to all parts. Bubbles will appear at the site(s) of the leak(s). A flame should never be used for this purpose.

Should a leak be found in the cylinder valve itself, it may be possible to tighten the packing nut by turning it slightly in a clockwise direction (see special handle in Fig. 1.5), unless the manufacturer recommends otherwise.

If the leak cannot be remedied by tightening connections without using excessive force, the valve should be closed, and the cylinder should be marked defective and returned to the supplier with a note indicating the fault.

17. Even if no hissing sound is audible when the valve is opened, a slow leak may be present and should be suspected if there is loss of pressure when no gas is being used. These leaks should be located and corrected.

18. A cylinder should be secured when in use but not to any movable object or heat radiator.

19. The valve should always be fully open

when the cylinder is in use. Marginal opening may result in failure to deliver adequate gas.

After Use

1. At the end of a work shift or any time an extended period of nonuse is anticipated the cylinder valve should be closed completely and all pressure vented (bled) from the system.

2. An empty or near-empty cylinder should not be left on an anesthesia machine. A defective check valve in the yoke could result in accidental filling if the valve is left open. In addition, the presence of an empty cylinder may create a false sense of security. Yokes should not be left empty. If a full cylinder is not available, a yoke plug (see page 55) should be in place. Some gas suppliers request that cylinders be returned with enough pressure (e.g., 25 psig) remaining to maintain the integrity of the cylinder (15).

3. Before removing a cylinder from a regulator or yoke the valve should be closed and all pressure released.

4. When a cylinder is empty, the lower part of the tag should be removed. A DOT green, yellow, or red label should be covered with an "Empty" label, or if the cylinder is provided with a combination label-tag, the lower portion should be removed.

5. Valves should be completely closed on all empty cylinders. Often cylinders are not completely empty and accidents have resulted from release of gas from a supposedly empty cylinder. If the valve is left open on an empty cylinder, debris and contaminants could be sucked into it when the temperature changes.

6. Valve protection caps should be replaced before shipment back to the manufacturer.

TRANSFILLING (1,2)

This practice should not be performed by unskilled, untrained persons. It is best performed by a gas manufacturer or distributor. If performed by a user, it should be in accordance with suggested procedures and not in a patient care area. There are several hazards.

1. Transfer of medical gases from one cylinder to another by inexperienced persons may adversely affect purity.

2. When small cylinders are transfilled from large cylinders containing gas at high pressure, rapid recompression of the gas in the small cylinder may cause the temperature to rise sufficiently to ignite combustible materials and oxidize metals rapidly.

3. The hazard of overfilling small cylinders is always present. Filling capacities may vary for cylinders even though their sizes appear to be the same. Overfilling may result in damage to the cylinder or dispensing equipment.

4. Cylinders used for one gas may accidentally be charged with a gas other than that originally contained in the cylinder, resulting in a dangerous mixture. If an oxygen cylinder were filled with a gas other than oxygen, hypoxia could occur with use.

5. Safety relief devices and other parts must be inspected at frequent intervals to ensure safe operation and repairs and to ensure that replacements are made when defects are found. If transfilling is performed by users, this may not be done.

HAZARDS

Incorrect Cylinder. In spite of almost universal use of the Pin Index Safety System, reports of incorrect tanks being connected to yokes continue to appear (16–25). Yokes or regulators may be poorly or incorrectly built or may be altered. Pins can be bent, broken, or forced into the yoke, pin index holes may become worn and more than one washer may be used. Some lasers have yokes that lack pins, allowing connection of an incorrect cylinder (26).

Incorrect Contents. A cylinder may not contain the gas for which it is indexed and labeled (27–30). In a cylinder with a mixture, the gases may not be mixed (31).

Incorrect Valve. Cylinders may be correctly labeled for the gas that they contain but have a valve for another gas (32–35). This usually will prevent their attachment to the dispensing apparatus. Industrial, rather than medical, gas cylinders are sometimes used to power surgical tools. These may have connections that fit equipment designed for other gases (36).

Incorrect Color. Cylinders may be painted with other than their standard color (33).

Incorrect Labeling. A cylinder with the correct color and valve may be delivered with an incorrect label (32,37).

Inoperable Valve. A cylinder may be delivered with an inoperable or blocked valve outlet (33,38).

Damaged Valve. If the retaining screw of the yoke is screwed into the safety relief device instead of the conical depression, the valve will be damaged. This may result in a leak of cylinder contents (8,9).

Suffocation. Sudden discharge of large quantities of gas from a cylinder into a closed space could displace the air from that space, creating a dangerous condition. If an oxygen-deficient atmosphere is suspected, an oxygen monitor should be used to check this.

Fires (2). Materials that burn in air will burn much more vigorously and at a higher temperature in oxygen at normal pressure and explosively in oxygen under pressure. Some materials that do not burn in air will burn in an oxygen-enriched atmosphere, particularly under pressure. Similarly, materials that can be ignited in air have lower ignition energies in oxygen. Many such materials may be ignited by friction at a valve seat or stem packing or by adiabatic compression produced when oxygen at high pressure is rapidly introduced into a system initially at low pressure. If pressurized oxygen equipment is contaminated with grease, oil, paraffin or other combustible substances, explosive rupture and burning of system components may occur (2,13,39,40). Oxygen regulators and cylinders contaminated with oil have been sold (41–43).

Explosion. Because gas in cylinders is under pressure, rapid escape of cylinder contents and rocketing of the cylinder are potential hazards (44–46). Cylinder are sometimes overfilled (32,33,47). A cylinder that has been incorrectly filled with the wrong gas may explode if the valve does not have the proper pressure relief device (46). Improper handling or storage of cylinders can cause them to fall over. If the valve protection cap is not present, the valve could snap off (2). If the packing nut rather than the stem is loosened, the stem may be ejected when the valve is opened (6).

Burns. A burn caused by freezing nitrous oxide when the cylinder valve was being cracked has been reported (7). In another case, a nitrous oxide cylinder with a leak was turned to the horizontal position and a small volume of liquid nitrous oxide fell on the user's hand, causing burns.

Contamination of Cylinder Contents. Medical gases in cylinders may contain contaminants (33,48–50). Medical-grade oxygen is required to be 99% pure (48,51). Of the remaining 1% (10,000 ppm), not more than 300 ppm of carbon dioxide, 10 ppm of carbon monoxide, or 5 ppm of oxides of nitrogen can be present. No other contaminants are specifically excluded from the other 9,685 ppm. Thus the possibility exists that oxygen or other gases may contain potentially dangerous amounts of other compounds and not be in violation of existing standards (48). CGA guidelines state that there should be no odor from the contents of compressed gas cylinders. An industrial-grade gas may not have the same requirements for purity as a medical-grade gas and may contain relatively large amounts of impurities (36). Accidental use of such gas could cause significant problems. Cases of poisoning by contamination of nitrous oxide cylinders with higher oxides of nitrogen have occurred (49).

Moisture may contaminate a cylinder and flow into the dispensing equipment if the cylinder is inverted (52). Adiabatic expansion of gas as it is released causes cooling, and the moisture could form ice and jam the regulator or yoke. In the past, this has been a significant problem with nitrous oxide.

Theft of Nitrous Oxide Cylinders. Theft of nitrous oxide cylinders for substance-abuse purposes can be a serious problem.

Liquid Oxygen Containers

Small, specially designed containers filled with liquid oxygen have become popular, especially for patient transfer. Another use is when anesthesia is administered outside a healthcare facility, e.g., by armed forces (53). Advantages include low gas pressure, compactness, low weight, portability, and simplicity.

EQUIPMENT

A stationary unit (reservoir, supply container) is kept in a suitable area and refilled by the gas supplier as needed (Fig. 1.15). The smaller, portable (receiving) units are filled from the stationary unit. The portable unit has a means of regulating oxygen flow. The amount of gas contained can be measured by weighing.

Liquid gas containers are manufactured, maintained, filled, and transported in accordance with DOT regulations. In comparison to cylinders, they are broader and less tall. Required markings include the specification number and service pressure for which the container is designed (1). Other marks, normally located beneath these markings, include an identifying mark of the original container owner and a serial number. The date of original manufacture and a symbol identifying the inspector are also present. Each container must have a pressure relief device and a means to limit the amount of liquid oxygen contained.

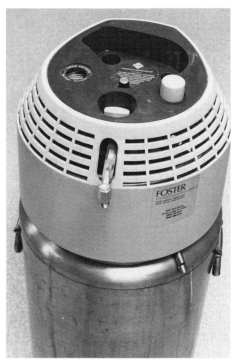
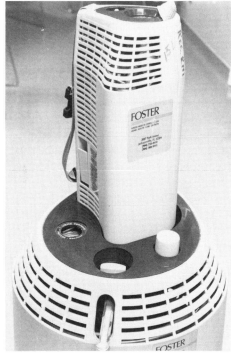

Figure 1.15.   Liquid oxygen containers. **Left,** The stationary unit, which is refilled by the gas supplier as needed. Note the pressure relief valve at right front. **Right,** the portable unit is attached to the stationary unit for transfilling.

When not in use, the pressure in the container is controlled by venting excess gas to atmosphere. This limits the time oxygen can be stored in the portable unit (54).

RULES FOR SAFE USE OF LIQUID OXYGEN CONTAINERS

1. If liquid oxygen is spilled, a considerable time must be allowed for the oxygen to dissipate.
2. Contact between the skin and liquid oxygen must be avoided.
3. Liquid oxygen equipment must be kept clean of organic or combustible materials. These materials can react violently with liquid oxygen under certain conditions.
4. Cryogenic transfilling devices must be kept free of moisture to prevent accumulation of frost on valves or couplings that may cause them to freeze open or shut.
5. Containers should not be subjected to extremes of heat or cold.
6. Containers should be handled so as to avoid physical damage.
7. Markings and labels on containers must be legible and must not be altered.
8. Under no circumstances should any attempt be made to loosen, tighten or otherwise tamper with the pressure relief device.

STORAGE (1)

1. Both the stationary and portable units should be kept in open, cool, well-ventilated areas. Containers should not be stored in a closed space such as a closet (2).
2. Liquid oxygen containers should be stored away from any heat source (1).
3. Containers should be protected from corrosive atmospheres.

4. Containers should be stored in an upright position.

TRANSFILLING (1)

Liquid oxygen may be transferred by means of a cryogenic flexible hose assembly or the manufacturer's noninterchangeable direct connection. If a flexible hose assembly is used, its end connections must conform with CGA regulations (1) or the manufacturer's noninterchangeable connections and must have a pressure relief device.

Transfilling must be performed in a well-ventilated location that is remote from patient care areas, has no sources of ignition, and is posted with "NO SMOKING" signs.

HAZARDS (1)

Fires. If liquid oxygen equipment becomes contaminated with hydrocarbons such as oil or grease, or other combustible materials, ignition may occur. Vaporization of spilled liquid oxygen will result in an oxygen-enriched atmosphere, increasing the fire hazard.

High Pressure. The large volume of gaseous oxygen resulting from vaporization of liquid oxygen has the potential, if trapped in a closed space not protected by adequate pressure relief devices, to generate pressures high enough to cause danger to life, limb, and property.

Burns. Liquid oxygen is at a very low temperature. Contact with cold liquid or frosted valves or couplings may cause cryogenic burns. Physical damage to or failure of liquid oxygen equipment can result in liquid spilling or spraying in an uncontrolled manner. Relief valves on portable containers may open prematurely and vent liquid oxygen during or immediately after the filling of the container (55).

Equipment Freezing. Valves or couplings may freeze shut if they are not kept free of moisture.

Inaccurate Flows. One study showed on a high percentage of portable liquid oxygen

devices measured flows differed substantially from those set (56).

REFERENCES

1. Compressed Gas Association. Handbook of compressed gases. 3rd ed. New York: Van Nostrand, Reinhold, 1990.
2. Klein BR. Health care facilities handbook. 3rd ed. Quincy, MA: National Fire Protection Association, 1990.
3. Russell WJ. Equipment for anaesthesia and intensive care. Adelaide, Australia: Author, 1983.
4. Petty C. The anesthesia machine, New York: Churchill Livingstone, 1987.
5. McPherson SP. Respiratory therapy equipment. 3rd ed. St Louis: CV Mosby, 1985.
6. Finch JS. A report on a possible hazard of gas cylinder tanks. Anesthesiology 1970;33:467.
7. Yamashita M, Motokawa K, Watanabe S. Do not use the "innovated" cylinder valve handle for cracking the valve. Anesthesiology 1986;64:658.
8. Fox JWC, Fox EJ. An unusual occurrence with a cyclopropane cylinder. Anesth Analg 1968;47:624–626.
9. Milliken RA. Correspondence. Anesth Analg 1971;50:775.
10. Jones PL. Some observations on nitrous oxide cylinders during emptying. Br J Anaesth 1974;46:534–538.
11. Kumar P, Mishra LD. Deviation from international colour codes. Anaesthesia 1986;41:1055–1056.
12. Czajka RJ. Cylinder caution: open slowly to minimize recompression heat. Anesthesiology 1978;49:226.
13. Anonymous. Oxygen regulator fire caused by use of two yoke washers. Technol Anesth 1990;11:1–2.
14. Anonymous. Understanding the fire hazard. Technol Anesth 1992;12:1–6.
15. Anonymous. Storage and handling of gas cylinders. MD DI 9:49–52, 1983.
16. Anonymous. Patient dies after oxygen tank is replaced with carbon dioxide; investigation clears hospital. Biomed Safe Stand 1983;13:5–6.
17. Anonymous. Misconnection of oxygen regulator to nitrogen cylinder could cause death. Biomed Safe Stand 1988;18:90–91.
18. Anonymous. Nonstandard user modification of gas cylinder pin indexing. Technol Anesth 1989;10:2.
19. Anonymous. Medical gas cylinders. Technol Anesth 1991;12:12.
20. Goebel WM. Failure of nitrous oxide and oxygen pin-indexing. Anesth Prog 1980;27:188–191.
21. Hogg CE. Pin-indexing failures. Anesthesiology 1973;38:85–87.

22. MacMillan RR, Marshall MA. Failure of the pin index system on a Cape Waine Ventilator. Anaesthesia 1981;36:334–335.

23. Mead P. Hazard with cylinder yoke. Anaesth Intensive Care 1981;9:79–80.

24. Orr IA, Hamilton L. Entonox hazard. Anaesthesia 1985;40:496.

25. Upton LG, Robert EC Jr. Hazard in administering nitrous oxide analgesia: report of a case. J Am Dent Assoc 1977;94:696–697.

26. Anonymous. Lack of pin-indexing for laser gas supplies. Technol Anesth 1987;8:1–3.

27. Anonymous. Medical gas cylinders. Technol Anesth 1986;7:8.

28. Anonymous. Nitrous oxide cylinders found to contain carbon dioxide. Biomed Safe Stand 1990;20:84.

29. Menon MRB, Lett Z. Incorrectly filled cylinders. Anaesthesia 1991;46:155–156.

30. Jawan B, Lee JH. Cardiac arrest caused by an incorrectly filled oxygen cylinder: A case report. Br J Anaesth 1990;64:749–751.

31. Anonymous. Cylinders with unmixed helium/oxygen. Technol Anesth 1990;10:4.

32. Boon PE. C-size cylinders. Anaesth Intensive Care 1990;18:586–587.

33. Feeley TW, Bancroft ML, Brooks RA, Hedley-Whyte J. Potential hazards of compressed gas cylinders: a review. Anesthesiology 1978;48:72–74.

34. Jayasuriya JP. Another example of Murphy's Law—mix up of pin index valves. Anaesthesia 1986;41:1164.

35. Steward DJ, Sloan IA. Additional pin-indexing failures. Anesthesiology 1973;39:355.

36. Russell WJ. Industrial gas hazard. Anaesth Intensive Care 1985;13:106.

37. Sawhney KK, Yoon YK. Erroneous labeling of a nitrous oxide cylinder. Anesthesiology 1983;59:260.

38. Blogg CE, Colvin MP. Apparently empty oxygen cylinders. Br J Anaesth 1977;49:87.

39. Garfield JM, Allen GW, Silverstein P, Mendenhall MK. Flash fire in a reducing valve. Anesthesiology 1971;34:578–579.

40. Ito Y, Horikowa H, Ichiyanagi K. Fires and explosions with compressed gases: report of an accident. Br J Anaesth 1965;37:140–141.

41. Anonymous. Medical gas cylinders. Technol Anesth 1985;6:17.

42. Anonymous. Oxygen regulators may be contaminated with oil. Biomed Safe Stand 1990;20:13.

43. Anonymous. Oxygen cylinders recalled because of oil contamination. Biomed Safe Stand 1991;21:20.

44. Anonymous. Medical Gas Cylinders. Technol Anesth 1987;7:10.

45. Morse HN. Legal case: who is responsible for the oxygen-tank explosion?—manufacturer or user. Med Elect Prod, Dec. 6, 1980, p. 6.

46. Tracey JA, Kennedy J, Magner J. Explosion of carbon dioxide cylinder. Anaesthesia 1984;39:938–939.

47. Gray WM, Richardson W. Filling CO_2 cylinders. Anaesthesia 1985;40:504.

48. Bassell GM, Rose DM, Bruce DL. Purity of USP medical oxygen. Anesth Analg 1979;58:441–442.

49. Clutton-Brock J. Two cases of poisoning by contamination of nitrous oxide with higher oxides of nitrogen during anaesthesia. Br J Anaesth 1967;39:388–392.

50. Herlihy WJ. Report: contamination of medical oxygen. Anaesth Intensive Care 1973;1:240–241.

51. Rendell-Baker L. Purity of oxygen, USP. Anesth Analg 1980;59:314–315.

52. Coveler LA, Lester RC. Contaminated oxygen cylinder. Anesth Analg 1989;69:674–676.

53. Bull PT, Merrill SB, Moody RA, et al. Anaesthesia during the Falklands campaign. The experience of the Royal Navy. Anaesthesia 1983;38:770–775.

54. Ramage CMH, Kee SS, Bristow A. A new portable oxygen system using liquid oxygen. Anaesthesia 1991;46:395–397.

55. Anonymous. Valves may open & release liquid oxygen. Biomed Safe Stand 1990;20:20–21.

56. Massey LW, Hussey JD, Albert RK. Inaccurate oxygen delivery in some portable liquid oxygen devices. Am Rev Respir Dis 1988;137:204–205.

Chapter 2

Medical Gas Distribution Systems

Most healthcare facilities use a piping system to deliver nonflammable gases such as oxygen, nitrous oxide, air, carbon dioxide, and nitrogen to operating rooms and other areas where they are used. In special care areas an alternative local source may be installed to supply these gases during a breakdown of the main system (1).

Usually, central piping systems are installed by mechanical contractors and maintained by the hospital engineering or maintenance department, with little input from the users. This not only neglects a potentially valuable contribution but, more important, leaves those who use the gases ignorant of how the system works. Because the system is mostly out of sight and usually functions well, it generally does not attract attention until a problem occurs.

When a new hospital or addition is being planned, anesthesia personnel should play a key role in designing the piping system. Their input is important in sizing the system and locating outlets (including remote parts of the hospital where patients are taken for diagnostic studies or various types of therapy). Careful planning may avoid expense and inconvenience at a later date.

Definitions

BULK OXYGEN SYSTEM (2)

Any assembly of equipment and interconnecting piping that has a storage capacity of more than 20,000 cubic feet of oxygen, including unconnected reserves on hand at the site.

BULK NITROUS OXIDE SYSTEM

An assembly of equipment that has a storage capacity of more than 28,000 cubic feet of nitrous oxide.

TERMINAL UNIT (STATION OUTLET)

The point in a piped medical gas distribution system at which the user normally makes connections and disconnections.

Standards and Sources of Information

The National Fire Protection Association (NFPA), the Compressed Gas Association (CGA), the International Standards Organization (ISO), and the Canadian Standards Association (CSA) have published a number of standards on safe practices related to hospital piping systems (2–6). These are incorporated into law in many locations. Compliance with these standards is one of the bases for accreditation by the Joint Commission on the Accreditation of Healthcare Organizations. These organizations do not approve, inspect or certify any installations, procedures, equipment, or materials. In most cases compliance with standards is left to the individual gas supplier and hospital. Lack of compliance with existing NFPA regulations is common (7). There are many state and local codes that preempt, and sometimes exceed, these standards.

Throughout this chapter, the recommendations and requirements will be those from the NFPA Handbook (2).

Components

A medical gas distribution system consists of a central supply with control equipment, piping extending to locations where the gas may be required, and terminal units at each point of use. Hoses that extend from terminal units to the anesthesia machine or other equipment, although not part of the piped system, are included because of their importance to anesthesia.

CENTRAL SUPPLIES

Central supplies may be located outdoors (with the control panel protected from the weather), in an enclosure used only for this purpose, or in a room or enclosure used only for this purpose that is situated within a building that is used for other purposes. Access to the central supply area should be restricted to individuals familiar with and responsible for the system, in light of reported thefts of nitrous oxide cylinders for substance-abuse purposes and to prevent unauthorized persons from creating a hazard or harming themselves.

A common type of central supply is shown in Figure 2.1. Two banks (or units) of cylinders are present. Each bank must have its own pressure regulator and must contain at least an average day's supply, with a minimum of two cylinders. Larger amounts may be necessary in areas remote from suppliers. The cylinders are connected to a common manifold (header) that converts them into one continuous supply. A check (nonreturn) valve is placed between each cylinder lead and the header to prevent loss of gas from the manifolded cylinders if there is a leak in an individual cylinder or lead. The primary (duty, running) supply is the portion actually supplying the system at any time, while the other bank is the secondary (standby) supply. When the primary supply is unable to supply the system, the secondary supply automatically becomes the primary supply. The switchover is accomplished by a pressure-sensitive switch, the manifold changeover device. This is a normal operating procedure. The primary plus the secondary supply is known as the operating supply. It is the portion that normally supplies the piping system.

Frequently, a reserve supply is added, as shown in Figure 2.2. A reserve supply is required with bulk medical gas systems.

The reserve consists of three or more manifolded cylinders and must either be equipped with a check valve between each cylinder lead and the header or be provided with an activating switch that operates the master signals when the reserve drops to one day's supply.

Check valves between each cylinder lead and the manifold header are not required on the primary and secondary supplies if there is

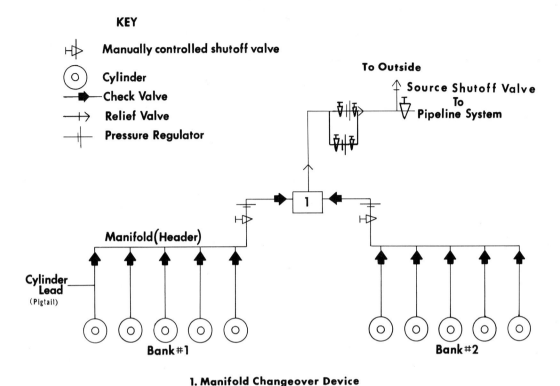

KEY

⊢▷ Manually controlled shutoff valve

Ⓞ Cylinder

──■► Check Valve

──┼► Relief Valve

──┼┼─ Pressure Regulator

To Outside

↑ Source Shutoff Valve
To
Pipeline System

Manifold (Header)

Cylinder Lead
(Pigtail)

Bank #1

Bank #2

1. Manifold Changeover Device

Figure 2.1. Cylinder supply system without reserve supply. This is known as an alternating supply system. The manual shutoff (on-off) valves permit isolation of either bank of cylinders. Fluctuations in the distribution pressure can be decreased by reducing the pressure in two stages, so a regulator is installed in the outgoing pipe. A manual shutoff valve must be located upstream of and a shutoff or check valve downstream of each regulator. This arrangement, plus having two regulators, makes it possible to service a regulator without shutting down the entire piped system. An actuating switch connected to the master signal panels must be present to indicate when, or just before, the changeover to the secondary bank occurs. Supply systems with different arrangements of valves and regulators are permissible if they provide equivalent safeguards. Redrawn from National Fire Protection Association. Nonflammable medical gas systems (NFPA 56F). Quincy, MA: NFPA, 1977.

a reserve supply, but a check valve in the primary supply main line upstream of the point of intersection with the secondary or reserve supply is required.

The reserve operates in the event that the operating supply is unable to furnish sufficient gas to the piping system. It functions only in an emergency and not as a normal operating procedure. It may be used when maintenance or repair of the operating supply is needed. An activating switch to indicate when, or just before, the reserve begins to supply the system must be connected to the master signal panels.

A pressure regulator is installed in the main supply line upstream of the pressure relief valve. Gases other than nitrogen are normally piped at a pressure of 50 psig. Nitrogen normally is delivered at 160 psig. Some systems have a second main line pressure regulator in case the first one should fail.

All final line regulators must be duplexed or placed in a valved bypass arrangement to permit service to the regulator without completely shutting down the piped gas system.

Oxygen

Oxygen may be stored either as a liquid at low pressures or as a compressed gas in cylinders. When large quantities are required,

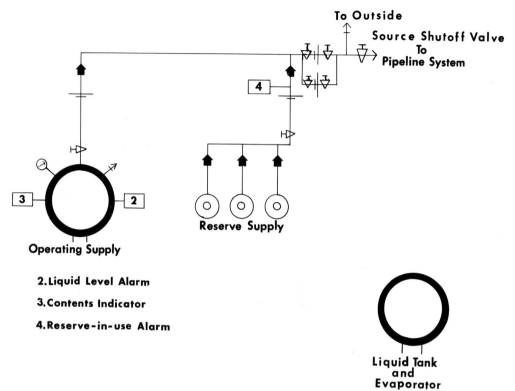

Figure 2.2.   Bulk supply system. A liquid oxygen container serves as the operating supply with cylinders constituting the reserve supply. The reserve supply may also be a cryogenic liquid oxygen container. Operation of the reserve should activate the reserve-in-use alarm. This is known as a continuous-type system, because under normal operating conditions one primary source (which is refilled periodically) always supplies the system. Redrawn from National Fire Protection Association. Nonflammable medical gas systems (NFPA 56F). Quincy, MA: NFPA, 1977.

liquid storage is usually preferred. Cylinder supplies are used for small hospitals, sections of hospitals not piped for oxygen, and auxiliary systems.

Gaseous Supply

Gaseous oxygen is most commonly supplied from G or H cylinders that are transported between the gas distributor and the central supply area or from cylinders that are permanently fixed at the site and refilled by the distributor. A third source is oxygen concentrators (8).

Liquid Supply (3,9–11)

When large amounts of oxygen are required, it is less expensive and more convenient to store it as a liquid: 1 cubic foot of liquid oxygen at a temperature of −300°F

yields approximately 860 cubic feet of gaseous oxygen at 70°F. Less storage space and fewer deliveries to the hospital are required, and there is less handling of individual gas containers. Most frequently, liquid oxygen containers are refilled from supply trucks without interruption of service. Fill hoses from supply trucks are indexed to prevent misfilling (3). Alternatively, filled liquid containers may be transported between the supplier and the healthcare facility.

Liquid oxygen containers are installed at ground level and outside so that they are readily accessible to supply trucks. They should be located where exposure to potential ignition sources is minimal. NFPA standards specify how far the container must be from sidewalks, parked vehicles, etc.

To prevent the liquid from evaporating,

it must be kept at or below its boiling point (−297°F). This is accomplished by keeping it in special insulated containers under low pressure. The containers vary in size and shape. They are constructed similar to thermos bottles with outer and inner metal jackets separated by insulation and a layer of near vacuum to retard heat transfer from the exterior into the cold liquid. Each container should have a contents indicator and low liquid level alarm.

Because liquid oxygen vaporizes at low temperatures and a small quantity of liquid will produce a large volume of gas, it is important that these containers be provided with devices to allow some of the gas on top of the liquid to escape if the pressure rises. A minimum vapor space must be maintained.

Although the insulation of such a tank is usually good, a small amount of heat will be absorbed continuously from the surroundings, causing evaporation of the liquefied gas. The amount of this uncontrolled evaporation is normally less than the demand for the piped system. If there is no flow from the container to the pipeline the pressure in the container will slowly increase until the safety relief valve opens and oxygen is vented to atmosphere. If a liquid system is left standing unused for long periods of time, a significant amount of oxygen will be lost. The use of liquid containers is economical only when there is a fairly constant high-volume demand. Having the proper size container will minimize venting.

Most of the time the oxygen is kept cold by the latent heat of vaporization as gaseous oxygen is removed and the temperature tends to fall. As the temperature falls, the pressure within the tank also falls. To maintain pressure, liquid oxygen must be removed from the tank and passed through a vaporizer (evaporator, vaporizing column, gasifier), which supplies heat. The liquid absorbs heat and is returned to the top of the tank as gas. The gaseous oxygen is drawn off as required and passed through a heater to bring it up to ambient temperature and raise its pressure.

Nitrous Oxide

Most hospitals use high-pressure nitrous oxide cylinders manifolded together in banks, in an arrangement similar to that described for oxygen cylinders. One problem with nitrous oxide cylinders is that the regulator may become so cold that it freezes. Nitrous oxide may also be stored as a liquid at low pressure in special insulated vessels.

Warning signs should be posted around areas where nitrous oxide tanks are located to warn that nitrous oxide is an asphyxiant and that if there is a leak a hypoxic mixture may be produced.

Compressed Air (2)

Air may be supplied from manifolded cylinders, a proportioning device that mixes gas from oxygen and nitrogen cylinders, or motor-driven compressors. Air from cylinders is usually cleaner and drier than that from compressors but is more expensive if a large amount is required.

The vast majority of piped air systems employ two or more compressors, which operate alternately or simultaneously, depending on demand. Each compressor must be capable of handling 100% of the estimated peak flow demand. When more than two compressors are provided, there must be the capability to meet the peak calculated demand with the largest compressor out of service. The reserve may be manifolded cylinders or a separate compressor system. A local audible and visual signal must be provided to indicate when the reserve or off-duty compressor is in operation. In some cases it may be appropriate to install a small local compressor for a particular department to avoid installing extensive piping.

Each compressor takes in ambient air, compresses it to above the working pressure and supplies it to one or more receivers (accumulators, reservoir tanks, storage receivers, reservoirs, receiver tanks) from which air can be withdrawn as needed. This allows a nonpulsatile air stream to be delivered to the regulator. It also serves to reduce wear on the compressor. The receiver must be equipped with a safety valve, automatic drain, sight glass to permit visual checking that the drain is operating properly, and a pressure gauge. A high water level alarm should be provided. The receiver must be provided with a bypass to permit servicing without shutting down the piped air system.

The location of the intakes is important in ensuring that the air will be as free of contaminants as possible. It is often situated outside the hospital in a location where it will take in air that is as free of dirt, fumes, and odors as possible. However, if a source is available that is equal to or better than outside air it may be used.

Treatment systems for medical air compressor systems are not mandated by NFPA (2), as it can be demonstrated that ambient air taken from a location free from auto exhausts or other sources of pollution is normally well within the limits required for compressed air (*U.S. Pharmacopoeia* [*USP*]) (2). Air quality does vary from place to place and from day to day and may in a few areas exceed the contaminant limits of USP air for unacceptably long periods. This can only be determined through knowledge of local conditions and testing at the intake.

Where the quality of the intake air is unreliable, specific air treatment devices may be desirable. When installed, these devices must be monitored and have alarms. Such devices add considerably to the purchase price and maintenance of the air system, but their use may offset even greater costs with respect to what untreated air may do to the piped air system.

One or more filters must be installed between the intake and the compressor. Other filters may be installed downstream of the compressor. Filters must be duplexed with appropriate valves to permit service without shutting down the system. Selection of filters should be made on the characteristics of the compressor, probable intake conditions, and other considerations.

To render air suitable for medical use, its water content must be reduced. An aftercooler in which the air is cooled and the condensed moisture removed is usually installed downstream of each compressor. More water may condense in the receiver. Additional water may be removed by running the air through a dryer located between the receiver and the line pressure regulator. Aftercoolers and dryers must be duplexed and valved to allow isolation and continued operation of the system in the event of failure of the unit in service.

Recommendations for monitoring air downstream of the dryers and upstream of the piping system for gaseous hydrocarbons, liquid hydrocarbons, carbon monoxide, carbon dioxide, particulate matter, and dew point (the temperature at which condensation occurs when a gas mixture is cooled) have been made by the NFPA.

It should be noted that although medical air is usually very clean, it is not sterile. Some manufacturers of devices using air recommend that filters be placed between the station outlet and the equipment and many incorporate filters in their apparatus.

Nitrogen

Central nitrogen supplies may consist of manifolded high-pressure cylinders or cryogenic liquid containers.

Carbon Dioxide

The source for piped carbon dioxide is high-pressure cylinders.

PIPED DISTRIBUTION SYSTEM

There are three general classes of piping:

1. *Main Lines.* Pipes connecting the source to risers or branch lines or both.
2. *Risers.* Vertical pipes connecting the main line with branch lines on various levels of the facility.
3. *Branch (Lateral) Lines.* The sections of the piping system that service a room or group of rooms on the same story of the facility.

Layouts of piped systems vary considerably. A typical one is shown in Figure 2.3. Distribution pipes are made of copper or brass. Identification of the pipes by labeling at least every 20 feet and at least once in every room and story traversed by the piping system is important to ensure that those installing and maintaining the pipeline are aware of its content. It is recommended that piping and manifolds for oxygen service be of a different size than those for other gases to prevent cross-connections. Generally oxygen is installed in ½ inch outer diameter (OD) and other gases in ⅜ inch OD pipes.

Permanently installed flexible hosing may be used near the station outlet (2). It is limited to 5 feet in length and may not penetrate walls, floors, ceilings, or partitions.

PRESSURE RELIEF VALVES

Each central supply system must have a pressure relief valve set at 50% above normal line pressure downstream of the line pressure regulator(s) and upstream of any shutoff valve. This is to prevent a buildup of pressure in the supply portion of a system if a shutoff valve is closed. The valve should close automatically when the excess pressure has been relieved.

SHUTOFF VALVES

Shutoff valves (zone, on-off, isolating, section valves) permit isolation of specific areas

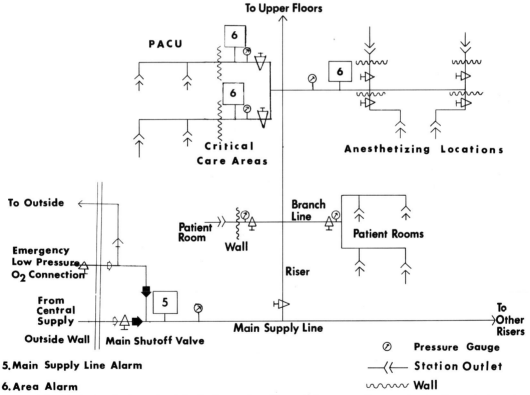

Figure 2.3. Typical medical gas piped distribution system. The main line runs on the same level as the central supply and connects it to risers or branch lines or both. In anesthetizing locations individual room shutoff valves are located downstream of the area alarm. Other locations have a single shutoff valve for the entire area with the area alarm actuator downstream from the shutoff valve. The main supply line alarm is activated by a 20% increase or decrease in line pressure. Area alarms must be installed in branch lines leading to intensive care units, postanesthesia care units, and anesthetizing locations to signal if the pressure increases or decreases 20% from normal operating pressure.

of the piping system in the event of a fire or other problem distal to the valve and allow parts of the system to be isolated for maintenance, repair, testing, or expansion without the whole system having to be switched off.

A quarter-turn shutoff valve with an indicating handle has become standard. Shutoff valves are installed in boxes with frangible or removable windows (Fig. 2.4). Each valve should be permanently marked to indicate function, gas, and area controlled as well as that it should be closed only in an emergency. Shutoff valves should be located where they will be readily accessible to those who need to use them in an emergency and where access is unlikely to be obstructed.

In the central supply there must be a manually operated shutoff valve upstream of each pressure regulator and a shutoff or check valve downstream.

A shutoff (source) valve is required at the outlet of the source of supply, upstream of

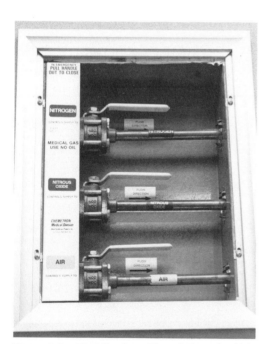

Figure 2.4. Shutoff valves. The window should be frangible or removable to permit manual operation of the valve. The valves should be labeled to show the gases and areas controlled.

the main line shutoff valve. This allows the entire source of supply, including all accessory devices, to be isolated from the pipeline system. The source valve must be located in the immediate vicinity of the source equipment.

The main supply line must be equipped with a shutoff valve near the entry into the building. This allows the entire supply to the hospital to be shut off. It should be at a location well-known and readily accessible to those responsible for maintenance of the system but where any attempt to tamper with it would be noticed.

Each riser must be equipped with a shutoff valve adjacent to the riser connection. Each branch (lateral) line except those supplying anesthetizing locations and other vital life support and critical areas, such as postanesthesia care units, intensive care units, and coronary care units must have a shutoff valve located near the connection of the branch line to the riser. A shutoff valve is required immediately outside each vital life support or critical care area, located so as to be readily accessible in an emergency. A separate shutoff valve is required for each anesthetizing location so that shutting off the supply of gas to one location will not affect other locations. The shutoff valve must be located outside the anesthetizing location so that in an emergency people inside the room will exit and so that staff outside the room, in addition to those inside, would be able to shut off gas supplies. A facility is not precluded from installing a shutoff valve inside an operating room, although additional alarms would be required.

EMERGENCY OXYGEN SUPPLY CONNECTOR

When the central oxygen supply is located outside of the building served, an emergency oxygen supply connection for connecting a temporary auxiliary source of supply for emergency or maintenance situations is required. The inlet must be located on the exterior of the building and must be protected from tampering and unauthorized access. The connection for this emergency supply is installed downstream of the shutoff valve on the main supply line (see Fig. 2.3). There must be a check valve in the main line between the connection and the main line shutoff valve and a check valve between the connection and the emergency supply shutoff valve. The connection must be provided with a pressure relief valve set to open if the pressure exceeds 50% above normal.

ALARMS

Master Alarm System

A master alarm system monitors the central supply and the pressure in the main line for all medical gas systems. This system may be connected to a centralized computer (e.g., building management system).

To ensure continuous responsible observation, master signal panels must be located in two separate warning locations, wired in parallel to a single sensor for each condition. One panel should be in the office or principal working area of the individual responsible for maintenance of the system and the other at the telephone switchboard, security office, or other suitable location.

An alarm should signal when a changeover from the primary supply to the secondary bank has occurred, when or just before the reserve supply goes into operation, under certain circumstances when the reserve supply is reduced to one average day's supply, when the pressure in the reserve is below that required to function properly, when the liquid level of a cryogenic supply has reached a certain level, or when the pressure in the main line increases or decreases from normal operating pressure. In the medical air system there must be alarms for malfunction of one or more of the compressors or dryers and when the dew point has been exceeded.

Area Alarm Systems

Special care areas such as operating rooms, postanesthesia care units, intensive care units, coronary care units, etc. must have an area (local) alarm system to indicate if the pressure increases or decreases 20% from normal operating pressure. In anesthetizing locations the alarm will be upstream of the shutoff valves to the individual rooms. In other areas it will be placed downstream of the shutoff valve for the area. An area alarm is sometimes placed in each anesthetizing location (2).

An appropriately labeled warning signal panel for area alarms must be installed at the nurses' station or other suitable location near the point of use that will provide responsible surveillance (Fig. 2.5).

General Requirements

Each alarm must be labeled for the gas and area it monitors. Signals should be both audible and visible. The visual signal should continue until the problem is corrected. Some systems allow the audible signal to be temporarily silenced. Each panel should contain a mechanism to test the function of the alarms. Alarms should be designed to function during an electrical power failure.

Clear, concise instructions should be given to the persons monitoring the alarms to ensure the signals are reported promptly to the proper parties. Cases have been reported in which a hospital employee did not know what to do when an alarm sounded (7). Activation of the signal should be reported immediately to the department responsible for operation and maintenance of the gas piping system. The action to be taken in response to an alarm will depend on the individual arrangements for each hospital. These should be recorded in a procedure manual, which is reviewed periodically, and new employees should be given clear instructions regarding actions to be taken.

PRESSURE GAUGES

A pressure gauge must be installed in the main line adjacent to the actuating switch for the main supply line pressure alarm and in

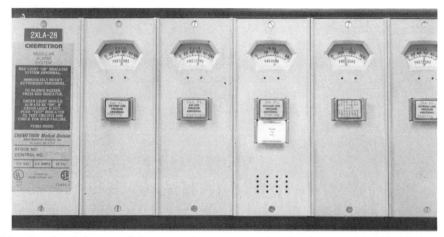

Figure 2.5.   Area (local) alarm panel. Pressures of gases are monitored and a warning provided if the pressure increases or decreases from the normal operating pressure. A button for testing the alarms is provided. Area alarm systems are provided for anesthetizing locations and other vital life support and critical care areas such as postanesthesia care units, intensive care units, and coronary care units.

each line being monitored at each area alarm panel.

TERMINAL UNITS (5,12)

The terminal unit (station outlet, pipeline outlet, end use terminal, service outlet, terminal outlet, outlet point, outlet station, outlet assembly, wall outlet) is the point in a piped gas distribution system at which the user normally makes connections and disconnections. Equipment may be connected to a terminal unit either directly or by means of a flexible hose.

Components

Base Block

The terminal unit base block is that part of a terminal unit which is attached to the pipeline distribution system.

Face Plate

The face plate should be permanently marked with the name and/or symbol of the gas it conveys. The identifying color may also be present. In some station outlets, the face plate and primary valve are an integral unit.

Primary Valve

The primary valve is also called the automatic shutoff valve; terminal unit valve or check valve; terminal valve; self-sealing valve, device, or unit; and primary check valve. Each station outlet contains a valve that opens and allows the gas to flow when the male probe is inserted and closes automatically when the connection is broken. This serves to prevent loss of gas when the nonfixed component is disconnected. Although often called a check valve it is not a unidirectional valve and will permit flow in either direction.

Secondary Valve (2)

The secondary valve (shutoff valve, terminal stop valve, maintenance valve, isolating valve, secondary valve, secondary shutoff valve, secondary check valve) is designed so that when the primary valve is removed (e.g., for cleaning or servicing) the flow of gas is shut off. When the primary valve is in place, the secondary valve stays open. With hose booms and pendants incorporating hoses, the secondary valve is fitted at or near the end of the permanent pipework.

Gas-Specific Connection Point (Socket Assembly)

Incorporated into each terminal unit is the receptor for a noninterchangeable gas-specific connector. This is either part of or attached to the base block. The connector may be a threaded Diameter Index Safety System or a proprietary (manufacturer-specific) nonthreaded, noninterchangeable quick connector. The corresponding male component of the noninterchangeable connection is attached to the equipment to be used or to a flexible hose leading to the equipment. The female component is called a socket or outlet connector. The male member is commonly called a plug, striker, probe, jack, or inlet connector.

Each quick connector or DISS connection must be equipped with a backflow check valve designed to prevent flow of gas from the anesthesia apparatus or other dispensing apparatus into the piping system.

The Diameter Index Safety System (3). The Diameter Index Safety System (DISS) was developed to provide noninterchangeable connections for medical gas lines at pressures of 200 psig or less. As shown in Figure 2.6, each DISS connection consists of a body, nipple, and nut combination. There are two concentric and specific bores in the body and two concentric and specific shoulders on the nipple. The small bore (BB) mates with the small shoulder (MM) and the large bore (CC) mates with the large shoulder (NN). To achieve noninterchangeability between different connections, the two diameters on each part vary in opposite directions, so that as one diameter increases, the other decreases. Only properly mated parts will fit together and allow thread engagement. A check valve may be added to the body portion of the connection (3). The American Society for Testing and Materials (ASTM) machine standard requires that every anesthesia machine have a DISS fitting for each pipeline inlet (13).

Quick Connectors. Because gases are frequently needed without delay, quick connectors (automatic quick couplers valves, quick connects, quick-connect fittings, quick couplers) have become popular. They allow the desired apparatus (hose, flowmeter, etc.) to be connected or disconnected by a single action using one or both hands without the use of tools or undue force.

Each quick coupler consists of a pair of nonthreaded, gas-specific male and female components. A releasable spring mechanism locks the components together. Insertion into an incorrect outlet is prevented by the use of different shapes for mating portions, different spacing of mating portions, or some combination of these. A national standard has not been developed for quick connectors. Therefore it is up to each manufacturer to ensure noninterchangeability between connections for different gases. Quick connectors are more convenient than DISS fittings, but because of the presence of O rings, seals and springs tend to leak more than the metal-to-metal DISS fittings.

Types

Wall Outlets

Wall outlets are mechanically simple, but the hoses to the machine frequently must be of considerable length and draped across the floor. This leads to problems with tripping, difficulty in moving equipment, wear and tear on the hose, and accumulation of debris along the hose. For large rooms two sets of wall outlets may be advisable. Terminal units should be installed at a height that makes them easily accessible but that minimizes the risk of damage from furniture and equipment.

Swinging Boom (Beam)

A wall- or ceiling-mounted boom with extendible arms is mechanically simple, relatively cheap, and avoids cluttering the floor. When mounted on a side wall, it can serve an anesthesia machine at either end or one side of the table. If an unusual placement of the

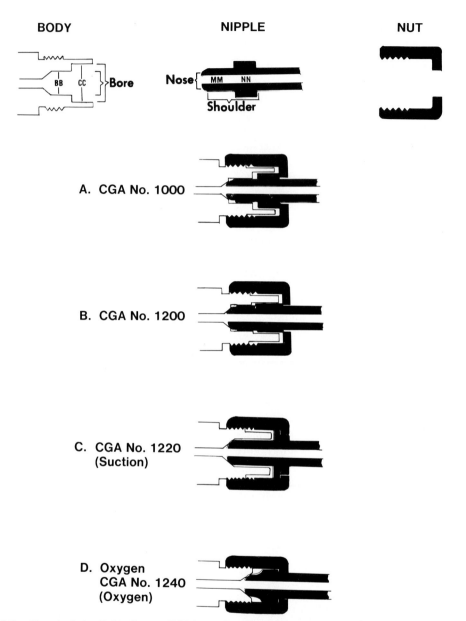

BODY   **NIPPLE**   **NUT**

Nose

Shoulder

A. CGA No. 1000

B. CGA No. 1200

C. CGA No. 1220
   (Suction)

D. Oxygen
   CGA No. 1240
   (Oxygen)

Figure 2.6. Diameter Index Safety System. With increasing CGA number, the small shoulder of the nipple becomes larger and the large diameter becomes smaller. If assembly of a nonmating body and nipple is attempted either MM will be too large for BB or NN will be too large for CC. Redrawn courtesy of the Compressed Gas Association.

operating table becomes necessary, the hoses can be temporarily unhooked from the boom. An effort should be made to keep the boom from passing over layouts of sterile equipment. Unfortunately, the outlets on a boom may be too high for short people to reach and tall people may hit their heads.

Rigid Column (14)

Columns mounted on the ceiling (Fig. 2.7) can provide connections for elec-

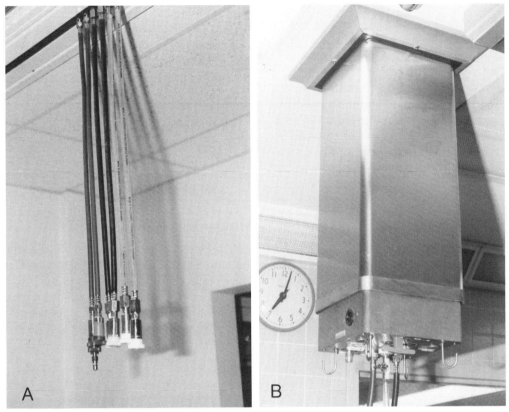

Figure 2.7. **A**, Hoses are on tracks so that they can be moved. **B**, The rigid column can be made retractable and can be put on a track.

trical outlets and monitoring channels as well as station outlets. This allows the majority of hoses and wires to approach the patient from one angle. They can be made movable by mounting them on overhead tracks. They can also be made retractable so that the column can be lowered for attachment/detachment of lines and then raised to keep it out of the way. Disadvantages include the possibility of people hitting their heads and the difficulty in gaining access to hoses inside the column.

Hoses (15)

A hose attached to the ceiling with the station outlet at its free end (see Fig. 2.7) is simple, cheap, and less of a danger than a rigid column. It should reach low enough that short people will be able to make connec-

tions easily. Retractable hoses or hose reels are desirable in this respect. Hoses can be put on tracks but care must be taken when they are moved not to get dust on the operating field.

Location in Anesthetizing Location

When a new anesthetizing location is being planned, it should be determined what the position of the operating room table will be most of the time, and station outlets should be placed near the expected position of the head of the table. Exceptions may be made for rooms to be used primarily for procedures on the head and neck, because the anesthesia machine is frequently at the side of the table. In situations for which it is undesirable or impossible to set up for all surgical procedures without changing the position of the operating table and anesthesia machine, a degree of flexibility can be obtained by installing two sets of station outlets on opposite sides of the room, using a boom, or installing columns or hoses on movable tracks (see Fig. 2.7). If the position of the operating table is optional and the room has a nonrecirculating air-conditioning system, consideration should be given to placing the station outlets near the outlet for the air-conditioning system so that it can be used for waste gas scavenging. If an overhead location is chosen, it should be established that the station outlet will not interfere with movement of the operating room light(s) under normal operating conditions.

In the postanesthesia care unit station outlets should be placed so as to facilitate access to the patient's head and to minimize the chances of equipment falling on a patient.

The Nitrogen Piping Station Outlet

Because the pressure required for nitrogen-driven tools varies, a means of adjusting the pressure at the station outlet is needed. An adjustable regulator of the type described in Chapter 3 is used. Figure 2.8 shows the regulator built into the wall. Two gauges are present, one indicating the distribution pressure and the other the reduced pressure. Figure 2.9 shows a different arrangement. A regulator and gauge to indicate the reduced pressure are attached to the station outlet.

HOSES (16)

Hoses (droplines, hose assemblies, low-pressure flexible connecting assemblies, flexible hose assemblies, pipeline pressure supply hoses, hose pipes) are used to connect anesthesia machines and other apparatus to terminal units. Each end should have a

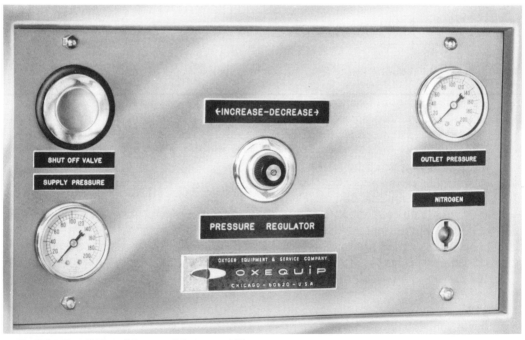

Figure 2.8. Termination of nitrogen piping system. Two gauges are present, one showing pipeline and one, reduced pressure. The reduced pressure can be altered using the pressure regulator. The station outlet is in the right lower corner. Courtesy of Oxequip Co.

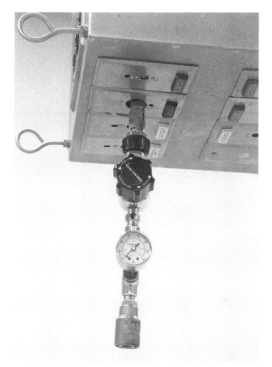

Figure 2.9. Another termination of nitrogen piping system. The pressure regulator and gauge are attached to the station outlet.

When an anesthesia machine is moved and a hose must be disconnected, this should be done quickly and preferably without opening the valve of a cylinder on the machine, because the cylinder may become depleted if the valve is not closed after the hose is reconnected. However, if it is necessary that the hose be disconnected for more than a few seconds, a cylinder should be opened and then closed as soon as the hose is reconnected.

The use of several extension hoses is undesirable. It is better to use one long hose, as resistance caused by multiple connections may interfere with flow. One long hose is less likely to leak because most leaks in hoses occur in the connectors or where the connector fits into the hose.

Hoses should be kept in good repair. They should be checked at least yearly for leaks. The hose should approach the anesthesia machine at a gentle curve, avoiding acute angulation or stretching.

permanently attached, noninterchangeable connector. The connector that attaches to a station outlet is called the supply (inlet) connector and the connector that attaches to equipment such as on an anesthesia machine is the equipment (outlet) connector.

Color coding of the hose and having the name and/or chemical symbol of the contained gas on each connector are desirable. The hose should be resistant to occlusion by external forces under normal conditions of use. Hoses should be kept away from any heat source, especially operating room lights, because contact may cause the hose to rupture (17,18). Whenever possible, they should be kept off the floor because of the danger of tripping, the added wear and tear on the hose, and difficulties with keeping such hoses clean and moving equipment over or around them.

Testing of Medical Gas Distribution Systems

INITIAL TESTING (2,19,20)

Because problems with medical gas systems are most likely to occur with a new system or one that has been modified or repaired, it is essential that such a system be thoroughly tested before being put into use. If a system is brand new, the entire system must be tested. For a new or modified portion of an existing system, the extent of testing will depend on how much of the existing system can be isolated and not affected by the work.

Confusion during installation of a medical gas piping system is compounded by a number of factors. There are usually a large number of people employed by different companies involved. Passage of time may require transfer of responsibility and information between a succession of individuals, each of whom is primarily concerned with his or her own area of involvement and less with whether the work before him or her has been performed according to specifications. Many workers at various stages of the enterprise know only what they themselves are to do and do not ask who is responsible for the rest or whether it is being done properly.

Responsibility

There has been controversy over who should carry out the final (commissioning) tests to make sure the piping system complies with regulations. Commercial services that inspect medical gas pipelines and offer certification are available. As there are currently no national certification or registration programs for installers, inspectors, or testers of medical piped gas systems, a facility should be careful in the selection of the person(s) or companies to perform these tasks.

There may be local or state requirements relative to the need for a permit before a piping system can be installed. The Canadian Standard (21) requires that the preoperational tests be made by a testing agency experienced in the field, independent of the contractor, gas and equipment suppliers, and the owner. It also requires that a member of the staff of the healthcare facility and a representative of the installer be present to witness testing.

Anesthesia personnel have an obligation to ensure that the system is properly designed and functions correctly. A member of the department should witness the tests performed, especially those for cross-connections. A personal independent check using an oxygen analyzer or other apparatus, such as Raman spectroscopy or mass spectrometer, is an excellent idea.

Test procedures and results of all tests, including room and area of testing, dates of tests, and names of persons conducting the tests, should be made part of the permanent records of the facility.

Procedures (20)

Pressure Testing (2,12,20)

Pressure testing is done to detect leaks. This is important because a leak in an oxygen line may create a fire hazard, a leak in a nitrous oxide line may cause health problems in exposed workers (see Chapter 11) and a leak in any line represents a waste of money.

Before attachment of system components (pressure-actuating switches for alarms, pressure gauges, or pressure relief valves) but after installation of the station outlets and before closing of the walls, each section of the piping system must be subjected to a test pressure of at least 150 psig with oil-free dry air or nitrogen with the source valve closed. This pressure is maintained until each joint has been examined for leakage using soapy water or some other safe means of leak detection. If any leaks are found, they must be corrected.

After all components of the system have been installed, the entire system is subjected to a 24-hr standing pressure test at 20% above the normal working pressure with the source valve closed. This permits testing without damaging system components or activating pressure-relief devices. Leaks, if any, must be located and repaired, and the test must be repeated until normal.

Testing for Cross-Connections (2)

Testing for cross-connections (anticonfusion test or continuity test) is to determine that the gas delivered at each station outlet is that shown on the outlet label and that the proper connecting fittings are present.

One gas system is tested at a time. Each gas is turned off at the source valve and the pressures reduced to atmospheric. The pipeline being tested is then filled with oil-free air or nitrogen at its working pressure. With appropriate adaptors matching outlet labels, each individual station outlet is checked to ensure that test gas emerges only from the outlets of the medical gas system being tested. Each additional gas system is tested in turn.

An alternative method of testing for cross-connections is as follows: The pressures of all medical gas systems are reduced to atmospheric. The pressures in all medical gas piping systems are increased to the following values:

Medical Gas	Psig	kPa Gauge
Gas mixtures	20	140
Nitrogen	30	210
Nitrous oxide	40	280
Oxygen	50	350
Compressed air	60	420
Carbon dioxide	70	490

Following adjustment of these pressures each station outlet for each medical gas is tested using a pressure gauge with a gas-specific connection. The pressure indicated on the test gauge must be that listed above.

An oxygen analyzer should be used to check the identity of the gas at each station outlet, giving readings of 0% for nitrous oxide, carbon dioxide, and nitrogen; 21% for air; and 100% for oxygen. If another means of analysis, such as mass spectrometry or Raman spectroscopy is available, this should be used to check the identity of all piped gases.

Tests of Individual Components (2)

The central supply should be checked for the following: changeover from one cylinder bank to the other and activation of the changeover signal; changeover from primary to secondary supply and activation of the changeover signal; operation of the reserve (if present) and the reserve-in-use warning signal; function of the activating signal on the reserve supply low alarm; function of the pressure relief valve set at 50% above normal line pressure to ensure that it opens at the correct pressure and reseats when the excess pressure is relieved; proper functioning of the safety valve, automatic drain, pressure gauge, and high water level sensors on the medical air compressor; proper functioning of the pressure regulator(s); and proper identification and activation of all signals at the master signal panels.

In the piped system, shutoff valves should be checked for tightness, that they control only those station outlets for which they are intended, and that they are properly labeled for the gas and area controlled. The test for tightness is performed by closing the valve, releasing the pressure downstream, and monitoring this pressure for 30 min. If the pressure rises, the valve is not tight.

Each station outlet should be checked for satisfactory operation by inserting appropriate equipment and verifying that it locks into position and releases properly. The station outlet should be checked for proper labeling and to ensure that it accommodates only connections for the gas for which it was designed. Pressures and flows should be checked to verify that the proper flow can be delivered (22). The Canadian Standard requires a flow of 120 liters/min with a maximum pressure drop of 4 psi for gases delivered at 50 psi. For nitrogen, the standard requires a flow of 400 liters/min with a maximum pressure drop of 10 psi for gas delivered at 180 psi (12).

Area alarm panels should be checked to ensure that they are properly labeled and are activated by a 20% increase or decrease in pressure in the piping system. Pressure relief devices should be tested to ensure that they open at the correct pressure and reseat when the excess pressure is relieved.

Cleaning, Purging, and Purity (2)

All pipes for medical gases must be thoroughly cleaned before installation, then the ends kept sealed until the actual installation. During installation, every effort must be made to keep tools free of contaminating materials and not to allow flux or metal to get inside the piping as it is being installed.

After installation of the piping, but before installation of the station outlets and other components the line must be blown clear using oil-free dry air or nitrogen.

After testing for cross-connections and

pressures, each gas is connected to its respective system and all outlets opened in a progressive order, starting nearest the source and completing the process at the outlet farthest from the source. This is done to remove the test gas and reduce particulate contamination. Satisfactory reduction of contamination by purging may require several days (23,24).

After purging, the flow from each station outlet is tested with an oxygen analyzer or other device to confirm the presence of the desired percentage of oxygen. Cases have been reported in which patients died from failure to purge the nitrogen from the oxygen pipeline before use in a new facility (21).

PERIODIC TESTING (2,4,13)

The installers of a piping system should be required to provide complete "as fitted" drawings, diagrams, charts, and maintenance instructions to be used as the foundation for a preventive maintenance program. These should be kept readily at hand in the department responsible for maintenance of the system.

Inspection and testing of piping systems should be performed on a regular basis, and the results recorded in a permanent log. If this involves shutting down parts of a pipeline system, the shutdown should be coordinated with the clinical staff in the area affected so that no patients are being served by the portion of the system being tested.

Shutoff valves should be tested to verify proper operation and rooms or areas they control. Pressure relief valves should be checked to determine the pressure at which relief occurs and that they close after the pressure is relieved. All alarms should be retested annually. If test buttons are provided, audible and visual signals should be tested monthly.

The location of the air intakes should be rechecked quarterly to ensure that they are as free from contamination as possible. Proper functioning of the pressure gauges and high water level alarms on the receivers should be checked at least annually. The receiver should be checked daily to determine if an excessive quantity of condensed water has accumulated.

At least annually, all hoses and station outlets in the anesthetizing locations and postanesthesia care units should be checked for wear, damage, and proper function. Terminal units should be checked for ease of insertion and locking of the connector; ease of unlocking and removal; leakage, wear, and damage; contamination; gas specificity; labeling; flow; and pressure (13).

Shutoff valves to anesthetizing locations can be checked for tightness and components downstream of the valve for leakage by the following test. An anesthesia machine with a pipeline pressure gauge is connected to the piping system. Cylinder valves on the machines are closed, the zone shutoff valves outside each operating room are closed, and gas is released until each pipeline pressure gauge reads 40 psig. This pressure is then monitored for 4 hr. It should remain at 40 psig. If the pressure rises, the shutoff valve is not working properly. If the pressure falls, there is a leak in the pipe to the room, the station outlet, or the hose to the anesthesia machine. This will not detect leakage in the primary valve or in the station outlet. It is essential that the shutoff valves be reopened after this test has been performed.

The main line pressure gauge and area pressure gauges should be checked daily. Pipeline pressure gauges are included on all new anesthesia machines. These should be checked before administration of anesthesia is begun. If a machine does not have a pipeline pressure gauge, the pressure should be checked on the local area pressure gauge (see Fig. 2.5).

Problems

Many problems in piping systems are the result of a lack of awareness among hospital personnel who have been lulled into believing that the piping system cannot fail and who are not sufficiently familiar with it to make emergency adjustments.

Lack of communication between clinical and maintenance departments and commercial suppliers may also be a contributing factor. Finally, lack of adherence to existing codes is responsible for many hazards.

INADEQUATE PRESSURE

This is the most frequently reported malfunction (10). Loss of pressure may result in a flow inadequate to power a ventilator but sufficient to provide adequate flow to the anesthesia machine.

Causes

Causes of inadequate pressure include damage, especially during hospital construction projects unrelated to the piping system (7), fires (19,25), vehicular accidents, theft of nitrous oxide tanks (7), environmental forces (earthquakes, excessive cold, tornadoes [26], lightning), depletion of or damage to the central supply (27,28), human error such as closure of a shutoff valve (7,29), inappropriate adjustment of the main line pressure regulator (10), equipment failures (leaks, activation of a shutoff valve [30–32]), failure of standby supply during routine maintenance (33), regulator malfunction (7,34,35), problems with automatic switching gear (34), obstruction of the pipeline (frequently by debris left following installation [7,36,37]), failure of a quick coupler to fit into a station outlet or to allow gas to flow (22,32,37–40), fracturing of a quick connect (41,42), plugging of a connector (36,43), detachment of a terminal unit (19), kinking or obstruction by external equipment (44,45), or a leak in a hose (17,46–48). Deliberate tampering with a system is a possibility that should not be overlooked.

Disaster Plan (10)

Because loss of oxygen or air pipeline pressure is not uncommon and because the consequences can be so severe, each hospital should have a plan to deal with it. Because no single plan is feasible for every healthcare facility, this section is intended only to provide guidance in the preparation and implementation of an individual plan.

The key to effective emergency preparedness planning is flexibility, which is attained by considering all possibilities and developing options for action that are maximally effective under each possibility. A key element of a disaster plan is that it be functional any time of day or night, any day of the year.

The organization of an effective response to the loss of a piped gas must include reliable communication pathways and individual responsibilities that take into account practical circumstances. The details of such a plan should be discussed and rehearsed in advance in the form of mock disaster drills if an effective response is to be expected during a real emergency. Each individual involved in patient support should be aware of his or her role under the plan. Locations of shutoff valves should be known by the staff, so that if the loss of pressure is caused by a large leak in one area, the pipeline to that section can be isolated to prevent further loss of gas.

The person discovering a fault in the piped supply should immediately inform the telephone operator who, in turn, should inform the department responsible for maintenance of the system, respiratory therapy, surgery, the postanesthesia care unit, obstetrics, the emergency room, special care units such as intensive care and nursery, the nursing supervisor, and the hospital administrator. Each department in turn should have carefully established procedures to deal with the emergency. These should be reviewed regularly, revised as necessary, and put in procedure manuals.

Because every anesthesia machine should have at least one emergency oxygen cylinder, there should be no immediate threat to life in the operating rooms but a prudent course of action would be to use low fresh gas flows and manual ventilation. Attention should be focused on the postanesthesia care unit (recovery room). It may be advantageous to move anesthesia machines not in use into the recovery room to supply oxygen until other sources can be obtained. Alternately, patients in the recovery room can be wheeled back into the operating rooms. Potential emergency oxygen sources other than compressed cylinders include portable liquid oxygen containers and oxygen concentrators and generators (49–56). For patients on ventilators it may be necessary to use manual ventilation.

The need for additional oxygen should be assessed and elective surgery postponed until adequate supplies can be ensured. Efforts should be coordinated with other departments to determine needs and supplies on hand and with the department responsible for the piping system to determine how long the loss of piped gas will last.

Emergency Auxiliary Supply

Because of the dangers associated with failure of piped oxygen and air systems, special areas such as intensive care units, recovery rooms, emergency rooms, etc. may add an auxiliary oxygen and/or air supply. These areas must be capable of being isolated by means of a shutoff valve. When an emergency arises, the shutoff valve is turned off and the auxiliary source is connected to an outlet within the zone not in use or by means of a specially installed T. All outlets within the area can then operate from the auxiliary source.

EXCESSIVE PRESSURE

Excessive pressure is also a relatively common problem (7). As shown in Figure 2.3, a pressure relief valve in the main supply line is required. This should offer some protection from excessive pressure. However, this can be set improperly or malfunction.

High pressures can result in damage to equipment, especially regulators (23,35) and may cause barotrauma to patients. Few anesthesia machines or ventilators have mechanisms to prevent damage from high pres-

sures. Some ventilators will not operate properly if the line pressure is too high.

The most common cause of high pressure is failure of a regulator. In humid atmospheres ice may form on the vaporizers in a liquid oxygen system. This will hamper heat transfer and may result in liquid oxygen passing into the piping system with resultant damage to the regulator and pressure relief valve. This also has been reported after the addition of liquid oxygen to the main tank (23). Other causes of high pressure include combustion of foreign material in a pipeline (7) and deliberately increasing the pressure setting of the main line regulator in an attempt to compensate for low pressure from the central system (35).

Whenever excessive pipeline pressure occurs it is best to disconnect apparatus from the pipeline system and use cylinders until the problem is corrected.

ALARM DYSFUNCTION

Failure, absence, or disconnection of an alarm is not uncommon (7,35,57). Another problem is that the alarm signal goes off but the person who hears it either does not know the proper course of action or fails to follow it (7,58).

False alarms are also a common problem. They may result from calibration drift in line pressure sensors (10). Repeated false alarms can cause complacency among personnel, which may have serious consequences if a real emergency occurs.

CROSS-CONNECTION OF GASES

Although an uncommon event, the accidental substitution of one gas for another can have devastating consequences. The most common cross-overs have been between nitrous oxide and oxygen, because they are the gases most frequently piped, but various other combinations have been reported. Pipeline alarms indicate only pressure faults and give no signal if an incorrect gas is present. Because the consequences are most severe when the cross-over results in hypoxia, it is essential that a reliable oxygen analyzer be included as a component of every breathing system.

Central Supply

Cases have been reported in which liquid oxygen tanks were filled with nitrogen (57,59) and argon (41,60). Incorrect tanks have been placed on the central supply manifold (37,41,61).

Distribution System

Crossing of pipelines usually occurs during installation of, alterations to, or repairs to a system (62–71). In one case a fistula was created between two pipes during construction (24).

Flooding of an oxygen line with nitrogen has occurred when nitrogen was used to test for leaks after making repairs or extensions to an existing system and the shutoff valve to that area did not prevent backflow (19,72). To prevent this, it is recommended that the section being modified be isolated from the sections in use.

Station Outlets

There are numerous reports of outlets labeled for one gas that delivered another (73–75). The wrong outlet connector may be installed (37,24,76). A terminal unit may accept an incorrect connector (77–80).

Hoses

Several cases have been reported in which the wrong connector was put on one or more hoses (7,72,81–83). Most of these have involved repairs to hoses performed by hospital personnel. Whenever a hose is altered or repaired, it should be checked carefully before it is put into service to make certain that the proper connectors are in each end. With extension hoses, this is easily performed by inserting one end of the hose into the other. Blue hoses turning green have been reported (84). This could result in attachment of an oxygen-specific fitting to one end of a green (previously blue) hose.

Peripheral Devices

Numerous cases have been reported in which an air/oxygen mixer or ventilator that used both air and oxygen had a defect such that the gas supplies became interconnected and oxygen flowed into the air pipeline (34,85–92) or air flowed into the oxygen piping (34,93,94). The faulty device often was not in use. The level of contamination depends on how long the defective device is plugged in and the difference in supply pressure between the two gases. It is suggested that respiratory equipment be disconnected from the pipeline supply when not in use (85).

CONTAMINATION OF GASES

Particulate

Particulate contamination can be a serious problem, particularly when a new pipeline system is opened. Metallic and hydrocarbon contaminants may be trapped inside the piping and will be present in the gas coming from the station outlets (23,24). Another source of contamination may be oil from an air compressor (72,95). These particles can damage equipment, especially ventilators, and may be harmful to a patient if inhaled. Particulate matter can cause a significant reduction in flow. Failure of a line pressure sensor owing to foreign material has been reported (10).

During installation every effort should be made to keep pipes, fittings, and valves as clean as possible. The majority of particles can be removed by purging, which may require several days, but particulate purging may never be complete, especially in tall buildings (72).

Gaseous

Inhalation of volatile hydrocarbons can be unpleasant and potentially harmful to the patient, may cause damage to equipment, or create a fire hazard. Volatile hydrocarbons in piped gas supplies may be the result of materials left in the pipes during construction

(23,24), even though the use of organic solvents to clean fittings and other components is prohibited. In one reported case, a cleaning solvent was not purged from the hose that connected the delivery truck to the hospital to maintain the oxygen supply during delivery of liquid oxygen to the main hospital storage tank (96).

The inlet to the air compressors can be a source of contamination (23). In one case, the intake for the air compressor was located at the ambulance entrance and exhaust gases were taken into the piped system (97). In another case, a piped air system became contaminated when a filter was soaked in cleaning fluid and replaced without allowing it to dry (98).

Water

Water contamination of the air supply is potentially damaging to equipment such as ventilators and may adversely affect their accuracy (99,100).

Bacterial

Piped medical gases are not sterile and bacterial contamination has been documented (101–103). A filter must be used to produce sterile gases.

Fires

Equipment used with a pipeline system for medical gases must be clean and free from oil, grease, and particulate matter to avoid fires. A hose that contains oxygen or nitrous oxide can rupture and burn if it comes in contact with a light (17,46,18).

The following steps listed in the approximate order of their importance should be taken if a fire occurs (2):

1. Remove the immediately exposed patient(s) from the site of the fire, if their hair or clothing are not burning. If they are burning, extinguish the flames first.
2. Sound the fire alarm.
3. Close off the supply of oxygen, nitrous oxide, and air to any equipment involved,

if this can be accomplished without injury to personnel. Zone shutoff valves usually allow this to be accomplished easily (19). Unfortunately, these are not always clearly labeled, nor are their positions always known to the hospital staff. Because each gas line to an operating room should have an individual zone valve, closing of the valve to one room would not endanger patients in other rooms. However, in other areas of the hospital, closure of the zone valve will cut off the supply to multiple patients.

4. Close doors to contain smoke and isolate the fire.
5. Remove patients threatened by the fire.
6. Attempt to extinguish or contain the fire.
7. Direct firefighters to the site of the fire.
8. Take whatever steps are necessary to protect or evacuate patients in adjacent areas.

LEAKS

Leaks are also a common problem (7). They may occur anywhere in the piping system from the central supply to the hose. Leaks are expensive and potentially hazardous if oxidizing gases are allowed to accumulate in closed spaces. Leaks of nitrous oxide may pose a health hazard to hospital personnel (see Chapter 11).

DEPLETION OF THE RESERVE SUPPLY (10,35)

Depletion of the reserve supply caused by failures of connections, pressure imbalances, and leaks has been reported.

THEFT OF NITROUS OXIDE CYLINDERS

Theft of nitrous oxide cylinders from a central supply area for substance-abuse purposes has occurred (104).

REFERENCES

1. Gjerde GE. Retrograde pressurization of a medical oxygen pipeline system: safety backup or hazard? Crit Care Med 1980;8:219–221.

2. Klein BR. Health care facilities handbook. 3rd ed. Quincy MA: National Fire Protection Association, 1990.

3. Compressed Gas Association, Inc. Handbook of compressed gases. 3rd ed. New York: Van Nostrand Reinhold, 1990.

4. Canadian Standards Association. Nonflammable medical gas piping systems (CSA Z305.1-M1984). Toronto: CSA, 1984.

5. International Organization for Standardization. Terminal units for use in medical pipeline systems (ISO 9170:1990(E)). Geneve, Switzerland: ISO, 1990.

6. International Organization for Standardization. Oxygen concentrators for medical use—safety requirements (ISO 8359:1988(E)). Geneve, Switzerland: ISO, 1988.

7. Feeley TW, Hedley-Whyte J. Bulk oxygen and nitrous oxide delivery systems: design and dangers. Anesthesiology 1976;44:301–305.

8. Friesen RM. Oxygen concentrators and the practice of anaesthesia. Can J Anaesth 1992;39:R80–R84.

9. McPherson SP. Respiratory therapy equipment. 3rd ed. St Louis: CV Mosby 1985.

10. Bancroft ML, du Moulin GC, Hedley-Whyte J. Hazards of hospital bulk oxygen delivery systems. Anesthesiology 1980;52:504–510.

11. Howell RSC. Low failure rate for medical gas line systems in United Kingdom. Anesthesiology 1981;54:526.

12. Canadian Standards Association. Medical gas terminal units (CAN/CSA-Z305.5-M86). Toronto: CSA, 1986.

13. American Society for Testing and Materials. Specification for minimum performance and safety requirements for components and systems of anesthesia gas machines (ASTM F1161-88). Philadelphia: ASTM, 1988.

14. Wilder RJ, Williams GR. The ceiling-retractable service column. JAMA 1981;246:1403–1404.

15. Zeller HR. Use of ceiling hose reels by anesthesiologists in the operating room. Anesth Analg 1961;40:413–417.

16. Canadian Standards Association. Low-pressure connecting assemblies for medical gas systems (CSA Z305.2-M1980). Toronto: CSA, 1980.

17. Anderson EF. A potential ignition source in the operating room. Anesth Analg 1976;55:217–218.

18. Anonymous. Unshielded radiant heat sources. Technol Anesth 1985;5:1.

19. Arrowsmith LWM. Medical gas pipelines. Eng Med 1979;8:247–249.

20. Anonymous. Modification of medical gas systems. Health Devices 1980;9:181–185.

21. Canadian Standards Association. Qualification requirements for agencies testing non-flammable medical gas piping systems (CSA Z305.4-1977). Toronto: CSA, 1977.

22. Morrison AB. Information letter. Medical gas station outlets and outlet connectors. Rexdale (Toronto), Canada: Health Protection Branch, Health and Welfare, January 14, 1981.

23. Eichhorn JH, Bancroft ML, Laasberg L, du Moulin GC, Saubermann AJ. Contamination of medical gas and water pipelines in a new hospital building. Anesthesiology 1977;46:286–289.

24. Tingay MG, Ilsley AH, Willis RJ, Thompson MJ, Chalmers AH, Cousins MJ. Gas identity hazards and major contamination of the medical gas system of a new hospital. Anaesth Intensive Care 1978;6:202–209.

25. Wright CJ, Bostock F. Pipeline hazards—a simple solution. Anaesthesia 1978;33:759.

26. Johnson DL. Central oxygen supply versus mother nature. Respir Care 1975;20:1043–1044.

27. Chi OZ. Another example of hypoxic gas mixture delivery. Anesthesiology 1985;62:543–544.

28. Russell WJ. Oxygen supply at risk. Anaesth Intensive Care 1985;13:216–217.

29. Anonymous: Mystery of turned-off hospital oxygen supply solved by Denver police. Biomed Safe Stand 1987;17:18–19.

30. Black AE. Extraordinary oxygen pipeline failure. Anaesthesia 1990;45:599.

31. Gibson OB. Another hazardous pipeline isolator valve. Anaesthesia 1979;34:213.

32. MacWhirter GI. An anesthetic pipe line hazard. Anaesthesia 1978;33:639.

33. Francis RN. Failure of nitrous oxide supply to theatre pipeline system. Anaesthesia 1990;45:880–882.

34. Carley RH, Haughton IT, Park GR. A near disaster from piped gases. Anaesthesia 1984;39:891–893.

35. Feeley TW, McClelland KJ, Malhotra IV. The hazards of bulk oxygen delivery systems. Lancet 1975;1:1416–1418.

36. Janis KM. Sudden failure of ceiling oxygen connector. Can Anaesth Soc J 1978;25:155.

37. Krenis LJ, Berkowitz DA. Errors in installation of a new gas delivery system found after certification. Anesthesiology 1985;62:677–678.

38. Craig DB, Culligan J. Sudden interruption of gas flow through a Schrader oxygen coupler unit. Can Anaesth Soc J 1980;27:175–177.

39. Chung DC, Hunter DJ, Pavan FJ. The quick-mount pipeline connector: failure of a "fail-safe" device. Can Anaesth Soc J 1986;33:666–668.

40. Mather SJ. Put not your trust in: a case of pipeline failure during routine anaesthesia. Anaesth Points West 1969;2:21–22.

41. Anonymous. Puritan-Bennett quick connect valves for medical gases: Canadian medical devices

alert warns of possible cracks. Biomed Safe Stand 1984;14:52–53.

42. Morrison AB. Puritan-Bennett quick connect valves for medical gases. Medical devices alert. Ottawa: Health and Welfare Canada, April 9, 1984.

43. Anderson B, Chamley D. Wall outlet oxygen failure. Anaesth Intensive Care 1987;15:468–469.

44. Anderson WR, Brock-Utne JG. Oxygen pipeline supply failure: a coping strategy. J Clin Monit 1991;7:39–41.

45. Muir J, Davidson-Lamb R. Apparatus failure—cause for concern. Br J Anaesth 1980;52:705–706.

46. Anonymous. Unshielded radiant heat sources. Technol Anesth 1984;5:1.

47. Ewart IA. An unusual cause of gas pipeline failure. Anaesthesia 1990;45:498.

48. Lacoumenta S, Hall GM. A burst oxygen pipeline. Anaesthesia 1983;38:596–597.

49. Carter JA, Baskett PJF, Simpson PJ. The "Permox" oxygen concentrator. Anaesthesia 1985;40:560–565.

50. de Sousa H. Use of an oxygen concentrator as the gas source for general anesthesia. Anesth Analg 1990;70:S82.

51. Easy WR, Douglas GA, Merrifield AJ. A combined oxygen concentrator and compressed air unit. Assessment of a prototype and discussion of its potential applications. Anaesthesia 1988;43:37–41.

52. Hall LW, Kellagher REB, Fleet KJ. A portable oxygen generator. Anaesthesia 1986;41:516–518.

53. Harris CE, Simpson PJ. The "Mini O2" and "Healthdyne" oxygen concentrators. Anaesthesia 1985;40:1206–1209.

54. Howell RSC. Oxygen concentrators. Br J Hosp Med 1985;34:221–223.

55. Lush D. Oxygen concentrators. Anaesthesia 1986;41:83.

56. Swar BB. Oxygen concentrators. Can J Anaesth 1987;34:538–539.

57. Sprague DH, Archer GW. Intraoperative hypoxia from an erroneously filled liquid oxygen reservoir. Anesthesiology 1975;42:360–362.

58. Paul DL. Pipeline failure. Anaesthesia 1989;44:523.

59. Holland R. Foreign correspondence: "wrong gas" disaster in Hong Kong. APSF Newslett 1989;4:26.

60. Smith FP. Multiple deaths from argon contamination of hospital oxygen supply. JFSCA 1987;32:1098–1102.

61. Anonymous. O_2-N_2O mix-up leads to probe into deaths of two patients. Biomed Safe Stand 1981;11:123–124.

62. Anonymous. Medical Gas Systems. Technol Anesth 1982;12:5.

63. Anonymous. Emergency room mixup, Deaths linked. Am Biomed News, Aug. 8, 1977, p. 3.

64. Anonymous. Interchanged oxygen and nitrous oxide lines caused death, suit charges. Biomed Safe Stand 1980;10:28–29.

65. Anonymous. Undetected crossed air-oxygen lines may have contributed to deaths of 7. Biomed Safe Stand 1982;12:41.

66. Anonymous. Cross-connected anesthesia supply lines allegedly result in two deaths: negligence suits filed. Biomed Safe Stand 1984;14:15–16.

67. Anonymous. Medical gas/vacuum systems. Technol Anesth 1987;7:1–2.

68. Deas T. A preventable tragedy. Items Top 1977;23:6–7.

69. Emmanuel ER, Teh JL. Dental anaesthetic emergency caused by medical gas pipeline installation error. Aust Dent J 1983;28:79–81.

70. LeBourdais E. Nine deaths linked to cross-contamination: Sudbury General inquest makes hospital history. Dimens Health Serv 1974;51:10–12.

71. Sato T: Fatal pipeline accidents spur Japanese standards. APSF Newslett 1991;6:14.

72. Dinnick OP. Medical gases-piping problems. Eng Med 1979;8:243–247.

73. Anonymous. Installation of oxygen system probed in nitrous oxide death suit. Biomed Safe Stand 1980;10:41–42.

74. Anonymous. Fittings, quick-connect. Technol Anesth 1982;3:4.

75. Anonymous. Crossed N_2O & O_2 lines blamed for outpatient surgery death. Biomed Safe Stand 1992;22:14.

76. Anonymous. Crossed connections in medical gas systems. Technol Anesth 1984;5:3.

77. Anonymous. Fittings/adapters, pneumatic, quick connect. Technol Anesth 1990;11:11.

78. Klein SL, Lilburn K. An unusual case of hypercarbia during general anesthesia. Anesthesiology 1980;53:248–250.

79. Lane GA. Medical gas outlets—a hazard from interchangeable "quick connect" couplers. Anesthesiology 1980;52:86–87.

80. Anonymous. Misconnection of O_2 line to CO_2 outlet claimed in death. Biomed Safe Stand 1991;21:92–93.

81. Anonymous. The Westminster inquiry. Lancet 1977;2:175–176.

82. Anonymous. Anesthesia units. Technol Anesth 1982;3:2.

83. Robinson JS. A continuing saga of piped medical gas supply. Anaesthesia 1979;34:66–70.

84. Anonymous. Hoses, compressed gas. Technol Anesth 1986;7:5.

85. Weightman WM, Fenton-May V, Saunders R, Lewis A, Wise CC. Functionally crossed pipelines. An intermittent condition caused by a faulty ventilator. Anaesthesia 1992;47:500–502.

86. Anonymous. Bourns Bear 1 ventilator. Health Devices 1983;12:167–168.
87. Bageant RA, Hoyt JW, Epstein RM. Error in a pipeline gas concentration: an unanticipated consequence of a defective check valve. Anesthesiology 1981;54:166–169.
88. Bedsole SC, Kempf J. More faulty Bear check valves. Respir Care 1984;29:1159.
89. Jenner W, George BF. Oxygen-air shunt syndrome strikes again. Respir Care 1982;27:604.
90. Shaw A, Richardson W, Railton R. Malfunction of air-mixing valves. Anaesthesia 1985;40:711.
91. Shaw R, Beach W, Metzler M. Medical air contamination with oxygen associated with the Bear 1 and 2 ventilators. Crit Care Med 1988;16:362.
92. Ziecheck HD. Faulty ventilator check valves cause pipeline gas contamination. Respir Care 1981;26:1009–1010.
93. Karmann U, Roth F. Prevention of accidents associated with air-oxygen mixers. Anaesthesia 1982;37:680–682.
94. Thorp JM, Railton R. Hypoxia due to air in the oxygen pipeline. Anaesthesia 1982;37:683–687.
95. Bushman JA, Clark PA. Oil mist hazard and piped air supplies. Br Med J 1967;3:588–590.
96. Gilmour IJ, McComb C, Palahniuk RJ. Contamination of a hospital oxygen supply. Anesth Analg 1990;71:302–304.
97. RB. Contaminated "medical" air. Respir Care 1972;17:125.
98. Lackore LK, Perkins HM. Accidental narcosis. Contamination of compressed air system. JAMA 1970;211:1846–1847.
99. Conely JIM, Railton R, MacKenzie AI. Ventilator problems caused by humidity in the air supplied from simple compressors. Br J Anaesth 1981;53:549–550.
100. McAdams SA, Barnes W. Air compressor failure complicating mechanical ventilation. Respir Care 1983;28:1601.
101. Bjerring P, Oberg B. Bacterial contamination of compressed air for medical use. Anaesthesia 1986;41:148–150.
102. Bjerring P, Oberg B. Possible role of vacuum systems and compressed air generators in cross-infection in the ICU. Br J Anaesth 1987;59:648–650.
103. Warren RE, Newsom SWB, Matthews JA, Arrowsmith LWM. Medical grade compressed air. Lancet 1986;1:1438.
104. Stein DW. Anesthetic agent misuse reported. ASA Newslett, June 1978.

Chapter 3

The Anesthesia Machine

The first apparatus resembling an anesthesia machine appeared in 1905. Until recently the development of anesthesia machines was a slow, relatively unstructured process. Changes in machines have been occurring at an escalating rate, with the number of controls, indicators, and alarms increasing rapidly. The prevailing trend is to incorporate ventilators and vigilance aids such as airway pressure monitors, respirometers, carbon dioxide monitors, pulse oximeters and automatic blood pressure monitors into the machine.

Machine Standards

In 1979, after many years of hard work, with input from both anesthesiologists and industry representatives, a standard for anesthesia machines was published by the American National Standards Institute (ANSI) (1). This document determined how machines would be constructed for the fol-

lowing 10 years. Most machines sold since 1979 comply with the standard. In 1988, the ANSI standard was superseded by a standard prepared under the auspices of the American Society for Testing and Materials (ASTM) (2). This defined basic design, performance, and safety requirements for anesthesia machines for the 1990s. All American anesthesia machine manufacturers have agreed that machines sold after 1988 will comply with the standard.

Some older machines that do not comply with all or part of these standards can still be serviced, but owners of machines from companies that have discontinued business or that have dropped particular machines from their product lines may find it difficult to have these machines serviced.

The Canadian Standards Association has published a standard (3) relating to anesthesia machines that set down requirements similar to those of the ANSI standard.

As shown in Figure 3.1, the anesthesia machine can be conveniently divided into three

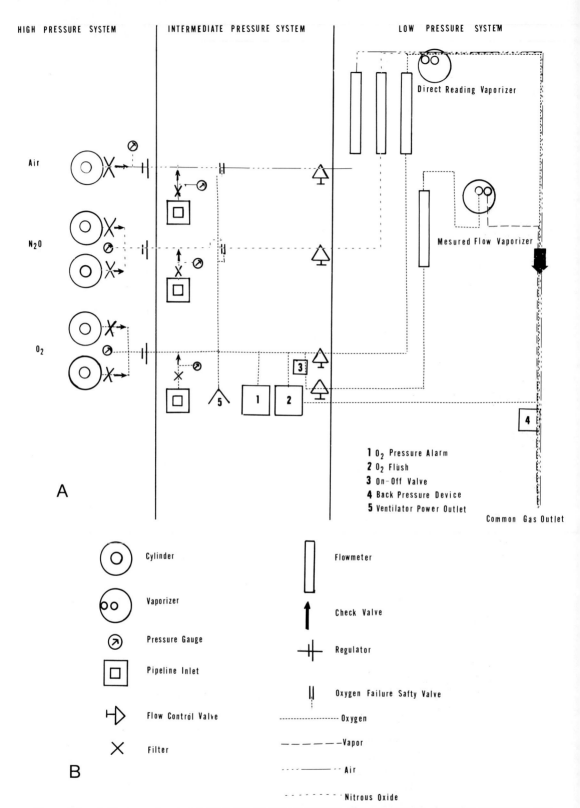

Figure 3.1. A, Diagram of a generic three-gas anesthesia machine. The components and their arrangement may differ somewhat with machines from different manufacturers. **B,** Key to components in part **A**.

parts: the high-pressure system, which receives gases at cylinder pressure, reduces the pressure, and makes it more constant; the intermediate pressure system, which receives gases from the regulator or hospital pipeline and delivers them to the flow control valves or oxygen flush valve; and the low-pressure system, which takes gases from the flow control valves to the common gas outlet.

The High-Pressure System

The high-pressure system consists of all parts of the machine that receive gas at cylinder pressure. These include the following: (*i*) the hanger yoke by which a cylinder is connected to the machine; (*ii*) the cylinder pressure gauge that indicates the gas pressure in the cylinder; and (*iii*) the pressure regulator that converts a high, variable gas pressure into a lower, more constant pressure suitable for use in the machine.

HANGER YOKE

The functions of the hanger yoke (connecting yoke) are to orient and support the cylinder, provide a gas-tight seal, and ensure a unidirectional flow of gas into the machine. It is composed of several parts: (*i*) the body, which is the principal framework and supporting structure; (*ii*) the retaining screw, which tightens the cylinder in the yoke; (*iii*) the nipple, through which gas enters the machine; (*iv*) the index pins, which prevent attachment of an incorrect cylinder; (*v*) the washer, which helps to form a seal between the cylinder and the yoke; (*vi*) a filter to remove dirt from the gas in the cylinder; and (*vii*) the check valve assembly, which ensures a unidirectional flow of gas through the yoke.

Each yoke assembly must be permanently identified with the name or chemical symbol of the gas it accommodates and should be marked with the color assigned to the gas (2).

Body

The body of the yoke is threaded into the frame of the machine. It provides support for the cylinder and prevents attachment of the cylinder at an angle. On the swinging gate (toggle handle, swivel gate) type (Fig. 3.2), the distal part of the yoke is hinged. The retaining screw is in the middle of this part.

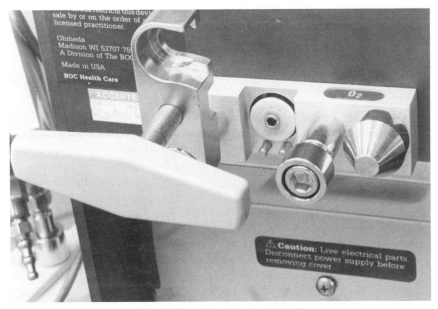

Figure 3.2. Swinging gate type yoke.

When a cylinder is being inserted into or removed from the yoke, the hinged part can be swung to the side.

The ASTM machine standard (2) requires that each yoke be fitted with a mechanism to prevent tightening of the clamping device until the pins of the Pin Index Safety System and the nipple are correctly engaged with appropriate recesses on the cylinder valve. Pins have been damaged and rendered inoperative by forceful attempts to seat an incorrect cylinder (4). A properly constructed swinging gate yoke meets this requirement, because the gate cannot be closed unless the cylinder valve is correctly in place.

Retaining Screw

The retaining screw (clamping device or retaining bar) is threaded into the distal end of the yoke (see Fig. 3.2). Tightening the screw presses the outlet of the cylinder valve against the washer and nipple so that a gas-tight seal is achieved. The cylinder is then supported by the retaining screw, the nipple of the yoke, and the index pins.

The conical point of the retaining screw is shaped to fit the conical depression on the cylinder valve. To prevent penetration of the safety relief device on the cylinder valve, it is important that the point not have an acute angle. The ASTM standard requires that it be tapered at an angle of 100° to 120° and be at least 7 mm in diameter.

Nipple

The nipple is the part of the yoke through which the gas enters the machine. It projects from the proximal part of the yoke and fits into the port on the cylinder valve. If the nipple is damaged, it may be impossible to create a tight seal with the cylinder valve.

Index Pins

The pins of the Pin Index Safety System are mounted into holes below the nipple. The holes into which the pins are fitted must be of a specific depth. If they extended too far into the body of the yoke, it might be possible to

insert an incorrect cylinder into the yoke (4). Tightening it would simply force the pins deeper into the yoke.

Washer

A washer (gasket) is used to achieve a seal between the cylinder valve and the yoke. Gas pressure on the inner circumference of the washer compresses and thickens it, creating a seal. A washer is generally supplied with each full cylinder.

When a cylinder is fitted to a yoke, care should be taken to ensure that the washer is present and in good condition. A broken or curled washer should not be used, because a leak could result. An extra washer should be kept in case one becomes damaged. No more than one washer should ever be used as that may prevent establishment of a tight seal or may nullify the Pin Index Safety System (4).

Filter

The ASTM standard (2) stipulates that a filter (100 μm maximum) be installed between the cylinder and regulator to prevent particulate matter from entering the machine where it could cause damage to other components.

Check Valve

The purpose of the check valve is to prevent retrograde flow of gases from the machine to the atmosphere when there is no cylinder in the yoke. In the case of a double yoke, the check valve prevents the transfer of gas from one cylinder to another with a lower pressure. It also allows an empty cylinder to be replaced with a full one without having to turn off the "in-use" cylinder.

A typical check valve is shown in Figure 3.3. It consists of a plunger that slides away from the side of the greater pressure. When cylinder pressure exceeds the pressure on the machine side, the plunger moves to the right and gas passes into the machine. When machine pressure exceeds cylinder pressure, the plunger moves to the left, blocking the flow of gases.

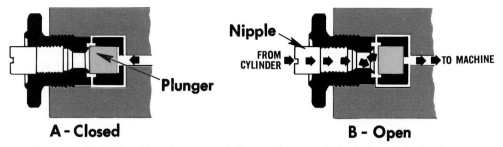

Figure 3.3.   Yoke check valve. When the pressure in the machine exceeds that in the cylinder the plunger moves to the left, preventing escape of gas from the machine. When cylinder pressure exceeds machine pressure, the plunger moves to the right and gas flows into the machine. From a drawing furnished by Ohmeda, a division of BOC, Inc.

These check valves are not designed to act as permanent seals for empty yokes and may allow a small amount of gas to escape. The ASTM standard (2) allows for a leak of up to 200 ml per minute at a pressure up to 2200 psig. To minimize such losses, yokes should not be left vacant. As soon as a cylinder is exhausted, it should be replaced by a full one. If a full cylinder is not available, a yoke plug (dummy cylinder block or plug) (Fig. 3.4) should be placed in the empty yoke. This is a solid piece of metal or other material that has a conical depression on one side to fit the tip of the retaining screw and a hollowed out area on the other side to fit over the nipple. When in place, it forms a seal to prevent the escape of gases from the machine. It also serves to keep the nipple clean and to prevent damage to the yoke. In the absence of a yoke plug a leak can occur through a flowmeter with an open flow control valve through the yoke (5). Machine manufacturers often chain yoke plugs to the machine (see Fig. 3.4).

To prevent transfilling between paired cylinders as a result of a defective check valve, only one cylinder should be open at a time.

Placing a Cylinder in a Yoke

Before a cylinder is placed in a yoke, the yoke should be checked to make certain that the two Pin Index Safety System pins are present. A missing pin can allow the safety system to be bypassed (6).

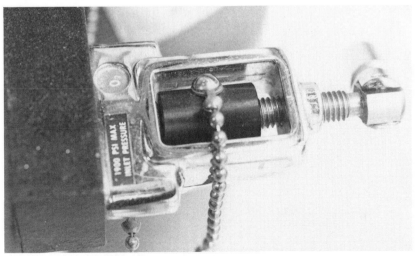

Figure 3.4.   Yoke plug in place. Note that it is chained to the machine.

The first step in placing a cylinder in a yoke is to retract the retaining screw as far as possible. With the gate-type yoke the gate is swung open. The washer is placed over the nipple. The cylinder is then supported with the tip of the toe and raised into the yoke (Fig. 3.5). The port of the cylinder valve is slid over the nipple and the index pins engaged in the appropriate holes. The gate is then closed. The retaining screw is tightened so that it contacts the conical depression on the cylinder valve and pushes the valve over the nipple and index pins. It is important to ensure that the cylinder is correctly in place before tightening the retaining screw. Otherwise it may be screwed into the safety relief device on the cylinder (7). The cylinder valve should be opened to make sure that the cylinder is full and that there is no leak (as evidenced by a hissing sound).

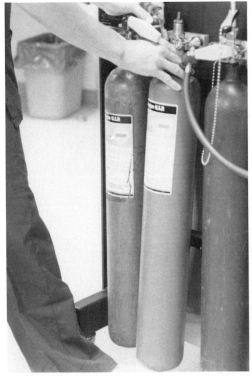

Figure 3.5. Placing cylinder in yoke. The cylinder is supported by the foot and guided into place manually.

CYLINDER PRESSURE GAUGE

The ASTM standard (2) requires that each hanger yoke or group of interconnected yokes be provided with a pressure gauge (indicator) or other quantitative contents indicator that will display the delivery pressure of cylinder-supplied gas. If there is more than one yoke for a gas, one gauge may be provided for each yoke or one gauge may be provided for a group of yokes.

If the gauge is circular, the diameter must be at least 38 mm with the lowest pressure indication between the 6 o'clock and 9 o'clock positions on a clock face (Fig. 3.6). The indicating end of the pointer must contrast with the background, whereas the tail end must be shorter than the indicating end and should blend into the background or be obscured from view. These requirements are designed to provide better resolution of the dial numbers and to facilitate recognition of the empty position on each gauge, which has been a problem in the past (8). The units of calibration are to be in kilopascals (kPa) but may also be in pounds per square inch (psig) (see Fig. 3.15).

The gauge must be clearly and permanently marked with the name or chemical symbol of the gas it monitors and should be identified by the color assigned to that gas.

These gauges are usually of the Bourdon tube (Bourdon spring) type, illustrated in Figure 3.6. A hollow metal tube is bent into a curve, sealed and linked to a clock-like mechanism. The other end is connected into the gas source and soldered into a socket. An increase in pressure of the gas inside the tube causes it to straighten. As the pressure falls, the tube resumes its curved shape. Because the open end is in a fixed position, the sealed end moves. Through the clock-like mechanism these motions are transmitted to the indicator, which moves on a scale calibrated in units of pressure.

In the event of a tight check valve in the yoke, the gauge may continue to display a reading even after the cylinder has been re-

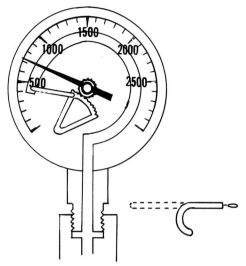

Figure 3.6. Bourdon pressure gauge. As gas pressure within the flexible tube increases, the tube tends to straighten. The motion is translated through the gearing mechanism so that the indicator shows a higher pressure. The tail end of the pointer is shorter than the indicating end and blends into the background. The lowest pressure indication is between the 6 o'clock and 9 o'clock positions on a clock face.

moved from the yoke, thus indicating a cylinder gas supply that does not exist (9).

PRESSURE REGULATOR

The pressure in a gas cylinder varies with the temperature and contents. To maintain constant flow with changing supply pressure, the anesthesia machine is fitted with pressure regulators. These devices—also called reducing valves, reducing regulators, and regulator valves—reduce the high and variable pressure found in a cylinder to a lower (usually

around 50 psig), more constant pressure suitable for use in an anesthesia machine. The ASTM standard (2) requires regulators for each gas supplied to the machine at a pressure in excess of 100 psig. Usually, there is a regulator for every double or single yoke. Separate yokes for the same gas may be connected to one regulator.

Physics

Pressure is defined as a force acting against a given area. One can increase force either by increasing the pressure or by increasing the area over which the pressure acts. To illustrate this, consider the simple balance shown in Figure 3.7.

A large pressure, Pc, acting on a small area, A1, is balanced by a smaller pressure, Pr, acting on a large area, A2. The force exerted by the higher pressure is

$$Pc \times A1$$

This is balanced by the force on the right:

$$Pr \times A2$$

Because these forces are equal, it follows that

$$Pr \times A2 = Pc \times A1$$

Solving for Pr,

$$Pr = \frac{A1}{A2} \times Pc$$

In a pressure regulator these same principles apply. Figure 3.8 shows a cylinder of gas under a high pressure, Pc (inlet pressure). R is the inside of a regulator containing gas

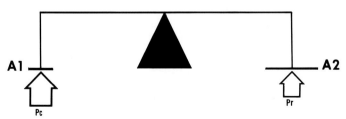

Figure 3.7. A large pressure acting over a small area is balanced by a smaller pressure acting over a large area. The relative sizes of the arrows represent the magnitudes of the pressures.

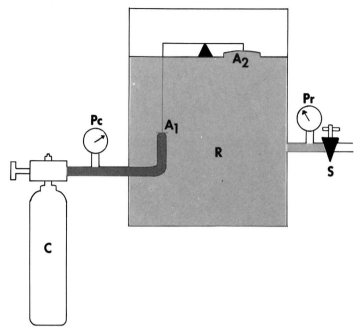

Figure 3.8.   The simplified pressure regulator is in the closed state (see text for details).

under a reduced pressure, Pr (outlet pressure). The opening between C and R is occluded by a seat of area A1. A2 is the area of a flexible diaphragm on which Pr acts. When the stopcock (S) is closed, the forces are in balance. The seat seals the opening from the cylinder so that no gas flows from C into R.

In Figure 3.9, the stopcock is open and gas flows from R, causing the pressure, Pr, to drop. The forces are no longer balanced because $Pc \times A1 > Pr \times A2$. The flexible diaphragm becomes flatter, the balance tips to the right and the seat no longer occludes the opening from the cylinder, so that gas flows from the cylinder into R. As long as the stopcock is open, the forces will be in balance and gas will continue to flow from the cylinder. This situation is analogous to opening the flow control valve on the anesthesia machine. When the stopcock is closed, gas will continue to flow briefly into R, until Pr increases to the point at which a balance of forces is restored. The small increase in Pr after the stopcock is closed is called the static increment.

The regulator shown in Figures 3.8 and 3.9 will yield a constant reduced pressure only if the supplied pressure, Pc, is constant. If Pc decreases, as when the cylinder pressure decays, Pr must decrease to preserve the balance of forces. With this type of regulator, the flowmeter would constantly need readjustment to compensate for the pressure drop.

To remedy this, a main spring (S1) is added (Fig. 3.10). This spring exerts a downward force on the flexible diaphragm. The magnitude of this force depends on an adjustable screw. Now the forces acting to push the diaphragm upward remain at

$$Pr \times A2$$

Forces acting to push the diaphragm downward are

$$(Pc \times A1) + F_{s1}$$

where F_{s1} is the force exerted by the spring. If the values for Pc, Pr, A1, and A2 remain unchanged, there would be an imbalance of forces, because the force of the main spring would be added to the force of Pc acting on

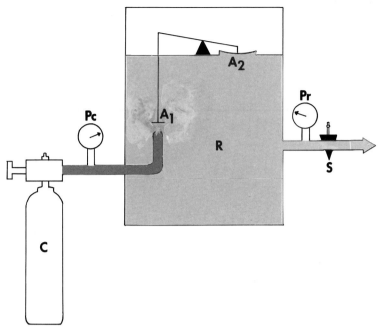

Figure 3.9. The pressure regulator with its stopcock (*S*) open. An imbalance of forces is created, allowing gas to pass from the cylinder into the regulator (see text for details).

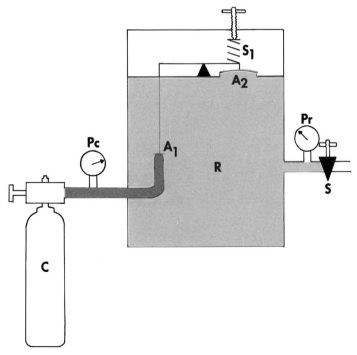

Figure 3.10. A mainspring (*S1*) and adjusting screw have been added to the pressure regulator (see text for details).

A1. To compensate for this imbalance, A1 may be reduced, A2 may be increased, or both. At equilibrium,

$$(Pc \times A1) + F_{s1} = Pr \times A2$$

Solving this equation for Pr,

$$Pr = (F_{s1}/A2) + Pc(A1/A2) \qquad (1)$$

The force exerted by Pr acting on the diaphragm, therefore, is opposed by two forces: a constant force from the spring ($F_{s1}/A2$) and a variable force from Pc acting on the seat, Pc(A1/A2). If the force exerted by the spring is large in comparison with the force exerted by Pc, large variations in Pc will cause only slight variations in Pr.

Example: Suppose Pc initially is 100 and is then reduced to 50. If F_{s1} is small (20), A2 is 10 and A1 is 2. When Pc is 100,

$$Pr = 20/10 + 100(2/10)$$
$$Pr = 2 + 20$$
$$Pr = 22$$

When Pc is reduced to 50

$$Pr = 20/10 + 50(2/10)$$
$$Pr = 2 + 10$$
$$Pr = 12$$

So the reduction in Pc is accompanied by a large change in Pr. However, if F_{s1} is large (1000) and A1 and A2 are adjusted appropriately (to 1 and 50, respectively), when Pc is 100,

$$Pr = 1000/50 + 100(1/50)$$
$$Pr = 20 + 2$$
$$Pr = 22$$

When Pc is reduced to 50,

$$Pr = 1000/50 + 50(1/50)$$
$$Pr = 20 + 1$$
$$Pr = 21$$

A large change in Pc has caused only a small change in Pr.

The value of Pr will depend on F_{s1}. The tension in the spring can be varied by means of the adjustable screw, and in this way, Pr may be varied. For this reason the main spring is sometimes called the adjusting spring.

One more addition to the regulator is necessary. In Figure 3.11 a sealing (shutoff) spring (S2) is added. This acts to force the seat against the opening from the cylinder. This prevents gas from flowing from C to R when the adjusting spring is completely relaxed and the stopcock open. Equation 1 then becomes

$$Pr = (F_{s1} - F_{s2})/A2 + Pc(A1/A2) \qquad (2)$$

The value of F_{s2} is considerably smaller than F_{s1} so that ($F_{s1} - F_{s2}$) is large compared with Pc, and Pr will remain relatively constant in spite of variations in Pc.

There will, however, be some variations in Pr with variations in Pc. A change, ΔPc, in the cylinder pressure will produce a change, ΔPr, in the reduced pressure. From Equation 2,

$$\Delta Pr = \Delta Pc(A1/A2)$$

As Pc decreases, Pr also decreases (pressure-proportioned reduction). The magnitude of the change in Pr is governed by the ratio A1:A2.

The regulator illustrated in Figures 3.8 to 3.11 is an example of a direct-acting regulator. This is because the components are arranged so that the cylinder pressure tends to open the valve.

An indirect-acting regulator is shown diagrammatically in Figure 3.12. In this case, Pc acts to close the valve. Equation 2 then becomes

$$Pr = (F_{s1} - F_{s2})/A2 - Pc(A1/A2)$$

The variation in Pr with variation in Pc is given by the equation

$$\Delta Pr = \Delta Pc(A1/A2)$$

As Pc decreases, Pr increases (pressure inversion).

The Modern Regulator

The modern regulator, depicted in Figures 3.13 and 3.14, functions on the same princi-

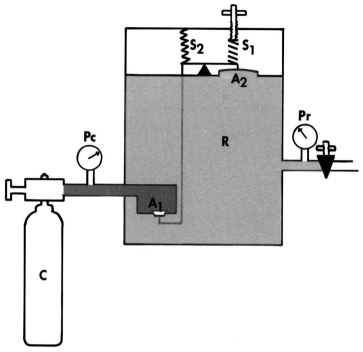

Figure 3.11. A sealing spring has been added to complete the pressure regulator (see text for details).

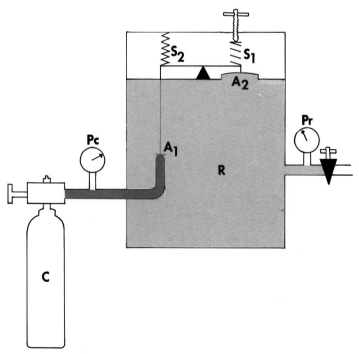

Figure 3.12. Indirect-acting regulator. The components are arranged so that cylinder pressure tends to close the valve (see text for details).

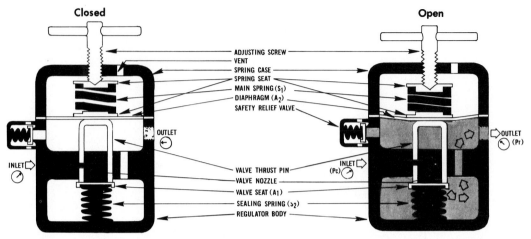

Figure 3.13.   Direct-acting regulator. The *darker shades* are used for gas under high pressure, whereas the *lighter shades* represent gas under reduced pressure. The *arrows* indicate the path of gas flow. The valve is opened by turning the adjusting screw (see text for details). Redrawn from a drawing furnished by Ohmeda, a division of BOC, Inc.

ples as the regulators shown in Figures 3.11 and 3.12. All of the components are present in the modern regulator, but their arrangement differs slightly.

A direct-acting regulator is shown in Figure 3.13. The valve's functioning is determined by a balance of forces acting to position the seat, A2. With the valve closed, the force of the sealing spring (S2), pushing the seat up against the nozzle, is greater than the

downward force exerted by the main spring (S1) and the inlet pressure (Pc) against the seat. No gas flows from the inlet into the regulator. Pr is 0.

When the valve is opened by tightening the adjusting screw, the downward force of the main spring (S1) is increased. This force is transmitted along the valve thrust pin to the seat and, in combination with the inlet pressure, overcomes the force of the sealing

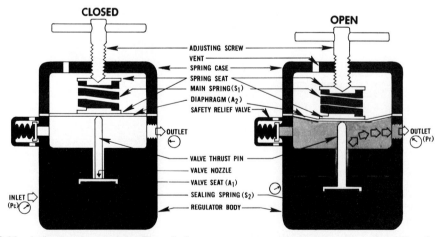

Figure 3.14.   Indirect-acting regulator. The cylinder pressure opposes the opening of the valve. When the adjusting screw is opened, gas flows from the lower to the upper chamber along the valve thrust pin. Redrawn from a drawing furnished by Ohmeda, a division of BOC, Inc.

spring. Gas at reduced pressure (Pr) flows into the space under the diaphragm and exerts an upward force on the diaphragm (Pr $\times$ A2). Gas then flows on to the outlet. The forces are not in balance, but Pr will remain constant, because a steady state is soon achieved. Gas will continue to flow until either the cylinder is exhausted or the gas flow is turned off at a point distal to the regulator. If it is turned off, gas will continue briefly to flow into the space under the diaphragm. Here, its pressure will increase (static increment) until the force of the reduced gas on the diaphragm (Pr $\times$ A2) plus the force of the sealing spring, S2, balance the force of the cylinder pressure and the main spring (Pc $\times$ A2 + F_{s2}), as in Equation 2.

Figure 3.14 illustrates an indirect-acting regulator. With the valve closed, gas enters the space surrounding the sealing spring (S2) and the valve seat (A1). Its own pressure (Pc) tends to hold the valve seat against the nozzle. When the adjusting screw is turned so that the main spring exerts a downward force on the diaphragm (F_{s1}),the valve thrust pin moves downward, opening the seat, so that gas at reduced pressure (Pr) expands through the holes for the thrust pin and into the cavity under the diaphragm. When the gas flow is turned off distal to the regulator, the gas continues to flow into the space under the diaphragm. Here its pressure increases (static increment), pushing the diaphragm upward until the seat closes against the nozzle, stopping further flow.

Regulators are of two types: adjustable and preset. An adjustable regulator has a means for easy user adjustment of the delivery pressure. With a preset regulator, tools are required to adjust the preset delivery pressure.

Regulators used in anesthesia machines are preset at the factory and should not be altered by the user. The ASTM (2) standard requires that they be adjusted so that the machine uses only gas from the pipeline when the pipeline inlet pressure is 345 kPa (50 psig) or greater. This is to prevent use of gas from a cylinder if the cylinder valve is open while the pipeline supply is in use. An important consequence of this is that if the user suspects that the piped oxygen system is delivering less than 100% oxygen, opening an oxygen cylinder will not correct the situation. It is also necessary to disconnect the oxygen pipeline hose.

Some anesthesia machines have two-stage regulators, which, as the name implies, are two single-stage regulators in tandem. The outlet of the first stage is the inlet of the second stage, so that the pressure reduction occurs in two steps instead of one. An advantage of this arrangement is reduced wear on the diaphragms, because their movement is reduced. In addition, variations in Pr secondary to variations in Pc are reduced.

Some modern machines have additional regulators downstream of both the pipeline inlets and the cylinder regulators. These reduce the pressure to approximately 16 psig. This minimizes bobbing of the flowmeter indicator, resulting from pressure fluctuations in the pipeline inlets.

When pipeline supplies of gases are being used, cylinder valves should be closed. This is because the machine will always use gas from the source that has the highest pressure. If the pipeline pressure drops below that supplied by the cylinder regulator and the cylinder valve is open, some gas will be withdrawn from the cylinder. Eventually, the cylinder will be depleted. In this case, the operator would be unaware that a changeover has occurred until the cylinder became exhausted. Knowing that the pipeline supply has failed allows the operator to make arrangements for additional cylinders to be supplied as those in use are exhausted.

To protect the rest of the machine from excessive pressure a regulator must be equipped with a relief valve that opens at not more than four times the normal inlet pressure and at not more than two thirds of the minimum burst pressure of the diaphragm (2). If there is a buildup of pressure, this valve opens and vents to atmosphere.

A defective regulator blocking the flow of gas from cylinders has been reported (10).

Intermediate Pressure System

The intermediate pressure system (see Fig. 3.1) contains the components of the machine that receive gases at reduced pressures (37–55 psig). These include the following: (*i*) pipeline inlet connections; (*ii*) pipeline pressure gauges; (*iii*) piping; (*iv*) the gas power outlet for a ventilator; (*v*) the master switch that provides both pneumatic and electrical power to the system; (*vi*) oxygen pressure failure devices that either interrupt the flow of anesthetic gases or provide an alarm when the oxygen pressure fails; (*vii*) the oxygen flush, which allows delivery of high flows of oxygen; (*viii*) additional regulators (if so equipped); and (*ix*) the flow control valves.

PIPELINE INLET CONNECTIONS

The ASTM standard (2) mandates pipeline inlets for oxygen and nitrous oxide. Suc-

tion and air inlets are usually available as options. These inlets are fitted with Diameter Index Safety System fittings (see Chapter 2).

Each inlet must contain a check valve to prevent flow of gas from the machine into the piping system or to atmosphere if no hose is connected. Some inlets contain filters. Problems have been reported with the check valve. In one case it stuck in the closed position, causing obstruction of oxygen flow (11), and there are reports of failure of the valve (12,13).

PIPELINE PRESSURE GAUGE

Gauges to monitor the pressure (Fig. 3.15) of each gas supplied by a pipeline to the machine are required by the ASTM standard (2). They are usually of the Bourdon tube type and must meet the same requirements relating to readability as cylinder pressure gauges.

The 1979 ANSI standard (1) required that the gauge be on the pipeline side of the check valve in the pipeline inlet. On older machines, the gauge may be attached on either

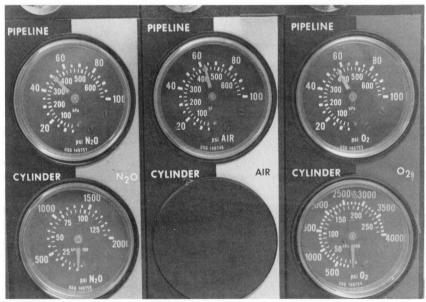

Figure 3.15. Cylinder and pipeline pressure gauges. Note that the lowest pressure indication is between the 6 o'clock and 9 o'clock positions on a clock face.

the pipeline or machine side of the check valve. If the gauge is on the pipeline side of the check valve, it will monitor pipeline pressure only. If the hose is disconnected or improperly connected it will read 0 even if a cylinder valve is open (14). If the gauge is on the machine side of the check valve, it cannot be depended on to give a true indication of the pipeline supply pressure unless the cylinder valves are turned off. If a cylinder valve is open and the pipeline supply fails, there will be no change in the pressure shown on the gauge until the cylinder is nearly empty (15).

The relationship of the gauge to the check valve is not obvious on inspection of the machine. The user can ascertain the location by disconnecting the pipeline hose and turning on the cylinder valve. If the reading on the pipeline gauge remains zero, the gauge is on the pipeline side of the check valve. If a reading is obtained, the gauge is connected on the machine side.

The indication of an adequate pressure on the pipeline gauge does not mean that gas is not being drawn from a cylinder. If for any reason the pressure of gas coming from a cylinder via a pressure regulator exceeds the pipeline pressure and a cylinder valve is open, gas will be drawn from the cylinder. It follows that cylinders should always remain closed when a pipeline supply is in use. Pipeline pressure gauges should always be checked before the machine is used. They should register between 45 and 55 psig (310 and 380 kPa). They should be observed repeatedly during use.

MACHINE PIPING

Connections between components inside the machine are usually made from metal tubing. They must be able to withstand four times the intended service pressure without rupturing.

Cases of cross-connections of piping inside the machine have been reported (16). To avoid this, the ASTM standard (2) requires that either connections be made noninter-changeable or the piping be labeled at each junction or where the piping joins a component.

The ASTM standard (2) specifies that leaks between the pipeline inlet or cylinder and the flow control valve not exceed 10 ml/min at normal service pressure.

GAS POWER OUTLET FOR VENTILATOR

Most machines are equipped with a connection to supply oxygen or air to power a ventilator. The gas power outlet (power outlet accessory) may be fitted with a DISS fitting or quick coupler. The ASTM standard (2) requires it to have a check valve so that gas can only flow from the machine. A spring-loaded valve prevents gas from flowing into atmosphere if the ventilator hose is not attached.

On machines equipped with a power outlet, the reduced pressure issuing from the regulator may be set just below 50 psig, because some ventilators will not function properly at lower pressures. On some machines it is possible to operate a ventilator only from pipeline supplies and not from cylinders.

MASTER SWITCH

One of the safety features of modern machines is the coordination of all the machine functions under a central control (Fig. 13.16). Turning on the master switch causes both the pneumatic and electronic functions of the machine to be activated. This has the advantage that all the alarms and safety devices as well as many of the monitors are automatically activated before the machine can be used. The oxygen flush is usually independent of this feature.

Modern anesthesia machines depend on an uninterrupted supply of electricity and have batteries to automatically power the machine should the main power fail or become disconnected.

The ASTM standard (2) requires alarms in machines to be of one of three categories: high priority (requiring immediate operator

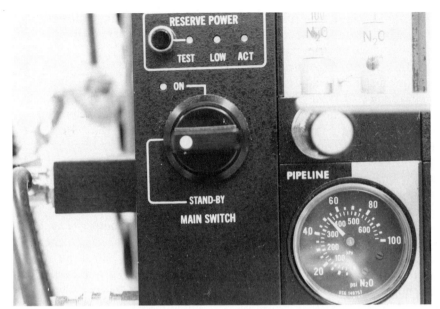

Figure 3.16. Master switch. Turning this on activates both pneumatic and electrical functions of the machines as well as certain alarms and safety features.

response), medium priority (requiring prompt operator response), and low priority (requiring operator awareness). There must be different visual and audible indications for each priority alarm. With each alarm, the audible indicator must reset automatically when the condition causing the alarm has cleared. The maximum time the audible indicator for a high or medium priority alarm can be silenced is 120 sec. The alarms may be incorporated into a central alarm system.

OXYGEN PRESSURE FAILURE PRECAUTIONS

One of the most serious mishaps that occurred with earlier machines was depletion of the oxygen supply (usually from a cylinder) without the user's noticing, so that there was delivery of 100% anesthetic gas. Prevention of such an accident has been the object of numerous inventions. Among these have been devices that (*i*) cut off the supply of gases other than oxygen (oxygen failure safety valves) or (*ii*) give an audible and/or visible warning (alarms) when oxygen pressure has fallen to a dangerous level.

Devices

Oxygen Failure Safety Valve (17)

The oxygen failure safety valve is also known as the low-pressure guardian system, oxygen pressure failure protection device, pressure sensor shutoff system or valve, Safe-T-Lor, fail safe, pressure sensor system, and nitrous oxide shutoff valve.

The ASTM standard (2) requires that an anesthesia machine be designed so that whenever the oxygen supply pressure is reduced below normal, the set oxygen concentration at the common gas outlet does not decrease. The oxygen failure safety device shuts off or proportionally decreases and ultimately interrupts the supply of nitrous oxide and other gases if the oxygen supply pressure decreases.

One such device is shown in Figure 3.17. It is similar to an indirect-acting pressure regulator with the adjusting spring replaced by oxygen pressure. The opening (B) is connected to the intermediate pressure oxygen system. If oxygen pressure is normal, the diaphragm and stem will be pushed downward,

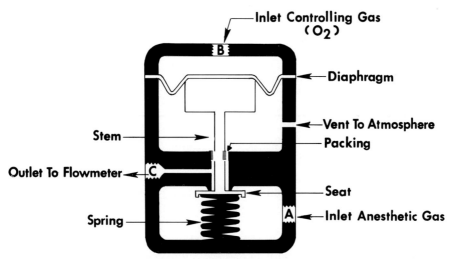

Figure 3.17. Oxygen failure safety valve. When oxygen pressure in the machine is normal, it will push the diaphragm and stem downward, opening the valve. The anesthetic gas then flows in at *A,* around the stem, and out at *C.* When the oxygen pressure falls, the stem moves upward, closing the valve. The middle chamber is vented to atmosphere to prevent mixing of anesthetic gas and oxygen in the event that the diaphragm ruptures or the packing leaks. Redrawn from a drawing furnished by Ohmeda, a division of BOC, Inc.

allowing the anesthetic gas to pass around the seat and on to the outlet. Should oxygen pressure drop, the combined force of the spring and the pressure of the anesthetic gas in the lower chamber will overcome the downward force from the oxygen and the valve will close, stopping the flow of anesthetic gas. This valve, therefore, is a simple on-off valve.

A leak in this valve has been reported (18,19). Oxygen was lost through the vent to atmosphere in the center chamber. This resulted in considerable noise, but no danger.

Another type of oxygen failure safety device is known as a gas-loaded regulator, because it acts both as a regulator for an anesthetic gas and an oxygen failure safety valve. The second stage of the regulator is modified so that as the oxygen pressure falls, the pressure of the anesthetic gas also falls. Eventually, the oxygen pressure will become so low that the flow of anesthetic gas will cease. This differs from the previous type in that instead of the anesthetic gas flow being either on or off, the flow is gradually reduced as oxygen pressure falls.

Cases have been reported in which a tear in the diaphragm of a gas-loaded regulator resulted in a direct communication between the oxygen and nitrous oxide systems inside the machine (20,21).

As shown in Figure 3.1, oxygen failure safety valves are located upstream of the flow control valves of all gases except oxygen, and on some machines, air. Oxygen pressure acts as a control for other gases. If it is normal, the gas in the associated line will proceed to its flow control valve. Should the oxygen pressure drop, the flow of the other gas is halted. Although this device performs an essential function, it does not warn the practitioner that it has shut down the flow of the other gas, except for the visual observation that the gas is not flowing.

Oxygen failure safety valves are now present on most anesthesia machines but may not be on some older machines or may be present for only one of several gases. To determine if a machine has a properly functioning oxygen failure safety valve, set midrange flows for oxygen and the other gas. Disconnect the oxygen supply hose and turn the oxygen cylinder off. If the oxygen failure safety valve is functioning properly, the flowmeter indicator for the other gas will fall to the bottom of the tube before the oxygen indicator descends. If a machine is lacking such a device for any gas except air, it should be modified or replaced.

Oxygen Supply Failure Alarm (22)

Another approach to the loss of oxygen pressure has been to develop alarms that give an audible and/or visible warning of loss of oxygen pressure. These are the oxygen supply failure alarms, or oxygen pressure depletion warnings or alarms.

The ASTM standard (2) specifies that whenever the oxygen supply pressure falls below a manufacturer-specified threshold, a medium priority alarm shall be annunciated within 5 sec. After the alarm has been activated, it may be silenced for a period not exceeding 120 sec.

A commonly used mechanism utilizes a pressurized canister that is filled with oxygen when the anesthesia machine is turned on. When the oxygen pressure falls below a certain value, the alarm directs a stream of oxygen through a whistle. The sound will continue until the reservoir is depleted. It is important to note that the ending of the whistle tone does not necessarily mean that the low oxygen pressure condition has ended. Other machines use a pressure-operated electrical switch that ensures a continuous audible alarm when the oxygen supply pressure falls below a set amount.

Some older machines in use may not have such a warning device. Frequently, such a device can be installed on an existing machine.

Limitations

Because both the oxygen failure safety valve and alarm depend on pressure and not flow, they have limitations that are not always fully appreciated by the user. These devices do not offer total protection against a hypoxic mixture being delivered, because they do not prevent anesthetic gas from flowing if there is no flow of oxygen. They do aid in preventing hypoxia caused by some prob-

lems (such as disconnected oxygen hoses, low oxygen pressure in the pipeline, and depletion of oxygen cylinders) occurring upstream in the machine circuitry. They do not guard against accidents owing to cross-overs in the pipeline system or wrong contents in a cylinder. Equipment problems (such as leaks) or operator errors (such as closed or partially closed oxygen flow control valves) that occur downstream are not prevented. Oxygen failure safety valves usually close the line at a pressure between 15 and 30 psig. If the machine is gas tight, the oxygen system may stay pressurized for weeks without being connected to a source of oxygen.

Some new devices have been developed to overcome the problems of having anesthetic gases but no oxygen flowing. These will be discussed in the section on flowmeters. Even these devices, however, do not guard against hypoxia caused by the wrong gas coming through a flowmeter. The use of an oxygen analyzer in the breathing system that is enabled and functioning whenever the machine is turned on is essential.

OXYGEN FLUSH VALVE

The oxygen flush valve (also called the oxygen bypass and emergency oxygen) receives oxygen from the pipeline inlet or cylinder regulator and directs a high unmetered flow to the common gas outlet (see Fig. 3.1). The ASTM standard (2) requires that the flow be between 35 and 75 liters/min. Flush valves for gases other than oxygen are not permitted by the ASTM standard.

The ASTM standard (2) requires that the oxygen flush be a single-purpose, self-closing device and that it be permanently marked to show its function and designed to minimize accidental activation. Barotrauma and cases of awareness caused by its activation have been reported (23).

The oxygen flush valve most commonly found in modern anesthesia machines is shown in Figure 3.18. It consists of a button and stem connected to a pin or ball. The pin or ball is in contact with the seat. When the button is depressed, the pin or ball is forced

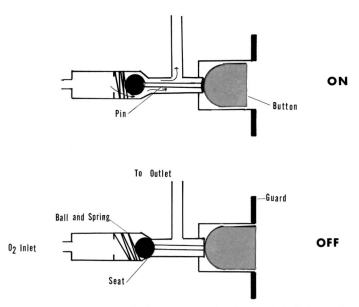

Figure 3.18. Oxygen flush valve. Depressing the button causes the pin to push the ball away from the seat, allowing oxygen to pass directly to the machine outlet. Redrawn from a diagram furnished by Ohmeda, a division of BOC, Inc.

away from the seat, allowing the oxygen to flow to the machine outlet. A spring opposing the ball or pin will close the valve and hold it closed when the button is not depressed. The button is commonly recessed or placed in a collar to prevent accidental activation (see Fig. 3.33*B*).

Activation of the oxygen flush may or may not result in other gas flows being shut off. Activation may result in either a positive or negative pressure in the machine circuitry, depending on the design of the inlet of the flush line into the common gas line. This pressure will be transmitted back to other structures in the machine, such as flowmeters and vaporizers, and may change the vaporizer output and the flowmeter readings. The effect of activation will depend on the pressure generated, the presence or absence of check valves in the machine, and the relationship of the oxygen flush valve to other components.

The ASTM standard (2) requires that the connection of the flush valve delivery line to the common gas outlet be designed so as to minimize pressure fluctuations that may produce a pumping effect on the vaporizer

(see Chapter 4), and in no case shall the pressure in the vaporizers increase by more than 100 cm water above its normal working pressure during use of the flush valve.

Reported hazards associated with the oxygen flush are mainly with valves not designed to the current machine standard (2). They include accidental activation by various objects (24–26) and internal leaking, which resulted in an oxygen-enriched gas mixture being delivered (27). There have been reports of modern oxygen flush valves sticking in the on position (28,29). There is a report of a flush valve sticking so that it obstructed flow of the anesthesia gases and oxygen from the flowmeters (30).

Use of the oxygen flush to ventilate a patient through a catheter inserted percutaneously has been investigated (31). Only the machine that delivered the gas at 55 psi was capable of providing effective ventilation.

SECOND-STAGE REGULATOR

Some machines have a regulator just upstream of the flowmeters. This receives gas from either the pipeline or the cylinder regulator and reduces it to 12 to 16 psig. It is similar in construction to those discussed previously. The purpose of this regulator is to eliminate fluctuations in pressure supplied to the flowmeter caused by fluctuations in pipeline pressure. By reducing the pressure below the normal fluctuation range, the flowmeter setting will remain constant.

FLOW CONTROL VALVE

The flow control valve (needle valve, pin valve, fine adjustment valve, flow adjustment control) controls the rate of flow of a gas through its associated flowmeter by manual adjustment of a variable orifice. Most flow control valves have both a control and an on-off function. On some machines the on-off control function may be a function of the master switch.

Components

Body

The body of the flow control valve screws into the base of the flowmeter.

Stem and Seat

The stem and seat are shown diagrammatically in Figure 3.19. The stem has fine threads so that it moves only a short distance when a complete turn is made. The pin at the end is conical. When the valve is closed, the pin fits into the seat and no gas can pass through the valve. When the stem is turned outward, an opening between the pin and the seat is created. This allows gas to flow through the valve. By turning the screw, one can increase or decrease the opening and thus control the flow of gas. To eliminate any looseness in the threads, the valve may be spring loaded (32). This also minimizes flow fluctuations from lateral or axial pressure applied to the flow control knob.

It is advantageous to have stops for the off and maximum flow positions. A stop for the off position avoids damage to the valve seat. A stop for the maximum flow position prevents the stem from becoming disengaged from the body.

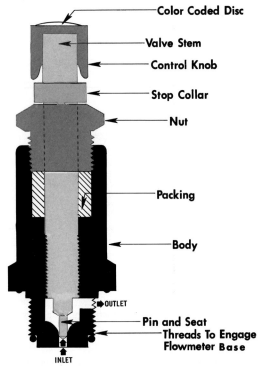

Figure 3.19. Flow control valve, shown in the closed position. Turning the stem creates a leak between the pin and seat so that gas flows to the outlet. The stop collar prevents overtightening of the pin in the seat. Redrawn from a drawing furnished by Foregger Co., a division of Puritan Bennett Co., Inc.

Control Knob

The control knob is joined to the stem. It should be large enough that it can be turned easily. The ASTM standard (2) requires the flow control knob to be marked with the name or chemical formula of the gas or gases it controls and it may have the color of that gas. The oxygen flow control knob must have a fluted profile (Figs 3.20 and 3.21) and be larger than that for any other gas. Such a touch-coded profile may reduce the possibility of an operator error (33). All other flow control knobs must be round. A touch-coated oxygen flow control knob can be installed on a machine that does not have it.

The close proximity of the flow control knobs on some machines contributes to the probability of errors. The ASTM standard (2) requires at least 25 mm between knobs and

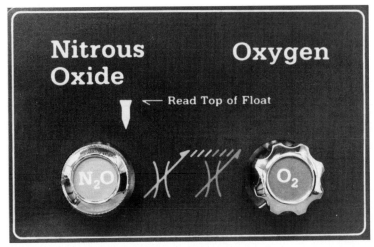

Figure 3.20.   Flow control valves. Note that the oxygen flow control valve is fluted and larger than the nitrous oxide flow control valve.

the knobs must be designed so as to minimize inadvertent change from a preset position. This can be accomplished by a shield, bar, or other protective barrier (see Fig. 3.21) and by placing them high enough above the working surface to lessen the likelihood of contact with objects on that surface.

Knobs are turned counterclockwise to increase flow and clockwise to decrease flow. Flow control knobs should operate smoothly and be easy to adjust, yet stiff enough to resist unintentional changes. The ASTM (2) standard requires that the control knob undergo a rotation of at least 90° to move the indica-

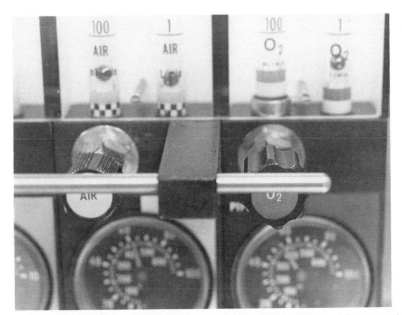

Figure 3.21.   Flow control knob guard. The bar serves to protect the flow control knobs from an accidental change. Note the fluted oxygen control valve and ball indicators.

tor through the upper 90% of the flow rates on the tube.

Use

The flow control valve is a delicate piece of equipment and can be damaged by misuse. When the valve is closed, it should be turned only until the flow of gas ceases, as further tightening may result in damage to the pin or seat. Some manufacturers provide a stop collar on the valve to prevent it from being closed too tightly. The stop, however, can be overridden or changed by overturning the knob.

Whenever a machine is not being used, the gas source (cylinder or pipeline) should be closed or disconnected. The flow control valves should be opened until the gas pressure is bled to zero, then closed.

Before use of the machine is resumed, the flow control valves should be checked to see that they are closed. Sometimes the habit develops of leaving the flow control valves open after the gas is bled out. In addition, the flow control valves may be opened when the machine is cleaned or moved by people not in a position to understand the possible consequences. If the gas supply to an open flow control valve is restored and the associated flowmeter is not observed, the indicator may rise to the top of the tube where its presence may not be noticed by the operator for some time. Even if no harm to the patient results, the sudden rise of the indicator may damage it and impair the accuracy of the flowmeter (34).

Performance

The performance of flow control valves has been investigated (35). It was found that under normal conditions of use, once the valve has been adjusted, the mass flow of gas through the valve is independent of downstream changes in resistance and compliance encountered in normal anesthetic practice. On the other hand, flow through the valve will vary directly with upstream pressure.

Problems with Flow Control Valves

Loose Knob

If the flow control valve knob is too loose or worn, it may respond to a light touch or even accidental brushing. It then becomes dangerously easy to inadvertently alter the flow rates of gases.

Absence of Fine Control

Cases have been reported in which only a small rotation of the control knob was required to achieve maximal flow.

Inability to Turn Control Knob

A case has been reported in which the stop pins for a flow control valve became locked so that the valve could not be turned on (36).

Leak Through Open Flow Control Valve

Flow control valves should be closed when not in use. If there is no yoke plug or cylinder in the yoke, gases from the flowmeter manifold can leak through an open valve (5,37–39).

Failure to Allow Adequate Gas Flow

In one case, the tip of the stem had become impacted in the inlet path (40). The shaft also had broken, allowing the flow control knob to turn freely. In another case, the soft metal seating into which the stem extended became detached and obstructed flow (41).

Low-Pressure System

The low-pressure system (see Fig. 3.1) is the part of the machine downstream of the flow control valve in which the pressure is slightly above atmospheric. The components found in the low-pressure system are flowmeters, vaporizer circuit control valves, back pressure safety devices, low-pressure piping, and the common gas outlet. Vaporizers, which are found in the low-pressure system, will be considered in Chapter 4.

FLOWMETERS

A flowmeter measures and indicates the rate of flow of a gas passing through it.

Physical Principles

Flowmeters used in modern anesthesia machines are of the variable orifice (variable area) type, also known as a Thorpe tube. The Thorpe tube (Fig. 3.22) consists of a vertical tapered tube that has its smallest diameter at the bottom. It contains an indicator that is free to move up and down inside the tube. When there is no flow of gas, the float rests at the bottom of the tube. As shown in Figure 3.22*B,* when the flow control valve is opened, gas enters at the bottom and flows up the tube, elevating the indicator. The gas passes through the annular opening between the float and the tube and on to the outlet at the top of the tube. The indicator floats freely in the tube at an equilibrium position where the downward force on it caused by gravity

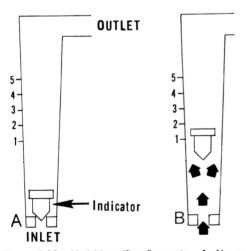

Figure 3.22. Variable orifice flowmeter. **A,** No gas flow. **B,** Gas enters at the base and flows through the tube, causing the indicator to rise. The gas passes through the annular opening around the float. The area of this annular space increases with the height of the indicator. Thus the height of the indicator is a measure of gas flow.

equals the upward force caused by gas molecules hitting the bottom of the float. As gas flow increases, the number of molecules hitting the bottom of the float increases and the float rises. Because the tube is tapered, the size of the annular opening around the indicator increases with height and more gas flows around the float. When the flow is decreased, gravity causes the indicator to settle to a lower level. A scale marked on or beside the tube shows the gas flow.

The rate of flow through this tube will depend on three factors: the pressure drop across the constriction, the size of the annular opening, and the physical properties of the gas.

Pressure Drop across the Constriction

As gas flows around the indicator, it encounters frictional resistance between the float and the wall of the tube. The flow also becomes less laminar and more turbulent. There is a resultant loss of energy reflected in a pressure drop. This pressure drop is constant for all positions in the tube and is equal to the weight of the float divided by its cross-sectional area.

Size of the Annular Opening

The larger the annular opening around the float, the greater the flow of gas. Because the pressure drop across the constriction is always balanced by the weight of the float, the increased or decreased area must be balanced by an increase or decrease in lifting force (P = F/A) caused by a change in the gas flow.

In the variable orifice flowmeter, the annular cross-sectional area varies while the pressure drop across the float remains constant for all positions in the tube. For this reason, these flowmeters are often called constant pressure flowmeters. Increasing the flow does not increase the pressure drop but causes the float to rise to a higher position in the tube, thereby providing greater flow area for the gas. The elevation of the float is a measure of the annular area for flow and, therefore, of the flow itself.

Physical Characteristics of the Gas

When a low flow of gas passes through the Thorpe tube, the annular opening between the float and the wall of the tube will be narrow. As flow increases, the annular opening becomes wider. The physical property that relates gas flow to the pressure difference on the two sides of the constriction varies with the form of the constriction. With a longer and narrower constriction (low flow), flow is a function of the viscosity of the gas (Poiseuille's law). When the constriction is shorter and wider (high flow), flow depends on the density of the gas (Graham's law).

Temperature and Pressure Effects

Flowmeters are calibrated at atmospheric pressure (760 torr) and room temperature (20°C). Temperature and pressure changes will affect both the viscosity and the density of a gas and so influence the accuracy of the indicated flow rate. Temperature changes as a rule are slight and do not induce significant changes.

In a hyperbaric chamber a flowmeter will deliver less gas than the setting indicates. With decreasing barometric pressure (as with increasing altitude), the actual flow rate will be higher than the flowmeter reading.

Conventional Flowmeter Blocks

The majority of anesthesia machines have individual flow control valves for each gas. Proportioning devices will be discussed later. The flowmeter assembly consists of the tube through which the gas flows, the indicator, a stop at the top of the tube, and the scale that indicates the flow. Lights are available on some machines. Each flowmeter assembly must be clearly and permanently marked with the appropriate color and name or chemical symbol of the gas or gas mixture it measures. The flowmeter assembly is usually protected by a plastic shield.

Tube

Flowmeter tubes are usually made of glass. In some flowmeter tubes, rib guides are

used. These are thickened bars running the length of the tube, spaced equally around the circumference. Figure 3.23 shows sections at upper and lower parts of the tube. Gas passes between the ball and the inner wall of the tube. Because the tube is tapered, this space increases from below upward. The area occupied by the rib guides varies with the height of the tube.

Indicator

The indicator (float or bobbin) is a free-moving float within the tube. The ASTM (2) standard requires that the point of reference for reading the indicator be marked on the flowmeter assembly (see Fig. 3.20).

Nonrotating Floats.   One type of indicator, the nonrotating float (Fig. 3.24), is designed so that gas flow keeps it in the center of the tube if the tube is kept vertical. The reading is taken at the upper rim.

Rotameters.   As shown in Figure 3.24, the rotating floats have an upper rim whose diameter is larger than that of the body.

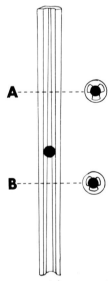

Figure 3.23.   Flowmeter tube with rib guides. This is used with ball indicators. The triangular thickening of the inside of the tube keeps the ball centered. The area through which the gas flows increases with increasing height in the tube. Redrawn courtesy of Fraser Harlake, Inc.

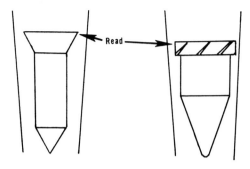

Nonrotating Float   Plumb Bob Float

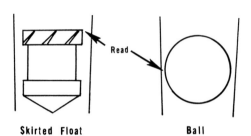

Skirted Float   Ball

Figure 3.24. Flowmeter indicators. The plumb bob and skirted floats are kept centered in the tube by constant rotation. The reading is taken at the top. The ball indicator is kept centered by rib guides. The reading is taken at the center. The nonrotating float does not rotate and is kept centered by gas flow. Redrawn partly from Binning R, Hodges EA. Flowmeters. Can they be improved? Anaesthesia 1967;22:643–646.

Slanted grooves, or flutes, are cut into the rim. When gas passes between the rim of the bobbin and the wall of the tube, it impinges on the flutes, causing the bobbin to rotate. If the tube is vertical, the free spinning maintains the float in the center of the tube. This prevents fluctuations, reduces wear and tear, assists the passage of small particles and reduces errors caused by friction between the tube and the float. A rotating bobbin is evidence that gas is flowing and the bobbin is not stuck. Deviations from the vertical position will result in the rotor striking the side of the tube. The reading is taken at the upper rim.

Ball Floats. A third type of indicator is the ball (see Fig. 3.24). The reading is taken at the center of the ball. The ball is kept in the center of the tube by rib guides. The ball may

rotate and sometimes has two colors so that the rotation can be easily seen.

It is important to observe the indicator frequently during use and especially in response to an adjustment of the flow control valve. Erratic movement of the indicator may mean that readings will be inaccurate.

Stop

The stop at the top of the flowmeter tube prevents the indicator from plugging the outlet, which could lead to damage to the tube (34). It also prevents the indicator from ascending to a point at which it is hidden. This is important, because a flowmeter with the indicator hidden looks much like one which is turned off.

Stops have been known to break off and fall down into the tube. If it descends far enough to rest on the indicator, it will cause the indicator to register less flow than is actually occurring.

Scale

The ASTM machine standard (2) requires that the flowmeter scale either be marked on the tube or be located on the right side of the tube as viewed from the front. On some older machines the scale may be on the left, so care must always be taken to read the correct scale.

The ASTM (2) standard requires that flowmeters be calibrated in liters per minute, except that for flows up to 1 liter/min, the flow may be expressed either in milliliters or in decimal fractions of a liter per minute with a zero before the decimal point. Flowmeter scales are individually calibrated. The scale, tube, and float should be regarded as an inseparable unit. Should any of the components need replacement, a complete new set must be obtained.

Lights

Flowmeter lights are offered as an option on most modern anesthesia machines. This enhances safety when the machine is used in a darkened room.

Arrangement of Flowmeter Tubes

On an anesthesia machine flowmeters tubes for different gases are grouped side by side as an integral assembly. The various gas flows meet at the common manifold at the top. Sometimes there are two flowmeters for the same gas: one for low flows and one for high flows. In such a case, the tubes may be arranged either parallel or in series (tandem).

Parallel

The parallel arrangement features two complete flowmeter assemblies with two flow control valves. The total flow of that gas to the common manifold is the sum of the flows on both flowmeters.

Because accidental use of a low-flow oxygen flowmeter when a high flow was intended is a hazard whenever two oxygen flow control knobs are fitted, the machine standard (2) requires that only one flow control valve be provided for each gas, so parallel flowmeters will not be available in the future. When fine and coarse flowmeters are desired, the series arrangement fulfills the requirements of the standard.

Series

With an in-series arrangement (Fig. 3.25), there is one flow control valve for the two flowmeter tubes. Gas from the flow control valve first passes through a tube calibrated up to 1 liter/min, then passes to a second tube that is calibrated for higher flows. The total flow is not the sum of the two tubes but that shown on the higher flow tube.

Sequence of Flowmeter Tubes

Flowmeter sequence can be a cause of hypoxia (42). Figure 3.26 shows four different arrangements for oxygen, nitrous oxide, and air flowmeters. Normal gas flow is from bottom to top in each tube and then from left to right at the top. A leak exists in the unused air flowmeter. Potentially dangerous arrangements exist in Figure 3.26*A* and *B* because the nitrous oxide flowmeter is located in the downstream position. A substantial

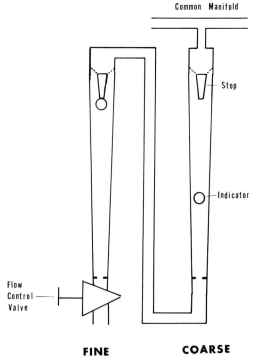

Figure 3.25. Flowmeter tubes in series. The total flow is that shown on the higher flow tube, not the sum of the two tubes.

portion of oxygen flow passes through the leak while all nitrous oxide is directed to the common gas outlet. Hypoxia from this has been reported (43). Safer configurations that comply with the ASTM standard (2) are shown in Figure 3.26*C* and *D*. By placing the oxygen flowmeter nearest the outlet a leak upstream from the oxygen results in a loss of nitrous oxide rather than oxygen.

Before discovering that the sequence of flowmeters was important in preventing hypoxia, there was no consensus on where the oxygen flowmeter should be in relation to flowmeters for other gases. Thus on older machines the oxygen flowmeter might be on the right, the left, or the center of the flowmeter assembly. This was dangerous, because users unfamiliar with a particular anesthesia machine might reach for the site where they were used to finding the gas controls, but because the controls' positions were

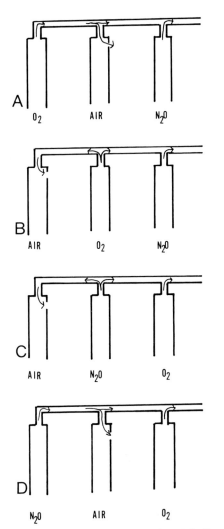

Figure 3.26. Flowmeter sequence. **A** and **B,** Potentially dangerous arrangements, with the oxygen flowmeter upstream. If a leak occurs, oxygen will be selectively lost. **C** and **D,** Oxygen is downstream from other gases, which is a safer situation because anesthetic gas rather than oxygen will be lost. *Arrows* represent flows of gases. Redrawn from Eger EI, Hylton RR, Irwin RH, Guadagni N. Anesthetic flow meter sequence—a case for hypoxia. Anesthesiology 1963;24:396–397.

reversed, they might turn off the oxygen rather than the nitrous oxide. To avoid such confusion the ASTM and the Canadian standards require that the oxygen flowmeter be placed on the right side of a group of flowmeters as viewed from the front. If a separate vaporizer flowmeter is placed to the right of the oxygen flowmeter, it must be separated by at least 10 cm.

It should be noted that having the oxygen flowmeter at the right side of the flowmeter bank is specific to North America and the market supplied by American manufacturers. An international standard for anesthesia machines under development calls for the oxygen flowmeter to be located at the left, and this is the arrangement in many countries. This sets the stage for operator error if a user administers anesthesia in a country other than that where he or she was trained.

Proper sequence of flowmeters is no guarantee that hypoxia from a broken flowmeter cannot occur. A leak in the oxygen flowmeter tube between the float and the manifold can cause selective loss of oxygen even when the oxygen flowmeter is in the downstream position (44,45).

Safety Devices

One of the hazards associated with flowmeters is the possibility that the operator will set the flows so that a hypoxic mixture will be delivered. Various devices have been developed to prevent this.

Mandatory Minimum Oxygen Flow

Some anesthesia machines require a minimum flow of oxygen before other gases will flow. This minimum flow is preset at the factory (sometimes to the customer's specifications). This may be activated when the main switch is turned on. On some machines, the mandatory minimum oxygen flow feature is disabled when the air flowmeter is used. This minimum flow may be provided by either a stop on the oxygen flow control valve or a resistor that permits a small flow to bypass a totally closed oxygen flow control valve (22). On some machines, an alarm is activated if the oxygen flow goes below a certain minimum (even if no other gases are being administered). This does not in itself prevent a hypoxic gas concentration from being delivered. A hypoxic gas mixture can be delivered with only modest anesthetic gas flows.

Minimum Oxygen Ratio

Another method of ensuring that a hypoxic mixture will not be delivered is to equip the machine with minimum oxygen ratio devices that either deliver a minimum flow of oxygen in proportion to the total gas flow or provide an alarm that is set off if this proportion is too low.

Minimum Oxygen Ratio Device. Flow control valves can be linked mechanically (Fig. 3.27) or pneumatically (Fig. 3.28) so that the operator cannot set the oxygen:nitrous oxide flow ratio below a factory-preset minimum (usually 25% or greater). This minimum oxygen ratio device (or proportioning system) permits independent control of each gas as long as the percentage of oxygen is above the minimum. If the operator attempts to increase the nitrous oxide flow too much, the oxygen flow is automatically increased. If the operator attempts to lower the oxygen flow too much, the flow of nitrous oxide is lowered proportionally. It should be noted that these devices only link two gases, normally nitrous oxide and oxygen. Administration of a third gas such as helium can result in a hypoxic mixture.

Problems have been reported with minimum oxygen ratio devices that rely on a chain-link mechanism between flow control valves. A loose set screw or the chain coming off the sprockets will invalidate the link between the flow control valves (46–49).

Alarms. Alarms are available on some machines to alert the operator when the oxygen:nitrous oxide flow ratio has fallen below a preset value. Such an alarm is often linked to the master switch (if present) so that it is activated whenever the switch is turned on (Fig. 3.29). The pressures downstream of the flow control valves are transmitted to diaphragms, which are linked together. If the O_2/N_2O flow ratio is low, the diaphragms move to the right, causing a leaf-spring contact to close and actuate an alarm.

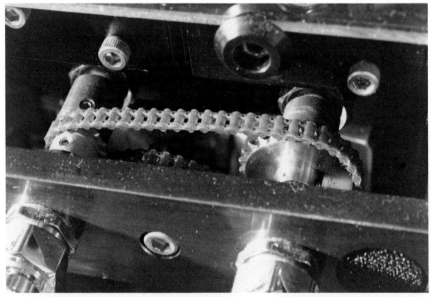

Figure 3.27. Mechanically linked flow control valves. Sprockets are secured to the stems of the oxygen and nitrous oxide flow control valves. A chain linking the sprockets limits the minimum oxygen concentration that can be set. Either nitrous oxide or oxygen flow can be adjusted independently, but the minimum oxygen concentration is maintained. If the nitrous oxide flow is increased beyond the maximum allowed, there is a proportional increase in oxygen flow. If the oxygen flow is lowered, there is a proportional decrease in nitrous oxide flow.

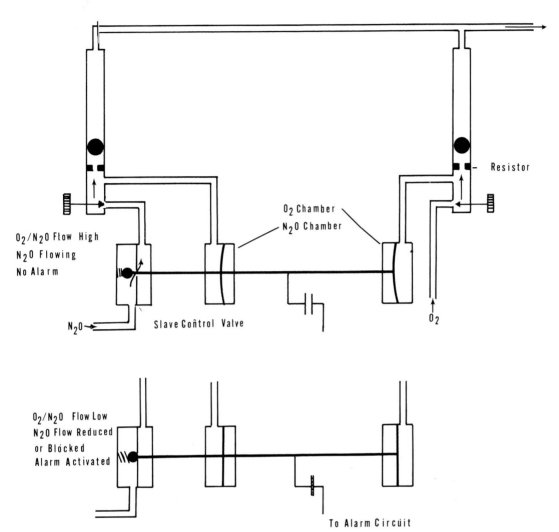

Figure 3.28. Oxygen ratio monitor controller. An oxygen chamber, a nitrous oxide chamber, and a nitrous oxide slave control valve are all interconnected by a mobile horizontal shaft. The nitrous oxide and oxygen flowmeters have resistors downstream from the flow control valves. These resistors create back pressures that are directed to the oxygen and nitrous oxide chambers. If the pressure in the oxygen chamber is low relative to that in the nitrous oxide chamber, the horizontal shaft moves to the right, decreasing the nitrous oxide delivery pressure to the nitrous oxide control valve and thus the nitrous oxide flow.

Oxygen-Nitrous Oxide Proportioning Devices

Proportioning devices (ratiometers) combine nitrous oxide and oxygen flowmeter assemblies so that the percentage of oxygen and the total fresh gas flow are dialed directly. The relative concentrations of nitrous oxide and oxygen are varied by adjusting a concentration dial, which is usually calibrated between 30% and 100% oxygen. Adjustment of the second dial, the flow control dial, causes the flows of both nitrous oxide and oxygen to increase or decrease, but they remain in the proportion set on the concentration dial. Total gas flow and oxygen proportion can be confirmed visually by observing the two flowmeter assemblies.

One such device, the 30/70 proportioner,

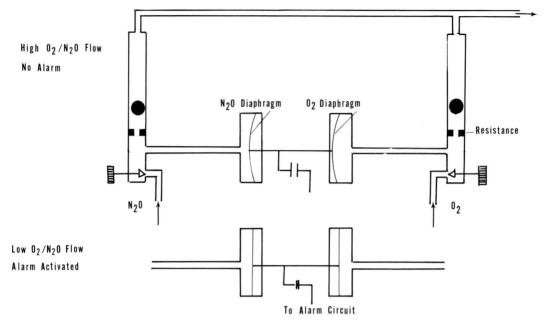

Figure 3.29. Oxygen ratio monitor. The gas flow through each resistor produces a back pressure that is proportional to flow. Each back pressure is transmitted to a diaphragm (*top*). The diaphragms are connected by a shaft that in turn connects to the switch to the alarm. If the ratio of oxygen flow to nitrous oxide flow is low (*bottom*), the shaft and switch lever will move toward the right and the leaf-spring contact for the alarm will be closed.

is shown in Figure 3.30. A flow control knob allows settings of total gas flow from 3 to 16 liters/min. The concentration dial allows administration of oxygen concentrations from 30% to 100%. The 30/70 proportioner device is shown diagrammatically in Figure 3.31. It has a number of interdependent components.

Components.

On-Off Valve. The on-off valve, which is mechanically linked to the total flow control valve, receives oxygen from the pipeline or cylinder and in the on position routes it to the reference regulator. It has a vent that permits rapid depressurization when it is switched to the off position.

Reference Regulator. The reference regulator, which receives oxygen from the on-off valve at approximately 50 psig, reduces the pressure to 12 psig and delivers it to the pro-

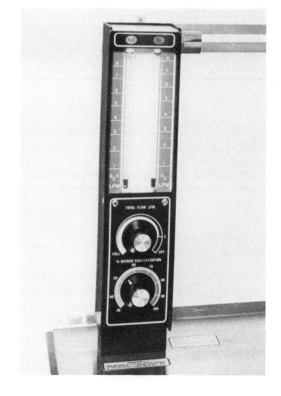

Figure 3.30. 30/70 proportioner machine. Courtesy of Ohmeda, a division of BOC, Inc.

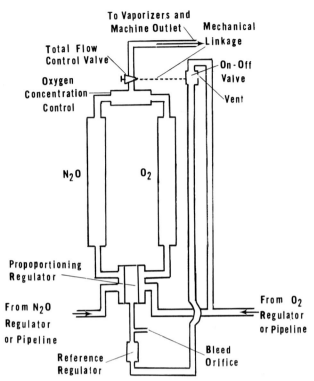

Figure 3.31. 30/70 proportioner machine (see text for details). Redrawn from a diagram furnished by Ohmeda, a division of BOC, Inc.

portioning regulator. A bleed orifice in the pressure line from the reference regulator to the proportioning regulator permits a rapid reduction in the pressure when the on-off valve is turned off or the oxygen pressure fails.

Proportioning Regulator. The proportioning regulator (Fig. 3.32) consists of three parts: a nitrous oxide section, an oxygen section, and a central control section. The central section is separated from the oxygen and nitrous oxide sections by flexible diaphragms that are connected to valve stems. These in turn contact throttling orifices.

Oxygen from the reference regulator enters the central control section and exerts pressure on the diaphragms. This causes the valve stems to move and open the orifices. Oxygen and nitrous oxide flow into their respective sections of the proportioning regulator. When the pressure in either section be-

comes greater than the pressure in the central control section (12 psig) the diaphragm will be pushed toward the center, pulling the valve stem and closing the orifice. Thus the proportioning regulator serves to maintain the pressures of both the nitrous oxide and oxygen sections at 12 psig. It also acts as an oxygen pressure failure device, because in the event the oxygen pressure fails, the central control section will depressurize and the flow of both oxygen and nitrous oxide to the flowmeters will cease.

Flowmeters. As shown in Figure 3.32, from the proportioning regulator the gases flow to standard flowmeter tubes, which provide a visual indication of the rate at which the gases are flowing and the proportion of oxygen.

Oxygen Concentration Control. From the flowmeters the gases flow to the oxygen concentration control (see Fig. 3.31). This

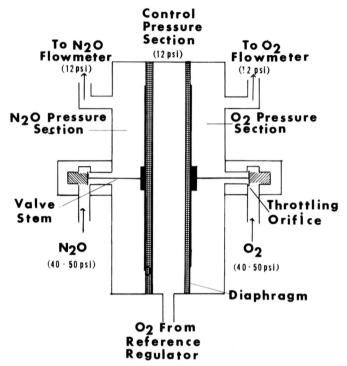

Figure 3.32.   Proportioning regulator of the 30/70 proportioner machine. The two flexible diaphragms separate the central control section from the oxygen and nitrous oxide sections. Attached to each diaphragm is a valve stem. When oxygen at 12 psig flows into the central control section, the diaphragms are pushed outward. This moves the valve stems and opens the throttling orifices. Redrawn from a diagram furnished by Ohmeda, a division of BOC, Inc.

has two flow control valves that are linked so that as one is opened the other automatically closes. The control is designed to prevent nitrous oxide from exceeding 70% of the total flow.

Total Flow Control Valve. The gases from the flowmeters flow into a common chamber where they are mixed and then to the total flow control valve. This needle valve is linked to the on-off valve so that when the on-off valve is in the off position, there will be no gas flow (2).

Evaluation of Proportioning Devices. Because the concentration dial cannot be set below 30% oxygen, a hypoxic mixture cannot be delivered. This is the main advantage of these devices. However, these devices are difficult to use for low-flow or closed system anesthesia because there is a limit to how low a flow can be obtained. Leak testing is more

difficult with these machines and requires a special device that must be supplied by the manufacturer. Only two gases can be metered with a proportioning device.

Problems with Flowmeters

Inaccuracy

Studies of flowmeters in daily use have shown that the percent of error increases as the flow decreases, and at flows below 1 liter/min, it becomes clinically significant (50–52). Inaccuracy at low flows is compounded by difficulty reading the low end of flowmeters. There are several causes of inaccuracy.

Improper Assembly or Calibration. Routine maintenance by manufacturers may not include flowmeter calibration checks and a new or recently serviced flowmeter may not be accurate (53).

The flowmeter tube, scale, and indicator are calibrated as a unit. If any parts are broken or damaged, the entire assembly must be replaced. Parts should never be interchanged. Cases have been reported in which indicators or tubes have been transposed (54,55). Differences in density and viscosity among different gases means that a tube calibrated for one gas will not necessarily be accurate for another.

Dirt. If dirt causes a decrease in the area around the indicator, the flowmeter will indicate higher than actual flow. Erratic movement of the float may indicate that its performance is affected by dirt. Dirt may cause the indicator to stick, giving a reading higher or lower than actual flow. Of the commonly used anesthetic gases, compressed air is most likely to contain dirt.

Back Pressure. Most flowmeters on anesthesia machines are not back-pressure compensated and are affected by pressure increases transmitted from the breathing system or from use of the oxygen flush valve. These pressure increases cause the gas within the flowmeter tube above the float to be compressed. The lifting effect from gas flowing into the tube at the bottom is reduced and the float drops to a lower position so that it reads less than actual flow. The effect of the pressure changes can be reduced by certain devices near the common gas outlet.

Improper Alignment. Flowmeters are designed to be kept in a vertical position. If the tube is not vertical the annular opening becomes asymmetrical and inaccuracy results. The indicator is more likely to stick if the tube is not vertical

Static Electricity. Another possible source of flowmeter inaccuracy with a metal indicator is static electricity (56–58). This can cause sticking or erratic movement of the indicator. As long as the indicator rotates in a normal manner there is no inaccuracy owing to electrostatic charges (57).

Often a change of gas flow will redistribute the electrical charges so that the indicator becomes steady. Putting a moist fingertip on the flowmeter tube and the machine metal or use of antistatic sprays will remove charges from the outside of the tube.

Problems with the Indicator. Indicator damage can result from the sudden projection to the top of the tube when a cylinder is opened or a pipeline hose connected with the flow control valve open. Floats can become worn or distorted by handling (59). The stop at the top of the flowmeter tube can became dislodged and rest on top of the float (60,61).

Indicator Unnoticed at Top of Tube

A flowmeter tube with the indicator at the top looks very much like one with the indicator at the bottom, so this problem can be easily missed.

Blockage of Tube Outlet

If the stop at the top of the tube is not replaced or breaks off, the float may close the outlet so there is no flow, although the flowmeter will indicate a very high flow. A leak or rupture of the tube may result.

Reading of Wrong Flowmeter

A user will occasionally turn a flow control valve without looking at the flowmeter. If the user follows up by merely glancing to make sure a float is at an elevation associated in his or her mind with the desired result and does not verify by inspection that it is the proper float, the user may find that he or she has used the wrong flow control valve entirely. Deaths have occurred when an indicator was read beside an adjacent but inappropriate scale. In machines that have parallel flowmeters, the fine control flowmeter may be used in place of the high-flow one and inadequate oxygen given (62).

Changes in Float Position

Floats should be observed at frequent intervals, particularly soon after the first setting. On some machines, the position of the float may change with a change in supply pressure.

Leaks

A leak in a flowmeter downstream of the indicator but upstream of the common manifold will result in a lower-than-expected concentration of that gas in the fresh gas mixture. A leak can be caused by a crack or chip in the flowmeter tube or a problem with the connections of the tube (43,45,63–66). Partial obstruction to gas flow downstream of the flowmeter head may cause the seal at the top of the flowmeter to rupture (67).

A leak may occur if a flow control valve is left open and there is no cylinder or yoke plug in the yoke (5,37,39). The indicator at the bottom of the tube does not produce a seal to prevent backflow of gases.

Care

Flowmeters should be protected by turning each flow control valve off when cylinder valves are opened or the pipeline hoses are connected to the machine. This prevents a sudden rise of the indicator to the top of the tube, which might damage the indicator or allow it to go unnoticed. In machines with an oxygen failure safety device, the flowmeter for an anesthetic gas or oxygen will register zero when the oxygen pressure is low, even if the flow control valve is open. When the oxygen pressure is restored, there will be a sudden rush of anesthetic gas through the flowmeter, which may cause the indicator to rise abruptly to the top.

VAPORIZER CIRCUIT CONTROL VALVE

The purposes of the vaporizer circuit control valve (also called the vaporizer selector switch and selector valve) are to (*i*) direct a flow of carrier gas, oxygen, to a measured-flow vaporizer when the vaporizer is in use; (*ii*) direct the vapor-laden oxygen to the common gas outlet; and (*iii*) isolate the vaporizer from the rest of the machine when it is not in use. It is important that the vaporizer circuit control valve be placed in the bypass position when the vaporizer is not in use, or there may

be leakage of vapor into the fresh gas line (68,69).

The ASTM (2) standard does not preclude the use of measured-flow vaporizers. It does preclude vaporizer circuit control valves that include a third position for the oxygen flush. On some older machines the flow of gas through the vaporizer flowmeter would be discharged to atmosphere. This is not permitted by either machine standard (1,2).

UNIDIRECTIONAL VALVE

When ventilation is controlled or assisted, positive pressure from the breathing system is transmitted back to the machine. Use of the oxygen flush valve may also create a positive pressure. Such an increase in pressure can affect the concentration of volatile anesthetic agents issuing from vaporizers in the machine (70). It can also increase leaks and cause inaccurate flowmeter readings. To minimize these problems a unidirectional (check) valve may be inserted between the vaporizers and the common gas outlet, most commonly upstream of where the oxygen flush flow joins the fresh gas flow. This will lessen the pressure increase, but not prevent it, because gas must still flow from the flowmeters during time of increased pressure.

These check valves are of great importance when checking the machine for leaks. Testing the breathing system for leaks will not detect a leak in a machine equipped with a check valve (71–73).

A hazard was reported in which a portion of this valve became dislodged and migrated downstream. This caused an obstruction, preventing gas from reaching the common gas outlet (74).

PRESSURE RELIEF DEVICE

Some machines have a pressure relief valve near the common gas outlet to prevent high pressure from being transmitted into the machine and to protect the patient from high pressures from the machine. This valve opens to atmosphere and releases fresh gas if a preset pressure is exceeded.

If a direct-reading vaporizer with high resistance is placed downstream of such a pressure relief valve the resistance of the vaporizer may result in a pressure in excess of the opening pressure of the valve, especially when the oxygen flush is activated (75). Such vaporizers should be located between the flowmeters and the common gas outlet.

Presence of a pressure relief valve can limit the ability of an anesthesia machine to provide adequate jet ventilation.

LOW-PRESSURE PIPING

The low-pressure gas piping is noteworthy because of the number of connections that are necessary. Components located within this area are subject to breakage and leaks (71). The ASTM standard (2) allows a maximum leak of 30 ml/min at a pressure of 30 cm H_2O between the flow control valve and the common gas outlet for any gas with the vaporizers turned off.

COMMON (FRESH) GAS OUTLET

The common gas outlet receives all the gases and vapors from the machine. Most machine outlets have a 15-mm female slip-joint connection (that will accept a tracheal tube connector), with a coaxial 22-mm male connection. They may also have a load-bearing fitting for secure attachment of accessory apparatus. Because the common gas outlet is a frequent location for a leak or disconnection, the ASTM standard (2) mandates that it be provided with a retaining device (Fig. 3.33). The fresh gas supply tube, which conveys gas to the fresh gas inlet in the breathing system, attaches to the common gas outlet.

The Anesthesia Workstation

A term that will be used frequently in the future is the *anesthesia workstation* (or work place), which integrates most of the components necessary for anesthesia into one unit. In the past, it was the practice to purchase an anesthesia machine, then add an oxygen analyzer, respirometer, CO_2 analyzer, pulse oximeter, and other monitors. The monitors were often from different manufacturers and were mounted onto the machine or a monitoring cart in whatever way they would fit. This resulted in a clutter of devices, cables, and hoses. Another problem was that it was sometimes difficult to find needed data. If an alarm sounded, it was often difficult to determine from which monitor the signal was coming, unless it had a distinctive sound. Fi-

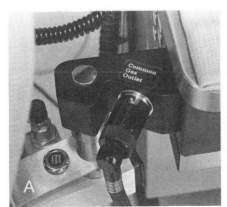 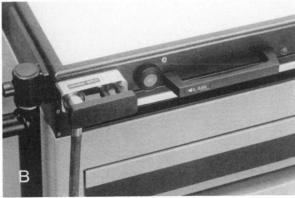

Figure 3.33. Common gas outlets with retaining devices. Note that the oxygen flush valve button is protected from inadvertent activation by the collar around it.

nally, the monitors did not communicate with one another.

The movement toward the anesthesia workstation began when manufacturers began making the oxygen analyzer and airway pressure monitor integral parts of the machine so that they were activated whenever the machine was turned on. These were followed by other monitors. Finally, central alarm displays and prioritized alarm systems were developed so that when an alarm sounded there was one place to look to determine which alarm had been activated and how serious the condition was. Other information such as the suggested checkout procedure is now commonly displayed.

One advantage of the workstation is that monitoring functions can be integrated. For example, if a blood pressure cuff is on the same arm as the pulse oximeter, inflation of the cuff will not result in the pulse oximeter alarm being activated. Another advantage is that data can be displayed on a single screen so that the user has an overview and can better assimilate the information. Data from different monitors may be analyzed. When a problem is sensed, potential causes and appropriate responses can be displayed. For example, if the problem is a leak or disconnection in the breathing system, the workstation might be able to determine the location of the problem or to advise the user where to look. These data can be displayed in icon form. Finally, the workstation takes up much less space than the anesthesia machine with monitors added onto it.

Automated Record Keeping

Automated record keeping (or an information management system), at present in an advanced developmental stage, is likely to become important in the future. The traditional anesthesia record has been handwritten. Problems include illegibility and incomplete and inaccurate data entry. Inaccuracies are especially likely when rapid changes are taking place and the user's attention is occupied with other things.

An automated record keeper may be a part of the anesthesia machine or a separate unit. It collects data from all the monitors and the anesthesia machine. Patient information can be added by connecting to the admissions computer. For drugs, fluids, intubation information, and miscellaneous details, data must be entered by keyboard, touch screen, or mouse. The information management system can be equipped with an alarm system that backs up the individual monitor alarms.

To have an automated record, the various monitors need to be able to communicate with each other. This is usually not a problem if they all come from the same manufacturer. Because this is often not the case, there needs to be a way for instruments of different companies to talk to each other. The primary monitors need to have the best possible sensing devices so as to provide clear output signals that are as free of artifact as possible.

Artifactual data can be addressed in two ways. The first is to prevent the artifact from appearing on the record by using algorithms that detect and eliminate artifactual data. The second way is to explain artifactual data on the record.

There are a number of advantages to an information management system. Data entry is rapid. Printouts can be made during or after the case. Retrospective analysis of data for research or quality assurance is facilitated. The record is legible, the data complete, and data are recorded during times when anesthesia personnel are too busy to make entries. Data can be used for billing purposes. Information on drug usage will be more accurate than with a handwritten record. What supplies were used can be documented. Data from an automated record may be more credible than a handwritten record. Some liability insurance carriers offer premium reductions if automated records are used.

Disadvantages include the time and effort

needed to learn to use the automated record. A major problem is artifactual data. The need for the user to make entries takes time and attention away from other tasks. These systems are expensive. The medicolegal implications are unclear. There are problems relating to access to, alteration of, and destruction of records.

Servicing

The Joint Commission on Accreditation of Healthcare Organizations requires a preventive maintenance procedure for anesthesia machines at least annually (76). A frequently asked question is who should service a machine. Because many anesthesiologists are gadgeteers at heart, the temptation to modify the machine or make one's own repairs may be great. Servicing an anesthesia machine requires a detailed knowledge of the components, how they function, and how they are fitted into the machine. In addition, it is necessary to have the proper replacement parts. It is recommended that the user not perform any service beyond those items that are in the manual that comes with the machine. Maintenance should not be attempted by hospital maintenance, respiratory therapy, or biomedical personnel who have no particular training with anesthesia machines. Serious hazards have resulted from repairs and alterations made to anesthesia machines by untrained personnel, and such actions will usually relieve the manufacturer of any responsibility. Some manufacturers will train and certify hospital biomedical personnel to work on machines. Some state laws specify that only certified personnel may work on anesthesia machines.

Most companies provide service contracts for maintenance of their machines. With such a contract, a service representative will inspect and perform routine maintenance (including testing, cleaning, lubrication, adjustments, and replacement of damaged parts) on the machine at regular intervals,

usually three or four times a year. There is great variation in the quality of service representatives. It should not be taken for granted that servicing has been performed correctly. Whenever a machine has been serviced, it should be thoroughly checked before use.

Servicing has important medicolegal implications. If a problem occurs with an anesthesia machine and a patient suffers harm, it is important to be able to show that proper servicing was performed. It should be noted, however, that routine servicing does not relieve the user of the responsibility of checking the machine before each use.

Records should be kept on each machine, including problems that occur, service performed, when it was performed, and by whom. Records on equipment are required by the Joint Commission on Accreditation of Healthcare Organizations, and they can be very helpful in the event of legal action.

Choice of Anesthesia Machine

Only machines that meet all the requirements of the ASTM standard (2) should be considered for purchase. Several things should be considered when choosing which anesthesia machine best suits your particular requirements. A trial period with a model of a new machine is desirable.

SERVICE

All machines that comply with the ASTM standard (2) should perform well when new. All machines, however, will require servicing. The quality of that service varies among companies and from area to area with the same company. If you are receiving satisfactory service from one company it would make sense to consider newer models of this company's machines first. If this is not the case, you should shop carefully, realizing that any sales representative will promise good service but you must determine whether that service will be provided. One way is by inquiring into the experiences of colleagues in the same area to determine whether they have long down times waiting for repairs, whether servicing is available locally, whether machines for loan are available, and whether service contracts are honored. The cost of servicing is also a factor.

SIZE

Some manufacturers offer compact machines for small operating rooms. A small machine will be easier to move if a machine needs to be transported outside the operating suite. Larger machines usually offer more drawers and a larger tabletop, which can be used as a work space.

SPECIAL FEATURES AND EQUIPMENT

Certain machines offer important safety features that may make them particularly desirable. Also, the ability to add additional equipment is important. One machine may be more user friendly than another.

REFERENCES

1. American National Standards Institute. Minimum performance and safety requirement for components and systems of continuous flow anesthesia machines for human use (ANSI Z-79. 8). New York: ANSI, 1979.
2. American Society for Testing and Materials. Specification for minimum performance and safety requirements for components and systems of anesthesia gas machines (ASTM F-1161-88). Philadelphia: ASTM, 1988.
3. Craig DB, Longmuir J. Implementation of Canadian Standards Association 2168.3-M 1980 anaesthetic gas machine standard: the Manitoba experience. Can Anaesth Soc J 1980;27:504–509.
4. Hogg CE. Pin-indexing failures. Anesthesiology 1973;38:85–87.
5. McQuillan PJ, Jackson IJB. Potential leaks from anaesthetic machines. Anaesthesia 1987;42:1308–1312.
6. Youatt G, Love J. A funny yoke. Tale of an unscrewed pin. Anaesth Intensive Care 1981;9:79–80.
7. Fox JWC, Fox EJ. Guest discussion. Anesth Analg 1968;51:790–791.
8. Blum LL. Equipment design and human limitations. Anesthesiology 1971;35:101–102.
9. Schreiber P. Anaesthesia systems. Boston: Merchants Press, 1984.
10. Allberry RAW. Minireg failure. Anaesth Intensive Care 1989;17:234–235.
11. Varga DA, Guttery JS, Grundy BL. Intermittent oxygen delivery in an Ohmeda Unitrol anesthesia machine due to a faulty O-ring check valve assembly. Anesth Analg 1987;66:1200–1201.
12. Bamber PA. Possible safety hazard on anaesthetic machines. Anaesthesia 1987;42:782.
13. Heine JF, Adams PM. Another potential failure in an oxygen delivery system. Anesthesiology 1985;63:335–336.
14. Craig DB, Longmuir J. Anaesthetic machine pipeline inlet pressure gauges do not always measure pipeline pressure. Can Anaesth Soc J 1980;27:510–511.
15. Dinnick OP. More problems with piped gases. Anaesthesia 1976;31:790–792.
16. Bonsu AK, Stead AL. Accidental cross-connexion of oxygen and nitrous oxide in an anaesthetic machine. Anaesthesia 1983;38:767–769.
17. Epstein RM, Rackow H, Lee ASJ, Papper EM. Prevention of accidental breathing of anoxic gas mixtures during anesthesia. Anesthesiology 1962;23:1–4.
18. Jones DE, Watson CB, Goetter C. Oxygen pressure sensor shutoff valve failure in the Ohio "wedge" anesthesia machine. Anesthesiology 1984;61:634–635.
19. Riddle RT. Oxygen pressure sensor shutoff valve failure in the Ohio "wedge" anesthesia machine. In reply. Anesthesiology 1984;61:635–636.
20. Craig DB, Longmuir J. An unusual failure of an oxygen fail-safe device. Can Anaesth Soc J 1971;18:576–577.
21. Puri GD, George MA, Singh H, Batra YK. Awareness under anaesthesia due to a defective gas-loaded regulator. Anaesthesia 1987;42:539–540.
22. Eisenkraft JB. The anesthesia delivery system—part I. Prog Anesth 1989;3(7):1–7.
23. Dodd KW. Inadvertent administration of 100% oxygen during anaesthesia. Br J Anaesth 1979;51:573.
24. Anderson CE, Rendell-Baker L. Exposed O_2 flush hazard. Anesthesiology 1982;56:328.
25. Cooper CMS. Capnography. Anaesthesia 1987;42:1238–1239.
26. Hanafiah Z, Sellers WFS. Nudging the emergency oxygen. Anaesthesia 1991;46:331.
27. Anonymous. Judge awards $219,000 in oxygen equipment case. Biomed Safe Stand 1980;10:42.
28. Bailey PL. Failed release of an activated oxygen flush valve. Anesthesiology 1983;59:480.
29. Puttick N. Hazard from the oxygen flush control. Anaesthesia 1986;41:222–224.
30. McMahon DJ, Holm R, Batra MS. Yet another machine fault. Anesthesiology 1983;58:586–587.

31. Gaughan SD, Benumof JL, Ozaki GT. Can an anesthesia machine flush valve provide for effective jet ventilation? Anesthesiology 1991;75:A130.

32. Emmett CP, Clutton-Brock TH, Hutton P. The Ohmeda Excel anaesthetic machine. Anaesthesia 1988;43:581–583.

33. Calverley RK. A safety feature for anaesthetic machines—touch identification of oxygen flow control. Can Anaesth Soc J 1971;18:225–229.

34. Cooper M, Ali D. Oxygen flowmeter dislocation. Anaesth Intensive Care 1989;17:109–110.

35. Hutton P, Boaden RW. Performance of needle valves. Br J Anaesth 1986;58:919–924.

36. Rung GW, Schneider AJL. Oxygen flowmeter failure on the North American Drager Narcomed 2a anesthesia machine. Anesth Analg 1986;65:211–212.

37. Russell WJ, Ward JB. Hypoxia with a third flowmeter tube on the anaesthetic machine. Anaesth Intensive Care 1978;6:355–357.

38. Lenoir RJ, Easy WR. A hazard associated with removal of carbon dioxide cylinders. Anesthesiology 1988;43:892–93.

39. Williams AR, Hilton PJ. Selective oxygen leak: a potential cause of patient hypoxia. Anaesthesia 1986;41:1133–1134.

40. Beudoin MG. Oxygen needle valve obstruction. Anesth Intensive Care 1988;16:130–131.

41. Fitzpatrick G, Moore KP. Malfunction in a needle valve. Anaesthesia 1988;43:164.

42. Eger EI, Hylton RR, Irwin RH, Guadagni N. Anesthetic flowmeter sequence—cause for hypoxia. Anesthesiology 1963;24:396–397.

43. Powell J. Leak from an oxygen flowmeter. Br J Anaesth 1981;53:671.

44. Chung DC, Jing QC, Prins L, Strupat J. Hypoxic gas mixtures delivered by anaesthetic machines equipped with a downstream oxygen flowmeter. Can Anaesth Soc J 1980;27:527–530.

45. Russell WJ. Hypoxia from a selective oxygen leak. Anaesth Intensive Care 1984;12:275–277.

46. Abraham ZA, Basagoitia J. A potentially lethal anesthesia machine failure. Anesthesiology 1987;66:589–590.

47. Davis TM. Failure of a new system to prevent delivery of hypoxic gas mixture. A reply. Anesthesiology 1981;54:437.

48. Malone BT. Failure of a new system to prevent delivery of hypoxic gas mixture. Anesthesiology 1981;54:436–437.

49. Richards C. Failure of a nitrous oxide-oxygen proportioning device. Anesthesiology 1989;71:997–999.

50. Sadove MS, Thomason RD, Thomason CL, Ries M. An evaluation of flowmeters. J Am Assoc Nurse Anesth 1976;44:162–165.

51. Waaben J, Stokke DB, Brinklov MM. Accuracy of

gas flowmeters determined by the bubble meter method. Br J Anaesth 1978;50:1251–1256.

52. Waaben J, Brinklov MM, Stokke DB. Accuracy of new gas flowmeters. Br J Anaesth 1980;52:97–100.

53. Kelley JM, Gabel RA. The improperly calibrated flowmeter—another hazard. Anesthesiology 1970;33:467–468.

54. Slater EM. Transposition of rotameter bobbins. Anesthesiology 1974;41:101.

55. Thomas D. Interchangeable rotameter tubes. Anaesth Intensive Care 1983;11:385–386.

56. Hagelsten J, Larsen OS. Static electricity in anaesthetic flowmeters eliminated by radioactive pistol. Br J Anaesth 1965;37:799–800.

57. Clutton-Brock J. Static electricity and rotameters. Br J Anaesth 1972;44:86–90.

58. Clutton-Brock J. Static electricity and rotameters. Br J Anaesth 1973;45:304.

59. Hodge EA. Accuracy of anaesthetic gas flowmeters. Br J Anaesth 1979;51:907.

60. Doblar DD, Hinkle JC. Flowmeter malfunction: effect on delivered anesthetic concentration. Anesthesiology 1984;61:220–222.

61. Luich RJ. Flowmeter malfunction: effect on delivered anesthetic concentration: a reply. Anesthesiology 1984;61:222.

62. Rendell-Baker L, Klein OL, Charles P. Hazard of separate low and high flow O_2 flowmeters: an interim solution. Anesthesiology 1982;56:155–156.

63. Dudley M, Walsh E. Oxygen loss from rotameter. Br J Anaesth 1986;58:1201–1202.

64. Gupta BL, Varshneya AK. Anaesthetic accident caused by unusual leakage of rotameter. Br J Anaesth 1975;47:805.

65. Hanning CD, Kruchek D, Chunara A. Preferential oxygen leak—an unusual case. Anaesthesia 1987;42:1329–1330.

66. Williams OA. Potential hazard of a cracked rotameter. Anaesthesia 1989;44:523.

67. Thompson JB, Fodor IM, Baker AB, Sear JW. Anaesthetic machine hazard from the Select-a-tec block. Anaesthesia 1983;38:175–177.

68. Cook TL, Eger EI, Behl RS. Is your vaporizer off? Anesth Analg 1977;56:793–800.

69. Greenhow DE, Barth RL. Oxygen flushing delivers anesthetic vapor—a hazard with a new machine. Anesthesiology 1973;38:409–410.

70. Hill DW, Lowe HJ. Comparison of concentration of halothane in closed and semiclosed circuits during controlled ventilation. Anesthesiology 1962;23:291–298.

71. Andrews JJ. The anatomy of modern anesthesia machines (ASA Refresher Course #174). New Orleans: ASA, 1989.

72. Berner MS. Profound hypercapnia due to disconnection within an anaesthetic machine. Can J Anaesth 1987;34:622–628.

73. Comm G, Rendell-Baker L. Back pressure check valve a hazard. Anesthesiology 1982;56:327–328.

74. Chang J, Larson CE, Bedger RC, Bleyaert AL. An unusual malfunction of an anesthetic machine. Anesthesiology 1980;52:446–447.

75. Kataria B, Price P, Slack M. Delayed filling of the breathing bag due to a portable vaporizer. Anesth Analg 1987;66:1055.

76. McMahon DJ. A synopsis of current anesthesia machine design. Biomed Instrum Technol 1991;25:190–199.

Vaporizers

Most of the inhalational anesthetic agents in use today are liquids under normal conditions and must be converted into vapors before they can be used. A vapor is the gaseous phase of a substance which is a liquid at room temperature and atmospheric pressure. A vaporizer is an instrument designed to facilitate the change of a liquid anesthetic into its vapor and to add a controlled amount of this vapor to the fresh gas flow. Up to three vaporizers are commonly attached to an anesthesia machine.

Physics

VAPOR PRESSURE

Figure 4.1 A shows a volatile liquid inside a container closed to atmosphere. Molecules of liquid break away from the surface and enter the space above, forming a vapor. If the container is kept at a constant temperature, a dynamic equilibrium is formed between the liquid and vapor phases so that the num-

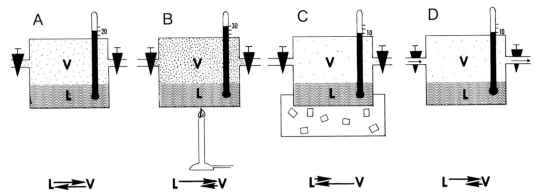

Figure 4.1. A–C, Vapor pressure changes with varying temperature. **A,** The liquid and vapor are in equilibrium. **B,** The application of heat causes the equilibrium to shift so that more molecules enter the vapor phase, as illustrated by the increased density of dots above the liquid. **C,** Lowering the temperature causes a shift toward the liquid phase and a decrease in vapor pressure. **D,** Passing a carrier gas over the liquid shifts the equilibrium toward the vapor phase. The heat of vaporization is supplied from the remaining liquid. This causes a drop in temperature.

ber of molecules in the vapor phase remains constant. These molecules bombard the walls of the container, creating a pressure. This is called the saturated vapor pressure and is represented by the density of dots above the liquid.

If heat is supplied to the container (see Fig. 4.1B), the equilibrium will be shifted so that more molecules enter the vapor phase and the vapor pressure will rise. If heat is taken away from the system (see Fig. 4.1C), more molecules will enter the liquid state and the vapor pressure will be lowered. It is meaningless, therefore, to talk about vapor pressure of a liquid without specifying the temperature. Vapor pressures of the commonly used anesthetic agents at 20°C are shown in Table 4.1.

Vapor pressure depends only on the liquid and the temperature. It does not depend on the barometric pressure within the range of pressures encountered in anesthesia.

BOILING POINT

The boiling point of a liquid is the temperature at which the vapor pressure is equal to the atmospheric pressure. The lower the atmospheric pressure, the lower the boiling point. The boiling points for some com-

monly used anesthetic agents at sea level (760 mm Hg) are shown in Table 4.1.

CONCENTRATION OF GASES

Two methods are commonly used to express the concentration of a gas or vapor: partial pressure and volumes percent.

Partial Pressure

A mixture of gases in a closed container will exert a pressure on the walls of the container. The part of the total pressure caused by any one gas in the mixture is called the partial pressure of that gas. The total pressure of the mixture is the sum of the partial pressures of the constituent gases. With most vaporizers, the total pressure will be equal to atmospheric pressure. The partial pressure exerted by the vapor of a liquid agent depends only on the temperature of that agent and is unaffected by the total pressure above the liquid. The highest partial pressure that can be achieved by a gas at a given temperature is its vapor pressure.

Volumes Percent

The concentration of a gas in a mixture can also be expressed as its percentage of the total volume. Volumes percent (vol %) is the

Table 4.1. Properties of Common Anesthetic Agents

Agent	Trade Name	Boiling Point (°C, 760 mm Hg)	Vapor Pressure (torr, 20°C)	Density of Liquid (g/ml)	Heat of Vaporization		Specific Heat of Liquid		MAC[a] in O$_2$ (%)
					cal/g	cal/ml	cal/ml	cal/g	
Halothane	Fluothane	50.2	243	1.86 (20°C)	35 (20°C)	65 (20°C)	0.35	0.19	0.75
Enflurane	Ethrane	56.5	175	1.517 (25°C)	42 (25°C)	63 (25°C)			1.68
Isoflurane	Forane	48.5	238	1.496 (25°C)	41 (25°C)	62 (25°C)			1.15
Desflurane	Suprane	23.5	664	1.45 (20°C)					6.0
Sevoflurane		58.5	160						2.0

[a]Minimum anesthetic concentration. From Quasha AL, Eger EI, Tinker JH. Determination and applications of MAC. Anesthesiology 1980;53:315–334.

number of units of volume of a gas in relationship to a total of 100 units of volume for the total gas mixture. In a mixture of gases, each constituent gas exerts the same proportion of the total pressure as its volume is of the total volume. In other words, volumes percent expresses the relative ratio of gas molecules in a mixture, whereas partial pressure expresses an absolute value.

$$\frac{\text{Partial pressure}}{\text{Total pressure}} = \frac{\text{Volumes percent}}{100} \quad (1)$$

Although gas and vapor concentrations are most commonly expressed in volumes percent, patient uptake and the level of anesthesia are directly related to partial pressure but only indirectly to volumes percent (1). Although a certain partial pressure represents the same anesthetic potency under various barometric pressures, this is not the case with volumes percent.

HEAT OF VAPORIZATION

It takes energy for the molecules in a liquid to break away and enter the gaseous phase. The heat of vaporization of a liquid is the number of calories necessary to convert 1 g of liquid into a vapor. Heat of vaporization can also be expressed as the number of calories necessary to convert 1 ml of liquid into a vapor (2). The heats of vaporization of the commonly used anesthetic agents are shown in Table 4.1.

Vaporization removes the more energetic molecules so that the remaining molecules have a lower mean kinetic energy. Therefore, the temperature of the liquid decreases as vaporization proceeds. As the temperature falls below that of the surroundings, a temperature gradient is created so that heat flows from the surroundings to the liquid. The lower the temperature, the greater the gradient and the greater the flow of heat from the surroundings. Eventually, an equilibrium is established so that the heat lost to vaporization is matched by the heat supplied from the

surroundings. At this point, the temperature ceases to drop.

The importance of heat of vaporization is illustrated in Figure 4.1D: A flow of gas (carrier gas) is passed through the container and molecules of vapor are carried away with it. This causes the equilibrium to shift so that more molecules from the liquid enter the vapor phase. Unless some means of supplying heat is available, the liquid will cool. As the temperature drops, so does the vapor pressure of the liquid and fewer molecules will be picked up by the carrier gas. This results in a decrease in concentration in gas flowing out of the container.

SPECIFIC HEAT

The specific heat of a substance is the quantity of heat required to raise the temperature of 1 g of the substance 1°C. The higher the specific heat, the more heat required to raise the temperature of a given quantity of that substance. A slightly different definition of specific heat is the amount of heat required to raise the temperature of 1 ml of the substance 1°C (2). Conversion from one quantity to the other may be made by use of the following formula:

$$\frac{\text{Specific heat}}{\text{gram}} \times \text{Density}$$
$$= \frac{\text{Specific heat}}{\text{ml}} \quad (2)$$

Water is the standard with a specific heat of 1 cal/g/°C or 1 cal/ml/°C.

Specific heat of anesthetic liquids is important when considering the amount of heat that must be supplied to a liquid to maintain a stable temperature when heat is lost as a result of vaporization. Values of specific heats for some liquid anesthetics are given in Table 4.1.

Specific heat is also important in the choice of material from which a vaporizer is constructed. A substance with a high specific heat will change temperature more slowly than one with a low specific heat. Thus a container constructed from a material with a high specific heat will provide a more stable temperature than one constructed of a material of low specific heat, if the masses are the same. The specific heats of some substances used in the construction of vaporizers are given in Table 4.2. Thermal capacity is the product of specific heat and mass, and represents the amount of heat stored in the vaporizer body (3).

THERMAL CONDUCTIVITY

Another consideration in choosing material from which to construct a vaporizer is the thermal conductivity of the material. Heat flows from an area of higher temperature to one of lower temperature. Thermal conductivity is a measure of speed with which heat flows through a substance (4). The higher the thermal conductivity, the better the substance conducts heat. The thermal conductivity of some substances used in vaporizers is shown in Table 4.2.

As seen in Table 4.2, copper has a moderate specific heat and a high thermal conductivity. For these reasons it has been used frequently in vaporizers.

THERMOSTABILIZATION (5)

Thermostabilization is achieved by constructing vaporizers of heavy-metal parts that act as heat reservoirs and prevent rapid temperature changes when the vaporizer is in use. In vaporizers containing wicks, it is important that the wicks be in contact with a metal part so heat lost as a result of vaporization can be replaced quickly.

Classification of Vaporizers

Many authors have attempted to classify vaporizers on the basis of a single characteristic. The wide variety of vaporizers available makes any single method of classification incomplete. The classification shown in Table 4.3 lists five characteristics that describe most of the important points about each vaporizer.

METHODS OF REGULATING OUTPUT CONCENTRATIONS

The vapor pressures of most anesthetic agents at room temperature are much greater than the partial pressure required to produce anesthesia. To produce clinically useful concentrations, a vaporizer must bring about dilution of the saturated vapor. This can be accomplished in one of two ways.

1. The total flow from the machine goes through the vaporizer and is divided into two parts. Some passes through the vaporizing chamber (the part of the vaporizer containing the liquid anesthetic agent) and the remainder goes through a bypass to the vapor-

Table 4.2. Materials Used in Construction of Vaporizers

Material	Specific Heat (cal/°C/g)	Thermal Conductivity $\left(\dfrac{cal/sec}{cm^2 \times °C/cm}\right)$
Copper	0.1	0.92
Aluminum	0.214	0.504
Glass	0.16	0.0025
Air	0.0003	0.000057
Steel	0.107	0.115
Brass	0.0917	0.260

Table 4.3. Classification of Vaporizers

A. Method of regulating output concentration
  1. Concentration calibrated
  2. Measured flow
B. Method of vaporization
  1. Flow over
  2. Bubble through
  3. Injection
C. Temperature compensation
  1. Thermocompensation
  2. Supplied heat
D. Specificity
  1. Agent specific
  2. Multiple agent
E. Resistance
  1. Plenum
  2. Low resistance

izer outlet. This is known as a concentrated-calibrated vaporizer.

2. A measured amount of gas is supplied to the vaporizer and all of the gas passes through the vaporizing chamber. It is then diluted by additional flow from the machine. This is known as a measured-flow vaporizer.

Concentration-Calibrated Vaporizers

Concentration-calibrated vaporizers are also called variable bypass, direct-reading, dial-controlled, automatic plenum, percent-age-type, and tec-type vaporizers and is sometimes referred to as a vaporizer chamber bypass arrangement. With these vaporizers, the total gas flow from the flowmeters goes through the vaporizer, picks up a predictable amount of vapor, then flows to the common gas outlet. Concentration is controlled by a single calibrated knob or dial that is an integral part of the vaporizer. This is usually calibrated in volumes percent. The machine standard requires that the control knob or dial open counterclockwise.

Figure 4.2 shows a vaporizer with a variable bypass. In the off position, the bypass mechanism (*dark squares*) occludes the inlet and outlet of the vaporizing chamber. Gas flows through the bypass to the outlet. In the on position, the incoming gas flow is divided into two portions: one part goes through the bypass and the other flows to the vaporizing chamber, where it is enriched with the vapor of the liquid anesthetic agent. Both gas flows rejoin downstream.

The ratio of bypass gas to gas going to the vaporizing chamber is called the splitting ratio (5,6) and depends on the ratio of resistances in the two pathways. This in turn depends on the variable (adjustable) orifice. This orifice may be in the inlet to the vaporizing chamber, but in most modern vaporizers, it is in the outlet (7). The splitting ratio also depends on the total flow to the vaporizer.

It has been observed that with many concentration-calibrated vaporizers carrier gas composition affected vaporizer output (vaporizer aberrance). Most vaporizers are calibrated using oxygen as the carrier gas. Generally, little change in output occurs if air is substituted for oxygen. When nitrous oxide is added to the carrier gas, both a temporary and a long-lasting effect on vaporizer output are seen. The temporary effect is almost always a reduction in concentration. The duration of this effect depends on the gas flow rate and the volume of liquid in the vapor-

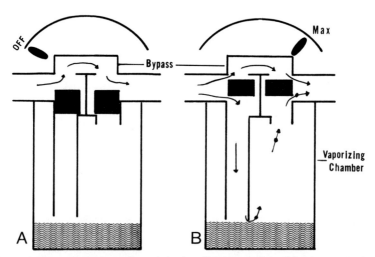

Figure 4.2. Concentration-calibrated vaporizer. **A,** In the off position, all the inflowing gas is directed through the bypass. **B,** In the on position, gas flow is divided between the bypass and the vaporizing chamber. In the max position, all of the gas flow allowed by the vaporizer goes to the vaporizing chamber.

izer. The permanent effect may be an increase or decrease, depending on the construction of the vaporizer (1).

Measured-Flow Vaporizers

Measured-flow vaporizers (also called kettle-type, flowmetered, and flowmeter-controlled vaporizer systems) use a measured flow of carrier gas, usually oxygen, to pick up anesthetic vapor. Each vaporizer system consists of three parts.

Vaporizer

The vaporizer includes the body that holds the liquid. It also has a window to view the liquid level, a filler port, and a thermometer to measure the temperature within the vaporizer.

A Flowmeter Assembly

The flowmeter may be calibrated either for the flow of gas through the flowmeter or for the vapor flow.

An On-Off Valve

The on-off valve's function is to isolate the vaporizer from the system.

To calculate the vaporizer output one must know the vapor pressure of the agent, the atmospheric pressure, the total flow of gases, the flow to the vaporizer, and the temperature. The formula is

% concentration

$$= \frac{\text{Vaporizer output of anesthetic}}{\text{Total flow}} \times 100$$

$$(4)$$

or

% concentration

$$= \frac{(VF)(V_{pa})}{AP(VF + DF) - (V_{pa})(DF)} \times 100 \quad (5)$$

where DF = diluent flow; VF = flow to the vaporizer; V_{pa} = vapor pressure of the liquid anesthetic; and AP = atmospheric pressure (8). By using this formula and making periodic adjustments for temperature changes, a

vaporizer of this type can be used accurately with a number of different anesthetic agents. Thus these vaporizers have the advantage of flexibility but the disadvantage that the vapor concentration must be calculated.

When calculating the concentration of gases in the outflow from a machine that uses a measured-flow vaporizer, the operator must make sure that the oxygen going through the vaporizer flowmeter is counted in addition to that metered on the other flowmeters.

METHODS OF VAPORIZATION

Flow-Over Vaporizers

In a flow-over vaporizer, a stream of carrier gas passes over the surface of the liquid. The efficiency of vaporization can be improved by increasing the area of the carrier gas-liquid interface. This can be done using baffles or spiral tracks to lengthen the pathway of the gas over the liquid. Another way is to employ wicks that have their bases in the liquid. The liquid moves up the wick by capillary action.

Bubble-Through Vaporizers

Another means of providing contact between the carrier gas and the volatile liquid is to bubble the gas through the liquid. Usually, there is some means to break the gas up into small bubbles, further increasing the gas-liquid interface.

Injection Vaporizers

If the volume of gas into which a known amount of liquid anesthetic or pure vapor is injected is known, accurate control of vapor concentration is possible (1). This mechanism is used in certain vaporizers.

TEMPERATURE COMPENSATION

As a liquid is vaporized, energy in the form of heat is lost. As the temperature of the liquid decreases, so does the vapor pressure. To maintain a constant vapor output with fluctuations in liquid anesthetic temperature, two methods have been employed.

Thermocompensation

Most concentration-calibrated vaporizers compensate for changes in vapor pressure with temperature by altering the splitting ratio so that the percentage of the carrier gas that is directed through the vaporizing chamber is changed (6). In measured-flow vaporizers, thermocompensation is performed manually by adjusting the flow through the vaporizer.

Supplied Heat

An electric heater can be used to supply heat to a vaporizer and maintain it at a constant temperature.

SPECIFICITY

Some vaporizers are designed to be used with a single agent, whereas others may be used with a variety of agents. A vaporizer should always be labeled to indicate its contents. The use of more than one agent in a vaporizer is not advisable, because a mixture of different agents can result. An agent-specific vaporizer should be used only with the agent for which it was designed. Even if a predictable concentration of another agent is possible, the incorrect agent could react with seals or gaskets inside the vaporizer, producing potentially harmful byproducts.

RESISTANCE

Plenum

Most modern vaporizers have a high resistance and depend on compressed gases driven under pressure over or through the liquid anesthetic. These vaporizers are commonly called plenum type—a plenum being a chamber in which the pressure within is greater than the pressure without (5).

Low-Resistance Vaporizers

Vaporizers with low resistance designed to be situated within the breathing system have been manufactured. Vaporization is a consequence of respiratory gas flow.

Effects of Altered Barometric Pressure

Most vaporizers are calibrated at standard (sea level) atmospheric pressure. Because vaporizers are sometimes used in hyperbaric chambers or at high altitudes, where atmospheric pressure is low, it is important to have some knowledge of how they will perform when the barometric pressure is changed. The ASTM machine standard requires that the effects of changes in ambient pressure on vaporizer performance be stated in operation manuals. Low boiling point, high-saturated vapor pressure anesthetic agents are more susceptible to the influence of barometric pressure variations than agents with higher boiling points (6).

LOW ATMOSPHERIC PRESSURE

Concentration-Calibrated Vaporizers

A concentration-calibrated vaporizer will deliver approximately the same partial pressure with decreases in barometric pressure, but will deliver increasing concentrations measured as volumes percent (7,9). The effect of a change in barometric pressure on the volumes percent output of this type of vaporizer may be calculated as follows:

$$c' = c(p/p')$$

where c' is the output concentration at a different barometric pressure in volumes percent; c is the dial setting of the vaporizer in volumes percent; p is the barometric pressure for which the vaporizer is calibrated; and p' is the barometric pressure for which c' is being established. Because partial pressure is the important factor in anesthetic depth, the clinical effect will be almost independent of atmospheric pressure. Small deviations in performance do occur owing to changes in the splitting ratio (6). The high-resistance pathway through the vaporizing chamber offers less resistance under hypobaric conditions, increasing vaporizer output slightly.

Measured-Flow Vaporizers

With measured-flow vaporizers the delivered partial pressure increases and volumes percent increases even more if the surrounding pressure is lowered (7). The amount of the increase depends on the barometric pressure and the vapor pressure of the agent (and thus the temperature). The closer the vapor pressure is to the barometric pressure, the greater the effect (7). Anesthetic depth may not change much if nitrous oxide is included in the inspired mixture, because the increased partial pressure of the potent agent will be offset by the decreased partial pressure of the nitrous oxide (10).

HIGH ATMOSPHERIC PRESSURES

Concentration-Calibrated Vaporizers

When atmospheric pressure is increased, the density of the gas changes. This causes more resistance to flow through the vaporizing chamber and a decrease in vaporizer output in both partial pressure and volumes percent (11). At two atmospheres, the concentration in volumes percent is halved (1). The effect on partial pressure (and hence anesthetic potency) is less dramatic.

Measured-Flow Vaporizers

A measured-flow vaporizer will deliver a lower concentration, expressed either as partial pressure or volumes percent, when atmospheric pressure is increased.

Effects of Intermittent Back Pressure

When assisted or controlled ventilation is used, the positive pressure generated during inspiration is transmitted from the breathing system back to the machine and some may be transmitted to the vaporizers. Another source of back pressure is use of the oxygen flush valve. Usually, the output from the oxygen flush valve enters the machine circuitry downstream of the vaporizers, and activating the oxygen flush valve produces high pressures. This back pressure may either increase (pumping effect) or decrease (pressurizing effect) the output of the vaporizer.

THE PUMPING EFFECT

Factors

Studies have shown that concentrations delivered by some vaporizers during controlled or assisted ventilation are considerably higher than when the vaporizer was used with free flow (12). This change is most pronounced when there is less agent in the vaporizing chamber, when carrier gas flow is low, when the pressure fluctuations are high and frequent and when the dial setting is low.

Mechanisms

Concentration-Calibrated Vaporizers

A proposed mechanism for the pumping effect for variable bypass vaporizers is shown in Figure 4.3*a–c*. Figure 4.3*a* shows the vaporizer during exhalation. Flows to the bypass and the vaporizing chamber are determined by the relative resistances of the outlets of the bypass and vaporizing chamber (points 3 and 4 in the figure).

Figure 4.3*b* shows inspiration. The positive pressure at point C prevents the outflow of gases and vapor. The pressure is transmitted to points A and B. This results in compression of gas in the vaporizing chamber and bypass. Because the bypass has a smaller volume than the vaporizing chamber, more molecules go to the vaporizing chamber. The normal ratio between the flow to the vaporizing chamber and the flow through the bypass is disturbed. There is, in effect, an increased flow to the vaporizing chamber, which then picks up anesthetic vapor.

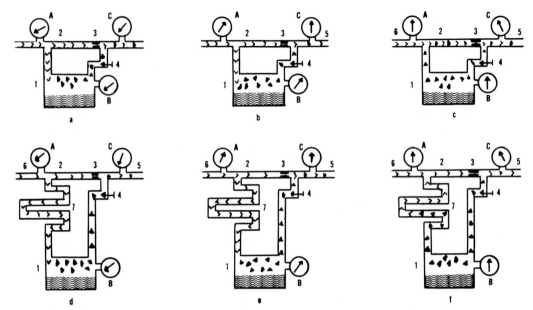

Figure 4.3.   The pumping effect in a concentration-calibrated vaporizer (see text for details). From Hill DW. The design and calibration of vaporizers for volatile anesthetic agents. Br J Anaesth 1968;40:656.

Figure 4.3*c* shows the situation just after the beginning of exhalation. The pressure at point C falls rapidly and gas flows suddenly from the vaporizing chamber and the bypass into the outlet. Because the bypass has less resistance than the vaporizing chamber outlet, the pressure in the bypass falls more quickly than that in the vaporizing chamber, and gas containing anesthetic vapor flows from the vaporizing chamber into the bypass. Because the gas in the bypass (which dilutes the gas from the vaporizing chamber) now carries anesthetic vapor and the gas flowing from the vaporizing chamber is still saturated, the vaporizer concentration is increased.

Measured Flow Vaporizers

As discussed previously, the gas flow to these vaporizers becomes saturated with anesthetic vapor and is joined by gas from other flowmeters, which dilutes its concentration. When back pressure is applied, there is a retrograde flow of gas so that the diluted gas mixture is forced back into the vaporizer. Because this gas is not saturated, it will then pick up anesthetic vapor. The result is an increase in vaporizer output.

Modifications to Minimize the Pumping Effect

Alterations in the Concentration-Calibrated Vaporizer (5)

Because the increase in output in variable bypass vaporizers is related to the relative sizes of the space above the liquid in the vaporizing chamber and the space in the bypass, keeping the size of the vaporizing chamber small or increasing the size of the bypass will decrease the effects of back pressure. Another method is to employ a long, spiral or large-diameter tube to lead to the vaporizing chamber (see Fig. 4.3*d–f*). The extra gas forced into this tube and subsequently returned to the bypass does not reach the vaporizing chamber. Another method is to exclude wicks from the area where the inlet tube joins the vaporizing chamber. Finally, an overall increase in resistance to gas flow through the vaporizer may be used.

Alterations to the Measured-Flow Vaporizer

Some measured-flow vaporizers have a relief valve at the outlet to limit the pressure.

Others have a check valve to prevent backward flow of gas. The outlet tube may be made longer so that unsaturated gas will have to pass farther back before picking up anesthetic vapor. Finally, keeping the vaporizing chamber small will result in less unsaturated gas being forced back into it.

Alterations to the Anesthesia Machine

These devices (pressurizing valve, unidirectional valve, and pressure relief device) were discussed in Chapter 3. A check valve at the machine outlet offers less protection from the pumping effect than a check valve at the outlet of a measured-flow vaporizer (13).

The ASTM machine standard (14) requires that the connections of the oxygen flush valve delivery line to the common gas outlet be designed so as to minimize pressure fluctuation that may produce a pumping effect on the vaporizer. The standard (14) also limits the pressure transmitted to the vaporizers during use of the flush valve to no more than 10 KPa (100 cm H_2O) above normal working pressure when the common gas outlet is open to the atmosphere and limits the change in concentration delivered by a vaporizer to not more than 20% with typical intermittent back pressures. Manufacturers are required to state in catalogs and operations manuals the extent to which back pressure affects a vaporizer's performance.

THE PRESSURIZING EFFECT

Factors

The output of some vaporizers used in conjunction with automatic ventilators has been found to be lower than during free flow to atmosphere (15,16). The effect is greater with high flows, large pressure fluctuations and low vaporizer settings.

Mechanism of the Pressurizing Effect

The explanation for the pressurizing effect is shown in Figure 4.4*A,B.* Figure 4.4*A* shows a vaporizer flowing free to atmosphere. The

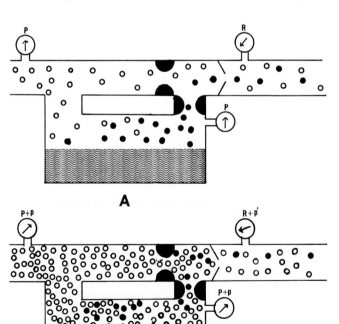

Figure 4.4. The pressurizing effect. An increase in pressure (p′) causes an increase in pressure (p) inside the vaporizer. The vapor pressure of the volatile anesthetic is unaffected by changes in the total pressure of the gas mixture above it. As a result, the concentration is reduced.

pressure in the vaporizing chamber and the bypass is P. As the gas flows to the outlet, the pressure is reduced to R. The number of molecules of anesthetic agent picked up by each milliliter of carrier gas depends on the density of the anesthetic vapor molecules in the vaporizing chamber. This, in turn, depends on the vapor pressure of the agent. The vapor pressure depends solely on the temperature and is not affected by alterations in the atmospheric pressure.

Figure 4.4*B* shows the situation when an increased pressure (p′) is applied to the vaporizer outlet and transmitted to the vaporizing chamber (p). The increased pressure in the vaporizer will compress the carrier gas so there will be more molecules per milliliter. The number of molecules of anesthetic vapor in the vaporizing chamber will not be increased, however, because this depends on the saturated vapor pressure of the anesthetic and not on the pressure in the container. The net result is a decrease in the concentration of anesthetic in the vaporizing chamber and the vaporizer outlet.

INTERPLAY BETWEEN PRESSURIZING AND PUMPING EFFECTS

The changes in vaporizer output caused by the pumping effect usually are greater in magnitude than those associated with the pressurizing effect. The pressurizing effect is seen with high gas flows and the pumping effect, at low flows.

Vaporizers and the 1988 Anesthesia Machine Standard

The 1988 ASTM machine standard (14) contains the following provisions regarding vaporizers:

1. A vaporizer must be capable of accepting a total gas flow of 15 liters/min from the anesthesia machine and, in turn, of delivering a gas flow with a predictable concentration of vapor.

2. The effects of the conditions of use (including variations in ambient temperature and pressure, back pressure, and input flow rates) on vaporizer performance must be stated in catalogs and operation manuals. The effect of carrier gas composition on vaporizer output should also be supplied.

3. The extent to which temperature and input flow rates influence the vapor concentration must be stated on the vaporizer or anesthesia machine or in a manual. If this information is provided in the manual only, a label must be placed on the vaporizer directing the user's attention to the manual.

4. A system that isolates the vaporizers from each other and prevents gas from passing through the vaporizing chamber of one vaporizer and then through that of another must be provided.

5. Controls must be provided to limit the escape of anesthetic vapor from the vaporizing chamber into the fresh gas supply when the vaporizer is in the off position. The delivered concentration must be less than 0.1% when the vaporizer is turned off.

6. All vaporizer control knobs must open counterclockwise.

7. The units of calibration must be marked on the control knob or on a scale.

8. The vaporizer must be equipped with a liquid level indicator visible from the front of the anesthesia machine.

9. The vaporizer must be designed so that it cannot be overfilled when in the normal operating position.

10. The vaporizer must permit maximal calibrated flows of oxygen and nitrous oxide simultaneously in the on and off positions with the vaporizer filled to the maximum safe indicated level without discharging liquid through the its outlet, when it is mounted and used in accordance with the manufacturer's instructions.

11. Vaporizers unsuitable for use in the

breathing system must have noninterchangeable proprietary or 23-mm fittings. 22-mm and 15-mm fittings cannot be used. When 23-mm fittings are used, the inlet of the vaporizer must be male and the outlet female and the direction of gas flow must be marked.

12. Vaporizers suitable for use in the breathing system must have standard 22-mm fittings or screw-threaded, weight-bearing fittings with the inlet female and the outlet male. The inlet and outlet ports must be marked, the direction of gas flow must be indicated by arrows, and the vaporizer must be marked "for use in the breathing system."

Specific Vaporizers

SIEMENS

Classification

Concentration calibrated, injection, no thermocompensation, agent specific (halothane, enflurane, or isoflurane), plenum.

Construction

The Siemens vaporizer (Fig. 4.5) is designed to be fitted to the Siemens 900D Ventilator. The on-off valve on the right side has a locking device that must be released before the vaporizer can be turned on. The concentration dial is at the front, above the vaporizing chamber window and liquid level scale. The vaporizing chamber can hold up to 125 ml of liquid agent.

The filling system (Figs. 4.6 and 4.7) consists of an adaptor that fits on a bottle with a collar and fits into the filling receptacle at the back of the vaporizer. Noninterchangeability is accomplished by using different-size collars to fit different-size filling ports on the vaporizers. Once the collar is fitted into the vaporizer filler, a gentle push will open the valve in the filling device to let agent enter the vaporizer. The adaptor is self-sealing so it can remain on the bottle when the vaporizer is not being filled.

The Siemens vaporizer is diagrammed in Figure 4.8. Gas from the mixing device passes the bellows valve, which is open when the bellows needs refilling and closed when

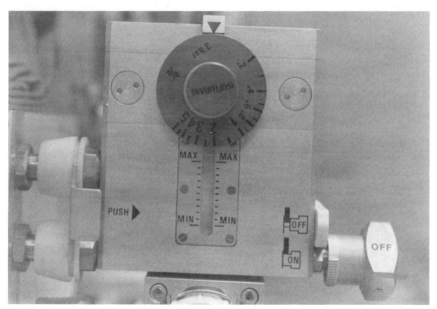

Figure 4.5. Siemens vaporizer. The on-off valve with the lock is at the right. In the center is the liquid scale and window, below the concentration dial. The filling mechanism is at the back.

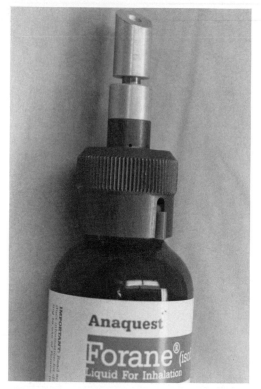

Figure 4.6. Bottle adaptor for Siemens vaporizer.

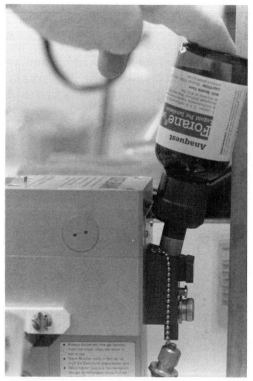

Figure 4.7. Filling the Siemens vaporizer. The adaptor is inserted into the filling receptacle. The bottle is pushed downward to allow the liquid to flow.

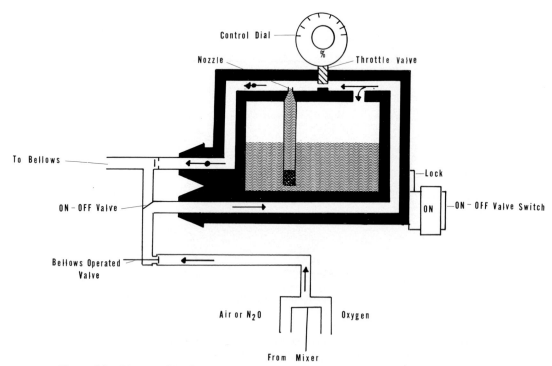

Figure 4.8. Diagram of the Siemens vaporizer. Redrawn from a drawing furnished by Siemens.

the bellows is full. When the vaporizer on-off valve is in the on position, gas from the mixing device passes through the vaporizer. The throttle valve, which is adjusted via the concentration dial, causes resistance to gas flow. This results in back pressure that is transmitted to the reservoir, which contains liquid anesthetic. The pressure causes liquid anesthetic to be pushed through the nozzle of the injector into the stream of gas flowing to the bellows. The liquid quickly vaporizes in this gas stream. The more the throttle valve constricts the channel, the higher the pressure in the reservoir and the more liquid pushed through the injector.

Evaluation

The manufacturer claims an accuracy of ± 10% of set value or ± 0.1 volume percent. A wide range of rapidly changing gas flow rates can be accommodated without loss of accuracy (1). The composition of carrier gas does affect output (Fig. 4.9). Output increases with increasing temperature.

Hazards

The vaporizer must not be turned upside down or sideways. One case has been reported in which a malfunctioning inlet control valve on the ventilator caused low concentrations to be delivered (17).

Maintenance

The external surface can be cleaned by wiping it with a cloth soaked in disinfectant solution. No other cleaning or disinfection should be attempted by the user. The vaporizer connections to the machine can be checked for leaks by turning the vaporizer on and using leak detection fluid. The manufacturer recommends that the halothane vaporizer be drained monthly or, if the vaporizer is out of use for a long time, the contents discarded and the vaporizer rinsed with a small amount of halothane.

The accuracy of vaporizer output should be checked periodically using an agent monitor. If none is available, the following test described in the operations manual can be used: Set the ventilator controls at the values marked in green and the preset inspiratory minute volume at 7.5 liters/min. Set the vaporizer to 3% for halothane, 3.5% for enflurane, and 3% for isoflurane. Set the ventilator to deliver 35% O_2 and 65% N_2O, The liquid level should drop two scale divisions in 18 to 24 min if the vaporizer is operating correctly.

TEC 3

Tec 3 vaporizers include the Fluotec Mark 3, Enfluratec 3, and Fortec 3. These vaporizers are no longer being manufactured.

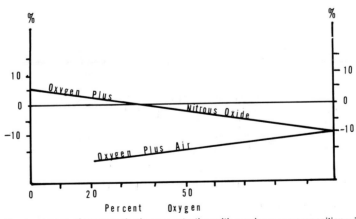

Figure 4.9. Deviation in percent of set anesthetic concentration with varying gas composition with the Siemens vaporizer. Redrawn from a drawing furnished by Siemens.

Classification

Concentration calibrated, flow over with wick, automatic thermocompensation, agent specific (halothane, enflurane, or isoflurane), plenum.

Construction

The vaporizer is diagrammed in Figure 4.10 and shown in Figure 4.11. It consists of a lower vaporizing chamber and an upper duct and valve system. Control of the delivered concentration is achieved by rotation of the knob at the top. This opens and closes ports and thus regulates the amount of gas passing through the vaporizing chamber.

In the off position (see Fig. 4.10, *left*), gas enters at the inlet, passes through a filter, and then flows to the outlet via two bypass channels. One of these channels directs a small stream of gas past a bimetallic temperature-sensitive element. This element is located concentrically within the vaporizing chamber so that its temperature is close to that of the anesthetic agent (18). The inlet and outlet of the vaporizing chamber are closed.

In the on position (see Fig. 4.10, *right*), the top bypass channel is closed and the channel to the vaporizing chamber and the control channel (from the vaporizing chamber to the vaporizer outlet) are open. Gas still flows past the temperature-sensitive element in the lower bypass channel. Gas travels down one vaporizing chamber channel and over the liquid, and by the wicks where it becomes saturated with vapor. It then flows out of the chamber via the other vaporizing chamber channel and enters the control channel. The size of the control channel is controlled by the position of the control knob.

The delivered concentration is determined by resistances to flow past the temperature-sensitive element and in the control channel. Cooling causes increased resistance to flow past the element, so that more gas flows through the vaporizing chamber.

The external design of a Tec 3 vaporizer is shown in Figure 4.11. The concentration dial turns on counterclockwise. To the left of the concentration dial is a locking lever that must be depressed to turn the vaporizer on. On the Enfluratec 3, the lever must also be

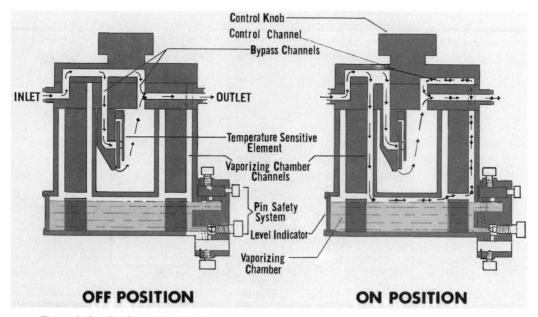

Figure 4.10.   Tec 3 vaporizer. The filter at the inlet is not shown Redrawn courtesy of Fraser Harlake.

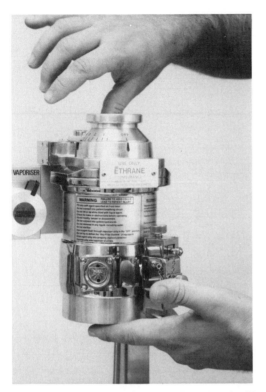

Figure 4.11. Enfluratec 3 vaporizer equipped with agent-specific filling device. The locking lever is at the left of the concentration dial. Note the front drain screw and dummy plug chained to the filling device. This vaporizer has a ring that extends the base below the filler block. This allows the vaporizer to be placed upright on a flat surface. A selector valve is to the left of the vaporizer. Courtesy of Fraser Harlake.

depressed to increase the concentration above 5%. At the bottom is a sight window on the left and a filling mechanism on the right.

Evaluation

The manufacturer's performance data are given in Figure 4.12. All are accurate at low dial settings. At higher settings, most put out higher-than-expected concentrations at low flow rates and lower-than-expected concentrations at high flow rates.

Several investigations have shown that these vaporizers are quite accurate (18–26). Most investigations of effects of carrier gas composition on output show that addition of nitrous oxide results in an initial decrease in

output followed by a slow increase to a new value that is less than that seen when the carrier gas is oxygen.

An investigation of the Fluotec 3 showed that in the 0% to 0.5% dial-setting range the output was governed mainly by the position of the concentration dial and was little affected by the fresh gas flow (27). For approximately the first half of the rotation of the dial from off to the 0.5% position, the output was 0. In the second half of the distance there was an almost linear increase in output to approximately 0.6% at a dial setting of 0.5%.

Manufacturer's data indicate no effect on vaporizer output from intermittent back pressure. Studies on the Fluotec 3 have confirmed this finding (18,20).

Hazards

The Fluotec 3 has been found to leak small amounts of vapor into the bypass in the off position (28,29). In one case a Fortec 3 delivered very high concentrations, even when turned off (30,31).

Several cases were reported of a Tec 3 vaporizer on which it was possible to turn the dial beyond the off position, resulting in delivery of vapor when none was desired (32–36). The manufacturer redesigned the vaporizer, and there have been no reports of this problem since 1984 (37).

A case was reported in which a damaged gasket in a Fluotec 3 caused a leak that allowed half the fresh gas flow to exit around the top of the vaporizer when the control dial was at a setting other than 0 (38).

One study showed that tipping these vaporizers to 30° or 90° had no effect on the concentration subsequently delivered (39). However, after inversion to 180° with the dial set at zero or higher the concentration delivered was much greater than shown on the dial, initially exceeding 12% for all agents. A study of the Fluotec 3 vaporizer filled and securely mounted on a gurney found that movements during normal motion did not cause an increase in delivered concentration (40).

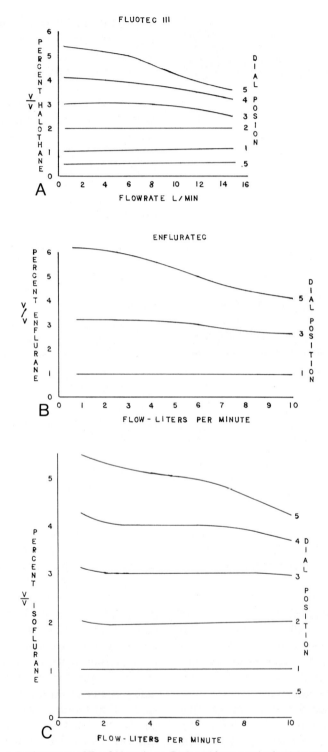

Figure 4.12.   A, Performance of Tec 3 Vaporizers. Redrawn from graphs furnished by Fraser Harlake.

Maintenance

Yearly return of the vaporizer for maintenance is recommended by the manufacturer. This includes disassembly, inspection, cleaning, and replacement of wicks and other components. After reassembly, the unit is tested for leaks and recalibrated. Product improvements may be made during maintenance.

TEC 4

Tec 4 vaporizers include the Fluotec 4, Enfluratec 4, and the Fortec 4.

Classification

Concentration calibrated, flow over with wick, automatic thermocompensation, agent specific (halothane, enflurane, or isoflurane), plenum.

Construction

The Fortec 4 is shown in Figure 4.13. At the top is a control dial that is turned counterclockwise to increase the concentration. The release button to the left of the control dial must be depressed before the vaporizer can be turned on. To the rear of the control dial is a locking lever. This is connected with the control dial so that the vaporizer cannot be turned on until it is locked on the manifold.

These vaporizers are available with either of two filling mechanisms. One is a screw cap, shown in Figure 4.13. Below the cap is a drain plug that extends up into the center of the cap. This plug is unscrewed to drain the vaporizer. The other filling device is a keyed system that has a single port for filling and emptying.

The Tec 4 vaporizers are designed to be attached to the back bar of the anesthesia machine by means of the Selectatec manifold system that allows for easy removal and mounting of vaporizers. Before mounting a vaporizer, any adjacent vaporizer must be turned off and the control dial must be in the

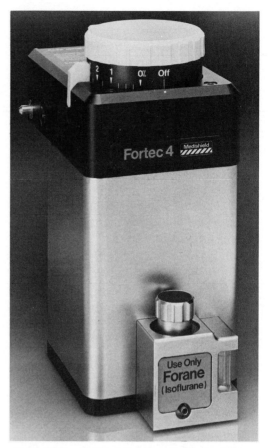

Figure 4.13. Fortec 4 vaporizer Courtesy of Fraser Harlake.

off position. The vaporizer is fitted onto the manifold and the locking lever turned clockwise to the locked position. To remove a vaporizer from the manifold, the control dial is turned off and the locking lever turned to the unlock position. The vaporizer can then be lifted off the manifold.

When the vaporizer is turned on, two plungers within the vaporizer open the valve ports in the back bar, connecting the vaporizer into the fresh gas stream. At the same time, two extension rods are extended and locked. These prevent operation of any adjacent vaporizer. The plungers cause the vaporizer to be isolated from the fresh gas flow when the vaporizer is turned off.

A diagram of the internal construction of the vaporizer is shown in Figure 4.14. When the vaporizer is in the off position, gas from the inlet flows through the bypass, and on to the outlet. When the vaporizer is turned on, the incoming gas is split into two streams by the rotary valve attached to the concentration dial. One stream is directed through the vaporizing chamber that surrounds the bypass chamber. After passing through the inner section, the gas flows along the sides of the vaporizer, where two concentric wicks enclose a copper helix. The wicks dip into the liquid and increase contact between the carrier gas and the anesthetic agent. Gas with vapor leaves the vaporizing chamber and flows past the rotary valve to the outlet. The balance of the fresh gas flow passes through the bypass chamber. Inside this chamber is a temperature-sensitive element that causes more gas to flow into the vaporizing chamber as cooling occurs.

Evaluation

The manufacturer's performance data for the vaporizers are given in Figure 4.15. One evaluation showed that at low and very high flow rates anesthetic delivery was less precise than in the median flow range (41). Another study found that at dial settings of 0.25%, the output was decreased by 40% between 0.2 and 1 liter/min (42). At dial settings between 0.4% and 0.5%, deviation in output concentration ranged from −5.5% for halothane and isoflurane to +22% for enflurane. Another evaluation found that the vaporizer was accurate in the proximity of an MRI magnet (43).

The vaporizers are calibrated at 21°C. Output tends to rise slightly with elevated ambient temperature, especially with higher dial settings. The variation in output from intermittent positive pressure is negligible. Steady back pressure will reduce the output but this effect is of such small magnitude that it can be ignored under normal clinical circumstances.

Changes in output with changes in carrier gas composition are normally less than 10% of setting, with output less when nitrous oxide is added to the carrier gas.

Hazards

Deviations from the upright position will not affect the output of the vaporizer but may give a misleading impression of the amount of agent in the vaporizing chamber. One study confirmed that the vaporizer could be tipped to 30°, 90°, or 180° without altering the concentration subsequently delivered (39).

The vaporizer should not be carried by the control dial. The vaporizer should not be used if it is visibly out of line on the manifold or can be lifted off when the locking lever is in the locked position.

A hazard in the attachment of a Tec 4 vaporizer to the back bar of an anesthesia machine has been reported (44). It was possible to lock the vaporizer in place when it was not correctly positioned. This resulted in a leak at the vaporizer–back bar junction when the vaporizer was turned on. Such a leak would not be detected unless the vaporizer was turned on when the machine was checked.

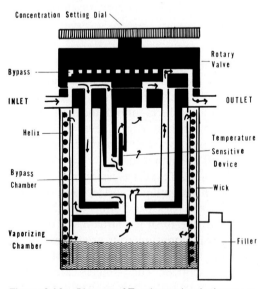

Figure 4.14. Diagram of Tec 4 vaporizer in the on position (see text for details). Redrawn from a diagram furnished by Fraser Harlake.

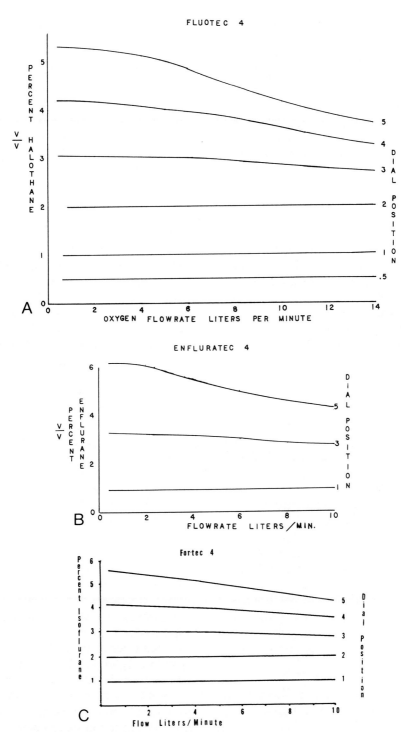

Figure 4.15. Performances of Tec 4 vaporizers at various flow rates and vaporizer settings. Redrawn from graphs furnished by Fraser Harlake and Ohmeda, a division of BOC Health Care, Inc.

The manufacturer has made modifications to eliminate this problem (45).

Leakage of liquid agent from the drain port caused by inadvertent loosening of the drain plug when the filler cap was removed has been reported (46). Consequences include loss of liquid agent, exposure of operating room personnel to anesthetic vapors, and damage to items below the vaporizer.

Maintenance

Although the manufacturer has recommended that vaporizers for halothane be drained at intervals not exceeding 2 weeks and less frequently for vaporizers for enflurane and isoflurane, studies show that draining every 6 months is probably sufficient (47).

The vaporizers should be sent to a service center yearly for disassembly, cleaning, and inspection for damage and wear. The wicks; seals; and damaged, worn, or outdated parts are replaced. The vaporizer is lubricated and calibrated before being returned to the owner.

In-house cleaning includes wiping the exterior surface with a damp cloth. No cleaning solution should be allowed to accumulate in the filler, the gas inlet, or around the control dial.

If an incorrect agent is put into the vaporizer, the vaporizer should be drained and the liquid discarded. The dial should be set to the highest setting and the vaporizer flushed with a 5 liter/min flow until no trace of the agent is detected. At least 2 hr should be allowed for the vaporizer temperature to stabilize before use. If water or a nonvolatile substance is placed in a vaporizer, the vaporizer must be returned to the manufacturer for service.

TEC 5

Tec 5 vaporizers include the Isotec 5, Fluotec 5, Enfluratec 5, and Sevofluratec.

Classification

Concentration calibrated, flow over with wick, automatic thermocompensation, agent specific (halothane, enflurane, isoflurane, or sevoflurane), plenum.

Construction

Tec 5 vaporizers are shown in Figure 4.16. On top is a control dial that is turned counterclockwise to increase the concentration. At the rear of the dial is a release button that must be pushed in before the vaporizer can be turned on. Operation of the dial release connects the vaporizer to the fresh gas flow and activates the interlock device. At the rear of the vaporizer is a locking lever that is connected to the control dial so that the vaporizer cannot be turned on until it is locked on the manifold. At the bottom right front of each vaporizer is a sight glass.

Tec 5 vaporizers are available with either of two filling devices. One is a keyed system (see Fig. 4.16). The filling-draining port is at the front of the vaporizer on the left near the bottom. A locking lever to secure the filler block is located to the left of the vaporizer. A small lever at the base allows the liquid to be added to or drained from the vaporizer. The other filling device is a screw cap that has a drain plug that can be loosened to drain the vaporizer.

The Tec 5 vaporizer is designed to be used with the Selectatec manifold. Before mounting a vaporizer, any adjacent vaporizer must be turned off and the control dial must be in the off position. The locking lever should be in the unlock position. The vaporizer is placed over the two manifold port valves. The locking lever is pushed down then turned clockwise to the locked position. If the vaporizer is visibly out of line with other vaporizers, or can be lifted off the manifold with the lever in the locked position, it has been improperly mounted. It should be possible to turn on only one vaporizer at a time. To remove a vaporizer from the manifold, the control dial is turned to off and the locking lever, to the unlocked position. The vaporizer can then be lifted off.

To turn a vaporizer on, the dial release must be pushed in. This causes two plungers

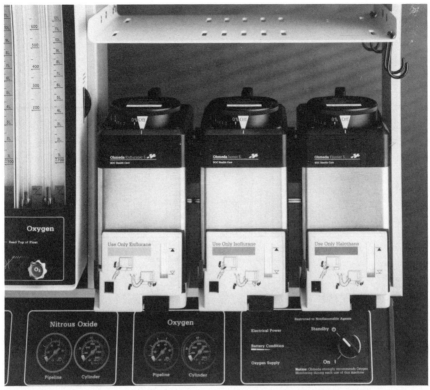

Figure 4.16. Tec 5 vaporizer. The locking lever for the filling device is to the left of each vaporizer. The lever for filling-draining is at the base, below the sight glass. To fill, the bottle adaptor is inserted into the port and clamped in place by pulling the locking lever down. The bottle is then lifted up and the filling-draining lever is pulled forward. When filling is completed, the filling-draining lever is returned to the closed position, the bottle is lowered, the clamping lever is pushed upward, and the bottle is removed. Draining of the vaporizer is accomplished using the same levers but lowering the bottle rather than lifting it. Courtesy of Ohmeda, a division of BOC Health Care, Inc.

within the vaporizer to open valves in the Selectatec manifold, connecting the vaporizer into the fresh gas stream. These valves cause the vaporizer to be isolated when it is turned off. Operation of the dial release also activates two interlock extension rods that prevent operation of any other vaporizer installed on the manifold.

A schematic diagram of a Tec 5 vaporizer is shown in Figure 4.17. The internal baffle system is designed to keep liquid from reaching the outlet if the vaporizer is tipped or inverted.

When the concentration dial is in the zero position, all incoming gas flows directly to the outlet via the bypass. When the dial is turned past zero, in-flowing gas is split into two streams by the rotary valve. One stream is directed to the vaporizing chamber, the other through the bypass.

Gas flowing through the bypass circuit flows down one side of the vaporizer and past the thermostat, a bimetallic strip in the base. As the temperature in the vaporizer decreases, the thermostat allows less gas to flow through the bypass so a greater proportion passes through the vaporizing chamber. From the thermostat, the gas flows up the other side of the vaporizer and joins the gas that has passed through the vaporizing chamber at the vaporizer outlet.

The gas flowing to the vaporizing chamber first passes through the central part of the rotary valve, after which it is directed through

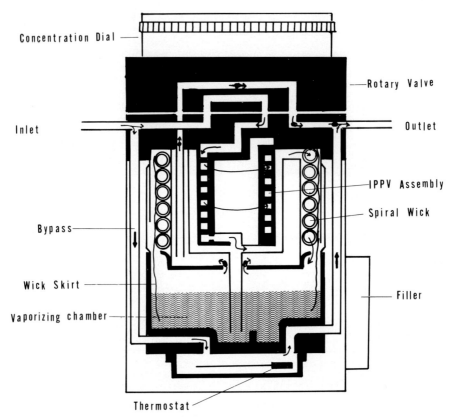

Figure 4.17. Diagram of Tec 5 vaporizer in the on position (see text for details). Redrawn from a drawing furnished by Ohmeda, a division of the BOC Health Care, Inc.

the helical intermittent positive pressure ventilation (IPPV) assembly and then past a spiral wick, which is designed to give maximum contact between carrier gas and liquid agent. The spiral wick is in contact with the wick skirt, which dips into the liquid agent. Gas with vapor leaves the vaporizing chamber via a channel in the rotary valve and flows to the outlet.

Evaluation

The manufacturer's performance curves are shown in Figure 4.18. Greatest accuracy is at a fresh gas flow at 5 liters/min and dial settings of less than 3%. At higher flows and higher dial settings, there is a decrease in output.

The greatest accuracy is between 15° and 35°C. The thermostat does not respond to temperatures below 15°C and the vaporizer output will be less than indicated on the dial. If the temperature is above 35°C, the vaporizer output will be unpredictably high.

These vaporizers are unaffected by fluctuating back pressures encountered under normal clinical conditions. Carrier gas composition affects the output of the Tec 5 vaporizers. At low flows, the output is less when air or nitrous oxide is used then when oxygen is the carrier gas. At high flows, a small increase in output will occur.

Hazards

Most of the hazards associated with direct-reading vaporizers can occur with this vaporizer. Specific hazards have not been reported.

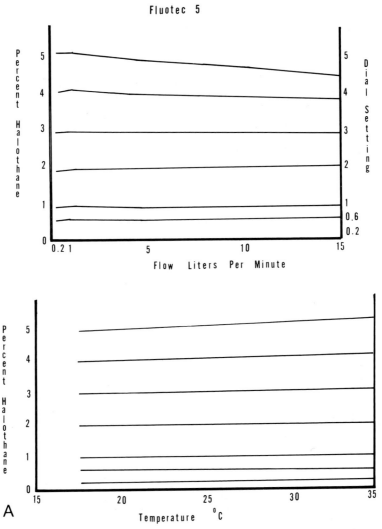

Figure 4.18. Performances of four Tec 5 vaporizers. Redrawn from drawings furnished by Ohmeda, a division of the BOC Health Care, Inc.

Maintenance

It is recommended by the manufacturer that the vaporizer be drained every 2 weeks or when the level is low if the agent contains additives or stabilizing agents. If these are not present the vaporizer can be drained at less frequent intervals.

Every 3 years the vaporizer should be returned to a service center for complete disassembly, cleaning, inspection for damage and wear, replacement of worn or damaged parts, updating, lubrication, and calibration. Agent monitoring is recommended if servicing is carried out at 3-year intervals.

The exterior of the vaporizer may be wiped with a damp cloth. No other cleaning or disinfection should be attempted.

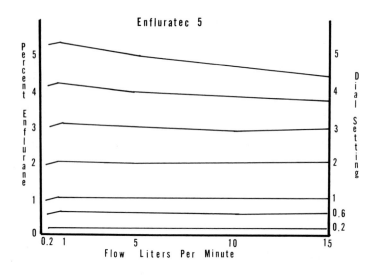

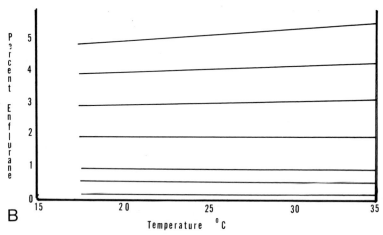

Figure 4.18—*continued.*

TEC 6

Classification

Concentration calibrated, injection, thermocompensation by supplied heat, agent specific (desflurane), plenum.

Construction

The Tec 6 vaporizer is shown in Figure 4.19. It is somewhat larger than the Tec 4 and Tec 5 vaporizers. It can be used on both Ohmeda and North American Drager anesthesia machines. The mounting is different for the North American Drager machines. For Ohmeda machines, the vaporizer mounts to the anesthesia machine by the Selectatec mounting system that ensures that a vaporizer cannot be turned on unless it is locked on the manifold and that gas flow enters a vaporizer only when that vaporizer is turned on. It also has interlocks to prevent more than one vaporizer from being turned on at a time. The Tec 6 can be interchanged with Tec 4 and 5 vaporizers, which mount with this system.

The concentration dial at the top is cali-

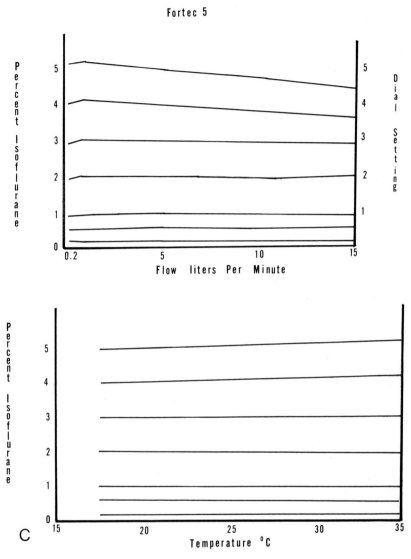

Figure 4.18—continued.

brated from 1% to 18% in gradations of 1% up to 10% and 2% between 10% and 18%. A dial release is at the back of the dial. This must be depressed to turn the dial from the standby position and to dial concentrations over 12%. This release cannot be depressed unless the operational light-emitting diode (LED) is illuminated.

The filler port is at the front on the left. It is keyed so that only a desflurane-specific bottle can be inserted into it. The power cord attachment and battery case are on the bottom of the vaporizer. A nonrechargeable battery provides power for the alarms and liquid crystal level indicator display during main power failure. The power cord comes out at the side of the vaporizer. The drain plug is also located at the base of the vaporizer. A draining kit is required to drain the vaporizer.

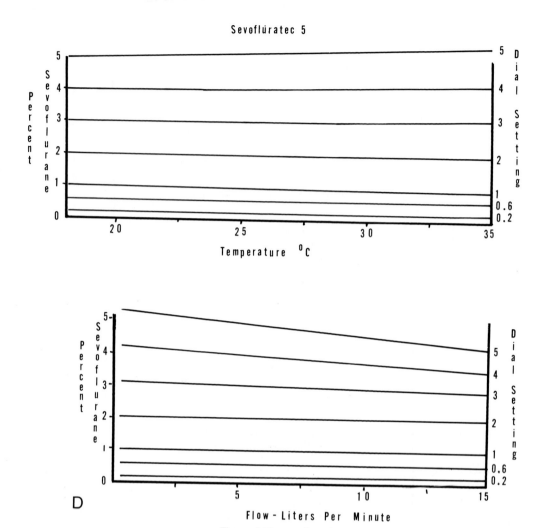

Figure 4.18—continued.

On the front lower right of the vaporizer is the display panel, which has visual indicators for monitors of vaporizer function (see Fig. 4.19). With the exception of the tilt condition there is a 10-sec delay between detection of a malfunction and alarm activation. An auditory alarm is mounted behind the upper part of the display panel. A mute button is located above the display panel.

The amber *warm-up* LED indicates an initial warm-up period after the vaporizer is first connected to the main power. Once warm-up is complete, the green *operational* LED lights, indicating that the vaporizer has

reached its operating temperature and that the concentration dial can be turned on. There are no audible signals for these modes except for a short tone that sounds at the transition from warmup to operational.

The red *no output* LED flashes and an auditory alarm of repetitive tones (0.5 sec on and 0.5 sec off) occurs if the vaporizer reaches a state in which it is no longer able to deliver vapor. This can be caused by an agent level less than 20 ml, tilting of the vaporizer, a power failure, or an internal malfunction. Turning the concentration dial to standby will mute this alarm and illuminate the red

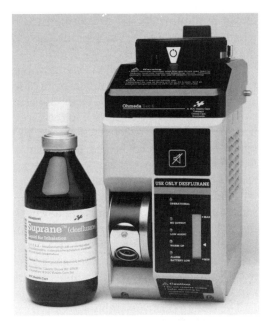

Figure 4.19. Tec 6 vaporizer. The filler port is at the bottom left. At the bottom right are the liquid level indicator and the visual signals for monitors of vaporizer function. A bottle of desflurane with the protection cap in place is to the left of the vaporizer. Courtesy of Ohmeda, a division of BOC Health Care, Inc.

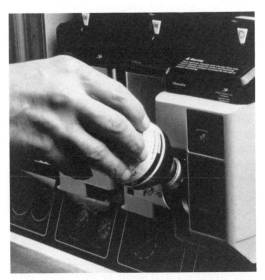

Figure 4.20. Filling Tec 6 vaporizer. The bottle is fitted to the filler port. After it is engaged in the filler port it is rotated upward. When it reaches the upper stop, agent will enter the vaporizer. Courtesy of Ohmeda, a division of BOC Health Care, Inc.

light continuously. If the no output alarm occurs while the concentration dial is in the standby position, it can be muted by pressing the mute button.

The amber *low agent* LED accompanied by an audible alarm of repetitive tones (1.5 sec on and 0.5 sec off) flashes to indicate that there is less than 50 ml of agent in the vaporizer. This alarm can be muted for 120 sec. If less than 20 ml remain in the vaporizer, the no output alarm is activated.

The amber *alarm battery low* LED illuminates to indicate that a new battery is required. There is no auditory signal for this condition.

The liquid level indicator has a liquid crystal display (LCD) that shows the amount of liquid in the vaporizer between 50 and 425 ml. The LCD is lit whenever the vaporizer is powered. There are 20 bars. A single bar corresponds to a volume of approximately 20 ml. An arrow on the side indicates the 250 ml refill mark. If the level is below this mark, the vaporizer will accept a full bottle (240 ml) of desflurane.

If the vaporizer is tilted more than 10°, the tilt switch is activated. This causes vapor output to cease and activates the red no output LED and auditory alarm.

When the unit is plugged in, the electronics go through a self-test. For 2 sec the alarm sounds and each LED and LCD display illuminates. This self-test can be repeated at any time by pressing the mute button for 4 sec or more. Once the vaporizer is plugged in the power is always on and the sump heaters are operational. Initially, the vaporizer will take 5 to 10 min to reach operating temperature. During this time, the dial is locked in the standby position. An internal shutoff valve is closed to prevent flow of vapor from the sump.

The Tec 6 filling system is shown in Figures 4.20 and 4.21. Because desflurane boils so close to room temperature, it cannot be poured into a funnel and allowed to drain into the vaporizer. The vaporizer can be filled with the vaporizer in operation but the

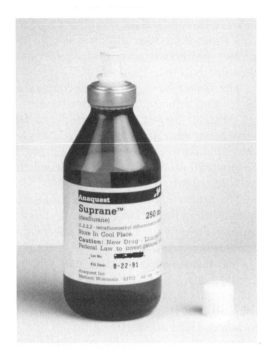

Figure 4.21. Bottle for filling Tec 6 vaporizer. The protection cap has been removed and is at the right. Courtesy of Ohmeda, a division of BOC Health Care, Inc.

fresh gas flow should be less than 8 liters/min and the concentration dial set at no more than 8% and the vaporizer should not be subjected to any high back pressure. The vaporizer can be filled when the vaporizer is in its warm-up cycle or at any time the vaporizer is in use.

The bottle (see Fig. 4.21) has a crimped-on adaptor. This adaptor has a spring-loaded valve that opens when the bottle is pushed into the filling port on the vaporizer. To fill the vaporizer, the bottle protection cap is removed and the bottle fitted to the filler port by holding it below and pushing it up against the spring. After the bottle fully engaged in the port, it is rotated upward (see Fig. 4.20). When the bottle reaches the upper stop, agent will enter the vaporizer. The bottle is held in this position while filling. When the LCD liquid level gauge indicates that the sump is full or when the bottle is empty, the bottle is rotated downward and removed from the vaporizer. The valve on the bottle

closes automatically to prevent spillage of agent. The filling port has a spring valve to prevent escape of agent.

The internal construction of this vaporizer is shown in Fig. 4.22. It differs from other vaporizers in that none of the fresh gas passes through a vaporizing chamber. In the vaporizer, desflurane is heated to 39°C (102°F), which is well above its boiling point. An external heat source is needed because the potency of desflurane requires that large amounts be vaporized and thermocompensation using the usual mechanical devices is impossible. Power for the heater, alarms and controls is furnished from a standard hospital electrical system. A transformer and AC to DC converter provide a DC supply for the vaporizer.

The heated sump assembly serves as a reservoir of desflurane vapor. It has an upper chamber that can contain up to 375 ml and a lower chamber that can hold up to 50 ml, providing a total capacity of 425 ml. Two heaters fitted into the base heat the agent to 39°C. The temperature is monitored and associated electronics act as a thermostat. There are also two heaters in the upper part of the vaporizer to prevent condensation of agent. The casing of the vaporizer is normally warm to the touch when it is connected to the electrical supply.

The level of liquid agent is sensed by a probe and sheath mounted in the sump assembly. These measure the capacitance using the agent as a dielectric. The display is on the front of the vaporizer.

When the electrical supply is first turned on, the amber warm-up light remains illuminated during the warm-up cycle, which may take up to 10 min. During that time, the shut-off valve between the sump assembly and the agent pressure regulating valve is closed. The solenoid interlock prevents the concentration dial from being turned until the vaporizer is ready for use.

When the proper temperature is attained, the green operational LED illuminates. A signal from the control electronics operates

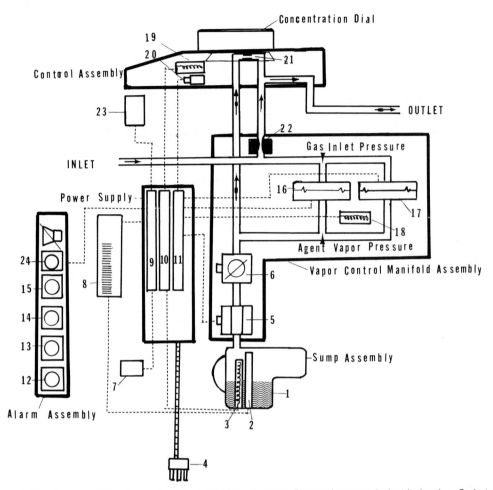

Figure 4.22. Diagram of Tec 6 vaporizer. *1*, agent; *2*, level sensor *3*, sump heaters; *4*, electrical mains; *5*, shut-off valve;*6*, agent pressure-regulating valve; *7*, battery for alarms; *8*, LCD level display; *9*, alarm electronics; *10*, heater electronics; *11*, control electronics; *12*, alarm battery low LED; *13*, warm-up LED; *14*, low agent LED; *15*, no output LED; *16*, pressure transducer; *17*, pressure monitor; *18*, heater in vapor manifold; *19*, heater in valve plate; *20*, solenoid interlock; *21*, variable resistor (controlled by rotary valve); *22*, fixed restrictor; *23*, tilt switch; *24*, operational LED. See text for details. Redrawn from a diagram furnished by Ohmeda, a division of BOC Health Care, Inc.

the solenoid interlock, allowing the dial and rotary valve to be turned. When the dial and rotary valve are turned, a signal from the control electronics opens the shut-off valve.

Fresh gas flow enters the vaporizer and encounters a fixed resistor. Electromechanical devices operate to maintain the agent vapor pressure at the variable resistor in the rotary valve at the same level as the fresh gas pressure at the fixed restrictor. This pressure balance between the desflurane and the diluent flow compensates for changes in tempera-

ture, vapor pressure or diluent flow rate. The pressures are sensed by a transducer that sends a signal of the difference to the control electronics, which in turn alters the agent pressure at the variable resistor by opening or closing the agent pressure regulating valve to balance the pressures.

With this balance of pressures maintained, the concentration delivered by the vaporizer depends only on the ratio of the fresh gas flow through the fixed restrictor and agent vapor flow through the variable resistor, which depends on the setting of the concentration dial. For example, when the concentration dial is turned to a higher value the resistance to desflurane flow decreases and the flow of desflurane increases. Similarly, with an increase in diluent flow the electronics will increase the flow in the desflurane limb to maintain the pressure balance. The vapor mixes with fresh gas in proportions consistent with the selected dial setting before flowing to the vaporizer outlet.

Evaluation

The manufacturer's data are shown in Figure 4.23. The vaporizer is calibrated for flows from 0.2 to 10 liters/min. The output is almost linear at the 3%, 7%, and 12% dial settings with slightly lower outputs at flows less than 5 liters/min and slightly greater outputs at higher flows. At a dial setting of 18%, the output is higher than setting at flows less than 5 liters/min and less at higher flows. The vaporizer is designed to be used at ambient temperatures from 18° to 30°C.

Fluctuating back pressure does not affect its output significantly. Small decreases in

output occur when either air or nitrous oxide is the carrier gas, compared to when oxygen is the carrier gas. The effect is greatest (up to 20% of setting) at low flows when nitrous oxide is employed.

Hazards and Precautions

Vapor can leak into the fresh gas. This will be minimized if the vaporizer is turned off. The battery must be replaced annually.

When the electrical supply is applied to the vaporizer, each LED and all the LCD agent level indicator bars on the front display panel should flash and the auditory alarm should be activated for approximately 1 sec. If any of the LEDs or level indicator bars do not illuminate, or the audible alarm is not heard, the vaporizer should not be used.

When filling the vaporizer, the bottle must be gripped tightly when it is rotated downward from the upper position to the lower stop position. Otherwise the bottle may be dropped when it is released under pressure at the lower position.

High dial settings and low fresh gas flows can result in the delivery of hypoxic mixtures.

Maintenance

This vaporizer requires a full service every year at an authorized service center. The external surface may be wiped using a cloth slightly dampened with a cleaning agent. No other cleaning or disinfection should be attempted.

OHIO CALIBRATED VAPORIZER

Classification

Concentration calibrated, flow-over with wick, automatic thermocompensation, agent specific (halothane, enflurane, or isoflurane), plenum.

Construction

A schematic view of the Ohio calibrated vaporizer is shown in Figure 4.24. Fresh gases enter the vaporizer and pass through a

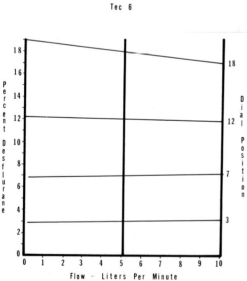

Figure 4.23. Performance of Tec 6 vaporizer, with oxygen as the carrier gas. From a graph furnished by Ohmeda, a division of BOC Health Care, Inc.

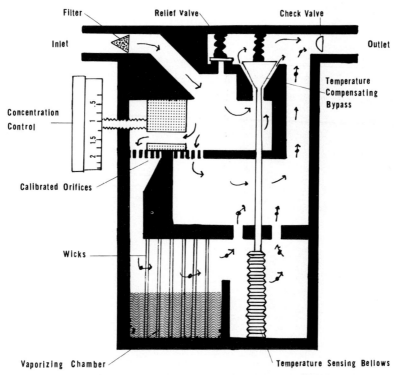

Figure 4.24. Schematic drawing of Ohio calibrated vaporizer. For the purpose of illustration the concentration control dial is shown at the left, although it is actually on top. Redrawn from a drawing furnished by Ohmeda, a division of the BOC Health Care, Inc.

filter. There are three possible paths for the gases to follow. The first is through the relief valve at the top, which opens when the pressure rises above a set amount.

Most of the gas flows past the temperature-compensating bypass to the outlet. The temperature of the gas leaving the vaporizing chamber is sensed by a bellows. When the vapor is warm, the bellows expands. This increases the size of the opening around the bypass so that more of the incoming gas goes directly to the outlet. When the vapor cools, the bellows contracts and partially closes the bypass. This forces a greater proportion of gas through the vaporizing chamber.

The remaining gas flows to the two sets of orifices. Flow through one set is directed to the vaporizer outlet. Flow through the other orifices is directed into the vaporizing chamber. Turning the concentration control dial simultaneously opens one set of orifices while closing the other set and so determines the ratio between gas flowing to the outlet and that going to the vaporizing chamber.

Gas entering the vaporizing chamber flows around a series of wicks where it becomes saturated with vapor. It then leaves the vaporizing chamber, flows around the temperature-sensing bellows and on to the outlet.

The vaporizer is shown in Figure 4.25. There are two sight windows: one with a *full* and one with an *empty* indication. The filling port can be either the funnel or keyed block type. The concentration dial is at the top. There are clicks at each increment on the dial. There is a locking button at the top rear that must be depressed before the dial can be turned on. On the enflurane vaporizer, the dial relocks at the 5% position, and the locking button must again be depressed to dial a concentration greater than 5%.

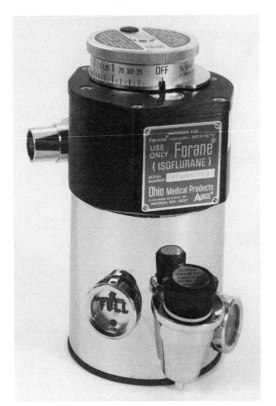

Figure 4.25. Ohio calibrated vaporizer. Courtesy of Ohmeda, a division of BOC Health Care, Inc.

Evaluation

Figure 4.26 shows the manufacturer's data for enflurane, halothane, and isoflurane. The vaporizers are accurate at fresh gas flows from 300 ml to 10 liters/min and between 16° and 32°C.

A study of the enflurane and halothane vaporizers at fresh gas flows from 100 to 5000 ml/min found they performed satisfactorily (20). There was a transient but significant increase in output when high flow was suddenly reduced. A transient reduction in output occurred when the flow was increased from low to high. Intermittent back pressures affected vaporizer output, but mean output was the same as with free flow to atmosphere. Use of the oxygen flush increased the output more than 10% at low fresh gas flows. Another evaluation showed these vaporizers to be reasonably accurate (48).

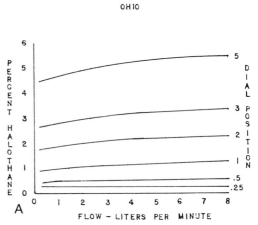

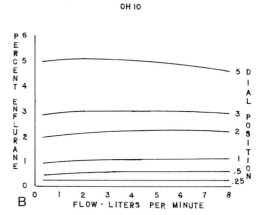

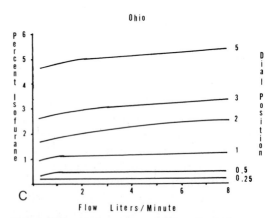

Figure 4.26. Performances of Ohio calibrated vaporizers. **A,** Halothane. **B,** Enflurane. **C,** Isoflurane. Redrawn courtesy of Ohmeda, a division of BOC Health Care, Inc.

The manufacturer's product literature indicates that the addition of nitrous oxide to the carrier gas will lower the output. Several authors (20,21,23,25,49,50) found this to be true at settings below 3%. At 3% and above, the addition of nitrous oxide may increase vapor output slightly (21,25).

Hazards

When the anesthesia machine is in use and the concentration knob is turned to off, a small amount of vapor can diffuse from the vaporizing chamber into the bypass circuit.

These vaporizers can be tilted up to 20° even while in use without effect. If not in use, they can be tilted up to 45° without effect. If tilted more than these amounts, liquid may enter the control head and a higher-than-expected concentration will be delivered, even after it has been restored to an upright position.

Discoloration of liquid enflurane and isoflurane was noted in early vaporizers of this type (51,52). This was traced to a reaction between the liquid and plastic wick spacers (53). No evidence of toxicity was found (54,55).

Maintenance

The company recommends that the vaporizer be sent to a service center once a year for calibrating, cleaning, checking for leaks, and replacing worn parts.

VAPOR 19.1

Classification

Concentration calibrated, flow over with wick, automatic thermocompensation, agent specific (halothane, enflurane, or isoflurane), plenum.

Construction

The Vapor 19.1 is shown in Figure 4.27. The *0* must be depressed before the concentration dial can be turned. A filling spout, sight glass, and drain are located at the bottom front of the vaporizer. The isoflurane

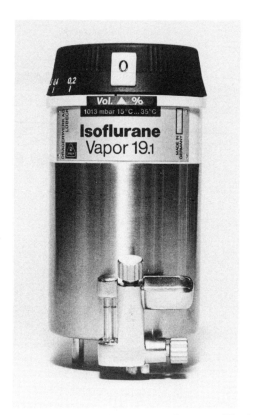

Figure 4.27. Vapor 19.1 vaporizer. Courtesy of North American Drager.

Vapor 19.1 has a concentration range from 0.2% to 5.0%; the enflurane, from 0.2% to 5% (or by special type up to 7%); and the halothane, from 0.2% to 5% (or 7% by special model).

The Vapor 19.1 is shown schematically in Figure 4.28. In the off position, the inlet and outlet of the vaporizing chamber are interconnected and vented to the outside. This prevents anesthetic agent from leaking into the fresh gases. Fresh gas passes directly through a bypass in the vaporizer.

In the on position, incoming gases are diverted past the bypass cone to the lower vaporizing section. Part of the fresh gas flows to the vaporizing chamber where it becomes saturated with agent while the balance is routed past the bypass cone where it mixes with gas from the vaporizing chamber and flows to the vaporizer output. Turning the

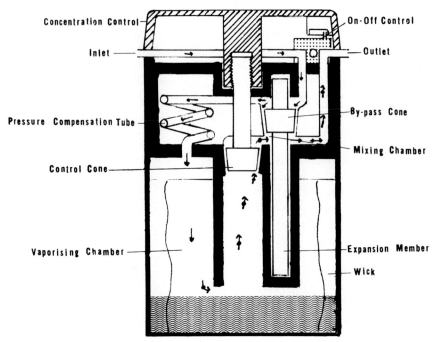

Figure 4.28. Vapor 19.1 vaporizer in the on position (see text for details). Redrawn from a drawing furnished by North American Drager.

concentration dial changes the position of the control cone at the vaporizing chamber outlet. A change in temperature changes gas flow to the vaporizing chamber by altering the position of the bypass cone.

Evaluation

The manufacturer's data for the three Vapor 19.1's are shown in Figure 4.29. Output is independent of fresh gas flow in the range of 0.3 to 15 liters/min with lower dial settings, but with high gas flows, total saturation of the gas flowing through the vaporizing chamber is not possible and output falls. An accuracy of ± 10% can be expected between 10° and 40°C. At temperatures outside this range, the vaporizer will be less accurate.

Investigations of Vapor 19.1 vaporizers for isoflurane, enflurane, and halothane with high and low flows have shown that they perform accurately (20,41,42).

The concentration delivered depends on the composition of the fresh gas. The Vapor

19.1 is calibrated using air as the carrier gas. When operated on 100% oxygen, the delivered concentration is 5% to 10% higher than the set concentration (20). When operated with 30% oxygen and 70% nitrous oxide, the concentration is 5% to 10% lower. Changing from 66% nitrous oxide in oxygen to 100% oxygen results in an increase in output followed by a decrease (26).

An investigation of the vaporizer at pressures up to 4 atmospheres showed a decrease in vaporizer output with increasing pressure, but the output remained within 20% of setting (11).

Hazards

If a Vapor 19.1 filled with agent is tilted, liquid agent may spill into the control device, irrespective of whether the vaporizer is turned on or off. This can result in either an increase or decrease in delivered concentration. If the vaporizer is tipped more than 45°, it should be flushed with a flow of 10 liters/min at a dial setting of 4% for at least 20 min.

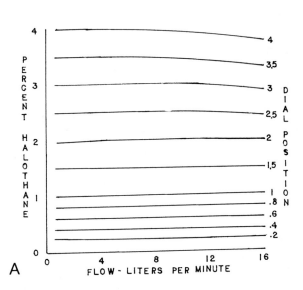

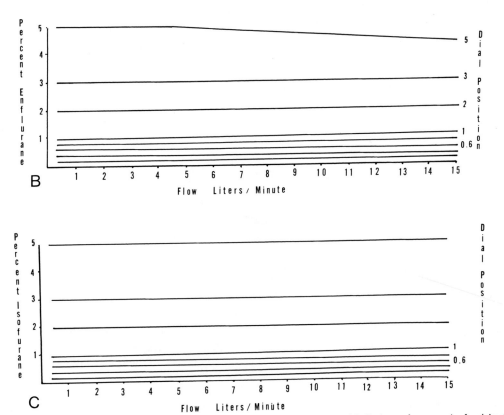

Figure 4.29. Output of Vapor 19.1 vaporizers at an ambient temperature of 22°C. Redrawn from graphs furnished by North American Drager.

Maintenance

The outer part of the vaporizer can be cleaned with a damp cloth soaked with a detergent. The manufacturer recommends that the halothane vaporizer be rinsed when the liquid in the site glass shows discoloration or dirt particles. This should be performed at least monthly. The discolored liquid is drained, the vaporizer filled with fresh halothane, then drained again.

Every 6 months the vaporizer should be inspected by trained personnel. The vaporizing chamber should be cleaned and the wicks changed every 2 years.

SIDE ARM VERNI-TROL

The side arm Verni-Trol vaporizer is no longer in production.

Classification

Measured flow, bubble through, thermocompensation by manual flow adjustment, multiple agent, plenum.

Construction

The side arm Verni-Trol is built into certain anesthesia machines. It has its own flowmeter assembly and an on-off valve.

A diagram of the complete vaporizer unit is shown in Figure 4.30. It has a thick-walled brass container for thermostability. Oxygen enters at the inlet and passes through a limiting valve that restricts flow to the vaporizer flowmeter. It functions to prevent the delivery of excessive unmetered quantities of oxygen and anesthetic vapor to the vaporizer outlet and to avoid damage to the vaporizer.

The oxygen next passes through the flowmeter assembly, enters the top of the vaporizer, passes through a filter and descends in a spiral-down tube to the bottom of the vaporizing chamber. It bubbles up through the liquid and leaves through the outlet tube.

At the base of the Verni-Trol, is an on-off valve that directs the flow of the gas with vapor either to the machine or to a vent to atmosphere. When the ring handle is pulled

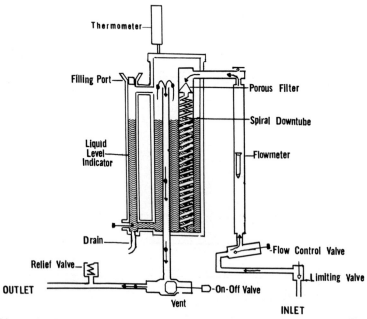

Figure 4.30. Older model side arm Verni-Trol vaporizer (see text for details). Redrawn courtesy of Ohmeda, a division of BOC Health Care, Inc.

toward the operator and turned in either direction, it is locked in the on position. On some machines with a back bar, this on-off valve is located to the right of the flowmeter assembly head and the ring is pulled down. Oxygen with vapor then passes a relief valve and flows to the machine where it is diluted by gases from other flowmeters. The relief valve limits the pressure in the flowmeter and vaporizer and prevents reverse flow of agent into the flowmeter tube or discharge of liquid anesthetic into the vaporizer outlet.

A glass tube at the left of the vaporizer indicates the liquid level. The filling port is at the top and there is a drain at the bottom. A thermometer is connected to the top.

Newer versions of this vaporizer (Figs. 4.31 and 4.32) have a knob that is pulled out and turned 90° to turn the vaporizer on. This is located upstream of the flowmeter assembly rather than downstream as in older models. Oxygen will not flow through the flowmeter unless the on-off valve is in the on position. On newer models, the filling port is at the side to prevent overfilling. Finally, on

newer models there is a check valve upstream of the relief valve to minimize loss of gases from the rest of the machine through the vaporizer, and to prevent intermittent back pressure from affecting vaporizer output or liquid anesthetic from entering the flowmeter tube.

Evaluation

Studies on the effects of back pressure on the older side arm Verni-Trol have shown that the output is increased by the pumping effect. The addition of the check valve should limit this, however.

Studies have shown that if the on-off valve is in the off position, there is no leakage of vapor into the fresh gas line (28). If the switch is in the on position but there is no flow through the vaporizer, trace concentrations can be detected in the machine outflow.

Hazards

Overfilling is possible in the older vaporizers with a top filling port. An accident resulting in overdose was reported in which liq-

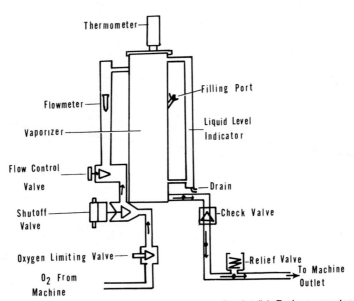

Figure 4.31. Newer model side arm Verni-Trol vaporizer (see text for details). Redrawn courtesy of Ohmeda, a division of BOC Health Care, Inc.

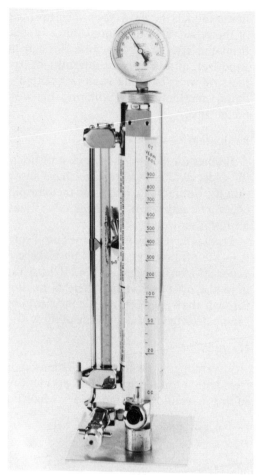

Figure 4.32. New version side arm Verni-Trol vaporizer. Note that the filling funnel is at the side rather than the top to prevent overfilling. Also the on-off valve at the base has been changed. Courtesy of Ohmeda, a division of BOC Health Care, Inc.

uid halothane was delivered as a result of a damaged flow control valve seat (56,57). Limiting valves are used to help prevent this problem.

There is a report of liquid anesthetic backing up into the flowmeter tube as a result of a loose cap at the top of the flowmeter (58). This did not present an immediate hazard to the patient. However, residue remaining in the tube could cause the indicator to stick and become inaccurate.

Errors in calculating output can be made.

Another common problem is forgetting to turn the on-off valve to the on position.

Maintenance

Service to this vaporizer is performed with routine machine maintenance and includes maintenance of the flowmeter and checks for leaks.

PENLON PPV SIGMA

Classification

Concentration calibrated, flow over with wick, automatic thermocompensation, agent specific (halothane, enflurane, or isoflurane), plenum.

Construction

The Penlon PPV vaporizer is shown in Figure 4.33. The top and the front bar on the

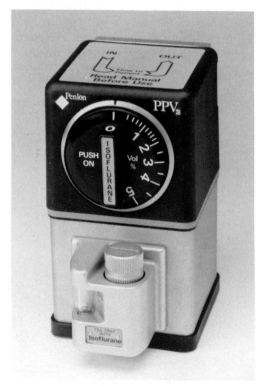

Figure 4.33. PPV Sigma vaporizer with screw cap filler and back entry connections. Courtesy of Penlon, Ltd.

concentration dial are color coded for the agent the vaporizer is designed for. A zero lock is part of the concentration control dial. To set a concentration, the dial assembly is pushed in and rotated counterclockwise. The dial is marked in intervals of 0.2% from 0% to 2% and intervals of 0.5% from 2% to 5%. The filling device can be either a screw cap or keyed filler type. The liquid level indicator has lines for minimum and maximum levels. The direction of gas flow through the vaporizer is shown on the top. The vaporizer can be fitted with cage-mount, 23-mm tapered adaptors for mounting to a back bar, a back entry mount, or a Selectatec mounting system.

The internal construction of the vaporizer is shown in Figure 4.34. Gas enters the vaporizer and is split into two streams, one passing through the bypass and the other through the vaporizing chamber. In the zero lock position, the bypass remains open, but the vaporizing chamber is completely shut off from gas flow. If the zero lock port is open, when the concentration control dial is pushed in, gas passes through a spiral tube into the vaporizing chamber that contains a stainless-steel wick. Gas saturated with vapor then exits the vaporizing chamber through the vapor control orifice. The size of this orifice is controlled by the setting of the concentration control dial. The gas saturated with vapor then joins the bypass gas and flows to the outlet.

Temperature compensation is provided by a liquid-filled expansion bellows operating a variable resistance valve in the bypass. Gas flowing through the bypass passes this variable resistance. As the vaporizing chamber cools, the orifice becomes smaller, so that a greater proportion of gas passes through the vaporizing chamber.

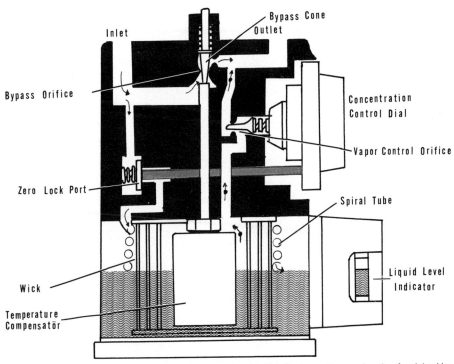

Figure 4.34. Diagram of PPV Sigma vaporizer (see text for details). Redrawn from a drawing furnished by Penlon, Ltd.

Evaluation

The performance characteristics supplied by the manufacturer are illustrated in Figure 4.35. The vaporizer is accurate at temperatures from 15° to 35°C (58° to 95°F). At higher temperatures vapor output is increased. If nitrous oxide is in the carrier stream, output will be increased slightly. Air or helium in the carrier stream causes the output to drop slightly. Intermittent back pressure may result in some increase in output.

Hazards

If the vaporizer is transported when filled, the control must be in the zero position and

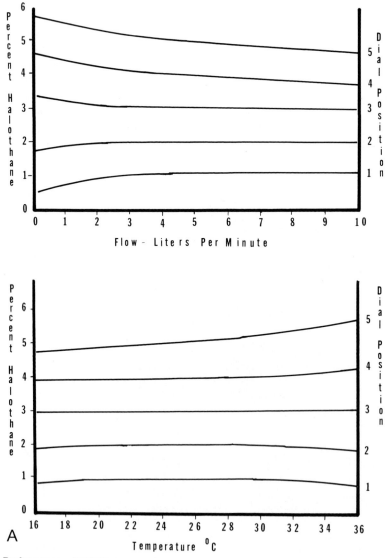

Figure 4.35. Performances of PPV Sigma vaporizers with oxygen as the carrier gas. Redrawn from graphs furnished by Penlon, Ltd.

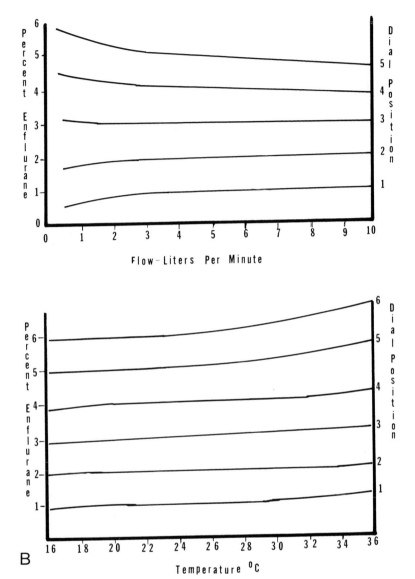

Figure 4.35—*continued.*

at least 2 min should elapse with the vaporizer in a secured upright position before use. If the vaporizer has been transported with the control in the open position, it must be flushed with gas at 4 liter/min for 2 min.

The concentration dial must be in the zero position during filling or draining and the vaporizer must be upright to avoid overfilling.

A vaporizer that has been overfilled should be withdrawn from use.

Maintenance

The vaporizer should be calibrated and tested for leaks every 3 to 6 months, with a major overhaul every 5 years. The exterior of the vaporizer should be kept clean with a dry cloth. No liquids, including water, should be

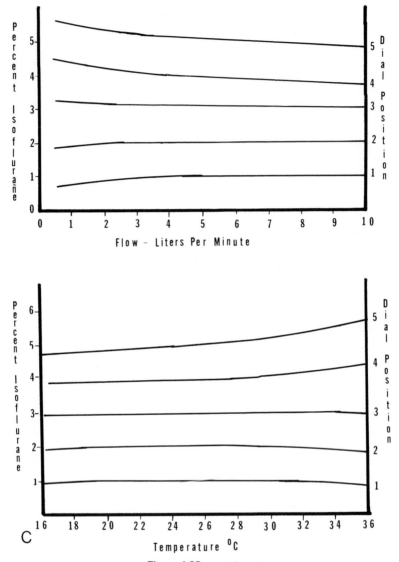

Figure 4.35—continued.

Agent-Specific Filling Systems

Agent-specific filling systems are also known as keyed filling systems, filler systems applied to the surface. The halothane vaporizer should be drained periodically and the liquid discarded to prevent buildup of thymol.

or devices, and pin safety systems. The ASTM machine standard (14) recommends, but does not require, that a vaporizer designed for a single agent be fitted with a permanently attached, agent-specific device to prevent accidental filling with the wrong agent. Such a device is available as an option on most modern vaporizers. Their use may result in less pollution of operating room air as spillage of liquid agent is reduced.

COMPONENTS

Bottle Collar

Each bottle of liquid anesthetic has a specially designed colored collar attached securely at the neck (Fig. 4.36). Each collar has two projections, one thicker than the other, which are designed to mate with corresponding indentations on bottle adaptor. The colors for the commonly used agents are red for halothane, orange for enflurane, and purple for isoflurane. These colors are also used on the bottle labels.

Bottle Adaptor

Bottle adaptors (also called adaptor tubes or assemblies, tube adaptors, and filler tubes) are shown in Figures 4.37 and 4.38. They are color coded. The adaptor shown in Figure 4.37 has at one end a bottle connector that has a screw thread to match the thread on the bottle and a skirt that extends beyond the screw threads and has slots that match the projections on the bottle collar. At the other end is the male adaptor that fits into the vaporizer filler receptacle. A short length of plastic tubing with two inner tubes connects the ends. The inner tube is for air and the concentric outer tube is for anesthetic fluid. The tubing allows the bottle to be held higher or lower than the vaporizer. Figure 4.38 shows a male adaptor (key, probe, tube

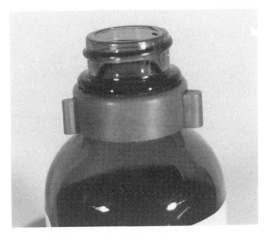

Figure 4.36. Bottle collar. The collar is color coded according to the bottle contents. It has two projections, one thicker than the other, which are designed to mate with corresponding indentations on the bottle adaptor.

block, filler plug, male adaptor). It consists of a rectangular piece of plastic with a groove on one side and two holes on another surface. The groove is designed to prevent the probe from being placed in an incorrect vaporizer. The larger hole is for the agent to enter or leave the vaporizer and the smaller hole is for air. There may be a ball valve to facilitate filling.

The bottle adaptor in Figure 4.39 is for use with vaporizers without an agent-specific filling system. The bottle connector is the same. The other end has a beveled tip.

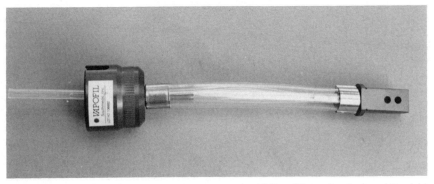

Figure 4.37. Bottle adaptor. The bottle connector is at left and the male adapter, at the right.

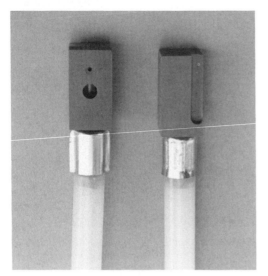

Figure 4.38. Male adaptor. The groove corresponds to a projection on the vaporizer filler receptacle. The larger hole is for anesthetic agent and the smaller hole, for air.

Filler Receptacle (59,60)

The vaporizer filler receptacle (filler socket or block, vaporizer filler unit, fill and drain system) must permit insertion of the intended agent-specific male adaptor only. There must be a means for tightening the male adaptor to form a seal when the adaptor is inserted. There must also be a means to seal the receptacle when the bottle adaptor is not inserted.

There may be a single port for both filling and draining or two ports (Figs. 4.40 and 4.41). A valve attached to a knob at the top controls the opening into the vaporizer. A ball valve in the air line occludes the air port after the vaporizer is filled. This prevents overfilling and flooding of the air line with liquid anesthetic.

USE

Filling

To fill a vaporizer, the cap from the appropriate bottle is removed and the bottle adaptor screwed to the collar until tight. If the connection is not tight, the vaporizer may be overfilled or a leak may occur. The vaporizer must be turned off before proceeding further. The plug, if present, is removed. The filler block is then inserted with the groove match-

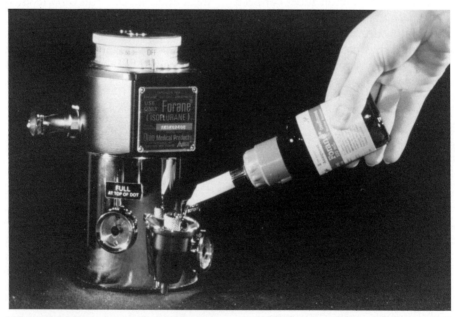

Figure 4.39. Bottle adaptor for vaporizers without agent-specific filling devices. It allows filling of a pour fill vaporizer without excessive spillage. Courtesy of Southmedic, Inc.

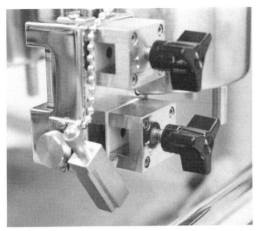

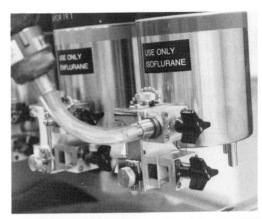

Figure 4.40. Dual-port vaporizer filler receptacle. Note the plug to prevent leaks, the drain valve at the bottom, and the two retaining screws at the right. If the plug is not reinserted and the screw tightened, the vaporizer will leak.

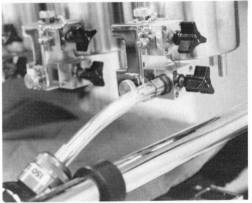

ing that on the vaporizer receptacle. During insertion, the tube should be bent slightly so that the bottle is below the level of the inlet. After the filler block is inserted, the retaining screw is tightened and the fill valve (vent) opened. The bottle is then held higher than the filler receptacle to drive the liquid through the outer concentric tube of the bottle adaptor into the vaporizer (see Fig. 4.41, *top*). The air inside the vaporizer, which is displaced by the liquid, moves through the inner tube and bubbles through the liquid in the bottle to the air space inside the bottle. Gentle up-and-down motion may help to clear air bubbles and facilitate filling.

For filling to be successful, the outer tube must contain liquid and the inner tube must remain filled with air. If the male adaptor is not placed securely in the filler receptacle or if there is a poor seal at the filler-vaporizer interface for other reasons, it is possible for the inner tube to become full of liquid. After the desired level of liquid in the vaporizer has been reached, the valve on the top is closed, the bottle lowered, and the retaining screw loosened. The bottle adaptor is removed, and

Figure 4.41. Keyed filling device with one front screw and top vent. **Top,** Filling the vaporizer. To fill, the plug is removed, the filler block inserted, and the retaining screw tightened. The vent is opened, and the bottle is tipped upward. **Bottom,** Draining the vaporizer. The filler block is inserted into the drain receptacle, the retaining screw is tightened, and the drain is opened. The bottle is held below the vaporizer.

the dummy plug reinserted and tightened in place.

Draining

To drain the vaporizer, the bottle adaptor is first attached to an appropriate bottle. In the dual port filler, the bottom socket is used. The filler plug is removed, the male adaptor inserted, and the retaining screw tightened. The bottle is held below the receptacle (see Fig. 4.41, *bottom*) and the drain valve (spool valve) opened. Fluid drains through the outer tube into the storage bottle and air moves upward from the bottle through the inner tube. After the vaporizer is drained, the drain valve is closed, the retaining screw loosened, and the bottle adaptor removed. The filler plug should be reinserted and the retaining screw tightened.

Storage

Usually the bottle adaptor is removed and replaced with a cap between fillings. If the bottle adaptor is not removed, leakage is minimal (61). This, however, may make storage difficult.

PROBLEMS WITH KEYED FILLING DEVICES

Difficulty in Filling

Causes of difficulty in filling include malalignment of the bottle adaptor in the filler receptacle, the adaptor not sealing at the bottle end, a leak in the bottle adaptor, and air bubbles (59).

Lost Bottle Adaptor

If the filler tube is lost, it is almost impossible to fill the vaporizer.

Vaporizer Tipping

The filler receptacle on some vaporizers extends below the base of the vaporizer and will prevent the vaporizer from being set upright on a flat surface, so it is necessary to set it at the edge of the surface with the block extending over the edge. This increases the possibility of the vaporizer being knocked to the floor. A useful addition is a ring fitted to the base of the vaporizer that extends the base below the projection of the filler block (see Fig. 4.11). This allows the vaporizer to be placed upright on a flat surface.

Failure of the Keyed System

This device should be regarded as a backup to the basic safety rule that labels should always be read before use. One case has been reported in which the bead on the filler receptacle on the vaporizer was too small to prevent incorrect filling (62). In an-

other case the bottle adaptor for one agent fit a bottle for another agent that did not have a collar (63). If the bottle collar for ethrane or halothane is upside down on the bottle, the bottle adaptor for the other agent will fit on it (64–67).

Poor Drainage

Causes of difficulty in draining the vaporizer include the bottle adaptor being wrongly positioned and the inner tube broken. Usually a new bottle adaptor will be needed to rectify these problems.

Liquid Leaks

Leakage of liquid can result from failure to tighten the retaining screw, failure to tighten the adaptor on the bottle, blockage of the fluid path inside the vaporizer, or a leakage in a valve (59). The filler block can leak from the overfill vent at the beginning or end of the filling cycle. If the fill or drain valve is not closed, liquid can leak (68). Frequent flexing of the tube on the bottle adaptor can result in a leak, usually at the male adaptor (59).

Incomplete Emptying of Bottle

With some filling devices, 0.9 to 6.3 ml of liquid agent may be left in the bottle after the vaporizer is filled (69).

Location

MEASURED-FLOW VAPORIZERS

All measured-flow vaporizers are part of the anesthesia machine, as described above.

CONCENTRATION-CALIBRATED VAPORIZERS

Between the Flowmeters and the Common Gas Outlet

The preferred location for concentration-calibrated vaporizers is between the flowmeters and the common gas outlet. On most machines, vaporizers are mounted to the right of the flowmeter tubes.

Between the Common Gas Outlet and Breathing System

Locating the vaporizer between the common gas outlet and the breathing system is not recommended for several reasons. It is difficult to secure such a vaporizer properly. This arrangement invites disconnections (70). Some machines have a relief valve in the machine, near the common gas outlet (see Chapter 3). This vents gas to atmosphere if a certain pressure is exceeded. If a vaporizer is inserted downstream of such a valve, the increased resistance to flow will cause an increase in pressure, especially with use of the oxygen flush. If the pressure exceeds the opening pressure of the relief valve, there will be a decrease in flow (71).

Another potential problem is reversed connection. Because the vaporizers have slip-on connections, it is possible to connect the vaporizer so that the flow of carrier gas is opposite to normal. In vaporizers studied this has resulted in an increase in output (72,73).

Another reason a vaporizer should not be placed in this location is because use of the oxygen flush may cause a high concentration to be delivered following the flush (74). Finally, such an installation allows more than one vaporizer to be turned on at a time.

IN-SYSTEM VAPORIZERS

Currently no vaporizers suitable for use in the breathing system on anesthesia machines are being manufactured in the United States. A number of vaporizers for use in remote locations that use air as the carrier gas are available in other parts of the world. Problems include resistance to flow and unpredictable output.

Arrangement of Vaporizers

If more than one vaporizer are present on an anesthesia machine, they may be mounted in parallel or in series.

PARALLEL

In a parallel arrangement, a selector valves direct gas from the flowmeters to one vaporizer while isolating all other vaporizers. Some selector valves have a bypass position in which all vaporizers are isolated (Fig. 4.42). In others, the flow is always directed to one vaporizer. A selector valve may be combined

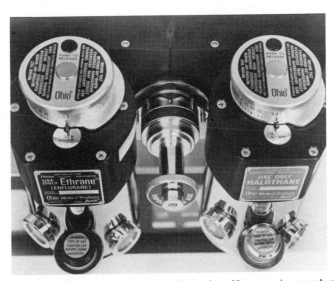

Figure 4.42.   Selector valve. This valve allows gas to be directed to either vaporizer or a bypass position in which both vaporizers are isolated. Courtesy of Ohmeda, a division of BOC Health Care, Inc.

with an interlock device so that only one vaporizer may be turned on at a time and/or a vaporizer can be turned on only if the selector valve is directing flow to it. Some selector valves block gas flow either to or from the vaporizers in the off position. Others control both the inlet and outlet of the vaporizers. With the first type, trace concentrations may diffuse into the fresh gas line.

Problems with these devices have been reported. In several cases, a defect in the device or improper seating of a vaporizer caused loss of most or all metered gases to atmosphere (75–80). In other cases, partial or complete obstruction to gas flow occurred (81,82). In one case, malfunction resulted in no output from the vaporizer, although metered gases continued to flow (83).

When a system designed to facilitate changing of vaporizers on the back bar is used, several checks should be made to ensure proper positioning after a vaporizer is mounted (78). These include sighting across the tops of the vaporizers to ensure that they are level and at the same height. An attempt should be made to lift each off the manifold without unlocking it. If the vaporizer can be removed, it is improperly positioned. Finally, the anesthesia machine must be checked for leaks as described in Chapter 18.

SERIES

In a series arrangement, gas from the flowmeters passes through more than one vaporizer. A hazard with this arrangement is that agent from the upstream vaporizer may be deposited in the downstream vaporizer if more than one vaporizer is turned on at the same time (85,86). This will result in changes in both the upstream and downstream agent concentrations. During subsequent use, the output of the downstream vaporizer will be contaminated with agent from the upstream vaporizer. For these reasons most modern machines with vaporizers in series have interlock devices that allow only one vaporizer to be turned on at a time (Figs. 4.43 and 4.44). Add-on devices are available (87).

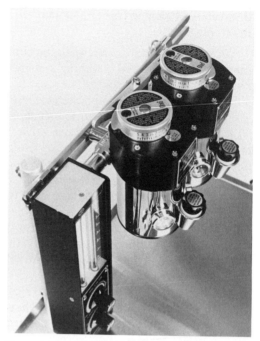

Figure 4.43.   Interlock device. Only one vaporizer may be turned on at a time. Courtesy of Ohmeda, a division of BOC Health Care, Inc.

Their use may require changes in the vaporizer as well as the machine. Failures of interlock devices have been reported (88–90). Diffusion of agent into the fresh gases is not prevented by an interlock device.

Hazards of Vaporizers

INCORRECT AGENT

A common hazard involves filling an agent-specific vaporizer with an agent other than the one for which it was designed (62,91,92). If an agent of low potency or low volatility is mistakenly placed in a vaporizer meant for an agent of higher potency or volatility, the effect will be a low concentration of anesthetic. Conversely, if an agent of high potency or volatility is accidentally used in a vaporizer intended for an agent or low potency or volatility, a dangerously high concentration may be delivered.

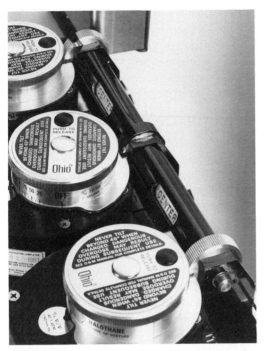

Figure 4.44. Interlock devices. The concentration dials on the left and right vaporizers cannot be turned on while the center one is in use. Courtesy of Ohmeda, a division of BOC Health Care, Inc.

The effects of a mixture of agents in a vaporizer depend on the potencies of each agent and the relative amounts in the mixture (93). If an ideal solution were formed, the vapor output would be proportional to the ratio of the number of moles of each agent in the solution. It is likely that enflurane and isoflurane do form an ideal solution. This is not the case with halothane and enflurane or isoflurane. Halothane facilitates vaporization of enflurane and isoflurane. In the process, it is itself somewhat more likely to vaporize. Thus a filling error involving both halothane and either isoflurane or enflurane will result in an increase in both agents.

Although halothane and isoflurane have similar vapor pressures, they cannot be used in agent-specific vaporizers without changing the concentration delivered. Use of isoflurane in a vaporizer intended for halothane will result in isoflurane concentrations as much as 25% to 50% more than expected (94,95). Using halothane in a vaporizer intended for isoflurane will result in delivery of a lower-than-expected concentration.

Placing similar vaporizers in a row on a machine may make filling a vaporizer with an incorrect agent more likely than when the vaporizers are different or not in proximity to each other (91).

In multiple-agent vaporizers, confusion can arise as to which agent is in the vaporizer. A vaporizer should always be clearly marked for the agent contained and should always be drained into a container labeled with the name of the drained agent and never into an unmarked container.

Some anesthetic agent monitors (see Chapter 17) will detect mixtures of agents (96). Smelling cannot be relied on to tell which agent is in a vaporizer, because the smell of a small amount of one agent can completely mask the odor of a less-pungent agent, even if the second agent is present in much higher concentration (97). Anesthesia personnel can detect the presence of a volatile agent but are not able to identify an agent by smell (98).

If a vaporizer is filled with the wrong agent, it must be completely drained and all liquid discarded. Gas should be allowed to flow through it until no agent can be detected in the outflow before the vaporizer is refilled. Draining cannot be relied on to completely empty a vaporizer (91).

TIPPING

As can be seen from the drawings and discussions of individual vaporizers, if a vaporizer is tipped sufficiently, liquid from the vaporizing chamber may get into the bypass or outlet. If this occurs, a high concentration of agent will be delivered when the vaporizer is again put into use.

Tipping can be prevented by mounting vaporizers securely and handling them with care when they are not mounted. Systems that allow easy removal of a vaporizer may be associated with tipping. Unless specifically designed to be transported with liquid in the vaporizing chamber, a vaporizer should be drained before being moved.

Should tipping occur, a high flow of gas should be run through the vaporizer with the concentration dial set at a low concentration until the output shows no excessive agent.

OVERFILLING

If a vaporizer is overfilled, liquid agent may enter the fresh gas line and lethal concentrations may possibly be delivered. This has been a problem mainly with vaporizers that are filled from the top. A clear sight glass may make the liquid level hard to see so that an overfilled vaporizer looks like an empty one. Most vaporizers now have the filling port on the side at the maximum safe level so that overfilling cannot occur. Liquid will pour over the edge of the funnel before the level inside the vaporizer rises to a dangerous level.

Agent-specific filling devices prevent overfilling by connecting the air intake in the bottle to the inside of the vaporizer chamber. Many users of keyed filling devices have found that by slightly unscrewing the bottle adaptor from the bottle during the filling process, air from atmosphere can enter the bottle and the speed of filling is increased. Turning the concentration dial of the vaporizer on during filling will accomplish the same end. Such practices should not be performed because they can override the safety features in the filler system that prevent overfilling.

REVERSED FLOW

Although the machine standard (14) requires that the vaporizer inlet be male and the outlet female, the direction of gas flow be marked, and the inlet and outlet parts be labeled, it is easy to connect the fresh gas delivery line of the anesthesia machine to the outlet side of the vaporizer and the delivery tube to the breathing system to the inlet side of the vaporizer (99). This is easily overlooked. Reversed flow through a vaporizer has been re-

ported after repairs to the selector valve resulted in a plumbing misconnection (100).

Investigations of Tec 3 vaporizers have found that reversed flow resulted in approximately double the concentration indicated on the concentration dial (72,100).

CONCENTRATION DIAL IN WRONG POSITION

It is not unusual that previous use of a vaporizer by a colleague or servicing by a technician results in a vaporizer concentration dial being left on (101–104). For this reason, checking vaporizer control dials as well as contents should be part of the preuse checking procedure.

The concentration dial may be changed during a case without the operator's knowledge, especially if the vaporizer has the concentration dial at the top. Operating room personnel moving a machine or simply passing by may grab the dial and change the setting.

LEAKS

With a leak in a vaporizer, the machine will function normally until the vaporizer is turned on. At that point, fresh gas flow from the machine will be reduced and may contain little or no vapor. In addition to affecting fresh gas composition and flow, leaks cause pollution of operating room air.

The consequences of a leak in a measured-flow vaporizer will depend on the size of the leak, its location, and whether or not there is a check valve at the vaporizer outlet. Most measured-flow vaporizers and some direct-reading vaporizers have such check valves. These will decrease the loss of gas caused by a leak inside a vaporizer. Anesthetic vapor delivery will still be less than expected.

A common cause of a leak is failure to replace the filler cap or to tighten it adequately. This is usually detected by spillage of liquid anesthetic from the vaporizer when it is turned on (105,106), but if the level is low, liquid may not be splattered (107,108). If the fill valve on a keyed filling system is not closed or if the plug is not replaced and tightened in place, a leak will occur (see Fig. 4.40).

Other locations for leaks include the on-off valve of a measured-flow vaporizer (109), a selector valve (110,111), the mounting mechanism (77,112), an interlock device (113), outlet connection (114), and various parts of direct-reading vaporizers (38). The fitting between a vaporizer and its inlet or outlet connection may become loose or broken (70, 115–117).

A leak should be suspected if a vaporizer appears to require filling with unusual frequency or when the odor of an agent can be detected. Splattering of liquid from the filling port may be observed if the cap is not tight. This may not be seen if a keyed filling device is in place and the filling screw is loose. Personnel responsible for filling vaporizers should be instructed always to close filler caps (or screws) tightly. These should be checked for tightness when the machine is checked before use or the liquid level is low.

A leak in a vaporizer can be detected when the anesthesia machine is tested before use, if each vaporizer is turned on (see Chapter 18). With measured-flow vaporizers it is necessary to turn the vaporizer on-off valve to the on position.

VAPOR LEAK INTO THE FRESH GAS LINE

Some direct-reading vaporizers leak small amounts of vapor into the bypass when turned off (28,29,118). One case was reported in which a vaporizer returned from service delivered 1.5% isoflurane when the dial was in the off position (30). With measured-flow vaporizers no leaks were found if the on-off valve was in the off position. If it was turned to the on position, vapor could be detected in the machine outflow, even with no flow through the vaporizer. The amount of vapor leak was increased by intermittent back pressure (119).

Interlock devices will not prevent this problem if the vaporizers are connected in series. A selector valve will not prevent it if there is still a diffusion pathway via the selector valve (29).

When a machine is not in use, anesthetic vapor will accumulate in the bypass of a vaporizer, so that when the fresh gas is initially turned on, a bolus of vapor will be swept out. This also occurs when the on-off valve of a measured-flow vaporizer is left in the on position. After the initial bolus is swept out, a very small amount of vapor will continuously enter the outlet circuit.

The extent of such contamination depends on the ambient temperature (and hence the vapor pressure of the liquid) as well as the size and configuration of the internal ports. Although the amounts delivered are usually too small to produce a clinical effect, a small leak might cause a "sensitized" individual to react to a halogenated agent or trigger an episode of malignant hyperthermia (120).

These leaks can be reduced by not turning a vaporizer from the off to 0 setting unless it is to be used. With measured-flow vaporizers, it is important to leave the on-off valve in the off position when the vaporizer is not in use.

Another possible source of vapor leaking into the fresh gas line is vaporizer malfunction. Cases have been reported in which a malfunction prevented a vaporizer from being turned off (121,122). Cases have been reported in which it was possible to turn the concentration dial past the off position (32,35). In this position, the vaporizer delivered concentrations of vapor high enough to produce clinical effects.

A large vapor leak can be detected by breathing through the breathing system after a small amount of fresh gas from the machine has flowed through it (see Chapter 18).

CONTAMINANTS IN THE VAPORIZING CHAMBER

Tap water or a detergent solution in a vaporizer can cause corrosion and result in excessive carrier gas passing through the vaporizing chamber, causing a greater-than-expected output (123,124).

The output of a halothane vaporizer is progressively reduced as the concentration of thymol increases (125,126). A 5% reduction in output requires a 650% increase in thymol concentration.

PHYSICAL DAMAGE

Shock or excessive vibration may lead to malfunction (127). Damage to vaporizers mounted on a machine is significantly less than with those that are disconnected (128). A sufficient number of vaporizers should be purchased so that they do not need to be moved around. If a vaporizer must be removed, care should be taken to protect it from physical damage.

OBSTRUCTION TO FRESH GAS FLOW

Problems with selector valves have led to obstruction of all or some fresh gas flow from the machine (75,76,81,82).

INCORRECT CALCULATIONS

With measured-flow vaporizers, calculations are necessary to achieve the desired delivered concentration. Errors resulting in overdosage and underdosage may be made.

Servicing

Vaporizers are precise instruments and require regular, skillful maintenance if they are to remain reliable and precise. Periodic draining and discarding of residual liquid may be advisable. Servicing should be carried out by the manufacturer or its certified service agent (129). Manufacturers occasionally make changes in the vaporizer at the time of service (130).

If an agent analyzer is in routine use, some manufacturers will lengthen the time between service and recalibration for certain vaporizers.

Because the number of facilities servicing vaporizers is limited, most vaporizers must be sent long distances. It is helpful to have at least one extra agent-specific vaporizer for each agent used so that servicing will result in a minimum of inconvenience. Some companies provide the loan of a vaporizer during servicing.

REFERENCES

1. White CD. Vaporization and vaporizers. Br J Anaesth 1985;57:658–671.
2. Macintosh R, Mushin WW, Epstein HG. Physics for the anaesthetist. Oxford, UK: Blackwell Scientific, 1963.
3. Eisenkraft JB: Vaporizers and vaporization of volatile anesthetics. Prog Anesth 1988;2:1–16.
4. Blackwood O, Kelly W: General physics. New York: Wiley, 1955.
5. Jones MJ: Breathing systems and vaporizers. In: Nimmo WS, Smith G, eds. Anaesthesia. Oxford, UK: Blackwell Scientific, 1989.
6. Leigh JM: Variations on a theme:splitting ratio. Anaesthesia 1985;40:70–72.
7. Schreiber P. Effects of barometric pressure on anesthesia equipment. Audio Digest 1975;17(14).
8. Schreiber P. Anesthesia equipment. Performance, classification, and safety. New York: Springer-Verlag, 1972.
9. James MFM, White JF. Anesthetic considerations at moderate altitude. Anesth Analg 1984;63:1097–1105.
10. Speer DL. Vaporization of anesthetic agents at high altitude. In: Aldrete JA, Lowe HJ, Virtue RW, eds. Low flow and closed system anesthesia. New York: Grune & Stratton, 1979:235–250.
11. Satterfield JM, Russell GB, Graybeal JM, Richard RB. Anesthetic vaporizers accurately deliver isoflurane in hyperbaric conditions. Anesthesiology 1989;71:A360.
12. Hill DW, Lowe HJ. Comparison of concentration of halothane in closed and semiclosed circuits during controlled ventilation. Anesthesiology 1962; 23:291–298.
13. Keet JE, Valentine GW, Riccio JS. An arrangement to prevent pressure effect on the Verni-Trol vaporizer. Anesthesiology 1963;24:734–737.
14. American Society for Testing and Materials. Standard specification for minimum performance and safety requirements for components and systems of anesthesia gas machines (ASTM F1161-88). Philadelphia: ASTM, 1988.
15. Cole JR. The use of ventilators and vaporizer performance. Br J Anaesth 1966;38:646–651.
16. Heneghan CPH. Vaporizer output and gas driven ventilators. Br J Anaesth 1986;58:932.

17. Slinger PD, Scott WAC, Kliffer AP. Intraoperative awareness due to malfunction of a Siemens 900B ventilator. Can J Anaesth 1990;37:258–261.
18. Paterson GM, Hulands GH, Nunn JF. Evaluation of a new halothane vaporizer: the Cyprane Fluotec Mark 3. Br J Anaesth 1969;41:109–119.
19. Noble WH. Accuracy of halothane vaporizers in clinical use. Can Anaesth Soc J 1970;17:135–143.
20. Lin C. Assessment of vaporizer performance in low-flow and closed-circuit anesthesia. Anesth Analg 1980;59:359–366.
21. Prins L, Strupat J, Clement J, Knill RL. An evaluation of gas density dependence of anaesthetic vaporizers. Can Anaesth Soc J 1980;27:106–110.
22. Steffey EP, Woliner M, Howland D. Evaluation of an isoflurane vaporizer: the Cyprane Fortec. Anesth Analg 1982;61:457–464.
23. Lin C. Enflurane vaporizer accuracy with nitrous oxide mixtures. Anesth Analg 1979;58:440–441.
24. Palayiwa E, Sanderson MH, Hahn CEW. Effects of carrier gas composition on the output of six anaesthetic vaporizers. Br J Anaesth 1983;55:1025–1038.
25. Stoelting RK, Nawaf K. Enflurane vaporizer accuracy with nitrous oxide mixtures. Anesth Analg 1979;58:441.
26. Synnott A, Wren WS. Effect of nitrous oxide on the output of three halothane vaporizers. Br J Anaesth 1986;58:1055–1058.
27. Latto IP. Administration of halothane in the 0–0.5% concentration range with the Fluotec Mark 2 and Mark 3 vaporizers. Br J Anaesth 1973;45:563–569.
28. Cook TL, Eger EI, Behl RS. Is your vaporizer off? Anesth Analg 1977;56:793–800.
29. Robinson JS, Thompson JM, Barratt RS. Inadvertent contamination of anaesthetic circuits with halothane. Br J Anaesth 1977;49:745–753.
30. Gill RS, Lack JA. Vaporizers—serviced and checked? Anaesthesia 1991;46:695–696.
31. Bridges RT. Vaporizers—serviced and checked? A reply. Anaesthesia 1991;46:696–697.
32. Davies JR. Enfluratec vaporizer. Br J Anaesth 1980;52:356–357.
33. Davies JR. Broken control on a selectatec vaporizer. Anaesthesia 1987;42:215.
34. Bar ZG. Inadvertent administration of halothane with the Fluotec Mk. 3 vaporizer. Anaesth Intensive Care 1984;12:378.
35. Miller JM, Cascorbi HF. Yet another vaporizer hazard. Anesth Analg 1980;59:805.
36. Novack GD, Ursillo RC. Malfunctioning halothane vaporizer. Anesth Analg 1981;60:121.
37. Smith B. Broken control on Selectatec vaporizer. A reply. Anaesthesia 1987;42:215.
38. Rosenberg M, Solod E, Bourke DL. Gas leak through a Fluotec Mark III vaporizer. Anesth Analg 1979;58:239–240.
39. Scott DM. Performance of BOC Ohmeda Tec 3 and Tec 4 vaporisers following tipping. Anaesth Intensive Care 1991;19:441–443.
40. Yemen TA, Nelson WW. Are vaporizers in motion safe? Anesth Analg 1992;74:S364.
41. Fitzal S, Gilly H, Steinbereithner K. Do modern plenum vaporizers provide accurate anesthetic mixtures irrespective of gas flow? Anesthesiology 1986;65:A168.
42. Gilly H, Fitzal S, Steinbereithner K. Low flow accuracy of vaporizers: a laboratory comparison between TEC and VAPOR systems. Eur J Anaesthesiol 1987;4:73–74.
43. Rao CC, Krishna G, Baldwin S, Robbeloth R. Ohmeda (R) Fluotec-4 vaporizer output near MRI magnet. Anesthesiology 1990;73:A476.
44. Carter JA, McAtteer P. A serious hazard associated with the Floutec mark 4 vaporizer. Anaesthesia 1984;35:1257–1258.
45. Gibson TJ. A serious hazard associated with the Fluotec mark 4 vaporizer. A reply. Anaesthesia 1984;35:1258.
46. Goldman DB, Mushlin PS. Leakage of anesthetic agent from an Ohmeda Tech IV vaporizer. Anesth Analg 1991;72:567.
47. Carter KB, Gray WM, Railton R, Richardson W. Long-term performance of Tec vaporizers. Anaesthesia 1988;43:1042–1046.
48. Anonymous. Anesthesia units. Health Devices 1980;10:31–51.
49. Gould DB, Lampert BA, MacKrell TN. Effect of nitrous oxide solubility on vaporizer aberrance. Anesth Analg 1982;61:938–940.
50. Knill R, Prins L, Strupat J, Clement J. Nitrous oxide and vaporizer outputs: transient or continuous effect? Anesth Analg 1980;59:808–809.
51. Gandolfi AJ, Blitt CD, Weldon S. Discoloration and impurities in isoflurane vaporizer. Anesth Analg 1983;62:366.
52. Wald A. Discoloration of enflurane. Anesth Analg 1981;60:843.
53. Gandolfi AJ, Weldon ST, Blitt CD. Production and characterization of impurities in isoflurane vaporizers. Anesthesiology 1983;59:A159.
54. Blitt CD, Weldon ST, Willians-Van Alstyne SI, Gandolfi AJ. Survey of impurities in isoflurane and enflurane vaporizers. Anesth Analg 1984;63:189.
55. Weldon ST, Williams-Van Alstyne SI, Gandolfi AJ, Blitt CD. Production and characterization of impurities in isoflurane vaporizers. Anesth Analg 1985;64:634–639.
56. Kopriva CJ, Lowenstein E. An anesthetic accident: cardiovascular collapse from liquid halothane delivery. Anesthesiology 1969;30:246–247.
57. Sharrock NE, Gabel RA. Inadvertent anesthetic overdose obscured by scavenging. Anesthesiology 1978;49:138.

58. Gabel RA, Danielsen JB. Backflow of liquid halothane into a flowmeter. Anesthesiology 1971; 34:492–493.

59. Richardson W, Carter KB. Evaluation of keyed fillers on TEC vaporizers. Br J Anaesth 1986; 58:353–356.

60. O'Carroll TM, Greenbaum R, Thornton PGN. Agent-specific filling devices. Anaesthesia 1980;35:807–810.

61. Davies JM, Strunin L, Craig DB. Leakage of volatile anaesthetics from agent-specific vapourizer filling devices. Can Anaesth Soc J 1982;29:473–476.

62. McBurney R. Letter to the editor. Can Anaesth Soc 1977;24:417–418.

63. Klein SL, Camenzind T. Hazards of bottle adaptors for vaporizers. Anesth Analg 1978;57:596–597.

64. Dickson JJ. Enflurane key filling system. Anaesth Intensive Care 1985;13:331.

65. George TH. Failure of keyed agent-specific filling devices. Anesthesiology 1984;61:228–229.

66. Mar J. A dangerous error in fluothane packaging. Can Med Assoc J 1980;122:990.

67. Riegle EV, Desertspring D. Failure of the agent-specific filling device. Anesthesiology 1990;73:353.

68. Urmey WF. Elliott W, Raemer DB. Vaporizer fill system leak. Anesth Analg 1988;67:711.

69. Wittmann PH, Wittmann FW, Connor T, Connor J. The "nonempty" empty bottle. Anaesthesia 1992;47:721–722.

70. Capan L, Ramanathan S, Chalon J, O'Meara JB, Turndorf H. A possible hazard with use of the Ohio ethrane vaporizer. Anesth Analg 1980;59:65–68.

71. Kataria B, Price P, Slack M. Delayed filling of the breathing bag due to a portable vaporizer. Anesth Analg 1987;66:1055.

72. Marks WE, Bullard JR. Another hazard of free-standing vaporizers, increased anesthetic concentration with reversed flow of vaporizing gas. Anesthesiology 1976;45:445–446.

73. Rosewarne FA, Duncan IN. Reversed connexions of free-standing vaporizers. Anaesthesia 1990; 45:338–339.

74. Kelly DA. Free-standing vaporizers. Another hazard. Anaesthesia 1985;40:661–663.

75. Childres WF. Malfunction of Ohio Modulus anesthesia machine. Anesthesiology 1982;56:330.

76. Jove F, Milliken RA. Loss of anesthetic gases due to defective safety equipment. Anesth Analg 1983;62:369–370.

77. Jablonski J. Reynolds AC: A potential cause (and cure) of a major gas leak. Anesthesiology 1985;62:842.

78. Riddle RT. A potential cause (and cure) of a major gas leak. A reply. Anaesthsiology 1985;62:842–843.

79. Wraight WJ. Another failure of Selectatec block. Anaesthesia 1990;45:795.

80. Pyles ST, Kaplan RF, Munson E. Gas loss from Ohio Modulus vaporizer selector-interlock valve. Anesth Analg 1983;62:1052.

81. Riendl J. Hypoxic gas mixture delivery due to malfunctioning inlet port of a select-a-tec vaporizer manifold. Can J Anaesth 1987;34:43.

82. Hogan TS. Selectatec switch malfunction. Anaesthesia 1985;40:66–69.

83. Duncan JAT. Selectatec switch malfunction. Anaesthesia 1985;40:911–912.

84. Murphy AS. Selectatec malfunction a reply. Anesthesia 1985;40:912.

85. Dorsch SE, Dorsch JA. Chemical cross-contamination between vaporizers in series. Anesth Analg 1973;52:176–180.

86. Murray WJ, Zsigmond EK, Fleming P. Contamination of in-series vaporizers with halothane-methoxyflurane. Anesthesiology 1973;38:487–489.

87. Browne RA, McDonald S. A vapourizer interlocking system. Can Anaesth Soc J 1983;30:653–654.

88. Anonymous. Improper setting of anesthesia vaporizer interlock system leads to safety alert. Biomed Safe Stand 1990;20:91.

89. Silvasi DL, Haynes A, Brown ACD. Potentially lethal failure of the vapor exclusion system. Anesthesiology 1989;71:289–291.

90. Anonymous. Anesthesia unit vaporizers. Technol Anesth 1989;9:4.

91. Karis JH, Menzel DB. Inadvertent change of volatile anesthetics in anesthesia machines. Anesth Analg 1992;61:53–55.

92. Martin ST. Hazards of agent-specific vaporizers: a case report of successful resuscitation after massive isoflurane overdose. Anesthesiology 201992;62:830–83.

93. Bruce DL, Linde HW. Vaporization of mixed anesthetic liquids. Anesthesiology 1984;42:342–346.

94. Deriaz H, Baras E, Duranteau R, Benmosbah L, Lienhart A. Can isoflurane be administered with an halothane vaporizer? Anesthesiology 1989;71:A362.

95. Shih A, Wu W. Potential hazard in using halothane-specific vaporizers for isoflurane and vice versa. Anesthesiology 1981;55:A115.

96. Munshi C, Dhamee S, Bardeen-Henschel A, Dhruva S. Recognition of mixed anesthetic agents by mass spectrometer during anesthesia. J Clin Monit 1986;2:121–124.

97. Paull JD, Sleeman KW. An anaesthetic hazard. Br J Anaesth 1971;3:1202.

98. Roberts SL, Forbes RB, Moyers JR, Tinker JH. Can olfaction identify and quantify volatile anesthetics? Anesthesiology 1985;63:A193.

99. Anonymous. Death from misconnected vaporizer leads to $750,000 settlement. Biomed Saf Stand 1992;22:78.

100. Railton R, Inglis MD. High halothane concentrations from reversed flow in a vaporizer. Anaesthesia 1986;41:672–673.
101. Austin TR. A warning device for the "Fluotec" Mark II and III. Anaesthesia 1971;26:368.
102. Coleshill GG. Safe vaporizers. Can J Anaesth 1988;35:667–668.
103. Petty C. Equipment safety: Vaporizer exclusion or interlock systems. APSF Newslett 1992;7:10.
104. Williams L, Barton C, McVey JR, Smith JD: A visual warning device for improved safety. Anesth Analg 1986;65:1364.
105. Rajah A, Zideman DA. A problem with the TEC 5 vaporizer. Anaesthesia 1992;47:271–272.
106. Bridges R. A problem with a TEC 5 vaporizer. A reply. Anaesthesia 1992;47:272.
107. Cooper PD. A hazard with a vaporizer. Anaesthesia 1984;39:935.
108. Mullin RA. Letter to the editor. Can Anaesth Soc J 1978;25:248–249.
109. Eldrup-Jorgensen S, Sprissler GT. Gas leaks in anesthesia machines. Anesthesiology 1977;46:439.
110. Anonymous. Ohmeda targets June 1 to complete FDA class II recall of vaporizer selector valves. Biomed Saf Stand 1985;15:50–51.
111. Loughnan TE. Gas leak associated with a Selectatec. Anaesth Intensive Care 1988;16:501.
112. Anonymous. Anesthesia unit vaporizers. Technol Anesth 1991;12:6–7.
113. Hartle AJ, Daum REO. Failure of Ohmeda Tec 4 safety interlock. Anaesthesia 1992;47:171.
114. Van Besouw JP, Thurlow AC. A hazard of free-standing vaporizers. Anaesthesia 1987;42:671.
115. Anonymous. Anesthesia unit vaporizers. Technol Anesth 1991;12:7.
116. Forrest T, Childs D. An unusual vaporiser leak. Anaesthesia 1992;37:1220–1221.
117. Marsh RHK, Thomas NF. A hazard of the Penlon off-line vaporizer mounting system. Anaesthesia 1986;41:438.
118. Ritchie PA, Cheshire MA, Pearce NH. Decontamination of halothane from anaesthetic machines achieved by continuous flushing with oxygen. Br J Anaesth 1988;60:859–863.
119. Greenhow DE, Barth RL. Oxygen flushing delivers anesthetic vapor—a hazard with a new machine. Anesthesiology 1973;38:409–410.
120. Varma RR, Whitsell RC, Iskandarani MM. Halothane hepatitis without halothane: role of inapparent circuit contamination and its prevention. Hepatology 1985;5:1159–1162.
121. Bahl CP. A cause of inaccuracy in vaporizer delivery. Anaesthesia 1977;32:1037.
122. Lewis JJ, Hicks RG. Malfunction of vaporizers. Anesthesiology 1966;27:324–325.
123. Anonymous. Water in halothane vaporizers. Technol Anesth 1985;5:2–3.
124. Anonymous. Vaporizer, anesthesia, nonheated. Biomed Saf Stand 1986;16:18.
125. Gray WM. Dependence of the output of a halothane vaporizer on thymol concentration. Anaesthesia 1988;43:1047–1049.
126. Rosenberg PH, Alila A. Accumulation of thymol in halothane vaporizers. Anaesthesia 1984;38:581–583.
127. Anonymous. FDA class I recall of pre-1980 Ohmeda vaporizers "overhalf done": involves testing, possible component replacement. Biomed Saf Stand 1985;15:50.
128. Anonymous. Concentration calibrated vaporizers. Technol Anesth 1987;7:2.
129. Smith B. Equipment malfunction: a possible hazard. A reply. Anaesthesia 1986;41:1271.
130. Carter RW. Enfluratec vaporizer. Br J Anaesth 1980;52:356–357.

Chapter 5

The Breathing System: General Principles, Common Components, and Classifications

General Principles	Sleeves	**Size and Type of Fittings**
Resistance	Connectors and Adaptors	**Classification of Breathing Systems**
Rebreathing	Reservoir Bag	Classification by Function
Discrepancy between Inspired and	Breathing Tubes	Classification by Equipment
Delivered Volumes	Adjustable Pressure Limiting (APL)	
Discrepancy between Inspired and	Valve	
Delivered Concentrations	Positive End Expiratory Pressure	
Common Components	(PEEP) Valves	
Bushings (Mounts)	Filters	

The breathing system (breathing or patient circuit, respiratory circuit or system) is a gas pathway in direct connection with the patient, through which gas flows occur at respiratory pressures, in which directional valves may be present, and into which a gas mixture of controlled composition may be dispensed (1). The function of the breathing system is to convey oxygen and anesthetic gases to the patient and remove waste and anesthetic gases from the patient. In practice, a breathing system is usually regarded as extending from the point of fresh gas inlet to the point at which gas escapes to atmosphere or a scavenging system. Scavenging equipment is not considered part of the breathing system.

General Principles

RESISTANCE

Physics

When gas passes through a tube, the pressure at the outlet will be lower than that at the

inlet. The pressure drop is a measure of the resistance that must be overcome when gas is forced or drawn through the tube. Resistance varies with the volume of gas passing through per unit of time. Therefore, flow rate must be stated when a specific resistance is mentioned.

The nature of the gas flow is important in determining resistance. There are two types of flow: laminar and turbulent. In clinical practice, flow is usually a mixture of the two.

Laminar Flow

Figure 5.1*A* shows a laminar flow of gas through a tube. The flow is smooth and orderly and particles of fluid move parallel to the walls of the tube. Flow is fastest in the center of the tube where there is less friction.

When flow is laminar, the Hagen-Poiseuille law applies. This law states that

$$\Delta P = (L \times v \times V)/r^4$$

where r is the radius of the tube, P is the pressure gradient across the tube, v is the viscosity of the gas, and V is the flow rate. Resist-

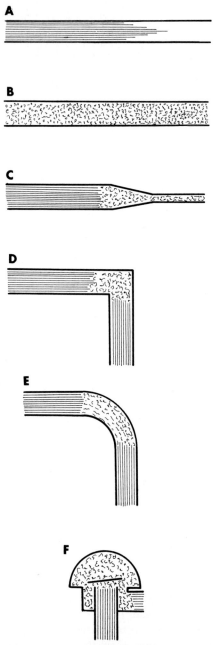

Figure 5.1. Laminar and turbulent flow. **A,** Laminar flow; the lines of flow are parallel and flow is slower near the sides of the tube, because of friction. **B,** Generalized turbulent flow, which occurs when the critical flow rate is exceeded. Eddies move across or opposite the general direction of flow. **C–F,** Localized turbulence, which occurs when there is change in direction or the gas passes through a constriction.

ance is directly proportional to flow rate with laminar flow.

Turbulent Flow

Figure 5.1*B* shows a turbulent flow of gas through a tube. The lines of flow are no longer parallel. Eddies, composed of fluid particles moving across or opposite the general direction of flow, are present. The flow rate is the same across the diameter of the tube.

For turbulent flow, the factors responsible for the pressure drop along the tube include those described for laminar flow, but also include gas density, which becomes more important than viscosity.

$$\Delta P = (L \times V^2 \times K)/r^5$$

where K is a constant, including such factors as gravity, friction, and gas density and viscosity. Resistance is proportional to the *square* of the flow rate with turbulent flow.

Turbulent flow can be generalized or localized.

Generalized Turbulent Flow. When the flow of gas through a tube exceeds a certain value, called the critical flow rate, generalized turbulent flow results.

Localized Turbulent Flow. As seen in Figure 5.1*C–F,* when gas flow is below the critical flow rate but encounters constrictions, curves, valves or other irregularities, an area of localized turbulence results. The increase in resistance will depend on the type and number of obstructions encountered.

Minimal apparatus resistance, therefore, dictates that gas-conducting pathways be of minimal length, maximal internal diameter, and without sharp bends or sudden variations in diameter.

Significance of Resistance

High resistance will place a burden on the spontaneously breathing patient. Changes in resistance tend to parallel changes in the work of breathing, which may be a more relevant parameter to study (2). Studies show that the tracheal tube is usually the source of more resistance and is a more important factor in determining the work of breathing than the breathing system (3). There is lack of agreement about what level of resistance is excessive (4,5). Anesthesia personnel should be aware of how much resistance components of breathing systems offer and to employ, wherever possible, those offering the least resistance.

For some patients, increased expiratory resistance may be desirable. It is suggested that this be achieved by using devices designed for this purpose.

REBREATHING

Rebreathing means to inhale previously respired gases from which carbon dioxide may or may not have been removed. There is a tendency to associate the word *rebreathing* with carbon dioxide accumulation. This is unfortunate because, although it is true that rebreathing can result in higher inspired carbon dioxide concentrations than normal, it is possible to have partial or total rebreathing without an increase in carbon dioxide. Total prevention of rebreathing is not always desirable.

Factors Influencing Rebreathing

The amount of rebreathing will depend on the fresh gas flow, the mechanical dead space, and the design of the breathing system.

Fresh Gas Flow

The amount of rebreathing varies inversely with the total fresh gas flow. If the volume of fresh gas supplied per minute is equal to or greater than the patient's minute volume, there will be no rebreathing, as long as provision is made for unimpeded expiration to atmosphere or a scavenging system at a point close to the patient's respiratory tract (5). If the total volume of gas supplied per minute is less than the minute volume, some exhaled gases must be rebreathed to make up the required volume (assuming no air dilution).

Mechanical (Apparatus) Dead Space

The mechanical dead space is the space in a breathing system occupied by gases that are rebreathed without any change in composition. The minimum volume of gas that can be rebreathed is equal to the volume of the mechanical dead space. An increase in dead space increases rebreathing. Apparatus dead space may be minimized by separating the inspiratory and expiratory gas streams as close to the patient as possible.

The mechanical dead space should be distinguished from the physiological dead space, which includes (*i*) anatomical dead space, consisting of the conducting airway of the patient down to the alveoli, and (*ii*) alveolar dead space, which is the volume of alveoli ventilated but not perfused.

The composition of gas in the mechanical dead space will vary according to whether it is occupied by anatomical dead space gas, alveolar gas or mixed expired gas. Gas exhaled from the anatomical dead space has a composition similar to inspired gas, but is saturated with water vapor and warmer. Alveolar gas is saturated with water vapor at body temperature and has less oxygen and more carbon dioxide than inspired gas. The concentration of anesthetic agent in alveolar gas will differ from that in the inspired gas. Mixed expired gas will have a composition intermediate between that of anatomical dead space and alveolar gas.

Design of the Breathing System

In addition to the above factors, the various components of a breathing system may be arranged so that there is more or less rebreathing. This will be discussed more fully under the individual systems.

Effects of Rebreathing

With no rebreathing, the composition of inspired gas is identical to that of the fresh gas delivered by the anesthesia machine. With rebreathing, the inspired gas is composed partly of fresh gas and partly of rebreathed gas.

Retention of Heat and Water

Fresh gas from the anesthesia machine is anhydrous and at room temperature. Exhaled gases are warm and saturated with water. Hence rebreathing reduces heat and water loss from the patient. In most breathing systems, heat is rapidly lost to atmosphere, and gas that is reinhaled has a lower temperature and water content than exhaled gas (6).

Alteration of Inspired Gas Tensions

The effects of rebreathing on inspired gas tensions will depend on what parts of the exhaled gases are reinhaled and whether these pass to the alveoli (and so influence gas exchange) or only to the anatomical dead space.

Oxygen. Rebreathing of alveolar gas will cause a reduction in the inspired oxygen tension due to patient uptake of oxygen and the addition of nitrogen, carbon dioxide, and water vapor to the gas.

Inhaled Anesthetic Agents. The rebreathing of alveolar gas exerts a "cushioning" effect on changes in inspired gas composition with changes in the fresh gas composition. During induction, when alveolar tensions are lower than those in the fresh gas flow, rebreathing of alveolar gas will reduce the inspired tension and prolong induction. During recovery, the alveolar tension exceeds that of the inspired gases and rebreathing slows the elimination of anesthetic agent.

Carbon Dioxide. Rebreathing of alveolar gas will cause an increase in inspired carbon dioxide tension unless the gas passes through an absorbent before being rebreathed. Because carbon dioxide is concentrated in the alveolar portion of expired gases, the efficiency with which it is eliminated from a breathing system varies. If the

circuit is designed so that alveolar gas is preferentially eliminated through the adjustable pressure limiting (APL) valve, carbon dioxide retention will be minimal, even with a low fresh gas flow. Circuits that do not maintain the separation between fresh gas, deadspace gas, and alveolar gas require high gas flows to eliminate carbon dioxide.

With spontaneous respiration, carbon dioxide retention is generally considered undesirable. Although the patient can compensate by increasing minute volume, a price must be paid in terms of increased work of breathing, and in some cases the compensation may not be adequate.

During controlled ventilation, some CO_2 in inhaled gases may be advantageous. An increase in dead space will allow normocarbia to be achieved despite hyperventilation (7). Thus hypocarbia is avoided and heat and moisture retained while the lungs are kept well expanded by large tidal volumes.

DISCREPANCY BETWEEN INSPIRED AND DELIVERED VOLUMES

The volume of gas discharged by a ventilator or reservoir bag usually differs from that which enters the patient during inspiration. The volume actually inspired may be less or greater than that delivered.

Causes of Increased Inspired Volume

When an anesthesia ventilator is in use and the fresh gas flow rate is greater than the rate at which it is absorbed by the patient or lost through leaks in the breathing system, the portion of the fresh gas flow delivered during inspiration adds to the tidal volume delivered by the ventilator (9–11). This augmentation increases with higher fresh gas flows and I:E ratios and decreased respiratory rates (9).

Causes of Decreased Inspired Volume

A reduction in tidal volume (wasted ventilation) will result from compression of gases and distension of the components of the breathing system (12,13). Wasted ventilation increases with the pressure during inspiration, PEEP, the volume and distensibility of components of the breathing system, and patient airway resistance (12,14,15). If a highly compliant adult system is used with a small patient, the volume lost to distension may exceed the tidal volume (12).

Tidal volume is also decreased by leaks in the breathing system. The amount lost will depend on the size and location of the leaks and the pressures during inspiration and expiration.

Tidal volumes are best measured between the patient and the breathing tubes (see Chapter 17). Measuring tidal volume at the end of the expiratory limb will reflect increases caused by fresh gas flow and decreases resulting from leaks but will miss decreases from compression of gases and distension of components (13).

DISCREPANCY BETWEEN INSPIRED AND DELIVERED CONCENTRATIONS

The composition of the gas mixture that exits the machine may be modified by the breathing system so that the mixture the patient inspires differs considerably from that delivered to the system. There are several contributing factors.

Rebreathing

The effect of rebreathing will depend on the volume of the rebreathed gas and its composition. This will depend on the factors discussed previously.

Air Dilution

If the fresh gas supplied per respiration is less than the tidal volume, negative pressure during spontaneous ventilation may result in air dilution if the inspiratory limb is open to atmosphere or there is a leak. The amount of air dilution will depend on the presence or absence of reservoirs in the system, the respiratory pattern and the total fresh gas flow.

Air dilution makes it difficult to maintain a stable anesthetic state. When it occurs, the concentration of anesthetic in the inspired mixture falls. This results in lighter anesthesia with attendant stimulation of ventilation. The increased ventilation causes more air dilution. The opposite also is true. Deepening anesthesia depresses ventilation. Depression of respiration decreases air dilution and thereby increases the inspired anesthetic agent concentration. This in turn leads to further depression of respiration.

Leaks

When a leak occurs, positive pressure in the system will force gas out of the system. The composition and amount of the gas lost will depend on the location and size of the leak, the pressure in the system, and the compliance and resistance of both the system and the patient.

Uptake of Anesthetic Agent by the Breathing System Components

Uptake of anesthetic agents by rubber, plastics, metal, and carbon dioxide absorbent will produce a lower inspired concentration. Uptake will be directly proportional to the concentration gradient between the gas and the components, the partition coefficient, the surface area, the diffusion coefficient, and the square root of time. The diffusion coefficients and partition coefficients are constant for any anesthetic agent. The surface area will depend on the system used and must include the delivery hose from the machine.

Release of Anesthetic from the System

Elimination of anesthetic agent from the breathing system will depend on the same factors as uptake. Of clinical significance is the fact that with some anesthetics the system may function as a low output vaporizer for many hours after the primary vaporizer has been turned off even if the rubber goods and absorbent are changed (16–18). This can result in unplanned exposure of a patient to the agent.

Common Components

Certain pieces of equipment are found in only one type of breathing system. These will be discussed under the individual systems. Other components (or breathing attachments) are common to more than one system so that their inclusion in a general chapter such as this is appropriate.

BUSHINGS (MOUNTS)

A bushing serves to modify the internal diameter of a component. Most often it has a cylindrical form and is inserted into and becomes part of a pliable component, such as a reservoir bag or a breathing tube.

SLEEVES

A sleeve alters the external diameter of a component.

CONNECTORS AND ADAPTORS

A connector is a fitting intended to join together two or more components. An adaptor is a specialized connector that establishes functional continuity between otherwise disparate or incompatible components.

An adaptor or connector may be distinguished by: (*i*) shape (straight, right-angle [or elbow], T, or Y); (*ii*) component(s) to which it is semipermanently attached; (*iii*) added features (with nipple or pop-off) and (*iv*) size and type of fitting at either end (15-mm male, 22-mm female).

All anesthesia systems terminate at the patient connection port, which is the opening at the patient end of the breathing system intended for connection to a tracheal tube connector, face mask, or elbow connector. All face masks, both adult and pediatric, have a 22-mm female opening and all tracheal tube connectors have a 15-mm male fitting. To facilitate the change from mask to tracheal tube and vice versa, a component having a 22-mm male fitting with a concentric 15-mm female opening to fit either a mask or a tracheal tube connector is used at the patient end of most systems. Often this component is a right-angle connector (Fig. 5.2) and may be known as an elbow adaptor, elbow joint, elbow connector, face mask angle piece, mask adaptor, or mask elbow.

Connectors and adaptors serve several purposes:

1. To extend the distance between the patient and the breathing system. This is especially important in head and neck surgery when the presence of the breathing system near the head may make it inaccessible to the anesthesia personnel and/or interfere with the surgical field.

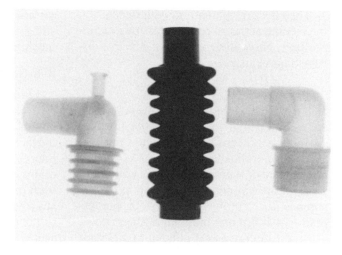

Figure 5.2. Typical connectors. The right-angle connectors at the right and left can connect the breathing system to either a mask or tracheal tube connector so that the change from mask to tracheal tube, and vice versa, is easily accomplished. This component may be known as an elbow adaptor, elbow joint, elbow connector, face mask angle piece, mask adaptor, or mask elbow. The connector on the left has a port for aspiration of gases from the system. In the middle is a flexible rubber connector with metal fittings at either end. It is commonly used to increase the distance between the patient and the breathing system and to increase dead space. Photograph by Duncan Sawyer.

2. To change the angle of connection between the tracheal tube and the breathing system.
3. To allow a more flexible and/or less kinkable connection between the tracheal tube and the breathing system.
4. To increase the dead space.

A variety of connectors are available commercially (see Fig. 5.2) and many more have been described in the literature. Connectors should have a 15-mm male (OD) fitting at the machine end and either a 22-mm male/15-mm female fitting for connection to either a tracheal tube connector or a mask or simply a 15-mm female fitting for connection to a tracheal tube connector.

In selecting a connector, several principles should be kept in mind.

1. Resistance increases markedly with sharp curves and rough sidewalls.
2. Connectors add dead space; in the adult patient this may not be of much significance, but in infants any increase in dead space may be excessive.
3. Addition of a connector(s) increases the number of possible locations at which disconnections can take place.

RESERVOIR BAG

The reservoir bag is also known as the respiratory bag, breathing bag, or somewhat erroneously, the rebreathing bag. Most bags are composed of rubber or neoprene. The neck of the bag is the part that connects with the breathing system. The tail is the end of the bag opposite from the neck. A hanging loop may be provided near the tail to facilitate drying. The neck of the bag must be a 22-mm female fitting (19).

The bag has the following functions:

1. It allows accumulation of gas during exhalation so that a reservoir is available for the next inspiration. This permits rebreathing, allows more economical use of gases and prevents air dilution.

2. It provides a means whereby anesthesia personnel may assist or control ventilation.
3. It can serve through visual and tactile observation as a monitor of a patient's spontaneous respirations.
4. It acts to protect the patient from excessive pressure in the breathing system (20–22).

The pressure-volume characteristics of rubber bags are shown in Figure 5.3. Adding volume to a bag causes a negligible rise in pressure until the nominal capacity is reached. As more volume is added, the pressure rises rapidly to a peak then attains a plateau. As the bag distends further, the pressure falls slightly. The peak pressure is of particular interest as this represents the maximal pressure that will develop in a breathing system. The ASTM standard for reservoir bags (19) requires that for bags of 1.5 liters or smaller the pressure shall be not less than 30 cm H_2O or exceed 50 cm H_2O when the bag is expanded to four times its capacity (19). For bags larger than 1.5 liters, the pressure shall be not less than 35 cm H_2O or exceed 60 cm H_2O when the bag is expanded to four times its size. One study found this pressure was often exceeded, especially if the bag was new and there was a high inflow rate (22).

New bags develop greater pressures when first overinflated than bags that have been overinflated several times or have been prestretched (20,22). It is good practice to overinflate or stretch a new bag before it is used. This will not limit the ability to produce high airway pressures by squeezing and will increase the margin of safety.

Disposable plastic bags are inelastic and do not stretch after full inflation. Excessively high pressure may develop within seconds when they are inadvertently overfilled (20).

The size of the bag that should be used will depend on the patient, the breathing system in which it is used, and the user's preference. A large bag may be difficult to squeeze and will make monitoring of the patient's spon-

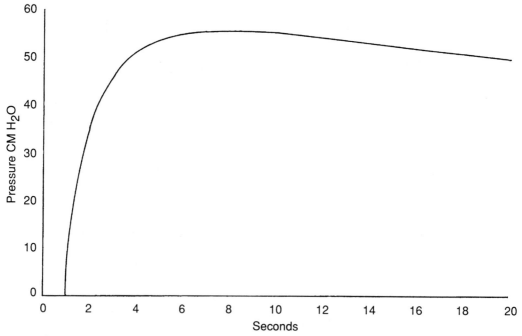

Figure 5.3. Pressure-volume characteristics of a reservoir bag. Flow rate 50 liter/min. Redrawn from Parmley JB, Tahir AN, Dascomb HE, et al. Disposable versus reusable rebreathing circuits: advantages, disadvantages, hazards and bacteriologic studies. Anesth Analg 1972;51:890.

taneous respiration difficult because the bag excursions will be smaller. A small bag, on the other hand, provides less of a safety factor for distention and may not provide a large enough reservoir.

A spare bag should always be kept immediately available. A bag may rupture at any time or become lost while a ventilator is in use. If a spare bag is not immediately available, the anesthesia personnel will be confronted with the problem of ventilating an apneic patient. This may be accomplished by occluding the bag attachment point while the oxygen flush is activated. The hand is removed for exhalation. This is a somewhat dangerous method and will not keep the patient anesthetized.

BREATHING TUBES

Large bore, nonrigid breathing (conducting) tubes, composed of rubber or plastic and usually corrugated, are used in most breathing systems to convey gases to and from the patient. Corrugations prevent obstruction from kinking and increase flexibility. Clear plastic tubes allow visualization of the interior and are more lightweight than rubber tubes, so that they cause less drag on the tracheal tube or mask. They absorb less of the halogenated agents than rubber tubes and have a lower compliance. The ASTM standard requires single breathing tubes to have 22-mm female fittings at either end (23). It also requires the patient end of the T piece to have a 22-mm male, 15-mm female coaxial fitting.

Breathing tubes have two functions. One is to act as a reservoir in certain systems. The second function is to provide a flexible, low-resistance, lightweight connection from one part of the system to another.

Breathing tubes have some distensibility but not enough to prevent excessive pressures from developing in the system (24). During spontaneous ventilation, breathing tubes tend to collapse on inspiration and bulge on exhalation. This is referred to as *backlash* and may cause some rebreathing. During controlled and assisted ventilation, the tubes tend to bulge on inspiration and return to a resting position on exhalation. This is referred to as *wasted ventilation,* because it results in less volume entering the patient than leaves the ventilator or reservoir bag.

ADJUSTABLE PRESSURE LIMITING (APL) VALVE

The APL valve is a user-adjustable valve that releases gases to atmosphere or a scavenging system and that is intended to provide control of the pressure in the breathing system (1). Other commonly used names for this component include pressure relief valve, venting port, relief valve, overspill valve, pop-off valve, overflow valve, dump valve, blow-off valve, safety relief valve, excess valve, Heidbrink valve, adjustable pressure limiter, excess gas venting valve, spill valve, exhaust valve, expiratory valve, excess gas valve, pressure release valve, and release valve.

Construction

The housing of most APL valves is metal. If the valve is to be used in an MRI environment, it should be constructed from aluminum.

Control Part

The control part serves to control the pressure at which the valve opens. Several types are available.

Spring-Loaded Disc. A commonly used APL valve uses a disc held onto a seat by a coiled spring (Fig. 5.4). A threaded screw cap over the spring allows the pressure exerted by the spring to be varied. When the cap is fully tightened, the disc will prevent any gas from escaping from the system. As the cap is loosened, the tension on the spring is reduced.

When the pressure in the breathing system increases, it exerts an upward force on the disc. When this force exceeds the downward force exerted by the spring, the disc rises and

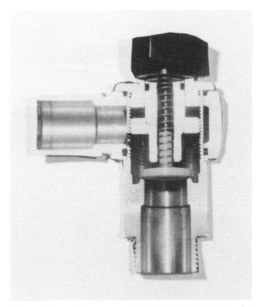

Figure 5.4. APL valve with spring-loaded disc. Gas from the breathing system enters at the base and passes into the collection device at left. Turning the control knob varies the tension in the spring and the pressure necessary to lift the disc off its seat.

gas flows out of the system. When the pressure in the system falls, the disc returns to its seat. When the cap is at its maximum upward position, there will be no pressure exerted by the spring. The weight of the disc ensures that the reservoir bag fills before the disc rises.

Stem and Seat. Another control part employed in APL valves is the stem and seat (Fig. 5.5). This is similar to a flow control valve in that a threaded stem allows variable contact with a seat. As the valve is opened, the opening at the seat becomes larger and more gas is allowed to escape. A disc or ball that must be moved to open the valve ensures that there will be sufficient pressure in the system to fill the reservoir bag before the valve opens.

Diaphragm. A diaphragm valve is shown in Figure 5.6. It works in a manner similar to the spring-loaded disc valve except that the cap and spring push on a diaphragm rather than on a disc. Increased pressure in the breathing system will push the dia-

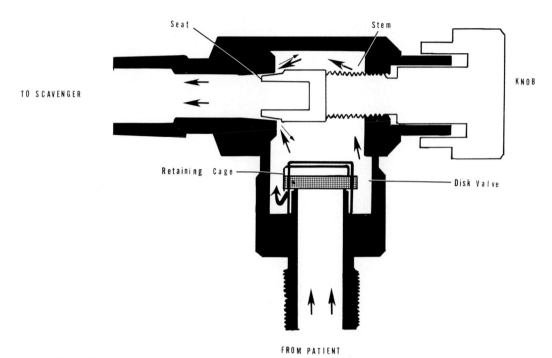

Figure 5.5. APL valve with stem and seat. Rotation of the control knob causes the opening between the stem and seat to vary. The disc ensures that the reservoir bag will fill before the valve opens. It also prevents transmission of positive pressure from the scavenging system to the breathing system. Redrawn courtesy of North American Drager, Inc.

phragm off its seat. Increasing or decreasing the tension of the spring controls the amount of gas that will escape through the valve.

If there is negative pressure in the scavenging system, the diaphragm is pulled onto the seat and the negative pressure is not transmitted to the breathing system. There is a danger associated with this valve. If the diaphragm is closed by negative pressure and gas continues to flow into the breathing system, it cannot escape. The only quick way to relieve pressure in the breathing system is to disconnect the scavenging system at some point until the source of the negative pressure in the scavenging system has been eliminated.

Control Knob

Most APL valves have a rotary control knob. The ASTM standard requires that valves with rotating controls be designed so that a clockwise motion increases the limiting pressure and ultimately closes the valve (1). It also requires an arrow or other mark-

ing to indicate the direction of movement required to close the valve. The standard also recommends that the full range of relief pressure be adjusted by less than one full turn of the control.

Exhaust Port

The exhaust port is the port through which excess gases are discharged to the scavenging system. It must have a 19- or 30-mm male connector (25).

Collection Device

Almost all APL valves are now fitted with collection devices that collect the gases that are vented and direct them to a scavenging system.

Use

Spontaneous Respiration

With spontaneous respiration, the APL valve remains closed during inspiration. During exhalation, it opens when its opening

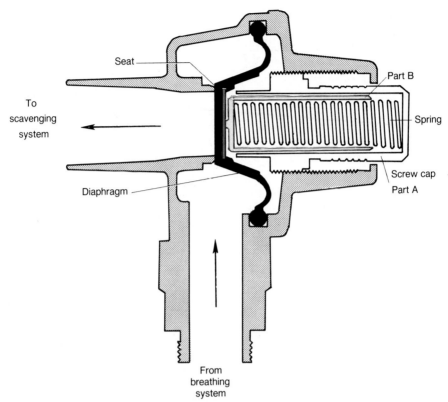

Figure 5.6. APL valve with diaphragm. Turning the control knob (screw cap) varies the tension in the spring and thus controls the amount of gas vented through the valve. Negative pressure in the scavenging system will pull the diaphragm onto its seat. Redrawn from a drawing furnished by Ohmeda, a division of BOC Health Care, Inc.

pressure is exceeded. Normally, the valve is left fully open during spontaneous ventilation. It should be closed slightly only if the reservoir bag collapses.

With spontaneous respiration, anesthesia personnel must be constantly aware of the amount of bag inflation. If attention is diverted, the bag may collapse or become overdistended. Negative pressure transmitted from the scavenging system may result in either closure of the valve or evacuation of gases from the system. An obstruction in the scavenging system may result in the bag becoming overdistended.

There is considerable variation in the resistance of APL valves when fully open (26–28) so they should be checked periodically. Fully open APL valves should have a pressure drop between 0.1 and 0.3 kPa (1.0 and 3.0 cm H_2O) at an air flow of 3.0 liters/min

and a pressure drop at 30 liters/min of not less than 0.1 kPA (1.0 cm H_2O) and not greater than 0.5 kPa (5.0 cm H_2O) (1).

Manually Controlled or Assisted Ventilation

During manually controlled or assisted ventilation, the valve is usually left partially open. During inspiration, the bag is squeezed and pressure is developed until the relief pressure is reached. Before this, the patient receives all of the gas displaced from the bag (less a small amount because of compression of the gases and expansion of the tubes). Once the APL valve opens, the additional volume the patient receives is determined by the relative resistances to flow exerted by the patient and the APL valve. Careful and frequent adjustments of the valve are necessary to achieve the desired level of ventilation and maintain adequate filling of the reservoir bag. If compliance of the lungs and thorax falls, the valve must be tightened to maintain the desired tidal volume. Adjustment should be made on the basis of chest movements and/or exhaled volume measurements.

An alternative method is to close the valve completely and open it periodically to release excess gas or set the fresh gas flow so low that it equals uptake by the patient and the system.

The resistance felt during bag compression ("the educated hand") cannot be relied on to ensure adequate ventilation of the patient (29). An increase in resistance to ventilating the patient will result in more gas being lost through the APL valve unless the valve setting is changed.

Mechanical Ventilation

When a ventilator is used the APL valve should be closed completely. Gas will be vented from the ventilator during expiration. If the valve is left open gas will be vented from the system during inspiration, and this may result in inadequate ventilation (30).

Bag-ventilator selector switches (selector valves) that facilitate the change from manual to automatic ventilation are available and are discussed in Chapter 7. Some of these automatically isolate the APL valve when the selector valve is turned to automatic ventilation.

POSITIVE END EXPIRATORY PRESSURE (PEEP) VALVES

Application of PEEP may be used to improve patient oxygenation. On most newer anesthesia machines a PEEP valve is incorporated into the CO_2 absorber assembly or ventilator. For older machines, a disposable PEEP valve can be placed in the exhalation limb for PEEP during manual or artificial ventilation or between the breathing system and the ventilator to provide PEEP during artificial ventilation. A number of different means have been used to achieve PEEP (31). A ball PEEP valve must be kept in an upright

position. Using a spring-loaded or magnetic PEEP valve eliminates this need.

Fixed pressure PEEP valves are marked to indicate the amount of PEEP they provide. More than one valve can be used to obtain an additive effect. Variable pressure valves have a means to adjust the amount of PEEP. Some valves have a scale that indicates the PEEP at a given setting. If no scale is present, a manometer must be used to measure the pressure.

PEEP valves can be divided into two types: unidirectional and bidirectional (32). A bidirectional valve has a second flow channel with its own one-way valve. It has been recommended that only bidirectional PEEP valves be used (33,34). Only a bidirectional valve should be used between the breathing system and the ventilator.

When inserting a disposable PEEP valve it is important that it be placed in the correct position and oriented correctly. The ASTM standard requires that a PEEP valve be marked with an arrow indicating the proper directional flow or the words *inlet* and *outlet* or both (1). Immediately after placement, the breathing system manometer should be checked to make certain PEEP is being delivered and the patient should be checked for effective ventilation. A unidirectional PEEP valve incorrectly oriented against the flow of gas in the inspiratory or expiratory limb will occlude gas flow (32,34,35). Incorrectly orienting a bidirectional PEEP valve in either the inspiratory or expiratory limb will not occlude flow, but no PEEP will be generated.

If a PEEP valve is used with an older model circle breathing system in which the pressure manometer is on the absorber side of the expiratory unidirectional valve, PEEP will not be indicated on the gauge (36,37). The user must depend on the accuracy of the valve markings to determine the level of PEEP or a second pressure manometer upstream of the PEEP valve may be used to determine the actual pressures (32). If the PEEP valve is placed between the breathing system and the ventilator, PEEP can be observed on the breathing system pressure gauge.

Certain precautions must be observed when using a PEEP valve. When the patient is breathing spontaneously without ventilatory assistance, use of a PEEP valve will result in increased exhalation effort. Use of PEEP in the breathing system with a pressure-limited ventilator or during manual ventilation may result in a substantial decrease in the tidal volume delivered to the patient, unless appropriate adjustments are made to ventilator settings or APL valve.

For ventilators that provide a control for setting the peak inspiratory pressure, the pressure setting must be set higher than the PEEP valve or inadequate tidal volume may be delivered.

FILTERS

Filters have three purposes:

1. Protection of the patient from pathogens and airborne particulate matter such as dirt, absorbent dust, and metallic flakes (38).
2. Protection of the anesthesia equipment and the hospital environment from exhaled contaminants.
3. Exchange of heat and moisture when placed between the patient and the breathing system (39).

A variety of materials has been used for the filter medium. Most have a hydrophobic coating. Filters with greater than 99% efficiency in blocking transmission of bacteria and viruses are available (40–42).

Filters for use in anesthesia are supplied in three forms: (*i*) attached to the breathing tube of a disposable circle system; (*ii*) attached to a ventilator hose; and (*iii*) as a separate component. Filters that are part of a disposable circle system have not been shown to be effective in reducing postoperative pulmonary infections and may be unnecessary if equipment is properly cleaned and sterilized after use (43–45).

A filter should be placed upstream of a humidifier or nebulizer because when wet it may become less efficient and allow bacteria to pass through. In addition, an increase in resistance, sometimes to a hazardous level, may be seen as the filter becomes wet (46–49).

Obstruction of filters caused by exhaled blood, edema fluid, a manufacturing defect, sterilization of a disposable filter, and inserting a unidirectional filter backward have all been reported (50–52). Aspiration of the filter medium may occur. A hole in a filter can cause a leak (see Fig. 12.8).

Size and Type of Fittings

The Compressed Gas Association and the American Society for Testing and Materials have published standards that specify the size and type of fittings for components in the breathing system. (1,19,23,53). Virtually all breathing system components manufactured in the United States in recent years conform to these. The safety provided by standardization of diameters of various connectors can be jeopardized by use of adaptors and adhesive tape.

Any component or accessory of the breathing system that permits only unidirectional flow or any device whose correct function depends on the direction of gas flow through it must be so labeled by the manufacturer and marked with an arrow indicating the proper direction of flow or the words *inlet* and *outlet* or both. *Distal* and *proximal* are used to designate the proximity of a component to the patient.

Connectors forming a part of components such as absorbers, Y pieces, and reservoir bag mounts, whose purpose is to permit attachment of these components to reservoir bags, breathing tubes, or masks must be male and "rigid." The breathing tube, mask and reservoir bag connectors must be female and nonrigid (resilient).

All connectors in an adult system are 22 mm. The component that is designed to connect to a tracheal tube connector must have a coaxial 15-mm female fitting at the patient end. The inspiratory and expiratory ports mounted on the absorber, and the reservoir bag connector must have male fittings. To avoid problems with connections between the breathing and scavenging systems, the exit port for the APL valve is shrouded and has either a 30- or 19-mm male fitting.

Classification of Breathing Systems

A favorite pastime among anesthesiology personnel has been the classification of breathing systems. The result has been a hopelessly confused terminology. In an attempt to provide some relief from this confusion, a description of various authors' classifications will be presented. Subsequently, a nomenclature will be described that the present authors believe is more useful.

CLASSIFICATION BY FUNCTION

Dripps, Echenhoff, and Vandam (54)

With this classification, techniques of anesthesia are divided into five categories according to the presence or absence of: (*i*) a reservoir bag in the breathing system; (*ii*) rebreathing; (*iii*) an absorber to remove expired carbon dioxide; and (*iv*) directional valves in the breathing system. The five techniques are insufflation, open, semiopen, semiclosed, and closed.

The insufflation system is one in which anesthetic gases and oxygen are delivered directly into the patient's airway. There are no valves, reservoir bag, or carbon dioxide absorption.

In the open system, the patient inhales only the anesthetic mixture delivered by the anesthesia machine. Valves direct each exhaled breath into atmosphere. A reservoir bag may or may not be present. Rebreathing is minimal and there is no carbon dioxide ab-

sorption. This includes systems used with intermittent flow machines and nonrebreathing valves.

In the semiopen system, exhaled gases flow into the surrounding atmosphere and also to the inspiratory line of the apparatus to be rebreathed. There is no chemical absorption of exhaled carbon dioxide. Rebreathing depends on the fresh gas flow. A reservoir bag and a directional valve are optional.

In the semiclosed system, part of the exhaled gases passes into atmosphere whereas part mixes with fresh gases and is rebreathed. Chemical absorption of carbon dioxide, directional valves, and a reservoir bag are present.

In the closed system, there is complete rebreathing of expired gas. Carbon dioxide absorption, a reservoir bag, and directional valves are present.

Moyers (55)

This classification is based on the presence or absence of a reservoir bag and rebreathing. An open system has no reservoir or rebreathing. The semiopen system has a reservoir but no rebreathing. The semiclosed system has a reservoir and partial rebreathing, and the closed system has a reservoir and complete rebreathing.

Collins (56)

This classification defines an open system as one in which an anesthetic agent is brought to the patient's respiratory tract with atmospheric air as the diluent. The respiratory tract has access to the atmosphere during both inspiration and expiration. There is no reservoir or rebreathing.

A semiopen system is one in which the patient's respiratory system is open to atmosphere during both inspiration and expiration. There is a reservoir that is open to atmosphere, rebreathing is absent, and atmospheric air either carries or dilutes the anesthetic agent.

The semiclosed system is one in which the

patient's respiratory system is completely closed to atmosphere on inspiration but open on expiration. A reservoir closed to atmosphere is present.

With a closed system, there is no access to atmosphere either during inspiration or expiration. Rebreathing is complete and a reservoir is required.

Adriani (57)

This classification divides systems into open vaporization, insufflation, semiclosed and closed (rebreathing). An open system is one employing an open-drop mask. With the insufflation technique a continuous stream of gas flows to the patient's nasopharynx, oropharynx, or trachea. The semiclosed system is one in which there is complete enclosure of the inspired atmosphere and no air dilution. The closed system permits complete rebreathing.

Conway (58)

With this classification, an open system is one with infinite boundaries and no restriction to fresh gas flow. The semiopen system is one partially bounded, with some restriction to fresh gas flow. The closed circuit is defined as having no provision for gas overflow. The semiclosed system is one allowing for overflow of excess gas. It is divided into semiclosed rebreathing, semiclosed absorption, and semiclosed nonrebreathing circuits.

Hall (59)

In this classification, an open system has no reservoir bag or rebreathing. The semiopen system also has no reservoir bag but has partial rebreathing. Semiclosed systems have a reservoir bag and partial rebreathing. They are divided into those with and without carbon dioxide absorption. The closed system has complete rebreathing and a reservoir.

McMahon (60)

This system used rebreathing as the basis for classification of breathing systems into open, semiclosed, and closed. An open technique is one in which no rebreathing is employed. This includes techniques in which gases are administered at a total flow rate equal to or greater than the respiratory minute volume. Techniques with flows less than the respiratory minute volume would also be considered as open if there were no increase in dead space. The semiclosed system would employ some rebreathing. The closed system employs total rebreathing.

Baraka (61)

This system classified breathing systems according to their mechanisms of carbon dioxide elimination. Carbon dioxide is eliminated from the circuit by either washout or absorption. Open systems are those that eliminate carbon dioxide by washout and have no reservoir bag. Semiopen systems also wash out carbon dioxide, but have a reservoir bag. Semiclosed systems use carbon dioxide absorption and have a fresh gas flow that exceeds patient uptake. Closed systems also use carbon dioxide absorption and have a fresh gas flow that equals patient uptake.

The International Standards Organization

The International Standards Organization (ISO 4135:1979) has devised a classification of breathing systems based on the amount of rebreathing that occurs. Systems are classified as nonrebreathing, partial rebreathing, and complete rebreathing.

Marini, Culver, and Kirk (62)

This system classifies breathing circuits on the basis of carbon dioxide elimination. Carbon dioxide is eliminated either by washout by fresh gas inflow or by absorption. The classification of carbon dioxide washout systems is further divided into open, which do not have a reservoir bag, and semiopen, which do have a reservoir bag. Examples of the open variety include the open drop mask, insufflation, and the T piece (Mapleson E). The semiopen systems include the Magill and Lack (Mapleson A), Bain (Mapleson D), Jackson-Rees (Mapleson F) Mera F, and the nonrebreathing valve systems (mostly used in resuscitation). The carbon dioxide absorption units include the circle system.

CLASSIFICATION BY EQUIPMENT

Hamilton (63) recognized the shortcomings of the nomenclatures described above and proposed that the terms open, semiopen, etc. be dropped in favor of a description of the equipment and the total fresh gas flow to the system. The description of the equipment will be familiar to the reader after reading the next two chapters. The fresh gas flow will determine the amount of rebreathing, if any, that takes place.

REFERENCES

1. American Society for Testing and Materials. Standard specifications for minimum performance and safety requirements for anesthesia breathing systems (ASTM F1208-89). Philadelphia: ASTM, 1989.
2. Bolder PM, Healy TEJ, Bolder AR, Beatty PCW, Kay B. The extra work of breathing through adult endotracheal tubes. Anesth Analg 1976;65:853–859.
3. Bersten AD, Rutten AJ, Vedig AE, Skowronski GA. Additional work of breathing imposed by endotracheal tubes, breathing circuits, and intensive care ventilators. Crit Care Med 1989;17:671–677.
4. Davies JM, Hogg MIJ, Rosen M. Upper limits of resistance of apparatus for inhalation analgesia during labour. Br J Anaesth 1974;46:136–144.
5. Hogg MIJ, Davies JM, Mapleson WW, Rosen M. Proposed upper limit of respiratory resistance for inhalation apparatus used in labour. Br J Anaesth 1974;46:149–152.
6. McMahon J. Rebreathing as a basis for classification of inhalation technics. J Am Assoc Nurse Anesth 1951;19:133–158.
7. Sykes MK. Rebreathing circuits. Br J Anaesth 1968;40:666–674.
8. Scott PV, Jones RP. Variable apparatus dead space. Anaesthesia 1991;46:1047–1049.
9. Aldrete JA, Castillo RA, Bradley EL. Changes of fresh gas flow affect the tidal volume delivered by anesthesia ventilators. Anesth Analg 1986;65:S4.
10. Ghani GA. Fresh gas flow affects minute volume during mechanical ventilation. Anesth Analg 1984;63:619.
11. Gravenstein N, Banner MJ, McLaughlin G. Tidal volume changes due to the interaction of anesthesia machine and anesthesia ventilator. J Clin Monit 1987;3:187–190.
12. Cote CJ, Petkau AJ, Ryan JF, Welch JP. Wasted ventilation measured in vitro with eight anesthetic circuits with and without inline humidification. Anesthesiology 1983;59:442–446.
13. Feldman JM, Muller J. Tidal volume measurement errors—the impact of lung compliance and a circuit humidifier. Anesthesiology 1990;73:A469.
14. Aarandia HY, Byles PH. PEEP and the Bain circuit. Can Anaesth Soc J 1981;28:467–470.
15. Elliott WR, Harris AE, Philip JH. Positive end-expiratory pressure: implications for tidal volume changes in anesthesia machine ventilation. J Clin Monit 1989;5:100–104.
16. Dykes MHM, Chir MB, Laasberg LH. Clinical implications of halothane contamination of the anesthetic circle. Anesthesiology 1971;35:648–649.
17. Murray WJ, Fleming P. Patient exposure to residual fluorinated anesthetic agents in anesthesia machine circuits. Anesth Analg 1973;52:23–26.
18. Samulksa HM, Ramaiah S, Noble WH. Unintended exposure to halothane in surgical patients: halothane washout studies. Can Anaesth Soc J 1972;19:35–41.
19. American Society for Testing Materials. Standard specification for anesthesia reservoir bags (ASTM F1204-88). Philadelphia: ASTM, 1988.
20. Parmley JB, Tahir AH, Dascomb HE, Adriani J. Disposable versus reusable rebreathing circuits: advantages, disadvantages, hazards, and bacteriologic studies. Anesth Analg 1972;51:888–894.
21. Johnstone RE, Smith TC. Rebreathing bags as pressure-limiting devices. Anesthesiology 1973;38:192–194.
22. Stone DR, Graves SA. Compliance of pediatric rebreathing bags. Anesthesiology 1980;53:434–435.
23. American Society for Testing Materials. Standard specification for anesthesia breathing tubes (ASTM F1205-88). Philadelphia: ASTM, 1988.
24. Parmley JB, Tahir AH, Adriani J. Disposable plastic breathing bags and tubes. JAMA 1971;217:1842–1844.
25. American Society for Testing Materials. Specification for anesthetic equipment-scavenging systems for anesthetic gases (ASTM F1343-91). Philadelphia: ASTM, 1991.
26. Mehta S, Behr G, Chari J, Kenyon D. A passive method of disposal of expired anesthetic gases. Br J Anaesth 1977;49:589–593.
27. Morgan BA, Nott MR. Wear in plastic exhaust valves. Anaesthesia 1980;35:717–718.
28. Nott MR, Norman J. Resistance of Heidbrink-type expiratory valves. Br J Anaesth 1978;50:477–480.
29. Egbert LD, Bisno D. The educated hand of the an-

esthesiologist: a study of professional skill. Anesth Analg 1967;46:195–200.

30. Conway CM, Schoonbee C. Factors affecting the performance of circle systems used without carbon dioxide absorption. Br J Anaesth 1981;53:115P.

31. Kacmarek RM, Dimas S, Reynolds J, Shapiro BA. Technical aspects of positive end-expiratory pressure (PEEP). Part I: physics of PEEP devices. Respir Care 1982;27:1478–1489.

32. Anonymous. Hazard: PEEP valves in anesthesia circuits. Technol Anesth 1983;4(5):1–2.

33. Morse HN. Who is liable when respiratory valve is installed erroneously? Med Elect Prod 1989; (October):32.

34. Lee D. Old equipment PEEP safety cited [Letter to the Editor]. APSF Newslett 1990;5:21.

35. Anonymous. Unidirectional PEEP valves and anesthesia. Technol Anesth 1986;6(9):1–2.

36. Mayle LL, Reed SJ, Wyche MQ. Excessive airway pressures occurring concurrently with use of the Fraser Harlake PEEP valve. Anesthesiol Rev 1990;17:41–44.

37. Cooper JB. Unidirectional PEEP valves can cause safety hazards. APSF Newslett 1990;4:28–29.

38. Davis R. Soda lime dust. Anaesth Intensive Care 1979;7:390.

39. Chalon J, Markham JP, Ali MM, Ramanathan S, Turndorf H. The Pall Ultipore breathing circuit filter—an efficient heat and moisture exchanger. Anesth Analg 1970;63:566–570, 1970.

40. Berry AJ, Nolte FS. An alternative strategy for infection control of anesthesia breathing circuits: a laboratory assessment of the Pall HME filter. Anesth Analg 1991;72:651–655.

41. Fargnoli JM, Arvieux CC, Coppo F, Girardet P, Eisele JH. Efficiency and importance of airway filters in reducing microorganisms. Anesth Analg 1992;74:S93.

42. Hedley RM, Allt-Graham J. A comparison of the filtration properties of heat and moisture exchangers. Anaesthesia 1992;47:414–420.

43. Pace NL, Webster C, Epstein B. Failure of anesthesia circuit bacterial filter to reduce postoperative pulmonary infections. Anesthesiology 1979;57:S362.

44. Garibaldi RA, Britt MR, Webster C, Pace NL. Failure of bacterial filters to reduce the incidence of pneumonia after inhalation anesthesia. Anesthesiology 1981;54:364–368.

45. Ping FC, Oulton JL, Smith JA, Skidmore AG, Jenkins LC. Bacterial filters—are they necessary

on anaesthetic machines? Can Anaesth Soc J 1979;26:415–419.

46. Buckley PM. Increase in resistance of in-line breathing filters in humidified air. Br J Anaesth 1984;56:637–643.

47. Dryden GE, Dryden SR, Brown DG, Schatzle KC, Godzeski C. Performance of bacteria filters. Respir Care 1980;25:1127–1135.

48. Loeser EA. Water-induced resistance in disposable respiratory—circuit bacterial filters. Anesth Analg 1978;57:269–271.

49. Mason J, Tackley R. An acute rise in expiratory resistance due to a blocked ventilator filter. Anaesthesia 1981;36:335.

50. Kopman AF, Glaser L. Obstruction of bacterial filters by edema fluid. Anesthesiology 1976;44:169–170.

51. Smith CE, Otworth JR, Kaluszyk P. Bilateral tension pneumothroax due to a defective anesthesia breathing circuit filter. J Clin Anesth 1991;3:229–234.

52. Grundy EM, Bennett EJ, Brennan T. Obstructed anesthetic circuits. Anesth Rev 1976;3:35–36.

53. Compressed Gas Association. Standard for 22 mm anesthesia breathing circuit connectors (Pamphlet M-1). New York: CGA, 1972.

54. Dripps RD, Echenhoff JE, Vandam LD. Introduction to anesthesia. 3rd ed. Philadelphia: WB Saunders, 1968.

55. Moyers J. A nomenclature for methods of inhalation anesthesia. Anesthesiology 1953;14:609–611.

56. Collins VJ. Principles of anesthesiology. Philadelphia: Lea & Febiger, 1966.

57. Adriani J. The chemistry and physics of anesthesia. Springfield, IL: Charles C Thomas, 1962.

58. Conway CM. Anaesthetic circuits. In: Scurr C, Feldman, S, eds. Foundations of anaesthesia. Philadelphia: FA Davis, 1970:37.

59. Hall J. Wright's veterinary anaesthesia. 6th ed. London: Bailliere, Tindall & Cox, 1966.

60. McMahon J. Rebreathing as a basis for classification of inhalation technics. J Am Assoc Nurse Anesth 1951;19:133–158.

61. Baraka A. Functional classification of anaesthesia circuits. Anaesth Intensive Care 1977;5:172–178.

62. Marini JJ, Culver BH, Kirk W. Flow resistance of exhalation valves and positive end-expiratory pressure devices used in mechanical ventilation. Am Rev Respir Dis 1984;131:850–854.

63. Hamilton WK. Nomenclature of inhalation anesthetic systems. Anesthesiology 1964;25:3–5.

Chapter 6

The Mapleson Breathing Systems

The Mapleson breathing systems are characterized by the absence of valves to direct gases to or from the patient. Because there is no device for absorbing CO_2, the fresh gas flow must wash CO_2 out of the circuit. For this reason, these systems are sometimes called carbon dioxide washout circuits or flow-controlled breathing systems.

These systems were classified by Mapleson (1) into five basic types: A through E . A sixth, the Mapleson F system, was added later (2). The classification is diagrammed in Figure 6.1. The arrangement of components differs among the various systems and this greatly influences the systems' performances. Some components are absent from certain systems. There are many variations of these systems and only the common ones will be discussed.

Because there is no clear separation of inspired and expired gases, when the inspiratory flow exceeds the fresh gas flow, some rebreathing will occur. The composition of the inspired mixture will depend on how much rebreathing takes place. A large number of studies to determine the fresh gas flow needed to prevent rebreathing with these systems have been performed. There is lack of agreement on the proper definition of rebreathing. Because of this and because variables such as minute ventilation, respiratory waveform, responsiveness to carbon dioxide, and physiological dead space may be unpredictable in anesthetized patients, recommendations for fresh gas flows should be viewed with caution. Monitoring of end-tidal CO_2 is the safest and most accurate approach to determine the optimal fresh gas flow.

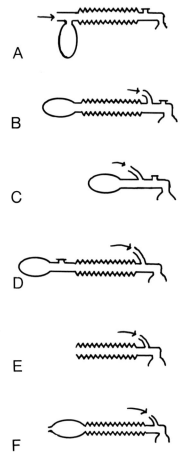

Figure 6.1. The Mapleson classification. Components include a reservoir bag, corrugated tubing, APL valve, fresh gas inlet, and patient connection. Redrawn from Mapleson WW. The elimination of rebreathing in various semiclosed anesthetic systems. Br J Anaesth 1954;26:323–332.

Mapleson A System

CONFIGURATIONS

Classic Form

The Mapleson A system (also called the Magill attachment or system) is shown diagrammatically in Figure 6.1A. It differs from the other Mapleson systems in that fresh gas does not enter the system near the patient connection, but near the reservoir bag at the other end of the system. A corrugated tubing connects the bag to the APL valve at the patient end of the system.

A sensor for a nondiverting respiratory gas monitor or the sampling site for a diverting monitor (see Chapter 16) may be placed between the APL valve and the corrugated tubing. In adults, it may be placed between the APL valve and the patient. In small patients, this location could result in excessive dead space. It could also be placed between the neck of the bag and its mount, between the bag and the corrugated tubing, or in the fresh gas supply tube, but in these locations the concentration shown on the monitor may differ substantially from the inspired concentration, especially during controlled ventilation.

Lack Modification (3,4)

The Lack modification of the Mapleson A system (Fig. 6.2) has an added "expiratory" limb, which runs from the patient connection to the APL valve at the machine end of the system. This makes it easier to adjust the valve and facilitates scavenging of excess gases.

The Lack system is available in both a dual tube (parallel) arrangement and a tube-within-a-tube (coaxial) configuration in which the expiratory limb runs concentrically inside the outer inspiratory limb. (5).

TECHNIQUES OF USE

For spontaneous ventilation, the APL valve is kept in the fully open position. Excess gas exits through it during the latter part of exhalation.

For controlled or assisted ventilation, intermittent positive pressure is applied to the bag. The APL valve is tightened so that when the bag is squeezed sufficient pressure is built up to inflate the lungs. The APL valve opens during inspiration.

FUNCTIONAL ANALYSIS

Spontaneous Respiration (6)

The sequence of events during the respiratory cycle using the Magill system with

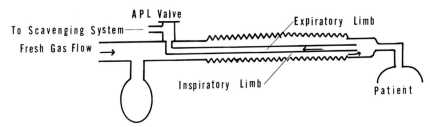

Figure 6.2. Lack modification of the Mapleson A system. The coaxial version is shown.

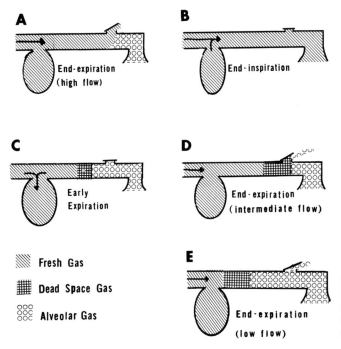

Figure 6.3. Magill system with spontaneous ventilation (see text for details). Redrawn from Kain ML, Nunn JF. Fresh gas economies of the Magill circuit. Anesthesiology 1968;29:964–974.

spontaneous ventilation is shown in Figure 6.3. As the patient exhales (*C*), first dead-space gas and then alveolar gas flow into the corrugated tubing toward the bag. At the same time, fresh gas flows into the bag. When the bag is full, the pressure in the system rises until the APL valve opens. The first gas vented will be alveolar gas. The remainder of exhalation—containing only alveolar gas— exhausts through the open valve. The continuing inflow of fresh gas reverses the flow of exhaled gases in the corrugated tubing. Some alveolar gas that had bypassed the APL valve now returns and exits through it. If the fresh gas flow is high (*A*), it will force the dead-space gas out also; if the fresh flow gas is intermediate (*D*), some dead-space gas will be retained in the system. If the fresh gas flow is low (*E*), alveolar gas will be retained.

At the start of inspiration, the first gas inhaled will be from dead space between the patient and the APL valve. The next gas will be either alveolar gas (if the fresh gas flow is low), exhaled dead-space gas (if the fresh gas flow is intermediate), or fresh gas (if the fresh gas flow is high) (see Fig. 6.3*B*).

If the fresh gas flow is so low that alveolar gas is reinhaled, the tidal volume or respiratory rate may increase, but this will not compensate because the increased volume of gas

A

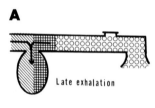

Late exhalation

B

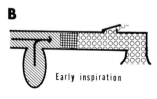

Early inspiration

C

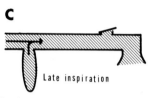

Late inspiration

Figure 6.4. Magill system with controlled ventilation (see text for details).

inhaled will contain more alveolar gas. Changes in respiratory flow pattern have been found to have no effect on rebreathing with the Mapleson A system (7). This analysis assumes little gas mixing. Placement of the APL valve at the point where alveolar and dead-space gas are separated is likely to disturb gas flow, resulting in mixing. It has been suggested that the geometrical arrangement of the Lack system allows better separation of gases before the APL valve is reached (8).

Investigators have found rebreathing to begin when the fresh gas flow is reduced to 56 to 82 ml/kg/min (8–14) or 60% to 75% of minute volume (6,15–18). When this critical flow is approached, normal variations in tidal volume and alveolar ventilation may cause a transient disparity between ventilatory requirements and the fresh gas flow. Should carbon dioxide accumulation occur, the patient will respond by increasing minute volume. This may set up a vicious circle, because increased ventilation will increase the fresh gas flow needed to prevent rebreathing. For this reason, it is suggested that the fresh gas flow be somewhat higher than the above values (19).

Studies comparing the Lack and Magill systems during spontaneous ventilation have found the Lack more efficient (8,16), equally efficient (13,20,21), and less efficient (17). Fresh gas flows of 51 to 85 mg/kg/min (8,13,20) and 51% to 88% of minute volume (16,20) have been recommended to avoid rebreathing with the Lack system.

Controlled or Assisted Ventilation

During controlled or assisted ventilation (Fig. 6.4), the pattern of gas flow changes. During exhalation (*A*), the pressure in the system will remain low and no gas will escape through the APL valve, unless the bag becomes distended. All exhaled gases, both dead space and alveolar, remain in the corrugated tubing, with alveolar gas nearest the patient. If the tidal volume is large, some alveolar gas may enter the bag (19).

At the start of inspiration (Fig. 6.4*B*), these exhaled gases flow to the patient. Because alveolar gases occupy the space nearest the patient, they will be inhaled first. As the pressure in the system rises, the APL valve opens so that gas both exits through the APL valve and continues to enter the patient. When all the exhaled gas has been driven from the tube, fresh gas reaches the APL valve and the patient (*C*). Some enters the patient but some is lost through the valve. Thus during controlled ventilation, some rebreathing of alveolar gases occurs and some fresh gas is wasted. The composition of the inspired gas mixture depends on the respiratory pattern (19,22). The system becomes more efficient as the expiratory phase is prolonged.

Most investigators believe that the Mapleson A is an illogical system to use for controlled ventilation and should not be used without a method to monitor expired carbon dioxide concentrations.

HAZARDS

A mechanical ventilator that relieves excess gases should not be used with this system, because the entire system then becomes dead space. The ventilators found on most anesthesia machines in the United States are unsuitable.

Earlier models of the Lack system had too small an inspiratory limb (23). This has been corrected (19,24).

A case has been reported in which a Lack circuit was incorrectly manufactured so that the inner expiratory tube that should have been connected to the APL valve was connected to the reservoir bag (25). This converted the entire tubing into dead space.

Misassembly of the Lack system so that the fresh gas inlet was mounted adjacent to the APL valve rather than the reservoir bag has been reported (26). This would result in a great increase in dead space. This problem has reportedly been corrected (27).

TESTS OF THE MAPLESON A SYSTEMS

The Mapleson A system is tested by occluding the patient end of the system, closing the APL valve, and pressurizing the system. Maintenance of the pressure confirms the integrity of the system. Opening the APL valve will confirm proper functioning of that component. In addition, the user or a patient should breathe through the system.

The coaxial Lack modification requires additional testing to confirm the integrity of the inner tube. One suggested method is to attach a tracheal tube to the inner tubing at the patient end of the system (28). Blowing down the tube with the APL valve closed will produce movement of the bag if there is leakage between the two limbs. Another method is to occlude both limbs at the patient connection with the APL valve open, then squeeze the bag (29). If there is a leak in the inner limb, the bag will collapse and gas will escape through the APL valve.

Mapleson B System

The Mapleson B system is shown in Figure 6.1*B*. The fresh gas inlet and APL valve are both located near the patient connection port. The reservoir bag is at the distal end of the system, separated from the fresh gas inlet by corrugated tubing. The sensor or sampling site for the respiratory gas analyzer can be placed between the corrugated tubing and the fresh gas inlet. It may also be placed in the fresh gas supply tube or, in adults, between the fresh gas inlet and the APL valve.

TECHNIQUES OF USE

To use the Mapleson B system with spontaneous respirations, the APL valve is opened completely. Excess gas is vented through the valve during exhalation.

Assisted or controlled ventilation is accomplished by tightening the APL valve sufficiently to allow the lungs to be inflated. Excess gases are vented during inspiration.

FUNCTIONAL ANALYSIS

Spontaneous Respiration

As the patient exhales, dead-space gas will pass down the corrugated tubing, along with fresh gas. At the end of exhalation, the part of the tube near the patient will be filled with fresh gas and some alveolar gas. When the bag reaches full capacity, the APL valve opens and both fresh gas and alveolar gas will exit from the system. When the patient begins to inspire, the APL valve closes and the patient inhales fresh gas and gas from the corrugated tubing. No gas should be inhaled from the bag if the volume of the corrugated tubing exceeds the tidal volume.

The amount of rebreathing will depend on the fresh gas flow. To avoid rebreathing completely, the fresh gas flow must be equal to peak inspiratory flow rate (normally 20 to 25 liters/min) (30). A fresh gas flow more than double minute volume has been recommended (1,30), but flows as low as 0.8 to 1.2 times minute volume may be sufficient (19).

Controlled or Assisted Ventilation

The behavior of the Mapleson B system during controlled or assisted ventilation is similar to that of the Mapleson A, but it is slightly more efficient because fresh gas accumulates at the patient end of the tubing during the expiratory pause (19,30). Because the composition of inspired gas is greatly influenced by the ventilatory pattern, this system has variable performance during controlled ventilation (19). A fresh gas flow of 2 to 2.5 times minute volume has been recommended (19,30,31).

Mapleson C System

The Mapleson C system is identical to the Mapleson B system except that the corrugated tubing is omitted (see Fig. 6.1C).

TECHNIQUES OF USE

Use of this system is similar to that described for the Mapleson B system.

FUNCTIONAL ANALYSIS

The Mapleson C system behaves similarly to the Mapleson B system. A fresh gas flow of 2 times minute volume has been recommended during spontaneous ventilation. During controlled ventilation, fresh gas flow should be 2 to 2.5 times minute volume (19,32).

Mapleson D System

The Mapleson D, E, and F systems all have a T piece near the patient and function similarly. The T piece is a three-way tubular connector with a patient connection port, a port for the fresh gas, and a port for connec-

tion to corrugated tubing. The Mapleson D system is popular because scavenging of excess gases is relatively easy and it is the most efficient of the Mapleson systems during controlled ventilation.

CONFIGURATION

Classic Form

The Mapleson D system is shown in Figures 6.1D and 6.5. The T piece with fresh gas inlet is at the patient end. A length of corrugated tubing connects the T piece to the APL valve and the reservoir bag adjacent to it. The length of the tubing has no importance as long as the volume of the tube and reservoir bag exceeds the patient's tidal volume (33), but it does determine the distance the user can be from the patient.

The sensor or sampling site for a respiratory gas monitor may be placed between the bag and its mount, between the corrugated tubing and the T piece, or between the corrugated tubing and the APL valve. In adults, it may be placed between the T piece and the patient connection port.

In the Bain modification, the fresh gas supply tube runs coaxially inside the corrugated tubing. This decreases the bulk of the system. The outer tubing of most commercially available versions of the Bain system is narrower than conventional corrugated tubing (19).

The Bain modification is available with a metal head with channels drilled into it (Fig. 6.6). This provides a fixed position for the reservoir bag and APL valve, and attachment of corrugated tubing. Some heads also have a pressure manometer.

Positive end expiratory pressure devices have been used with the Mapleson D system. A bidirectional PEEP valve may be placed between the corrugated tubing and the APL valve (35). This permits PEEP to be admin-

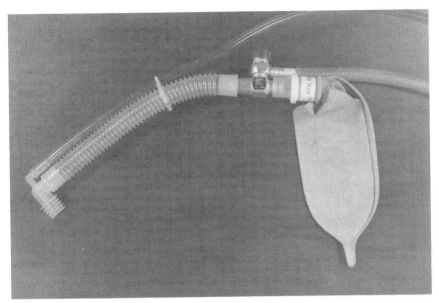

Figure 6.5.   Mapleson D system. A tube leading to the scavenging system is attached to the APL valve.

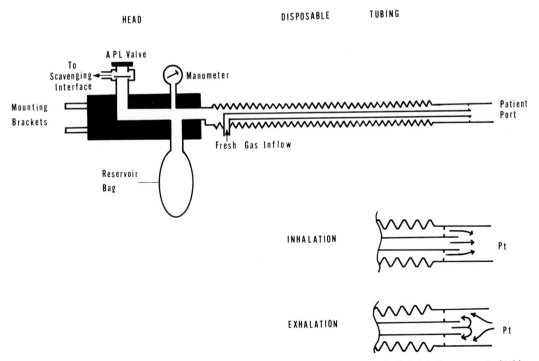

Figure 6.6.   Bain modification of the Mapleson D system. The fresh gas supply tube is inside the corrugated tubing.

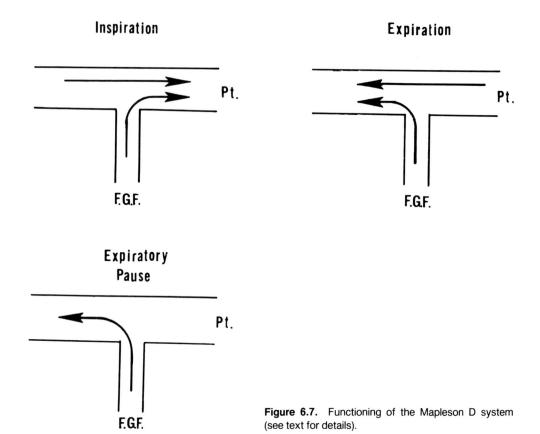

Figure 6.7. Functioning of the Mapleson D system (see text for details).

istered during manually or mechanically controlled ventilation. However, some PEEP valves will close when a negative pressure is applied. Spontaneous breathing is impossible with such a valve in the system. To eliminate this danger the PEEP valve may be placed in the hose leading to the anesthesia ventilator. In this location it will be effective only during mechanical ventilation. A unidirectional PEEP valve can be used at the bag attachment site using special connectors and unidirectional valves (36). Such an arrangement allows application of PEEP during spontaneous or mechanical but not manual ventilation (35,37,38).

TECHNIQUES OF USE

For spontaneous respirations, the APL valve is left completely open and excess gases are discharged during expiration.

Manually controlled or assisted ventilation is performed by partially closing the APL valve and squeezing the bag. Mechanically controlled ventilation is achieved by connecting the hose of an anesthesia ventilator in place of the reservoir bag and closing the APL valve. Excess gases are vented through the ventilator.

FUNCTIONAL ANALYSIS

Spontaneous Breathing

During exhalation (Fig. 6.7), exhaled gases mix with fresh gases and move through the corrugated tube away from the patient toward the bag. After the bag has filled, the mixture exits via the APL valve. During the expiratory pause, fresh gas flows down the corrugated tubing, pushing exhaled gases in front of it.

During inspiration, the patient will inhale gas from the fresh gas inlet and the corrugated tubing. If the fresh gas flow is high, all the gas drawn from the corrugated tube will be fresh gas. If the fresh gas flow is low, some exhaled gas containing CO_2 will be reinhaled. The ventilatory pattern may help to determine the amount of rebreathing (39). Factors that tend to decrease rebreathing include a high inspiratory:expiratory time ratio, a slow rise in inspiratory flow rate, a low flow rate during the last part of exhalation, and a long expiratory pause (7,40–42).

As gas containing CO_2 is reinhaled, the end-tidal CO_2 will rise. If the patient's spontaneous respiration then increases, the end-tidal CO_2 will fall while inspired CO_2 will increase (43). Provided rebreathing is not extreme, a normal end-tidal CO_2 can be achieved but only at the cost of increased work on the part of the patient. The end-tidal CO_2 tends to reach a plateau. At that point, no matter how hard the patient works, the end-tidal CO_2 cannot be lowered further (44). If the patient's respiration is depressed, end-tidal CO_2 will rise further (43). Patient responsiveness and stimulation have varied widely among studies, so it should not be surprising that recommendations for fresh gas flows also differ considerably.

Minute Volume

End-tidal CO_2 depends on both the ratio of minute volume and fresh gas flow and their absolute values (43,45). If expired volume is greater than fresh gas flow, end-tidal CO_2 will be determined mainly by fresh gas flow. If fresh gas flow is greater than minute volume, end-tidal CO_2 will be determined mainly by minute volume.

Most studies have recommended that the fresh gas flow be 1.5 to 3.0 times the minute volume to prevent significant rebreathing (2,17,20,21,46–49). However, one study in anesthetized patients showed that rebreathing was usually small if the fresh gas flow equaled minute volume (50).

Body Weight

Recommendations include 100 ml/kg (51), greater than 150 ml/kg (8,9,14), and 200 to 300 ml/kg (20,45,52).

Body Surface Area

Fresh gas flows of 4000 to 4700 ml/m^2/min have been recommended (52,53).

Flows higher than recommended should be used (or ventilation controlled) in patients with an increase in carbon dioxide production (fever and hyperalimentation), those with an increased dead space (including mask ventilation), and patients with decreased minute ventilation (44,53).

Controlled Ventilation

During exhalation, gases flow from the patient down the corrugated tubing. At the same time, a steady flow of fresh gas enters the tubing. During the expiratory pause, the fresh gas flow continues and pushes the exhaled gases down the tubing. During inspiration, fresh gas and gas from the corrugated tubing enter the patient. Thus most of the fresh gas enters the patient.

If the fresh gas flow is low, some expired gases may be forced back through the corrugated tubing. Prolonging the inspiratory time, increasing the respiratory rate, or adding an inspiratory plateau all increase rebreathing (41,54). Rebreathing can be decreased by allowing a long expiratory pause so that the fresh gas flow can flush exhaled gases from the tubing.

In analyzing the performance of these systems with controlled ventilation, two relationships become evident (44,55). (*i*) When the fresh gas flow is very high, the patient does not rebreathe exhaled gases and the end-tidal CO_2 is determined by minute ventilation (56). (*ii*) When the minute volume substantially exceeds the fresh gas flow, the fresh gas flow is the controlling factor for carbon dioxide elimination. The higher the fresh gas flow, the lower the end-tidal CO_2.

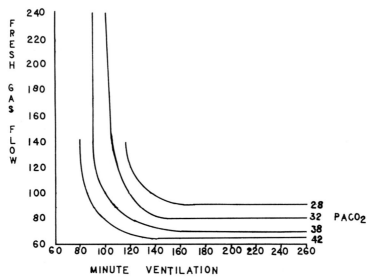

Figure 6.8.   Mapleson D system used with controlled ventilation. Each isopleth represents a constant level of $PaCO_2$. Note that essentially the same $PaCO_2$ is achieved for fresh gas flows from 100 to 240 ml/kg/min. Redrawn from Froese AB. Anesthesia circuits for children (ASA Refresher Course). Park Ridge, IL: ASA, 1978.

Combining fresh gas flow, minute volume and arterial CO_2 levels, a graph can be constructed (Fig. 6.8). An infinite number of combinations of fresh gas flow and minute volume can be chosen to produce a given $PaCO_2$. One can use high fresh gas flows and low minute volumes or high minute volumes and low fresh gas flows or combinations in between. In Figure 6.8, at the left, with a high fresh gas flow, the circuit is a nonrebreathing one and end-tidal CO_2 depends only on ventilation. Such high flows are uneconomical and associated with heat loss and low humidity. End-tidal CO_2 becomes dependent on minute volume, which is difficult to adjust accurately, especially in small children (44). On the right is the region of hyperventilation and partial rebreathing. End-tidal CO_2 is regulated by adjusting the fresh gas flow. Lower fresh gas flows (and increased rebreathing) are associated with higher humidity, less heat loss, and greater economy of fresh gases. Hyperventilation can be used without inducing hypocarbia. Individual differences in dead space:tidal volume are minimized at high levels of minute volume (44). For these rea-

sons, it would seem advantageous in most cases to aim for the right side of the graph. Exceptions might be patients with stiff lungs, poor cardiac performance, or hypovolemia.

Formulas to predict fresh gas flow requirements have been based on body weight (44,57–62), minute volume (44,63) and body surface area (64). Slightly higher fresh gas flows should be used when respiration is assisted (65). In many of the studies, emphasis has been placed on the prevention of rebreathing rather than carbon dioxide retention. With controlled ventilation, normocarbia or hypocarbia may be achieved despite the occurrence of considerable rebreathing. Frequently, the inspired carbon dioxide concentration will be above zero. Increases in CO_2 production, minute volume, and dead space will increase the fresh gas flow requirements. Because of the many factors involved, it is suggested that monitoring of end-tidal CO_2 always be performed.

HAZARDS OF THE BAIN SYSTEM

Special hazards are associated with the Bain system. The system should not be used with an intermittent-flow machine unless the machine is set for continuous flow (66,67). If the inner tube becomes detached from its connections or develops a leak at the machine end (68–71), or the fresh gas supply tube becomes kinked or twisted (72–74), the entire exhalation limb becomes dead space. Incorrect assembly can also cause this (75).

An incident of improper assembly has been reported in which the large bore tubing was connected to the common gas outlet of the anesthesia machine and the small bore tube was attached to the APL valve (76). High inflation pressures were needed for ventilation.

In departments that use both a Bain circuit and other circuits such as the Mapleson A, a conventional wide-bore tubing may be attached to the system (77). This will result in total rebreathing. Another problem is that two standard length coaxial tubings may be connected together (78).

High inflation pressures may result in opening of the safety-relief valve on the ventilator, resulting in a leak (79,80).

TESTING BEFORE USE

The Mapleson D System is tested for leaks by occluding the patient end, closing the APL valve, and pressurizing the system. If there is no leak, the pressure will be maintained. The APL valve is then opened. The bag should deflate easily if the valve and scavenging system are working properly (81). In addition, either the user or a patient should breathe through the system to detect any obstructions.

The Bain modification of the Mapleson D requires special testing to confirm the integrity of the inner tubing. This can be performed by setting a low flow of oxygen on a flowmeter and occluding the inner tube (with a finger or the barrel of a small syringe) at the patient end while observing the flowmeter indicator. If the inner tube is intact and correctly connected, the indicator will fall (82,83).

The integrity of the inner tube can also be confirmed by activating the oxygen flush and observing the bag (84). A Venturi effect caused by the oxygen flow at the patient end will create a negative pressure in the outer exhalation tubing, and this will cause the bag to deflate. If the inner tube is not intact, this maneuver will cause the bag to inflate slightly. However, this test would not expose a faulty Bain system in which the inner tube was omitted or did not extend to the patient port or one that had holes at the patient end of the inner tube (85–87).

CONTINUOUS POSITIVE AIRWAY PRESSURE

In the operating room, application of continuous positive airway pressure (CPAP) to the up (nondependent, unventilated) lung is often used to enhance oxygenation during one-lung ventilation. This can be accomplished by attaching a Mapleson D system to the lumen of tube leading that lung.

A number of configurations have been suggested in the literature (88–99). One is shown in Figure 6.9. A source of oxygen is connected to the system and set to deliver 1 to 2 liters/min. The APL valve is set so that the desired pressure, which is read from the manometer, is maintained. A PEEP valve may be added to function as a high-pressure pop-off safety device (100). Another arrangement is shown in Figure 6.10. A PEEP valve is connected to one end of a corrugated tube. A source of oxygen is connected at the other end.

Mapleson E (T Piece) System

Use of the Mapleson E system for anesthesia has decreased because of difficulties in scavenging excess gases, but it is still commonly used to administer oxygen or humidified gas to an intubated patient breathing spontaneously.

The Mapleson E system is shown in Figure 6.1E. A length of tubing may be attached to the T piece to form a reservoir. The expiratory port is sometimes enclosed in a plastic

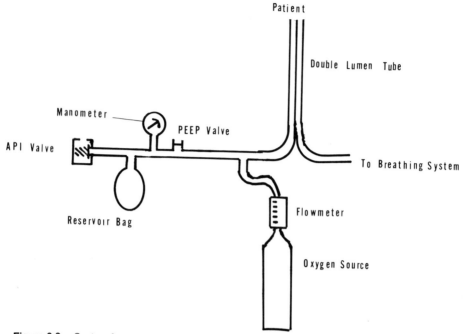

Figure 6.9.   System for continuous positive airway pressure. The PEEP valve is added for safety.

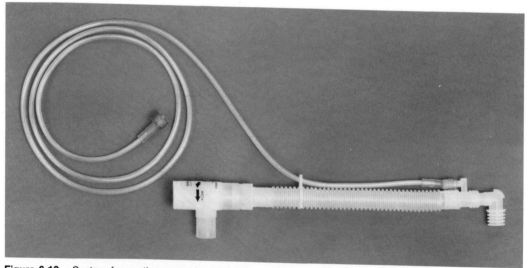

Figure 6.10.   System for continuous positive airway pressure. The elbow connection at right is connected to the lumen of the double-lumen tube leading to the up lung. The amount of CPAP is determined by the PEEP valve at the left. Courtesy of Vital Signs, Inc.

chamber from which excess gases are evacuated.

The sensor or sampling site for the respiratory gas monitor may be placed between the expiratory port and the expiratory tubing. In larger patients, it may be placed be-

tween the T piece and the patient, but this should be avoided in small patients because it increases dead space.

Numerous modifications of the original T piece have been made. Many have the fresh gas inlet extending inside the body of the T piece toward the patient connection to minimize dead space. A pressure-limiting device may be added to the system.

TECHNIQUES OF USE

For spontaneous ventilation, the expiratory limb is left open. Controlled ventilation can be performed by intermittently occluding the expiratory limb and letting the fresh gas flow inflate the lungs. Satisfactory assisted respiration is difficult to achieve.

FUNCTIONAL ANALYSIS

The sequence of events during the respiratory cycle is similar to that of the Mapleson D system shown in Figure 6.7. The presence or absence and the amount of rebreathing or air dilution will depend on the fresh gas flow, the patient's minute volume, the volume of the exhalation limb, the type of ventilation (spontaneous or controlled) and the respiratory pattern (101).

Rebreathing

With spontaneous ventilation, if there is no exhalation limb, no rebreathing can occur. If there is an expiratory limb, the fresh gas flow needed to prevent rebreathing will be the same as for the Mapleson D system.

During controlled ventilation, there can be no rebreathing, because only fresh gas will inflate the lungs.

Air Dilution

No air dilution can occur during controlled ventilation. During spontaneous ventilation air dilution cannot occur if the volume of the exhalation tubing is greater than the patient's tidal volume. If there is no expiratory limb or if the volume of the expiratory limb is less than the patient's tidal volume, air dilution can be prevented by providing a fresh gas flow that exceeds the peak inspiratory flow rate, normally 3 to 5 times the minute volume. A fresh gas flow of 2 times minute volume and a reservoir volume one-third of the tidal volume will prevent air dilution (102).

HAZARDS OF BAROTRAUMA WITH THE T PIECE SYSTEM

Controlling ventilation by intermittently occluding the expiratory limb may lead to overinflation and barotrauma (103). This is particularly a danger with this system because the user does not have the "feel" of inflation that he or she has with a system containing a bag, the pressure-buffering effect of the bag is absent, and there is no APL valve. To overcome this potential hazard, it has been recommended that a pressure-limiting device be placed in the system (104–108).

Mapleson F System (109)

The Mapleson F system also is called the Jackson-Rees, the Rees system, or the Jackson-Rees modification of the T piece system. It has a bag with a mechanism for venting excess gases on the exhalation limb (Fig. 6.1*F*). The mechanism is most commonly a hole in the tail of the bag. It may be fitted with a device to prevent the bag from collapsing while at the same time allowing excess gases to escape. Alternately, the hole may be in the side of the bag so the user can place his or her finger over it. An anesthesia ventilator may be used in place of the bag (110).

Scavenging can be performed by enclosing the bag in a plastic chamber from which waste gases are suctioned or by attaching various devices to the relief mechanism in the bag.

TECHNIQUES OF USE

For spontaneous respiration the relief mechanism is left fully open. For assisted or controlled respiration the relief mechanism is occluded sufficiently to distend the bag. This may result in some positive end expiratory pressure (111). Respirations can then be controlled or assisted by squeezing the bag. Alternately, the hole in the bag can be occluded by the user's finger during inspiration. If it is desired to use a mechanical ventilator, the bag is replaced by the hose from the ventilator.

FUNCTIONAL ANALYSIS

The Mapleson F system functions much like the Mapleson D system. The flows required to prevent rebreathing during spontaneous and controlled respiration are the same as those required with the Mapleson D system. Two authors have found higher carbon dioxide levels with manually than with mechanically controlled ventilation (112,113).

PEEP does not affect end-tidal carbon dioxide during controlled respiration but causes an increase during spontaneous breathing when fresh gas flows are less than three times minute volume (114). PEEP should not be applied using an underwater seal (115).

HAZARDS

The hazards of the Mapleson F system are the same as those described for the Mapleson E system. Excessive pressure is somewhat less likely to develop, because there is a bag in the system.

Combination Systems

None of the above-described systems is ideal for every situation. Some systems are better for spontaneous breathing and others are more efficient with controlled ventilation. When comparing the systems during spontaneous ventilation, the relative order of merit is A, D, F, E (with an expiratory limb), C, and B. During controlled ventilation, the order becomes D, F, E (with an expiratory limb), B, C, and A. In an attempt to develop a universal system a number of combination systems have been introduced.

HUMPHREY ADE SYSTEM (116)

Description of Equipment

The ADE system can be used in different configurations. In the A configuration, it is similar to the Lack variation of the Mapleson A system. In the D configuration, it resembles the Bain modification of the Mapleson D system. It also allows the APL valve to be bypassed in the D configuration so that it resembles the Mapleson E system.

The system is shown in Figure 6.11. It is available in both coaxial and noncoaxial versions. It has two levers whose positions determine the functioning of the system. A self-locking mechanism prevents accidental displacement of either lever from its selected position. In the coaxial version, the expiratory tubing runs concentrically inside the inspiratory limb. In the noncoaxial version, the two tubes are held together by a metal bridge at the machine end.

The inspiratory limb consists of a fresh gas inlet, a reservoir bag with a lever, and a length of corrugated tubing that runs to the patient connection port. When the lever is vertical, gases can flow in and out of the bag. When the lever is horizontal, gas flow into the bag is blocked, making the inspiratory limb a simple tube.

The expiratory limb consists of a length of tubing running from the patient connection, an APL valve, a valve bypass outlet, and a lever that directs the flow of gases through either the APL valve or valve bypass outlet. When the lever is vertical, the gases pass through the APL valve. When it is horizontal, the APL valve is isolated and gases flow through the valve-bypass outlet. Both outlets have 30-mm external diameters for attachment of scavenging devices. The valve-by-pass outlet also has a 22-mm internal diameter for attachment of a hose leading to a ventilator or reservoir bag. A pressure-limiting device may be fitted near the APL valve (11).

A single-lever Humphrey ADE system has been developed (11). It is also available in coaxial and parallel forms. The lever controls a single rotating cylinder that passes through both the inspiratory and expiratory limbs. When the lever is upright, the reservoir bag and APL valve are in circuit, and the valve bypass outlet is excluded. When the lever is turned down, the bag and APL valve are ex-

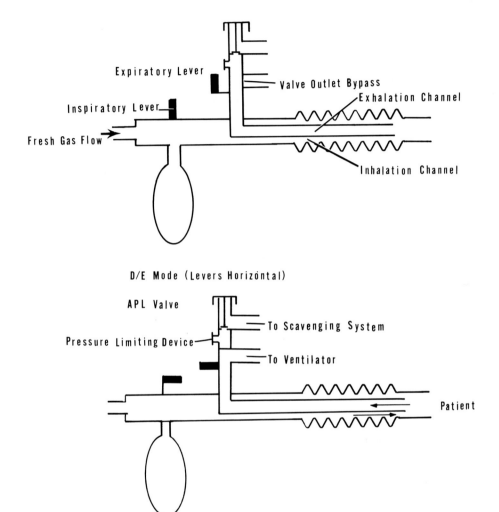

A Mode (Levers Vertical)

Expiratory Lever

Valve Outlet Bypass

Exhalation Channel

Inspiratory Lever

Fresh Gas Flow

Inhalation Channel

D/E Mode (Levers Horizóntal)

APL Valve

To Scavenging System

Pressure Limiting Device

To Ventilator

Patient

Bag

Figure 6.11. Humphrey ADE system. The dual-lever coaxial version is shown.

cluded from the system, and the valve bypass outlet is connected into the system.

Techniques of Use

To use the system in the A mode (for spontaneous ventilation), both levers (or the lever in the single-lever version) are placed vertical and the APL valve is left open (Fig. 6.11, *top*). The ventilator hose can be left connected and ready for use, because it will be excluded when the levers are vertical. If manual ventilation is desired, the bag is squeezed and the leak is controlled by adjusting the APL valve. However, this system should not be used very long in this manner, as the Mapleson A system is very inefficient with controlled ventilation.

To use the system in the D/E mode (for controlled ventilation), both levers are moved to the horizontal position (Fig. 6.11, *bottom*). For the single-lever version, the lever is turned downward. If mechanical ventilation is desired, the hose from a ventilator is attached to the valve-bypass outlet. Excess gases are scavenged through the ventilator. The APL valve does not need to be closed because it is bypassed.

To use manual ventilation in the D/E mode, a length of flexible tubing with a bag is attached to the valve bypass outlet. The bag is squeezed to ventilate the patient. The leak is adjusted by rotating the expiratory lever between vertical and horizontal with the APL valve fully open.

To use spontaneous ventilation in the D/E mode, the expiratory lever is placed horizontal and the valve-bypass outlet is connected to the scavenging system.

Functional Analysis

A Mode

When placed in the A mode, the system functions like the Lack modification of the Mapleson A. Mean fresh gas flows ranging from 46 to 56 ml/kg/min have been found to prevent rebreathing (10,11,116,117). If the APL valve is excluded by placing the expiratory lever horizontal, dead-space gas can escape without hindrance at the beginning of expiration, so the system is less efficient and fresh gas flows need to be increased up to one-third (116).

If the ADE system is used in the A mode with controlled ventilation, it is more efficient than the Magill (118) (but still very inefficient).

D or E mode

For spontaneous ventilation, one-third of the fresh gas flow necessary for a Mapleson F system is required (116). The only difference between the ADE system in the D configuration and the Bain are the positions of the inspiratory and expiratory tubes. Most studies have found that when controlled ventilation is used with the system in the D mode, fresh gas flow requirements are similar to

those of the Mapleson D (117,119,120), although one study has found the Bain system to be more efficient (121).

Hazards

With the dual-lever system, incorrect positioning or accidental displacement of the expiratory lever from a vertical to a horizontal position or obstruction of the expiratory port in the A mode may result in a dangerous rise in pressure (122, 123).

If a ventilator is used and the sensor for the low airway pressure monitor is in the inspiratory limb, the alarm may fail to provide a warning if there is a disconnection (124).

THE MULTICIRCUIT SYSTEM (125)

The multicircuit system (Fig. 6.12) is available in both dual-tube and coaxial versions. It has a single lever for switching between modes. A lock prevents the lever from being moved accidentally. The inspiratory part of the system, which receives the fresh gas flow, has a bag mount for the A mode. Gas flows from this part through a corrugated tube to the patient. The expiratory portion, which receives gas from the patient, has connections for a pressure-limiting valve and a hose to a ventilator.

In the A mode (selector control lever down), the reservoir bag is connected into the system. On the expiratory side, gas flow is directed through the APL valve. The ventilator is excluded from the system.

When the selector control is set to the D/E position, the bag is excluded from the inspiratory side of the circuit. The APL valve and the ventilator are both connected into the system on the expiratory side. The APL valve must be closed when the ventilator is used. If manual ventilation is desired, a bag is attached at the ventilator connection and the APL valve adjusted to provide adequate ventilation.

An evaluation of this system in the A mode found its function comparable to that of the Magill system (126–128). Studies on anesthetized patients using the dual-tube

A   Mode (Spontantaneous Ventilation)

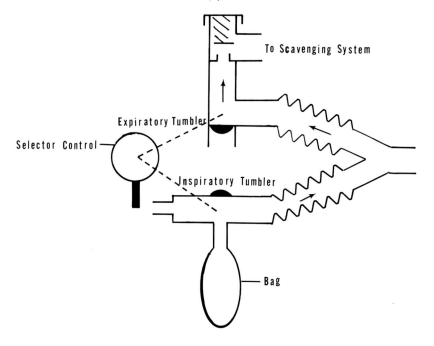

D/E Mode (Controlled Ventilation)

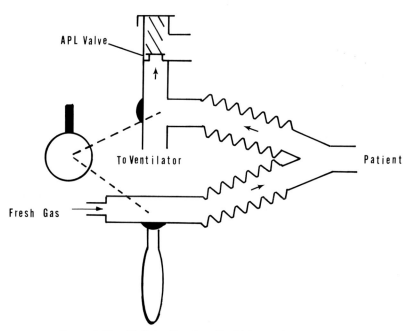

Figure 6.12.   Multicircuit system. Dual-tube version.

unit showed that a normal $PaCO_2$ could be achieved with a fresh gas flow of 70 ml/kg in both the A and D modes, provided the patient's CO_2 response was not compromised.

Respiratory Gas Monitoring and the Mapleson Systems

All the Mapleson systems except the A have the fresh gas inlet near the patient connection port. For this reason it may be difficult to get a reliable sample of exhaled gases. One study examined four sampling sites (Fig. 6.13): at the junction of the breathing system and elbow connector, at the corner of the elbow connector, 2 cm distal in the elbow connector and in the tracheal tube connector (129). It was found that if sampling were carried out at the two sites closest to the patient, values were accurate. Significant errors were noted when samples were taken from the corner of the elbow connector, but only if a high fresh gas flow was used. Significant errors were noted when sampling was performed at the junction of the breathing system and elbow connector even if low fresh gas flows were used.

In another study involving infants and children, sampling at the junction of the tracheal tube and breathing system resulted in falsely low end-tidal CO_2 values in patients weighing less than 8 kg (54). The accuracy of measurements can be improved by insertion of a small heat and moisture exchanger between the breathing system and the tracheal tube connector (130)

Advantages of the Mapleson Systems

1. The equipment is simple and inexpensive.

2. All parts can be disassembled and disinfected or sterilized in a variety of ways.

3. The equipment is rugged. With the ex-

ception of the APL valve, there are no moving parts.

4. The Mapleson systems provide a buffering effect so that variations in minute volume affect end-tidal CO_2 less than in a circle system or nonrebreathing circuit (20).

5. Rebreathing will result in retention of heat and moisture. In coaxial systems (Lack, Bain, Humphrey ADE) the inspiratory limb is heated by the warm exhaled gas in the coaxial expiratory tubing (131,132).

6. Resistance to airflow is usually within the recommended ranges at flows likely to be experienced in normal clinical practice (133). A commonly held view is that the work of breathing during spontaneous ventilation is significantly less with these systems than with the circle system. However, studies indicate this is not always the case (134–137) The work of breathing will be increased if the APL valve is not oriented properly (135).

7. These systems are lightweight and not bulky. They are not likely to cause excessive drag on the mask or tracheal tube, facial distortion, or accidental extubation. They are easy to position conveniently. A long Mapleson D system may be used to provide oxygenation and ventilation for a patient undergoing MRI (138). The APL valve should be made from aluminum.

Disadvantages of the Mapleson Systems

1. These systems require high gas flows. This results in higher costs, loss of heat and humidity, increased atmospheric pollution and difficulties in assessment of spontaneous ventilation.

2. The optimum fresh gas flow may be difficult to determine. It is necessary to change the flow when going from spontaneous to controlled ventilation or vice versa.

3. Anything that causes the fresh gas flow to be lowered presents a hazard, because dangerous rebreathing may occur. This has been

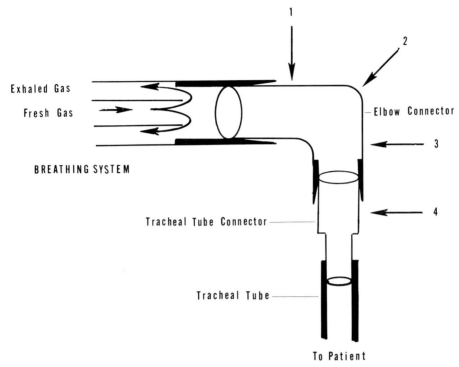

Figure 6.13.   Respiratory gas sampling with a Mapleson system. Accurate values for expiratory concentrations can be obtained by sampling at sites 3 and 4. Sampling at site 2 will yield accurate values only if the fresh gas flow is not high. Sampling at site 1 will yield inaccurate values even at low fresh gas flows. Redrawn from Gravenstein N, Lampotang S, Beneken JEW. Factors influencing capnography in the Bain circuit. J Clin Monit 1985;1:6–10.

reported with emptying of a nitrous oxide tank (139), loss of gas through a loose vaporizer filler cap (140,141), and a leak in a humidification device (142).

4. In the Mapleson A, B, and C systems the APL valve is located close to the patient where it may be inaccessible to the user. In addition, scavenging is difficult to perform. This disadvantage can be overcome by using the Lack modification of the Mapleson A.

5. The Mapleson E and F systems are difficult to scavenge and air dilution can occur with the Mapleson E system.

6. Mapleson systems are not suitable for patients with malignant hyperthermia, because it may not be possible to increase the fresh gas flow enough to remove the increased carbon dioxide load (143).

REFERENCES

1. Mapleson WW. The elimination of rebreathing in various semiclosed anaesthetic systems. Br J Anaesth 1954;26:323–332.
2. Willis BA, Pender JWM, Mapleson WW. Rebreathing in a T-piece: volunteer and theoretical studies of the Jackson-Rees modification of Ayre's T-piece during spontaneous respiration. Br J Anaesth 1975;47:1239–1246.
3. Lack JA. Pollution control by co-axial circuits. Anaesthesia 1976;31:561–562.
4. Lack JA. Theatre pollution control. Anaesthesia 1976;31:259–262.
5. Robinson DA, Lack JA. The Lack parallel breathing system. Anaesth 1985;40:1236–1237.
6. Kain ML, Nunn JF. Fresh gas economies of the Magill circuit. Anesthesiology 1968;29:964–974.
7. Jonsson LO, Zetterstrom H. Influence of the respiratory flow pattern on rebreathing in Mapleson

A and D circuits. Acta Anaesthesiol Scand 1987;31:174–178.

8. Humphrey D. The Lack, Magill and Bain anaesthetic breathing systems: a direct comparison in spontaneously-breathing anesthetized adults. J R Soc Med 1982;75:513–524.

9. Alexander JP. Clinical comparison of the Bain and Magill Anaesthetic systems during spontaneous respiration. Br J Anaesth 1982;54:1031–1036.

10. Dixon J, Charabarti MK, Morgan M. An assessment of the Humphrey ADE anaesthetic system in the Mapleson A mode during spontaneous ventilation. Anaesthesia 1984;39:593–596.

11. Humphrey D, Brock-Utne JG, Downing JW. Single lever Humphrey A.D.E. low flow universal anaesthetic breathing system. Can Anaesth Soc J 1986;33:698–709.

12. Millar SW, Barnes PK, Soni N. Comparison of the Magill and Lack anaesthetic breathing systems in anaesthetized patients. Br J Anaesth 1987;59:930P.

13. Millar SW, Barnes PK, Soni N, Tennant R. Comparison of the Magill and Lack anaesthetic breathing systems in anaesthetized patients. Br J Anaesth 1989;62:153–158.

14. Ungerer MJ. A comparison between the Bain and Magill anaesthetic systems during spontaneous breathing. Can Anaesth Soc J 1978;25:122–124.

15. Soni N, Ooi R, Pattison J. Rebreathing in the Magill breathing system. Br J Anaesth 1992;69:215P–216P.

16. Ooi R, Pattison J, Soni N. Parallel Lack breathing system: fresh gas flow requirements during spontaneous ventilation. Br J Anaesth 1992;69:216P.

17. Chan ASH, Bruce WE, Soni N. A comparison of anaesthetic breathing systems during spontaneous ventilation. An in-vitro study using a lung model. Anaesthesia 1989;44:194–199.

18. Miller DM, Couper JL. Comparison of the fresh gas flow requirements and resistance of the preferential flow system with those of the Magill system. Br J Anaesth 1983;55:569–574.

19. Conway CM. Anaesthetic breathing systems. Br J Anaesth 1985;57:649–657.

20. Jonsson LO, Zetterstrom H. Fresh gas flow in coaxial Mapleson A and D circuits during spontaneous breathing. Acta Anaesthesiol Scand 1986;30:588–593.

21. Nott MR, Walters FJM, Norman J. The Lack and Bain systems in spontaneous respiration. Anaesth Intensive Care 1982;10:333–339.

22. Tyler CKG, Barnes PK, Rafferty MP. Controlled ventilation with a Mapleson A (Magill) breathing system: reassessment using a lung model. Br J Anaesth 1989;62:462–466.

23. Barnes PK, Seeley HF, Gothard JWW, Conway CM. The Lack anaesthetic system. Anaesthesia 1976;31:1248–1253.

24. Norman JF, Nott M, Walters F. Performance of the Lack circuit. Anaesthesia 1977;32:673.

25. Muir J, Davidson-Lamb R. Apparatus failure; cause for concern. Br J Anaesth 1980;52:705–706.

26. Jones PL. Hazard: single-use parallel Lack breathing system. Anaesthesia 1991;46:316–317.

27. Williams SK. Hazard: single-use parallel Lack breathing system. A reply. Anaesthesia 1991;46:317.

28. Furst B, Laffey DA. An alternative test for the Lack system. Anaesthesia 1984;39:834.

29. Martin LVH, McKeown DW. An alternative test for the Lack system. Anaesthesia 1985;40:80–81.

30. Sykes MK. Rebreathing circuits. Br J Anaesth 1968;40:666–674.

31. Christensen KN, Thomsen A, Hansen OL, Jorgensen S. Flow requirements in the Hafnia modification of the Mapleson circuits during spontaneous respiration. Acta Anaesthesiol Scand 1978;22:27–32.

32. Christensen KN. The flow requirement in a nonpolluting Mapleson C circuit. Acta Anaesthesiol Scand 1976;20:307–312.

33. Bain JA, Spoerel WE. Low flow anesthesia utilizing a single limb circuit. In: Aldrete JA, Lowe JH, Virtue RW, eds. Low Flow and Closed System Anesthesia. New York: Grune & Stratton, 1979:151–164.

34. Bain JA, Spoerel WE. A streamlined anaesthetic system. Can Anaesth Soc J 1972;19:426–435.

35. Arandia HY, Byles PH. PEEP and the Bain circuit. Can Anaesth Soc J 1981;28:467–470.

36. Erceg GW. PEEP for the Bain breathing circuit. Anesthesiology 1979;50:542–543.

37. Arandia HY. Bain PEEP. Anesthesiology 1980;52:193–194.

38. Erceg GW. Bain PEEP. A reply. Anesthesiology 1980;52:194.

39. Byrick RJ, Janssen EG. Respiratory waveform and rebreathing in T-piece circuits: a comparison of enflurane and halothane waveforms. Anesthesiology 1980;53:371–378.

40. Dorrington KL, Lehane JR. Minimum fresh gas flow requirements of anaesthetic breathing systems during spontaneous ventilation: a graphical approach. Anaesthesia 1987;42:732–737.

41. Gabrielsen J, van den Berg JT, Dirksen H, Ruben H. Effect of inspiration-expiration ratio on rebreathing with the Mapleson D system (Bain's modification; coaxial system). Acta Anaesthesiol Scand 1980;24:336–338.

42. Stenqvist O, Sonander H. Rebreathing characteristics of the Bain circuit. An experimental and theoretical study. Br J Anaesth 1984;56:303–310.

43. Spoerel WE. Rebreathing and end-tidal CO₂ during spontaneous breathing with the Bain circuit. Can Anaesth Soc J 1983;30:148–154.

44. Froese AB. Anesthesia circuits for children (ASA Refresher Course). Park Ridge, IL: ASA, 1978.

45. Goodwin K. Letter to the editor. Can Anaesth Soc J 1976;23:675.

46. Dean SE, Keenan RL. Spontaneous breathing with a T-piece circuit. Anesthesiology 1982; 56:449–452.

47. Conway CM, Seeley HF, Barnes PK. Spontaneous ventilation with the Bain anaesthetic system. Br J Anaesth 1977;49:1245–1249.

48. Lindahl SGE, Charlton AJ, Hatch DJ. Accuracy of prediction of fresh gas flow requirements during spontaneous breathing with the T-piece. Eur J Anaesth 1984;1:269–274.

49. Lindahl SGE, Charlton AJ, Hatch DJ. Ventilatory responses to rebreathing and carbon dioxide inhalation during anaesthesia in children. Br J Anaesth 1985;57:1188–1196.

50. Meakin G, Coates AL. An evaluation of rebreathing with the Bain system during anaesthesia with spontaneous ventilation. Br J Anaesth 1983; 55:487–495.

51. Spoerel WE. Aitkieh RR, Bain JA. Spontaneous respiration with the Bain breathing circuit. Can Anaesth Soc J 1978;25:30–35.

52. Soliman MG, Laberge R. The use of the Bain circuit in spontaneously breathing paediatric patients. Can Anaesth Soc J 1978;25:276–281.

53. Rayburn RL. Pediatric anaesthesia circuits. (ASA Refresher Course). Park Ridge, IL: ASA, 1981.

54. Badgwell JM, Heavner JE, May WS, Goldthorn JF, Lerman J. End-tidal PCO₂ monitoring in infants and children ventilated with either a partial-rebreathing or a non-rebreathing circuit. Anesthesiology 1987;56:405–410.

55. McIntyre JWR. Anesthesia breathing circuits. Can Anaesth Soc J 1986;33:98–105.

56. Bain JA, Spoerel WE. Flow requirements for a modified Mapleson D system during controlled ventilation. Can Anaesth Soc J 1973;20:629–636.

57. Bain JA, Spoerel WE. Prediction of arterial carbon dioxide tension during controlled ventilation with a modified Mapleson D system. Can Anaesth Soc J 1975;22:34–38.

58. Bain JA, Spoerel WE. Carbon dioxide output and elimination in children under anaesthesia. Can Anaesth Soc J 1977;24:533–539.

59. Chu YK, Rah KH, Boyan CP. Is the Bain breathing circuit the future anaesthesia system? An evaluation. Anesth Analg 1977;56:84–87.

60. Henville JD, Adams AP. The Bain anaesthetic system: an assessment during controlled ventilation. Anaesthesia 1976;31:247–256.

61. Kneeshaw JD, Harvey P, Thomas TA. A method for producing normocarbia during general anaesthesia for caesarean section. Anaesthesia. 1984;39:922–925

62. Rose DK, Froese AB. The regulation of PaCO₂ during controlled ventilation of children with a T-piece. Can Anaesth Soc J 1979;26:104–113.

63. Badgwell JM, Wolf AR, McEvedy BAB, Lerman J, Creighton RE. Fresh gas formulae do not accurately predict end-tidal PCO₂ in paediatric patients. Can J Anaesth 1988;35:581–586.

64. Rayburn RL, Graves SA. A new concept in controlled ventilation of children with the Bain anesthetic circuit. Anesthesiology 1978;48:250–253.

65. Shah NK, Bedford RF. Conservation of anesthetic gases using the Bain circuit. Anesthesiology 1987;67:A212.

66. Padfield A, Perks ER. Misuse of coaxial circuits. Anaesthesia 1978;33:77–78.

67. Sugg BR. Misuse of coaxial circuits. A reply. Anaesthesia 1978;33:78.

68. Breen M. Letter to the editor. Can Anaesth Soc J 1975;22:247.

69. Hannallah R, Rosales JK. A hazard connected with reuse of the Bain's circuit: a case report. Can Anaesth Soc J 1974;21:511–513.

70. Wildsmith JAW, Grubb DJ.Defective and misused co-axial circuits. Anaesthesia 1977;32:293.

71. Williams AR, Hasselt GV. Adequacy of preoperative safety checks of the Bain breathing system. Br J Anaesth 1992;68:637.

72. Goresky GV. Bain circuit delivery tube obstructions. Can J Anaesth 1990;37:385.

73. Inglis MS. Torsion of the inner tube. Br J Anaesth 1980;52:705.

74. Mansell WH. Bain circuit: the hazard of the hidden tube. Can Anaesth Soc J 1976;23:227.

75. Paterson JG, Vanhooydonk V. A hazard associated with improper connection of the Bain breathing circuit. Can Anaesth Soc J 1975;22:373–377.

76. Pfitzner J. Apparatus misconnection: Mapleson D systems and scavenging. Anaesth Intensive Care 1981;9:396–397.

77. Boyd CH. Another hazard of coaxial circuits. Anaesthesia 1977;32:675.

78. Robinson DN. Hazardous modification of Bain breathing attachment. Can J Anaesth 1992; 39:515–516.

79. Nichols PKT. Higher pressure ventilation and the Bain coaxial breathing system. Anaesthesia 1991;46:994.

80. Sedwards BJ. Higher pressure ventilation and the Bain coaxial breathing system. A reply. Anaesthesia 1991;46:994.

81. Cooper CMS. A test for breathing systems. Anaesthesia 1987;42:1019.

82. Foex P, Crampton-Smith A. A test for coaxial circuits. Anaesthesia 1977;32:294.

83. Ghani GA. Safety check for the Bain circuit. Can Anaesth Soc J 1984;31:487.

84. Pethick SL. Correspondence. Can Anaesth Soc J 1975;22:115.

85. Beauprie IG, Clark AG, Keith IC, Spence D, Eng P. Pre-use testing of coaxial circuits: the perils of Pethick. Can J Anaesth 1990;37:S103.

86. Peterson WC. Bain circuit. Can Anaesth Soc J 1978;25:532.

87. Robinson S, Fisher DM. Safety check for the CPRAM circuit. Anesthesiology 1983;59:488–489.

88. Baraka A, Sibai AN, Muallem M, Baroody M, Haroun S, Mekkaoui T. CPAP oxygenation during one-lung ventilation using an underwater seal assembly. Anesthesiology 1986;65:102–103.

89. Brown DL, Davis RF. A simple device for oxygen insufflation with continuous positive airway pressure during one-lung ventilation. Anesthesiology 1984;61:481–482.

90. Benumof JL, Gaughan S, Ozaki GT. Operative lung constant positive airway pressure with the Univent blocker tube. Anesth Analg 1992;74:406–410.

91. Cook CE, Wilson R. Dangers of using an improvised underwater seal for CPAP oxygenation during one-lung ventilation. Anesthesiology 1987;66:707–708.

92. Capan LM, Turndorf H, Patel C, Ramanathan S, Acinapura A, Chalon J. Optimization of arterial oxygenation during one-lung anesthesia. Anesth Analg 1980;59:847–851.

93. Galloway DW, Howler BMR. A simple CPAP system during one-lung anaesthesia. Anaesthesia 1988;43:708–709.

94. Hannenberg AA, Satwicz PR, Dienes RS, O'Brien JC. A device for applying CPAP to the nonventilated upper lung during one-lung ventilation. II. Anesthesiology 1984;60:254–255.

95. Lyons TE. A simplified method of CPAP delivery to the nonventilated lung during unilateral pulmonary ventilation. Anesthesiology 1984;61:216–217.

96. Shah JB, Skerman JH, Till WJ, Nossaman BD. Improving the efficacy of a CPAP system during one-lung anesthesia. Anesth Analg 1988;67:715–716.

97. Slinger P, Triolet W, Chang M. CPAP circuit for non-ventilated lung during thoracic surgery. Can J Anaesth 1987;34:654–655.

98. Scheller MS, Varvel JR. CPAP oxygenation during one-lung ventilation using a Bain circuit. Anesthesiology 1987;66:708–709.

99. Thiagarajah S, Job C, Rao A. A device for applying CPAP to the nonventilated upper lung during one-lung ventilation. I. Anesthesiology 1984;60:253–254.

100. Hensley FA, Martin F, Skeehan TM. High pressure pop-off safety device when using the Bain circuit for CPAP oxygenation during one-lung ventilation. Anesthesiology 1987;67:863.

101. Harrison GA. Ayre's T-piece: a review of its modifications. Br J Anaesth 1964;36:115–120.

102. Naunton A. The minimum reservoir capacity necessary to avoid air-dilution. Br J Anaesth 1985;57:803–806.

103. Arens JF. A hazard in the use of an Ayre T-Piece. Anesth Analg 1971;50:943–946.

104. Freifeld S. Modification of the Ayre T-piece system. Anesth Analg 1963;42:575–577.

105. Inkster JS. Kinked breathing systems. Anaesthesia 1990;45:173.

106. Keuskamp DHG. Automatic ventilation in paediatric anaesthesia using a modified Ayre's T-piece with negative pressure during expiratory phase. Anaesthesia 1963;18:46–56.

107. Ramanathan S, Chalon J, Turndorf H. A safety valve for the pediatric Rees system. Anesth Analg 1976;53:741–743.

108. Taylor C, Stoelting VK. Modified Ayre's T-tube technic—anesthesia for cleft lip and palate surgery. Anesth Analg 1963;42:55–62.

109. Rees GJ. Anaesthesia in the newborn. Br Med J 1950;2:1419–1422.

110. Hatch DJ, Yates AP, Lindahl SGE. Flow requirements and rebreathing during mechanically controlled ventilation in a T-piece (Mapleson E) system. Br J Anaesth 1987;59:1533–1540.

111. Kacmarek RM, Dimas S, Reynolds J, Shapiro BA. Technical aspects of positive end-expiratory pressure (PEEP). Part I: physics of PEEP devices. Respir Care 1982;27:1478–1489.

112. Akkineni S, Patel KP, Bennett EJ, Grundy EM, Ignacio AD. Fresh gas flow to limit $PaCO_2$ in T and circle systems without CO_2 absorption. Anesthesiol Rev 1977;4:33–37.

113. Kuwabara S, McCaughey TJ. Artificial ventilation in infants and young children using a new ventilator with the T-piece. Can Anaesth Soc J 1966;13:576–584.

114. Dobbinson TL, Fawcett ER, Bolton DPG. The effects of positive end expiratory pressure on rebreathing and gas dilution in the Ayre's T-piece system—laboratory study. Anaesth Intensive Care 1978;6:19–25.

115. Lawrence JC. PEEP and the Ayre's T-piece system. Anaesth Intensive Care 1978;6:359.

116. Humphrey D. A new anaesthetic breathing system combining Mapleson A, D, and E principles. A simple apparatus for low flow universal use without carbon dioxide absorption. Anaesthesia 1983;38:361–372.

117. Shulman MS, Brodsky JB. The A.D.E. system—a new anesthetic breathing system. Anesth Analg 1984;63:273.

118. Humphrey D, Brock-Utne JG. Manual ventilation with the Humphrey ADE system. Can J Anaesth 1987;34:S128–S129.

119. Humphrey D, Brock-Utne JG, Downing JW. Single lever Humphrey A.D.E. low flow universal anaesthesia breathing system. Part II: comparison with Bain system in anaesthetized adults during controlled ventilation. Can Anaesth Soc J 1986;33:710–718.

120. Criswell J, McKenzie S, Day S, Disley J, Bruce WE, Soni N. The Bain, ADE, and enclosed Magill breathing systems. A comparative study during controlled ventilation. Anaesthesia 1990;45:113–117.

121. Shah NK, Loughlin CJ, Bedford RF. Comparison of the Bain and the ADE systems during controlled ventilation in adults. Br J Anaesth 1989;62:150–152.

122. Taylor MB. A suggestion. Anaesthesia 1983;38:906.

123. Newton N, Cundy JM. The ultimate goal? Anaesthesia 1983;38:906–907.

124. Murphy PJ, Rabey PG. The Humphrey ADE breathing system and ventilator alarms. Anaesthesia 1991;46:1000.

125. Salkield IM. The Multicircuit system 1. Description of a device providing several Mapleson functions. Anaesth Intensive Care 1985;13:153–157.

126. Bradley JP, Marsland A, Salkfield I. The MCS system (multi-circuit system) Can Anaesth Soc J 1985;32:S102–S103.

127. Bradley JP, Marsland AR, Massang JR. The MultiCircuit System. 2. A study during spontaneous ventilation in awake volunteers using the Mapleson A mode. Anaesth Intensive Care 1985;13:158–162.

128. Zavattaro M, Marsland AR. The multicircuit system and spontaneous respiration. Anaesth Intensive Care 1987;15:358.

129. Gravenstein N, Lampotang S, Beneken JEW. Factors influencing capnography in the Bain circuit. J Clin Monit 1985;1:6–10.

130. Brock-Utne JC, Humphrey D. Multipurpose anaesthetic breathing systems—the ultimate goal. Acta Anaesthesiol Scand Suppl 1985;80:67.

131. Ramanathan S, Chalon J, Capan L, Patel C, Turndorf H. Rebreathing characteristics of the Bain anesthesia circuit. Anesth Analg 1977;56:822–825.

132. Rayburn RL, Watson RL. Humidity in children and adults using the controlled partial rebreathing anaesthesia method. Anesthesiology 1980;52:291–295.

133. Martin DG, Kong KL, Lewis GTR. Resistance to airflow in anaesthetic breathing systems. Br J Anaesth 1989;62:456–461.

134. Conterato JP, Lindahl GE, Meyer DM, Bires JA. Assessment of spontaneous ventilation in anesthetized children with use of a pediatric circle or a Jackson-Rees system. Anesth Analg 1989;69:484–490.

135. Gravenstein N, Gallagher RC. External flow-resistive, circuit-related work of breathing: Bain vs circle. Anesthesiology 1985;63:A183.

136. Kay B, Beatty PCW, Healy TEJ, Accoush MEA, Calpin M. Change in the work of breathing imposed by five anesthetic breathing systems. Br J Anaesth 1983;55:1239–1247.

137. Rasch DK, Bunegin L, Ledbetter, Kaminskas D. Comparison of circle absorber and Jackson-Rees systems for paediatric anaesthesia. Can J Anaesth 1988;35:25–30.

138. Boutros A, Pavlicek W. Anesthesia for magnetic resonance imaging. Anesth Analg 1987;66:367.

139. Dunn AJ. Empty tanks and Bain circuits. Can Anaesth Soc J 1978;25:337.

140. Mullin RA. Letter to the editor. Can Anaesth Soc J 1978;25:248–249.

141. Mullin RA. Bain circuit (a reply). Can Anaesth Soc J 1979;26:239.

142. Nimocks JA, Modell JH, Perry PA. Carbon dioxide retention using a humidified "nonrebreathing" system. Anesth Analg 1975;54:271–273.

143. Rogers KH, Rose DK, Byrick RJ. Severe hypercarbia with a Bain breathing circuit during malignant hyperthermia reaction. Can J Anaesth 1987;34:652–653.

Chapter 7

The Circle Absorption System

In the circle system gases flow in a circular pathway through separate inspiratory and expiratory channels. The direction of flow is determined by two unidirectional valves. A typical circle absorption system is diagrammed in Figure 7.1. A U.S. standard for breathing systems with particular emphasis on circle absorption systems was published in 1989 (1).

Components

CARBON DIOXIDE ABSORBER

The absorber is a heavy, bulky component that is usually attached to the anesthesia machine but may be a separate unit. An absorber assembly has an absorber and may include two ports for connection to breathing tubes, a fresh gas inlet, inspiratory and expi-

ratory unidirectional valves, an APL valve, and a bag mount. Disposable absorbers and absorber assemblies are available.

Canisters

Construction

The canisters (carbon dioxide absorbent containers, chambers, units, or cartridges), which hold the absorbent, make up the main part of the absorber. The sidewalls are usually constructed of a transparent material. A screen at the bottom of each canister holds the absorbent in place.

Modern absorbers use two canisters in apposition (Fig. 7.2). With fresh absorbent in both chambers, carbon dioxide is absorbed mostly in the upstream chamber. As that absorbent becomes exhausted, carbon dioxide will enter the downstream chamber where absorption will continue.

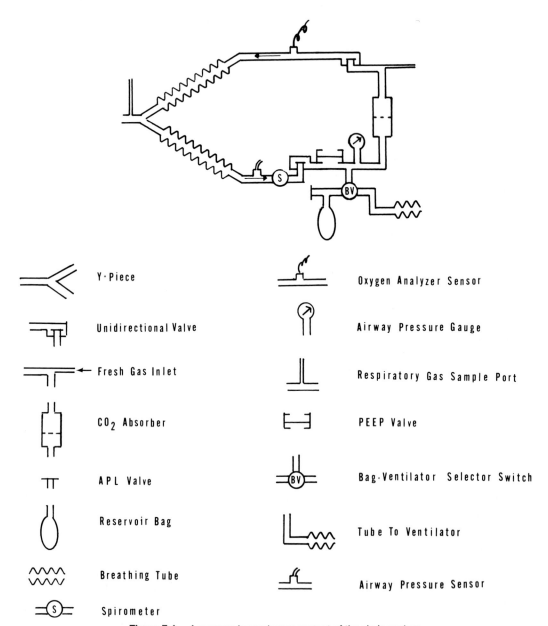

Y·Piece		Oxygen Analyzer Sensor	
Unidirectional Valve		Airway Pressure Gauge	
Fresh Gas Inlet		Respiratory Gas Sample Port	
CO_2 Absorber		PEEP Valve	
APL Valve		Bag·Ventilator Selector Switch	
Reservoir Bag		Tube To Ventilator	
Breathing Tube		Airway Pressure Sensor	
Spirometer			

Figure 7.1. A commonly used arrangement of the circle system.

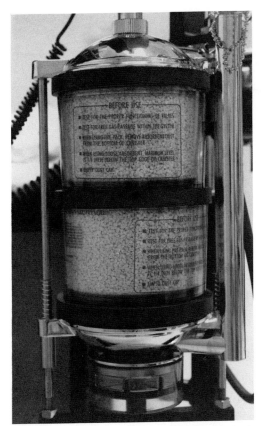

Figure 7.2. Absorber with two canisters, a dust/moisture trap at the bottom and a side tube at the right.

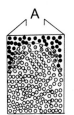 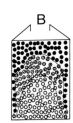 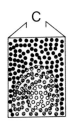

Figure 7.3. Pattern of carbon dioxide absorption in a canister. *Darkened circles* represent exhausted absorbent. It makes no difference whether the gases enter at the top or bottom of the absorber. **A,** After limited use; absorption has occurred primarily at the inlet and to a lesser extent along the sides. **B,** After extensive use; the granules at the inlet and along the sides are exhausted. **C,** Carbon dioxide is filtering through the canister; in the distal third of the canister a spot remains where the granules are still capable of absorbing carbon dioxide. Redrawn from Adriani J, Rovenstein EA. Experimental studies on carbon dioxide absorbers for anesthesia. Anesthesiology 1941;2:10.

Disposable canisters are available. They eliminate the need for emptying and refilling but can be a source of obstruction if a label or wrap is not removed (2).

Size

Canisters of varying capacity have been used. Modern canisters are much larger than older ones. Advantages of large canisters include better utilization of absorbent and longer intervals between absorbent changes. Use of a canister with a large cross-sectional area results in lower flows through it, so that resistance and absorbent dust migration are reduced.

Pattern and Direction of Flow

The pattern of absorption within a correctly packed canister is shown in Figure 7.3. It makes no difference whether the gases enter at the top or bottom. The first absorption occurs at the inlet and along the sides. The tendency of gases to travel along the periphery of the canister is known as the wall effect.

Flow through the canister is pulsatile. The direction of flow during the respiratory cycle will depend on the location of other components of the circle system. In the configuration shown in Figure 7.1, with the reservoir bag upstream of the absorber and the fresh gas inlet downstream, gases upstream of the absorber move through it during inhalation. During the expiratory pause, fresh gases from the anesthesia machine will push gases retrograde through the absorber.

Housing

The head and base of the absorber are usually constructed of metal. Gaskets at the bottom and top fit against the interposed canisters. The housing (or canister support) and canisters are tightened together by raising the base of the housing so that the upper canister seals against the upper gasket. Lowering the base creates a gap between the rim of the upper canister and the upper gasket.

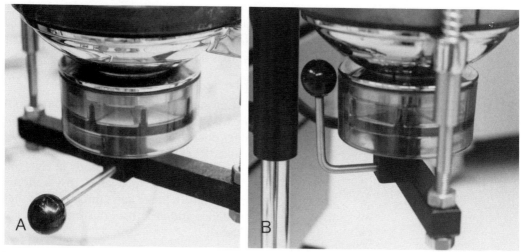

Figure 7.4. The lever connects to a geared arrangement at the base of the absorber and is used to lower or raise the bottom. **A,** The lever projects straight out, making it susceptible to accidental displacement. **B,** The lever is bent to prevent accidental displacement. Note the dust and moisture trap at the bottom of the absorber.

Two methods have been employed to raise and lower the base. One uses a screw or wing nut. This often does not turn freely and is difficult to operate. Most of the newer absorbers have a lever-actuated cam (Fig. 7.4). The lever may be accidentally displaced (3,4). To prevent this, a lever that points toward the front of the absorber can often be altered to face upward and toward the side (see Fig. 7.4) or toward the rear of the absorber, making it less susceptible to inadvertent displacement.

There are spaces at the top and bottom of the absorber for incoming gases to disperse before passing through the absorbent or for outgoing gases to collect before passing on through the circle. This promotes even distribution of flow through the absorber (5). In the base, this space allows dust and condensed water to accumulate (see Figs. 7.2 and 7.4). This helps to prevent caking in the bottom layers of absorbent. Some bases have a means of draining water from the bottom.

Baffles

Baffles, annular rings that serve to direct gas flow toward the central part of the canister, are frequently placed at the top and bottom of the absorber. This increases the path

of travel for gases along the sides and compensates for the reduced resistance to flow along the walls of the canister (5).

Side Tube

A side tube external to the canisters is employed to move gases either to or from the bottom of the absorber (see Fig. 7.2). The main flow of gases passing through the absorber will be in the opposite direction to that of gases passing through the side tube.

Bypass (6)

An older absorber may be equipped with a bypass controlled by a manually operated valve. The bypass is also called the cutout control, rebreathing valve, and bypass channel or control. Bypasses are no longer available in the United States but are used in many countries around the world. When the valve is in the on position, gas flows through the absorber. With the valve in the off position, some or all gas flow is diverted around the absorber. A complete bypass diverts all of the gases entering the absorber to the outlet without passing through the absorbent. A partial bypass allows a portion of the incoming gas to bypass the absorbent. A complete bypass allows the absorbent to be changed

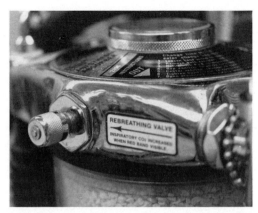

Figure 7.5. Partial bypass at side of the absorber. This is located on the opposite side of the absorber from where the user normally stands and is easily overlooked.

during a case, whereas a partial bypass does not, because there would be a loss of integrity of the circuit if the canisters were loosened.

A hazard with a bypass is that if it is in the bypass position and the fresh gas flow is low, carbon dioxide accumulation can occur. On one absorber the bypass is located on the side of the absorber opposite from where the operator normally stands or sits and is not easily seen (Fig. 7.5).

CARBON DIOXIDE ABSORPTION

Absorbents

Carbon dioxide absorption employs the general principle of a base neutralizing an acid. The acid is carbonic acid formed by the reaction of carbon dioxide with water. The base is the hydroxide of an alkali or alkaline earth metal. The end products of the reaction are water and a carbonate.

There are two absorbents in common use today: soda lime and barium hydroxide lime.

Soda Lime

Composition. The composition of soda lime has varied over the years. Most soda lime used today is the "wet," or "high-moisture," variety. By weight it is 4% sodium hydroxide, 1% potassium hydroxide, 14% to 19% water, and enough calcium hydroxide to make 100%. Small amounts of silica and kie-

selguhr are added for hardness, and indicators are added to allow assessment of absorption capacity.

The water is present as a thin film on the granule surface (7). Moisture is essential because the reactions take place between ions that exist only in the presence of water. Absorbents with low moisture exhaust rapidly. On the other hand, those with high moisture have a slower rate of absorption, stickiness, and increased resistance (8). The humidity of the gas does not affect the capacity of soda lime to absorb carbon dioxide (9). Absorption is as effective when the gases are dry as when they are humidified, provided the soda lime has a high moisture content.

Chemistry. To initiate the chemical reaction, carbon dioxide must first react with the water on the surface of the granule to form carbonic acid:

$$CO_2 + H_2O \rightleftharpoons H_2CO_3$$

This is a weak acid and is incompletely dissociated into its ions:

$$H_2CO_3 \rightleftharpoons H^+ + HCO_3^-$$
$$\downarrow$$
$$H^+ + CO_3^{-2}$$

Sodium hydroxide and calcium hydroxide are likewise dissociated into their ions:

$$NaOH \rightleftharpoons OH^- + Na^+$$
$$Ca(OH)_2 \rightleftharpoons 2OH^- + Ca^{2+}$$

The sodium and calcium ions combine with the carbonate ions, forming as end products sodium carbonate and calcium carbonate:

$$2NaOH + 2H_2CO_3 + Ca(OH)_2 \rightleftharpoons$$
$$CaCO_3 + Na_2CO_3 + 4H_2O$$

Water is formed from the hydrogen and hydroxyl ions. Heat is liberated at the rate of 13,700 calories per mole of water produced (or CO_2 absorbed). This heat does not affect absorption efficiency (10).

A phenomenon known as *peaking* or *regeneration* is seen with soda lime. The soda lime appears to be reactivated with rest. The amount of regeneration depends on the length of the period of rest (11). After a number of such periods of efficient absorption with intervening periods of rest, terminal exhaustion occurs. Regeneration is probably owing to the fact that sodium hydroxide is more soluble and active than calcium hydroxide and combines preferentially with carbon dioxide to form sodium carbonate. Sodium carbonate, because it is soluble, will dissolve in the moisture on the granules and can then penetrate into the granule and react with the less active and less soluble calcium hydroxide to form calcium carbonate, which is insoluble, and sodium hydroxide. The regenerated sodium hydroxide then imparts renewed activity to the absorbent. There is general agreement that with modern "wet" soda lime the absorption capacity regenerated with rest is slight and affords no appreciable improvement in the overall life of the absorbent (12,13).

Regeneration does have some importance when indicators are used. Soda lime that shows an exhausted color, if allowed to rest, will often show a reversal of color. The absorption capacity of that soda lime will be low and the exhausted color will reappear after only a brief exposure to carbon dioxide.

Shape and Size of Granules. Soda lime is supplied in granules that have irregular surfaces to provide maximum area for absorption. The size of the granules is important. Small granules provide greater surface area and decrease channeling, the passage of gas occuring preferentially along low-resistance pathways and bypassing the bulk of the absorbent (14,15). However, they cause more resistance and caking (14–17). Larger granules cause less resistance to air flow but offer less surface area. Studies have shown that a blend of larger and smaller granules has the effect of minimizing resistance with little sacrifice in absorption efficiency (18).

Granule size is measured by mesh number. A 4-mesh strainer has four openings per inch whereas one of 8 mesh has eight openings per inch. Soda lime granules graded 4 mesh will pass through the 4-mesh strainer but not through a strainer with smaller holes. In other words, the higher the mesh number, the smaller the particles. Soda lime used in anesthesia today consists of granules in the size range of 4 to 8 mesh (7).

Hardness. Soda lime granules fragment easily, producing dust (*fines*). There may be variations in the dust content of different brands of absorbent (19). Excessive powder produces channeling, resistance to flow, and caking. Dust may be blown through the system to the patient (20,21). To prevent this, small amounts of silica are added to increase hardness (7). Silica tends to clog the pores of the soda lime and reduce its efficiency, a drawback overcome by the addition of kieselguhr (22). Some manufacturers coat the outside of the granules with a film to which dust particles adhere.

Hardness is tested by placing a weighed amount of absorbent in a pan with steel ball bearings and agitating it. The soda lime is then sifted onto an 8-mesh screen. The percentage of the original sample remaining on the screen is the hardness number, which should be greater than 75 (7).

Barium Hydroxide Lime

Composition. Barium hydroxide lime is a mixture of approximately 20% barium hydroxide and 80% calcium hydroxide. It may also contain some potassium hydroxide and an indicator (22). Barium hydroxide is the more active component, acting much as sodium hydroxide in soda lime.

Moisture is incorporated into the structure of the barium hydroxide as an octahydrate: $Ba(OH)_2 \cdot 8H_2O$. Some moisture is also present on the surface. Compared with soda lime, the water content is less variable and less likely to be lost through evaporation. Water will be lost, however, if barium hydroxide lime is heated over 100°C.

Chemistry. The reactions between barium hydroxide lime and carbon dioxide are as follows:

$$Ba(OH)_2 \cdot 8H_2O + CO_2 \rightarrow$$
$$BaCO_3 + 9H_2O$$
$$9H_2O + 9CO_2 \rightarrow 9H_2CO_3$$
$$9H_2CO_3 + 9Ca(OH)_2 \rightarrow$$
$$9CaCO_3 + 18H_2O$$
$$2KOH + H_2CO_3 \rightarrow K_2CO_3 + 2H_2O$$
$$Ca(OH)_2 + K_2CO_3 \rightarrow CaCO_3 + 2KOH$$

Heat and water formation vary little from soda lime under identical conditions (23). There is some regeneration with barium hydroxide lime (13).

Size and Shape. Barium hydroxide lime is supplied in granular form (4 to 8 mesh) similar to soda lime. In the past it was supplied in the form of pellets, which had shorter lives than granules.

Hardness. It is not necessary to add a hardening agent to barium hydroxide lime, because the water of crystallization present imparts sufficient hardness to prevent dust formation (13,16).

Compatibility of Absorbents and Anesthetic Agents

Sevoflurane, isoflurane, desflurane, and halothane have been shown to be degraded by absorbent to some extent (24–28). The rate of degradation is increased with increased temperature and decreased as the concentration of water or exhausted absorbent is increased (25,28,29). Sevoflurane is degraded more by baralyme than soda lime (26).

The rate of degradation is too small to affect the requirements for clinical anesthesia even in a low-flow system but is of concern because of the potential for toxic breakdown products. One study found that when halothane reacts with soda lime, a metabolite toxic to mice is produced (27). However, even with a system closed for 4 hr, the concentration of this metabolite remained quite low. One of the degradation products of sevoflurane is lethal in very high concentrations (30), but these concentrations were far above those expected during anesthesia.

High concentrations of carbon monoxide have been reported in filled absorbers that have not been used for at least 24 hr, possible the result of a slow chemical reaction between the anesthetic agent or a compound present in the anesthetic and the absorbent (31,32).

Absorbents can absorb volatile anesthetic agents (25,26,33–36). This can slow anesthetic induction and result in exposure of subsequent patients to volatile agents. Dry absorbent absorbs more agent than wet (25,34,35,37).

Indicators

An indicator is an acid or base whose color depends on pH and that is added to the absorbent to signify when exhaustion has occurred. The indicator does not affect absorption. Some of the commonly used indicators and their colors are shown in Table 7.1. Confusion may result because one indicator is white when fresh whereas another is white when exhausted.

Ethyl violet undergoes deactivation even if stored in the dark (38). Deactivation is accelerated in the presence of light, especially high-intensity light.

Contents

Granular Space

The granular space is occupied by solid absorbent.

Air Space

The air space occupies 48% to 55% of the volume of the canister (13). It is divided into the void space and the pore space.

Table 7.1. Indicators for Absorbents

Indicator	Color When Fresh	Color When Exhausted
Phenolphthalein	white	pink
Ethyl violet	white	purple
Clayton yellow	red	yellow
Ethyl orange	orange	yellow
Mimosa Z	red	white

Void Space. The void (intergranular or interstitial) space is between the granules. It varies with the size of the granules and how tightly they are packed. The smaller the granules and the closer they fit together, the smaller the void space. The void space of soda lime is 40% to 47% of its volume (13). For barium hydroxide lime, it is 45%.

Pore Space. The pore (intragranular) space is within the pores of the granules. The pore volume for fresh absorbent is 8% of the total volume. As absorption proceeds, the pore space decreases (7).

Storage and Handling of Absorbents

Absorbents are supplied in several types of containers: resealable packages, pails, cans, cartons, and disposable prefilled containers. Once opened, containers should be resealed as soon as possible to prevent reaction of the absorbent with carbon dioxide in the air, deactivation of the indicator, and moisture loss. High temperatures will have no effect on absorbents if the containers are sealed, but any temperature below freezing is harmful because the moisture will expand and cause fragmentation of the granules.

Absorbents should always be handled gently to avoid fragmentation and dust formation. All personnel involved in the handling of absorbents should be periodically warned that absorbent dust is irritating to the eyes and respiratory tract and that absorbents are caustic to the skin, particularly when damp.

When a canister is emptied, care should be taken to remove dust particles along the rubber surfaces as they will cause the seals to warp, making it difficult to achieve a tight fit. Screens should be cleared to reduce resistance to respiration.

Filling of the canister should always be performed with care. The canister should be held over a suitable container to avoid getting particles on the floor. The absorbent should be slowly poured into the canister while the canister is rotated, stopping occasionally to tap the sides to settle the granules (39). The canister should be filled completely but not overfilled. A small space should be left at the top to promote even flow of gases through the canister. The upper layer of the absorbent should be level.

With disposable, prefilled containers, it is important to remove the top and bottom labels or plastic wrap, if present, before insertion. If this is not done, gas cannot flow through the container (2).

Changing the Absorbent

Measuring the carbon dioxide concentration in the inspiratory gas is the only reliable method to detect absorbent exhaustion. The following methods are less reliable.

Indicator Color Change

Confidence should not be placed on indicator color change, because this does not reliably demonstrate CO_2 breakthrough (40). The following should be kept in mind when using a color indicator:

1. When the exhausted color shows strongly, the absorbent is at or near the point of exhaustion. When little or no color change shows, active absorbent may be present, but the amount is indeterminate and may be quite small.

2. When a canister is rested, the color may revert back to its preexhaustion color even when the absorbent is sufficiently exhausted to be of no value clinically. Upon reuse, the indicator color will rapidly return to its exhausted state. The rested canister, therefore, can give a false impression of its usefulness.

3. When channeling occurs, the absorbent along the channels will become exhausted and carbon dioxide will filter through the canister. If the channeling occurs at other sites than the sides of the canister, the color change along the channels may not be visible.

4. Use of absorbent without indicators has been reported (41).

5. Ethyl violet undergoes deactivation even if it is stored in the dark (38). Light, especially ultraviolet, accelerates this process.

Heat in the Canister

The chemical reaction of carbon dioxide with absorbent produces heat, and changes in absorbent temperature occur earlier than changes in the color of the indicator. Periodically checking the temperature of the canisters is useful. Some heat production should be apparent unless very high fresh gas flows are used.

One study suggested that when the temperature of the downstream canister exceeds that of the upstream chamber the absorbent in the upstream canister should be changed (42).

To change the absorbent, the base of the absorber housing is lowered and the canister is removed. The absorbent in the upstream canister is discarded and the canister is filled with fresh absorbent. Care should be taken when placing the last of the absorbent into the canister. If excessive dust is present, the remaining absorbent should be discarded and filling completed from a new container (43). The canisters are then reversed in position so that the canister that was downstream is placed in the upstream position.

UNIDIRECTIONAL VALVES

Unidirectional valves are also known as flutter valves, one-way valves, check valves, directional valves, dome valves, flap valves, nonreturn valves, and inspiratory and expiratory valves. Two unidirectional valves are used in each circle system to ensure that the gases flow toward the patient in one breathing tube and away in the other. They are usually part of the absorber assembly. The 22-mm male connector next to the inspiratory unidirectional valve is called the inspiratory port and that next to the expiratory unidirectional valve is called the expiratory port. The ASTM standard requires that the direction of intended gas flow be permanently marked on the valve housing or near its associated hose terminal with either a directional arrow or with the marking *inspiration* or *expiration* so that it is visible to the user (1).

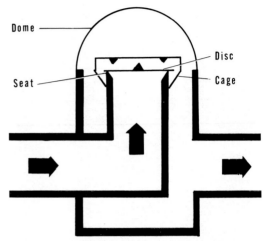

Figure 7.6. Unidirectional valve. Gas flowing into the valve raises the disc from its seat, then passes through the valve. Reversing the gas flow causes the disc to contact its seat, stopping further retrograde flow. The guide (cage) prevents lateral or vertical displacement of the disc. The transparent dome allows observation of disc movement.

A typical unidirectional valve is shown diagrammatically in Figure 7.6. A disc (leaflet or poppet) seats horizontally on an annular seat. A cage or guide mechanism (such as projections from the seat and dome) serves to prevent the disc from becoming dislodged laterally or vertically (Fig. 7.7). A transparent dome allows observation of disc movement. Gas enters at the bottom and flows through the center of the valve, raising the disc from its seat. The gas then passes under the dome and on through the breathing system. Reversing the gas flow will cause the disc to contact the seat, stopping further retrograde flow. Unidirectional valves are positional and must be vertical for the disc to seat properly.

As can be seen in Figure 5.1*F*, turbulence results from gas flow through a unidirectional valve. Although this was a significant problem with older valves, modern valves have light discs and present only slight resistance.

Incompetence of one or both unidirectional valves is not uncommon (44). The disc

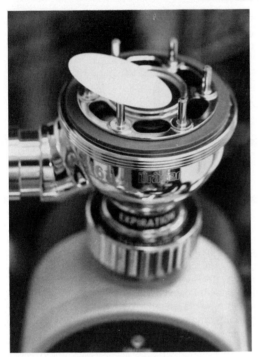

Figure 7.7. Unidirectional valve with dome removed. The disc is displaced from its seat. The projections on the seat prevent lateral displacement of the disc.

may adhere to the dome unless a guard is present. Moisture may cause the disc to stick (45). Electrostatic charges may cause the disc to be attracted to the top of the valve (46). An unsecured cage may allow the disc to move laterally (47). The disc may catch on a pin of a cage (46). Foreign material such as absorbent granules may hold the valve open (47). Because an open valve offers less resistance to flow than one that must open, the flow of gas will be primarily through the incompetent side, resulting in rebreathing.

A unidirectional valve may jam, obstructing gas flow (48). In one reported case, the disc was lost during cleaning and not recovered (49). It was later found out of sight below the seat, where it had moved into such a position that it covered the opening to the bag mount and functioned as a one-way valve. Gas could flow into the system, but not back out again.

INSPIRATORY AND EXPIRATORY PORTS

The inspiratory port of the circle system is the opening through which gases pass during inspiration. The expiratory port is the opening through which gases pass during expiration. These are traditionally mounted on the absorber. The ASTM standard requires that each port be a 22-mm conical male fitting (1).

Y PIECE

The Y piece (Y connector, Y yoke, Y adaptor, and three-way breathing system connector) is a three-way tubular connector with two 22-mm male ports for connection to the breathing tubes and a 15-mm female patient connection port. The patient connection port may have a coaxial 22-mm male fitting to allow direct connection between the Y piece and face mask. In most disposable systems, the Y piece and breathing tubes are permanently attached. The Y piece may be designed so that the patient port swivels. A septum may be placed in the Y piece to decrease the dead space.

Y pieces on some disposable systems may become detached from the breathing tubes (50) and many are prone to leak (51).

FRESH GAS INLET

The fresh gas inlet is the point at which gas from the anesthesia machine enters the system. Most commonly it is connected to the common gas outlet on the anesthesia machine by a flexible rubber tubing—the fresh gas supply tube (delivery hose). The ASTM standard requires that the fresh gas inlet port, or nipple, have an inside diameter of at least 4.0 mm and that the fresh gas delivery tube have an inside diameter of at least 6.4 mm (1).

APL VALVE

APL valves were discussed in Chapter 5. During spontaneous breathing the valve should be fully open. It will open after the bag has become distended during expiration or the expiratory pause. When manually assisted or controlled ventilation is used, the APL valve should be closed enough that the desired inspiratory pressure can be achieved. When this pressure is attained, the valve opens and excess gas is vented.

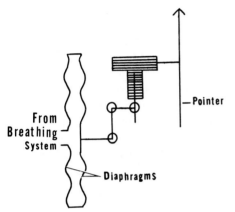

Figure 7.8. Diaphragm-activated pressure gauge. Two thin metal diaphragms are sealed together, with a space between them. This space is connected to the breathing system. Variations in pressure in the breathing system are transmitted to the diaphragms, which bulge outward or inward. A series of levers is activated, moving the pointer, which records the pressure.

PRESSURE GAUGE (MANOMETER)

Most circle systems have a pressure gauge attached to the absorber. The ASTM standard (1) requires that they be marked in units of kPa and/or cm water or both.

The gauge is usually of the diaphragm type shown in Figure 7.8. Changes in pressure in the breathing system are transmitted to the space between two diaphragms, causing them to move inward or outward. Movements of one diaphragm are transmitted to the pointer, which moves over a calibrated scale.

BREATHING TUBES

Most breathing tubes in use today are made of plastic. Unfortunately, they are sometimes defective. Problems include kinking, indentations, leaks, and separation of components (50,51). Plastic breathing tubes are less compliant than rubber ones (52). The length of the tubes does not affect the amount of dead space or rebreathing in the circle system. There is an ASTM standard that covers specifications for breathing tubes (53).

A coaxial breathing system, the Mera-F, has been developed (54). As shown in Figure 7.9, the tubings attach to a conventional

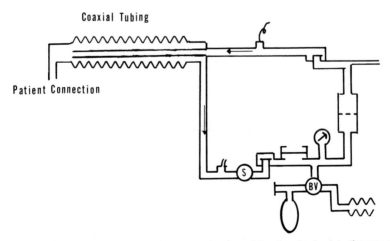

Figure 7.9. Mera F system. Gases pass through the inspiratory unidirectional valve into the smooth inner tube of the coaxial tubing and on to the patient. Exhaled gases flow to the expiratory unidirectional valve via the outer corrugated tube.

valved absorber assembly. The inner tube is connected to the inspiratory port and the outer tube to the expiratory port. Gases flow through the smooth inner tube to the patient and exhaled gases flow to the absorber via the outer corrugated tube. The inspired gas is warmed in the process. Advantages of this system include small size, increased inspired heat and humidity, and light weight. Disadvantages include increased resistance (55). Problems include kinking of the inner tube, misassembly (resulting in obstruction of the outer tube), reversed attachment to the absorber (allowing condensed water to accumulate in the inner tube), and elongation of the outer tube (resulting in an increase in dead space) (56–58).

RESERVOIR BAG

Bags were discussed in Chapter 5. Specifications for reservoir bags are covered by an ASTM standard (59). Bag size should be suited to the size of the patient and the anesthesia provider's hand. Bags of 3 to 5 liters' capacity are generally used for adults.

The bag is attached to the bag port (bag mount or extension), a 22-mm male port. A case has been reported in which the bag mount broke off, preventing use of the system (60).

BAG/VENTILATOR SELECTOR SWITCH

A selector switch provides a convenient method to shift rapidly between manual and automatic ventilation, without removing the bag or the ventilator hose from its mount. The bag/ventilator selector switch is also called the switch valve, mode selector valve, selector valve, bag-ventilator switch valve, switching valve, switchover valve, manual/automatic selector valve, and ventilator valve assembly.

As shown in Figure 7.10, the selector switch is essentially a three-way stopcock. One port connects to the breathing system. The second is attached to the bag mount. The third attaches to the ventilator hose. The handle or knob used to select the position indicates the position in which the switch is set (Fig. 7.11). There are two types of selector switches (see Fig. 7.10).

Without APL Valve (Figure 7.10 A and B)

The selector switch without an APL valve (see Fig. 1.10A,B) is found on some older anesthesia machines. Operation of the selector switch does not affect the APL valve. It is necessary to close the valve when switching from bag to ventilator. Failure to close the valve in the ventilator mode may result in inadequate ventilation.

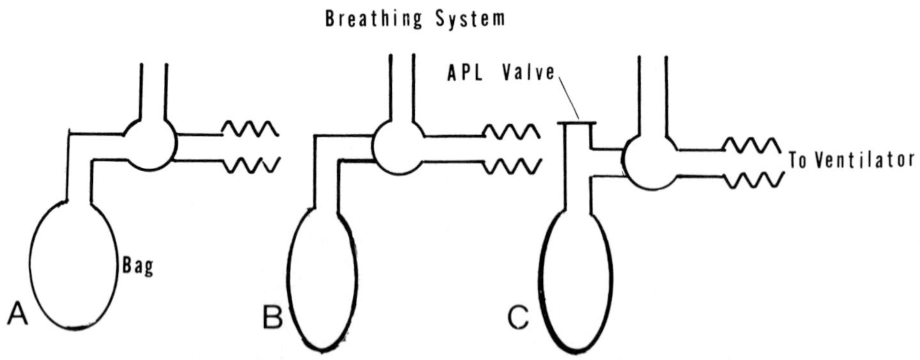

Figure 7.10. Bag/ventilator selector switch. **A and B,** Older type. In **A** the switch is set for manual or spontaneous ventilation. The bag is connected to the breathing system. **B** shows the switch set for automatic ventilation; the APL valve is still connected to the system and must be closed. **C,** Newer type. The APL valve is on the bag side of the valve. When the switch is set for automatic ventilation, the APL valve is excluded from the system, so it is not necessary to close it.

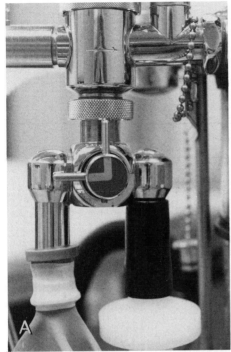
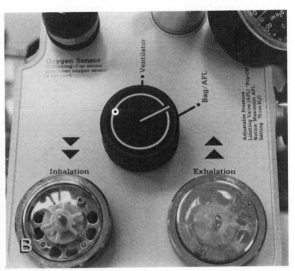

Figure 7.11. Bag/ventilator selector switches **A,** Older style. The APL valve is not excluded from the breathing system when the valve is set for ventilator use. The position of the handle indicates whether the valve is set for manual or automatic ventilation. **B,** Newer style. When the switch is in the ventilator position the APL valve is excluded from the circuit.

With APL Valve

The selector switch with an APL valve (see Fig. 7.10*C*) is the only type allowed by the ASTM standard (1) and is on newer anesthesia machines. The APL valve is located near the bag mount. When the switch is in the ventilator position, the APL valve is isolated along with the reservoir bag, so it does not need to be closed. Switching to the bag mode causes the APL valve to be connected to the breathing system.

A hazard with one of these valves has been reported. A missing retainer ring allowed the valve handle to be positioned so that when the bag was squeezed, gas escaped toward the ventilator (61).

RESPIRATORY GAS MONITOR SENSOR OR CONNECTOR

Respiratory gas monitor sensors are discussed in Chapter 16. Both mainstream and sidestream devices can be used with the circle system, but care must be taken when selecting the best position within the system.

SENSOR FOR AIRWAY PRESSURE MONITOR

Airway pressure monitors are discussed in Chapter 17. The sensor can be inserted into the circle system using a T-shaped adaptor or it may be incorporated into the absorber assembly.

OPTIONAL EQUIPMENT

PEEP Valve

Positive end expiratory pressure valves are integral parts of some absorbers assemblies. One can also be added to a circle system. If the PEEP valve is a separate component, it usually has a fixed pressure. It is essential that such a valve be placed in the expiratory limb and that it be oriented correctly. Placing a

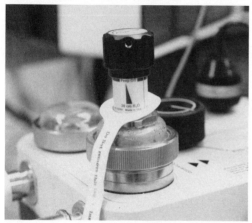

Figure 7.12.   PEEP valve built into absorber assembly. The amount of PEEP is dialed by turning the knob and is read on the manometer. A hazard with this valve is that it may be left on and a subsequent user may be unaware of this. Another hazard is that it may be accidentally altered.

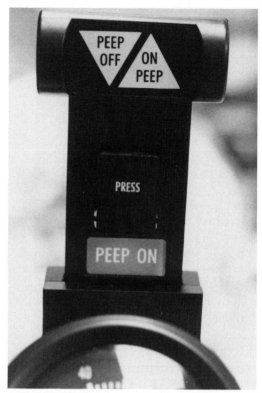

Figure 7.13.   PEEP on-off indicator. The handle must be raised before the PEEP can be dialed. This alerts the user that the PEEP is being applied.

unidirectional PEEP valve backward will occlude gas flow. If a bidirectional PEEP valve is placed backward, gas flow will not be occluded, but no PEEP will be produced.

PEEP valves that are an integral part of the absorber assembly are usually of the variable pressure type. The amount of PEEP is dialed on the valve and read on the manometer (Fig. 7.12). A hazard with this device is that if it is not returned to zero at the end of a case the next user may not notice this. Some of the newer PEEP valves have a method to indicate when they are on (Fig. 7.13).

Filters

One of the disadvantages of the circle system is that it is difficult to clean and/or sterilize certain components, particularly the absorber, ventilator, and unidirectional valves. To avoid transmission of pathogens, filters may been used. These were discussed in Chapter 5.

Heated Humidifier

A heated humidifier is often placed in the inspiratory limb of the circle system. These will be discussed more fully in Chapter 9.

Respirometer

A respirometer to measure ventilatory volumes is commonly used in the circle system. These are discussed in Chapter 17.

Arrangement of Components

The relative placement of components comprising the circle system influences its function. Figure 7.1 illustrates a commonly used arrangement.

OBJECTIVES

1. Maximum inclusion of fresh and dead-space gases in the inspired mixture and maximum venting of alveolar gas (62,63). Fresh gas should be preferentially included in the

inspired mixture so that the inspired concentrations approach those in the fresh gas. This will result in faster inductions and emergences. The lower the fresh gas flow, the more important this objective becomes, because one of the effects of using lower fresh gas flows is that changes in concentration in the fresh gas flow are reflected more slowly in inspired concentrations.

Faster induction and emergence will also be aided by selective venting of alveolar gases. During induction when the concentration of anesthetic agent in the fresh gas is higher than in inspired mixtures, it is advantageous that alveolar gases containing low concentrations of anesthetic agents, rather than fresh or dead-space gases containing higher concentrations, be eliminated through the APL valve. During emergence, the opposite is true.

2. Minimal consumption of absorbent (64). For efficient absorbent use, the gas vented through the APL valve should have the highest possible concentration of carbon dioxide. This will occur when (*i*) exhaled gas does not pass through the absorber before being vented, (*ii*) exhaled gas is diluted as little as possible before venting, and (*iii*) the vented gas is that exhaled late in exhalation, as the first gas exhaled is that from the dead space and contains a low concentration of carbon dioxide.

As fresh gas flow is reduced, more gas must pass through the absorbent, so this objective becomes less important. When using a closed system, the arrangement of components should have no effect on the utilization of absorbent, because all exhaled gases will pass through the absorber.

3. Accurate readings from a respirometer placed in the system (65–67). If the fresh gas inlet is positioned so that the fresh gas continuously flows through the respirometer, measured ventilatory volumes will not be accurate.

4. Meaningful pressures on a manometer or transmitted by the sensor for an airway pressure monitor.

5. Maximal humidification of inspired gases.

6. Minimal dead space.

7. Low resistance.

8. Avoidance of hazards. Components should not exert pull on the tracheal tube or mask.

9. Convenience. Components should be so arranged that they do not create difficulties during use. Tubings and wires should not become tangled.

There is no one arrangement of components that will meet all of the above objectives. In some cases objectives may conflict. For example, venting carbon dioxide upstream of the absorber will conserve absorbent but will tend to reduce inspired humidity, because the amount of heat and humidity produced are directly proportional to the volume of carbon dioxide entering the canister. In certain clinical situations particular objectives need to be given priority. For example, in pediatric patients, dead space and humidification are more significant than in adults.

CONSIDERATION OF INDIVIDUAL COMPONENTS

Fresh Gas Inlet

Figure 7.14 shows possible locations of the fresh gas inlet. It is most commonly placed upstream of the inspiratory unidirectional valve and downstream of the absorber (position A). In this position, during exhalation and the expiratory pause fresh gas will flow into the absorber and then into components between the expiratory unidirectional valve and the absorber. At low fresh gas flows, no gas vented through the APL valve will have passed through the absorber. With higher flows, some gas that has been in the absorber may be vented. At very high flows, some fresh gas may be vented.

Placing the fresh gas inlet upstream of the absorber (position B) would result in less fresh gas in the inspired mixture. Anesthetic agent in the fresh gas would be retained in the absorber, resulting in a slower induction

Figure 7.14. Possible locations for the fresh gas inlet (see text for details).

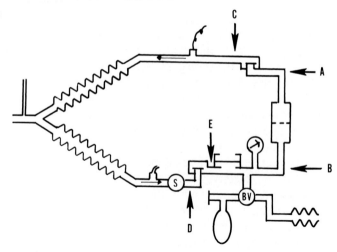

(68). Another problem with placing the fresh gas inlet in position B is that absorbent dust may be blown into the inspiratory limb when the oxygen flush is activated. Because of the proximity to the APL valve, fresh gas would be vented.

Placing the fresh gas inlet in position B will improve humidification of inspired gases (69–71), but will result in more drying of the absorbent. Because dry absorbent absorbs more anesthetic agent than moist, more agent will be retained in the absorbent, slowing induction (34). Subsequent patients will be exposed to more volatile agent as it is released by the absorbent.

Placing the fresh gas inlet in position B will prevent gas that has passed into the absorber from being vented through the APL valve, resulting in more efficient use of absorbent.

Placing the fresh gas inlet upstream of the bag and the APL valve (position E) would have all the disadvantages of position B and would result in more venting of fresh gas and more dilution of exhaled gas before it is vented.

Placing the fresh gas inlet upstream of the expiratory unidirectional valve (position D) has all the disadvantages of positions B and E. In addition, during inspiration the fresh gas flow would force exhaled gases back toward the patient, causing rebreathing.

Position C, downstream of the inspiratory unidirectional valve, was originally advocated to reduce the dead space by sweeping exhaled gases out of the Y piece during exhalation (64). However, if the unidirectional valves are competent, there will be only slight retrograde flow at the Y piece. With an incompetent valve, even a high inflow cannot prevent rebreathing of exhaled gases (64).

With the inflow in position C, during exhalation fresh gas would join exhaled gases and escape though the APL valve without reaching the patient. This would result in poor economy of fresh gas (72) and inefficient use of absorbent, because fresh gas would dilute the concentration of carbon dioxide in the gas vented through the APL valve.

Another disadvantage of position C is that a respirometer placed on the exhalation side of the circuit will not record tidal or minute volumes accurately (65–67,73) During exhalation, both exhaled and fresh gas will pass through the respirometer. The respirometer will register flow even if the patient is apneic. Accurate respirometer readings can still be obtained by turning off the fresh gas flow temporarily (66) or by placing the respirometer between the Y piece and the mask or tracheal tube connector (67).

A final disadvantage of position C is that if the oxygen flush were used and if there

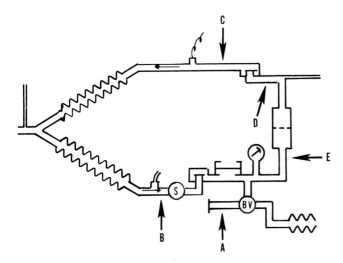

Figure 7.15. Possible locations for the reservoir bag (see text for details).

were an obstruction in the exhalation limb of the breathing system, the patient would be exposed to a sudden rapid increase in pressure (74). With the fresh gas inlet in other positions, the increase in pressure would be slower because gas could exit through the APL valve and the pressure increase would be buffered by the bag.

Use of position C would cause changes in the fresh gas composition to appear more rapidly in the inspired gases. If the Y piece has a septum, placement of the fresh gas inlet in this position will wash out dead space under a mask. This might be especially useful for mask inductions, when a respirometer would have little accuracy anyway.

Position C was found to be advantageous compared with position A in an experimental model using controlled ventilation without carbon dioxide absorption (75).

Reservoir Bag

Figure 7.15 shows possible locations for the reservoir bag. It is most commonly placed between the exhalation unidirectional valve and the absorber (position A).

During spontaneous ventilation, absorbent use is equally efficient if the bag is downstream (position D) or upstream (position A or E) of the absorber (64). With manually controlled or assisted ventilation, more efficient use occurs with the bag upstream of the absorber. If the bag were in position D, exhaled gases would pass through the absorber to the bag during exhalation. Squeezing the bag during inhalation would cause the gases to reverse flow and pass retrograde through the absorber, to be vented through the APL valve. This would result in inefficient absorbent use, because gases cleared of carbon dioxide would be vented.

When a mechanical ventilator is used, the APL valve is closed and excess gases are vented through the ventilator, so the position of the bag will determine which gas is vented. If the bag is placed in position D during mechanical ventilation, exhaled gases must pass through the absorber before being vented.

A disadvantage of placing the bag upstream of the absorber is that a sudden increase in pressure from squeezing the bag may force dust from the absorber into the inspiratory tubing (76).

Another possible position for the bag is position E, at the bottom of an absorber. An advantage may be better humidification as the fresh gas would flow over water condensed in the space below the absorbent. A disadvantage is that absorbent dust may collect in this area and a hard squeeze of the bag could force a cloud of this dust into the inspiratory limb (21).

If the bag is placed between the patient and either of the unidirectional valves (posi-

Figure 7.16. Possible locations for the APL valve (see text for details).

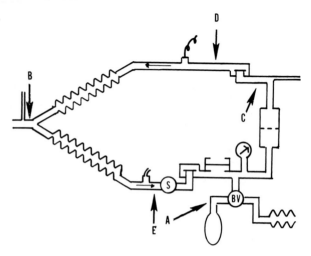

tion B or C), it would form a reservoir for exhaled gases that would then be rebreathed.

Unidirectional Valves

Two locations have been used for the unidirectional valves: in the Y piece and attached to the absorber. Valved Y pieces are no longer available commercially and are not permitted by the ASTM standard (1).

Placing the valves in the Y piece offers the advantage of eliminating backflow of exhaled gases into the inspiratory tubing. However, under normal circumstances backflow into this tubing is insignificant. With controlled ventilation, placing the valves in the Y piece results in more efficient absorbent use (64).

Disadvantages of placing the valves in the Y piece include the fact that they are bulky and difficult to see and have a higher resistance than unidirectional valves at the absorber (62). Serious accidents have occurred when a valved Y piece was placed into a circle system containing absorber-mounted valves (77–80). If this error occurs, there is a 50% chance that the valves in the Y piece will be opposed to those on the absorber and there will be no gas flow through the breathing system. For this reason, it is recommended that they not be used.

APL Valve

Figure 7.16 shows possible locations for the APL valve.

Spontaneous Ventilation

During spontaneous respiration, the most efficient use of absorbent will be with the APL valve on the Y piece (position B) (62,64). This is because during spontaneous respiration overflow occurs in the latter part of exhalation. Gas exhaled during the first part of exhalation is dead-space gas with a low concentration of carbon dioxide. Because the APL valve is not open, this gas passes by it. When the bag is filled, the pressure in the system rises and the APL valve opens. Because this opening occurs during the latter part of exhalation, the gas being expelled through the APL valve is mainly alveolar gas (with a high carbon dioxide content). No such discrimination is possible when the APL valve is distant from the patient (62).

With the APL valve at the Y piece, the added weight (especially when scavenging apparatus is added) may increase the incidence of disconnections. Transfer tubing to the scavenging interface may become entangled with other objects. The valve will be difficult to adjust during head and neck surgery. Finally, placing the valve at position B will cause a decrease in inspired heat and humidity (81).

Absorbent use is inefficient if the APL valve is downstream of the absorber (positions C and D) because vented gas would have passed through the absorber. If the APL valve is placed between the patient and the absorber (position E or B) only gas that has not passed through the absorber will be vented.

If the APL valve is placed at position C, fresh gas will be vented. Fresh gas will be vented if the APL valve is at position A only if the fresh gas flow is high (82).

If the APL valve were in position D, exhaled gases would move retrograde into the inspiratory tubing during exhalation, causing an increase in dead space.

Manually Controlled or Assisted Ventilation

During manually controlled or assisted ventilation, overflow of excess gases occurs during inspiration. If the APL valve were at the Y piece (position A), fresh gas and gas that had passed through the absorber would be vented, resulting in inefficient use of absorbent (62,64). The same holds true if the APL valve were located at position C or D. Locating the APL valve between the patient and the absorber (position E or B) would result in more efficient use of absorbent, although some fresh gas may dilute the gases vented at position E, and at position B, gases that have contacted absorbent will be vented (82).

Considerable venting of fresh gas will occur with the APL valve at position C, D, or A. There will be some venting if it is located at position E. Fresh gas will be vented at position B only if the fresh gas flow is quite high.

Locating the APL valve at the reservoir bag with an extender hose between the bag and the bag mount has been suggested (83). This location allows fresh gas that travels ret-

rograde through the absorber during exhalation more space in which to collect. This is the site to which excess gases are vented when an anesthesia ventilator is used with the circle system.

Automatic Ventilation

During automatic ventilation the APL valve is closed or isolated, so its location is of no significance.

Filters

Figure 7.17 shows five possible positions within the circle system for placement of a filter. Most disposable systems do not allow the interposition of a filter at position A or B. If the filter is placed in position A, C, or E, loose particles associated with the filter may be inhaled.

Position A is between the inhalation tubing and the Y piece. A filter here will protect the patient from contamination and absorbent dust, but does not protect the absorber or the operating room environment. If the filter is heavy or bulky, placing it in this position may be awkward. A filter should not be placed in this location if a humidifier is located upstream.

Position B is between the Y piece and the exhalation tubing. In this position the absorber, exhalation tubing and operating room environment will be protected. Water, mucus, or edema fluid can collect in the filter in this position, causing an increase in resistance or obstruction to gas flow (84,85). The bulk and weight of a filter may make it unsuitable for this location.

Position C is between the inspiratory tubing and the inspiratory unidirectional valve. A filter in this position will protect the patient from contamination from the absorber and its attached parts but not the inhalation tubing. It will catch absorbent dust (76). It will not protect the absorber or the operating room air from contamination from the patient. The size or weight of the filter is not a problem in this position. If a humidifier is

Figure 7.17. Possible locations for filters (see text for details).

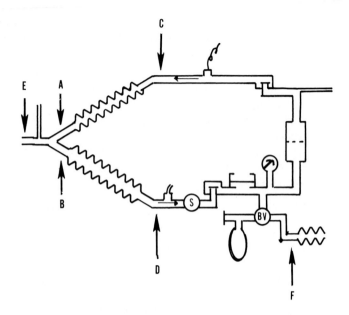

used, it should be downstream of the filter. Use of a filter in this position has been shown not to reduce the incidence of pneumonia after inhalation anesthesia (86).

Position D is between the exhalation unidirectional valve and the exhalation tubing. In this position, the filter will protect the internal parts of the absorber and other components from contamination but the exhalation tubing will become contaminated. Because the filter is on the expiratory side, obstruction from fluid is possible, although less likely than with position B.

Position E is between the Y piece and the tracheal tube or mask. In this position, the filter will protect the patient from the equipment and the equipment from the patient. It will also act as a heat and moisture exchanger (87). This suggests a strategy for infection control in anesthesia (88). Using a new filter between the patient and the breathing system with each patient would permit reuse of the breathing system. Potential problems with this site include increased dead space, increased possibility of disconnections and increased resistance. The filter may become clogged with blood, secretions, or edema fluid.

Position F is in the hose leading to the ven-

tilator. Disposable hoses with a filter are available for this purpose.

Respiratory Gases Monitor

Mainstream Devices

Oxygen Monitor. An oxygen monitor sensor may be fitted into the dome of a unidirectional valve, the top of the absorber or a T-shaped adapter. The sensor should be placed so that the tip points downward to prevent water from accumulating on the membrane.

Figure 7.18 shows possible locations for an oxygen monitor. Most disposable systems do not permit the sensor to be placed at position F or G. In positions H and I the sensor is inserted into the dome of a unidirectional valve.

Positions F, A, and H are on the inspiratory side, whereas positions G, E, I, and C are on the exhalation side. Placing the sensor on the expiratory side will usually expose it to more humidity, but with most sensors this is not a problem. If low fresh gas flows are used, the reading on the expiratory side will be lower than on the inspiratory side, but even with a closed system the inspired-expired difference is only 4% to 6% (89).

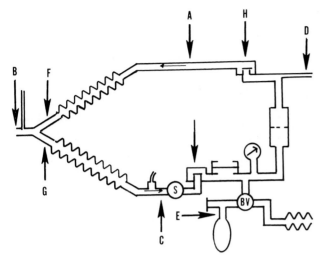

Figure 7.18. Possible locations for oxygen monitor sensor (see text for details).

It has been advocated that the oxygen analyzer be placed near the Y piece (position G, F or B), so that it will alarm in the event of a disconnection between the breathing system and the tracheal tube. However, an oxygen analyzer should not be relied on as a disconnect alarm. Although this is the most common site for disconnections, they occur in other locations. Furthermore, with a high fresh gas flow, the oxygen concentration may not fall sufficiently for the alarm to sound.

Placing the sensor in position B, F, or G may make it difficult to maintain in an upright position. In addition, the cable to the monitor may become entangled with other tubings or stretched, resulting in a pull on the Y piece. Placing the sensor in position B, between the Y piece and the tracheal tube or mask, will increase dead space.

Position D is in the fresh gas line. This position is not recommended, because the monitor will indicate only the concentration of oxygen in the gas mixture delivered to the breathing system and not in that inspired by the patient.

Mainstream CO$_2$ Monitor. To obtain satisfactory exhaled values, the sensor must be between the patient and the breathing system (position B in Fig. 7.18), as close as possible to the patient.

Sidestream Devices

Gases can be aspirated from a T adaptor in the breathing system or from a hole in a component such as an elbow adaptor. To obtain satisfactory samples of inhaled and exhaled gases, the sampling site should be close to the patient, in the elbow attached to the Y piece, in the Y piece itself, or in an adaptor between the Y piece and the patient.

Respirometer

Figure 7.19 shows possible locations for a respirometer in the circle system. Some have special adaptors for attaching them securely at particular locations.

A spirometer is usually placed on the expiratory side (position A), between the breathing tube and the expiratory unidirectional valve. During spontaneous respiration, the volumes recorded will be accurate. During controlled respiration, the spirometer will overread inspired volume, because of expansion of the breathing tubes and compression of gases (66,67).

A spirometer placed between the patient and the Y piece (position B) will record accurately with both spontaneous and controlled ventilation, but most are too bulky to place in this position and the increase in dead

Figure 7.19. Possible locations for a spirometer (see text for details).

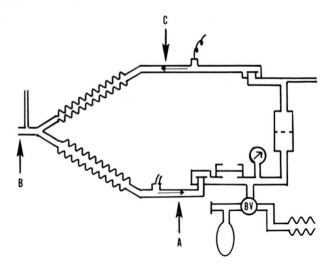

space may be significant. Use of this position may result in increased damage to the spirometer.

If the spirometer is placed on the inspiratory side (position C), during controlled or assisted ventilation it will overread volumes caused by expansion of the tubings and leaks between the spirometer and the patient.

Sensor for Airway Pressure Monitor

The sensor for an airway pressure monitor can be placed anywhere in the breathing system that the oxygen sensor can be placed (see Fig. 7.18). Most disposable systems do not allow placement at position F or G. Position B has the same disadvantages as placing the oxygen sensor at that point. To place the pressure sensor in the fresh gas line (position D) a special adaptor would be needed. In addition, the small diameter of the tubing and high flow of gas might result in falsely high pressures being sensed so that a low pressure in the breathing system might be missed.

Positions A, C, I, E, and H provide stable locations for the sensor. To use position I or H a special modification must be made to the dome of a unidirectional valve. T adaptors could be used in positions A, E, and C.

Positions on the expiratory side have an advantage over those on the inspiratory side. If there is obstruction to flow in the inspiratory limb and the sensor for airway pressures is located upstream of the obstruction, the low pressure at the patient will not be sensed. If the sensor is located downstream from the obstruction or on the expiratory side the low pressure will be detected.

PEEP Valve

The positive end expiratory pressure valve must be placed in the expiratory side of the breathing system. A disposable PEEP valve should be placed between the expiratory breathing tube and the expiratory unidirectional valve (position B in Fig. 7.20). Built-in PEEP valves are usually situated downstream of the expiratory unidirectional valve and upstream of the absorber (position A in Fig. 7.20). A bidirectional PEEP valve may be inserted between the anesthesia ventilator and breathing system.

Pressure Manometer

To measure PEEP accurately, the pressure manometer must be on the same side (patient or absorber) of the expiratory unidirectional valve as the PEEP valve (90). On most older absorber assemblies the manometer is on the absorber side of the unidirectional valve. If a PEEP valve is added to the expiratory limb on the patient side of the unidirectional valve PEEP will not register on the manometer gauge. Most newer absorber assemblies have a built-in PEEP valve located

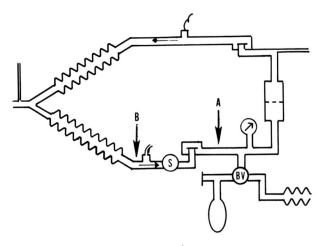

Figure 7.20. Possible locations for a PEEP valve (see text for details).

on the absorber side of the unidirectional valve with the pressure manometer in close proximity.

Resistance and Work of Breathing in the Circle System

In the past, one of the objections to using a circle system with small children was that it had a high resistance. However, investigations have shown that the resistance or work of breathing with the circle system is not significantly greater than with other breathing systems and may be less in some cases (55,91–95).

There are no studies to indicate that there is any greater problem in letting an infant breathe spontaneously with a circle system as opposed to a nonrebreathing system (96).

Use of coaxial tubings increases resistance (55).

Dead Space of the Circle System

In the circle system, dead space extends into the Y piece as far as the partition. Use of a Y piece with a septum will decrease dead space. When exhalation or inhalation starts, the gases in the breathing tubes move in the opposite direction from their usual flow until stopped by closure of one of the unidirec-

tional valves. This is referred to as *backlash* and causes a slight increase in dead space. If the unidirectional valves are competent, however, backlash will be clinically insignificant.

Heat and Humidity

In the circle system moisture is available from three sources: exhaled gases, the water content of the absorbent granules, and water liberated from the neutralization of carbon dioxide. Most inspired humidity is supplied by the absorbent; exhaled water vapor makes a small contribution (97). The amount derived from the neutralization of carbon dioxide is negligible.

Gases in the inspiratory limb of a circle system are near room temperature (98,99). Even with low fresh gas flows, gases reach the Y piece only 1° to 3°C above ambient temperature (100,101).

The humidity of a standard adult circle system using a fresh gas flow of 5 liters/min is shown in Figure 7.21. The initial inspired humidity was 30%. This rose to 61% in 90 min, stabilizing at this level. These values may be altered by the following factors.

1. Changing the fresh gas flow: Higher humidity results when lower fresh gas flows are used (81,100–103).

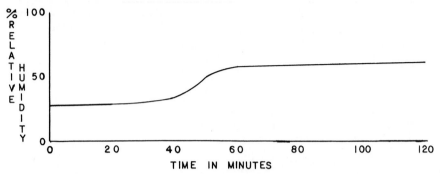

Figure 7.21. Humidity changes in the circle system. Fresh gas flow 5000 ml/min; CO_2 inflow 200 ml/min; respiratory rate 12/min; and tidal volume 500 ml. From Chalon J, Kao ZI, Dolorico VN, Atkin DH. Humidity output of the circle absorber system. Anesthesiology 1973;38:462.

2. Changes in carbon dioxide output by the patient: A reduction in the patient's carbon dioxide output will cause a decrease in the initial and final humidity (98).
3. Changes in minute ventilation: Increasing ventilation will increase the inspired humidity (98,88).
4. Prior use of the system: This results in an initially higher humidity that stabilizes in the same period of time at the same final humidity (98).
5. Position of components of the system (81): An increase in humidity of inspired gas occurs when the fresh gas inlet is upstream of the absorber (71,104).
6. Wetting the inspiratory tubing (105,106) or using a humidifier: Humidifiers will be discussed in Chapter 9.
7. Heating the canister (104) or the breathing tubes (107): This will increase both the inspired temperature and humidity.
8. Use of smaller canisters (81).
9. Modifications to the circle system: These include coaxial tubings (81,108–110) and the use of the heat of reaction to vaporize water (109,111,112).

Relationship between Inspired and Delivered Concentrations

In a system with no rebreathing, the concentrations of gases and vapors in the in-spired mixture will be close to those in fresh gas. With rebreathing, however, the concentrations in the inspired mixture may differ considerably from those in the fresh gas.

NITROGEN (113)

The importance of nitrogen lies in the fact that it hinders the establishment of high concentrations of nitrous oxide and may cause low inspired oxygen concentrations. Before any fresh gas is delivered, the concentration of nitrogen in the breathing system is approximately 80%. Nitrogen enters the system from exhaled gases and leaves through the APL valve or ventilator and leaks.

Using high fresh gas flows for a few minutes to eliminate most of the nitrogen in the system and much of that in the patient is called *denitrogenation*. Different methods have been described, with varying flows and times. A fresh gas flow of 10 liters/min for 1 min followed by 5 liters/min for 6 min after intubation suffices to wash out most nitrogen in the system (114).

After denitrogenation, nitrogen elimination by the patient will proceed at a slower rate. In a closed system, the nitrogen concentration will gradually rise. Provided denitrogenation has been carried out, even if all the body's nitrogen is exhaled, the concentration in the breathing should not increase to more than 18% in the average adult (114–119).

CARBON DIOXIDE

With Absorbent

The inspired carbon dioxide concentration should be near zero unless there is failure of one or both unidirectional valves (120,121), exhausted absorbent, or the bypass mechanism is left in the off position. If one of these conditions exists, a high fresh gas flow will limit the increase in inspired carbon dioxide concentration.

Without Absorbent

A number of studies using the circle system without absorbent have been published (75,122–130), with varying recommendations for fresh gas flow and ventilation. The arterial carbon dioxide level achieved will depend on the fresh gas flow, the arrangement of circle system components, and ventilation. Advantages of not using absorbent include the ability to achieve the desired level of arterial carbon dioxide with hyperventilation, lack of danger of inhaling absorbent dust, lack of dependence on absorbent to eliminate CO_2, and low resistance. Disadvantages include the need for uneconomical high flows and lower heat and humidity.

OXYGEN

The following factors influence the concentration of oxygen in the inspired mixture: rate of uptake by the patient; uptake and elimination of other gases by the patient; arrangement of the components of the circle; ventilation; fresh gas flow; volume of the system; and the concentration of oxygen in the fresh gas. Because so many of these are unpredictable and uncontrollable, use of a reliable oxygen analyzer in the breathing system should be mandatory.

ANESTHETIC AGENT (131)

The following factors influence the concentration of anesthetic agent in the inspired mixture: uptake by the patient; uptake by components of the system; arrangement of system components; uptake and elimination of other gases by the patient; volume of the system; concentration in the fresh gas flow; and fresh gas flow. Because of these many factors, it is not possible to predict the concentration accurately unless a high fresh gas flow is used. The greatest variation occurs during induction, when anesthetic uptake is high and nitrogen excretion by the patient dilutes the gases in the circuit. For this reason, most authors recommend that anesthesia be begun with high fresh gas flows. Several devices are now available to measure the inspired anesthetic agent concentration (see Chapter 16).

Use of Circle System with Low Fresh Gas Flows

DEFINITIONS

Low-flow anesthesia has been variously defined as an inhalation technique in which a circle system with absorbent is used with a fresh gas inflow of (*i*) less than the patient's alveolar minute volume, (*ii*) 1 liter/min or less (132), (*iii*) 3 liters/min or less (133), (*iv*) 0.5 to 2 liters/min (100), and (*v*) less than 4 liters/min (134). Closed system anesthesia is a form of low-flow anesthesia in which the fresh gas flow equals uptake of anesthetic gases and oxygen by the patient and system. No excess gas is vented through the APL valve.

EQUIPMENT

Anesthesia Machine

A standard anesthesia machine can be used, but it must have flowmeters that will provide low flows.

Circle System

A standard circle system with the absorber filled with active absorbent is used. If the absorber has a bypass this should be removed or the absorber should be replaced with one that does not have a bypass. Should the bypass be inadvertently left in the on position during low-flow anesthesia, extreme hypercarbia could result.

The system must have low leakage. Intubation with a cuffed tube (or a gas-tight fit if using a mask) is required.

Vaporizers

Anesthetic agent can be added to the circle in two ways.

Direct Injection into the Expiratory Limb (135–140)

If direct injection is used, care must be taken that only small amounts are injected at a time and that the syringe containing the liquid agent is not confused with those containing agents for intravenous injection. Another problem is that the liquid agent may cause deterioration of components in the system (141).

Calibrated Vaporizers (135)

Vaporizers capable of delivering high concentrations are required for low-flow anesthesia. Settings may need to be as high as 5% for halothane and isoflurane and 7% for enflurane (142). Some vaporizers cannot deliver high concentrations, and some are not accurate at low flows (143).

Ventilator

A ventilator whose bellows rises during exhalation will result in easier detection of disconnections and large leaks than one whose bellows descends (144,145). If a ventilator whose bellows descends during exhalation is used, leaks may lead to entrainment of driving gas or air.

Respiratory Gas Monitor(s)

Analysis of the major gaseous constituents will make low-flow anesthesia safer. Continuous measurement of oxygen concentrations should be mandatory. Monitoring of other gases is helpful. Lower flows can be used with mainstream analyzers, but with aspirating types, the fresh gas flow must be increased to compensate for the gases removed by the

monitor unless the gases are returned to the breathing system (146).

TECHNIQUES

Induction

Induction using low fresh gas flows can be accomplished by injecting measured amounts of liquid anesthetic directly into the expiratory limb of the circuit. Problems associated with this include the following: (*i*) Large body stores of nitrogen will be released into the breathing system and will dilute concentrations of other gases. (*ii*) If nitrous oxide is being used, it will take a prolonged period of time to establish concentrations high enough to have a clinical effect. (*iii*) Rapidly changing uptake of nitrous oxide and volatile agent as well as high oxygen consumption during this period mean that the anesthesia practitioner will have to make frequent injections and adjustments at a time when he or she is likely to be busy with other tasks.

More commonly, induction is accomplished using high flows to allow denitrogenation, establishment of anesthetic agent concentrations, and provide oxygen well in excess of consumption. After gas exchange has stabilized, low flows are used.

Maintenance

During maintenance, nitrous oxide and oxygen flows and vaporizer settings should be adjusted to maintain a satisfactory oxygen concentration and the desired level of anesthesia. If closed system anesthesia is used, a constant circuit volume is achieved by one of the following methods (142,147).

Constant Reservoir Bag Size

If the bag decreases in size, the fresh gas flow rate is increased. If bag increases in size, the flow must be decreased.

Ventilator with Ascending (Upright or Standing) Bellows

Constant volume can be achieved by adjusting the fresh gas flow so that the bellows is below the top of its housing at the end of exhalation. It is important that no negative pressure be transmitted to the bellows from the scavenging system, as this could cause the bellows to be held aloft in the presence of inadequate fresh gas flow (148).

Ventilator with Descending (Inverted or Hanging) Bellows

The fresh gas flow should be adjusted so that the bellows just reaches the bottom of its housing at the end of exhalation.

If a rapid change in any component of the inspired mixture is desired, the fresh gas flow should be increased. If, for any reason, the integrity of the circle is broken, high flows with desired inspired concentrations should be used for several minutes before returning to low flows. If closed system anesthesia is used, it is recommended that high flows be used for 1 to 2 min at least once an hour to eliminate gases such as nitrogen and carbon monoxide that accumulate in the system.

Emergence

Recovery from anesthesia will be extremely slow when low flows are used. High flows are usually needed at least briefly to clear nitrous oxide. Coasting, in which anesthetic administration is stopped toward the end of the operation and the circuit is maintained closed with enough oxygen flow to maintain a constant end-tidal volume of the ventilator or reservoir bag, is often used (149). A charcoal filter placed in the inspiratory limb will cause a rapid decrease in volatile agent concentration (150–152).

ADVANTAGES

Economy (153–159)

Significant savings can be achieved with lower flows of nitrous oxide and oxygen, but the greatest savings occurs with the potent volatile agents. These savings are partly offset by increased absorbent usage, but this is small (160–162). Because the amount of excess gases and vapors that must be removed

from the operating room is reduced, there will be a savings in energy if an active scavenging system is used.

Reduction of Operating Room Pollution

With lower flows, there will be less anesthetic agent put into the operating room. One study showed that with nitrous oxide flows of 300 ml/min the concentrations inhaled by operating room personnel were within the OSHA limits without scavenging (163). However, use of low-flow techniques does not eliminate the need for scavenging, because high flows are still necessary at times. Because a less volatile agent is used, vaporizers have to be filled less frequently so exposure of personnel to anesthetic vapors during filling is decreased.

Reduced Environmental Pollution

Fluorocarbons and nitrous oxide attack the earth's ozone layer (164–167). Nitrous oxide contributes to the greenhouse effect (165). With low flows, the ecological dangers are reduced.

Estimation of Anesthetic Agent Uptake and Oxygen Consumption (114,168,169)

In a closed system without significant leaks, fresh gas flow is matched by the patient's uptake of oxygen and anesthetic agents. Changes in volume may be attributed to changes in uptake of oxygen or nitrous oxide, because the volume contributed by the potent inhalational agents is not significant.

Buffering of Changes in Inspired Concentrations

The lower the fresh gas flow, the longer it takes for a change in concentration in the fresh gas flow to result in a comparable change in the inspired concentration.

Conservation of Heat and Humidity (100,102,103)

With lower gas flows, inspired humidity will be increased (81,100–103).

Less Danger of Barotrauma

High pressures in the breathing system take longer to develop with lower flows.

DISADVANTAGES

More Attention Required

With closed system anesthesia fresh gas flow into the system must be kept in balance with uptake. This could lead to insufficient attention to other aspects of the patient's care.

Inability to Alter Quickly Inspired Concentrations

This inability is a significant disadvantage only if the user insists on using low flows at all times. The user of low flows should accept that when it is necessary to change inspired concentrations rapidly, higher flows should be used.

Danger of Hypercarbia

The degree of hypercarbia from inactive absorbent, incompetent unidirectional valves, or the bypass on the absorber being left in the off position will be greater when low flows are used.

Greater Knowledge Required

Use of low-flow anesthesia requires knowledge of uptake. However, it is arguable whether the need to acquire this knowledge is a disadvantage.

Accumulation of Undesirable Gases in the System

The accumulation of undesirable gases is probably only a problem with closed circuit anesthesia, because low flows provide a continuous flush of the system. With closed system anesthesia flushing with high fresh gas flows once an hour will decrease the concentration of most of these substances. To date, there have been no cases reported of patient harm from breathing any of these substances.

Carbon Monoxide

Carbon monoxide from the breakdown of hemoglobin can accumulate in the closed circle system (170). However, the levels reported were unlikely to cause clinically significant effects. One study found that carboxyhemoglobin concentrations actually decreased during closed circuit anesthesia (135). Although the levels reported with normal patients should be innocuous, patients with severe hemolytic anemia, high COHb levels and/or a reduced total hemoglobin may be at some risk (171).

Acetone, Methane, Hydrogen, and Ethanol

Hydrogen, methane, and acetone accumulate during closed system anesthesia (117,172,173). However, dangerous levels are reached only after hours of closed system anesthesia (174). The common intoxicant ethanol can also accumulate. Flushing with high flows will decrease the concentrations of methane and hydrogen, but will not significantly affect the concentration of ethanol or acetone (117).

Toxic Metabolites of Anesthetic Agents

One study showed that low concentrations of two volatile metabolites of halothane and a metabolic decomposition product—which has been shown to be mutagenic in one study (175) but not in another (176)—could be found in exhaled gases of patients anesthetized with halothane using a circle system but not a system without absorbent (27). However, the levels found were well below those demonstrated to be toxic in laboratory animals (177). Maintenance of closed system anesthesia with isoflurane for 48 hr without evidence of toxicity has been reported (178).

Argon

If oxygen is supplied from an oxygen concentrator, there will be an accumulation of argon (179). Also USP oxygen contains argon (117). The importance of argon is that it lowers the concentration of oxygen and anesthetic agents.

Nitrogen

Even with denitrogenation, nitrogen will accumulate in the closed breathing circuit (114,115,117,135). If oxygen is being supplied by an oxygen concentrator, malfunction of one of the concentrator modules can cause nitrogen to appear in the product gas (179).

Uncertainty about Inspired Concentrations

One of the effects of rebreathing is that the inspired concentrations cannot be predicted accurately. However, absolute or near-absolute knowledge of inspired concentration of anesthetic agents is not necessary for safe conduct of anesthesia, because patients' responses to drugs vary widely.

Use of Circle System for Pediatric Anesthesia

In the past, special pediatric circle systems with small absorbers were used. These are no longer available commercially. What is referred to as a pediatric circle system is usually a standard absorber assembly with short, small-diameter tubings and a small bag attached. The circle system can be used with low flows with pediatric patients (180–184).

Advantages of Circle System

1. Low fresh gas flows can be used.
2. Pa_{CO_2} depends only on ventilation, not fresh gas flow.
3. Normocarbia can be achieved when a malignant hyperthermia syndrome develops.
4. The lengths of the tubings can be varied so that the machine can be placed away from the patient to allow optimal surgical exposure in head and neck surgery (185)

5. An easy and rapid changeover from an adult to a pediatric system can be made; smaller breathing tubes are attached to the inspiratory and expiratory ports and a 0.5- or 1-liter bag is attached to the bag mount (96).

Disadvantages of Circle System

1. It is composed of many parts that can be arranged incorrectly or may malfunction.
2. Some components are difficult to clean.
3. The system is bulky and not easily moved.
4. Minute volume must be limited to avoid profound hypocarbia.

REFERENCES

1. American Society for Testing and Materials. Standard specification for minimum performance and safety requirements for anesthesia breathing systems (ASTM F1208-89). Philadelphia: ASTM, 1989.
2. Anonymous. Sodasorb prePak CO_2 absorption cartridges. Health Devices 1988;17:35–36.
3. Anonymous. North American Drager Narkomed 2A carbon dioxide absorbers. Health Devices 1986;15:178–179.
4. Anonymous. Anesthesia machine owners alerted to potential breathing circuit leak. Biomed Safe Stand 1989;19:122.
5. Elam JO. The design of circle absorbers. Anesthesiology 1958;19:99–100.
6. Neufeld PD, Johnson DL. Results of the Canadian Anaesthetists' Society opinion survey on anesthetic equipment. Can Anaesth Soc J 1983; 30:469–473.
7. Adriani J. Disposal of carbon dioxide from devices used for inhalational anesthesia. Anesthesiology 1960;21:742–758.
8. Brown ES, Bakamjian V, Seniff AM. Performance of absorbents: effect of moisture. Anesthesiology 1959;20:613–617.
9. Miles G, Adriani J. Carbon dioxide absorption. Anesth Analg 1959;38:293–300.
10. Adriani J, Rovenstine EA. Experimental studies on carbon dioxide absorbers for anesthesia. Anesthesiology 1941;2:1–19.
11. Foregger R. The regeneration of soda lime following absorption of carbon dioxide. Anesthesiology 1948;9:15–20.

12. Jorgensen B, Jorgensen S. The 600 gram CO_2 absorption canister: an experimental study. Acta Anaesthesiol Scand 1977;21:437–444.

13. Sato T. New aspects of carbon dioxide absorption in anesthetic circuits. Med J Osaka Univ 1971;22:173–206.

14. Bracken A, Sanderson DM. Some observations on anaesthetic soda lime. Br J Anaesth 1955;27:422–427.

15. Lund I, Lund O, Erikson H. Model experiments on absorption efficiency of soda lime. 1957;Br J Anaesth 29:17–20.

16. Adriani J, Batten DH. The efficiency of mixtures of barium and calcium hydroxides in the absorption of carbon dioxide in rebreathing appliances. Anesthesiology 1942;3:1–10.

17. Hunt HK. Resistance in respiratory valves and canisters. Anesthesiology 1955;16:190–205.

18. Adriani J. The removal of carbon dioxide from rebreathing appliances. J Aviation Med 1941;12:304–309.

19. Maycock E. Soda lime dust. Anaesth Intensive Care 1980;8:217.

20. Davis R. Soda lime dust. Anaesth Intensive Care 1979;7:390.

21. Lauria JI. Soda-lime dust contamination of breathing circuits. Anesthesiology 1975;42:628–629.

22. Hale DE. The rise and fall of soda lime. Anesth Analg 1967;46:648–655.

23. Adriani J. Rebreathing in anesthesia. South Med J 1942;35:798–804.

24. Eger EI II. Stability of I-653 in soda lime. Anesth Analg 1987;66:983–985.

25. Eger EI, Strum DP. The absorption and degradation of isoflurane and I-653 by dry soda lime at various temperatures. Anesth Analg 1987;66:1312–1315.

26. Liu J, Laster MJ, Eger EI II, Taheri S. Absorption and degradation of sevoflurane and isoflurane in a conventional anesthetic circuit. Anesth Analg 1991;72:785–789.

27. Sharp JH, Trudell JR, Cohen EN. Volatile metabolites and decomposition products of halothane in man. Anesthesiology 1979;50:2–8.

28. Strum DP, Johnson BH, Eger EI II. Stability of sevoflurane in soda lime. Anesthesiology 1987;67:779–781.

29. Wong DT, Lerman J. Factors affecting the rate of disappearance of sevoflurane in baralyme. Can J Anaesth 1992;39:366–369.

30. Hanaki C, Fujii K, Morio M, Tashima T. Decomposition of sevoflurane by soda lime. Hiroshima J Med Sci 1987;36:61–67.

31. Moon RE, Ingram C, Brunner EA, Meyer AF. Spontaneous generation of carbon monoxide within anesthetic circuits. Anesthesiology 1991;75:A873.

32. Moon RE, Sparacino C, Meyer AF. Pathogenesis of carbon monoxide production in anesthesia circuits. Anesthesiology 1992;77:A1061.

33. Grodin WK, Epstein MAF, Epstein RA. Enflurane and isoflurane adsorption by soda lime. Anesthesiology 1981;55:A124.

34. Grodin WK, Epstein RA. Halothane adsorption complicating the use of soda-lime to humidify anaesthetic gases. Br J Anaesth 1982;54:555–559.

35. Grodin WK, Epstein MAF, Epstein RA. Mechanisms of halothane adsorption by dry soda-lime. Br J Anaesth 1982;54:561–565.

36. Tanifuji Y, Takagi K, Kobayashi K, Yasuda N, Eger EI. The interaction between sevoflurane and soda lime or baralyme. Anesth Analg 1989;68:S285.

37. Grodin WK, Epstein MAF, Epstein RA. Soda lime adsorption of isoflurane and enflurane. Anesthesiology 1985;62:60–64.

38. Andrews JJ, Johnston RV, Bee DE, Arens JF. Photodeactivation of ethyl violet: a potential hazard of Sodasorb. Anesthesiology 1990;72:59–64.

39. Elam JO. Channeling and overpacking in carbon dioxide absorbers. Anesthesiology 1958;19:403–404.

40. Lamb KSR, Cummings GC, Asbury AJ. Comparison of three commercially available preparations of soda-lime. Br J Anaesth 1988;60:329P–330P.

41. Detmer MD, Chandra P, Cohen PJ. Occurrence of hypercarbia due to an unusual failure of anesthetic equipment. Anesthesiology 1980;52:278–279.

42. Tsuchiya M, Ueda W. Heat generation as an index of exhaustion of soda lime. Anesth Analg 1989;68:683–687.

43. Anonymous. Soda lime in anaesthesia. Aust Ther Device Bull 1990;90(2):3.

44. Kim J, Kovac AL, Mathewson HS. A method for detection of incompetent unidirectional dome valves. Anesth Analg 1985;64:745–747.

45. Nunn BJ, Rosewarne FA. Expiratory valve failure. Anaesth Intensive Care 1990;18:273–274.

46. Schreiber P. Anaesthesia Equipment. Performance, classification, and safety. New York: Springer-Verlag, 1974.

47. Rosewarne F, Wells D. Three cases of valve incompetence in a circle system. Anaesth Intensive Care 1988;16:376–377.

48. Amir M. Caught by a cage. Anaesth Intensive Care 1992;20:389–390.

49. Dean HN, Parsons DE, Raphaely RC. Case report: bilateral tension pneumothorax from mechanical failure of anesthesia machine due to misplaced expiratory valve. Anesth Analg 1971;50:195–198.

50. Cottrell JE, Bernhard W, Turndorf H. Hazards of

disposable rebreathing circuits. Anesth Analg 1976;55:743–744.

51. Wang JS, Hung WT, Lin CY. Leakage of disposable breathing circuits. J Clin Anesth 1992;4:111–115.
52. Anonymous. Disposable anesthesia patient circuits. Health Devices 1979;9:3–15.
53. American Society for Testing and Materials. Standard specification for anesthesia breathing tubes (ASTM F1205-88). Philadelphia: ASTM, 1988.
54. McIntyre JWR. Anaesthesia breathing circuits. Can Anaesth Soc J 1986;33:98–105.
55. Shandro J. A coaxial circle circuit: comparison with conventional circle and Bain circuit. Can Anaesth Soc J 1982;29:121–125.
56. Crowhurst P. Mishaps with the Mera-F circuit. Anaesth Intensive Care 1987;15:121–122.
57. Evans IEH. Mera circuit. Anaesth Intensive Care 1985;13:105–106.
58. Sims C, Cullingford DWJ. Kinking of the Mera-F-circuit. Anaesth Intensive Care 1988;16:243.
59. American Society for Testing and Materials. Standard specification for anesthesia reservoir bags (ASTM F1204-88). Philadelphia: ASTM, 1988.
60. Stevenson PH, McLeskey CH. Breakage of a reservoir bag mount, an unusual anesthesia machine failure. Anesthesiology 1980;53:270–271.
61. Warren PR, Gintautas J. Problems with Dupaco ventilator valve assembly. Anesthesiology 1980; 53:524–525.
62. Eger EI, Ethans CT. The effects of inflow, overflow and valve placement on economy of the circle system. Anesthesiology 1968; 29:93–100.
63. Zbinden AM, Feigenwinter P, Hutmacher M. Fresh gas utilization of eight circle systems. Br J Anaesth 1991;67:492–499.
64. Brown ES, Seniff AM, Elam JO. Carbon dioxide elimination in semiclosed systems. Anesthesiology 1964;25:31–36.
65. Briere C, Patoine JG, Audet R. Inaccurate ventimetry by fresh gas inlet position. Can Anaesth Soc J 1974;21:117–119.
66. Campbell DI. Volumeter attachment on Boyle circle absorber, Br J Anaesth 1971;43:206–207.
67. Purnell RJ. The position of the Wright anemometer in the circle absorber system. Br J Anaesth 1968;40:917–918.
68. Grodin WK, Epstein RA. Halothane adsorption by soda lime. Anesthesiology 1979;51:S317.
69. Berry FA, Hughes-Davies DI. Methods of increasing the humidity and temperature of the inspired gases in the infant circle system. Anesthesiology 1972;37:456–462.
70. Shanks CA, Sara CA. Estimation of inspiratory-limb humidity in the circle system. Anesthesiology 1974;40:99–100.

71. Weeks DB. Higher humidity, an additional benefit of a disposable anesthesia circle. Anesthesiology 1975;43:375–377.
72. Harper M, Eger EI. A comparison of the efficiency of three anesthesia circle systems. Anesth Analg 1976;55:724–729.
73. Campbell DI. Change of gas inflow siting on Boyle MK3 absorbers. Anaesthesia 1971;26:104.
74. Russell WJ, Drew SE. A potential hazard with an inspiratory valve of a circle system. Anaesth Intensive Care 1977;5:269–271.
75. Schoonbee CG, Conway CM. Factors affecting carbon dioxide homeostasis during controlled ventilation with circle systems. Br J Anaesth 1981;53:471–477.
76. Amaranath L, Boutros AR. Circle absorber and soda lime contamination. Anesth Analg 1980; 59:711–712.
77. Dogu TS, Davis HS. Hazards of inadvertently opposed valves. Anesthesiology 1970;33:122–123.
78. LeBourdais E. Doctors say connector units are dangerous. Dimens Health Serv 1976;(Feb):10–11.
79. Rendell-Baker L. Another close call with crossed valves. Anesthesiology 1969;31:194–195.
80. White CW. Hazards of the valved Y-piece. Anesthesiology 1970;32:567.
81. Bengtson JP, Bengtson A, Stenqvist O. The circle system as a humidifier. Br J Anaesth 1989;63:453–457.
82. Varma YS, Puri GD. Location of the adjustable pressure limiting valve. Anaesthesia 1986;41:773–774.
83. Puri GD, Varma YS. A new site for the adjustable pressure limiting valve on a circle absorber. Anaesthesia 1985;40:889–891.
84. Kopman Aaron F. Obstruction of bacterial filters by edema fluid. Anesthesiology 1976;44:169–170.
85. Mason J, Tackley R. An acute rise in expiratory resistance due to a blocked ventilator filter. Anaesthesia 1981;36:335.
86. Garibaldi RA, Britt MR, Webster C, Pace NL. Failure of bacterial filters to reduce the incidence of pneumonia after inhalation anesthesia. Anesthesiology 1981;54:364–368.
87. Chalon J, Markham JP, Ali MM, Ramanathan S, Turndorf H. The Pall Ultipor breathing circuit filter—an efficient heat and moisture exchanger. Anesth Analg 1984;63:566–570.
88. Berry AJ, Nolte FS. An alternative strategy for infection control of anesthesia breathing circuits: a laboratory assessment of the Pall HME filter. Anesth Analg 1991;72:651–655.
89. MacKrell TN. Intravenous anesthesia plus nitrous oxide in a closed system. In: Aldrete JA, Lowe HJ, Virtue RW, eds. Low flows and closed system an-

esthesia. New York: Grune & Stratton, 1979:99–101.

90. Mayle LL, Reed SJ, Wyche MQ. Excessive airway pressures occurring concurrently with use of the Fraser Harlake PEEP valve. Anesthesiol Rev 1990;17:41–44.

91. Conterato JP, Lindahl GE, Meyer DM, Bires JA. Assessment of spontaneous ventilation in anesthetized children with use of a pediatric circle or a Jackson-Rees system. Anesth Analg 1989;69:484–490.

92. Gravenstein N, Gallagher RC. External flow-resistive, circuit-related work of breathing: Bain vs circle. Anesthesiology 1985;63:A183.

93. Kay B, Beatty PCW, Healy TEJ, Accoush MEA, Calpin M. Change in the work of breathing imposed by five anaesthetic breathing systems. Br J Anaesth 1983;55:1239–1246.

94. Rasch DK, Bunegin L, Ledbetter, KIaminskas D. Comparison of circle absorber and Jackson-Rees systems for paediatric anaesthesia. Can J Anaesth 1988;35:25–30.

95. Shandro J. Resistance to gas flow in the "new" anaesthesia circuits: a comparative study. Can Anaesth Soc J 1982;29:387–390.

96. Berry FA. Clinical pharmacology of inhalational anesthetics, muscle relaxants, vasoactive agents, and narcotics, and techniques of general anesthesia. In: Berry FA, ed. Anesthetic management of difficult and routine pediatric patients. 2nd ed. New York: Churchill Livingstone, 1990:83–84.

97. Dery R, Pelletier J, Jacques A, Clavet M, Houde JJ. Humidity in anaesthesiology II. Evolution of heat and moisture in the large carbon dioxide absorbers. Can Anaesth Soc J 1967;14:205–219.

98. Chalon J, Kao ZL, Dolorico VN, Atkin DH. Humidity output of the circle absorber system. Anesthesiology 1973;38:458–465.

99. Dery R, Pelletier J, Jacques A, Clavet M, Houde JJ. Humidity in anaesthesiology. Heat and moisture patterns in the respiratory tract during anaesthesia with the semi-closed system. Can Anaesth Soc J 1967;14:287–298.

100. Aldrete JA, Cubillos P, Sherrill D. Humidity and temperature changes during low flow and closed system anaesthesia. Acta Anaesthesiol Scand 1981;25:312–314.

101. Shanks CA, Sara CA. Airway heat and humidity during endotracheal intubation. III: rebreathing from the circle absorber at low fresh gas flows. Anaesth Intensive Care 1973;1:415–417.

102. Aldrete JA. Closed circuit anesthesia prevents moderate hypothermia occurring in patients having extremity surgery. Circular 1987;4:3–4.

103. Kleeman PP, Jantzen FP, Erdmann W. Fresh gas flow effects on airway climate: a controlled clinical study. Circular 1988;5:11.

104. Berry FA, Ball CG, Blankenbaker WL. Humidification of anesthetic systems for prolonged procedures. Anesth Analg 1975;54:50–54.

105. Chase HF, Kilmore MA, Trotta R. Respiratory water loss via anesthesia systems: mask breathing. Anesthesiology 1961;22:205–209.

106. Shanks CA, Sara CA. Airway heat and humidity during endotracheal intubation. 4: connotations of delivered water vapour content. Anaesth Intensive Care 1974;2:212–220.

107. Kadim MY, Lockwood GG, Chakrabarti MK, Whitwam JG. A low-flow to-and-fro system. Laboratory study of mixing of anaesthetic and driving gases during mechanical ventilation. Anaesthesia 1991;46:948–951.

108. Chalon J, Patel C, Ramanathan S, Turndorf H. Humidification of the circle absorber system. Anesthesiology 1978;48:142–146.

109. Chalon J, Goldman C, Amirdivani M, Rothblatt A, Ramanathan S, Turndorf H. Humidification in a modified circle system. Anesth Analg 1979; 58:216–220.

110. Ramanathan S, Chalon J, Turndorf H. Compact well-humidified breathing circuit for the circle system. Anesthesiology 1976;44:238–242.

111. Chalon J, Ramanathan S. Water vaporizer heated by the reaction of neutralization of carbon dioxide. Anesthesiology 1974;41:400–404.

112. Paspa P, Tang CK, Dwarkmanath R, Ramanathan S, Chalon J, Fischgrund GK, Turndorf H. A percolator vaporizer heated by reaction of neutralization of lime by carbon dioxide. Anesth Analg 1981;60:146–149.

113. Conway CM. Gaseous homeostasis and the circle system. Validation of a model. Br J Anaesth 1986;58:337–344.

114. Bengtson JP, Sonander H, Stenqvist O. Gaseous homeostasis during low-flow anaesthesia. Acta Anaesthesiol Scand 1988;32:516–521.

115. Barton F, Nunn JF. Totally closed circuit nitrous oxide/oxygen anaesthesia. Br J Anaesth 1975; 47:350–357.

116. Anonymous. Action required on scavenging systems. Br J Anaesth 1976;48:397.

117. Morita S, Latta W, Hambro K, Snider MT. Accumulation of methane, acetone, and nitrogen in the inspired gas during closed-circuit anesthesia. Anesth Analg 1985;64:343–347.

118. Philip JH. Nitrogen build-up in a closed circuit. J Clin Monit 1991;7:89.

119. Luttropp H, Rydgren G, Thomasson R, Werner O. A minimal-flow system for xenon anesthesia. Anesthesiology 1991;75:896–902.

120. Kerr JH, Evers JL. Carbon dioxide accumulation: valve leaks and inadequate absorption. Can Anaesth Soc J 1958;5:154–160.

121. Schultz EA, Buckley JJ, Oswald AJ, Van Bergen

FH. Profound acidosis in an anesthetized human: report of a case. Anesthesiology 1960;21:285–291.

122. Akkineni S, Patel KP, Bennett EJ, Grunty EM, Ignacio AD. Fresh gas flow to limit PaCO$_2$ in T and circle systems without CO$_2$ absorption. Anesthesiol Rev 1977;4:33–37.

123. deSilva AJC. Normocapnic ventilation using the circle system. Can Anaesth Soc J 1976;23:657–666.

124. Gibb DB, Prior G, Pollard B. Methods of conserving carbon dioxide in artificially ventilated patients. A clinical investigation. Anaesth Intensive Care 1977;5:122–127.

125. Harris PHP, Kerr JH, Edmonds-Seal J. Artificial ventilation using a circle circuit without an absorber. Anaesthesia 1975;30:269–270.

126. Keenan RL, Boyan CP. How rebreathing anaesthetic systems control PaCO$_2$ studies with a mechanical and mathematical model. Can Anaesth Soc J 1978;25:117–121.

127. Ladegaard-Pedersen HJ. A circle system without carbon dioxide absorption. Acta Anaesthesiol Scand 1978;22:281–286.

128. Patel K, Bennett EJ, Grundy EM, Ignacio A. Relation of PaCO$_2$ to fresh gas flow in a circle system. Anesth Analg 1976;55:706–708.

129. Scholfield EJ, Williams NE. Prediction of arterial carbon dioxide tension using a circle system without carbon dioxide absorption. Br J Anaesth 1974;46:442–445.

130. Snowdon SL, Powell DL, Fadl ET, Utting JE. The circle system without absorber. Anaesthesia 1975;30:323–332.

131. Conway CM. Gaseous homeostasis and the circle system. Factors influencing anaesthetic gas exchange. Br J Anaesth 1986;58:1167–1180.

132. Stone SB, Greene NM. Low-flow anesthesia. Curr Rev Clin Anesth 1981;1:114.

133. Spence AA, Alison RH, Wishart HY. Low flow and closed systems for the administration of inhalation anaesthesia. Br J Anaesth 1981;53:69S–73S.

134. Cotter SM, Petros AJ, Barber ND, White DC. Cost of low flow anaesthesia. Br J Anaesth 1991;66:408P–409P.

135. Lowe HJ, Ernst EA. The quantitative practice of anesthesia. Use of closed circuit. Baltimore: Williams & Wilkins, 1981.

136. Weingarten M, Lowe HJ. A new circuit injection technic for syringe-measured administration of methoxyflurane. A new dimension in anesthesia. Anesth Analg 1973;52:634–642.

137. Boulogne P, Demontoux MH, Colin D, Feiss P. Isoflurane requirements during low and high flow anesthesia. Circular 1988;5:10–11.

138. Dennison PH. Coaxial tubing for conventional anesthetic systems. Anaesthesia 1984;39:841.

139. O'Callaghan AC, Hawes DW, Ross JAS, White DC, Wloch T. Uptake of isoflurane during clinical anaesthesia. Servo-control of liquid anaesthetic injection into a closed-circuit breathing system. Br J Anaesth 1983;55:1061–1064.

140. El-Attar AM. Guided isoflurane injection in a totally closed circuit. Anaesthesia 1991;46:1059–1063.

141. Ferderbar PJ, Kettler RE, Jablonski J, Sportiello R. A cause of breathing system leak during closed circuit anesthesia. Anesthesiology 1986;65:661–663.

142. Ernst EA. A clinical approach to closed circuit anesthesia. Circular 1985;2:5–7.

143. Lin C. Assessment of vaporizer performance in low-flow and closed-circuit anesthesia. Anesth Analg 1980;59:359–366.

144. Graham DH. Advantages of standing bellows ventilators and low-flow techniques. Anesthesiology 1983;58:486.

145. Lin CY, Mostert JW, Benson DW. Closed circle systems. A new direction in the practice of anesthesia. Acta Anaesthesiol Scand 1980;24:354–361.

146. Huffman LM, Riddle RT. Mass spectrometer and/or capnograph use during low-flow closed circuit anesthesia administration. Anesthesiology 1987;66:439–440.

147. Lowe HJ. The anesthetic continuum. In: Aldrete JA, Lowe HJ, Virtue RW, eds. Low flow and closed system anesthesia. New York: Grune & Stratton, 1979:11–37.

148. Blackstock D. Advantages of standing bellows ventilators and low-flow techniques. Anesthesiology 1984;60:167.

149. El-Attar AM. Closed-circuit coasting from high flow isoflurane anesthesia. J Clin Monit 1992;8:182–183.

150. Baumgarten RK. Simple charcoal filter for closed circuit anesthesia. Anesthesiology 1985;63:125.

151. Ernst EA. Use of charcoal to rapidly decrease depth of anesthesia while maintaining a closed circuit. Anesthesiology 1982;57:343.

152. Jan-Peter AH, Jantzen DEAA. More on black and white granules in the closed circuit. Anesthesiology 1988;69:437–438.

153. Aldrete JA, Hendricks PL. Differences in costs: how much can we save? Anesthesiology 1986;64:656–657.

154. Bengtson JP, Sonander H, Stenqvist O. Comparison of costs of different anaesthetic techniques. Acta Anaesthesiol Scand 1988;32:33–35.

155. Christensen KN, Thomsen A, Jorgensen S, Fabricius J. Analysis of costs of anaesthetic breathing systems. Br J Anaesth 1987;59:389–390.

156. Cotter SM, Petros AJ, Dore CJ, Barber ND, White DC. Low-flow anaesthesia. Anaesthesia 1991;46:1009–1012.

157. Herscher E, Yeakel AE. Nitrous oxide-oxygen

based anesthesia: the waste and its cost. Anesthesiol Rev 1977;4:29–31.

158. Matjasko J. Economic impact of low-flow anesthesia. Anesthesiology 1987;67:863–864.

159. Virtue RW. Comparison of cost of high and low flows of anaesthetic agents. Can Anaesth Soc J 1981;28:182–184.

160. Virtue RW, Aldrete JA. Costs of delivery of anesthetic gases reexamined. II. Anesthesiology 1981;55:711.

161. Spain JA. Cost of delivery of anesthetic gases reexamined. III. Anesthesiology1981; 55:711–712.

162. Patel A, Milliken RA. Costs of delivery of anesthetic gases re-examined. I. Anesthesiology 1981;55:710.

163. Virtue RW, Escobar A, Modell J. Nitrous oxide levels in operating room air with various gas flows. Can Anaesth Soc J 1979;26:313–318.

164. Logan M, Farmer JG. Anesthesia and the ozone layer. Br J Anaesth 1989;63:645–647.

165. Sherman SJ, Cullen BF. Nitrous oxide and the greenhouse effect. Anesthesiology 1988;68:816–817.

166. Westhorpe R, Blutstein H. Anaesthetic agents and the ozone layer. Anaesth Intensive Care 1990; 18:102–109.

167. Brown AC, Canosa-Mas CE, Parr AD, Pierce JMT, Wayne RP. Tropospheric lifetimes of halogenated anaesthetics. Nature 1989;341:635–637.

168. Cohen AT, Beatty PCW, Kay B, Healy TEJ. Measurement of oxygen uptake: a method for use during nitrous oxide in oxygen anaesthesia. Eur J Anaesth 1984;1:63–75.

169. Ernst EA, Spain JA. Closed-circuit and high flow systems: examining alternatives. In: Calkins JM, ed. Future anesthesia delivery systems. Philadelphia: FA Davis, 1984.

170. Middleton V, Poznak AV, Artusio JF, Smith SM. Carbon monoxide accumulation in closed circle anesthesia systems. Anesthesiology 1965;26:715–719.

171. Spiess W. To what degree should we be concerned about carbon monoxide accumulation in closed circuit anesthesia? Circular 1984;1:8.

172. Morita S. Inspired gas contamination by non-anesthetic gases during closed circuit anesthesia. 1985;Circular 2:24–25.

173. Rolly G, Versichelen L. Methane accumulation during closed circuit anesthesia. Anesth Analg 1992;74:S253.

174. Baumgarten RK, Reynolds WJ. Much ado about nothing: Trace gaseous metabolites in the closed circuit. Anesth Analg 1985;64:1029–1030.

175. Garro AJ, Phillips RA. Mutagenicity of the halogenated olefin, 2-bromo-2-chloro-1,1-difluoroethylene, a presumed metabolite of the inhalation anesthetic, halothane. Environ Health Perspect 1977;21:65–69.

176. Waskell L. Lack of mutagenicity of two possible metabolites of halothane. Anesthesiology 1979;50:9–12.

177. Eger EI. Dragons and other scientific hazards (editorial). Anesthesiology 1979;50:1.

178. Kofke WA, Snider MT, Young RSK, Ramer JC. Prolonged low flow isoflurane anesthesia for status epilepticus. Anesthesiology 1985;62:653–656.

179. Parker CJR, Snowdon SL. Predicted and measured oxygen concentrations in the circle system using low fresh gas flows with oxygen supplied by an oxygen concentratior. Br J Anaesth 1988; 61:397–402.

180. Aldrete JA. . . . and the frog turned into a prince: closed circuit in pediatric anesthesia. Circular 1985;2:13.

181. Aldrete JA. Closed circuit and the pediatric patient. Circular 1988;5:12–13.

182. da Silva JMC, Tubino PJ, Vieira ZEG, Saraiva A. Closed circuit anesthesia in infants and children. Anesth Analg 1984;63:765–769.

183. Pappas ALS, Santos E, Sukhani R, Aldrete JA. Low flow closed circuit anesthesia in pediatrics—its safety and applicability. Circular 1988;5:13.

184. Pappas AS, Santos E, Sukhani R, Aldrete JA. Applicability and safety of low flow closed circuit anesthesia in pediatrics. Anesthesiology 1988; 69:A783.

185. Boyd GL, Funderberg BJ, Vasconez LO, Guzman G. Long-distance anesthesia. Anesth Analg 1992;74:477.

Chapter 8

Manual Resuscitators

Introduction

Breathing systems using nonrebreathing valves have largely disappeared from anesthesia practice. However, these valves are still used in small portable manual resuscitators, which are used principally for patient transport and at the site of emergencies. They can also be used to administer anesthesia. A manual resuscitator may be adapted for manual ventilation during magnetic resonance imaging (1).

Manual resuscitators are known by many different terms. Some of these terms are the following: bag ventilators; bag-assist devices; bag-type resuscitators; bag-valve devices, units, or resuscitators; bag-valve-mask units, resuscitators, or ventilators; emergency manual ventilators; hand ventilators; hand-operated bag resuscitators; hand-operated emergency ventilators; hand- or operator-powered resuscitators; handbag resuscitators; manual bag ventilators; manually operated resuscitators; manual pulmonary re-

suscitators; respiratory bags; resuscitator or resuscitation bags; self-inflating manual resuscitators; self-inflating respirator bags or resuscitators; ventilator bags; and self-inflating bag-valve devices. U.S., Canadian, and international standards for resuscitators have been published (2–4). These devices are frequently supplied in three sizes: adult; child; and infant. The U.S. standard classifies those delivering a tidal volume of 600 ml and over as adult resuscitators and notes that resuscitators designed to deliver a tidal volume of 20 to 50 ml are usually suitable for use with neonates. Disposable manual resuscitators that avoid the inconvenience and hazards associated with reprocessing and sterilizing of reusable resuscitators are available and in common use.

Components

A typical manual resuscitator is shown in Figure 8.1. Manual resuscitators have a compressible self-expanding bag, a bag refill

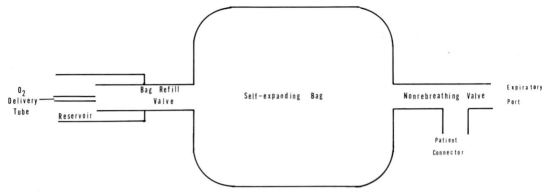

Figure 8.1. Components of a manual resuscitator. The nonrebreathing valve directs the gas from the bag to the patient during inspiration. During expiration, the nonrebreathing valve directs exhaled gases from the patient to atmosphere through the expiratory port and the bag refill valve opens to allow the bag to fill. An open reservoir is attached to the bag refill valve.

valve, and a nonrebreathing valve. In some units the two valves are combined. Optional components include a pressure-limiting device, oxygen enrichment device, PEEP valve, and mechanism for scavenging anesthetic gases.

SELF-EXPANDING BAG

The self-expanding bag (ventilating or ventilation bag, self-inflating bag, compressible unit, or compressible reservoir) is constructed so that in its resting state it is inflated. It may be cylindrical or football shaped. Some bags collapse like an accordion for storage.

During expiration the bag expands. If the volume of oxygen from the delivery source is inadequate to fill the bag, the difference is made up by intake of air. The rate at which the bag reinflates will determine the maximum respiratory rate.

NONREBREATHING VALVE

The nonrebreathing valve is sometimes referred to as the directional control valve, exhalation valve, expiratory valve, inflating valve, inhalation-exhalation valve, inflating-exhalation valve, inspiratory-expiratory valve, nonreturn valve, patient valve, routing valve, or one-way inflating valve.

Body

It is preferable that the housing be constructed so that operation of the mechanism can be observed by the operator.

Most nonrebreathing valves are T-shaped. The expiratory port is the opening through which exhaled gases pass to the atmosphere. A PEEP valve may be connected at this point (5). The expiratory port may have a tapered 19- or 30-mm connector for attachment of the transfer tube of a scavenging system. The ASTM standard (2) requires that such a connector have ridges in its internal lumen so that it cannot accept a 22-mm male connector.

The patient connector is the part that connects to either a tracheal tube or a face mask. It has 15-mm female and 22-mm male coaxial fittings. It may be designed to swivel.

The inspiratory port is the opening through which gas enters the valve from the bag. It may be permanently attached to the bag. During inspiration, the nonrebreathing valve directs gas from the bag to the patient connection port. At the same time, the expiratory port is blocked. As exhalation begins, the expiratory port opens and the patient exhales to atmosphere. Simultaneously, gas flow from the bag is blocked. The valve may have a means to prevent air intake so that the

CLOSED

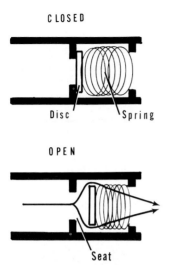

Disc   Spring

OPEN

Seat

Figure 8.2. Spring-disc unidirectional valve. In the closed position, the spring holds the disc against the seat. When the pressure to the left of the disc increases above the pressure of the spring, the disc is forced away from the seat. When the pressure to the left of the disc drops, the valve closes.

CLOSED

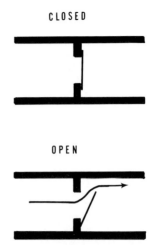

OPEN

Figure 8.3. Edge-mounted flap unidirectional valve. Increased pressure upstream of the flap pushes the flap away from the seat, opening the valve. When the pressure downstream of the flap increases above the pressure upstream, the flap is forced back against the seat, blocking the flow of gas.

spontaneously breathing patient will inhale only from the bag.

Unidirectional Valves

A nonrebreathing valve usually contains at least two of the following unidirectional valves (also called moving mechanisms and active parts). One ensures unidirectional flow from the bag to the patient, another from the patient to atmosphere.

Spring-Disc Valve

A spring-disc valve is shown in Figure 8.2. A spring holds the disc against a seat. When the pressure on the disc is great enough to overcome the force of the spring, the valve opens. As the pressure drops, the spring causes the disc to move to the left. Some unidirectional valves have a ball in place of the disc. The ball or disc may be held in place by gravity rather than a spring. An example of a spring-disc valve is shown in Figure 8.6.

CLOSED

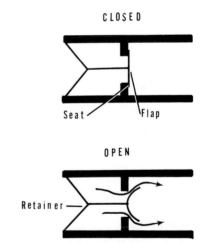

Seat   Flap

OPEN

Retainer

Figure 8.4. Center-mounted flap unidirectional valve. The flap valve is secured by a tab at the center. The tab is secured by a retainer, which is part of the valve body.

Flap Valve

The flap (leaf) valve has a rigid or flexible flap that moves. The flap may be fixed at the center or the edge (Figs. 8.3 and 8.4).

CLOSED

OPEN

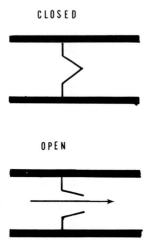

Figure 8.5. Fishmouth unidirectional valve. As pressure to the left increases, the leaflets open, allowing gas to flow through the valve. An increase in pressure to the right pushes the leaflets together, closing the valve and preventing backflow of gas.

Fishmouth Valve

The fishmouth (duckbill) valve is so named because it opens and closes like a fish's mouth (Fig. 8.5). As the pressure upstream of the valve increases, it opens at the slit in the center. An increase in pressure downstream pushes the leaflets together, closing the valve.

Diaphragm Valve

A diaphragm valve has a flexible diaphragm attached at the side. When pressure is applied to one side of the diaphragm, the central part moves, which causes the gas path to be opened or occluded (Fig. 8.7).

Mushroom Valve

A mushroom valve is a hollow balloon-like device that occludes an opening when inflated (Fig. 8.8).

Several representative nonrebreathing valves are shown in Figure 8.3 and Figure 8.6 through Figure 8.11.

Figure 8.6 shows a valve with a spring disc. In the resting position, the spring holds the disc away from the expiratory port and against the inspiratory port so that a spontaneously breathing patient may inhale room

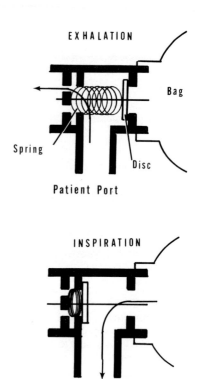

Figure 8.6. Spring-disc nonrebreathing valve. The disc is held on the seat by the spring. When the bag is squeezed, the disc moves to the left, closing the expiratory port. At the end of inspiration, the spring forces the disc to the right, so that the patient exhales to atmosphere and not into the bag. A guide pin keeps the disc in the center. A spontaneously breathing patient can inhale room air unless a valve is placed over the expiratory port to prevent air entrainment.

air through the exhalation port. When the bag is compressed, the disc is pushed across the valve, connecting the inspiratory port with the patient port and at the same time occluding the expiratory port. When the bag is released, the disc moves back toward the bag and exhaled gases pass out through the expiratory port. A guide pin keeps the disc centered. If the patient is breathing spontaneously, the disc will not close the exhalation port and air will be inhaled.

Figure 8.7 shows a diaphragm-flap valve. The diaphragm is attached at its periphery. When the bag is squeezed the diaphragm is pushed to the left and occludes the expiratory port. Flap valves at the side of the diaphragm open, allowing the gas from the bag to flow to

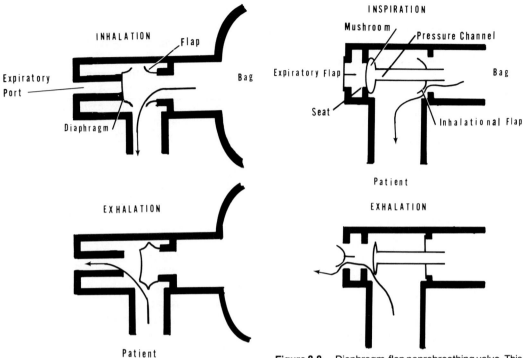

Figure 8.7. Diaphragm-flap nonrebreathing valve. During inspiration when the bag is squeezed, the pressure to the right increases and the diaphragm is pushed to the left, closing the exhalation channel. At the same time, the flaps at the edge of the diaphragm open, allowing gas from the bag to flow to the patient connector. When inspiration ends, the diaphragm moves away from the exhalation channel and the flaps close, blocking the inspiratory port.

Figure 8.8. Diaphragm-flap nonrebreathing valve. This valve has one diaphragm and two flap valves. During inspiration the diaphragm is inflated and blocks the expiratory channel, preventing flow of gas to atmosphere. At the same time, the inhalation flap valve opens so that gas flows to the patient. At the end of inspiration, the diaphragm collapses, opening the exhalation channel. The inhalational flap valve prevents flow of gas back into the bag. The expiratory flap opens during exhalation. It prevents room air from being inspired during spontaneous ventilation.

the patient. When inhalation ends, the diaphragm returns to its resting position, and the flap valves close so the patient can exhale through the expiratory port. A spontaneously breathing patient may inhale room air through the exhalation port.

The valve illustrated in Figure 8.8 combines one mushroom and two flap valves. The inside of the mushroom is connected to a pressure channel. During inspiration, the mushroom is inflated against the seat, preventing flow of gas through the expiratory port and the inhalational flap opens. During expiration, the inhalational flap prevents flow back into the bag. The mushroom col-

lapses and opens the exhalation channel. A flap valve over the expiratory port prevents the inhalation of room air during spontaneous ventilation.

The valve diagrammed in Figure 8.9 and pictured disassembled in Figure 8.10 is a combination of fishmouth and two flap valves. The fishmouth and circular flap valves are combined into one piece, with the flap surrounding the central fishmouth. Outside the main body of the valve is another circular flap valve. During inspiration with either spontaneous or controlled ventilation, the fishmouth opens and the circular flap valve closes the exhalation ports. The outside flap valve prevents room air from entering the valve during spontaneous respiration. During expiration, the fishmouth section closes. The circular flap valve attached to it is

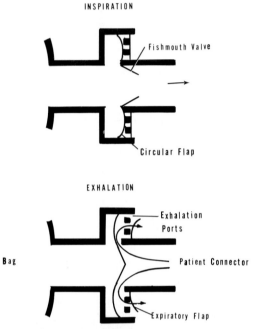

INSPIRATION

Fishmouth Valve

Circular Flap

EXHALATION

Bag

Exhalation Ports

Patient Connector

Expiratory Flap

Figure 8.9. Fishmouth-flap nonrebreathing valve. The circular flap and fishmouth valves are attached, with the diaphragm around the periphery. When the bag is squeezed, the diaphragm is seated against the exhalation ports and the fishmouth portion of the valve opens. During expiration, the fishmouth closes and the flap falls away from the exhalation channel. A second flap valve over the exhalation ports prevents air from being inspired during spontaneous respiration.

lifted off the expiratory apertures, allowing exhaled gas to escape.

Figure 8.11 shows a nonrebreathing valve that incorporates flap and diaphragm valves. During inspiration, the center-mounted flap valve moves to the right. The diaphragm is inflated and covers the exhalation ports. During exhalation, the flap valves moves to the left, preventing gas from entering the bag and the diaphragm deflates, opening the exhalation ports. The diaphragm prevents inhalation of room air in the spontaneously breathing patient.

BAG REFILL VALVE

The bag refill (inlet) valve is a one-way valve that is opened by negative pressure inside the bag. When the bag is squeezed, the valve closes to prevent escape of gas back through the inlet. A simple flap valve (see Figs. 8.3 and 8.4) is most commonly used. A spring disc (see Fig. 8.2) may also be used. This valve is usually located at the opposite end of the bag from the nonrebreathing valve (see Fig. 8.1) but may be at the same end and may be combined with the nonrebreathing valve.

PRESSURE-LIMITING DEVICE

The pressure-limiting device is also called the pressure relief device, valve, or system; overpressure limiting system; overpressure valve; pop-off valve; and pressure-limiting system. The ASTM standard (2) requires a

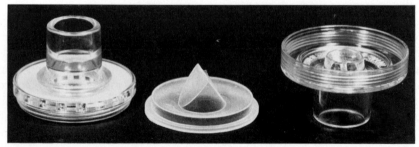

Figure 8.10. Components of the fishmouth-flap nonrebreathing valve. At the left is the patient connection with the expiratory flap. In the center is the fishmouth with its concentric flap. The right piece is the part of the housing closest to the bag.

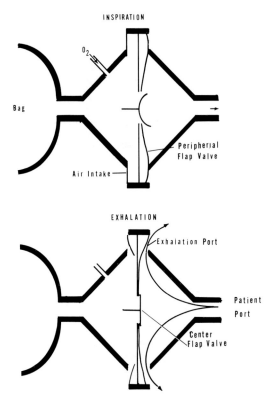

INSPIRATION

O_2

Bag

Peripherial
Flap Valve

Air Intake

EXHALATION

Exhalation Port

Patient
Port

Center
Flap Valve

Figure 8.11. Nonrebreathing valve with two flap valves. During inspiration, the center-mounted flap valve opens and the peripheral flap closes over the exhalation ports. During exhalation, the central flap valve closes and the peripheral flap falls away from the exhalation ports. This valve has an oxygen inlet and two bag refill valves, which open if the oxygen flow is not sufficient to prevent a negative pressure from developing in the space to the left.

pressure-limiting system with an opening pressure of 45 cm water with the option of an override for infant and child resuscitators. For adult resuscitators, the standard requires that if there is a device that limits the pressure to below 60 cm H_2O there be an override mechanism. If the override mechanism can be locked, the pressure override mechanism must be designed so that the operating mode, i.e., on or off, is readily apparent to the user. It recommends that if a resuscitator is equipped with a pressure-limiting system, there be an audible or visible warning to the operator when the pressure-limiting system is operating. It also requires that with a pres-

sure-limiting system set at one fixed pressure the nominal pressure setting at which the system is activated must be marked on the resuscitator.

A variety of devices have been used. One is a spring-loaded disc with the tension on the spring adjusted so that it opens at the desired pressure. Another is a magnetic device, with the force of the magnet adjusted to open at the desired pressure. Some systems provide a small hole. The maximum pressure depends on the size of the hole and how firmly the bag is compressed (6). Another resuscitator employs a double-bag design. An inner bag with elastic recoil properties similar to most resuscitation bags is contained within a thin outer bag. As pressure within the bags builds up, holes in the inner bag allow gas to enter the outer bag, causing it to balloon.

Many resuscitators with a pressure-limiting mechanism provide a means to override it. Often all that is required is to place a finger over the device. However, even such a simple action may be difficult when ventilating a patient, especially if a mask is being used. Another problem is that an override mechanism may cause confusion.

The means to create a higher inflation pressure is especially important in a resuscitator designed for infants. The first few breaths in neonatal resuscitation may require pressures as high as 50 to 70 cm H_2O and the pressure needed to overcome the resistance to flow in a narrow tracheal tube and to expand the stiff lungs of a premature infant may exceed 30 to 40 cm H_2O (7).

OXYGEN ENRICHMENT DEVICE

The ASTM standard (2) requires resuscitators to be equipped with a device to increase the inspired oxygen concentration when a source of oxygen is available.

Delivery of Oxygen near the Bag Refill Valve

Attachment of a tubing from an oxygen flowmeter near the bag refill valve is a simple means of increasing the concentration of oxygen in the bag. The oxygen does not enter the bag directly. The increase in oxygen concentration is limited, because air will still be drawn into the bag. The delivered oxygen concentration can be increased by increasing the oxygen flow, but because most flowmeters do not deliver over 15 liters/min, this is of limited value. The higher the minute volume and the greater the I:E ratio, the lower the delivered oxygen concentration.

Delivery of Oxygen Directly into the Bag

Delivery of oxygen directly into the bag will result in high delivered oxygen concentrations without making the resuscitator cumbersome. If the oxygen flow is less than the filling rate of the bag, the bag refill valve will open and admit air. However, provision must be made for venting excess oxygen to minimize the danger of the nonrebreathing valve locking in the inspiratory position.

Reservoir

Some units have a reservoir (accumulator) into which oxygen flows when the bag is not filling. It may be a tube or a bag. When the bag refill valve opens, oxygen from the reservoir enters the bag.

The size of the reservoir may limit the oxygen concentration delivered. If the volume of the reservoir is less than that of the bag, the inflowing oxygen may not be sufficient to make up the difference and room air will be drawn in. On the other hand, a large reservoir makes a resuscitator more cumbersome.

Open Reservoir

An open reservoir is shown in Figure 8.12. A piece of corrugated tubing or other material open to atmosphere at its distal end is placed like a sleeve around the bag refill valve. When the bag is not filling, oxygen flows into the reservoir. If the flow is high, oxygen will flow into atmosphere at the open end of the reservoir.

Closed Reservoir

A closed reservoir is shown in Figure 8.13. It has two valves: an overflow valve that vents

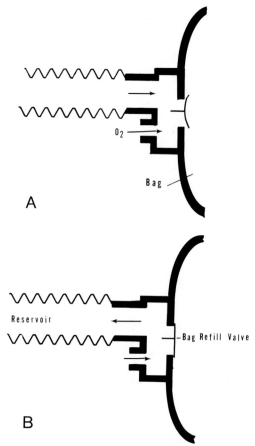

Figure 8.12. Open reservoir. **A,** The bag is filling. Oxygen from the delivery tubing as well as that in the reservoir flows into the bag. If the volume entering the bag exceeds that in the reservoir and flowing through the delivery tubing, room air will make up the difference. The size of the reservoir is, therefore, important. **B,** The bag refill valve is closed. Oxygen from the delivery tubing flows into the reservoir. Because the reservoir is open to atmosphere, some oxygen will be lost if the flow is high.

excess gases and an air intake valve that draws in ambient air if there is insufficient oxygen flow. A bag provides a visual indication that the reservoir is receiving sufficient oxygen flow. A deflated reservoir bag means there is a problem with the oxygen supply or a hole in the bag.

Demand Valve

A demand valve connecting a compressed gas source to the self-expanding bag will consistently provide a high inspired oxygen concentration (8). A negative pressure in the bag

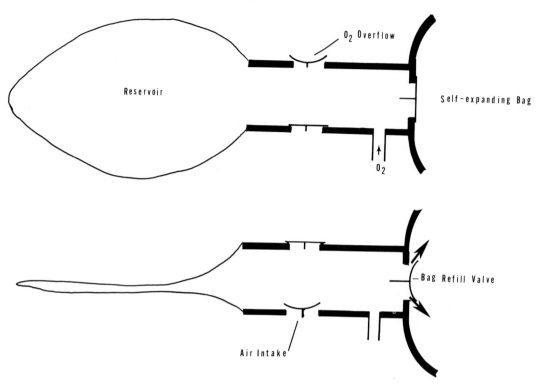

Figure 8.13. Closed reservoir. **Top,** The reservoir is full and the pressure increases. Oxygen flows through the overflow valve.**Bottom,** The resuscitator bag is filling. Because there is insufficient gas in the reservoir, air enters through the intake valve.

triggers the flow of oxygen, which stops at a preset pressure. A demand valve provides warning of problems with supplemental oxygen. Should the demand valve become stuck or the oxygen supply depleted, the bag will not refill.

PEEP DEVICE

A PEEP valve (see Chapter 5) is available on some resuscitators and can be added to the expiratory port on others (5,9).

SCAVENGING MECHANISM

A means for scavenging expired gases (see Chapter 11) can be mounted on the expiratory port of some resuscitators.

Functional Analysis

MINUTE VOLUME

The minute volume will be determined by the tidal volume and the respiratory rate.

These will be determined not only by the performance of the resuscitator but also by the skill of the operator. The volume delivered when the bag is compressed will vary with the size of the user's hand and whether one or two hands are used (10–18). Tidal volume may be increased by compressing the bag against a solid surface such as a thigh. The respiratory rate may be limited by how fast the bag reexpands, which in turn depends on the construction of the bag and the size of the refill valve inlet. The maximum compression rate may be reduced at low temperatures (16,19,20) and with the use of certain oxygen input adapters (20).

DELIVERED OXYGEN CONCENTRATION

The ASTM standard (2) states that a resuscitator for use with adults shall be capable, when an oxygen source is available, of delivering an inspired oxygen concentration of at least 40% when connected to an oxygen source supplying not more than 15 liters/min and at least 85% with an attachment made available by the manufacturer.

The delivered oxygen concentration is limited by size of the reservoir and the oxygen flow. If the volume of the reservoir is greater than the tidal volume of the bag and the oxygen flow is greater than the minute volume, the delivered oxygen concentration may approach 100%. If the tidal volume is greater than the reservoir volume plus the volume of oxygen delivered during inspiration, then air will be drawn into the unit and reduce the percentage of oxygen delivered (21).

Controlled Ventilation

The oxygen concentrations delivered during controlled ventilation have been investigated under a variety of conditions with and without enrichment devices (8,19,20–29). Because modifications to these devices are made frequently, it is suggested that only the most recent evaluations be considered.

The delivered oxygen concentration will be determined by the minute volume; the size of the reservoir, if present; the oxygen flow; and the technique of bag squeezing and release. If bag filling is allowed to proceed at its most rapid rate, all the oxygen in the reservoir may be exhausted and air drawn in. If bag filling is manually retarded, the delivered oxygen concentration will be higher (8,30). Manually restricting bag refill may be useful when low oxygen flows must be used or when a reservoir is small or not present, but it limits the respiratory rate and thus the minute volume that can be achieved. Furthermore, this maneuver may cause the nonrebreathing valve to jam in the inspiratory position (19).

Activation of the pressure-limiting device may cause the delivered oxygen concentration to be decreased (7,29).

Spontaneous Ventilation

With spontaneous ventilation inspired gas may come from the exhalation port as well as the bag. The portion coming from the bag may vary from 0% to 97% (20,21).

REBREATHING

If the nonrebreathing valve is competent, mixing of inhaled and exhaled gases should not occur. If the valve is incompetent, back leak will allow exhaled gases to pass back into the resuscitator and be reinhaled by the patient.

Use

A size bag and mask appropriate for the patient should be selected. For adults, an oxygen flow of 10 to 15 liter/min is most commonly used. For children and infants, lower flows are recommended.

If anesthetic gases are to be administered, the transfer tube from a scavenging system should be attached to the expiratory port.

A manual resuscitator can be adapted for manual ventilation during MRI by inserting an extension tube long enough to cover the distance between the patient and the person squeezing the bag between the nonrebreathing valve and the bag (1).

Hazards

HIGH AIRWAY PRESSURE

High airway pressure is a hazard only if the patient is intubated, because it is very difficult to achieve a dangerously high pressure using a mask.

Sticking of the Nonrebreathing Valve in the Inspiratory Position

If the nonrebreathing valve sticks (valve lockup) in the inspiratory position, the patient will be attempting to exhale against a closed outlet and continued inflow can cause a continuous and dangerous increase in pressure in a short period of time. A variety of conditions can cause this, including cessation of manual ventilation for observation of spontaneous respiratory efforts, manually restricting bag refill, contamination of the valve with foreign material, a squeeze or bump on the bag, the patient coughing, improper assembly of the nonrebreathing valve, attachment of an oxygen inlet nipple without vent holes directly to the resuscitator, and kinking of the reservoir tail (2,22,31–41). In several cases a sliding ball separated into two halves and one half wedged in the expiratory outlet (42–44).

High Oxygen Inflow

The ASTM resuscitator standard (2) requires that the valve not jam at an input flow of up to 30 liters/min. Obstruction can occur with as little as 5 liters/min. Infant resuscitators are more prone to obstruction with high flows because the bag is so small.

Use of a Demand Valve

Manual activation of a demand valve while the patient is exhaling can cause dangerously high pressures (8).

Failure of the Pressure-Limiting Device

Studies show that pressure-limiting devices often malfunction, opening well above an acceptable pressure (29,45,46).

REBREATHING

Rebreathing of exhaled gases can occur if the valve is not competent or is improperly assembled (39,47).

HYPOVENTILATION

A defective nonrebreathing valve may have forward leak, so that during inspiration part of the tidal volume expelled from the bag escapes through the expiratory port (47–49). Obstruction of the part of the valve that closes the expiratory port can cause unwanted venting (50). Unrecognized venting through the pressure relief device may result in hypoventilation (51,52).

Squeezing the bag may require considerable physical effort. During extended use, performance often deteriorates as the operator becomes fatigued. Operators with small hands may have difficulty delivering adequate tidal volumes. Adequate tidal volumes are frequently not delivered when a mask is used, unless two persons participate, one holding the mask and one squeezing the bag (15). Squeezing the bag using one hand instead of two tends to lower the delivered volume (14).

Because resuscitators are used away from the hospital, it is possible that they will be subjected to low temperatures. In this situation the maximum cycling rate is often greatly reduced and the units may become inoperable (19,20,31,34).

Cases have been reported in which it was possible to connect the patient connector into the bag (47,53), the tracheal tube to a part of the resuscitator other than the patient connector (19), and the expiratory port to the mask (54). In all these cases when the bag was squeezed, the contents were exhausted to atmosphere. The bag can become detached from the nonrebreathing valve (55).

If a resuscitator with an oxygen reservoir bag does not have an auxiliary air intake valve or patent air intake port, it can become nonfunctional during use if there is not enough oxygen flow to inflate the compressible bag.

DELIVERY OF LOW OXYGEN CONCENTRATIONS

Delivery of low oxygen concentrations may be the result of insufficient oxygen flow, detachment of the oxygen tubing, or problems with the oxygen enrichment device. The reservoir may be too small for the tidal volume. Incorrect assembly of a nonrebreathing valve can result in ambient air rather than gas from the bag being inhaled (56).

During spontaneous ventilation, the patient may inhale room air from the expiratory port as well as oxygen-enriched gas from the bag. Studies have shown that percentage of ventilation coming through the bag varies from 0% to 97% (20,21).

HIGH RESISTANCE

Some nonrebreathing valves offer high resistance to flow, so that high negative pressures must be generated during spontaneous ventilation (21).

CONTAMINATION (57,58)

Because these devices are often used on patients who have respiratory infections, they frequently become contaminated. Oxygen flowing through the valve may aerosolize bacteria and spread them into the surrounding air. For these reasons and because these devices are somewhat difficult to clean, disposable units have become popular.

INHALATION OF FOREIGN SUBSTANCES

Some of the early resuscitator bags were filled with a sponge that would deteriorate and small particles could be inhaled (59). These units are no longer produced. Rubber particles coming from the inside of the bag have also been reported. Parts of the resuscitator may break off and be inhaled (60–62).

Advantages

1. The equipment is compact, lightweight, and mobile, allowing it to be placed throughout the hospital and to be used outside the hospital.
2. The equipment is inexpensive, yet rugged.
3. The equipment is simple with a small number of parts. Disassembly and reassembly are usually easy to perform.
4. Dead space and rebreathing are minimal if the valve functions properly. Resistance is generally low.
5. With proper attention to the oxygen enrichment device, oxygen flow, and technique of ventilation, it is possible to administer close to 100% oxygen with most resuscitators.
6. In emergency situations in which a connection to a gas source is not readily available, the resuscitator can be used with room air until such a source becomes available.
7. The operator has some feel for pressures and volumes delivered. Barotrauma is less likely with these devices than with gas-powered resuscitators, which do not

allow the operator to sense when the patient's lungs are fully inflated.

Disadvantages

1. Some of the valves are noisy and stick, particularly when wet.
2. There may be considerable loss of heat and humidity from the patient.
3. The feel of the bag is different from that in other breathing systems. The user's hand must be reeducated.
4. The valve must be located at the patient's head. Its bulk may be troublesome and its weight may cause the tracheal tube to kink or be displaced downward.

REFERENCES

1. Taylor WF, Pangburn PD, Paschall A. Manual ventilation during magnetic resonance imaging. Respir Care 1991;36:1207–1210.
2. American Society for Testing and Materials. Proposed draft specification for minimum performance and safety requirements for resuscitators intended for use with humans (Rev ASTM F920-85). Draft 2. Philadelphia: ASTM, March 1992.
3. Canadian Standards Association. Resuscitators (Can Z168.7-M83) Rexdale, Ont., Canada: CSA, 1983.
4. International Organization for Standardization. Resuscitators intended for use with humans (ISO 8382). Geneva: ISO, 1988.
5. Perel A, Eimerl D, Grossberg M. A PEEP device for a manual bag ventilator. Anesth Analg 1976;52:745.
6. Anonymous. Manually operated infant resuscitators. Health Devices 1973;2:240–248.
7. Breivik H. A safe multipurpose pediatric ventilation bag. Crit Care Med 1976;4:32–39.
8. Campbell TP, Stewart RD, Kaplan RM, DeMichiei RV, Morton R. Oxygen enrichment of bag-valve-mask units during positive-pressure ventilation: a comparison of various techniques. Ann Emerg Med 1988;17:232–235.
9. Anonymous. A simple PEEP system for the Laerdal resuscitation bag. Respir Ther 1981;12:120.
10. Augustine JA, Seidel DR, McCabe JB. Ventilation performance using a self-inflating anesthesia bag: effect of operator characteristics. Am J Emerg Med 1987;5:267–270.

11. Elling R, Politis J. An evaluation of emergency medical technicians' ability to use manual ventilation devices. Ann Emerg Med 1983;12:765–768.

12. Hess D, Baran C. Ventilatory volumes using mouth-to-mouth, mouth-to-mask, and bag-valve-mask techniques. Am J Emerg Med 1985;3:292–296.

13. Hess D, Goff G, Johnson K. The effect of hand size, resuscitator brand, and use of two hands on volumes delivered during adult bag-valve ventilation. Respir Care 1989;34:805.

14. Hess D, Goff G. The effects of two-hand versus one-hand ventilation on volumes delivered bag-valve ventilation at various resistances and compliances. Respir Care 1987;32:1025–1028.

15. Jesudian MCS, Harrison RR, Keenan RL, Maull KI. Bag-valve-mask ventilation; two rescuers are better than one: preliminary report. Crit Care Med 1985;13:122–123.

16. Kissoon N, Nykanen D, Tiffin N, Frewen T, Brasher P. Evaluation of performance characteristics of disposable bag-valve resuscitators. Crit Care Med 1991;19:102–107.

17. Law GD. Effects of hand size on Ve, Vt, and FIO$_2$ during manual resuscitation. Respir Care 1982;27:1236–1237.

18. Tiffin NH, Kissoon N, Clarke G, Frewen TC. An evaluation of eight disposable and two nondisposable adult resuscitators. Can J Respir Ther 1989;25:13–19.

19. Anonymous. Manual resuscitators. Health Devices 1979;8:133–146.

20. LeBouef LL. 1980 Assessment of eight adult manual resuscitators. Respir Care 1980;25:1136–1142.

21. Mills PJ, Baptiste J, Preston J, Barnas GM. Manual resuscitators and spontaneous ventilation—an evaluation. Crit Care Med 1991;19:1425–1431.

22. Anonymous. Manually operated resuscitators. Health Devices 1974;3:164–176.

23. Barnes TA, Watson ME. Oxygen delivery performance of old and new designs of the Laerdal, Vitalograph and AMBU adult manual resuscitators. Respir Care 1983;28:1121–1128.

24. Barnes TA, Watson ME. Oxygen delivery performance of four adult resuscitation bags. Respir Care 1982;27:139–146.

25. Barnes TA, Potash R. Evaluation of five adult disposable operator-powered resuscitators. Respir Care 1989;34:254–261.

26. Eaton JM. Adult manual resuscitators. Br J Hosp Med 1984;31:67–70.

27. Fitzmaurice MW, Barnes TA. Fractional delivered oxygen concentrations of resuscitation bags. Respir Care 1981;26:581–583.

28. Fitzmaurice MW, Barnes TA. Oxygen delivery performance of three adult resuscitation bags. Respir Care 1980;25:928–933.

29. Finer NN, Barrington KJ, Al-Fadley F, Peters KL. Limitations of self-inflating resuscitators. Pediatrics 1986;77:417–420.

30. Priano LL, Ham J. A simple method to increase the FIO$_2$ of resuscitator bags. Crit Care Med 1978;6:48–49.

31. Anonymous. Manually operated resuscitators. Health Devices 1971;1:13–17.

32. Anonymous. New component designed for resuscitator valve sticking problem. Biomed Saf Stand 1991;21:123.

33. Anonymous. Resuscitators, pulmonary manual reusable. Technol Anesth 1991;12:9.

34. Carden E, Hughes T. An evaluation of manually operated self-inflating resuscitation bags. Anesth Analg 1975;54:133–138.

35. Dolan PF, Shapiro S, Steinbach RB. Valve misassembly—manually operated resuscitation bag. Anesth Analg 1981;60:66–67.

36. Hillman K, Albin M. Pulmonary barotrauma during cardiopulmonary resuscitation. Crit Care Med 1986;14:606–609.

37. Hunter WAH, Duthie RA. Malfunction of a Laerdal resuscitation valve. Anaesthesia 1991;46:505–506.

38. Klick JM, Bushnell LS, Bancroft ML. Barotrauma, a potential hazard of manual resuscitators. Anesthesiology 1978;49:363–365.

39. Kelly MP. Ventilation equipment. Br Med J 1968;2:176.

40. Newton NI, Adams AP. Excessive airway pressure during anaesthesia. Anaesthesia 1978;33:689–699.

41. Tucker J, Hanson CW, Chen L. Pneumothorax reexacerbated by a self-inflating bag-valve device. Anesthesiology 1992;76:1067–1068.

42. Anonymous. Ohio Hope II resuscitators. Health Devices 1981;10:199.

43. Anonymous. Resuscitator ball valve alert extended: germicidal solutions may crack new component. Biomed Saf Stand 1988;18:43.

44. Jumper A, Desai S, Liu P, Philip J. Pulmonary barotrauma resulting from a faulty Hope II resuscitation bag. Anesthesiology 1983;58:572–574.

45. Barnes TA, McGarry WP. Evaluation of ten disposable manual resuscitators. Respir Care 1990;35:960.

46. Kissoon N, Connors R, Tiffin N, Frewen TC. An evaluation of the physical and functional characteristics of resuscitators for use in pediatrics. Crit Care Med 1992;20:292–296.

47. Munford BJ, Wishaw KJ. Critical incidents with nonrebreathing valves. Anaesth Intensive Care 1990;18:560–563.

48. Anonymous. Valve component on resuscitation kits may leak. Biomed Saf Stand 1989;19:35–36.

49. Anonymous. Pulmonary resuscitators. Health Devices 1989;18:333–352.

50. Holland R. Special committee investigating deaths under anaesthesia: memorandum on the dangers of nonrebreathing valves. Med J Aust 1970;2:46–47.
51. Hirschman AM, Kravath RE. Venting vs ventilating. A danger of manual resuscitation. Chest 1982;82:369–370.
52. Kain ZN, Berde CB, Benjamin PK, Thompson JE. Performance of pediatric resuscitation bags assessed with an infant lung simulator. Anesthesiology 1992;77:A509.
53. Oliver JJ, Pope R. Potential hazard, with silicone resuscitators. Anaesthesia 1984;39:933–934.
54. Anonymous. Mismating of Laerdal exhalation diverters and intertech masks. Technol Anesth 1988;8:1–2.
55. Anonymous. Inspiron disposable adult manual pulmonary resuscitators. Technol Anesth 1987;8:2–3.
56. Cramond T, Mead P. Non-rebreathing valve assembly. Anaesth Intensive Care 1986;14:465.
57. Hartstein AI, Rashad AL, Liebler JM, et al. Multiple intensive care unit outbreak of *Acinetobacter colcoaceticus* subspecies *anitratus* respiratory infection and colonization associated with contaminated, reusable ventilator circuits and resuscitation bags. Am J Med 1988;85:624–631.
58. Thompson AC, Wilder BJ, Powner DJ. Bedside resuscitation bags: A source of bacterial contamination. Infect Control 1985;6:231–232.
59. Loveday R, Hurter DG. Hazard of self-inflating resuscitation bags. Br Med J 1969;4:111.
60. Anonymous. Resuscitators, pulmonary manual. Technol Anesth 1985;7:11.
61. Anonymous. Nonrebreathing valves. Biomed Saf Stand 1986;16:19.
62. Pauca AL, Jenkins TE. Airway obstruction by breakdown of a nonrebreathing valve: how foolproof? Anesth Analg 1981;60:529–531.

Chapter 9

Humidification Methods

General Considerations

HUMIDITY

Terminology

Humidity is a general term used to describe the amount of water vapor in a gas. It may be expressed several ways.

Absolute Humidity

Absolute humidity is the mass of water vapor present in a volume of gas. It is usually expressed in milligrams of water per liter of gas.

Humidity at Saturation

The maximum mass of water vapor that can be carried in a given volume of gas is the humidity at saturation. This will vary with the temperature. Table 9.1 shows the absolute humidity of saturated gas at various temperatures.

Relative Humidity

Relative humidity, or percent saturation, is the ratio of absolute humidity to the humidity at saturation and is expressed as a percentage.

Water Vapor Pressure

Humidity may also be expressed as the pressure exerted by water vapor in a gas mixture. Table 9.1 shows the vapor pressure of water in saturated gas at various temperatures.

Body Humidity

Body humidity refers to the humidity of saturated gas at body temperature. At a body temperature of 37°C it is 44 mg H_2O/liter.

Interrelationships

If a gas saturated with water vapor is heated, it can hold more water. Relative humidity falls, but its absolute humidity remains unchanged. Gas that is 100% saturated at room temperature and warmed to body temperature without additional humidity will be only about 40% saturated.

If gas saturated with water vapor is cooled, it will condense (rainout) the amount of water vapor it held at the original temperature less the amount it can hold at the lower

Table 9.1. Water Vapor Pressure and Absolute Humidity in Moisture-Saturated Gas

Temperature °C	mg H_2O/liter	mm Hg
0	4.84	4.58
1	5.19	4.93
2	5.56	5.29
3	5.95	5.69
4	6.36	6.10
5	6.80	6.54
6	7.26	7.01
7	7.75	7.51
8	8.27	8.05
9	8.81	8.61
10	9.40	9.21
11	10.01	9.84
12	10.66	10.52
13	11.33	11.23
14	12.07	11.99
15	12.82	12.79
16	13.62	13.63
17	14.47	14.53
18	15.35	15.48
19	16.30	16.48
20	17.28	17.54
21	18.33	18.65
22	19.41	19.83
23	20.57	21.07
24	21.76	22.38
25	23.04	23.76
26	24.35	25.21
27	25.75	26.74
28	27.19	28.35
29	28.74	30.04
30	30.32	31.82
31	32.01	33.70
32	33.79	35.66
33	35.59	37.73
34	37.54	39.90
35	39.57	42.18
36	41.53	44.56
37	43.85	47.07
38	46.16	49.69
39	48.58	52.44
40	51.03	55.32
41	53.66	58.34
42	56.40	61.50

temperature. Absolute humidity will fall, but relative humidity will remain 100%.

If inspired gas is to have a relative humidity of 100% at body temperature, it must be maintained at body temperature after humidification or heated above body temperature at the humidifier and allowed to cool to body temperature as it flows to the patient.

Physics

The specific heats of gases are low. As a consequence, they quickly assume the temperature of the surrounding environment. Inhaled gases quickly approach body temperature and gases in corrugated tubes rapidly approach room temperature.

The heat of vaporization of water is relatively high (580 cal/g). Vaporization of water, therefore, requires considerably more heat than warming of gases. Likewise, condensation of water yields more heat than cooling of gases.

Considerations for Anesthesia

NORMAL MECHANICS OF HUMIDIFICATION

In its passage to the alveoli, inspired gas is brought to body temperature (either by heating or cooling) and 100% relative humidity (either by evaporation or condensation). In the unintubated patient, the upper respiratory tract (especially the nose) functions as the principal heat and moisture exchanger. Normally, water is lost by the body as saturated vapor in expired gases and heat is lost primarily because the heat of vaporization of that water must be supplied by the body.

EFFECTS OF ANESTHESIA

Water is intentionally removed from medical gases—piped or from cylinders—to prevent corrosion and condensation in regulators and valves. Gases emerging from the anesthesia machine are dry and at room temperature. The breathing system may add some humidity to the inspired gas mixture.

Tracheal intubation bypasses the upper airway, modifying the pattern of heat and moisture exchange, so that the tracheobronchial mucosa must assume more of the burden of heating and humidifying gases before they reach the alveoli. To a considerable extent, the tracheal tube performs the function of the upper airway in alternately condensing expired moisture and adding it to inhaled gases (1). Apparatus dead space also functions as a heat and moisture exchanger, but of rather low efficiency.

EFFECTS OF INHALING DRY GASES

Damage to the Respiratory Tract

As the respiratory mucosa dries and its temperature drops, secretions thicken, ciliary function is reduced, surfactant activity is impaired and the mucosa becomes more susceptible to injury. Dried secretions can cause plugging of the tracheal tube. If secretions are not cleared, atelectasis or obstruction of the airway can result. There may be a fall in functional residual capacity and compliance and a rise in the alveolar-arterial oxygen difference (2,3). Thickened plugs may provide loci for infection. In sensitive individuals, dry gases can cause bronchoconstriction, further compromising respiratory function.

There is no agreement as to the minimum humidity necessary to prevent pathological changes. Recommendations have ranged from 12 to 35 mg water/liter (1,4–10). The international standard on humidifiers considers 30 mg/liter the minimum amount necessary to prevent inspissation of secretions and mucosal damage (11). Complete cessation of ciliary activity occurs following prolonged exposure to inspired gas with an absolute humidity below 22 mg/liter (12).

Many believe that inspired gases should be heated to body temperature with 100% relative humidity. However, others have suggested that conditions in the respiratory system should mimic normal breathing from the atmosphere and the output of a humidification device should match the conditions at the point of entry into the respiratory system (normally 34 to 37 mg H_2O/liter) (13).

The duration of exposure must be considered. It is unlikely that a brief exposure of the tracheobronchial tree to dry inspired gases will result in damage, but as exposure time increases, the likelihood of a significant effect rises.

Several studies have shown a decrease in postoperative pulmonary complications when gases are humidified (14–17), but one study showed no difference (18). Humidification may decrease the incidence of respiratory complications associated with inhalation induction with isoflurane (19).

Loss of Body Heat

Body temperature is lowered as evaporative cooling of the lower airways brings the inspired gas into temperature equilibrium and saturates it with water. This is especially a problem with pediatric patients. A low body temperature may result in shivering, an increase in oxygen demand, and high cardiac output during the immediate postoperative period.

Use of a humidification device can decrease the heat loss that normally occurs during anesthesia and on occasion may provide heat input (15,20–28).

In summary, the importance of humidification in anesthesia remains uncertain. It is of greatest benefit in pediatric patients, patients at increased risk for developing pulmonary complications, and in procedures of long duration. The benefits of deliberately increasing humidity must be weighed against its hazards and cost.

Sources of Humidity

CARBON DIOXIDE ABSORBENT

The reaction of absorbent with carbon dioxide liberates water. Water is also contained in the absorbent granules. This will provide some humidity (see Chapter 7).

EXHALED GASES

In systems that allow rebreathing, the humidity and temperature of inspired gases depend on the relative proportions of fresh gases and expired gases reinhaled. This will depend on the system and the amount of rebreathing it allows. As the fresh gas flow is increased, the temperature and humidity of inspired gases are reduced.

Previous use of a system on other patients can increase the initial inspired humidity caused by water condensed in parts of the system that are not changed between cases (29).

MOISTENING THE BREATHING TUBES AND RESERVOIR BAG

Rinsing the inside of the breathing tubes and reservoir bag with sterile water before use increases the inspired humidity (30). This has the advantage of simplicity, but there is a limit to the increase in humidity that can be achieved.

HEAT AND MOISTURE EXCHANGER

A heat and moisture exchanger (HME) conserves some of the exhaled water and heat and returns them to the inspired gases. The HME is also called the condenser humidifier, Swedish nose, artificial nose, passive humidifier, regenerative humidifier, moisture exchanger, and vapor condenser.

Description

Typical HMEs are shown in Figure 9.1. The size and configuration vary. Each has a 15-mm female connection port at its proximal (patient) end and a 22-mm male port at the distal end. The patient port may also have a concentric 22-mm male fitting (see Fig. 9.1*C* and *D*). There may be a port for aspiration of respiratory gases (see Fig. 9.1*B* and *D*).

The earliest type of HME consisted of a wire mesh screen or metal tubes encased in a metal housing. The next generation had disposable devices with paper-based condensation surfaces enclosed in a plastic housing.

A significant advance was made with the introduction of hygroscopic HMEs. These consist of wool, foam, or a paper-like material coated with moisture-retaining chemi-

cals (31). The medium of a hygroscopic HME may be impregnated with a bacteriocide (32). The hygroscopic layer may be combined with a large-pore felt layer to improve filtration efficiency (31). The latest development is the hydrophobic HME with a pleated membrane. These are efficient microbial filters (31,33,34). They allow the passage of water vapor but not liquid water.

The dead space of HMEs varies widely (4,35–37). Pediatric and neonatal HMEs with less dead space and resistance than adult models are available (38,39).

Action

The mechanism of action in an HME is the exchange of heat and moisture between a gas and the surface over which it flows. Expired gas is normally saturated. When it comes into contact with a surface at a lower temperature, the gas is cooled and some of the vapor condenses onto the surface. At the same time, the surface is warmed. When inspiration begins, gas at ambient temperature comes into contact with the same surface and, being dry by comparison, takes up as vapor some of the water previously deposited. It is also warmed. Hence, some of the heat and water in the exhaled gas is transferred to the inspired gas.

Performance

The inspired humidity achieved using an HME will depend on the humidity of gases passing through it during inspiration, the inspiratory and expiratory flows, and the efficiency of the HME. Increasing the fresh gas humidity will increase the inspired humidity (40,41). The faster gas passes through the HME, the less time there is to absorb and deposit moisture so an increased tidal volume causes the humidity of inspired gas to fall (32,37,42,43).

Many comparative investigations of the efficiency of HMEs have been performed (4,32,35–37,43--47), but the results vary with the experimental design. HMEs containing hygroscopic or hydrophobic materi-

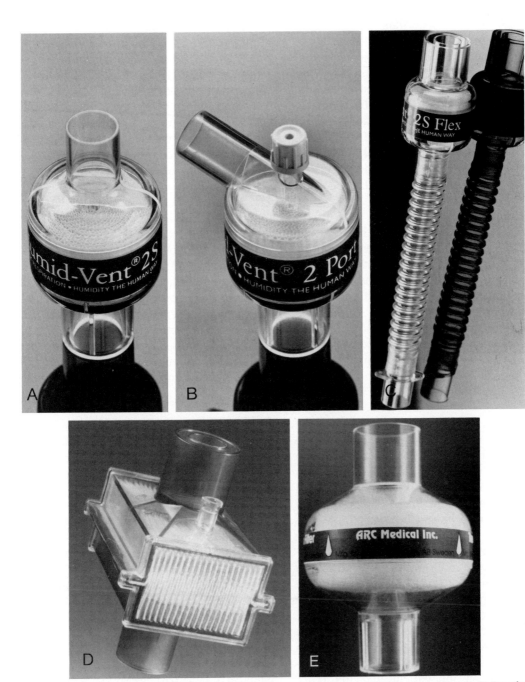

Figure 9.1.   Heat and moisture exchangers. **A,** Straight variety. **B,** Right-angle HME with port for aspiration of respiratory gases on the breathing system side. **C,** The flexible tube attached to the HME extends the distance between the patient and the breathing system and allows the angle between the breathing system and the patient to be altered. Because this HME has significant dead space, it should be used only with high tidal volumes and controlled ventilation with monitoring of inspired and expired CO_2. **D,** Hydrophobic HME with respiratory gas aspiration port. **E,** ThermoFlo filter. Parts **D** and **E,** courtesy of Gibeck Respiration, Pall Biomedical Products Corp., and ARC Medical Inc.

als are more efficient than those without these materials (4,32,37,45,48,49).

The time taken for HMEs to reach equilibrium can vary from 5 to 27 min (45). Most HMEs yield a declining performance with the passage of time, although this is not significant in the first 2 or 3 hr (32,44).

Connecting more than one HME in series will improve performance (4,50). Care must be taken that the units are pushed firmly together and the increase in dead space is not excessive.

A leak around the tracheal tube, or between the tracheal tube and the HME will result in a decrease in inspired humidity (32,38,51). The magnitude of this decrease increases as tidal volume and the proportion of expired volume lost through the leak increase.

Hygroscopic and hydrophobic HMEs both provide some bacteriologic protection, but the hydrophobic type is more efficient in this regard.

Use

The HME should be placed between the patient and the breathing system, as close to the patient as possible. It can be used with any breathing system or ventilator. They may be especially useful during transport of an intubated patient. Such ventilation rarely exceeds 1 or 2 hr and transport ventilators frequently have no means for humidifying inspired gases.

The pressure-sensing line for an airway pressure monitor should be between the patient and the HME. If it is placed between the breathing system and the HME, the HME may cause a back pressure high enough to prevent the low pressure alarm from being activated if there were a disconnection between the patient and the HME (52,53).

If a nebulizer is used to deliver medication, it should be inserted between the HME and the tracheal tube. (54) A respiratory gas sampling port should be located on the breathing system side of the HME (see Fig. 9.1*B* and*D*).

An HME may be used as the sole source of humidity or may be combined with another source such as an unheated humidifier (55). However, some HMEs should not be used with a humidifier or nebulizer. Some HMEs can be moistened before use to increase efficiency (56). A hygroscopic unit should not be moistened because this reduces its efficiency (44). The directions with each device should be read carefully before use.

Hazards

An HME can become obstructed due to fluids, blood, secretions, or a manufacturing defect or if nebulized drugs are passed through it (57-59). The weight of an HME may cause the tracheal tube to kink. Some HMEs contain materials that may be released in the form of particles or dust and are then inhaled by the patient (4,60,61). Separation of its parts may result in a large leak. The dead space of the HME may cause excessive rebreathing, especially with small tidal volumes.

Advantages

HMEs reproduce the fluctuating temperatures and humidities in the normal respiratory tract. They are inexpensive, easy to use, small, lightweight, reliable, simple in design, and silent in operation; they have low compliance and resistance when dry. Disposable ones require no cleaning or sterilization. They do not require water, an external source of energy, or temperature monitors or alarms. There is no danger of overhydration, burns of the skin or respiratory tract, or electrical shock.

All HMEs present a barrier to the passage of bacteria and some are efficient bacterial and viral filters (21,36,62). They prevent inhalation of large particles.

Disadvantages

The main disadvantage of HMEs is the limited humidity these devices can deliver. Some loss of water from the tracheobronchial tree will still occur. Therefore, an HME may not provide an acceptable humidity for lengthy cases with high flows of nonhumidified gases or for long-term intubation (63). They are not suitable for patients with copious or thickened secretions, poor hydration, or airway injury (64,65).

HMEs have not proved beneficial in reducing recovery time in patients having short operative procedures (66).

Placing an HME between the breathing system and patient increases dead space. This may necessitate an increase in tidal volume in small patients (67) and can lead to dangerous rebreathing (68). Use of an HME increases resistance to respiration, especially as it becomes saturated (33,39,69–75). The presence of viscous secretions can increase resistance greatly (76).

HUMIDIFIERS

A humidifier (vaporizer or vaporizing humidifier) is an instrument that passes a stream of gas over water or across wicks dipped in water (passover or blow-by) or through water (bubble or cascade).

Unheated Humidifiers

Unheated humidifiers are usually disposable, bubble-through containers that are used to increase the humidity of oxygen supplied to patients via a face mask or nasal cannulae. They cannot deliver more than about 9 mg H_2O/liter.

Heated Humidifiers

Heated humidifiers designed for use in anesthesia are available from a number of manufacturers. Most are supplied with adapters for mounting. Most heated humidifiers use electricity to supply heat.

Description

Humidification Chamber. The humidification chamber is the part from which water is immediately derived for humidification of inspired gases. It may be disposable or reusable. It may be detachable for filling. Some humidifiers have a reservoir that supplies liquid water to the humidification chamber.

Heat Source. Heat may be supplied by heated rods immersed in the water or a heated plate at the bottom of the humidification chamber (Fig. 9.2).

Delivery Tube. The delivery tube conveys humidified gas from the humidifier outlet. It may be heated. Methods of heating have included an electric wire inside the tube (see Fig. 9.2) (20,77), heating tape or orthopedic cast padding or an air or water jacket around the tube (78–81), and placing the inspiratory limb inside the expiratory limb (82,83).

The heating wire has the advantage of still allowing visualization of the tube (see Fig. 9.2). It should extend as close to the patient connection as possible. Disposable wires are present in preassembled disposable breathing systems. A reusable wire must be inserted manually into the delivery tube using a draw wire (84).

Temperature Monitors. Most heated humidifiers have a means to measure the delivered gas temperature (the temperature of the gas at the patient end of the breathing system). In systems using a heated wire, there is usually a second probe to measure the temperature at the humidifier outlet.

Thermostats. *Servo-Controlled Units.* A servo-controlled unit regulates power to the heating element in response to the temperature sensed by a probe near the patient connection or at the humidifier outlet (12,85).

Nonservo-Controlled Units. A nonservo-controlled unit provides power to the heating element according to the setting of a control, irrespective of the delivery temperature. A nonservo-controlled unit may include a servo-controlled circuit, but this maintains heater temperature rather than delivery temperature (12).

Usually, there are two thermostats in series, so that if one fails, the other will still cut off the power supply before a dangerous temperature is reached.

Controls. Most humidifiers allow selection of different temperatures at the end of the delivery tube or the humidification

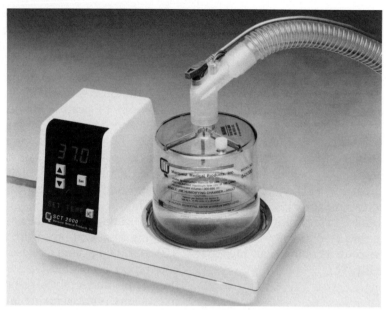

Figure 9.2.   Heated humidifier. Heat is supplied from a heated plate below the humidification chamber. Note the probe for monitoring the temperature of gas leaving the humidification chamber. A heating wire is inside the delivery tube. Courtesy of Marquest Medical Products, Inc.

chamber outlet, and some allow less than 100% relative humidity to be delivered (86). Some models generate saturated vapor only at a preset temperature (3).

Alarms.   Alarms warn when the temperature at the patient end of the circuit deviates from the set temperature by a fixed amount and when the temperature probe has not been placed correctly in the delivery tube or has become dislodged. An alarm may warn when the heater wire is not connected.

Action

Some humidifiers heat the gas to a temperature exceeding the desired patient airway temperature (superheating) so that the cooling that occurs as it flows to the patient will result in the desired temperature at the patient connection. In other units, temperature increases as it passes through the delivery tube, so that gas with less than 100% relative humidity is delivered.

In any humidifier in which the delivery tube is not heated, the temperature will drop as it flows to the patient. The magnitude of the drop depends on many factors, including the ambient temperature; gas flow; and the length, diameter, and thermal mass of the breathing system. Cooling can be reduced by shortening or insulating the delivery tube and using higher inspiratory flows (87). If the gas is saturated at the humidifier outlet, the temperature drop will cause condensation of water vapor (rainout) to occur.

Standard Requirements

An international standard on humidifiers has been published (11). The standard contains the following provisions.

1. The gas reaching the patient should contain at least 30 mg of water vapor per liter of gas if intended for an intubated patient and at least 10 mg/liter if it is to be presented to the upper airway.

2. If the humidifier includes a servo-controlled mechanism the average temperature at the delivery tube outlet shall not fluctuate by more than 2°C from the set temperature during any 5-min period after the manufacturer's stated warm-up period.

3. If the humidifier is heated, the gas temperature at the delivery tube outlet shall not exceed 41°C or the gas temperature at the humidifier outlet shall be indicated continuously and the temperature measuring device shall activate auditory and visual alarms when the temperature exceeds 41°C. If failure of the temperature-control system can constitute a thermal hazard, an additional nonself-resetting thermal cutout must be provided. The thermal cutout should activate a visual signal independently from the temperature monitoring system.

4. The temperature of any accessible surface (one that can be touched during normal use) shall not exceed 55°C if metal or 75°C if nonmetal. The accessible surface temperature of the delivery tube must not exceed 41°C within 50 mm of the delivery tube outlet.

5. When the humidifier is tilted 20° from its normal operating position, there shall be no spillage of water into the breathing system.

6. All operator controls and digital indicators shall be accurate to within 10% of their full-scale value.

7. If the humidifier is capable of producing a water content greater than 44 mg/liter, there must be a warning on the humidifier that excessive quantities of water can be delivered.

8. If the humidifier is intended to be placed in a breathing system, the connectors must be 22 mm if intended for adult use and 15 mm if intended for pediatric use.

The ASTM standard for breathing systems requires a humidifier whose correct function depends on the direction of gas flow through it to be marked with an arrow indicating the proper directional flow, and/or the words *inlet* and *outlet* (88).

Use

A heated humidifier is most commonly used in the circle system, connected into the inspiratory limb downstream from the inspiratory unidirectional valve. If a bacterial filter is used, it should be upstream of the humidifier to prevent it from becoming clogged.

Use of a heated humidifier in systems other than the circle has been described (81,89–92). It is usually placed in the fresh gas supply tube. Water condensation in this tube can be a problem, causing noise and requiring drainage or installation of a water trap to avoid obstruction of gas flow or patient aspiration. Using a large-diameter tubing and placing the humidifier near the end of the tube will decrease condensation (90). However, this may cause problems in mounting. The delivery tube temperature probe may be placed either between the fresh gas supply tube and the T piece or between the T piece and the patient (90).

The humidifier should always be kept at a lower level than the patient so that there is less risk of water running down the tube into the patient. Clear tubing should be used so this water can be seen. Condensed water should be drained periodically or a water trap inserted in the dependent part of the delivery tubing to prevent blockage of a breathing tube or aspiration of water. The humidification chamber and delivery tube should always be changed between patients.

Advantages

Most heated humidifiers are capable of delivering saturated gas at body temperature or above, even with high flow rates.

Disadvantages

Humidifiers are bulky and may be difficult to mount. They are somewhat complex and may be difficult to clean and sterilize. They are more costly than HMEs. The level of water in the humidifier chamber must be checked periodically. The need for electrical power means one more cord that operating room personnel may trip over.

Hazards

1. Bacterial contamination can be a problem in bubbling heated humidifiers (93).

2. Reported breathing system problems include sticking valves, leaks, disconnections, incorrect connections, obstruction of the fresh gas line or inspiratory limb, noise, and clogging of bacterial filters (90,94–101). Overfilling, misassembly, or malfunction can cause water to enter the breathing system (102–105). Melting of the delivery tubing by the humidifier or heater wire may occur, resulting in obstruction or a leak (84,98,106–108).

3. If the humidifier is placed in the fresh gas line, a sudden obstruction may result in water splashing back into the anesthesia machine (109).

4. Adding a humidifier may change the breathing system volume and compliance significantly (110). This can complicate delivery of small tidal volumes.

5. Use of a humidifier can produce a positive water balance and even overhydration. Although most anesthetics are of sufficiently short duration that this is not significant, it can be a problem with infants. Undesirable effects of overhydration include increased airway resistance; decreased ciliary function, surfactant activity, functional residual capacity, and static compliance; and atelectasis (3).

6. Undesirable heat gain may occur.

7. There is danger of water entering the tracheal tube and drowning the patient or causing a burn of the respiratory tract. These risks can be decreased by configuring the breathing system in a manner that does not allow condensate to drain into the patient, installing a water trap into the dependent portion of the breathing tube, draining condensate frequently, and placing the humidifier and breathing tubes below the level of the operating room table.

8. Fires caused by short-circuiting of heated wires and internal heating coils and defects in heated wires have been reported (12,111,112). Charring of the breathing system may result in fumes entering the patient's lungs (84).

9. High humidity can cause problems with sidestream (aspirating) respiratory gas monitors (113). Inserting a filter between the sampling line and the sensing port in the breathing system may help.

10. Halothane may be altered by passage through a humidifier whose heating element is in direct contact with the gas at a temperature of 68°C (114).

11. A humidifier may add enough resistance to prevent activation of a low airway pressure alarm if the sensor is upstream of the humidifier (53).

12. Hyperthermia, tracheitis and respiratory tract burns may occur if the inspiratory temperature exceeds 40°C (115–118). Burns to the skin have been reported from heated oxygen administered nasally (119). Skin contact with heated breathing circuits may cause burns (120,121).

Overheating of the inspired gas may be caused by omitting, misplacing, or dislodging the airway temperature probe or by not fully inserting it (12,119,122,123). This risk can be reduced by using an airway pressure monitor, CO_2 monitor, or respirometer with an alarm that will be activated if the probe is omitted or becomes dislodged. Many humidifiers have an alarm that is activated if the airway temperature probe does not sense an increase in temperature within a certain time after activation or if the probe temperature is a certain amount below the selected value.

A servo-controlled unit may overheat if turned on with a low gas flow through it or if the temperature probe is not placed in the patient airway (12,124). A nonservo-controlled unit can deliver overheated gas if its controls are improperly set or if gas flow is abruptly reduced.

A temporary increase in inspired gas temperature may occur following a period of interrupted flow or an increase in flow rate (124,125).

NEBULIZERS

Description

Nebulizers are also called aerosol generators, atomizers, and nebulizing humidifiers.

A nebulizer is an instrument that emits water in the form of an aerosol mist (water vapor plus liquid particulate water). The most commonly used are the pneumatic (gas driven, jet, high pressure, or compressed gas) and the ultrasonic. Both can be heated. In addition to providing humidification, these devices may be used to deliver drugs to the breathing system (126).

In a pneumatic nebulizer, a jet of high-pressure gas encounters the liquid, inducing shearing forces and breaking the water up into fine particles. An ultrasonic nebulizer produces a fine mist by subjecting the liquid to a high-frequency resonator. There is no need for a driving gas. The frequency of oscillation determines the size of the droplets. Ultrasonic nebulizers create a denser mist than pneumatic nebulizers (85).

Use

Because a high flow of gas must be used with a pneumatic nebulizer, it should be placed in the fresh gas line (127). An ultrasonic nebulizer can be used in the fresh gas delivery line or the inspiratory limb (17).

Hazards

Nebulized drugs may cause obstruction of an HME (57,58). Nebulization may have deleterious effects on the lungs if used for prolonged periods (128). Bronchospasm can result from their use (129). Overhydration can occur. If the droplets are not warmed, hypothermia may occur. Transmission of infection can be a significant problem, because bacteria can be suspended in the water droplets (130,131)

Advantages

Nebulizers can deliver gases saturated with water without heat and, if desired, can produce gases carrying more water.

Disadvantages

Nebulizers are somewhat costly. Pneumatic nebulizers require high gas flows. Ultrasonic nebulizers require a source of elec-

tricity and may present electrical hazards. There may be considerable water deposition in the tubings, requiring frequent draining and posing the dangers of water draining into the patient and blockage of the tubing.

REFERENCES

1. Dery R, Pelletier J, Jacques A, Clavet M, Houde JJ. Humidity in anesthesiology. Heat and moisture patterns in the respiratory tract during anaesthesia with the semi-closed system. Can Anaesth Soc J 1967;14:287–298.
2. Rashad K, Wilson K, Hurt HH, Jr, Graff TD, Banson DW. Effect of humidification of anesthetic gases on static compliance. Anesth Analg 1967;46:127–133.
3. Shelly MP, Lloyd GM, Park GR. A review of the mechanisms and methods of humidification of inspired gases. Intensive Care Med 1988;14:1–9.
4. Anonymous. Heat and moisture exchangers. Health Devices 1983;12:155–167.
5. Chamney AR. Humidification requirements and techniques. Including a review of the performance of equipment in current use. Anaesthesia 1969;24:602–617.
6. Chalon J, Loew DAY, Malebranche J. Effects of dry anesthetic gases on tracheobronchial ciliated epithelium. Anesthesiology 1972;37:338–343.
7. Forbes AR. Humidification and mucus flow in the intubated trachea. Br J Anaesth 1973;45:874–878.
8. Noguchi H, Takumi Y, Aochi O. A study of humidification in tracheostomized dogs. Br J Anaesth 1973;45:844–848.
9. Tsuda T, Noguchi H, Takkumi Y, Aochi O. Optimum humidification of air administered to a tracheostomy in dogs. Scanning electron microscopy and surfactant studies. Br J Anaesth 1977;49:965–977.
10. Weeks DB. Humidification during anesthesia. NY State J Med 1975;75:1216–1218.
11. International Organization for Standards. Humidifiers for medical use—safety standard (ISO 8185:1988). Geneva: ISO, 1988.
12. Anonymous. Heated humidifiers. Technol Anesth 1987;8:1–5.
13. Chatburn RL, Primiano FP. A rational basis for humidity therapy. Respir Care 1987;32:249–254.
14. Chalon J, Patel C, Ali M, et al. Humidity and the anesthetized patient. Anesthesiology 1979;50:195–198.
15. Fonkalsrud EW, Calmes S, Barcliff LT, Barrett CT. Reduction of operative heat loss and pulmonary secretions in neonates by use of heated and humidified anesthetic gases. J Thorac Cardiovasc Surg 1980;80:718–723.

16. Gawley TH, Dundee JW. Attempts to reduce respiratory complications following upper abdominal operations. Br J Anaesth 1981;53:1073–1078.

17. Stevens HL, Kennedy RL. The ultrasonic approach to humidification of anesthesia gases. J Asthma Res 1968;5:325–333.

18. Knudsen J, Lomholt N, Wisborg K. Postoperative pulmonary complications using dry and humidified anaesthetic gases. Br J Anaesth 1973;45:363–368.

19. Van Heerden PV, Wilson IH, Marshall FPF, Cormack JR. Effect of humidification on inhalation induction with isoflurane. Br J Anaesth 1990;64:235–237.

20. Baker JD, Wallace CT, Brown CS. Maintenance of body temperature in infants during surgery. Anesthesiol Rev 1977;4:21–25.

21. Chalon J, Markham JP, Ali MM, Ramanathan S, Turndorf H. The Pall ultipore breathing circuit filter—an efficient heat and moisture exchanger. Anesth Analg 1984;63:566–570.

22. Haslam KR, Nielsen CH. Do passive heat and moisture exchangers keep the patient warm? Anesthesiology 1986;64:379–381.

23. Morton GH, Flewellen EH. Prevention of intraoperative hypothermia in geriatric patients. Anesth Analg 1989;68:S204.

24. Pflug AE, Aasheim GM, Foster C, Martin RW. Prevention of post-anaesthesia shivering. Can Anaesth Soc J 1991;25:41–47.

25. Rashad KF, Benson DW. Role of humidity in prevention of hypothermia in infants and children. Anesth Analg 1967;46:712–718.

26. Stone DR, Downs JB, Paul WL, Perkins HM. Adult body temperature and heated humidification of anesthetic gases during general anesthesia. Anesth Analg 1981;60:736–741.

27. Tausk HC, Miller R, Roberts RB. Maintenance of body temperature by heated humidification. Anesth Analg 1976;55:719–723.

28. Wallace CT, Baker JD, Brown CS. Heated humidification for infants during anesthesia. Anesthesiology 1978;48:80.

29. Chalon J. Low humidity and damage to tracheal mucosa. Bull N Y Acad Med 1980;56:314–322.

30. Chase HF, Trotta R, Kilmore MA. Simple methods for humidifying nonrebreathing anesthesia gas systems. Anesth Analg 1962;41:249–256.

31. Hedley RM, Allt-Graham J. A comparison of the filtration properties of heat and moisture exchangers. Anesthesia 1992;47:414–420.

32. Anonymous. Evaluation report: heat and moisture exchangers. J Med Eng Technol 1987;11:117–127.

33. Berry AJ, Nolte FS. An alternative strategy for infection control of anesthesia breathing circuits: a laboratory assessment of the Pall HME filter. Anesth Analg 1991;72:651–655.

34. Lee MG, Ford JL, Hunt PB, Ireland DS, Swanson PW. Bacterial retention properties of heat and moisture exchange filters. Br J Anaesth 1992;69:522–525.

35. Weeks DB, Ramsey FM. Laboratory investigation of six artificial noses for use during endotracheal anesthesia. Anesth Analg 1983;62:758–763.

36. Shelly M, Bethune DW, Latimer RD. A comparison of five heat and moisture exchangers. Anaesthesia 1986;41:527–532.

37. Mebius C. A comparative evaluation of disposable humidifiers. Acta Anaesthesiol Scand 1983;27:403–409.

38. Gedeon A, Mebius C, Palmer K. Neonatal hygroscopic condenser humidifier. Crit Care Med 1987;15:51–54.

39. Wilkinson KA, Cranston A, Hatch DJ, Fletcher ME. Assessment of a hygroscopic heat and moisture exchanger for paediatric use. Anaesthesia 1991;46:296–299.

40. Usuda Y, Suzukawa M, Yamaguchi O, Kaneko K, Okutsu Y. Increased moisture output from heat and moisture exchangers combined with an unheated humidifier. Crit Care Med 1989;17:S35.

41. Shanks CA. Clinical anesthesia and multiple-gauze condenser humidifier. Br J Anaesth 1974;46:773–777.

42. Hay R, Miller WC. Efficacy of a new hygroscopic condenser humidifier. Crit Care Med 1982;10:49–51.

43. Ogino M, Kopotic R, Mannino FL. Moisture-conserving efficiency of condenser humidifiers. Anaesthesia 1985;40:990–995.

44. Oh TE, Thompson WR, Hayward DR. Disposable condenser humidifiers in intensive care. Anaesth Intensive Care 1981;9:331–335.

45. Turtle MJ, Ilsley AH, Rutten AJ, Runciman WB. An evaluation of six disposable heat and moisture exchangers. Anaesth Intensive Care 1987;15:317–322.

46. Walker AKY, Bethune DW. A comparative study of condenser-humidifiers. Anaesthesia 1976;31:1086–1093.

47. Weeks DB. A laboratory evaluation of recently available heat-and-moisture exchangers. Anesth Rev 1986;8:33–36.

48. Stoutenbeek Ch, Miranda D, Zandstra D. A new hygroscopic condenser humidifier. Intensive Care Med 1982;8:231–234.

49. Gedeon A, Mebius C. The hygroscopic condenser humidifier. A new device for general use in anaesthesia and intensive care. Anaesthesia 1979;34:1043–1047.

50. Shanks CA, Sara CA. A reappraisal of the multiple gauze heat and moisture exchanger. Anaesth Intensive Care 1973;1:428–432.

51. Tilling, SE, Hayes B. Heat and moisture exchang-

ers in artificial ventilation. Br J Anaesth 1987;59:1181–1188.

52. Milligan KA. Disablement of a ventilator disconnect alarm by a heat and moisture exchanger. Anaesthesia 1992;47:279.

53. Slee TA, Pavlin EG. Failure of low pressure alarm associated with the use of a humidifier. Anesthesiology 1988;69:791–793.

54. Leigh JM, White MG. A new condenser humidifier. Anaesthesia 1984;39:492–493.

55. Suzukawa M, Usuda Y, Numata K. The effects on sputum characteristics of combining an unheated humidifier with a heat-moisture exchanging filter. Respir Care 1989;34:976–984.

56. Duncan A. Use of disposable condenser humidifiers in children. Anaesth Intensive Care 1985; 13:330–337.

57. Anonymous. Heat/moisture exchange humidifiers. Technol Anesth 1991;11:5.

58. Anonymous. Humidifiers, heat/moisture exchange. Technol Anesth 1991;12:5.

59. Martin C, Perrin G, Gevaudan MJ, Saux P, Gouin F. Heat and moisture exchangers and vaporising humidifiers in the intensive care unit. Chest 1990;97:144–149.

60. Anonymous. Humidifiers, heat/moisture exchange. Technol Anesth 1985;6:8.

61. James PD, Gothard JWW. Possible hazard from the inserts of condenser humidifiers. Anaesthesia 1984;39:70.

62. Bygdeman S, von Euler C, Nystrom B. Moisture exchangers do not prevent patient contamination of ventilators. A microbiological study. Acta Anaesthesiol Scand 1984;28:591–594.

63. Roustan JP, Kienlen J, Aubas S, du Cailar J. Heat and moisture exchanger vs heated humidifier during prolonged mechanical ventilation. Anesthesiology 1989;71:A214.

64. Demers B. Endotracheal tube occlusion associated with the use of heat and moisture exchangers in the intensive care unit. Crit Care Med 1989;17:845–846.

65. Gilston A. Hygroscopic condenser humidifiers. Anaesthesia 1984;39:1030–1031.

66. Goldberg ME, Jan R, Gregg CE, Berko R, Marr AT, Larijani GE. The heat and moisture exchanger does not preserve body temperature or reduce recovery time in outpatients undergoing surgery and anesthesia. Anesthesiology 1988;68:122–123.

67. Raju R. Humidifier-induced hypercarbia. Anaesthesia 1987;42:672–673.

68. Mason DG, Edmondson L, McHugh P. Humidifier-induced hypercarbia. Anaesthesia 1987; 42:672–673.

69. Buckley PM. Increase in resistance of in-line breathing filters in humidified air. Br J Anaesth 1984;56:637–642.

70. Chung R, Soni NC. Work of ventilating heat and moisture exchangers. Br J Anaesth 1991;67:647P–648P.

71. Jones BR, Ozaki GT, Benumof JL, Saidman LJ. Airway resistance caused by a pediatric heat and moisture exchanger. Anesthesiology 1988;69:A786.

72. Ploysongsang Y, Branson R, Rashkin MC, Hurst JM. Pressure flow characteristics of commonly used heat-moisture exchangers. Am Rev Respir Dis 1988;138:675–678.

73. Ploysongsang Y, Branson RD, Rashkin MC, Hurst JM. Effect of flowrate and duration of use on the pressure drop across six artificial noses. Respir Care 1989;34:902–907.

74. Rodes WD, Banner MJ, Gravenstein N. Variations in imposed work of breathing with heat and moisture exchangers. Anesth Analg 1991;72:S226.

75. Steward DJ. A disposable condenser humidifier for use during anaesthesia. Can Anaesth Soc J 1976;23:191–195.

76. Kong KL, Rainbow C, Ford DB. Heat and moisture exchanging bacterial filters. Anaesthsia 1988;43:254.

77. Shanks CA, Gibbs JM. A comparison of two heated water-bath humidifiers. Anaesth Intensive Care 1975;3:41–47.

78. Berry FA, Hughes-Davies DI, Difazio CA. A system for minimizing respiratory heat loss in infants during operation. Anesth Analg 1973;52:170–175.

79. Epstein RA. Humidification during positive pressure ventilation of infants. Anesthesiology 1971; 35:532–536.

80. Mizutani AR, Ozaki G, Rusk R.Insulated circuit hose improves heated humidifier performance in anesthesia ventilation circuits. Anesth Analg 1991;72:566–567.

81. Racz GB. Humidification in a semiopen system for infant anesthesia. Anesth Analg 1971;50:995–1002.

82. Ramanathan S, Chalon J, Turndorf H. A compact, well-humidified breathing circuit for the circle system. Anesthesiology 1976;44:238–242.

83. Chalon J, Patel C, Ramanathan S, Turndorf H. Humidification of the circle absorber system. Anesthesiology 1978;48:142–146.

84. Anonymous. Heated wires can melt disposable breathing circuits. Technol Anesth 1989;9:2–3.

85. Anonymous. Heated humidifiers. Health Devices 1987;16:223–250.

86. Cook RI, Potter SS, Woods DD, McDonald JS. Evaluating the human engineering of microprocessor-controlled operating room devices. J Clin Monit 1991;7:217–226.

87. Anonymous. Heated humidifiers. Health Devices 1980;9:167–180.

88. American Society for Testing and Materials. Stan-

dard specifications for minimum performance and safety requirements for anesthesia breathing systems (ASTM F1208-89). Philadelphia: ASTM, 1989.

89. Garg GP. Humidification of the Rees-Ayre T-piece system for neonates. Anesth Analg 1973; 52:207–209.

90. Hannallah RS, McGill WA. A practical way of using heated humidifiers with pediatric T-piece systems. Anesthesiology 1983;59:156–157.

91. Kovac AL, Filardi JP, Goto H. Water trap for fresh gas flow line of Bain or CPRAM circuit. Can J Anaesth 1987;34:102–103.

92. Weeks DB. Provision of endogenous and exogenous humidity for the Bain breathing circuit. Can Anaesth Soc J 1976;23:185–190.

93. Rhame FS, Streifel A, McComb C, Boyle M. Bubbling humidifiers produce microaerosols which can carry bacteria. Infect Control 1986;7:403–407.

94. Anonymous. Humidifierrs, heat/moisture exchange. Technol Anesth 1985;6:7.

95. Bancroft ML. Problems with humidifiers. In: Randell-Baker L, ed. Problems with anesthetic and respiratory therapy equipment [Special issue]. Int Anesth Clin 1982;20(3):93–102.

96. McNulty S, Barringer L, Browder J. Carbon dioxide retention associated with a humidifier defect. Can J Anaesth 1987;34:519–521.

97. Nimocks JA, Modell JH, Perry PA. Carbon dioxide retention using a humidified "nonrebreathing" system. Anesth Analg 1975;54:271–273.

98. Patil AR. Melting of anesthesia circuit by humidifier. Another cause of "ventilator disconnect." Anesth Prog 1989;36:63–65.

99. Shroff PK, Skerman JH. Humidifier malfunction—a cause of anesthesia circuit occlusion. Anesth Analg 1988;67:710–711.

100. Shampaine EL, Helfaer M. A modest proposal for improved humidifier design. Anesth Analg 1991; 72:130–131.

101. Wang J, Hung W, Lin C. Leakage of disposable breathing circuits. J Clin Anesth 1992;4:111–115.

102. Poulton TJ. Humidification hazard. Chest 1984; 85:583–584.

103. Poplak TM, Leiman BC, Braude BM. A hazardous humidifier misconnexion. Anaesthesia 1984; 39:937.

104. Railton R, Shjaw A. Filling humidifiers. Avoiding a hazard. Anaesthesia 1982;37:105–106.

105. Ward CF, Reisner LS, Zlott LS. Murphy's law and humidification. Anesth Analg 1983;62:457–461.

106. Wong DHW. Melted delivery hose—a complication of a heated humidifier. Can J Anaesth 1988;35:183–186.

107. Wood D, Boyd M, Campbell C. Insulation of heated wire circuits. Anesth Analg 1992;74:471.

108. Sprague DH, Maccioli GA. Disposable circuit tubing melted by heated humidifier. Anesth Analg 1986;65:1247.

109. Amirdivani M, Siegel D, Chalon J, Ramanathan S, Turndorf H. A heated water humidifier with a rotating wick. Anesth Analg 1979;58:244–246.

110. Cote CJ, Petkau AJ, Ryan JF, Welch JP. Wasted ventilation measured in vitro with eight anesthetic circuits with and without inline humidification. Anesthesiology 1983;59:442–446.

111. Anonymous. "Potential fire hazard" from nebulizers reported. Biomed Saf Stand 1988;18:58.

112. Anonymous. Breathing circuit heating component could short and cause fire. Biomed Saf Stand 1990;20:67–68.

113. Sprung J, Cheng EY. Modification to an anesthesia breathing circuit to prolong monitoring of gases during the use of humidifiers. Anesth Analg 1991;72:264–265.

114. Karis JH. Alteration of halothane in heated humidifiers. Anesth Analg 1980;59:518.

115. Kirch TJ, DeKornfeld TJ. An unexpected complication (hyperthemia) while using the Emerson postoperative ventilator. Anesthesiology 1967;28: 1106–1107.

116. Klein EF, Graves SA. "Hot pot" tracheitis. Chest 1974;65:225–226.

117. Spurring PW, Shenolikar BK. Hazards in anaesthetic equipment. Br J Anaesth 1978;50:641–644.

118. Sims NM, Geoffrion CA, Welch JP, Jung W, Burke JF. Respiratory tract burns caused by heated humidification of anesthetic gases in intubated, mechanically ventilated dogs—a light microscopic study. Anesthesiology 1986;65:A490.

119. Anonymous. Heated humidifiers can burn infants during CPAP. Health Devices 1987;16:404–406.

120. Anonymous. Possible burn from heated breathing circuit. Biomed Safe Stand 1991;21:147.

121. Whiteley SM. A hazard of heated humidifiers. Anaesthesia 1992;47:909.

122. Anonymous. Heated humidifiers can burn infants during CPAP. Technol Anesth 1988;8:7–9.

123. Anonymous. Safety action bulletin. Anaesthesia 1992;47:547.

124. Steward DJ, Volgyesi GA. Heated humidifiers may deliver hot gases. Anesthesiology 1983; 59:A430.

125. Smith HS, Allen R. Another hazard of heated water humidifiers. Anaesthesia 1986;41:215–216.

126. Weeks DB. Micronebulizer for anesthesia circuits. Anesth Analg 1981;60:537–538.

127. Fortin G, Blanc VF. Miniature ventilators with interrupted non-rebreathing circle systems and other anaesthetic circuits. Can Anaesth Soc J 1970; 17:613–623.

128. Modell JH, Giammona ST, Davis JH. Effect of chronic exposure to ultrasonic aerosols on the lung. Anesthesiology 1967;28:680–688.

129. Burke RD, Kosanin RM, Riefkohl R. Bronchospasm caused by unheated nebulized oxygen. Anesthesiol Rev 1986;13:24–25.

130. Spaepen MS, Berryman JR, Bodman HA, Kundsin RB, Fenel V. Prevalence and survival of microbe contaminants in heated nebulizers. Anesth Analg 1978;57:191–196.

131. Vesley D, Anderson J, Halbert MM, Wyman L. Bacterial output from three respiratory therapy humidifying devices. Respir Care 1979;24:228–234.

Chapter 10

Anesthesia Ventilators

A ventilator (breathing machine) is an automatic device that is connected to the patient's airway and is designed to provide or augment the patient's ventilation. It is an essential component of the modern anesthesia delivery system.

Terminology (1,2)

TIDAL VOLUME

The tidal volume is the volume of gas entering or leaving the patient during the inspiratory or expiratory phase time.

MINUTE VOLUME

The minute volume is the sum of all the tidal volumes within 1 min.

VENTILATORY RATE OR FREQUENCY

The number of respiratory cycles per minute is called the ventilatory rate or frequency.

INSPIRATORY FLOW TIME

The period between the beginning and end of inspiratory flow is known as the inspiratory flow time.

INSPIRATORY PAUSE TIME

The inspiratory pause time is the period from the end of inspiratory flow to the start of expiratory flow.

INSPIRATORY PHASE TIME

The inspiratory phase time is the period of time between the start of inspiratory flow and the beginning of expiratory flow. It is the sum

255

of the inspiratory flow and inspiratory pause times.

EXPIRATORY FLOW TIME

The time between the beginning and end of expiratory flow is the expiratory flow time.

EXPIRATORY PAUSE TIME

The expiratory pause time is the interval from the end of expiratory flow to the start of inspiratory flow.

EXPIRATORY PHASE TIME

The time between the start of expiratory flow and the start of inspiratory flow is called the expiratory phase time. It is the sum of the expiratory flow and expiratory pause times.

INSPIRATORY:EXPIRATORY PHASE TIME RATIO

The I:E ratio is the ratio of the inspiratory phase time to expiratory phase time.

INSPIRATORY FLOW RATE

The volume of gas per unit time that passes from the patient connection of the breathing system to the patient is the inspiratory flow rate. It will not be constant.

EXPIRATORY FLOW RATE

The expiratory flow rate is the volume of gas per unit of time returned from the patient during the expiratory phase. It may not be constant.

RESISTANCE

Resistance is defined as the pressure difference per unit flow across the airway. Resistance is usually not constant but increases as flow increases.

COMPLIANCE

The ratio of a change in volume to a change in pressure is called compliance.

Relationship of the Ventilator to the Breathing System

A ventilator replaces the reservoir bag in the breathing system. It may be connected to the breathing system at the bag mount or at the bag/ventilator selector valve. If there is a selector valve, the switch from mechanical to manual ventilation is made by turning the valve. If no switch valve is present, the reservoir bag must be removed from its mount and the ventilator hose attached. Newer anesthesia ventilators are connected to the breathing system without a hose.

During automatic ventilation, the APL valve in the breathing system must be closed or isolated. Some selector valves when turned for ventilator operation isolate the APL valve from the rest of the system. With these, it is not necessary to close the APL valve when the ventilator is used. The APL valve must be opened when manual ventilation is used unless a closed system technique is being used.

Most anesthesia ventilators have a *bellows in a box* (bag in a bottle or double circuit) design (Fig. 10.1). In this design, the bellows is housed in a chamber and the inside of the bellows is connected to the breathing system. The bellows can be thought of as an interface between the breathing system and the ventilator driving gas, just as the reservoir bag acts as an interface between the breathing system and the anesthesiologist's hand. It separates breathing system gases from driving gas. The pressure of the anesthesiologist's hand is replaced by the pressure of driving gas.

During inspiration, driving gas is delivered into the space between the bellows and its housing. This causes pressure to be exerted on the bellows, causing it to be compressed. At the same time, the spill valve (which vents excess gases to the scavenging system) and exhaust valve (which vents driving gas) are closed. The compression of the bellows causes gas to flow into the breathing system.

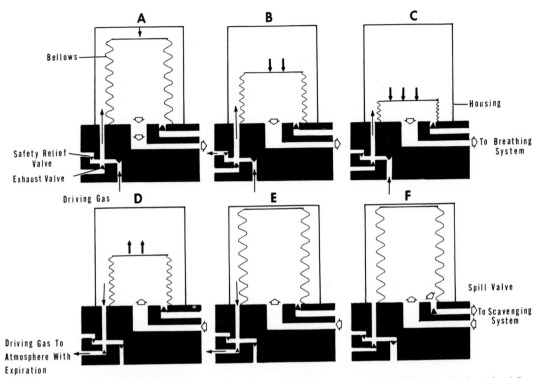

Figure 10.1. Functioning of the bellows-in-box ventilator. **A,** Beginning of inspiration. Driving gas begins to be delivered into the space between the bellows and its housing. The exhaust valve (which connects the driving gas pathway with atmosphere) is closed. The spill valve (which vents excess breathing system gases to the scavenging system) is also closed. **B,** Middle of inspiration. As driving gas continues to flow into the space around the bellows, its pressure increases, exerting a force that causes the bellows to be compressed. This pushes the gas inside the bellows toward breathing system. The exhaust and spill valves remain closed. If the pressure of the driving gas exceeds the opening pressure of the safety-relief valve, the valve will open and vent driving gas to atmosphere. **C,** End of inspiration. The bellows is fully compressed. The exhaust and spill valves remain closed. **D,** Beginning of expiration. Breathing system (exhaled and fresh) gases flow into the bellows, which begins to expand. The expanding bellows displaces driving gas from the interior of the housing. The exhaust valve opens and driving gas flows through it to atmosphere. The spill valve remains closed. **E,**Middle of expiration. The bellows is nearly fully expanded. Driving gas continues to flow to atmosphere. The spill valve remains closed. **F,** End of expiration. Continued flow of gas into the bellows after it is fully expanded creates a positive pressure that causes the spill valve at the base of the bellows to open. Breathing system gases are vented through the spill valve into the scavenging system.

During expiration the bellows reexpands as breathing system gases flow into it. Driving gas is vented to atmosphere through the exhaust valve. After the bellows is fully expanded, excess gases from the breathing system are vented to the scavenging system through the spill valve. Thus during mechanically controlled or assisted ventilation, excess gases are vented during expiration, in contrast to manually assisted or controlled ventilation, when they are vented during inspiration.

Components

A standard for ventilators intended for use during anesthesia has been published by the American Society for Testing and Materials (2). It sets down basic performance and safety requirements for components.

DRIVING GAS SUPPLY

The driving gas supply is also called the power gas supply. All currently available an-

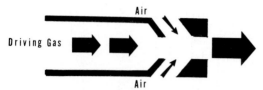

Figure 10.2. Injector (Venturi). Gas flows through the constricted area at a high velocity. The pressure around it drops below atmospheric and air is entrained. The net result is an increase in total gas flow leaving the outlet of the injector.

esthesia ventilators are pneumatically powered, most often by oxygen. The ventilator standard specifies that the ventilator shall continue to function within the manufacturer's specifications throughout a range of supply pressures of 55 psig +20% and −25%. Most ventilators are supplied with DISS oxygen connections.

INJECTOR

Some ventilators use a device called an injector (or Venturi mechanism) to increase the flow of driving gas. An injector is shown in Figure 10.2. As the gas flow meets a restriction, its lateral pressure drops (Bernoulli principle). When the lateral pressure drops below atmospheric, air will be entrained. The end result is an increase in the total gas flow leaving the outlet of the injector, but no increase in consumption of driving gas.

CONTROLS

The ventilator controls regulate the flow, volume, timing, and pressure of the driving gas that compresses the bellows. This is done indirectly via the pneumatic circuitry (see Fig. 10.1). Ventilator controls may be pneumatic, fluidic, or electronic.

Pneumatic

Pneumatic control uses pressure changes to initiate changes in the respiratory cycle.

Fluidic

Some modern anesthesia ventilators utilize fluidic logic, also known as fluidics. This technology uses moving streams of gas that flow through channels cut into a block of solid material to perform sensing, logic, am-

plification, and control functions. There are no electronics (and, therefore, no problems with electrical interference or static charges) and no moving parts (and, therefore, no wear). The latter feature, along with the ability to function in extremes of temperature and humidity, vibration, radiation, and electrical noise makes these systems highly reliable. They require little maintenance. Fluidic circuits are modular, easy to maintain, and because they are generally made of materials that are practically inert, can be autoclaved (3). Fluidic controls allow for a compact ventilator. Disadvantages of fluidic devices include sensitivity to dirt and consumption of a large amount of driving gas.

Electronic

Newer ventilators have a wider variety of controls and alarms than older ones. Such complexity requires use of computer chips and electronic controls. This type of ventilator requires electrical power as well as a source of driving gas. If there is an electrical power failure, it must be operated on batteries.

ALARMS

The ventilator standard (2) groups alarms into three categories: high, medium, and low priority, depending on whether the condition requires immediate action, prompt action, or operator awareness but not necessarily action.

The only alarm required by the standard is for loss of main power supply, and this is designated a high-priority alarm. The alarm must have a duration of at least 2 min and a means of silencing it following disconnection from the main power supply must be provided. If an alarm is provided to indicate loss of main power with backup power functioning, it shall be assigned to the low-priority category.

Most ventilators have other alarms. These will be mentioned when individual ventilators are discussed. The reader is also referred to the section on airway pressure alarms in Chapter 17.

SAFETY-RELIEF VALVE

The safety-relief valve is also called the pressure-limiting valve, maximum limited pressure mechanism, and driving gas pressure relief valve. A pressure-limiting valve is built into every ventilator to vent driving gas when a certain pressure is reached. On some ventilators this is preset (usually 65 to 80 cm H_2O); on others, the pressure is adjustable. Appropriate excessive pressure relief is difficult to define. Patients with high airway resistance or low compliance may require peak pressures well in excess of 60 cm H_2O, whereas those pressures may cause serious injuries with other patients. An adjustable safety-relief valve carries the hazard of operator error, whereas a factory-adjusted valve will prevent use of high peak pressures during artificial ventilation.

There are two types (4): The first is a spring-loaded valve assembly. When the pressure exceeds the closing force of the spring, the disc lifts and excess pressure is vented to atmosphere. During this time, the lungs are held inflated at the set pressure until the cycling mechanism terminates the inspiratory phase.

The second type has a diaphragm and two electrical contacts suspended by rigid metal strips. With this type, once the pressure-limiting device is activated, the inspiratory phase time is immediately terminated.

BELLOWS ASSEMBLY

The bellows assembly may be attached to the rest of the ventilator or separate from it. It consists of two parts: the bellows and its housing.

Bellows

The bellows (concertina bellows) is an accordian-like device that is attached either at the top or bottom of the bellows assembly. There are two types of bellows, distinguished by their motion during exhalation: ascending (standing, upright) and descending (hanging, inverted).

With a descending bellows (Fig. 10.3), the bellows is attached at its top and is compressed upward during inspiration. Inside

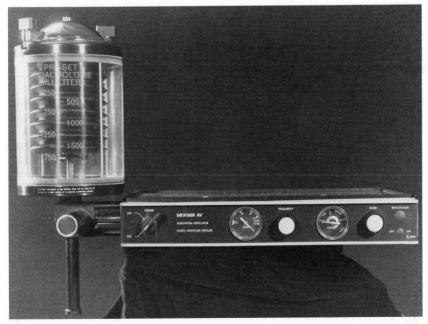

Figure 10.3. Drager AV ventilator. This model has a hanging bellows. The controls and gauges are on the front of the anesthesia machine, below the shelf. The alarms, not shown here, are to the left of the flowmeters on the anesthesia machine. Courtesy of North American Drager.

the dependent portion of the bellows is a weight that facilitates reexpansion downward during exhalation. As the weight descends, it is possible for negative pressure to be developed in the bellows and breathing system. Tidal volume is controlled by limiting the excursion of the bellows on filling. One method is to use a chain inside the bellows. When the control at the top of the bellows is turned, the length of the chain is altered. Another means is to have an adjustable footplate that contacts the lower end of the bellows and limits its excursion.

With an ascending bellows, the bellows is attached at the base of the assembly and the bellows is compressed downward during inspiration. During exhalation, the bellows expands upward. This results in a slight positive end expiratory pressure. Tidal volume may be regulated by adjusting the inspiratory time and flow or by a footplate that limits upward excursion of the bellows.

An important difference between the two types of bellows is that when there is a disconnection or major leak, the ascending bellows will usually collapse unless this is prevented by the scavenger system (5). When a disconnection occurs with a descending bellows ventilator, the ventilator will continue its upward and downward movements, drawing in room air and driving gas during its descent and discharging it during the upward movement. Gas flow during the upward movement may generate sufficient pressure that the low airway pressure alarm is not activated.

With an ascending bellows, the pressure in the bellows is always positive. PEEP of 2 to 4 cm H_2O will be exerted on the breathing system (6). With a descending bellows, the weight of the bellows results in a negative airway pressure during exhalation until the bellows has refilled.

Housing

The bellows is surrounded by a clear plastic cylinder that allows the bellows's movement to be observed. A scale on the side of the housing provides a rough approximation of the tidal volume being delivered. The housing is also called the canister and bellows chamber or cylinder.

EXHAUST VALVE

The exhaust valve (also referred to as the exhalation valve, patient system relief valve, ventilator relief valve, and compressed gas exhaust) communicates with the bellows housing. It is closed during inspiration. During expiration, it opens to allow driving gas inside the housing to be exhausted to atmosphere.

SPILL VALVE

The spill valve has been given many names, including the following: vent valve; dump valve; overflow valve; expired gas outlet; expiratory valve or port; safety dump valve; pop-off valve; relief valve; flapper valve; pressure relief valve; overspill valve; gas evacuation outlet valve; exhaust gas valve; gas evacuation or evacuator valve; and expiratory pressure relief valve.

Because the APL valve in the breathing system is either closed or isolated during ventilator operation, each ventilator must contain a spill valve for venting excess gases into the scavenging system. It is usually located within the bellows. During inspiration, this valve closes. During expiration it remains closed until the bellows is fully expanded. Then it opens to vent excess breathing system gases.

With an ascending bellows design the spill valve has a minimum opening pressure of 2 to 4 cm H_2O (7). This enables the bellows to fill during exhalation. This amount of PEEP is applied to the breathing system.

The scavenging transfer means connects the exhalation port of the spill valve to the scavenging system interface. Its connections must be either 19 or 30 mm.

CONNECTION FOR VENTILATOR HOSE

The ventilator standard requires that the fitting for the tubing that connects the ventilator to the breathing system be a standard 22-mm male conical fitting. A filter may be used on the tubing to lessen the transmission of pathogens.

Control of Parameters of Ventilation

TIDAL VOLUME

Most anesthesia ventilators are designed so that tidal volume is set directly. On others, tidal volume is determined indirectly by setting minute volume and respiratory rate. The minute volume divided by the respiratory rate gives the tidal volume. With time-cycled ventilators, tidal volume is set indirectly by varying the inspiratory time and flow.

Tidal volume is controlled by limiting the excursion of the bellows in its housing. The tidal volume control may be separate from other controls and part of the bellows assembly.

MINUTE VOLUME

Minute volume may either be set directly or determined indirectly by the product of tidal volume and respiratory rate. The ventilator standard requires that delivered volumes of the ventilator be indicated to the operator and must be accurate to ± 15%.

FREQUENCY (RATE) CONTROL

Frequency may be controlled directly or indirectly. Indirect control is achieved by varying the inspiratory time and expiratory pause. The ventilator standard requires that calibrated devices controlling frequency be accurate to within one breath per minute or 10% of set value, whichever is smaller.

I:E RATIO

The I:E ratio can be varied directly on some ventilators. On others, it is fixed and cannot be varied. On still others, it is determined indirectly by the settings of other controls.

It is essential that there be sufficient inspiratory time for the desired tidal volume to be delivered and sufficient expiratory time to allow full expiration. Insufficient inspiratory time may be indicated by a bellows that does not make a full excursion or a respirometer that indicates a less-than-expected tidal volume. Insufficient expiratory time may be indicated by a bellows that does not expand fully.

INSPIRATORY FLOW RATE

On some anesthesia ventilators, inspiratory flow rate is set directly. On others, it is determined indirectly by setting the minute volume, respiratory rate, and I:E ratio.

If the inspiratory flow is too low to provide the set tidal volume, the bellows will not complete its excursion. If the flow is set at a faster rate than is needed to provide the tidal volume, there will be an inspiratory pause time.

MAXIMUM WORKING PRESSURE CONTROL

The maximum working pressure control (pressure limit controller or inspiratory pressure limit) limits the highest pressure that can be attained during the inspiratory phase when the ventilator is functioning normally. It may limit the tidal volume.

Specific Ventilators

DRAGER AV ANESTHESIA VENTILATOR

Introduction

Controls

The Drager AV is fluidic with an on-off switch.

Ventilatory Rate

The ventilatory rate is 6 to 18 or 10 to 30 breaths/min. Higher rates may be obtained with settings beyond the maximum calibration mark on the dial.

Tidal Volume

The tidal volume is 250 to 1750 ml. A pediatric bellows is available for smaller tidal volumes

Inspiratory Flow Rate

Alarms

Low-Pressure (Apnea) Alarm. The low-pressure alarm is activated if a pressure greater or equal to the preset threshold (7.5, 12.5, or 25 cm H_2O) is not sensed within 15 sec.

Subatmospheric-Pressure Alarm. The subatmospheric-pressure alarm is activated if a pressure of less than or equal to -10 cm H_2O is sensed.

Continuing-Pressure Alarm. The continuing-pressure alarm is activated if a pressure equal to or greater than 15 cm H_2O is sensed for more than 10 sec.

High-Pressure Alarm. The high-pressure alarm is activated if a pressure above 60 cm H_2O is sensed.

The audio portion of the subatmospheric pressure and high pressure alarms can be disabled. A delay of 30 sec can be put on the audio portion of the low-pressure and continuing-pressure alarms.

Safety Features

The maximum pressure is limited to 60 cm H_2O when the inspiratory flow is in the low area; to 90 cm H_2O, in the medium area; and to 120 cm H_2O, in the high area. When the limit is reached, inflation pressure is held constant for the preset time before the exhalation phase begins.

Description

The Drager AV ventilator is shown in Figure 10.3. The controls are incorporated into the anesthesia machine. A few ventilators were sold separate from anesthesia machines. At the left is the on-off switch. The dial at the middle is the frequency (respiratory rate) control. The frequency gauge is to its left. To the right are the flow control valve and gauge. The gauge is divided into three sections labeled *low* (green), *medium* (yellow), and *high* (orange).

The bellows assembly is to the left of the controls. It has a chrome-plated dome. A volume scale is on the side of the housing. The bellows may be either hanging or upright. A footplate limits the bellows ascent or descent. The position of the footplate is controlled by turning a knob immediately below the bellows assembly. A self-locking mechanism prevents inadvertent movement of the knob. The alarms are to the left of the flowmeters on the anesthesia machine.

Internal Construction

A diagram of the ventilator is shown in Figure 10.4. When the on/off switch is in the on position, driving gas is supplied to two adjustable pressure regulators: the frequency regulator and the flow regulator. The frequency regulator, whose setting is determined by the frequency control, adjusts the input pressure to the pneumatic timer. A pilot line connects the timer to the manifold (on/off) valve. This valve, which consists of a piston operating against a spring, opens and closes with a frequency determined by the timer. The ratio of open time to closed time is always 1:2. The flow pressure regulator controls the pressure of driving gas delivered to the manifold valve. The pressure adjusted at this regulator is displayed on the flow control gauge on the front of the machine.

During inspiration, driving gas flows through the open manifold valve to the injector and into the bellows housing. This causes the bellows to be compressed. The chamber relief (exhaust) valve, which is parallel to the injector and consists of a piston operating against a spring, is held closed. Changing the setting of the flow regulator results in alteration of both flow rate into the housing and the maximum pressure in it. A pilot line connects the housing with the spill valve. As long as the pressure in the housing is greater than the pressure in the breathing system, this valve will be closed.

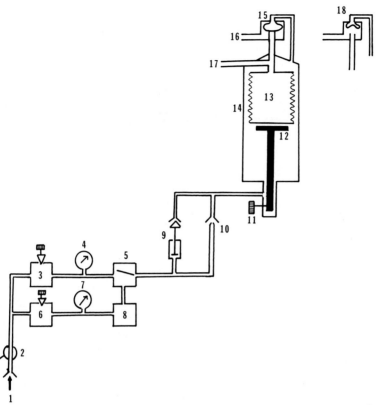

Figure 10.4. Internal construction of the Drager AV ventilator. *1,* driving gas; *2,* on-off switch; *3,* flow regulator and control; *4,* flow gauge; *5,* manifold (on-off) valve; *6,* frequency regulator and control; *7,* frequency gauge *8,* timer valve; *9,* chamber relief (exhaust) valve; *10,* injector; *11,* tidal volume control; *12,* tidal volume adjustment plate; *13,* bellows; *14,* bellows housing; *15,* spill valve; *16,* to scavenging system; *17,* to breathing system; *18,* spill valve open at end expiration. Redrawn from a diagram furnished by North American Drager.

After all the gas contained in the bellows has been discharged into the ventilator hose, the pressure in the housing rises until it reaches a value that causes the injector to cut off the flow of driving gas to the bellows housing and discharge it to atmosphere via the intake opening of the injector.

After a time determined by the setting of the frequency control, the timer closes the manifold valve and the flow of gas to the injector stops. The pressure on the chamber relief valve falls and it opens, so that driving gas flows from the bellows housing to atmosphere. Exhaled gases flow through the ventilator hose into the bellows, which reexpands. During this time, the pressure in the housing remains higher than the pressure in the breathing system, so that the spill valve remains closed. When the bellows is fully expanded, the spill valve opens and excess gases are vented to the scavenging system.

After a time determined by the frequency control setting, the manifold valve is again opened by the timer and another inspiration begins.

Control of Ventilation

The ventilator is volume preset and time cycled. Tidal volume is adjusted by altering the position of the footplate in the bellows assembly. The inspiratory flow rate has only a secondary effect on tidal volume. If the flow rate is set too low, it may not provide the full tidal volume in the allotted time. Minute volume is the product of tidal volume and respiratory rate. The I:E ratio is fixed at 1:2, and the unit has a fixed inspiratory phase time. An increase in tidal volume will result in a lengthening of inspiratory flow time and a shortening of the inspiratory pause. An increase in frequency will result in shortening of the inspiratory pause time.

Hazards

Either air or oxygen must be provided at a pressure between 40 and 60 psig. A supply pressure below 40 psi but higher than 20 psi will reduce the maximum minute volume obtainable but will not affect the functioning of the ventilator. The use of air as a driving gas will reduce the frequency by approximately 10% from the setting of the frequency gauge.

If the bellows is of the hanging type, a negative pressure may be generated during the early part of the expiratory phase, especially if a low fresh gas flow is used.

DRAGER AV-E ANESTHESIA VENTILATOR

Introduction

Controls

The Drager AV-E ventilator is electronic with an on-off switch.

Tidal Volume

The tidal volume is 250 to 1750 ml for the hanging bellows type and 200 to 1600 ml for the upright bellows type. Smaller volumes are available with the use of pediatric bellows.

Frequency

The frequency is 0 to 99 breaths/min.

I:E Ratio

The I:E ratios are from 1:1 to 1:4.5 in 0.5 increments.

Inspiratory Flow Rate

The pediatric bellows attachment incorporates a fine flow control valve downstream of the regular flow control valve. This can be used to fine tune the inspiratory flow but cannot increase the inspiratory flow beyond that set on the ventilator.

Pressure Limit Controller

The pressure limit controller is available as an add-on accessory. This provides a means to limit the peak inspiratory pressure to a preselected value, which can be as low as 15 cm H_2O. When the preselected inspiratory pressure is reached, a valve opens and bleeds off some of the driving gas into the atmosphere for the remainder of the inspiratory phase time.

Alarms

Low-Pressure Alarm. The low-pressure alarm is activated if the chosen peak inspiratory pressure (8, 12.5, or 25 cm H_2O) is not sensed within 15 sec. On later models, the pressure is user adjustable with a default value of 12 cm H_2O. The on-off control can be set so that the alarm will not be activated unless the chosen peak pressure is not sensed within 60 sec.

Subatmospheric-Pressure Alarm. The subatmospheric-pressure alarm is activated if a pressure of less than -10 cm H_2O is sensed.

High-Pressure Alarm. The high-pressure alarm is activated if a pressure greater than 60 cm H_2O is sensed. On later models, the high-pressure alarm is adjustable from 30 to 70 cm H_2O, with a default value of 50 cm H_2O.

Continuing-Pressure Alarm. The continuing-pressure alarm is activated if a pressure greater than the low-pressure alarm setting is sensed for more than 15 sec.

PEEP Advisory. If PEEP is set at greater than 4 cm H_2O the PEEP advisory is activated.

Excessive PEEP Caution. If PEEP is set at greater than 25 cm H_2O, the excessive PEEP caution is activated.

Safety Features

Maximum pressure within the bellows can vary from 25 to 100 cm H_2O, depending

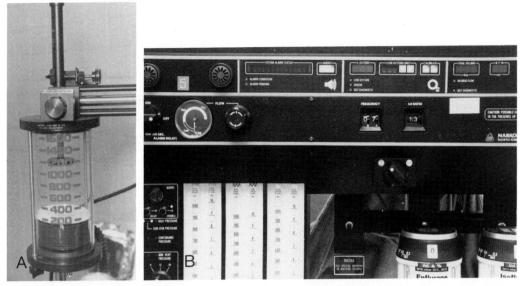

Figure 10.5. Drager AV-E ventilator **A,** Bellows assembly with upright bellows. Turning the knob at the top alters the position of the footplate and so limits the tidal volume. **B,** Ventilator controls and gauges. Note that the on-off switch has two on positions. Placing this switch in the six o'clock position results in a 60-sec delay in the low airway pressure alarm.

on the inspiratory flow setting. When the high-pressure alarm value is reached, the inflation pressure is held constant for the preset time before switching to the exhalation phase.

Special Feature

A PEEP (2 to 18 cm H_2O) valve is available.

Description

The Drager AV-E anesthesia ventilator is shown in Figure 10.5. The bellows may be upright or hanging. A volume scale is marked on the side of the bellows housing. A pediatric bellows is available. Control of tidal volume is by means of a self-locking knob immediately above or below the bellows assembly.

The controls are built into a shelf above the anesthesia machine. The on-off switch is to the left. On some models, this switch has two on positions: at the six and twelve o'clock positions. Placing it in the six o'clock position increases the time until the low-pressure alarm is activated to 60 sec. This al-

lows use of respiratory rates of less than 4/min.

The frequency (rate) control is a handwheel at the right on the control panel. The I:E ratio control is on the right. The flow control is located to the right of the on-off switch, and the flow rate indicated on an adjacent gauge. It is divided into low, medium, and high flow ranges.

Internal Construction

The internal construction of the Drager AV-E ventilator is shown in Figure 10.6. The primary electrical supply is a 120-V alternating current. The secondary supply is a 5-V direct current battery. Pneumatic power is by oxygen or air.

When the on-off switch is in the on position, electric power is supplied to the electronic control module and gas is supplied to the pneumatic portion of the ventilator. The gas switch supplies pressure to a transducer, which acts as an electronic on-off switch. A solenoid valve, which is controlled by the electronic circuits, delivers a pressure signal to the pneumatic control valve that opens

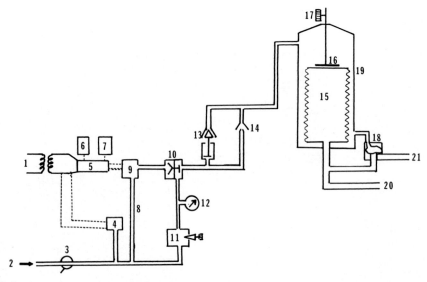

Figure 10.6. Internal construction of a Drager AV-E ventilator. *1,* electrical power supply; *2,* driving gas; *3,* on-off switch; *4,* transducer; *5,* electronic control module; *6,* I:E phase time ratio control; *7,* frequency control; *8,* pilot pressure line; *9,* solenoid valve; *10,* control valve; *11,* flow regulator; *12,* flow gauge; *13,* ventilator relief (exhaust) valve; *14,* injector; *15,* bellows; *16,* tidal volume adjustment plate; *17,* tidal volume adjustment control knob; *18,* spill valve; *19,* bellows housing; *20,* to breathing system; *21,* to scavenging system. Redrawn from a drawing furnished by North American Drager.

and closes with a frequency determined by the settings of the frequency and I:E ratio controls.

Driving gas passes through the flow regulator and on to the control valve. During inspiration, the solenoid valve opens the control valve and driving gas flows into the injector where it entrains ambient air and flows into the bellows housing, compressing the bellows. The flow regulator controls the pressure of gas delivered to the control valve, which is indicated on the flow gauge. While gas is flowing to the bellows housing, the relief (exhaust) valve is actuated and closed. The increased pressure within the housing closes the spill valve.

Exhalation begins when the solenoid valve causes the control valve to close. The exhaust valve opens and driving gas from the housing exits the bellows chamber and is vented to atmosphere through a muffler. The bellows expands until it is stopped by the footplate. The spill valve remains closed until the bellows is fully expanded. Further gas inflow causes the pressure inside the bellows to increase until the spill valve opens

and excess gases are vented into the scavenging system.

Control of Ventilation

The ventilator is time cycled. Tidal volume is dialed directly, and minute volume is the product of tidal volume and respiratory rate. An increase in flow rate with no change in tidal volume will result in an increase in the inspiratory pause time. An increase in the I:E ratio will result in a lengthening of the inspiratory pause time and a decrease in the expiratory phase time but will not affect the respiratory rate.

Hazards

Downward movement of the bellows in a hanging bellows ventilator may create a flow through a respirometer even with a total disconnection. The low airway pressure alarm may not sound.

A case has been described in which the muffler placed over the driving gas exhaust became saturated with water and obstructed the flow from the bellows chamber during expiration (8). This prevented exhalation, and high airway pressures resulted as gas continued to flow into the ventilator.

In another reported case, malfunction of the control valve resulted in the ventilator becoming stuck in the inspiratory mode (9). High airway pressures resulted as closure of the spill valve prevented venting of excess gas.

The delivered minute volume decreases with high resistance or low compliance (10,11).

There has been a report of the exhaust valve becoming incompetent, resulting in hypoventilation (12). In another reported case, the pilot line connecting the bellows chamber to the spill valve became kinked during inspiration so that the valve could not close (13). This caused a rapid increase in pressure in the breathing system. If the line became occluded during expiration, hypoventilation would result, because the spill valve would not close.

Prolongation of the inspiratory phase owing to insufficient lubrication of parts has been reported (14)

OHMEDA 7000 ANESTHESIA VENTILATOR

Introduction

Control

The Ohmeda 7000 ventilator is electronic with a power switch that turns the AC electrical power on or off.

Minute Volume

The minute volume is 2 to 30 liters/min for the adult bellows assembly and 2 to 12 liters/min for the pediatric bellows assembly.

Respiratory Rate

The respiratory rate is 6 to 40 breaths/min.

I:E Ratio

The I:E ratio is 1.1 to 1.3 for minute volumes from 2 to 15.5 liters/min. Above this range, the actual I:E ratio may be less than the dial setting.

Sigh

The sigh is 150% of tidal volume to a maximum of 1500 ml every 64 breaths.

Manual Cycle

There is a manual cycle that allows the operator to initiate an inspiration manually. The cycle can be activated only during the expiratory phase.

Alarms

Seven alarms plus a test button are provided. Six of the alarms are both visible and audible. The seventh, power failure, is audible only. In addition to the alarms, there is a lamp test. When it is pushed, all alarm lamps should light and all audible alarms sound.

1. Ventilator Failure Alarm. The ventilator failure alarm monitors the electronic circuitry of the ventilator. If a problem develops, the lamp will blink and the audible alarm will sound intermittently. The alarm will also be activated if a pressure exceeding 65 cm H_2O is sensed. Use of the ventilator must be discontinued when this alarm is actuated.

2. Set Volume Not Delivered Alarm. The set volume not delivered alarm is activated when the control settings require a tidal volume greater than 1500 ml or when a pressure over 65 cm H_2O is sensed. The light blinks and the audible alarm sounds intermittently. This alarm does not function when the pediatric bellows assembly is used.

3. Low Drive Gas (Oxygen) Supply Pressure Alarm. The low drive gas supply pressure alarm warns when the driving gas pressure is less than 40 psig. The lamp blinks and the audible alarm sounds. When this alarm is activated, ventilator use should be discontinued.

4. Low Airway Pressure Alarm. The low airway pressure alarm is triggered by inability to sense a pressure of at least 6 cm H_2O after two or three breathing cycles. The lamp blinks and the audible alarm sounds intermittently.

5. Actual I:E Less Than Dial Setting Alarm. The I:E alarm is activated when the control settings are adjusted to exceed the ventilator's operational limits. The lamp lights steadily and the audible alarm has a constant sound. The operator must change the settings to stop the alarm.

6. Vent Failure Alarm. The vent failure alarm activates all the alarm lamps as well as the audible alarm. This indicates a failure of the internal circuitry. Use of the ventilator must be discontinued.

7. Power Failure Alarm. The power failure alarm is activated if the power switch is turned to the on position but there is no electrical power. The alarm is audible only. It is powered by a battery that is automatically recharged when the ventilator is plugged in and the power switch is turned on.

All alarms except the ventilator failure alarm are self-canceling, which means that correction of the abnormal condition will cancel the alarm. No alarm can be turned off manually.

On earlier models only five alarms were provided: ventilator failure, set volume not delivered; set parameters out of range (or actual I:E less than dial settings); low oxygen supply pressure; and low airway pressure.

Safety Features

Pressure in the bellows housing is limited to 65 cm H_2O. When this pressure is sensed, some of the driving gas is vented. The maximal tidal volume is 1500 ml for the adult bellows and 300 ml for the pediatric bellows. Inspiratory flow limited to a maximum of 62 liters/min.

The ventilator will stop cycling if a pressure of 65 cm H_2O is sensed. The vent failure alarm will be activated and the ventilator must be turned off, then on again.

Description

The Ohmeda 7000 ventilator is shown with both adult and pediatric bellows assemblies in Figure 10.7. It consists of two parts: the bellows assembly and the control module. They may be attached to each other with the bellows assembly mounted on top or sep-

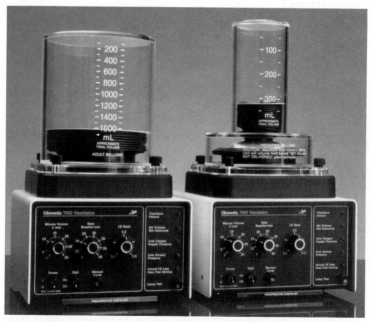

Figure 10.7. Ohmeda 7000 ventilators. The stand-alone ventilator is shown with both adult **(left)** and pediatric **(right)**bellows. Courtesy of Ohmeda, a division of BOC Health Care, Inc.

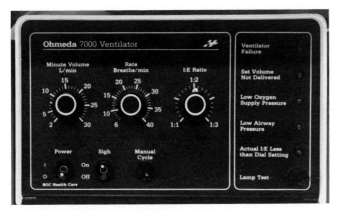

Figure 10.8. Control module of the Ohmeda 7000 ventilator.

arate and connected by flexible hoses. The bellows assembly may be mounted behind a carbon dioxide absorber assembly.

The bellows is of the standing variety. The housing is clear plastic and has a volume scale marked on the front.

The control module (Fig. 10.8) contains the controls and monitoring and alarm functions. The power and sigh controls have toggle switches, whereas the manual cycle has a push button. Each of the three control dials has a linear scale. The alarms are arranged vertically to the right of the control panel. The lamp test button is located below the alarms. An abbreviated preoperative checklist, which can be pulled out, is situated just below the front of the control module.

Internal Construction

The internal construction of this ventilator is shown in Figure 10.9. Driving gas (oxygen) at 50 psig enters the ventilator and passes through a filter enroute to the pressure regulator. Here the pressure is reduced to 38 psig at a flow of 24 liters/min. From here, the gas flows to five solenoid flow control valves.

During inspiration, the electronically controlled solenoid valves direct gas flow through orifices calibrated for flows of 2, 4, 8, 16, and 32 liters/min. The range of flow is from 4 to 62 liters/min in steps of 2 liters/min. The exhaust valve closes during inspiration so that the flow from the selected valves is delivered into the space between the

housing and the bellows. This compresses the bellows. A safety-relief valve limits the pressure in the bellows housing to approximately 65 cm H_2O.

At the end of inspiration, the solenoid valves close and the exhaust valve opens. Gas from the breathing system enters the bellows. As the bellows expands, driving gas from the housing is discharged through the exhaust valve to atmosphere. When the bellows is fully expanded, the spill valve opens and vents excess gas to the scavenging system. The opening pressure of the spill valve is approximately 2.5 cm H_2O.

The pressure of the driving gas upstream of the pressure regulator is monitored. If a pressure of less than 40 psig is sensed, the low supply pressure switch sends a signal to the control circuitry and the low oxygen supply pressure alarm is actuated. Pressure in the breathing system is also monitored. If a pressure of at least 6 cm H_2O is not sensed after three consecutive cycles, a signal is sent to the control circuitry and the low airway pressure alarm is activated.

Control of Ventilation

The three controls (minute volume, respiratory rate, and I:E ratio) are noninteractive. If the minute volume is increased and the ventilatory rate held constant, the tidal volume will increase. If the rate is increased and the minute volume is held constant, the tidal volume will decrease. Changes in the

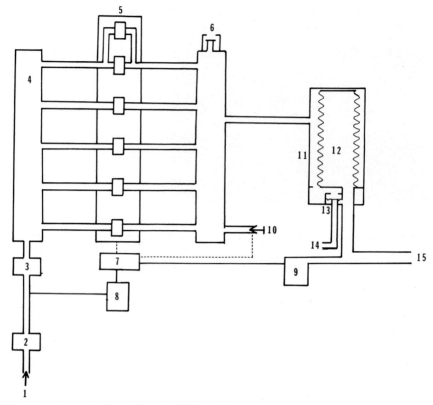

Figure 10.9. Internal construction of Ohmeda 7000 ventilator. *1,* driving gas; *2,* filter; *3,* pressure regulator; *4,* regulated gas supply; *5,* solenoid flow valves; *6,* safety-relief valve; *7,* control circuitry; *8,* low supply pressure switch; *9,* pressure switch; *10,*exhaust valve; *11,* bellows housing; *12,* bellows; *13,* spill valve; *14,* to scavenging system; *15,* to breathing system.

I:E ratio have no effect on tidal volume, minute volume, or frequency.

Hazards

The ventilator is designed to be powered by oxygen only. Use of any other gas will cause inaccurate operation and may damage the ventilator. Low driving gas pressure will cause the ventilator to deliver less than the set minute volume.

Because the low pressure alarm is not adjustable, it is possible that a disconnection could occur and an alarm not sound if there were high delivery circuit resistance and/or high inspiratory flow rates.

The delivered minute volume decreases with high resistance or low compliance

(10,11). The sigh control may inadvertently be left in the on position (15).

OHMEDA 7800 SERIES ANESTHESIA VENTILATORS

The Ohmeda 7800 may be a stand-alone ventilator or an accessory to the Excel anesthesia machine or can be fitted to a Modulus II machine. The 7810 is integrated into the Modulus II Plus machine, and the 7850 is integrated into the Modulus CD machine. On the 7810 and 7850 ventilators, the control module and bellows assembly are separate from each other; the control module is above the flowmeters on the machine and the bellows assembly is mounted on the absorber arm (Fig. 10.10) or to the left of the machine.

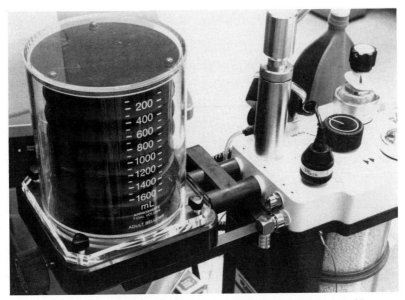

Figure 10.10. Ohmeda 7800 ventilator mounted on absorber assembly.

With the 7850, the ventilator's liquid crystal screen is blank unless one of the controls is altered or pressed. If the display pod is not functional, certain information will be displayed on the ventilator's liquid crystal screen.

Introduction

Controls

The Ohmeda 7800 is electronic with an on-off switch.

Tidal Volume

Tidal volume is 50 to 1500 ml. As the dial is turned, the tidal volume is displayed. The tidal volume setting can be checked without changing the volume by depressing the tidal volume dial.

Respiratory Rate

The respiratory rate is 2 to 100 breaths/min. The rate is displayed when the dial is turned or depressed.

Inspiratory Flow

The inspiratory flow is 10 to 100 liters/min. Touching or adjusting the inspiratory flow dial will cause the I:E ratio to be displayed.

Inspiratory Pressure Limit

The inspiratory pressure limit is 20 to 100 cm H_2O. Both the maximum inspiratory pressure and sustained pressure alarm limits are set using this dial. For inspiratory pressure limits from 20 to 60 cm H_2O, the ventilator sets the sustained pressure limit at one-half the inspiratory pressure limit. Any inspiratory pressure limit setting higher than 60 cm H_2O results in a sustained pressure limit of 30 cm H_2O. As the dial is turned, the maximum pressure limit and sustained pressure limit settings are displayed. To see the pressure limit displayed, the inspiratory pressure limit dial must be pressed and turned. Both the inspiratory limit and the sustained pressure limit will be displayed. The maximum inspiratory pressure limit is active during both mechanical and manual ventilation.

Inspiratory Pause

An inspiratory pause that is 25% of the set inspiratory time can be added to the inspiratory cycle. The expiratory time is decreased by the same amount. The I:E ratio is also changed, and the new value is displayed.

Alarms

Vent Set Error Alarm. The vent set error alarm is activated if the controls are set at a level that the ventilator cannot deliver.

High-Pressure Alarm. The high-pressure alarm is activated if the pressure set on the inspiratory pressure limit is exceeded. This is active during mechanical or manual ventilation.

Low-Pressure Alarm. The low-pressure alarm is activated if the airway pressure fails to change for at least 20 sec by a value that varies with the setting of the inspiratory flow control. The pressure change required to prevent triggering of the alarm will vary from 4

to 9 cm H_2O. This alarm is active only when mechanical ventilation is being used.

An alarm silence button is present on the 7800 and 7810 ventilators and on the display pod on the 7850 ventilator. When pressed, the audible alarm is silenced for 30 sec. Above the alarm silence button on the 7800 and 7810 are red and yellow light-emitting diodes that indicate the status of alarms. When an alarm condition occurs, a message will appear on the screen, a tone will sound, and an LED will flash. Once the alarm silence button is pressed, the ventilator will light the LED continuously.

Safety Features

If the high inspiratory pressure limit is reached, the ventilator terminates the inspi-

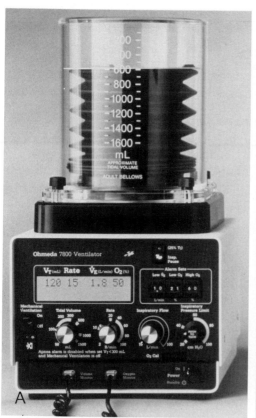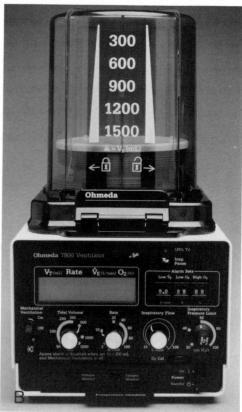

Figure 10.11. Ohmeda 7800 ventilators. **B,** This model has an autoclavable bellows assembly. Courtesy of Ohmeda, a division of BOC Health Care, Inc.

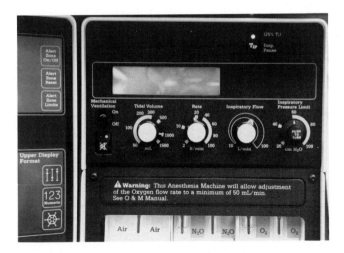

Figure 10.12. Control module of the Ohmeda 7850 ventilator. Courtesy of Ohmeda, a division of BOC Health Care, Inc.

ratory cycle. The ventilator displays a reminder if the inspired pressure is set above 60 cm H_2O, even if the ventilator is not turned on.

Description

The control module front panel of the 7800 and 7850 ventilators are shown in Figures 10.11 and 10.12. The control panel has a liquid crystal display that provides numeric readouts for tidal volume, respiratory rate, minute volume, and I:E ratio. The on-off control is a toggle switch. The tidal volume, respiratory rate, inspiratory flow, and inspiratory pressure limits have dial knobs and the inspiratory pause is a push button.

The alarm set points are determined with a series of setwheels on the front of the ventilator. In addition to set points for the oxygen concentration, there is a low exhaled volume alarm. To increase a value, the user pushes the button over the value that is to be changed, and to decrease a value the user depresses the button beneath the value. The ventilator will not accept oxygen set points below 18%. If the setwheels are set below this level, a *limit set error* message is displayed. There is a similar message if the high alarm limit is set equal to or below the low limit. The high oxygen alarm limit can be disabled by setting the alarm to zero.

Some alarms can be silenced for 30 sec and some permanently. Those that can be permanently silenced include power failure, oxygen sensor failure, low battery, ventilator failure, and oxygen calibration error. If the mechanical ventilation switch is off, the alarm silence button cancels and resets the apnea and low minute volume alarms and a *vol mon standby* message is displayed.

Two light-emitting diodes are part of the alarm system. When an alarm sounds, an LED flashes in addition to the message on the screen and the sound. If the alarm silence is activated, the LED is lighted continuously to remind the user that the alarm condition still exists. The red LED indicates that immediate operator response is required. The yellow LED indicates prompt operator response or awareness.

The control module contains the control dials and, in some versions, the alarms and set points. In addition, there is a pressure-sensing input for the low airway pressure alarm.

Internal Construction

Control Module

The internal parts of the ventilator control module are shown diagrammatically in Figure 10.13. When the ventilator is turned on, the gas inlet solenoid is energized, allowing the gas inlet valve to open and supplying

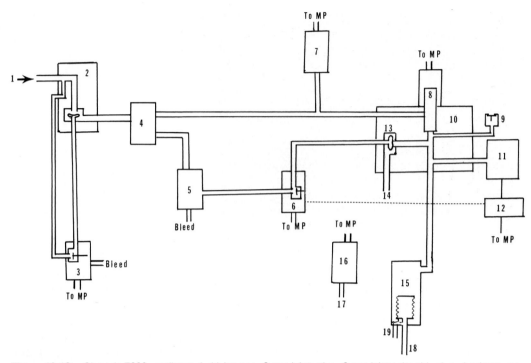

Figure 10.13. Ohmeda 7800 ventilator. *1,* driving gas; *2,* gas inlet valve; *3,* gas inlet solenoid valve; *4,* primary regulator; *5,* secondary regulator; *6,* exhalation solenoid valve; *7,* high-pressure transducer; *8,* flow control valve; *9,* air inlet valve; *10,* pneumatic manifold; *11,* high-pressure safety switch; *12,* relay; *13,* exhaust valve; *14,* exhaust port for driving gas; *15,* bellows assembly; *16,* low-pressure transducer; *17,* to breathing system for pressure monitoring; *18,* to breathing system; *19,* to scavenging system; *MP,* microprocessor. *Bleed,* used to reduce the pressure in a component.

driving gas to the primary regulator. The output of the primary regulator is monitored by the high-pressure transducer. If the driving gas pressure is greater than or equal to 30 psig, the microprocessor will not allow ventilation and an error message is displayed. The primary regulator connects directly to the pneumatic manifold. The driving gas flow is controlled by a flow control valve inside the pneumatic manifold. The flow control valve varies an orifice in proportion to the current supplied to the valve, producing a controlled flow rate. The amount of current supplied to the flow control and the time it is applied are determined by the microprocessor, based on the control settings.

Just before inspiration begins, the exhaust valve is supplied with pressure from the secondary regulator through the exhalation so-

lenoid, closing the valve. This valve remains closed during the inspiration phase when driving gas is being delivered into the bellows housing. It opens at the end of the inspiratory phase to provide an outlet for the driving gas that is being displaced from the bellows housing during expiration.

After the inspiratory phase time is ended, the flow control valve deenergizes and is returned to the closed position by its internal spring. Simultaneously, the exhalation solenoid is deenergized. This allows the exhaust valve to open and exhaust to atmosphere through the exhaust port. When the expiratory phase time is completed, the cycle is repeated by energizing the exhalation solenoid (closing the exhaust valve) and opening the flow control valve to begin the next inspiratory cycle.

If the patient is breathing spontaneously while connected to the ventilator, the air inlet valve in the pneumatic manifold will open.

Control of Ventilation

After the tidal volume and respiratory rate have been set, the inspiratory flow control can be used to set the desired I:E ratio. The I:E ratio will be changed whenever the inspiratory flow, tidal volume, or respiratory rate is altered or when the inspiratory pause is activated. The I:E ratio can be varied from 1:0.5 to 1:999.

Hazards

Electromagnetic interference or power line disturbances may cause the ventilator to stop ventilating, the monitoring functions to cease, or unintelligible messages to be displayed (16). If any of these problems occurs, manual ventilation should be instituted and the on-off switch on the front control panel of the anesthesia machine should be turned off for approximately 5 sec.

General Hazards

HYPOVENTILATION

Ventilator Dysfunction

Most anesthesia ventilators perform reliably for long periods of time. Nevertheless, one can and occasionally will fail to perform properly. Some problems may be insidious and result in less than total failure. Accuracy of any of the controls on a ventilator can result in inadequate ventilation.

Malfunction may not be readily apparent. A false sense of security may be generated by the constant noise the ventilator makes.

Cycling Failure

Causes of cycling failure include disconnection from or failure of the power source and an internal mechanical dysfunction (17–19)

Inadequate Design

Some anesthesia ventilators are not capable of delivering adequate volumes to patients with high airway resistance and/or poor compliance (10,20).

Leak of Driving Gas

If the bellows housing is not tightly secured, driving gas can leak, causing a reduction in the tidal volume (21,22). The housing may hit ceiling columns or other objects as the ventilator is moved. Operating room personnel may attempt to move a ventilator by grabbing the housing. These maneuvers may loosen the housing or cause it to break.

Loss of Breathing System Gas

Because most anesthesia ventilators are either volume or time cycled they have no means of compensating for loss of gas in the breathing system. This can be an insidious problem.

A ventilator may cycle but fail to occlude the exit port of the spill valve, thereby blowing part or all of the tidal volume into the scavenging system (12,13,17,23,24). Other reported sites of leaks are the spirometer box (25), the pole connecting the ventilator to the ventilator hose (26), and connections within the ventilator (27). The operator may fail to connect the ventilator hose to the breathing system. A leak, disconnection, or open APL valve in the breathing system can cause loss of gas.

If there is loss of breathing system gas and an ascending bellows ventilator is in use, the bellows may not return to its fully expanded position. This will usually be obvious (28). However, it should be noted that with the introduction of scavenging systems the bellows may stay expanded if there is a disconnection (5). There may be a change in the sound of the ventilator, although some of the newer ventilators are so quiet that this may not be apparent.

A descending bellows ventilator may appear to function normally in the face of loss of breathing system gas. Upward movement of the bellows may generate sufficient pressure to fool a low airway pressure alarm and/or a respirometer.

Incorrect Settings

In a crowded anesthetizing area, ventilator switches or dials may be inadvertently changed as personnel move about (29). An operator may fail to adjust respiratory rate and/or volumes with a new case, as when an adult follows a pediatric case. For ventilators that provide a control for setting the peak inspiratory pressure, setting that pressure too low may result in an inadequate tidal volume being delivered.

Ventilator Turned Off

There are times during administration of anesthesia when the ventilator must be turned off, such as during radiologic procedures for which movement would compromise the quality of the picture. The operator may forget to turn it back on.

Some on-off ventilator switches can be placed in an intermediate position. The potential exists for reverting to the off position with only a slight impact (30).

On most older ventilators, shutting the ventilator off also turned off the built-in alarms. Newer anesthesia machines have alarms that are activated if a minimal pressure, volume, or CO_2 concentration is not sensed within a preset time period after the ventilator is turned off. These alarms must be turned off separately from the ventilator.

Obstruction to Flow

As pointed out in Chapter 12, occlusion to gas flow to the patient can occur in a variety of sites and because of a variety of mechanisms. One is failure to change the position of the bag-ventilator selector valve when converting to automatic ventilation. If the valve is left in the bag position, the ventilator will operate against a dead end.

With obstruction to flow, the excursion of the bellows will be reduced but not totally

eliminated. The pressure shown on the system pressure gauge will vary, depending on the locations of the obstruction and the gauge.

HYPERVENTILATION

With a hole in the bellows or a loose connection between the bellows and its base assembly, driving gas from the housing can enter the bellows, causing an unexpectedly high tidal volume (31,32). This can be accentuated by a high inspiratory flow rate (17).

HYPEROXIA

A hole or tear in the bellows with oxygen as the driving gas can result in an increase in the inspired oxygen concentration and a lower-then-expected anesthetic depth (32–37).

EXCESSIVE AIRWAY PRESSURE

Excessive airway pressure can develop very rapidly, especially if high fresh gas flows are being used. Quick action may be required to prevent damage to the patient.

Because the spill valve is closed during inspiration and the APL valve in the breathing system is closed or isolated, oxygen flushing during the inspiratory phase can result in barotrauma (6). A hole in the bellows or a loose connection between the bellows and its base may allow driving gas to enter the bellows, resulting in a higher-than-expected pressure during inspiration. If the spill valve becomes stuck in the closed position, the pressure in the breathing system will continue to rise as fresh gas flows into the system (13, 38–40). Excessive suction applied to the scavenging attachment can hold the spill valve closed (22,41).

In one reported case, a muffler designed to silence the exhaust of driving gas from the ventilator became saturated with water and prevented gas from exiting from the bellows housing (8). Malfunction of a control valve can result in the ventilator becoming stuck in the inspiratory position (42).

A properly set pressure relief valve on a

ventilator should reduce the risk of barotrauma but will not eliminate it (22). Some ventilators have adjustable high-pressure alarms. On others the alarms are preset. Such an alarm may give warning of a problem in time to prevent harm to the patient. If a ventilator does not have a high-pressure alarm, it is suggested that this be added to the breathing system.

When there is high airway pressure while a ventilator is in use, a disconnection at the tracheal tube should be made immediately. Taking time to find the source of the problem may result in damage to the patient. Manual ventilation should be instituted using the reservoir bag in the breathing system.

NEGATIVE PRESSURE DURING EXPIRATION

Negative pressure is considered undesirable under most circumstances because of adverse effects on pulmonary function and increased risk of air embolism. Ventilators with weighted hanging bellows can generate subatmospheric pressure during the early part of expiration if expiratory flow is not impeded (17). This will be accentuated if the fresh gas flow is low. Some ventilators are equipped with a control to supply negative pressure during expiration.

ALARM FAILURE

Low airway pressure alarms that do not depend on the bellows's collapsing may fail to alarm if there is failure of the cycling mechanism (43) or a negative pressure is transmitted from the scavenging system to the bellows housing (44). Although low-pressure alarms have significantly advanced patient safety, they can fail (45,46).

When the low airway pressure alarm threshold is adjustable, it should be set just below the peak inspiratory pressure. Cases have been reported where resistance (from tracheal tube connectors, Y pieces, bacterial filters, and other components or from the patient port of the breathing system being pressed against the patient or a pillow) cou-

pled with high inspiratory flow rates created sufficient back pressure to generate a false-positive signal at the sensing site when the threshold was set too low.

Use of a PEEP valve in the breathing system may cause a low-pressure alarm not to sound if the PEEP valve raises the pressure above the alarm threshold pressure.

Because of these problems, other means of monitoring ventilation such as capnometry, respirometry, observing chest movement and listening to breath sounds should be used to detect problems before harm can come to the patient.

Advantages

1. Use of a ventilator allows anesthesia personnel to devote time and energy to other tasks and eliminates the fatigue resulting from squeezing a bag (47). It may help reduce human error.
2. A ventilator produces more regular ventilation with respect to rate, rhythm, and tidal volume than manual ventilation.
3. Compared with critical care ventilators, anesthesia ventilators are relatively simple in design and have fewer controls.

Disadvantages

1. Probably the greatest disadvantage to the use of ventilators is the loss of contact between the anesthesiologist and the patient. The feel of the bag can reveal such things as disconnections, changes in resistance or compliance, continuous positive pressure, and spontaneous respiratory movements. With mechanical ventilation these may go undetected for a considerable period of time.
2. A ventilator may induce a false sense of security in the user if it continues to make the appropriate sounds even when it malfunctions.
3. Use of a ventilator adds one more piece

of equipment that can malfunction and requires servicing and maintenance.

4. Some ventilators are large and cumbersome.

5. Some older ventilators lack proper monitoring and alarm capabilities.

6. Most anesthesia ventilators do not include the newer modes of ventilation such as pressure support. Some cannot develop high enough inspiratory pressures or flows or PEEP to ventilate certain patients adequately (10,20). It may be necessary to take a critical care ventilator into the operating room to provide adequate ventilation for critically ill patients.

7. Components that are subject to contamination are not always easy to remove or clean. Disinfection and sterilizing procedures may take considerable time and effort.

8. Some ventilators lack user friendliness. There is often room for improvement in the design and grouping of controls.

9. Some ventilators are disturbingly noisy.

10. Some ventilators require relatively high flows of driving or fresh gas (48). Oxygen consumption increases with increased minute volume and with some ventilators, an increased I:E ratio.

REFERENCES

1. Schreiber P. Anaesthesia equipment: performance, classification and safety. Berlin: Springer-Verlag, 1979.
2. American Society for Testing and Materials. Standard specification for ventilators intended for use during anesthesia (ASTM F1101-90). Philadelphia: ASTM, 1990.
3. Smith RK. Respiratory care applications for fluidics. Respir Ther 1979;9:29–32.
4. Dupuis YG. Ventilators, theory and clinical application. St. Louis: CV Mosby, 1986.
5. Blackstock D. Advantages of standing bellows ventilators and low-flow techniques. Anesthesiology 1984;60:167.
6. Andrews JJ. Understanding anesthesia ventilators (ASA Refresher Course No. 242). Park Ridge, IL: ASA, 1990.
7. Eisenkraft JB. The anesthesia delivery system. Part II. Prog Anesth 1989;3:1–12.
8. Roth S, Tweedie E, Sommer RM. Excessive airway pressure due to a malfunctioning anesthesia ventilator. Anesthesiology 1986;65:532–534.
9. Sprung J, Samaan F, Hensler T, Atlee JL, Kampine JP. Excessive airway pressure due to ventilator control valve malfunction during anesthesia for open heart surgery. Anesthesiology 1990;73:1035–1038.
10. Marks JD, Schapera A, Kraemer RW, Katz JA. Pressure and flow limitations of anesthesia ventilators. Anesthesiology 1989;71:403–408.
11. Marks JD, Katz JA, Schapera, MB, Kraemer RW. Evaluation of a new operating room ventilator: the Ohmeda 7810. Anesthesiology 1989;71:A462.
12. Sommer RM, Bhalla GS, Jackson JM, Cohen MI. Hypoventilation caused by ventilator valve rupture. Anesth Analg 1988;67:999–1001.
13. Eisenkraft JB. Potential for barotrauma or hypoventilation with the Drager AV-E ventilator. J Clin Anesth 1989;1:452–456.
14. Anonymous. Anesthesia unit ventilators. Technol Anesth 1990;11:6.
15. Beahan PG. A hazardous sigh. Anaesth Intensive Care 1989;17:515.
16. Anonymous. Anesthesia unit ventilators. Technol Anesth 1992;13:8–9.
17. Wyant GM, CraigDB, Pietak SP, Henkins LC, Dunn AJ. A panel discussion: safety in the operating room. Can Anaesth Soc J 1984;31:287–301.
18. Sarnquist FH, Demas K. The silent ventilator. Anesth Analg 1982;61:713–714.
19. Gruneberg A. Ventilator hazard identified and rectified. Br Med J 1984;288:1763.
20. Pinchak AC, Hancock DE, Shepard LS. Limitations of anesthesia ventilators in severe lung injury. Anesthesiology 1986;65:A149.
21. Lee K. Leak of driving gas from Air-Shields ventilator. Can Anaesth Soc J 1986;33:263–264.
22. Feeley TW, Bancroft ML. Problems with mechanical ventilators. In: Rendell-Baker L, ed. Problems with anesthetic and respiratory therapy equipment [Special issue] Int Anes Clin 1982;20(3):83–93.
23. Choi JJ, Guida J, Wu W. Hypoventilatory hazard of an anesthetic scavenging device. Anesthesiology 1986;65:126–127.
24. Khalil SN, Gholston TK, Binderman J, Antosh S. Flapper valve malfunction in an Ohio closed scavenging system. Anesth Analg 1987;66:1334–1336.
25. Judkins KC, Sage M. Routine servicing of the Cape-Wane ventilator. Anaesthesia 1983;38:1102.
26. Rolbin S. An unusual cause of ventilator leak. Can Anaesth Soc J 1977;24:522–524.
27. Anonymous. Valves, positive end expiratory pressure. Technol Anesth 1991;11:7.
28. Graham DH. Advantages of standing bellows ven-

tiators and low-flow techniques. Anesthesiology 1983;58:486.

29. Wald A, Neidzwski TJ. Front panel cover for Frazer Harlake ventilator. Anesth Analg 1983;62:619–620.

30. Ciobanu M, Meyer JA. Ventilator hazard revealed. Anesthesiology 1980;52:186–187.

31. Waterman PW, Pautler S, Smith RB. Accidental ventilator-induced hyperventilation. Anesthesiology 1978;48:141.

32. Rigg D, Joseph M. Split ventilator bellows. Anaesth Intensive Care 1985;13:213.

33. Baraka A, Muallem M. Awareness during anaesthesia due to a ventilator malfunction. Anaesthesia 1979;34:678–679.

34. Longmuir J, Craig DB. Inadvertent increase in inspired oxygen concentration due to defect in ventilator bellows. Can Anaesth Soc J 1976;23:327–329.

35. Love JB. Missassembly of a Campbell ventilator causing leakage of the driving gas to a patient. Anaesth Intensive Care 1980;8:376–377.

36. Marsland AR, Solomos J. Ventilator malfunction detected by O_2 analyser. Anaesth Intensive Care 1981;9:395.

37. Ripp CH, Chapin JW. A bellow's leak in an Ohio anesthesia ventilator. Anesth Analg 1985;64:942.

38. Anonymous. Wrongful death suit dismissal overturned. Am Med News, November 13, 1981, p. 19.

39. Henzig D. Insidious PEEP from a defective ventilator gas evacuation outlet valve. Anesthesiology 1982;57:251–252.

40. Hilton PJ, Clement JA. Surgical emphysema resulting from a ventilator malfunction. Anaesthesia 1983;38:342–345.

41. Anonymous. Pre-use testing prevents "helpful" reconnection of anesthesia components. Technol Anesth 1987;8:1–2.

42. Murray AW, Easton JC. Another problem with an expiratory valve. Anaesthesia 1988;43:891–892.

43. Sarnquist FH, Demas K. The silent ventilator. Anesth Analg 1982;61:713–714.

44. Heard SO, Munson ES. Ventilator alarm nonfunction associated with a scavenging system for waste gases. Anesth Analg 1983;62:230–232.

45. Mazza N, Wald A. Failure of battery-operated alarms. Anesthesiology 1980;53:246–248.

46. Lahay WD. Defective pressure/flow alarm. Can Anaesth Soc J 1982;29:404–405.

47. Amaranath L, Boutros AR. Circle absorber and soda lime contamination. Anesth Analg 1980;59:711–712.

48. Raessler KL, Kretzman WE, Gravenstein N. Oxygen consumption by anesthesia ventilators. Anesthesiology 1988;69:A271.

Chapter 11

Controlling Trace Gas Levels

In the past, the usual practice was to discharge excess anesthetic gases and vapors directly into room air. As a consequence, operating room personnel were exposed to low concentrations of these drugs. Such exposure resulted in the presence of these substances in every medium available for study, ranging from expired gas to breast milk (1), induction of drug-metabolizing enzymes, and increased biodegradation of the gases. For many decades operating room personnel worked in this environment without regard for any detrimental effects that might result from such exposure. In recent times, however, questions have been raised about possible hazards from exposure to trace amounts of anesthetic gases and vapors. (Throughout the remainder of this chapter anesthetic gases and vapors will be referred to as *gases,* because most vapors behave as gases.)

A trace level of an anesthetic gas is a level far below that needed for clinical anesthesia or that can be detected by smell (2). Trace gas levels are usually expressed in parts per million (ppm), which is volume/volume (100% of a gas is 1,000,000 ppm; 1% is 10,000 ppm).

Reported trace gas concentrations found in the absence of control measures vary greatly, depending on the fresh gas flows in use, the ventilation system, the length of time that anesthesia has been administered, the measurement site, and other variables.

Nitrous Oxide. In unscavenged rooms levels up to 7000 ppm have been found (3–20). In postanesthesia care units levels from 15 to 1660 ppm have been found (8,10,13,14,21).

Halothane. Levels in operating rooms usually fall between 1 and 10 ppm, with many higher and lower values being reported (3–5,8,9,12–15,22–33) In postanesthesia care units, levels from 0 to 8.2 ppm have been found (8,13,14,34).

Enflurane. Levels in operating rooms from 5 to 46 ppm have been reported (35).

Data for newer agents are not available, because they were introduced into use after control measures had been widely instituted.

Methods of Study (36)

Despite many studies and much discussion, opinions differ on whether or not a problem exists and what levels should be allowed in the working environment. To better interpret the data it is first necessary to understand how they were gathered. Four basic methods of study have been used. All have major limitations and disadvantages.

ANIMAL INVESTIGATIONS

In animal studies, laboratory animals are exposed to varying levels of gases for varying periods of time and studied to determine effects. These studies must be interpreted warily. Large numbers of animals need to be studied to achieve statistical significance (37). It has been shown in animals that diet affects tumor susceptibility and stress affects reproductive abilities (37). Toxicity usually depends on both exposure time and concentration, and it is difficult to correlate exposure time in animals with that in humans, because the lifespans are so different. Finally, variations in drug effects among species create uncertainty about the relevance of these findings to humans.

HUMAN VOLUNTEER STUDIES

Human volunteers have been used to study the effects of trace gases on skilled performance, immune responses, and patterns of drug metabolism.

EPIDEMIOLOGICAL STUDIES OF EXPOSED HUMANS

A number of epidemiological studies of exposed personnel have been made. All have serious flaws. Most were retrospective and used questionnaires that were sent through the mail. They suffer from low response rates, inappropriate control groups, poor recollections and biases on the part of the respondents, poor wording, failure to include significant points in the questionnaires, and misinterpretations because of differences in education and experience on the part of the respondents (1,37–40). Interpretation of the data is hampered by a lack of agreement as to what level of significance to accept (37,41). Finally, the studies have not been designed to test the cause-and-effect relationship between trace gases and problems in exposed personnel. Some show increased risk for specific groups but not for other equally exposed groups (42). Others have shown problems in groups with and without exposure to trace gases, suggesting that the risk may be related to some other factor. Finally, many of the studies were performed before scavenging and other methods to control trace gas levels were implemented. Prospective studies are needed to determine whether there is a relationship between current levels of occupational exposure to anesthetic gases and adverse outcomes.

MORTALITY STUDIES

Studies on the causes of death and the age at which death occurred among anesthesiologists have provided interesting and valuable data, despite some questions about the appropriateness of the control group and rather small numbers.

Problems

SPONTANEOUS ABORTIONS

Epidemiological Studies

Several retrospective studies have shown higher rates of spontaneous abortion in operating room and dental operatory personnel than women in different environments (43–50). The validity of these studies has been questioned (37,40–42,51,52). One study found that residents specializing in anesthesia had a higher rate of spontaneous abortion than most other residents (53).

Other studies have failed to find significant increases in spontaneous abortions in exposed personnel (54–60). One study found that the frequency of miscarriages among nurses working in intensive care units was approximately equal to that of nurses in the operating room, suggesting that psychic and/or physical stress may be the causative factors (49).

If anesthetic gases caused spontaneous abortions, a higher rate of miscarriage would be expected in those with greatest exposure. Statistics show that the incidence of miscarriage among operating room staff is higher in the United States than in the United Kingdom, despite the fact that routine use of carbon dioxide absorption and low flow rates plus air-conditioning in the United States probably result in lower average atmospheric contamination than in the United Kingdom where high flow rates are commonplace and air-conditioning is less common.

In summary, while most of the epidemiological studies on spontaneous abortions are flawed and subject to reporting bias, there are some data to support the contention that there is a slightly increased risk of spontaneous abortions among women exposed to trace anesthetics (61).

Animal Studies

All inhalation anesthetics in current use when administered to pregnant animals at anesthetic or near-anesthetic concentrations for sufficient time can produce toxic effects in embryos. However, this does not infer that similar results will follow exposure to trace concentrations.

Isoflurane.   Investigations have found no evidence of increased spontaneous abortion in mice exposed to up to 10,500 ppm isoflurane (62,63).

Enflurane.   Several investigations failed to show any toxic effects to fetuses in animals exposed to concentrations as high as 16,500 ppm (63–66).

Halothane.   Investigations have shown no lethal effects to embryos from exposures of up to 8000 ppm (63,67,68).

Nitrous oxide.   One study found that prolonged exposure to 1000 ppm nitrous oxide caused fetal death and resorption, but no effect was seen when 500 ppm was used (69). A later study found that the threshold for fetal death was higher (between 1000 and 5000 ppm) with intermittent exposure (70).

Mixtures.   Investigations using mixtures of halothane and nitrous oxide found no effect with concentrations as high as 1,600 ppm halothane plus 100,000 ppm nitrous oxide (68). Nitrous oxide 500,000 ppm plus isoflurane 3500 ppm had no effect on spontaneous abortions (71).

In summary, with the possible exception of nitrous oxide, animal studies indicate that if a threshold concentration of inhalation anesthetics causing increased spontaneous abortions exists, it is 10 to 100 or even 1000 times that commonly found in operating rooms. A finding of some interest in one study (68) was that animals stressed by experimental handling had dramatically higher fetal losses.

SPONTANEOUS ABORTION IN SPOUSES

Although several studies have shown an increased spontaneous abortion rate in wives of exposed males (45,50,72,73), results from the majority of studies suggest there is no increase (40,43,47 60).

One study found no changes in sperm concentration or morphology in male anesthesiologists working in hospitals with scavenging equipment (74). Studies have failed to show any adverse effect on reproductive processes of male animals exposed to up to 5000 ppm enflurane (63,75) or 10 ppm halothane plus 500 ppm nitrous oxide (76).

INFERTILITY

Epidemiological Studies

Two studies noted higher-than-expected rates of involuntary infertility among exposed personnel (46,50). Interpretation of these data has been questioned (42). One study found no effect from paternal exposure (47), and no changes in sperm count or morphology have been found in male anesthesiologists working in scavenged operating rooms (74).

Animal Studies

Isoflurane. Exposure of female mice to up to 4,000 ppm isoflurane had no effect on fertility (62). Exposure of male mice to 10,000 ppm caused no increase in percentage of abnormal spermatozoa (77). No effect on fertility was seen in flies exposed to 160,000 ppm.

Enflurane. No effect on fertility in male or female mice was found from exposure to up to 5,000 ppm (64,75). One study did find an increase in abnormal spermatozoa in mice exposed to 12,000 ppm (77). No effect on fertility was seen in male or female flies exposed to as high as 160,000 ppm (78).

Halothane. Studies show no effect on male fertility with exposure of up to 160,000 ppm halothane (78–80). Exposure of male mice to 8,000 ppm halothane caused no increase in percentage of abnormal spermatozoa (77).

In studies on female fertility, one found a decrease in fertility in rats exposed to 3,000, but not 1,000, ppm halothane (79). Other studies found no effect from exposure to 14,000 ppm in rats (80) or 160,000 ppm in flies (78).

Nitrous Oxide. No changes in male fertility and no sperm abnormalities were found in mice after exposure to up to 800,000 ppm (77,81). However, prolonged exposure of male rats to 200,000 ppm resulted in abnormalities in spermatogenic cells (82). One study found that male rats mated after exposure to 5,000 ppm nitrous oxide produced significantly smaller liters (83). This was reversible with time. Exposure to up to 800,000 ppm caused no changes in fertility in male or female flies (78).

Mixtures. Decreased fertility was seen in female rats exposed to halothane 10 ppm plus nitrous oxide 500 ppm before mating (76). Male rats exposed to these concentrations showed greater frequency of chromosomal aberrations in spermatogenic cells, but the aberrations were probably too infrequent to cause decreased fertility (78).

Overall, these studies indicate that anesthetics have mild toxic effects on male germ cells that are unlikely to be associated with infertility (78).

BIRTH DEFECTS

Epidemiological Studies

Several studies in humans have found an increase in congenital abnormalities in children of exposed personnel (43,45,46,50, 54,57,59,73,84). Interpretations of the data have been questioned (37,41,42,84,85), and several investigators have suggested there is no increase in birth defects among the offspring of exposed parents (40,47–49,56,60).

No increase in chromosomal abnormalities in exposed nurses or changes in sperm morphology in male anesthesiologists working in operating rooms have been found (74,86).

Animal Studies

Isoflurane. Exposures to concentrations up to 10,500 failed to cause any significant teratogenic effect (71,63).

Enflurane. Studies have found no teratogenic effects of exposure to up to 16,500 ppm (63,64,87). However, one study found changes in spermatozoa after exposure to 12,000 ppm (77).

Halothane. Several investigations have found exposure of pregnant rats to concentrations of halothane of up to 8000 ppm produced no effects that could be expected to result in permanent abnormalities or decreased survival (63,66–68,88,89). Chronic exposure of rats to 10 and 12.5 ppm of halothane in utero has been shown to produce later deficits in learning (90,91). However, the interpretation of these data have been questioned (42).

Nitrous Oxide. Studies have shown no gross abnormalities in animals exposed to up to 750,000 ppm (63,69,81,92).

Mixtures. No major teratogenic effects were seen with exposure to halothane 10 ppm and nitrous oxide 500 ppm (76). Decreases in fetal weight and slight developmental retardation have been found with exposure to mixtures of as high as 100,000 ppm nitrous oxide and 1600 ppm halothane, but this was unaccompanied by evidence of gross abnormalities (68,76).

In summary, studies of laboratory animals show that concentrations of inhalation agents that produce gross malformations are well above those found in even unscavenged operating rooms. The question of learning deficits, however, deserves more study.

IMPAIRMENT OF SKILLED PERFORMANCE

Operating room personnel are subjected to many stimuli that require precise, rapid, and complicated responses. Because the patient's survival depends on the alertness and performance of the professional team, anything that interferes with its ability to perceive changes in signals and react quickly and appropriately may cause harm to a patient.

Studies that have tested operating room personnel exposed to trace gases have failed to demonstrate decreased performance in exposed personnel (26,93–96).

Although a few early studies found exposure of volunteers to trace concentrations of nitrous oxide, halothane, or enflurane caused significant decreases in performance (97–99) subsequent efforts by other researchers to duplicate their results have failed (100–104). These studies found that the concentrations needed to decrease performance were hundreds of times greater than the average

levels found in unscavenged operating rooms.

In laboratory tests, exposure of adult rats to 10 ppm halothane failed to affect learning (105).

In summary, the current balance of data suggests that trace gases in the operating room have no effect on performance (106).

CANCER

Epidemiological Studies

A large study found no increase in cancer in exposed males but indicated that females in the operating room were at higher risk for cancer than nonexposed females (43). The significance of these data has been questioned (41,42). Similar results have been reported for female dental operatory assistants (45). Two studies of dentists have shown that the incidence of cancer is not significantly different among those exposed and those not exposed to trace concentrations of anesthetics (45,73). A review of combined data from six studies found an increased cancer risk among women but not men (61).

It should be pointed out that the lag time for industrial carcinogens is 20 years. Thus, the carcinogenic effects of some of the halogenated agents, if any, may only be starting to become manifest.

Mortality Studies

There is no increased death rate from cancer in male anesthesiologists (107–110). The death rate from cancer among female anesthesiologists is high compared with male anesthesiologists and control groups (109), but the numbers are too small to permit any strong conclusions. Also, new therapeutic modalities have resulted in higher cancer cure rates, so that assessment of the incidence of cancer cannot be inferred using only mortality data.

Animal Studies

Halothane. Studies have found no evidence of increased carcinogenicity in animals exposed to up to 5000 ppm halothane (111,112).

Enflurane. Mice exposed to up to 10,000 ppm enflurane have been found to have no increased risk of neoplasms (112,113).

Isoflurane. One study found hepatic neoplasms in mice exposed during gestation and early life to 1000 to 5000 ppm isoflurane (35), but the validity of this study has been questioned and it appears that the increased incidence of liver tumors may have been the result of other factors. In later studies, no evidence of increased carcinogenicity could be found in animals exposed to up to 6000 ppm isoflurane (112,114)

Nitrous Oxide. No evidence of increased carcinogenicity in mice has been found with exposure to up to 800,000 ppm (115,112).

Mixtures. No increase in neoplasms has been found in rats exposed to 10 ppm halothane plus 500 ppm nitrous oxide (116).

Mutagenicity Testing

Testing for carcinogenicity requires large numbers of animals and a great expenditure of money and effort. A more rapid and inexpensive method is to look for an increase in mutagens in a bacterial system exposed to an inhalational anesthetic. One of the mechanisms by which environmental agents are thought to produce cancer involves mutation of DNA (117). Because the DNA of all organisms is chemically similar, a study of mutagenic effects in a simpler organism may predict carcinogenicity in humans.

Cytogenetic methods are used increasingly for monitoring exposure to potential mutagens in the environment. Examination of sister chromatid exchanges in peripheral lymphocytes has been used to study anesthetic agents.

Although mutagenicity tests have predictive value in detecting carcinogens, lack of mutagenicity does not exclude the possibility that an agent may be carcinogenic to chronically exposed operating room personnel. Furthermore, there is the possibility that an anesthetic agent could increase the carcinogenic effect of other chemical and physical factors.

Human Studies

One study did find increased mutagenic activity in the urine of anesthesiologists (118), but another study found no difference in mutagenic activity in the urine of individuals working in scavenged and unscavenged operating rooms (119). Also, the urines of individuals collected before and after beginning training in anesthesia had similar mutagenic activity.

Monitoring of sister chromatic exchanges in lymphocytes in operating room personnel have shown no evidence of a mutagenic effect (120–122). A study of operating room personnel in unscavenged rooms did find an increase in the percentage of chromosome aberrations and sister chromatid exchanges (123).

Animal Studies

Halothane. Several studies have found halothane and its metabolites not mutagenic (117,124–128). Others have found it and/or its metabolites weakly mutagenic (129–133).

Enflurane. Several investigations (124, 134,135) were unable to demonstrate mutagenic effects from enflurane.

Isoflurane. Several investigations (124, 126,135) have found isoflurane not to be mutagenic.

Nitrous Oxide. Investigations (124,136) have found nitrous oxide not to be mutagenic.

Mixtures. One investigation found that halothane plus nitrous oxide did not increase mutagenesis (127). Another found that nitrous oxide had no effect on the mutagenicity of halothane (129). The same study found no mutagenicity with mixtures of nitrous oxide and enflurane or isoflurane.

LIVER DISEASE

Epidemiological Studies

Studies have found that operating room personnel have higher-than-expected rates of hepatic disease (43,36,137). Interpretation of these data has been questioned (41). Similar results have been reported in male dentists (45,73) and female chair-side assistants (45). Analysis of the data suggests that there is an increased risk of developing liver disease, especially among men (61).

Anesthesia personnel working in unscavenged operating rooms have been found to have normal levels of hepatic enzymes (138).

Recurrent hepatitis on exposure to halothane has been demonstrated in a few individuals (139–142), and exposure to trace anesthetic agents enhances hepatic metabolism of some drugs (143,144). The relevance of these facts to the effects of trace concentrations is not clear.

Mortality Studies

No increase in the death rate as a result of liver disease among anesthesiologists has been found (109).

Animal Studies

Exposure to halothane in concentrations as low as 20 ppm may be associated with mild toxic effects to the liver in rats (145–147). No evidence of such effects have been found from enflurane (145,147) or isoflurane (145).

RENAL DISEASE

Epidemiological Studies

The ASA National Study found that male and female operating room nurses and technicians and female anesthesiologists had a higher risk of kidney disease than did comparable groups outside the operating room (43). These differences were not found in male anesthesiologists. These results have been questioned (41). Another study failed to find any increase in kidney disease in male anesthesiologists (36). An early study in exposed dentists showed no increase in renal disease (72), but a later study showed an increase in both exposed dentists and female chair-side assistants (45). An analysis of sev-

eral studies found an increased risk of renal disease only among women (84).

Mortality Studies

No increase in deaths caused by renal disease among anesthesiologists has been found (109).

HEMATOLOGICAL STUDIES

Several studies have shown that inhalation of nitrous oxide inactivates vitamin B_{12} which may lead to impaired synthesis of DNA in the bone marrow (148). Changes can occur in patients exposed to nitrous oxide over prolonged periods, after multiple short-term exposures, and in the period immediately after operation.

Epidemiological Studies

In one study a higher-than-expected rate of leukemia was found in female anesthesiologists, but the small data base makes any valid conclusions difficult (43). Other studies have found no significant alterations in hematologic function in exposed individuals (6,138,149,150). However, 3 of 20 dentists exposed to concentrations of nitrous oxide higher than those normally found in operating rooms showed abnormalities in their bone marrows (151). Two had abnormalities in their peripheral blood.

Animal Studies

Halothane. No hematological effects were found from exposure of mice to 500 ppm halothane (111).

Enflurane. Exposure to 3000 ppm enflurane had no effect on hematopoiesis in mice (152).

Nitrous Oxide. Exposure to 10,000 ppm nitrous oxide caused no changes in hematopoiesis in rats (153).

Mixtures. Cytogenetic damage to bone marrow was found in rats exposed to 10 ppm halothane plus 500 ppm nitrous oxide (75).

NEUROLOGICAL SYMPTOMS

Two studies found an increase in neurological symptoms (numbness, tingling, and/

or muscle weakness) in dentists and female chair-side assistants exposed to anesthetic gases (45,154). Another study showed no difference in neurological symptoms or signs, sensory perception, or nerve conduction between dentists using nitrous oxide extensively and those using it sparingly or not at all (155).

A nonspecific polyneuropathy following chronic exposure to nitrous oxide has been described (156). Two of the patients were dental surgeons exposed to high concentrations. In animals, high levels of nitrous oxide have not been shown to cause neuromuscular or neurological abnormalities (155).

ALTERATIONS IN IMMUNE RESPONSE

Several studies have found that work in operating rooms does not change the immunologic profile of individuals (157–160).

CARDIAC DISEASE

Studies have shown a greater-than-expected frequency of hypertension and dysrhythmias (36,161), and there is one case report of atrial fibrillation secondary to halothane exposure (162). However, mortality studies give no evidence that anesthesiologists have a higher-than-expected risk of dying from heart disease (107–110).

MISCELLANEOUS

Various studies have reported higher-than-expected incidences of bone and joint disease (36), ulcers (36,161), ulcerative colitis (161), gallbladder disease (36), and migraine (161) in exposed personnel.

Case reports of exposed personnel who developed asthmatic symptoms (163), laryngitis (164), ophthalmic hypersensitivity (165), conjunctivitis (166), exacerbation of myasthenia gravis (167), and skin eruptions (168,169) have been published. Mortality statistics show a high incidence of suicide among anesthesiologists (107,109).

SUMMARY

More than two decades after widespread concern about operating theater pollution and health first emerged, the overwhelming majority of researchers believe that the hazard, if it exists, is not great and is more properly regarded as disquieting than alarming. Researchers who systematically examined the published epidemiological data found that adverse reproductive outcomes in women directly exposed to anesthetic gases during pregnancy were the only health effects for which there was reasonably convincing evidence (38). It is somewhat reassuring to note that studies have shown that anesthesiologists have a mortality rate less than that expected for physicians or the general population (108–110). However, reproductive problems such as spontaneous abortion and congenital anomalies are not reflected in mortality data and high cure rates may be responsible for the lack of increased mortality from health problems. Furthermore, one study showed an increased rate of early retirement as a result of permanent ill health and an high rate of deaths while working among anesthesia personnel (170).

A cause-and-effect relationship between occupational exposure and the problems described has not been established. If there is an increased risk, it may be related to other factors such as mental and physical stress; strenuous physical demands; disturbed night rest; need for constant alertness; long and inconvenient working hours often interfering with domestic life; irregular routine; exposure to transmissible infections, solvents, propellants, cleaning solutions, laser beams, methylmethacrylate, radiation, or ultraviolet light; preexisting health and reproductive problems; hormonal or dietary disturbances; the physical or emotional makeup of those who choose to work in operating rooms; socioeconomic factors; or some other as yet undefined factor. Causes may be multiple. Final proof that trace amounts of anesthetic gases contribute to the increased risk must await demonstration that measures to reduce their levels in operating room air also reduce the risk.

While reducing trace gas levels appears to be of little benefit to the patient (other than perhaps resulting in a healthier person administering the anesthesia), definite hazards to the patient have been created by the introduction of scavenging equipment (see "Hazards of Scavenging Equipment," in this chapter). Use of scavenging equipment and/or changing work practices also may be inconvenient or awkward for anesthesia personnel.

The authors of this text believe that the most prudent approach is to take action to reduce the levels of trace anesthetics to the lowest level consistent with reasonable cost, risk to the patient, and inconvenience.

The Committee on Occupational Health of Operating Room Personnel suggests that through some formal process, healthcare institutions bring to the attention of operating and recovery room personnel pertinent information on the claimed risks of excess anesthetic gases and ways by which these risks can be minimized (171). A sample letter is available (172).

Control Measures

Complete elimination of all anesthetic molecules from the operating room atmosphere is an impossible task. The goal should be to reduce concentrations to the lowest level consistent with a reasonable expenditure of effort and money. To achieve this goal, attention must be focused on four areas: scavenging, leaks, work techniques, and the room ventilation system. If anesthetic pollution is to be effectively controlled, attention must be paid to all of these areas.

SCAVENGING SYSTEMS

Scavenging is defined as the collection of excess gases from equipment used in administering anesthesia or exhaled by the patient and removal of these gases to an appropriate place of discharge outside the working environment. Scavenging systems are also called evacuation systems, waste anesthetic gas-disposal systems, and excess anesthetic gas-scavenging systems. The flowmeters on the

anesthesia machine are usually adjusted to deliver more gases than the patient can take up. In the absence of scavenging, these gases will flow into the operating room air. Installation of an efficient scavenging system is the most important step in reducing trace gas levels, because it will lower ambient concentrations by up to 90% (5,8,11,13,16,32, 33,173–176).

A scavenging system consists of five basic components (Fig. 11.1): a gas-collecting assembly, which captures gases at the site of emission; a transfer means, which conveys them to the interface; the interface, which provides positive (and sometimes negative) pressure relief and may provide reservoir capacity; the gas-disposal tubing, which conducts the gases from the interface to the gas-disposal assembly; and the gas-disposal assembly, which conveys them to a point where they can be discharged safely. Frequently, some or all of these components are combined.

A U.S. standard for scavenging systems has been published (177), and an international standard is in preparation. It differs from the U.S. standard in that only 30-mm fittings are permitted and some fittings are male rather than female and vice versa.

Gas-Collecting Assembly

The gas-collecting assembly collects excess gases from their source or sources and delivers them to the transfer means. It may attach to, or be an integral part of, a source. Frequently the outlets of two or more sources are joined together. This assembly is also referred to as the gas-capturing assembly, device, or valve; scavenging trap or valve; collecting or collection valve; scavenging exhale valve; evacuator; antipollution valve; ducted expiratory valve; collecting system exhaust valve, and scavenging trap.

The ASTM standard (177) specifies that the outlet connection must be either a 30- or 19-mm male fitting. The proposed international standard allows only a 30-mm fitting, and it is probable that this will be the only size available on future U.S. machines. The

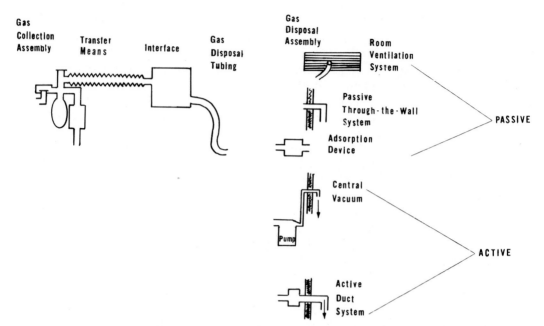

Figure 11.1. Complete scavenging system. The gas-collecting assembly may be an integral part of the breathing system, ventilator, or extracorporeal pump oxygenator. The interface may be an integral part of the gas-collecting assembly or some other portion of the scavenging system.

size is important because it should not be possible to connect components of the breathing system to the outlet. Some early assemblies had a 22-mm fitting and cases of misconnection with breathing system hoses occurred (178,179). Adapters are available to change 22-mm fittings to 19- or 30-mm and this should be done to prevent assembly errors.

Breathing Systems

Systems Containing an Adjustable Pressure-Limiting Valve. Systems with an adjustable pressure-limiting valve include the circle system and the Mapleson A, B, C, and D systems. The APL valve is fitted with a shroud (Fig. 11.2). With the circle and Mapleson D systems and the Lack variant of the Mapleson A system, the weight of the assembly can be supported by the anesthesia machine and the transfer means can be quite short, two distinct advantages. Smaller and lighter APL valves with gas-collecting assemblies are available for the Mapleson A, B, and C systems.

APL valves sometimes have a mechanism built into them that will prevent positive or negative pressure from the scavenging system from being transmitted to the breathing system (180).

T Piece Systems without an APL Valve. Numerous devices have been described for removing gases exhausted through the tail of the bag (181–198). One device has been described that evacuates gases when the hole is in the side of the bag (189).

Other methods use a container attached to suction (199,200). The waste gases are discharged into the container from the bag. A high-volume disposal system removes them before they can enter the room.

Resuscitation Equipment

A nonrebreathing valve with a scavenging adapter is commercially available. It is fairly simple to devise a means to attach transfer means to the exhalation port of some existing nonrebreathing valves without affecting valve function.

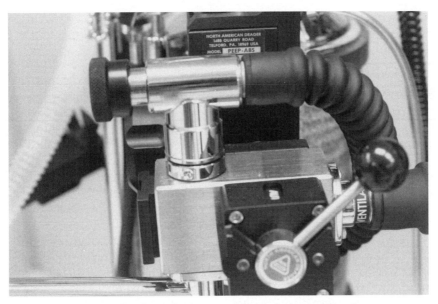

Figure 11.2. Gas-collecting assembly attached to an APL valve.

Masks or Nasal Cannulae

It is common practice in some institutions to administer nitrous oxide to patients through a nasal cannula or face mask for sedation. Placing a tent or hood around the patient's face and attaching a suction source can reduce the ambient nitrous oxide concentrations (18,201).

A double mask consisting of an inner smaller mask separated from an outer larger mask by a slot connected to a scavenging device will reduce exposure to anesthetic gases (202).

Ventilators

Most anesthesia ventilators are now equipped with gas-collecting assemblies, and most also come with an interface and gas-disposal assembly.

For a ventilator with only a gas-collecting assembly, it is useful to attach the assembly outlet to a Y that joins the effluent from the APL valve in the breathing system (see Fig. 11.6). With some ventilators, it is necessary to have a unidirectional valve between the ventilator and the Y to prevent flow of gases back into the ventilator and the operating room air when the ventilator is not in use.

With some older ventilators, the exhaust includes not only the excess breathing system gases but also the driving gas for the ventilator, so that a disposal system with high flows is required. Thus a scavenging system that functions efficiently with spontaneously breathing patients may fail to do so when used with some automatic ventilators (203).

Extracorporeal Pump Oxygenators

The outlet port of an extracorporeal pump oxygenator is a potential source of anesthetic pollution. Gas-collecting assemblies are available. It is important to provide an effective interface with these devices because significant positive or negative pressure alterations at the outflow port can markedly alter function (204).

Respiratory Gas Monitors

Some respiratory gas monitors that withdraw a sample of gas from the breathing system expel this sample into the room. These constitute a source of room contamination that is often ignored (205,206). Many monitors are now equipped so that the aspirated sample travels either back to the breathing system or to a scavenging system (207).

Cryosurgical Units

Many cyrosourgical units use nitrous oxide. These can contribute to operating room contamination (208). These units should be fitted with scavengers when possible or carbon dioxide should be used instead of nitrous oxide (209).

Leak Sites

When there is a definite leak site (as when a face mask or laryngeal mask is used or a vaporizer is filled), close (local) scavenging of contaminated air through a separate scavenging device or a low negative pressure hood can be used to lower ambient concentrations (210–213).

Transfer Means

The transfer means (also called the exhaust tubing or hose and transfer system) conveys gas from the collecting assembly to the interface when the interface is not an integral part of the gas-collecting assembly.

It is most commonly a length of tubing with a connector at either end. The inlet and outlet fittings should be either 30- or 19-mm. It should be as short as possible (this is facilitated by mounting the interface on the anesthesia machine) and of large enough diameter to carry a high flow of gas without a significant increase in pressure. It should be resistant to kinking. If the transfer means is not kink-resistant, a pressure relief valve can be added to the collector to prevent pressure increases that could result from occlusion of the tubing between the collector and the interface. If it must run along the floor it must be designed to prevent occlusion (171). It should be easily seen and easy to disconnect from the gas-collecting assembly in the event of malfunction or occlusion of the scavenging system. To discourage misconnections it is desirable that it be different (by color and/

or configuration) from breathing system tubing.

Interface

The interface serves to prevent pressure increases or decreases in the scavenging system from being transmitted to the breathing system, ventilator, or extracorporeal oxygenator. (The interface is also called the balancing valve or device, pressure balancing valve or device, interface system or block, intermediate site, safety block, air break receiver, receiving system, interface valve, and scavenging valve.) The American standard requires that the interface limit pressures immediately downstream of the gas-collecting assembly to between -0.5 and $+10$ cm H_2O during normal operating conditions and up to $+15$ cm H_2O with obstruction of the scavenging system for scavenging from a breathing system or ventilator (171). In the proposed international standard these limits are -0.5 cm H_2O and $+3.5$ cm H_2O. For scavenging from an extracorporeal oxygenator, the recommended limits are -0.25 to 0 cm H_2O (171).

The inlet should be a 30- or 19-mm male connection. The size of the outlet connection is optional, but should be different from breathing system connections and from the inlet connection if the device is sensitive to the direction of flow (171).

The interface may be part of the gas-collecting assembly in a breathing system, incorporated into a ventilator, or an independent device. It should be situated as close to the gas-collecting assembly as possible, preferably fitted onto the anesthesia machine, and where it can be readily observed and reached by anesthesia personnel.

There are three basic elements to an interface: positive pressure relief, negative pressure relief, and reservoir capacity. Irrespective of what type of disposal system is used, positive pressure relief must be provided to protect the equipment and patient if occlusion of the scavenging system occurs. If an active disposal system is used, negative pressure relief is needed to limit subatmospheric pressure and a reservoir is necessary to match the intermittent flow from the gas-collecting assembly to the continuous flow of the disposal system. A device that gives an audible signal may be fitted to the interface to indicate operation of the positive or negative pressure relief device. A flow indicator may be provided to monitor flow from the interface to the gas-disposal system (Fig. 11.4).

The reservoir may be a rigid container, wide tubing, a bag, or a combination of these. A distensible bag allows monitoring of the scavenging system. It should only be used with active disposal systems and should be of a different color from, and situated away from, the breathing system reservoir bag.

Interfaces can be divided into two types: open and closed, depending on the means to provide positive and negative pressure relief.

Open Interfaces (214,215)

An open interface (or air break receiver unit) is one that is open to atmosphere (allowing positive and negative pressure relief) and contains no valves. It should be used only with an active disposal system.

Because the discharge of waste gases is usually intermittent and flow through an active disposal assembly is continuous, a reservoir is needed to hold the surges of gas that enter the interface at an inflow greater than the disposal system flow until the disposal system removes them. The reservoir allows the flow rate in the disposal system to be kept just above the average, rather than at the peak flow rate of gases from the gas-collecting assembly.

It is important that the reservoir have adequate capacity, especially if a ventilator in which the driving gas mixes with waste gases is used or if high tidal volumes or high nitrous oxide flows are used (216). If a large amount of turbulence occurs, leakage into the atmosphere can occur before the volume of excess gas entering the interface equals the reservoir volume (214).

The safety afforded by an open system depends on the patency of the vents to atmosphere so it is good to have considerable redundancy in case some are accidentally blocked (217,218). Regular checking and cleaning of the vents is also necessary.

With any open interface, it is important that the inlet for waste gases, the disposal system connection, and the opening to atmosphere be arranged so that waste gases are removed preferentially before room air is entrained.

T Tube (219). An example of a simple type of open interface, known as a T tube, is shown in Figure 11.3*A*. One limb of the T attaches to the transfer means with the side limb leading to the active disposal system. The third limb of the T is fitted with a piece of tubing that serves as a reservoir. Surges of gases flowing out of the transfer means flow partly into the disposal system and partly into the reservoir tubing. They can then be removed from the reservoir by the disposal system.

As long as the free end of the reservoir remains open to atmosphere there is no danger that significant negative or positive pressure will be applied to the breathing system. It is important that a guard be placed at the free end to prevent occlusion or that holes be provided near the end (see Fig. 11.3*A*) so that an opening to atmosphere is still present if the end of the tubing is occluded.

Tube-within-a-Tube. A second type of open interface, known as the tube-within-a-tube (or coaxial), is shown in Figure 11.3*B*. It consists of two coaxial tubes. The proximal end of the inner tube is open to the outer tube and the distal end is connected to the active disposal device. The outer tube is connected to the transfer means proximally and the distal end is open to atmosphere. A variation of this is shown in Figure 11.3*C*. A distensible bag has been added so that the adequacy of scavenging can be monitored.

Another variation of this type of open interface is shown in Figure 11.3*D*. Anesthetic gases from the transfer means enter at the top and are conducted to the base where they are

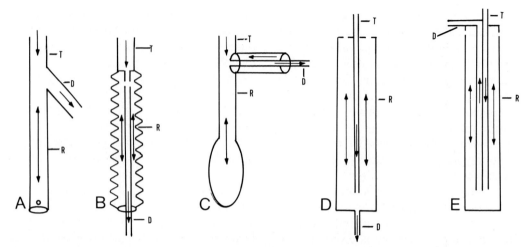

Figure 11.3. Open interfaces. **A,** T tube interface. Note the escape-inlet hole near the free end of the reservoir tubing. **B,** Tube-within-a-tube interface. **C,** Tube-within-a-tube interface with distensible bag for monitoring efficiency of scavenging. **D,** Tube-within-a-tube with the escape holes at top. **E,** Two parallel tubes are inside the canister, which acts as a reservoir. Gases from the breathing system travel down in one and are removed by suction applied to the other tube. The relief ports provide positive and negative pressure relief. *T,* transfer means; *R,* reservoir; *D,* active disposal system. Partly redrawn from a drawing furnished by Boehringer Laboratories, Inc.

dispersed by wire mesh. The mesh acts as a silencer, reducing the hiss generated by flow into the disposal tubing (220). Suction is applied to the base, and this serves to remove the gases. Gases are stored in the reservoir between exhalations. The holes at the top are open to atmosphere.

A commonly used open interface is shown in Figures 11.3*E* and 11.4. Gases from the transfer tubing enter at the top and travel to the base in a tube. A parallel tube is connected at the top to the active disposal system. The space around both tubes acts as a reservoir. Holes at the top are open to atmosphere.

The open interface is simple, but is fraught with the danger of polluting the atmosphere should the reservoir not have sufficient volume to contain the boluses of waste gases. Turbulence will increase the size of the reservoir, which contains air contaminated with anesthetic gases (214). Turbulence is greatest when gases from the breathing system flow against the disposal system flow and least when flow is in the same direction. In addi-

tion, anesthesia staff may forget to turn on the suction to evacuate gases.

Closed Interfaces

A closed interface is one in which the connection(s) with the atmosphere are through valve(s). A positive pressure relief valve is always required to allow release of gases into the room if there is obstruction of the scavenging system downstream of the interface. If an active disposal system is to be used, a negative pressure relief valve (known as a dumping valve, pop-in valve, or inlet relief valve) is necessary to allow entrainment of air when the pressure falls below atmospheric.

A reservoir is not required with a closed interface and should not be used unless an active disposal system is used, in which case a distensible bag is useful for monitoring the functioning of the scavenging system, as described above.

Positive Pressure Relief Only. A positive pressure relief only type of closed interface is used only with passive disposal sys-

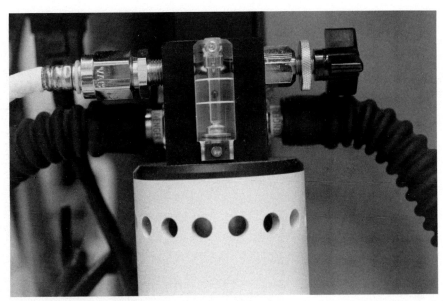

Figure 11.4. Open interface. The open ports in the reservoir provide positive and negative pressure relief. The adjustable needle valve regulates the suction flow. The flowmeter indicates whether or not the suction flow is within the range recommended by the manufacturer.

tems. An example is shown in Figure 11.5*A*. The positive pressure relief valve is closed unless there is a problem downstream of the interface. The device may be spring loaded or work by gravity.

Positive and Negative Pressure Relief. If one plans to use an active disposal system, a negative pressure relief valve must be present. Subatmospheric pressures greater than -0.5 H_2O water can raise or lower the opening pressure of some APL valves (221).

Examples of this type of closed interface are shown in Figures 11.5*B* and 11.6. When a passive disposal system is used, the negative pressure relief will remain closed at all times. If an active disposal system is used, it should close during high peak flow rates from the gas-collecting assembly and open when the gas-disposal assembly flow is greater than the flow of gases from the gas-collecting assembly.

The rate of flow into the gas-disposal assembly should be adjusted to the optimal level by observing the bag (if present) and the positive and negative relief valves. In an optimally adjusted system, the scavenger reser-

Pos
Relief

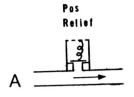

A

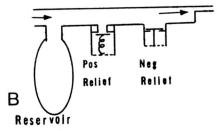

Pos
Relief

Neg
Relief

B

Reservoir

Figure 11.5. Closed interfaces. **A**, Without reservoir or negative relief device; for use with passive disposal systems only. **B**, With reservoir bag and negative pressure relief valve; for use with either a passive or active disposal system. If an active disposal system is used, the bag will be collapsed, except during periods of high flow from the gas collection assembly, and inadequate outflow will be indicated by bag distention.

Figure 11.6. Closed interface. There are three inlet ports to accommodate evacuation from an APL valve and ventilator joined by a Y connection (*A*) and from another gas collection assembly (*B*). A means to regulate suction flow is at top left (*C*). The reservoir bag (*D*) allows monitoring of the scavenging efficiency and permits adjustment of suction flow to the minimum necessary. *E* is a test button and *F* is the negative and positive pressure relief. If a passive disposal system is used, the reservoir bag is removed and the mount capped. The needle valve is closed and a tubing is attached from *B* to the gas disposal system. Courtesy of Ohmeda, a division of BOC Health Care, Inc.

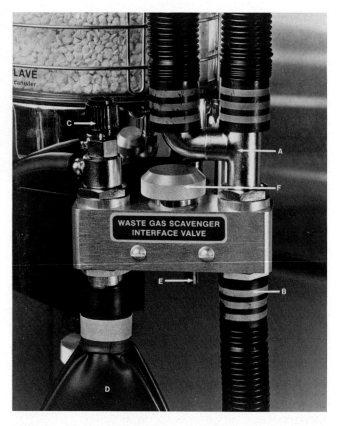

voir bag increases in size only when excess gas is released from the gas-collecting assembly and decreases in size during the rest of the ventilatory cycle (222). If the bag is continually collapsed or the negative pressure relief valve opens frequently, the flow should be lowered. If the bag becomes distended or the positive pressure relief valve opens frequently, flow should be increased.

A closed interface can be used with any type of disposal system but valves add to the complexity. They must be designed so that they do not stick or leak. Interfaces with two negative pressure relief valves are available and add a margin of safety.

Gas-Disposal Assembly Tubing

The gas-disposal assembly tubing (or disposal tubing) connects the interface to the disposal assembly (see Fig. 11.1). It should be different in size and appearance from the breathing system hoses to avoid misconnec-

tions. It should be as collapse proof as possible and free of leaks. With a passive gas-disposal assembly it is important that the hose be as short and wide as practical to minimize resistance.

Ideally, the gas-disposal tubing should be run overhead to minimize the risk of occlusion and to avoid the dangers of personnel tripping over it or other apparatus becoming entangled in it. Should the disposal point be a significant distance from the anesthesia machine or the tubing obstruct personnel or equipment movement, it may be hidden in a false ceiling (196). If the tubing must be run across the floor, it should be routed where it is least likely to be stepped on or have equipment rolled onto it. If it must pass a doorway, it should follow the door frame.

Gas-Disposal Assembly

The gas-disposal assembly consists of the components used to remove waste gases from the operating room; it is also referred to as the elimination system or route, disposal-exhaust route, and disposal system. The gases must be vented at a point that is isolated from personnel and any air intakes.

Disposal assemblies are of two types: active, in which a mechanical flow-inducing device moves the gases, and passive, in which the pressure is raised above atmospheric by the patient exhaling, manual squeezing of the reservoir bag, or a ventilator. With an active system there will be a negative pressure in the gas disposal tubing. With a passive system, this pressure will be positive.

Active systems are usually more effective in keeping operating room pollution levels low, because most leaks will be inward (8,223,224). They have the advantage that small-bore gas-disposal tubing can be used and excessive resistance is not a problem. They also aid room air exchange. They are, however, expensive in terms of energy costs. They are not automatic and must be turned on and off. If they are not turned on, air pollution will occur; if they are not turned off, there will be needless waste of energy. Active systems are more complex than passive ones. Their use requires that the interface have negative pressure relief.

Passive systems are simpler, but may not be as effective in lowering trace gas levels, because the positive pressure encourages outward leaks. They are less expensive to operate than active systems.

Passive Systems

Room Ventilation System (173,196, 225,226). Ventilation systems used in operating rooms are of two types: nonrecirculating (also called one-pass, single pass, and 100% fresh air) and recirculating. In the proposed international standard the room ventilation system is classified as an active disposal system, because a powered device is used for removal. It has also been called assisted-passive (227).

A nonrecirculating system takes in exterior air and processes it by filtering and adjusting the humidity and temperature. The processed air is circulated through the operating room and then all of it is exhausted to atmosphere. This type of ventilation system can be used for waste gas disposal by securing the disposal tubing to a convenient exhaust grill. The sweeping effect of air flowing into the ventilation system will remove the gases from the operating room.

Concern for fuel economy has increased the use of systems that recirculate air. With a recirculating system, a small amount of air is taken in from the atmosphere. Most of the gases exhausted from the operating room are shunted back into the intake and recirculated, while a volume of circulated air equal to the fresh air is exhausted. With this type of system waste gases must be vented beyond the point of recirculation, because venting gases upstream of this point would result in contamination of all rooms on the common manifold.

The hospital engineer should know which type of ventilation system is present. If not, absence of recirculation can be determined by sampling the room air inlet to see if it is free of trace gases after they have been released in another room.

An important consideration in using the room ventilation system for waste gas disposal is the increase in negative pressure downstream in the exhaust duct, away from the grille. If the waste gases are introduced at the exhaust grille, the negative pressure is usually low and its effect negligible (217). If waste gases are introduced at a distance downstream in the duct (as they must be with a recirculating system), negative pressure relief must be provided in the interface.

Using the room ventilation system is economical because an existing structure is used and no expenditure of energy is necessary. It is automatic, so there is no need to turn anything on or off or make adjustments.

In many operating rooms, the exhaust grilles are not located close to the anesthesia machine. Tubing should not lie on the floor because this greatly increases the risk of occlusion. In some cases, the disposal tubing can be extended to a wall- or ceiling-mounted connection that leads to a pipe in the wall (173). The pipe connects to the exhaust duct, preferably near the exhaust grille to avoid excessive negative pressure.

Piping Direct to Atmosphere (223,228). Piping direct to the atmosphere is also known as a direct duct or vent, specialized duct system, direct disposal line, and through-the-wall system. With this system, excess gases are vented through the wall, window, ceiling, or floor to the outside, using only the slight pressure of the gases leaving the gas-collecting assembly to provide the flow. To prevent cross-flow between rooms, each room must have its own duct.

The inlet to the system in each room should be close to the anesthesia machine. There should be a means to cap the opening to the duct when it is not connected to the gas-disposal tubing. The duct should be constructed of a material resistant to anesthetic gases and should be relatively short and of large diameter if excessive back pressure is to be avoided. Hence this type of system is not suitable for an operating room far from an outside wall (217). A unidirectional valve may be placed in the duct to prevent outside air from entering the operating room and to minimize the effects of wind pressure on the disposal system (229). The duct should be inclined so that water will not accumulate.

The discharge point on the outside should be selected so that it is away from wind pressures, ignition hazards, windows, and the inlets for the ventilation system. It may be advantageous to attach a short T piece as a terminal (230). The open end(s) should point downward to minimize the entry of water and dirt and be fitted with netting to prevent insects, rodents, and foreign matter from entering the pipe.

Such a disposal assembly is easy to use, but it requires a special installation. In redesigning an existing operating room or designing a new room, construction of a separate scavenging system should be considered. If the operating rooms are not near the outside of the building, this type of disposal assembly may not be practical.

Problems that can occur with this system include both positive and negative pressure caused by wind currents, obstruction from ice buildup (231) and accumulation of foreign matter at the outlet. There needs to be a means to determine the patency of the system. It is important to do trace gas monitoring under conditions of use with this system, to make sure a flow-inducing device is not needed.

Adsorption Device (32,232–240). An adsorption device removes some or all excess anesthetic agents by adsorbing them or converting them to harmless substances. Canisters of varying shape and capacity filled with activated charcoal have been used as waste gas disposal assemblies, by directing the gases from the gas-disposal tubing through them. The effectiveness of individual canisters and various brands of charcoal vary widely (232,233). Some can be regenerated by autoclaving (241). Different volatile agents are adsorbed with varying efficiency. The efficiency of adsorption also depends on the rate of flow through the canister (242).

Charcoal canisters have the advantages of being simple and portable and not requiring expensive installation or maintenance. An additional advantage is that halogenated anesthetic vapors are not released to the ozone layer (242).

They also have a number of disadvantages. At present, there is no adsorption device for removal of nitrous oxide. They are fairly expensive and effective for only relatively short periods of time. They must be replaced regularly and pose problems of storage and disposal. Determination that the adsorber is saturated requires continuous monitoring or weighing of the adsorber. Finally, a large canister may impose significant resistance (232).

It is recommended that use of these devices be limited to situations in which nitrous oxide is not being employed and in which no other means of eliminating waste gases are available.

Active Systems

Piped Vacuum (196,219,243). The central vacuum system is a popular method for gas disposal because no new equipment or installation is required.

The system should be capable of providing high volume (30 liters/min) flow, but only slight negative pressure is needed. There should be a means to allow the user to control the suction flow (see Figs. 11.4 and 11.6). This will conserve energy, cut down the wear and tear on the central pumps, and reduce the noise level in the operating room. For some units, this is done by observing the bag and the positive and negative pressure relief valves. Others have a means to allow the user to adjust the flow to that recommended by the manufacturer (see Fig. 11.4). A restrictive orifice may be placed in the suction nipple to limit the flow (244).

There are a number of problems associated with its use.

Inadequate Number of Outlets. Many operating rooms have only two suction outlets. This is barely enough for some surgical procedures, let alone anesthesia requirements. Ideally, anesthesia personnel should have two suction outlets available, one for suctioning the airway and one for scavenging waste gases.

If there are not enough outlets, a Y may be inserted into the suction line to create two lines. Unfortunately, this may reduce the flow so that it is inadequate for either purpose.

Some anesthesiologists use a single suction line for scavenging and patient suctioning. The suction line remains attached to the interface most of the time and is detached when needed for patient suctioning. If the flow of anesthesia gases is not turned off, there will be escape of anesthetic gases into the operating room air.

Inconvenient Outlets. If a suction outlet is not near the anesthesia machine, long tub-

ings must reach across the floor, with the dangers of occlusion, tripping of personnel, and entanglement with other apparatus.

Overload of the System. Because scavenging requires high flows, it is possible to overload the central vacuum system if too many devices are in use at once. This is especially likely with older systems, which over the years have had added to them more capacity than they were designed to handle. Overcoming this problem may require a major renovation of the system. The drain can be reduced if anesthesia personnel will adjust the flow down to that necessary to prevent spillage of gases into room air and turn off the suction after use.

Damage to the Suction Pump. Wear and tear on the suction pump can be expected to increase if the central vacuum system is used for disposal of waste gases. Widespread use of central vacuum systems for disposal of anesthetic gases and the paucity of reports of problems suggest that this is not a great problem.

Personnel Exposure. If the exhaust from the central vacuum pump goes to an area frequented by personnel or is situated near an air intake, open window, or door, use of the system for gas disposal will result in additional exposure of personnel to waste gases. It may be necessary to relocate the pump exhaust.

Inconvenience. To conserve energy, the suction system should be turned on just before anesthesia is begun and turned off at the termination of a procedure. For further energy conservation, the anesthesiologist should regulate the suction flow according to the volume of waste gases. These extra duties may be neglected and there will be either wasted energy or operating room pollution.

Active Duct System (217,223,245,246). The other type of active disposal assembly is a dedicated duct system that leads to the outside and employs a flow-inducing device (fan, pump, or Venturi) that can move large volumes of gas at low pressures. This active duct system also is known as the independent velocity specialized duct system, dedicated vacuum or exhaust system, and dedicated air mover. Each operating room is supplied with a duct, two or three of which are connected together to a common duct that leads outside. The flow-inducing device is located in the common duct and provides movement of gases at a low negative pressure. The negative pressure ensures that cross-contamination between operating rooms will not occur and prevents atmospheric conditions from affecting the outflow from the system. It has been recommended that two flow-inducing devices be provided and arranged so that if one fails to start the second one will run. Also, it is recommended that there be a pilot light at the operating room control desk to indicate that the scavenging system is running. Balancing dampers may be provided for each operating room to prevent pressure imbalances from developing between the operating rooms that are connected to the system (221). The outlet to atmosphere must be away from windows and ventilation intakes.

A means to adjust the flow and/or a flowmeter may be incorporated into the common duct. Unlike the interface, which is user balanced, these systems are balanced in the piping or ducting and the user makes no adjustments, other than to turn the system on and off.

The advantages of this system are that resistance is not a problem and wind currents do not affect the system. However, it requires a special installation, which should be considered during renovation or when a new operating room is being designed.

Disadvantages include those of any active system: added complexity and the need for negative pressure relief and reservoir capacity in the interface. The flow-inducing device means added energy consumption and requires regular maintenance. Installing the system is fairly expensive.

ALTERED WORK PRACTICES (38,247–249)

A number of work practices allow anesthetic gases to enter room air. Most of this

pollution can be prevented. Continuous trace gas monitoring can be used to demonstrate to anesthesia personnel the techniques needed to protect themselves and their colleagues from exposure to high concentrations of anesthetic agents.

Adherence to the following practices will significantly reduce contamination. Most of them can be followed without compromising safety and some of them are beneficial to the patient. However, adherence to them must not distract from the comfort and safety of the patient. For example, in pediatric anesthesia leakage of anesthetic agents around uncuffed tracheal tubes may be needed to avoid trauma to the trachea and holding the mask tightly against the face may be frightening to a child.

Checking before Use

Before starting an anesthetic, secure connection and proper operation of all components of the breathing and scavenging systems should be verified. If an active gas disposal assembly is to be used, the flow should be turned on. Nitrous oxide should be turned on only momentarily during preuse checkout of equipment. All other tests should be conducted using oxygen.

Using Scavenging Equipment

Failure to use available scavenging equipment is commonplace (250). In some cases, the reasons relate to equipment design and difficulty in scavenging in specific circumstances. Commonly, however, lack of concern causes this omission.

Proper Mask Fit

Obtaining a good mask fit requires skill, but is critical to maintain low levels of anesthetic gases in the operating room, especially during assisted or controlled ventilation, when higher pressures will magnify the leak between the patient and the mask. Anesthesia by face mask causes the highest levels of pollution in the operating room (212). Most investigators have found it difficult to keep trace anesthetic levels within safe limits unless the face mask was strapped extremely tightly (251,252). Sometimes a small change in mask angle can make a dramatic difference in fit. Several types and sizes of masks should be available.

Reduction of high levels of anesthetic gases in the operating room associated with poor mask fit can be reduced by placing a separate active scavenging device near the mask (195,213,253). A double mask for scavenging has been described (254).

Prevention of Flow from the Breathing System into Room Air

Nitrous oxide or a vaporizer should not be turned on until the mask is fitted to the patient's face or the patient is intubated and connected to the breathing system.

Disconnections can be prevented by making certain that all connections are tight before use. An airway pressure monitor (see Chapter 5) will aid in early detection of disconnections. Nonessential disconnections for activities such as taping the tracheal tube or positioning the patient should be kept to a minimum.

If it is necessary to make a disconnection, flow of anesthetic gases into the room can be avoided if the reservoir bag is first emptied (gradually rather than violently dumping it) into the scavenging system and all flowmeters turned off. Alternately, the patient port can be occluded and the APL valve opened so that the gases will enter the scavenging system (255). If a ventilator (which has its own spill valve) is being used in place of a reservoir bag, the APL valve, which is normally closed during ventilator operation, need not be opened.

Washout of Anesthetic Gases at the End of a Case

At the end of a case, 100% oxygen should be administered before extubation or mask removal, so the scavenging system can eliminate the bulk of excess anesthetic gases.

Prevention of Liquid Agent Spillage

It is easy to spill liquid agent when filling a vaporizer, so care should be exercised. Use of a pin-indexed vaporizer (see Chapter 4) will reduce spillage. Close scavenging will reduce contamination associated with filling and draining of vaporizers (212).

Keeping Keyed Filler on the Bottle

It has been found that there is less loss of agent if the keyed filler remains on the bottle after a vaporizer is filled (256). However, this may present storage problems.

Avoidance of Certain Techniques

Insufflation techniques in which an anesthetic mixture is introduced into the patient's respiratory system on inhalation are still widely used for laryngoscopy and bronchoscopy (257,258). High flow rates are required to avoid dilution with room air and result in a cloud of anesthetic gases escaping into the room air.

Proper Use of Tracheal Tubes

Cuffed tracheal tubes should always be used in adults and the cuff inflated until there is no leak. Only small leaks should be permitted around uncuffed tubes in pediatric patients. Reduction of contamination with an uncuffed tube can be achieved by placing a suction catheter in the mouth (259,260) and using a throat pack (261).

Disconnection of Nitrous Oxide Sources

Nitrous oxide and oxygen pipeline hoses leading to the machine should be disconnected at the end of the operating schedule. The disconnection should be made as close to the wall outlet as possible and not at the back of the anesthesia machine, so that if there is a leak in the hose, no gases will escape to room air while the hose is disconnected. This will result in lower levels of nitrous oxide in the operating room and will conserve gases.

When cylinders are used, the cylinder

valve should be closed at the end of the operating schedule. Gas remaining in the machine should be "bled out" and evacuated through the scavenging system.

Use of Low Fresh Gas Flows (20,262)

Use of low fresh gas flows will reduce the volume of anesthetic gases added to the room by reducing the pollution resulting from disconnections in the breathing system and from inefficient scavenging. It also allows use of low removal flows with active disposal assemblies, resulting in energy conservation and reduced wear and tear on the disposal device. Use of low flows does not make scavenging unnecessary, because high flows must still be used at times (see Chapter 8).

Use of Intravenous Agents and Regional Anesthesia

Use of an intravenous induction technique significantly reduces trace gas exposure (263).

LEAKAGE CONTROL (38,182,247,249,264–266)

Leakage of gases from equipment has been reported to account for 2.5% to 87% of total contamination (267). Some leakage is unavoidable, but it should be minimized. Control of leakage may require replacement of equipment that cannot be made gas tight.

Most anesthesia machines are under contract to undergo servicing by a manufacturer's representative at regular intervals, usually quarterly. Unfortunately, experience has shown that this servicing does not always identify or correct all leak points. In addition, leakage in some equipment develops fairly frequently so that quarterly servicing is not sufficient. In-house monitoring and maintenance are necessary to minimize leakage.

Initially, elimination of significant leakage will take a fair amount of time and effort, but following this, anesthesia equipment can usually be maintained in an acceptable state with a minimum of effort. It is recommended that one individual supervise leakage control.

Pressure Terminology

Some confusion exists in the literature as to the terminology of various pieces of anesthesia equipment. Some literature on scavenging has referred to all equipment upstream of the flow control valves as the high-pressure system and all equipment between the flow control valves and the patient plus the scavenging equipment as the low-pressure system (249,268,269). However, older terminology established by the National Fire Protection Association defines high pressure as more than 200 psig.

In this book (see Chapter 3), the high-pressure system refers to those components that contain gas whose pressure is normally above 50 psig. This includes the components between the cylinder and the regulator. The intermediate-pressure system includes components normally subjected to a pressure of approximately 50 psig. This includes the hospital pipeline pipes and hoses and the components of the machine between the regulators or pipeline inlets and the flow control valves. The low-pressure system consists of components downstream of the flow control valves to the patient, plus the scavenging system. Pressures in this system vary, but seldom exceed 40 cm H_2O.

Identification of Leak Sites

Once it has been determined that significant leakage exists, there are several techniques for precisely locating the leak sites. A continuous infrared nitrous oxide analyzer can be used. The equipment under test is pressurized with nitrous oxide and the sampling probe directed at suspected leak sites. The meter reading indicates the presence or absence of leakage. This will identify most leaks. An exception would be leakage in a vaporizer. Use of an infrared analyzer is the only way to find leakage in complicated pieces of equipment such as ventilators.

Leak sites can be identified by application

of a solution of 50% liquid soap and 50% water or a commercial leak test solution to a piece of equipment under pressure. Leakage will be revealed by bubbling.

Leakage can be assessed by testing the capacity of the equipment to sustain pressurization. The total leak rate for a system is determined, after which a component of the system is excluded and the leak rate redetermined. The difference is the leak rate for that piece of equipment.

High-Pressure System

To test for leakage in the high-pressure system, the pipeline hoses should be disconnected and the flow control valves closed. The valve on a nitrous oxide cylinder should be opened fully, the pressure recorded, and the cylinder valve closed. The pressure should be recorded again 1 hr later. If little or no pressure drop has occurred, there is no significant leakage. If it falls, the high-pressure system is not tight. The test should be repeated with the other nitrous oxide cylinder if there is a double yoke.

If significant leakage is found, the most common site is the yoke, and application of a leak test solution will demonstrate a poor seal. Tightening the cylinder in its yoke will often seal off the leak. Other easily correctable causes include double, absent, or deformed washers. If found, these should be replaced. If fixing these problems does not cause the pressure to hold, the leak is inside the machine or at the flow control valve and must be corrected by the manufacturer's service representative.

Because leakage in this area does not occur often, checking every 2 to 4 months and after a cylinder has been changed should be sufficient (186,247,249).

Intermediate-Pressure System

Leakage in the intermediate-pressure system components can be determined by measuring the nitrous oxide concentrations in the operating room when no anesthesia is being administered (249). The survey should be begun at least 1 hr after administration of anesthesia has been discontinued. If a recirculating air-conditioning system is in use, a longer period may be required. The early morning is an excellent time to perform this test.

Flow control valves should be closed, pipeline hoses connected, and cylinder valves closed. Any of the area sampling and monitoring methods (dosimetry, grab samples in bags or cartridges, or IR analysis) can be applied. Room air should be sampled from the anesthesia breathing zone (4 to 5 feet above the floor within 3 feet of the front of the anesthesia machine) and the room air intake and outlet. Nitrous oxide concentrations should be less than 5 ppm (1,204). If a higher level is found, the pipeline hoses should be disconnected and the measurements repeated. If a high level is still present, this indicates a leak in the nitrous oxide pipe leading into the operating rooms or the station outlet and should be reported to the hospital engineer. If the level falls, this indicates a leak in the pipeline hose or the anesthesia machine.

Common problems with pipeline hoses include worn wall connections, loose connections (especially quick-connects), deformed compression fittings, and holes. These should be corrected or the hoses replaced. Leaks inside the anesthesia machine require correction by a service representative.

Once leakage is corrected, it is suggested that testing of the intermediate pressure system be performed every 2 to 4 months (182,204,247,249).

Low-Pressure System

The low-pressure portion of the system develops leaks more frequently than other parts. The preuse test for leaks in the breathing system (described in Chapter 14) is sufficient for the safe conduct of anesthesia, yet can miss leaks that emit large amounts of anesthetic gases into room air.

One way to quantify leakage in most of the

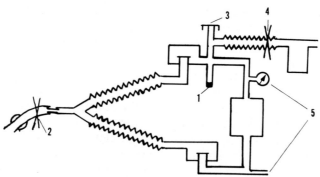

Figure 11.7.   Test for quantifying low-pressure leakage. *1,* The reservoir bag is removed and the bag mount is occluded. *2,* The patient port is occluded. *3,* The APL valve is opened fully. *4,* The transfer means is occluded just upstream of the interface. *5,* Oxygen flow is turned on and adjusted to maintain a pressure of 30 cm H_2O on pressure gauge in breathing system.

low-pressure system is shown in Figure 11.7. The breathing system is assembled as for clinical use. Components that are normally used should be present in their usual positions. The patient port is occluded. The bag is removed and the bag mount occluded. This is necessary because the bag's compliance makes it hard to quantitate low leak rates. The bag should be tested separately for leaks by pressurization. A vaporizer on the anesthesia machine should be turned on. The APL valve should be fully open and the scavenging system occluded upstream of the interface. The oxygen flow control valve is now opened sufficiently to establish and maintain a steady pressure of 30 cm H_2O on the pressure gauge in the breathing system. The flow on the oxygen flowmeter is the leak rate and should be less than 1000 ml/min (270). Leakage of 1000 ml/minute of nitrous oxide would result in a mean concentration of only 30 ppm in a 4000 cubic foot room with 15 air changes per hour (221). If the leak rate is greater than 1 liter/min the machine should not be used. The leakage test should be repeated with other vaporizers on the machine turned on.

If the leak rate exceeds 1000 ml/min, the APL valve should be closed and the leak rate redetermined. The difference is the leak rate in the scavenging system. The remaining leakage can be divided into that associated with the machine and that associated with the breathing system by attaching a sphygnomanometer bulb to the common gas outlet of the anesthesia machine and determining the oxygen flow necessary to achieve and maintain a pressure of 22 mm Hg. This is the portion of the low-pressure leakage associated with the machine. The machine leakage can be further divided by turning off the vaporizer and redetermining the leak rate.

Problems in the scavenging system may be as simple as a hole in a tubing (especially where it gets kinked) or a poor connection.

The breathing system is the most common location of significant low-pressure leakage, and the most common site in the breathing system is the absorber. Common causes include defective gaskets or seals, improper closure, inadequate tightening, and open or leaking drain cocks. Absorbent on the gaskets can prevent a tight seal. Many of these problems are easily corrected. Complicated repairs should be done by the manufacturer's representative.

Valve covers over unidirectional valves may become cracked or loose and should be replaced or tightened. Fittings for oxygen analyzer sensors that leak should be replaced.

The above test does not check for leakage in the ventilator. The ventilator and the low-pressure system can also be tested using an IR nitrous oxide analyzer. The anesthesia machine and breathing system are set up as for clinical use. The patient port outlet is occluded and the bag-ventilator selector switch is put in the bag mode. The APL valve is closed. Using the flowmeters, the breathing system is pressurized to 30 cm H_2O with a 50% mixture of nitrous oxide and oxygen. The machine and breathing system are scanned for nitrous oxide leakage. The selector valve is then put in the ventilator mode and the flowmeters set to deliver 2 liters/min oxygen and 2 liters/min nitrous oxide. The ventilator is turned on and set to a tidal volume such that a peak pressure of 30 cm H_2O is reached, with an I:E ratio of 0.5 at a rate of 10 to 20 breaths per minute. The scavenger system is activated. The machine, ventilator, breathing system, and scavenging system are scanned. Readings should not be greater than 25 ppm nitrous oxide.

Considerable controversy exists as to how often the low-pressure system should be tested for leakage. Suggested intervals vary from daily (204,247), to every other week (249) to monthly (182). It should be repeated with new equipment and when the absorbent is changed.

ROOM VENTILATION SYSTEM (15,267, 271,272)

An effective room ventilation system serves as an important adjunct to trace gas control by diluting and removing anesthetic gases resulting from leaks, errors in technique, and scavenging system malfunctions. Most building codes require 15 to 25 air exchanges per hour.

The concentration of an anesthetic gas can be calculated as

$$(60 \times L \times 1{,}000{,}000)/NV(1 - r)$$

where L is the leakage of anesthetic gas in liters/min, N is the number of room air changes per hour, r is the fraction of air changes recirculated, and V is the volume of room air in liters (269). A rule of thumb is that in a typical operating room with 10 fresh air exchanges per hour, a 100 ml/min leak of gas leads to less than 5 ppm in the atmosphere (177).

Recirculating systems are less effective in removing trace gases than nonrecirculating systems. A downward displacement ventilation system is more effective than a turbulent flow system (11,270).

The anesthesia machine should be placed as close to the exhaust grille as possible. This will ensure maximum removal of gases by the ventilation system and make it easy to use the ventilation system as the gas-disposal assembly. This should be taken into consideration when constructing a new operating room or renovating an older one.

Hazards of Scavenging Equipment

MISSASEMBLY

The additional equipment that scavenging adds provides opportunities for misconnections of components. To guard against this, most scavenging equipment has 19- or 30-mm connections rather than the 15- and 22-mm sizes found in breathing systems. This will not completely prevent misconnections, because there may be other apparatus in the room that will accept 19- or 30-mm connections (267). The safety potential provided by 19- and 30-mm connectors can be eliminated by using cheater adapters or tape for making connections.

Connection of a circle system hose to the outlet of the APL valve has been reported (178,179,273,274). Measures to prevent this include turning the exhaust port of the gas-collecting assembly so it points in the opposite direction from the breathing system ports, use of transfer and gas-disposal hoses of different colors and/or configurations from breathing system hoses, and using either 19- or 30-mm connections in the scavenging system.

PRESSURE ALTERATIONS IN THE BREATHING SYSTEM

The scavenging system extends the breathing system all the way to the disposal point. When a scavenging system malfunctions or is misused, positive or negative pressure can be transmitted to the breathing system, with potential harm to the patient.

Measures to prevent these untoward incidents include employing a collapse-proof material in all disposal lines, making the transfer means easy to disconnect, incorporation of positive and negative pressure relief mechanisms in the interface (and regular checking of these for proper functioning), and use of airway pressure monitors (see Chapter 17).

Positive Pressure

Positive pressure in the scavenging system can result from occlusion of the gas disposal assembly tubing or gas-disposal assembly by a wheel of an anesthesia machine (179,275,276), ice (231), insects, and other foreign matter. Another cause is defective components (277). Misassembly of the connection to the exhaust grille (278), and failure to include an opening between the inner and outer tubes of a tube-within-a-tube interface (279) have all been reported.

These malfunctions may not result in a pressure buildup if a positive pressure relief mechanism is incorporated into the interface. However, the positive pressure relief mechanism may be incorrectly assembled, may not open at a low pressure, or may be blocked (280). Obstruction of the transfer means may occur (281) and misconnection of the transfer means to the relief valve on the interface have been reported. The transfer means from a ventilator may be connected to that from an APL valve in the breathing system (282,283). Because these problems are on the patient side of the interface, disconnection of the transfer means from the gas-collecting assembly may be necessary to prevent a dangerous increase in pressure. In one

reported case, kinking of the transfer means caused back pressure to develop in the gas jacket of an extracorporeal oxygenator. This resulted in gas being forced into the blood (284).

Application of subatmospheric pressure to some APL valves can result in a buildup of positive pressure in the breathing system (279). In one reported case, subatmospheric pressure in the scavenging system drew a ventilator relief valve diaphragm to its seat and closed the valve, resulting in a buildup of pressure in the system (285).

Negative Pressure

In systems with an active disposal assembly, there is the danger that subambient pressure will be applied to the breathing system. Monitoring expired volumes (but not airway pressure) may fail to detect a disconnection in the breathing system because the scavenging system may draw a considerable flow of room air through the expiratory pathway (286,287).

Gas can be evacuated from the breathing system if the APL valve in the breathing system allows gas to be drawn through it at a pressure less than that needed to open the negative pressure valve on the interface (288,289). This can be overcome by partially closing the APL valve (290), increasing the fresh gas flow into the breathing system, or lowering the flow in the gas disposal assembly.

A malfunction of the negative pressure relief mechanism may occur. In one case, the valve disc became stuck in the closed position (291). In another, the valve was covered by a plastic bag so that air could not be entrained (292). In still another case, the opening to atmosphere of an open interface was taped over (280). Blockage of the opening to atmosphere as a result of dust and other material have been reported (293). With some scavenging systems that use a central vacuum, a restrictive orifice is incorporated into the vacuum hose fitting to limit the evacuation of gas, regardless of the pressure applied by the central vacuum source (244). Should this orifice be omitted or become damaged, full vacuum would be applied to the interface and the capacity of the negative pressure relief mechanism could be exceeded.

Prevention of these problems include provision of one or more negative relief mechanisms in the interface with an active disposal system (294), adjustment of gas disposal assembly flow to the minimum necessary, and protection of the openings to atmosphere from accidental occlusion with a passive system.

LOSS OF MEANS OF MONITORING

Use of a scavenging system may mask the strong odor of an inhalation anesthetic, delaying recognition of an overdose (281,295). Increasing use of agent monitoring should largely eliminate this problem.

Adding a gas-collecting assembly to an APL valve has the effect of silencing it, thereby removing one means of monitoring a patient's ventilation. The sounds emitted by a mechanical ventilator can be appreciably altered when scavenging lines are attached.

VENTILATOR FUNCTION DISRUPTION

A case has been reported in which negative pressure from the scavenging interface prevented the bellows of a ventilator from collapsing when a disconnection in the breathing system occurred (296). The low airway pressure alarm in the ventilator was not activated.

Monitoring Trace Gases

RATIONALE

Air monitoring is the best indicator of the success of a waste gas control program. It reflects how well leaks and errors in technique are being controlled plus the efficiency of the scavenging and room ventilation systems and documents that low trace levels are being maintained.

Monitoring is necessary because a scavenging system that appears adequate in design may perform inefficiently in use. Sites of gas leakage are diverse, frequently obscure and sometimes inaccessible (269). Even relatively large leaks may be inaudible. Nitrous oxide is odorless and the threshold for smelling potent agents such as halothane varies from 5 to 300 ppm (25,297). Without monitoring, operating room personnel may be unaware that atmospheric contamination is at unacceptable levels. A properly conducted monitoring program provides a constructive method of reminding anesthesia personnel to avoid careless work habits.

Although such a program will increase a healthcare facility's operating expense, it will help to reduce the institution's liability to claims by employees alleging overexposure to waste gases. Also, correction of leakage in nitrous oxide lines will result in a savings to the facility.

IN-HOUSE VERSUS COMMERCIAL LABORATORY (269)

The monitoring program should be directed by an interested and qualified person, preferably from the anesthesia department. Samples may be analyzed either by hospital-based personnel or by outside commercial laboratories. Use of outside laboratories avoids the cost of purchasing, operating, maintaining. and calibrating a gas analyzer. The responsibility for recordkeeping is shared. The chief disadvantage is the delay in reporting results. The precise circumstances of sampling are likely to have been forgotten and the effect of corrective measures cannot be immediately assessed. In addition, analysis of a large number of samples is expensive.

Advantages of in-house analysis include a virtually unlimited number of analyses at modest cost and immediate on-site reporting. Specific leaks can be found quickly and the effectiveness of the repair assessed immediately. An on-site continuous monitor is useful for demonstrating the effects of technique errors on trace gas levels.

A small hospital might periodically lease an instrument or share one with other hospitals in the area rather than purchase its own.

EQUIPMENT FOR DETERMINING TRACE GAS CONCENTRATIONS

Infrared Analyzers (269,298)

Each anesthetic gas has a unique set of absorption peaks in the infrared (IR) spectrum. In an infrared analyzer, a light beam of a certain wavelength is passed through a cell containing the sample to be analyzed. The concentration of the gas can be determined by measuring the amount of light absorbed. These monitors are the most practical for the average hospital because they are reliable, relatively inexpensive, and easy to use. They are very useful for pinpointing of leaks, especially those in unusual locations. They give continuous measurements so that exposed personnel and those responsible for air monitoring are given an immediate reading. When operated on battery power, a number of locations can be sampled quickly. A recording attachment may be helpful.

These instruments are most often used for monitoring nitrous oxide concentrations. Unfortunately, carbon dioxide and water vapor in high concentrations will interfere with the analysis. This can be avoided by sampling 6 to 10 inches away from personnel (268). Analyzers capable of measuring halogenated anesthetics are available but have many technical difficulties; alcohols and other substances in the operating room cause interference (9,22,298).

Dosimeter (269)

Passive dosimeters measure the amount of nitrous oxide that diffuses into a molecular sieve. Analysis (usually by the manufacturer) requires extraction of the nitrous oxide.

Passive dosimeters have many advantages. They can give a time-weighted average concentration for as long as a month. They are convenient to use. They can be made lightweight and compact so that they can be worn for personal sampling.

A variant of the passive dosimeter is the gas cartridge sampler, which is actually a small container that is filled with a sample of operating room air and then sent to the laboratory for analysis.

Active dosimeters depend on energy outside of the absorbing medium to obtain the sample. A pump is used to take in area gases that are then stored in a gas-tight bag in an absorbing medium. The samples are aspirated into an analyzer.

Ionizing Leak Detector (182,299,300)

The ionizing leak detector (leak meter) consists of three components: an electron capture detector housed within a hand piece and fitted with a probe; a control unit that processes the signal from the detector and displays the output on a meter; and a carrier gas supply. The instrument is compact, is relatively inexpensive, is portable, and can be operated on batteries.

It is suitable for measuring low concentrations of halogenated agents. However, there may be interference from other halogenated agents in the area, including antibiotic and skin-protection sprays. It is not useful for nitrous oxide detection. It is somewhat unstable in use, requiring frequent zeroing and recalibration (15,182).

Thermocamera (301-303)

Because nitrous oxide has the ability to absorb IR light, it will absorb the light liberated by a heat screen. An infrared camera with a filter allows visualization of dispersed or leaking nitrous oxide. It is sensitive to 100 ppm or more of nitrous oxide. This is not a quantitative meter and is primarily of use when constructing and evaluating scavenging equipment and in producing educational material.

Oxygen Analyzer

An oxygen monitor can be used to check the scavenging system. Using 100% oxygen the sensor is positioned at the interface where overflow would exit into the room. Any increase indicates that anesthetic gas will be released during normal use.

CO_2 Analyzer

The efficacy of scavenging with an open interface can be checked by analyzing the open end of the reservoir for CO_2 (215). If any of the patient's expired gases overflow, CO_2 will be detected.

SAMPLING METHODS

Instantaneous Sampling

Instantaneous sampling (also called grab, single-shot, periodic, and snatch sampling) is performed by drawing a sample of air into a container and subsequently measuring the trace gas concentration. The container must not adsorb or absorb the contaminant or leak. Nylon bags are the preferred storage container when nitrous oxide levels are measured (304).

This method is relatively inexpensive, quick and simple to perform, and does not involve taking bulky equipment into the operating room, but it has some serious disadvantages. A long interval between sampling and reporting makes it difficult to remember the precise circumstances that were in effect when the sample was taken. The effect of corrective measures cannot be immediately assessed. It is of limited value in determining leak sites and assessing correction of leaks. Another serious disadvantage is that each sample represents the level at one location in a relatively small volume and over a very short time period. Failure to sample in the right place at the right time can produce low-exposure level results that are optimistically misleading (38). Similarly, a report of a high-exposure level may lead to costly corrective action when, in fact, the measured levels were only momentarily high. One investigation concluded that gradients in operating rooms were sufficiently large to invalidate estimation of personnel exposure from instantaneous samples (19). This disadvantage can be decreased by taking multiple samples, but this increases the expense.

The instantaneous sample is probably best employed for analysis of steady-state contamination, i.e., sampling before starting anesthesia for intermediate pressure leaks or when an equilibrium has been achieved. If good techniques are employed and leakage has been controlled, trace gas levels tend to rise in a fluctuating pattern during the early part of an anesthetic, then roughly equilibrate, reaching a level that represents the net effects of leaks, air conditioning flow, inflow gas rate, scavenging efficiency and personnel movement (19). Under these circumstances an instantaneous sample 30 to 45 min after induction is probably a good index of the average trace gas levels (19,204). If poor techniques are employed and/or no attempt has been made to eliminate leakage, pollution levels will vary markedly and instantaneous samples may be quite misleading. If unacceptable high levels are found, one cannot be sure whether the cause is a leak, poor technique, or a fault in the scavenging system.

When an instantaneous sample is taken, it is important to record the date and time of collection, the work practices (breathing system, fresh gas flow rate, use of mask or tracheal tube, use of ventilator, spontaneous or manually controlled ventilation), location of sampling site, and the person administering anesthesia.

Time-Weighted Average Sampling

The toxicity of anesthetics is probably a function of both dose and exposure time. Hence a method that gives an average exposure level during a period of time (an integrated sample) is of interest. Time-weighted average sampling is sometimes called integrated and time-integrated sampling.

Time-weighted average (TWA) samples can be obtained using active dosimetry in which gases are pumped continuously over a period of time into an inert container

(4,22,305,306) or a tube or other device containing a sorbent (307–312).

Passive dosimetry, which depends on diffusion of gas into a molecular sieve, can be used to obtain time-weighted averages (313,314). Small, rugged, lightweight dosimeters (diffusive samplers) are available (262,313,315). They are unobtrusive, easily attached, and require a minimum of maintenance (8). They can be used either as personal or area monitors for periods of up to 40 hr (315). They have been found to be quite accurate (313,315,316). Separate sampling media have to be used for nitrous oxide and the halogenated agents (2). However, more than one halogenated agent can be measured from one sampler.

Other ways of obtaining a time-weighted average are to average the results of many instantaneous samples, average the concentrations measured at equal time intervals throughout the recorded tracing of a continuous analyzer, and integrate the output of a continuous analyzer (317).

By eliminating errors due to temporal fluctuations, time-weighted average sampling reflects personnel exposure better than instantaneous sampling. It requires only a modest capital investment, and there is a considerable savings of time and labor compared with taking and analyzing multiple instantaneous samples.

There are several disadvantages to this method. One is that it does not help in leak detection or improving work techniques. Delayed results make it difficult to correlate with activities at the time of collection. If concentrations in excess of those recommended are found, one cannot tell whether the problem is technique errors, leaks, or inadequate scavenging.

Continuous

Continuous (also called direct-reading and real-time) monitoring is carried out using an infrared analyzer or leak meter. Use of a battery-powered instrument allows for easy movement within and between rooms.

If a writer is attached and the analyzer is run over a period of time, a time-weighted average sample is obtained (317).

A continuous monitor can be used to detect leaks (by probing about the machine, hoses, wall sockets, etc.) and to determine if a leak has been reduced or eliminated. Furthermore, a continuous analyzer operated while anesthesia is being administered can be used to demonstrate the effects of improper work habits on trace levels and the improvement from modifying those practices.

The convenience and immediate feedback of continuous monitoring are distinct advantages over instantaneous or time-weighted average sampling. When high readings are obtained the causes can usually be determined immediately and corrective measures taken.

One disadvantage of continuous monitors is that the time and expense required to maintain one may make it unsatisfactory for a small hospital. In such circumstances, several hospitals might consider sharing an instrument or a manufacturer's service representative might use one during routine quarterly maintenance calls. This method tends to disrupt the operating room routine more than instantaneous or time-weighted average sampling. Finally, rapidly changing concentrations are difficult to interpret in terms of personnel exposure unless integration over time is employed.

End-Tidal Sampling (10,14,19,25,319)

End-tidal samples of gases may be taken from exposed personnel after a period of exposure. With high levels of agents in the atmosphere, some agent may be detectable in the morning from the previous day's exposure (10,14,33,319–321). End-tidal samples are inherently time weighted and show less scatter than time-weighted average samples (322). This method is most suitable for potent halogenated agents. Nitrous oxide is so rapidly absorbed and excreted that its level in end-tidal gas reflects only the most recent exposure of the subject.

The main disadvantage is that collecting end-tidal samples may be disruptive to operating room personnel performing their duties.

Blood or Urine Sampling (10,11,14,25, 321,323)

Samples of venous blood can be drawn from exposed personnel at the end of an exposure period and analyzed. Urinary nitrous oxide has been shown to be a good monitor of the agent in the blood (324,325).

In personnel exposed to high concentrations of potent agents, a detectable amount may be present in the blood or urine in the morning from the previous day's exposure (14,321).

AGENTS TO BE MONITORED

Ideally, all gases employed in the conduct of an anesthetic should be measured. Analyzers are available that can scan the infrared spectrum and are programmable to distinguish individual inhalational agents. Likewise, mass spectrometry and gas chromatography can measure all agents. However, it is simpler to monitor a single gas. The NIOSH criteria document (247) does not recommend monitoring of all anesthetic agents but only the one most frequently used.

Nitrous Oxide

Many people believe that nitrous oxide is the most logical agent to monitor because it is administered in higher concentrations than other agents, is easy to measure, and is more likely to be subject to occult leakage than potent agents (268).

Because nitrous oxide and other agents are not separated by buoyancy effects (15,182), they will be present in a room in the same ratio in which they are introduced. Because of this, many people contend that nitrous oxide can serve as a tracer of other agents administered with it to a degree of accuracy sufficient for routine appraisal of occupational exposure (326). This tracer concept works best under steady-state conditions and low equipment leakage. It does not work well when a vaporizer is being filled or drained, during cardiopulmonary bypass, during induction of or recovery from anesthesia, or when there is a nitrous oxide leak or a leak in a vaporizer.

Potent Agents

Monitoring of other agents can be worthwhile (327,338). Volatile halogenated agents can leak independently of nitrous oxide. Analyzers that measure potent agents are more expensive than those that measure only nitrous oxide (269).

SITES TO BE MONITORED

Monitoring should be scheduled so that the work of each anesthesia person and of each operating room is checked while using a mask and a tracheal tube and while using a ventilator. Monitoring should also be performed during spontaneous, manually assisted, and manually controlled ventilation. The results of the monitoring should be analyzed and discussed with all parties concerned.

Personal Monitoring

Sampling the zone of exposed personnel is usually considered the preferred method. Anesthesia personnel are considered the most important to monitor, because they usually are exposed to higher concentrations than other operating room personnel (329) and are more likely to remain in the room for the entire duration of anesthesia administration.

Passive dosimeters can be attached to the person's clothing and worn for prolonged periods. Sampling directly in the pathway of the subject's expired air must be avoided if measurement of nitrous oxide by infrared analysis is used.

Area (Room) Sampling

The exhaust grille of the air-conditioning system or the open door will be representative of average personnel exposure if gases are evenly distributed in the room. A total of 15 or more air exchanges per hour are sufficient to produce near homogeneity of anesthetic concentrations in all locations except those close to the source of leakage (15,269,330). At lower exchange rates, mixing may not be complete and localized areas of high concentrations (hot spots) and low concentration (cold spots) may occur. Area sampling may be less disruptive to the operating room routine than personal monitoring.

Postanesthesia Care Units

One study measured concentrations 24 inches over the patient's head (34). A more elaborate method is to take samples 50 cm above the patient's thorax, at the foot end of the bed, and 2 m from the foot end of the bed, all at 180 cm above floor level (21), and multiply these concentrations by how long personnel remained in the different areas. It is suggested that concentrations be measured during the "peak load period" when there are a maximum number of patients exhaling gases.

FREQUENCY OF MONITORING

At the initiation of a waste gas control program, frequent monitoring under actual working conditions will be necessary. As experience is gained and equipment is maintained leak tight, the frequency can be decreased. However, whenever concentrations higher than acceptable are found, new equipment is installed, or old equipment is modified, monitoring should be repeated.

The following have been suggested (38):

1. An annual comprehensive survey in which exposure levels are measured, leaks detected and corrected, and time-weighted average exposure levels are calculated or measured.
2. Quarterly follow-up with a less-detailed survey; if there appears to be a problem, a comprehensive survey should be performed to determine causes and assess corrective actions.
3. A repeat comprehensive survey in the

event of major changes to the ventilation system, anesthesia equipment, or scavenging systems.

Time-weighted average monitoring of each member of the staff for a short period, such as a week, repeated on a 6-month basis also has been suggested (22).

Role of the Federal Government (38,331,332)

In 1970 the U.S. Congress passed the Occupational Safety and Health Act. It created two separate executive-branch agencies to carry out the provisions of the act: the National Institute for Occupational Safety and Health (NIOSH), an agency with the Centers for Disease Control and Prevention under the Department of Health and Human Services, and the Occupational Safety and Health Administration (OSHA), under the Department of Labor.

OSHA is responsible for enacting job safety and health standards, establishing reporting and recordkeeping procedures, inspecting workplaces, and enforcing the requirements of the act using citations and fines.

NIOSH is responsible for conducting and funding research and education and for preparing criteria documents to be used for the development of standards. Criteria documents prepared by NIOSH are transmitted to the secretary of labor for review by the OSHA staff.

Such a criteria document on trace gases was published and transmitted to OSHA in 1977 (247). The following are important aspects of this document.

1. Although it was maintained that a safe level of exposure to waste anesthetic gases could not be defined, maximum concentrations to which a worker in the operating room should be exposed were recommended. For halogenated agents used alone this was 2 ppm time-weighted average. For nitrous oxide alone, a time-weighted average

exposure limit of 25 ppm was recommended. When halogenated agents are used in combination with nitrous oxide the recommended limits were 25 ppm nitrous oxide and 0.5 ppm of the halogenated agent. For dental facilities a level of 50 ppm nitrous oxide was recommended. The Ad Hoc Committee of the American Society of Anesthesiologists has suggested that less than 180 ppm nitrous oxide is satisfactory with mask techniques (204). The American Conference on Governmental Industrial Hygienists has suggested limits for some halogenated agents that are higher than those proposed by NIOSH (38).

The Swedish Occupational Health Standards specify that maximum exposure as a time-weighted average over 8 hr must not exceed 100 ppm for nitrous oxide, 5 ppm for halothane, and 10 ppm for enflurane and isoflurane (333). Norway, Denmark, and Italy have set a maximum limit of TWA of 100 ppm for nitrous oxide (334–336), while in the Netherlands it is 25 ppm (385). For halothane the limits are 5 ppm in Germany and 2.5 ppm in the Commonwealth of Independent States (8).

2. Monitoring of exposure levels is recommended in all areas with potential for worker exposure on a quarterly basis and following changes to ventilation systems, anesthetic equipment, or scavenging techniques. Breathing zone or immediate work area samples are most desirable.

3. Results of monitoring and corrective measures are to be maintained and retained for 20 years.

4. Recommendations were made regarding scavenging, ventilation systems, leak testing, and work practices aimed at minimizing employee exposure.

5. Medical surveillance, including comprehensive employee preplacement medical and occupational histories, annual updating of employee medical histories and preplacement, and annual physical examinations of employees exposed to waste anesthetic gases is recommended.

6. Employees are to be informed on as-

signment and at least yearly thereafter of the possible health effects of exposure to trace anesthetics, especially possible effects on reproduction. Appropriate signs and labeling were recommended.

7. Any abnormal outcome of the pregnancies of employees or of their spouses must be documented as part of the employees medical record.

NIOSH participation came to a halt after the transmittal of this document to OSHA. To promulgate this as a standard, OSHA would have to go through an extensive rulemaking procedure, including a public comment period. This has not occurred to date.

Joint Commission on the Accreditation of Healthcare Organizations

The Joint Commission on Accreditation of Healthcare Organizations in 1983 recommended, but did not require, that each anesthesia machine be equipped with a gas-scavenging device. It now recommends, but does not yet require, that monitoring be performed.

Medicolegal Considerations (337)

Because the NIOSH document does not constitute a promulgated OSHA standard, employers are not obligated to comply with its recommendations. However, the general duty clause of the 1970 act gives OSHA the authority to inspect workplaces to determine whether employers are providing a workplace free from hazards, even in the absence of a relevant standard.

The act gives each employee the right to request an OSHA inspection if the employee believes he or she is in imminent danger from a hazard or OSHA standards are being violated. Several inspections in response to employee complaints were carried out in the 1970s. Fines and citations were issued because employees were exposed to concentrations of nitrous oxide in excess of the NIOSH recommended levels or because exposure was not reduced to the lowest feasible level (332,338).

The ASA legal counsel has advised that it is within the right of an employer to refuse to permit an OSHA representative to enter the premises of the hospital or operating room unless such individual has either a search warrant or a court order compelling the inspection. OSHA would need to seek a search warrant from a federal court and show probable cause for making an inspection (338). If faced with a visit from an OSHA representative, obtaining legal counsel is advisable. Failure to demand a search warrant or court order normally would constitute a waiver of any later right to object to the validity of an inspection.

All states have workers' compensation laws so that individuals suffering occupational diseases can collect benefits, irrespective of whether or not the employer's negligence caused the disease. It is possible that a workers' compensation case could arise from an operating room employee suffering from one of the problems described in the first section of this chapter, provided the employee could show that the illness was work connected and that employment in the operating room subjected him or her to special risk in excess of those experienced by the general public.

In most states workers' compensation laws preclude private lawsuits by an employee against his or her employer. However, in addition to making a claim for workers' compensation, an employee can bring a civil suit for damages against a third party (such as an anesthesiologist) whom the employee claims caused injury.

REFERENCES

1. Spence AA. Environmental pollution by inhalation anaesthetics. Br J Anaesth 1987;59:96–103.
2. Ilsley AH, Plummer JL, Runciman WB, Cousins MJ. Anaesthetic gas analysers for vaporiser calibration, patient circuit monitoring and determi-

nation of environmental waste anaesthetic gas levels. Anaesth Intensive Care 1988;16:35–37.
3. Cohen EN. Anesthetic exposure in the workplace. Littleton, MA: PSG, 1980.
4. Davenport HT, Halsey MJ, Wardley-Smith FB, Wright BM. Measurement and reduction of occupational exposure to inhaled anaesthetics. Br Med J 1976;2:1219–1221.
5. Davenport HT, Halsey MJ, Wardley-Smith B, Bateman PE. Occupational exposure to anaesthetics in 20 hospitals. Anaesthesia 1980;35:354–359.
6. DeZotti R, Negro C, Gobbato F. Results of hepatic and hemopoietic controls in hospital personnel exposed to waste anesthetic gases. Int Arch Occup Environ Health 1983;52:33–41.
7. Flowerdew RMM, Brummitt WM. Reduction of nitrous oxide contamination in a paediatric hospital. Can Anaesth Soc J 1979;26:370–374.
8. Gardner RJ. Inhalation anaesthetics—exposure and control: a statistical comparison of personal exposures in operating theatres with and without anaesthetic gas scavenging. Ann Occup Hyg 1989;33:159–173.
9. Halliday MM, Carter KB, Davis PD, MacDonald I, Collins L, McCreaddie G. Survey of operating room pollution with an N.H.S. district. Lancet 1979;1:1230–1232.
10. Korttila K, Pfaffli P, Ertama P. Residual nitrous oxide in operating room personnel. Acta Anaesthesiol Scand 1978;22:635–639.
11. Krapez JR, Saloojee Y, Hinds CJ, Hackett GH, Cole PV. Blood concentrations of nitrous oxide in theatre personnel. Br J Anaesth 1980;52:1143–1148.
12. Linde HW, Bruce DL. Occupational exposure of anesthetists to halothane, nitrous oxide and radiation. Anesthesiology 1969;30:363–368.
13. Nikki P, Pfaffli K, Ahlman K, Ralli R. Chronic exposure to anaesthetic gases in the operating theatre and recovery room. Ann Clin Res 1972;4:266–272.
14. Pfaffli P, Nikki P, Ahlman K. Halothane and nitrous oxide in end-tidal air and venous blood of surgical personnel. Ann Clin Res 1972;4:273–277.
15. Piziali RL, Whitcher C, Sher R, Moffat RJ. Distribution of waste anesthetic gases in the operating room air. Anesthesiology 1976;45:487–494.
16. Sass-Kortsak AM, Wheeler IP, Purdham JT. Exposure of operating room personnel to anaesthetic agents. An examination of the effectiveness of scavenging systems and the importance of maintenance programs. Can Anaesth Soc J 1981;28:22–28.
17. Trefisan A, Gori GP. Biological monitoring of nitrous oxide exposure in surgical areas. Am J Ind Med 1990;17:357–362.

18. Bernow J, Bjordal J, Wiklund KE. Pollution of delivery ward air by nitrous oxide. Effects of various modes of room ventilation, excess and close scavenging. Acta Anaesthesiol Scand 1984;28:119–123.

19. Beynen FM, Knopp TJ, Rehder K. Nitrous oxide exposure in the operating room. Anesth Analg 1978;57:216–223.

20. Virtue RW, Escobar A, Modell J. Nitrous oxide levels in operating room air with various gas flows. Can Anaesth Soc J 1979;26:313–318.

21. Berner O. Concentration and elimination of anaesthetic gases in recovery rooms. Acta Anaesthesiol Scand 1978;22:55–57.

22. Campbell D, Davis PD, Halliday MM, MacDonald I. Comparison of personal pollution monitoring techniques for use in the operating room. Br J Anaesth 1980;52:885–892.

23. Gelbicova-Ruzickova J, Novak J, Janak J. Application of the method of chromatographic equilibration to air pollution studies. The determination of minute amounts of halothane in the atmosphere of an operating theatre. J Chromatogr 1972;64:15–23.

24. Gothe CZ, Ovrum P, Hallen B. Exposure to anesthetic gases and ethanol during work in operating rooms. Scand J Work Environ Health 1976;2:96–106.

25. Hallen B, Ehrner-Samuel H, Thomason M. Measurements of halothane in the atmosphere of an operating theatre and in expired air and blood of the personnel during routine anaesthetic work. Acta Anaesthesiol Scand 1970;14:17–27.

26. Korttila K, Pfaffli P, Linnoila M, Blomgren E, Hanninen H, Hakkinen S. Operating room nurses' psychomotor and driving skills after occupational exposure to halothane and nitrous oxide. Acta Anaesthesiol Scand 1978;22:33–39.

27. Thompson JM, Barratt RS, Hutton P, Robinson JS, Belcher R, Stephen WI. Ambient air contamination in a dental outpatient theatre. Br J Anaesth 1979;51:845–855.

28. Mehta S, Cole WJ, Chari J, Lewin K. Operating room air pollution. influence of anaesthetic circuit, vapour concentration, gas flow and ventilation. Can Anaesth Soc J 1975;22:265–274.

29. Nicholson JA, Sada T, Aldrete JA. Residual halothane: patient and personnel exposure. Anesth Analg 1975;54:449–454.

30. Ramanthan PS, Srivastava OP, Venkateswarlu CH, Walvekar AP. Study of anaesthetic vapour concentrations in operation theatres by gas chromatography. Indian J Med Res 1978;67:656–661.

31. Usubiaga L, Aldrete JA, Fiserova-Bergerova V. Influence of gas flows and operating room ventilation on the daily exposure of anesthetists to halothane. Anesth Analg 1972;51:968–974.

32. Yoganathan S, Johnston IG, Parnell CJ, Houghton IT, Restall J. Determination of contamination of a chemical warfare-proof operating theatre with volatile anaesthetic agents and assessment of anaesthetic gas scavenging systems. Br J Anaesth 1991;67:614–617.

33. Whitcher CE, Cohen EN, Trudell JR. Chronic exposure to anesthetic gases in the operating room. Anesthesiology 1971;35:348–353.

34. Bruce DL, Linde HW. Halothane content in recovery room air. Anesthesiology 1972;36:517–518.

35. Corbett TH. Cancer and congenital anomalies associated with anesthetics. Ann N Y Acad Sci 1976;271:58–66.

36. Spence AA, Knill-Jones RP. Is there a health hazard in anaesthetic practice? Br J Anaesth 1978;50:713–719.

37. Ferstandig LL. Trace concentrations of anesthetic gases. Acta Anaesthesiol Scand 1982;75:38–43.

38. Anonymous. Personnel exposure to waste anesthetic gases. Health Devices 1983;12:169–177.

39. Mazze RI, Lecky JH. The health of operating room personnel. Anesthesiology 1985;62:226–228.

40. Tannenbaum TN, Goldberg RJ. Exposure to anesthetic gases and reproductive outcome. J Occup Med 1985;27:659–668.

41. Walts LF, Forsythe AB, Moore G. Critique. Occupational disease among operating room personnel. Anesthesiology 1975;42:608–611.

42. Ferstandig LL. Trace concentrations of anesthetic gases. a critical review of their disease potential. Anesth Analg 1978;57:328–345.

43. Ad Hoc Committee on the Effects of Trace Anesthetics on the Health of Operating Room Personnel, American Society of Anesthesiologists. Occupational disease among operating room personnel: a national study. Anesthesiology 1974;41:321–340.

44. Cohen EN, Bellville JW, Brown BW. Anesthesia, pregnancy and miscarriage: a study of operating room nurses and anesthetists. Anesthesiology 1971;35:343–347.

45. Cohen EN, Brown BW, Wu ML, et al. Occupational disease in dentistry and chronic exposure to trace anesthetic gases. J Am Dent Assoc 1980;10:21–31.

46. Knill-Jones RP, Rodrigues LV, Moir DD, Spence AA. Anaesthetic practice and pregnancy. Lancet 1972;1:1326–1328.

47. Knill-Jones RP, Newman BJ, Spence AA. Anaesthesia practice and pregnancy. Lancet 1975;2:807–809.

48. Mirakhur RK, Badve AV. Pregnancy and anaesthetic practice in India. Anaesthesia 1975;30:18–22.

49. Rosenberg P, Kirves A. Miscarriages among operating theatre staff. Acta Anaesthesiol Scand Suppl 1973;53:37–42.

50. Tomlin PJ. Health problems of anaesthetists and their families in the West Midlands. Br Med J 1979;1:779–784.

51. Ferstandig LL. Trace concentrations of anesthetics are not proved health hazards. In: Eckenhoff JE, ed. Controversy in anesthesiology. Philadelphia: WB Saunders, 1979:56–69.

52. Rushton DI. Anaesthetics and abortions. 1976; Lancet 2:141.

53. Klebanoff MA, Shiono PH, Rhoads GG. Spontaneous and induced abortion among resident physicians. JAMA 1991;265:2821–2825.

54. Axelsson G, Rylander R. Exposure to anaesthetic gases and spontaneous abortion: response bias in a postal questionnaire study. Int J Epidemiol 1982;11:250–256.

55. Ericson A, Kallen B. Survey of infants born in 1973–1975 to Swedish women working in operating rooms during their pregnancies. Anesth Analg 1979;58:302–305.

56. Ericson HA, Kallen AJB. Hospitalization for miscarriage and delivery outcome among Swedish nurses working in operating rooms 1973–1978. Anesth Analg 1985;64:981–988.

57. Hemminki K, Kyyronen P, Lindbohm M. Spontaneous abortions and malformations in the offspring of nurses exposed to anaesthetic gases, cytostatic drugs, and other potential hazards in hospitals, based on registered information of outcome. J Epidemiol Community Health 1985;39:141–147.

58. Lauwerys R, Siddons M, Misson CB, et al. Anaesthetic health hazards among Belgian nurses and physicians. Int Arch Occup Environ Health 1981;48:195–203.

59. Pharoah POD, Alberman E, Doyle P. Outcome of pregnancy among women in anaesthetic practice. Lancet 1977;1:34–36.

60. Rosenberg PH, Vanttinen H. Occupational hazards to reproduction and health in anaesthetists and paediatricians. Acta Anaesthesiol Scand 1978;22:202–207.

61. Buring JE, Hennekens CH, Mayrent SL, Rosner B, Greenberg ER, Colton T. Health experiences of operating room personnel. Anesthesiology 1985;62:325–330.

62. Mazze RI. Fertility, reproduction, and postnatal survival in mice chronically exposed to isoflurane. Anesthesiology 1985;63:663–667.

63. Mazze RI, Fujinaga M, Rice SA, Harris SB, Baden JM. Reproductive and teratogenic effects of nitrous oxide, halothane, isoflurane, and enflurane in Sprague-Dawley rats. Anesthesiology 1986; 64:339–344.

64. Wharton RS, Mazze RI, Wilson AI. Reproduction and fetal development in mice chronically exposed to enflurane. Anesthesiology 1981;54:505–510.

65. Strout CD, Nahrwold ML, Taylor MD, Zagon IS. Effects of subanesthetic concentrations of enflurane on rat pregnancy and early development. Environ Heath Perspect 1977;21:211–214.

66. Halsey MJ, Green CJ, Monk SJ, Dore C, Knight JF, Luff NP. Maternal and paternal chronic exposure to enflurane and halothane. fetal and histological changes in the rat. Br J Anaesth 1981;53:203–215.

67. Lansdown ABG, Pope WDB, Halsey MJ, Bateman PE. Analysis of fetal development in rats following maternal exposure to subanesthetic concentrations of halothane. Teratology 1976;13:299–303.

68. Pope WDB, Halsey MJ, Phil HD, Lansdown ABG, Simmonds A, Bateman PE. Fetotoxicity in rats following chronic exposure to halothane, nitrous oxide, or methoxyflurane. Anesthesiology 1978;48:11–16.

69. Vieira E, Cleaton-Jones P, Austin JC, Moyes DG, Shaw R. Effects of low concentrations of nitrous oxide on rat fetuses. Anesth Analg 1980;59:175–177.

70. Vieira E, Cleaton-Jones P, Moyes D. Effects of low intermittent concentrations of nitrous oxide on the developing rat fetus. Br J Anaesth 1983;55:67–69.

71. Fujinaga M, Baden JM, Yhap EO, Mazze RI. Reproductive and teratogenic effects of nitrous oxide, isoflurane, and their combination in Sprague-Dawley rats. Anesthesiology 1987;67:960–964.

72. Askrog VF, Harvald B. Teratogen effekt of inhalatiosanaestetika. Nord Med 1970;83:498–500.

73. Cohen EN, Brown BW, Bruce DL, et al. A survey of anesthetic health hazards among dentists. J Am Dent Assoc 1975;90:1291–1296.

74. Wyrobek AJ, Brodsky J, Gordon L, Moore DH, Watchmaker G, Cohen EN. Sperm studies in anesthesiologists. Anesthesiology 1981;55:527–532.

75. Baden JM, Land PC, Egbert B, Kelley M, Mazze RI. Lack of toxicity of enflurane on male reproductive organs in mice. Anesth Analg 1982;61:19–22.

76. Coate WB, Kapp RW Jr., Lewis TR. Chronic exposure to low concentrations of halothane-nitrous oxide: reproductive and cytogenetic effects in the rat. Anesthesiology 1979;50:310–318.

77. Land PC, Owen EL, Linde HW. Morphologic changes in mouse spermatozoa after exposure to inhalational anesthetics during early spermatogenesis. Anesthesiology 1981;54:53–56.

78. Kundomal YR, Baden JM. Inhaled anaesthetics have no effect on fertility in Drosophila melanogaster. Br J Anaesth 1985;57:900–903.

79. Wharton RS, Mazze RI, Baden JM, Hitt BA, Dooley JR. Fertility, reproduction and postnatal survival in mice chronically exposed to halothane. Anesthesiology 1978;48:167–174.

80. Kennedy GL Jr., Smith SH, Keplinger ML, Calandra JC. Reproductive and teratologic studies with halothane. Toxicol Appl Pharmacol 1976;35:467–474.

81. Mazze RI, Wilson AI, Rice SA, Baden JM. Reproduction and fetal development in mice chronically exposed to nitrous oxide. Teratology 1982;26:11–16.

82. Kripke BJ, Kelman AD, Shah NK, Balogh K, Handler AH. Testicular reaction to prolonged exposure to nitrous oxide. Anesthesiology 1976;44:104–113.

83. Vieira E, Cleaton-Jones P, Moyes D. Effects of intermittent .5% nitrous oxide/air (v/v) on the fertility of male rats and the post–natal growth of their offspring. Anaesthesia 1983;38:319–323.

84. Corbett TH, Cornell RG, Endres JL, Leiding K. Birth defects among children of nurse-anesthetists. Anesthesiology 1974;41:341–344.

85. Cote CJ. Birth defects among infants of nurse anesthetists. Anesthesiology 1975;42:514–515.

86. Rosenberg PH, Kallio H. Operating-theatre gas pollution and chromosomes. Lancet 1977;2:452–453.

87. Green CJ, Monk SJ, Knight JF, Dore C, Luff NP, Halsey MJ. Chronic exposure of rats to enflurane 200 ppm: no evidence of toxicity or teratogenicity. Br J Anaesth 1982;54:1097–1104.

88. Pope WDB, Halsey MJ, Lansdown ABG, Bateman PE. Lack of teratogenic dangers with halothane. Acta Anaesthesiol Belg 1975;26 (suppl):169–173.

89. Wharton RS, Wilson AI, Mazze RI, Baden JM, Rice SA. Fetal morphology in mice exposed to halothane. Anesthesiology 1979;51:532–537.

90. Levin ED, Bowman RE. Behavioral effects of chronic exposure to low concentrations of halothane during development in rats. Anesth Analg 1986;65:653–659.

91. Quimby KL, Katz J, Bowman RE. Behavioral consequences in rats from chronic exposure to 10 ppm halothane during early development. Anesth Analg 1975;54:628–633.

92. Baden JM, Rice SA, Serra M, Kelley M, Mazze R. Thymidine and methionine syntheses in pregnant rats exposed to nitrous oxide. Anesth Analg 1983;62:738–741.

93. Gamberale F, Svensson G. The effect of anesthetic gases on the psychomotor and perceptual functions of anesthetic nurses. Work Environ Health 1974;11:108–113.

94. Gambill AF, McCallum RN, Henrichs TF. Psychomotor performance following exposure to trace concentrations of inhalation anesthetics. Anesth Analg 1979;58:475–482.

95. Stollery BT, Broadbent DE, Lee WR, Keen RI, Healy TEJ, Beatty P. Mood and cognitive functions in anaesthetists working in actively scavenged operating theatres. Br J Anaesth

96. Ayer WA, Russell EA, Ballinger ME, Muller T. Failure to demonstrate psychomotor effects of nitrous oxide oxygen exposure in dental assistants. Anes Prog 1978;25:186–187.

97. Bruce DL, Bach MJ. Psychological studies of human performance as affected by traces of enflurane and nitrous oxide. Anesthesiology 1975;42:194–196.

98. Bruce DL, Bach MJ, Arbit J. Trace anesthetic effects on perceptual cognitive and motor skills. Anesthesiology 1974;40:453–458.

99. Bruce DL, Bach MJ. Effects of trace anaesthetic gases on behavioural performance of volunteers. Br J Anaesth 1976;48:871–875.

100. Smith G, Shirley AW. Failure to demonstrate effect of trace concentrations of nitrous oxide and halothane on psychomotor performance. Br J Anaesth 1977;49:65–70.

101. Cook TL, Smith M, Winter PM, Starkweather JA, Eger EI. Effect of subanesthetic concentrations of enflurane and halothane on human behavior. Anesth Analg 1978;57:434–440.

102. Cook TL, Smith M, Starkweather JA, Winter PM, Eger EI. Behavioral effects of trace and subanesthetic halothane and nitrous oxide in man. Anesthesiology 1978;49:419–424.

103. Frankhuizen JL, Vlek CAJ, Burm AGL, Rejger V. Failure to replicate negative effects of trace anaesthetics on mental performance. Br J Anaesth 1978;50:229–234.

104. Allison RH, Shirley AW, Smith G. Threshold concentration of nitrous oxide affecting psychomotor performance. Br J Anaesth 1979;51:177–180.

105. Quimby KL, Aschkenase LJ, Bowman RE, Katz J, Chang LW. Enduring learning deficits and cerebral synaptic malformation from exposure to 10 ppm of halothane per million. Science 1974;185:625–627.

106. Smith G, Shirley AW. A review of the effects of trace concentrations of anaesthetics on performance. Br J Anaesth 1978;50:701–712.

107. Bruce DL, Eide KA, Smith NJ. A prospective survey of anesthesiologist mortality: 1967–1971. Anesthesiology 1974;41:71–74.

108. Doll R, Peto R. Mortality among doctors in different occupations. Br Med J 1977;1:1433–1436.

109. Lew EA. Mortality experience among anesthesiologists: 1954–1976. Anesthesiology 1979;51:195–199.

110. Linde HW, Mesnick PS, Smith NJ. Causes of

death among anesthesiologists: 1930–1946. Anesth Analg 1981;60:1–7.

111. Baden JM, Mazze RI, Wharton RS, Rice SA, Kosek JC. Carcinogenicity of halothane in Swiss/ICR mice. Anesthesiology 1979;51:20–26.

112. Eger EI II, White AE, Brown CL, Biava CG, Corbett TH, Stevens WC. A test of the carcinogenicity of enflurane, isoflurane, halothane, methoxyflurane and nitrous oxide in mice. Anesth Analg 1978;57:678–694.

113. Baden JM, Egbert B, Mazze RI. Carcinogen bioassay of enflurane in mice. Anesthesiology 1982;56:9–13.

114. Baden JM, Kundomal YR, Mazze RI, Kosek JC. Carcinogen bioassay of isoflurane in mice. Anesthesiology 1988;69:750–753.

115. Baden JM, Kundomal YR, Luttropp ME, Mazze RI, Kosek JC. Carcinogen bioassay of nitrous oxide in mice. Anesthesiology 1986;64:747–750.

116. Coate WB, Ulland BM, Lewis TR. Chronic exposure to low concentrations of halothane-nitrous oxide. Anesthesiology 1979;50:306–309.

117. Baden JM, Brinkenhoff M, Wharton RS, Hitt BA, Simmon VF, Mazze RI. Mutagenicity of volatile anesthetics: halothane. Anesthesiology 1976; 45:311–318.

118. McCoy EC, Hankel R, Rosenkranz HS, Giuffrida JG, Bizzari DV. Detection of mutagenic activity in the urines of anesthesiologists: a preliminary report. Environ Health Perspect 1977;21:221–223.

119. Baden JM, Kelley M, Cheung A, Mortelmans K. Lack of mutagens in urines of operating room personnel. Anesthesiology 1980;53:195–198.

120. Husum B, Wulf HC. Sister chromatid exchanges in lymphocytes in operating room personnel. Acta Anaesthesiol Scand 1980;24:22–24.

121. Husum B, Wulf HC. Niebuhr E. Monitoring of sister chromatid exchanges in lymphocytes of nurse-anesthetists. Anesthesiology 1985;62:475–479.

122. Holmberg K, Lambert B, Lindsten J, Soderhall S. DNA and chromosome alterations in lymphocytes of operating room personnel and in patients before and after inhalation anaesthesia. Acta Anaesthesiol Scand 1982;26:531–539.

123. Natarajan D, Santhiya ST. Cytogenetic damage in operation theatre personnel. Anaesthesia 1990; 54:574–577.

124. White AE, Takehisa S, Eger EI, Wolff S, Stevens WC. Sister chromatid exchanges induced by inhaled anesthetics. Anesthesiology 1979;50:426–430.

125. Waskell L. Lack of mutagenicity of two possible metabolites of halothane. Anesthesiology 1979;50:9–12.

126. Waskell L. A study of the mutagenicity of anesthetics and their metabolites. Mutat Res 1978; 57:141–153.

127. Sturrock J. Lack of mutagenic effect of halothane or chloroform on cultured cells using the azaguanine test system. Br J Anaesth 1977;49:207–210.

128. Basler A, Rohrborn G. Lack of mutagenic effects of halothane in mammals in vivo. Anesthesiology 1981;55:143–147.

129. Baden JM, Kundomal YR. Mutagenicity of the combination of a volatile anaesthetic and nitrous oxide. Br J Anaesth 1987;59:772–775.

130. Kramers PGN, Burm AGL. Mutagenicity studies with halothane in *Drosophila melanogaster.* Anesthesiology 1979;50:510–513.

131. Edmunds HN, Baden JM, Simmon VF. Mutagenicity studies with volatile metabolites of halothane. Anesthesiology 1979;51:424–429.

132. Garro AJ, Phillips RA. Mutagenicity of the halogenated olefin, 2-bromo-2-chloro-1,1-difluoroethylene, a presumed metabolite of the inhalation anesthetic halothane. Environ Health Perspect 1977;21:65–69.

133. Sachdev K, Cohen EN, Simmon VF. Genotoxic and mutagenic assays of halothane metabolites in *Bacillus subtilis* and *Salmonella typhimurium.* Anesthesiology 1980;53:31–39.

134. Sturrock JE. No mutagenic effect of enflurane on cultured cells. Br J Anaesth 1977;49:777–779.

135. Baden JM, Kelley M, Wharton RS, Hitt BA, Simmon VF, Mazze RI. Mutagenicity of halogenated ether anesthetics. Anesthesiology 1977;46:346–350.

136. Baden JM, Kelley M, Mazze RI, Simmon VF. Mutagenicity of inhalation anesthetics: trichlorethylene, divinyl ether, nitrous oxide, and cyclopropane. Br J Anaesth 1979;51:417–421.

137. Knill-Jones RP. Comparative risk of hepatitis in doctors working within hospitals and outside hospitals. Digestion 1974;10:359–360.

138. Nunn JF, Sharer N, Royston D, Watts WE, Purkiss P, Worth HG. Serum methionine and hepatic enzyme activity in anaesthetists exposed to nitrous oxide. Br J Anaesth 1982;54:593–597.

139. Belfrage S, Ahlgren I, Axelson S. Halothane hepatitis in an anaesthetist. Lancet 1966;2:1466–1467.

140. Johnston CI, Mendelsohn F. Halothane hepatitis in a laboratory technician. Aust N Z J Med 1971;2:171–173.

141. Klatskin G, Kimberg DV. Recurrent hepatitis attributable to halothane sensitization in an anesthetist. N Engl J Med 1969;280:515–522.

142. Lund I, Skulberg A, Helle I. Occupation hazard of halothane. Lancet 1974;2:528.

143. Ghoneim MM, Delle M, Wilson WR, Ambro JJ. Alteration of warfarin kinetics in man associated with exposure to an operating-room environment. Anesthesiology 1975;43:333–336.

144. Harman AW, Russell WJ, Frewin DB, Priestly BG. Altered drug metabolism in anaesthetists ex-

posed to volatile anaesthetic agents. Anaesth Intensive Care 1978;6:210–214.

145. Plummer JL, Hall P de la M, Jenner MA, Ilsley AH, Cousins MJ. Effects of chronic inhalation of halothane, enflurane, or isoflurane in rats. Br J Anaesth 1986;58:517–523.

146. Plummer JL, Hall P de la M, Cousins MJ, Bastin FN, Ilsley AH. Hepatic injury in rats due to prolonged sub-anaesthetic halothane exposure. Acta Pharmacol Toxicol 1983;53:16–22.

147. Clark GC, Kesterson JW, Coombs DW, Cherry CP, Prentice DE, Kohn FE. Comparative effects of repeated and prolonged inhalation exposure of beagle dogs and cynomolgus monkeys to anaesthetic and subanaesthetic concentrations of enflurane and halothane. Acta Anaesthesiol Scand Suppl 1979;71:1–11.

148. Nunn JF. Clinical aspects of the interaction between nitrous oxide and vitamin B_{12}. Br J Anaesth 1987;59:3–13.

149. Salo M, Rajamaki A, Nikoskelainen, J. Absence of signs of vitamin B12-nitrous oxide interaction in operating theatre personnel. Acta Anaesthesiol Scand 1988;28:106–108.

150. Armstrong P, Rae PWH, Gray WM, Spence AA. Nitrous oxide and formiminoglutamic acid: excretion in surgical patients and anaesthetists. Br J Anaesth 1991;66:163–169.

151. Sweeney B, Bingham RM, Amos RJ, Petty AC, Cole PV. Toxicity of bone marrow in dentists exposed to nitrous oxide. Br Med J 1985;291:567–569.

152. Baden JM, Egbert B, Rice SA. Enflurane has no effect on haemopoiesis in mice. Br J Anaesth 1980;52:471–474.

153. Cleaton-Jones P, Austin JC, Banks D, Vieira E, Kagan E. Effect of intermittent exposure to a low concentration of nitrous oxide in haemopoiesis in rats. Br J Anaesth 1977;49:223–226.

154. Brodsky JB, Cohen EN, Brown BW, Wu ML, Whitcher CE. Exposure to nitrous oxide and neurologic disease among dental professionals. Anesth Analg 1981;60:297–301.

155. Dyck P, Grina A, Lambert EH, et al. Nitrous oxide neurotoxicity studies in man and rat. Anesthesiology 1980;53:205–208.

156. Layzer RB. Myeloneuropathy after prolonged exposure to nitrous oxide. Lancet 1978;2:1227–1230.

157. Beall GN, Nagel EL, Matsui Y. Immunoglobulins in anesthesiologists. Anesthesiology 1975;42:232.

158. Bruce DL. Immunologically competent anesthesiologists. Anesthesiology 1972;37:76–78.

159. Salo M, Vapaavuori M. Peripheral blood t- and b-lymphocytes in operating theatre personnel. Br J Anaesth 1970;48:877–880.

160. Ziv Y, Shohat B, Baniel J, Ventura E, Levy E,

Dintsman M. The immunologic profile of anesthetists. Anesth Analg 1988;67:849–851.

161. Spence AA, Cohen EN, Brown BW, Knill-Jones RP, Himmelberger DU. Occupational hazards for operating room-based physicians. Analysis of data from the United States and the United Kingdom. JAMA 1977;238:955–959.

162. Lattey M. Halothane sensitization. A case report. Can Anaesth Soc J 1970;17:648–649.

163. Schwettmann RS, Casterline CL. Delayed asthmatic response following occupational exposure to enflurane. Anesthesiology 1976;44:166–169.

164. Pitt EM. Halothane as a possible cause of laryngitis in an anaesthetist. Anaesthesia 1974;29:579–580.

165. Boyd CH. Ophthalmic hypersensitivity to anaesthetic vapours. Anaesthesia 1972;27:456–457.

166. Dadve AV, Mirakhur RK. Ophthalmic hypersensitivity to anaesthetic vapours. Anaesthesia 1973;28:338–339.

167. Elder BF, Beal H, DeWald W, Cobb S. Exacerbation of subclinical myasthenia by occupational exposure to an anesthetic. Anesth Analg 1971;50:383–387.

168. Bodman R. Skin sensitivity to halothane vapour. Br J Anaesth 1979;51:1092.

169. Soper LE, Vitez TS, Weinberg D. Metabolism of halogenated anesthetic agents as a possible cause of acneiform eruptions. Anesth Analg 1973;52:125–127.

170. McNamee R, Keen RI, Corkill CM. Morbidity and early retirement among anaesthetists and other specialists. Anaesthesia 1987;42:133–140.

171. Arnold WP. Application of OSHA standard to waste anesthetic gases. ASA Newslett 1992;56(8):23.

172. Lecky JH. Anesthetic pollution in the operating room: a notice to operating room personnel. Anesthesiology 1980;52:157–159.

173. Oulton JL. Operating-room venting of trace concentrations of inhalation anesthetic agents. Can Med Assoc J 1977;116:1148–1151.

174. McIntyre JWR, Pudham JT, Jhsein HR. An assessment of operating room environment air contamination with nitrous oxide and halothane and some scavenging methods. Can Anaesth Soc J 1978;25:499–505.

175. Parbrook GD, Still DM, Halliday MM, Davis PD, Macdonald I. The reduction of nitrous oxide pollution in relative analgesia. Br Dent J 1981;150:128–130.

176. Henry RJ, Primosch RE. Influence of operatory size and nitrous oxide concentration upon scavenger effectiveness. J Dent Res 1991;70(9):1286–1289.

177. American Society for Testing and Materials. Standard specification for anesthetic equipment—

scavenging systems for anesthetic gases (ASTM F1343-91). Philadelphia: ASTM, 1991.

178. Flowerdew RMM. A hazard of scavenger port design. Can Anaesth Soc J 1981;28:481–483.

179. Tavakoli M, Habeeb A. Two hazards of gas scavenging. Anesth Analg 1978;57:286–287.

180. Gill-rodriguez JA. A modified MIE Superlite exhaust valve incorporating a positive pressure safety relief valve. Anaesthesia 1984;39:1237–1239.

181. Albert CA, Kwan A, Kim C, Shibuya J, Albert SN. A waste gas scavenging valve for pediatric systems. Anesth Analg 1977;56:291–292.

182. U.S. Department of Health Education and Welfare. Development and evaluation of methods for the elimination of waste anesthetic gases and vapors in hospitals (DHEW (NIOSH) Publication No. 75-137). Washington, DC: USGPO, 1975.

183. Brinklov MM, Andersen PK. Gas evacuation from paediatric anaesthetic systems. Br J Anaesth 1978;50:305.

184. Cestone KJ, Ryan WP, Loving CD. An anesthetic gas scavenger for the Jackson-Rees system. Anesthesiology 1976;55:881–882.

185. Emralino CQ, Bernhard WN, Yost L. Overflow-gas scavenger for Jackson-Rees anesthesia system. Respir Care 1978;23:178–179.

186. Flowerdew RMM. Coaxial scavenger for paediatric anaesthesia. Can Anaesth Soc J 1979;26:367–369.

187. Houghton A, Taylor PB. Problems with high-flow scavenging system. Anaesthesia 1983;38:292.

188. Keneally JP, Overton JH. A scavenging device for the T-piece. Anaesth Intensive Care 1977;5:267–268.

189. Karski J, Sych M. A simple device designed to protect operating theatres against atmospheric pollution by volatile anaesthetics. Anaesth Res Intensive Ther 1976;4:61–64.

190. Maver E. Extractors for anaesthetic gases. Anaesth Intensive Care 1975;3:348–350.

191. Oh TH, McGill WA, Becker MJ, Epstein BS. Scavenging pediatric circuits through an adult circle system. Anesthesiology 1980;53:S324.

192. Paul DL. An antipollution device for use with the Jackson-Rees modification of the Ayre's T-piece. Anaesthesia 1987;42:439–440.

193. Nott MR. A paediatric scavenging valve. Anaesthesia 1988;43:67–68.

194. Spargo PM, Apadoo A, Wilton HJ. An improved antipollution device for the Jackson-Rees modification of the Ayre's T-piece. Anaesthesia 1987;42:1240–1241.

195. Sik MJ, Lewis RB, Eveleigh DJ. Assessment of a scavenging device for use in paediatric anaesthesia. Br J Anaesth 1990;64:117–123.

196. Whitcher C. Waste anesthetic gas scavenging—indications and technology (ASA Refresher Course No. 126). Park Ridge, IL: ASA, 1974.

197. Whitcher CE. Control of occupational exposure to inhalational anesthetics—current status (ASA Refresher Course No. 205). Park Ridge, IL: ASA, 1977.

198. Weng J, Smith RA, Balsamo JJ, Gooding JM, Kirby RR. A method of scavenging waste gases from the Jackson-Rees system. Anesth Rev 1980;7:35–38.

199. Hatch DJ, Miles R, Wagstaff M. An anaesthetic scavenging system for paediatric and adult use. Anaesthesia 1980;35:496–499.

200. Steward DJ. An anti-pollution device for use with the Jackson Rees modification of the Ayre's T-Piece. Can J Anaesth 1972;19:670–671.

201. Nitka AC, O'Riordan EF, Julien RM. A new technique of scavenging exhaled nitrous oxide. Anesthesiology 1986;65:314–316.

202. Weber GM, Unterberger J, Gangoly W. Reduced exposure to halothane and nitrous oxide by operating personnel during induction of anesthesia in children using double mask system. Anesthesiology 1991;75:A927.

203. Railton R, Fisher J. Low flow active antipollution systems. An evaluation of two systems with automatic ventilators. Anaesthesia 1984;39:904–907.

204. Ad Hoc Committee on Effects of Trace Anesthetics on Health of Operating Room Personnel, American Society of Anesthesiologists. Waste gases in operating room air: a suggested program to reduce personnel exposure. Park Ridge, IL: ASA, 1981.

205. Lawson D, Jelenich S. Capnographs: a new operating room hazard? Anesth Analg 1985;64:378.

206. Yamashita M, Shirasaki S, Matsuki A. A neglected source of nitrous oxide in operating room air. Anesthesiology 1985;62:206–207.

207. Conley RJ. Scavenging of capnometers. Anesth Analg 1986;65:102–103.

208. Wray RP. A source of nonanesthetic nitrous oxide in operating room air. Anesthesiology 1980;52:88–89.

209. Anonymous. Update: nitrous oxide exhausted from cryosurgical units. Health Devices 1981;9:180.

210. Abadir AR. A simple gas scavenging hood for anesthesia machines. J Clin Monit 1992;8:168.

211. Sarma VJ, Leman J. Laryngeal mask and anaesthetic waste gas concentrations. Anaesthesia 1990;45:791–792.

212. Carlsson P, Ljungqvist B, Hallen B. The effect of local scavenging on occupational exposure to nitrous oxide. Acta Anaesthesiol Scand 1983;27:470–475.

213. Nilsson K, Sonander H, Stenqvist O. Close scavenging of anaesthetic gases during mask anaesthesia. Acta Anaesthesiol Scand 1981;25:421–426.

214. Houldsworth HB, O'Sullivan JO, Smith M. Dy-

namic behavior of air break receiver units. Br J Anaesth 1983;55:661–670.

215. Paloheimo M, Salanne SO. Open scavenging systems. Acta Anaesthesiol Scand 1979;23:596–602.

216. Jorgensen S, Jacobsen F. Uncalibrated anaesthetic scavenging systems with open reservoirs. Anaesthesia 1982;37:833–835.

217. Gray WM. Scavenging equipment. Br J Anaesth 1985;57:685–695.

218. Mostafa SM, Natrajan KM. Hydrodynamic evaluation of a new anaesthetic gas scavenging system. Br J Anaesth 1983;55:681–686.

219. Enderby DH, Booth AM, Churchill-Davidson HC. Removal of anaesthetic waste gases. An inexpensive antipollution system for use with pipeline suction. Anaesthesia 1978;33:820–826.

220. Houldsworth HB, O'Sullivan J, Smith M. An improved air break receiver unit. A design suited to high–vacuum scavenging systems. Br J Anaesth 1983;55:671–680.

221. Anonymous. Anesthesia scavengers. Health Devices 1983;11:267–286.

222. Eisenkraft JB, Sommer RM. Flapper valve malfunction. Anesth Analg 1988;67:1132.

223. Asbury AJ, Hancox AJ. The evaluation and improvement of an anti-pollution system. Br J Anaesth 1977;49:439–446.

224. Armstrong RF, Kershaw EJ, Bourne SP, Strunin L. Anaesthetic waste gas scavenging systems. Br Med J 1977;1:941–943.

225. Bruce DL. A simple way to vent anesthetic gases. Anesth Analg 1973;52:595–598.

226. Bethune DW, Collis JM. Anaesthetic practice. Pollution in operating theatres. Biomed Eng 1974;9:157–159.

227. Hawkins TJ. Anaesthetic gas scavenging systems. Anaesthesia 1984;39:190.

228. Mehta S, Behr G, Chari J, Kenyon D. A passive method of disposal of expired anaesthetic gases. Br J Anaesth 1977;49:589–593.

229. Mehta S. Terminal gas-exhaust valve for a passive disposal system. Anaesthesia 1977;32:51–52.

230. Vickers MD. Pollution of the atmosphere of operating theatres. Important notice. Anaesthesia 1975;30:697–699.

231. Hagerdal M, Lecky JH. Anesthetic death of an experimental animal related to a scavenging system malfunction. Anesthesiology 1977;47:522–523.

232. Alexander KD, Stewart NF, Oppenheim RC, Brown TCK. Adsorption of halothane from a paediatric T-piece circuit by activated charcoal. Anaesth Intensive Care 1977;5:218–222.

233. Enderby DH, Bushman JA, Askill S. Investigations of some aspects of atmospheric pollution by anaesthetic gases. II: aspects of adsorption and emission of halothane by different charcoals. Br J Anaesth 1977;49:567–573.

234. Hawkins TJ. Atmospheric pollution in operating theatres. Anaesthesia 1973;28:490–500.

235. Kim BM, Sircar S. Adsorption characteristics of volatile anesthetics on activated carbons and per-

236. Murrin KR. Atmospheric pollution with halothane in operating theatres. A clinical study using activated charcoal. Anaesthesia 1975;30:12–17.

237. Maggs FAP, Smith ME. Adsorption of anaesthetic vapours on charcoal beds. Anaesthesia 1976;31:30–40.

238. Murrin KR. Adsorption of halothane by activated charcoal. Further studies. Anaesthesia 1974;29:458–461.

239. Vaughan RS, Mapleson WW, Mushin WW. Prevention of pollution of operating theatres with halothane vapour by adsorption with activated charcoal. Br Med J 1973;1:727–729.

240. Vaughan RS, Willis BA, Mapleson WW, Vickers MD. The Cardiff Aldavac anaesthesic-scavenging system. Anaesthesia 1977;32:339–343.

241. Capon JH. A method of regenerating activated charcoal anaesthetic adsorbers by autoclaving. Anaesthesia 1974;29:611–614.

242. Hojkjaer V, Larsen VH, Severinsen I, Waaben J. Removal of halogenated anaesthetics from a closed circle system with a charcoal filter. Acta Anaesthesiol Scand 1989;33:374–378.

243. Wright BM. Vacuum pipelines for anaesthetic pollution control. Br Med J 1978;1:918.

244. Abramowitz M, McGill WA. Hazard of anesthetic scavenging device. Anesthesiology 1979;51:276.

245. Parbrook GD, Mok IB. An expired gas collection and disposal system. Br J Anaesth 1975;47:1185–1193.

246. Lai KM. A flow-inducer for anaesthetic scavenging systems. Anaesthesia 1977;32:794–797.

247. U.S. Department of Health Education and Welfare. Criteria for a recommended standard: occupational exposure to waste anesthetic gases and vapors (DHEW (NIOSH) Publication No. 77-140). Washington, DC: USGPO, 1977.

248. Ilsley AH, Crea J, Cousins MJ. Assessment of waste anaesthetic gas scavenging systems under simulated conditions of operation. Anaesth Intensive Care 1980;8:52–64.

249. Lecky JH. The mechanical aspects of anesthetic pollution control. Anesth Analg 1977;56:769–774.

250. Stone PA, Asbury AJ, Gray WM. Use of scavenging facilities and occupational exposure to waste anaesthetic gases. Br J Anaesth 1988;61:111P.

251. Torda TA, Jones R, Englert J. A study of waste gas scavenging in operating theatres. Anaesth Intensive Care 1978;6:215–221.

252. Hovey TC. A gas scavenger system. J Am Assoc Nurse Anesth 1977;45:170–177.

253. Cramond T, Mead P. Non-rebreathing valve assembly. Anaesth Intensive Care 1986;14:465–468.

254. Reiz S, Gustavisson A-S, Haggmark S, et al. The double mask—a new local scavenging system for anaesthetic gases and volatile agents. Acta Anaesthesiol Scand 1986;30:260–265.

255. Tharp JA. A simple way to limit anesthetic pollution during anesthetic induction. Anesth Analg 1987;66:198.

256. Davies JM, Strunin L, Craig DB. Leakage of volatile anaesthetics from agent-specific keyed vapourizer filling devices. Can Anaesth Soc J 1982; 29:473–476.

257. Sorensen BH, Thomsen A. Bronchoscopy and nitrous oxide pollution. Eur J Anaesth 1987;4:281–285.

258. Carden E, Vest HR. Further advances in anesthetic technics for microlaryngeal surgery. Anesth Analg 1974;53:584–587.

259. Becker MJ, McGill WA, Oh TH, Epstein BS. The effect of an airway leak on nitrous oxide contamination of the operating room. Anesthesiology 1981;55:A335.

260. Laucks SO. Scavenging waste gases in pediatric patients. Anesthesiology 1983;59:602.

261. Vickery IM, Burton GW. Throat packs for surgery. An improved design based on anatomical measurements. Anaesthesia 1977;32:565–572.

262. Kim JS, Aldrete JA, Kullavanijaya T. Measurements of exposure to N_2O by personal dosimeters: comparison using different gas flows. Circular 1987;4:31–33.

263. Ewen A, Sheppard SD, Goresky GV, Strunin L. Occupational exposure to nitrous oxide during paediatric anaesthesia: a comparison of two induction techniques. Can J Anaesth 1989;36:S132–S133.

264. Albert SN, Kwan AM, Dadisman JW Jr. Leakage in anesthetic circuits. Anesth Analg 1977;56:878.

265. Berner O. Concentration and elimination of anaesthetic gases in operating theatres. Acta Anaesthesiol Scand 1978;22:46–54.

266. Whitcher CE. Methods of control. In: Cohen EN, ed. Anesthetic exposure in the workplace. Littleton, MA: PSG, 1980:117–148.

267. Stringer BW. Scavenging adaptor misconnection. Anaesth Intensive Care 1982;10:169.

268. Berner O. Anaesthetic apparatus leakages. A possible solution. Acta Anaesthesiol Scand 1973; 17:1–7.

269. Whitcher C, Piziali RL. Monitoring occupational exposure to inhalation anesthetics. Anesth Analg 1977;56:778–785.

270. Whitcher C. Controlling occupational exposure to nitrous oxide. In: Eger EI, ed. Nitrous oxide/N_2O. New York: Elsevier, 1985:3133–337.

271. Langley DR, Steward A. The effect of ventilation system design on air contamination with halothane in operating theatres. Br J Anaesth 1974;46:736–741.

272. Male CG. Theatre ventilation. A comparison of design and observed values. Br J Anaesth 1978;50:1257–1263.

273. Mann ES, Sprague DH. An easily overlooked malassembly. Anesthesiology 1982;56:413–414.

274. Holly HS, Eisenman TS. Hazards of an anesthetic scavenging device. Anesth Analg 1983;62:458–460.

275. Davies G, Tarnawsky M. Letter to the editor. Can Anaesth Soc J 1976;23:228.

276. Mantia AM. Gas scavenging systems. Anesth Analg 1982;61:162–164.

277. Burns THS. Pollution of operating theatres. Anaesthesia 1979;34:823.

278. Hamilton RC, Byrne J. Another cause of gas-scavenging-line obstruction. Anesthesiology 1979; 51:365–366.

279. Malloy WF, Wightman AE, O'Sullivan D, Goldiner PL. Bilateral pneumothorax from suction applied to a ventilator exhaust valve. Anesth Analg 1979;58:147–149.

280. Rendell-Baker L. Hazard of blocked scavenge valve. Can Anaesth Soc J 1982;29:182–183.

281. O'Connor DE, Daniels BW, Pfitzner J. Hazards of anaesthetic scavenging: case reports and brief review. Anaesth Intensive Care 1982;10:15–19.

282. Sainsbury DA. Scavenging misconnection. Anaesth Intensive Care 1985;13:215–216.

283. Phillips S. Scavenging hazard. Anaesth Intensive Care 1991;19:615.

284. Anonymous. Scavenging gas from membrane oxygenators. Technol Anesth 1987;8:6–7.

285. Schreiber P. Anesthesia systems. Telford, PA: North American Drager, 1984.

286. Smith DG. Anaesthetic gas scavenging systems. Anaesthesia 1985;40:90.

287. Gray WM, Hall RC, Carter KB, Shaw A, Thompson WJ. Medishield AGS system and servo 900 ventilators. Anaesthesia 1984;39:790–794.

288. Blackstock D, Forbes M. Analysis of an anaesthetic gas scavenging system hazard. Can J Anaesth 1989;36:204–208.

289. Lanier WL. Intraoperative air entrainment with Ohio Modulus anesthesia machine. Anesthesiology 1986;64:266–268.

290. Mostafa SM, Sutclffe AJ. Antipollution expiratory valves. A potential hazard. Anaesthesia 1982; 37:468–469.

291. Mor ZF, Stein ED, Orkin LR. A possible hazard in the use of a scavenging system. Anesthesiology 1977;47:302–303.

292. Patel KD, Dalal FY. A potential hazard of the Drager scavenging interface system for wall suction. Anesth Analg 1979;58:327–328.

293. Seymour A. Possible hazards with an anaesthetic gas scavenging system. Anaesthesia 1982; 37:1218–1219.

294. Milliken RA. Hazards of scavenging systems. Anesth Analg 1980;59:162.

295. Sharrock NE, Gabel RA. Inadvertent anesthetic overdose obscured by scavenging. Anesthesiology 1978;49:137–138.

296. Heard SO, Munson ES. Ventilator alarm nonfunction associated with a scavenging system for waste gases. Anesth Analg 1983;62:230–232.

297. Halsey MJ, Chand S, Dluzewski AR, Jones AJ, Wardley-Smith BS. Olefactory thresholds: detection of operating room contamination. Br J Anaesth 1977;49:510–511.

298. Ilsley AH, Crea J, Cousins MJ. Evaluation of infrared analysers used for monitoring waste anaesthetic gas levels in operating theatres. Anaesth Intensive Care 1980;8:436–440.

299. Holmes CM. Pollution in operating theatres. Part 2. The solution. N Z Med J 1978;87:50–53.

300. Knights KM, Strunin JM, Strunin L. Measurement of low concentrations of halothane in the atmosphere using a portable detector. Lancet 1975;1:727–728.

301. Allander C, Carlsson P, Hallen B, Ljungqvist B, Nordlander O. Thermocanera, a macroscopic method for the study of pollution with nitrous oxide in operating theatres. Acta Anaesthesiol Scand 1981;25:21–24.

302. Carlsson P, Ljungqvist B, Allander C, Hallen B, Nordlander O. Thermocamera studies of enflurane and halothane vapours. Acta Anaesthesiol Scand 1981;25:315–318.

303. Carlsson P, Hallen B, Hallonsten A, Ljungqvist B. Thermocamera studies of nitrous oxide dispersion in the dental surgery. Scand J Dent Res 1983;91:224–230.

304. Austin JC, Shaw R, Crichton R, Cleaton-Jones PE, Moyes D. Comparison of sampling techniques for studies of nitrous oxide pollution. Br J Anaesth 1978;50:1109–1112.

305. Gray WM, Burnside GW. The evacuated canister method of personal sampling. An assessment of its suitability for routine monitoring of operating theatre pollution. Anaesthesia 1985;40:288–294.

306. Austin JC, Shaw R, Moyes D, Cleaton-Jones PE. A simple air sampling technique for monitoring nitrous oxide pollution. Br J Anaesth 1981;53:997–1003.

307. Burm AG, Spierdijk J. A method for sampling halothane and enflurane present in trace amounts in ambient air. Anesthesiology 1979;50:230–233.

308. Carter KB, Halliday MM. A personal air sampling pump for hospital operating staff. J. Med Eng Technol 1978;2:310–312.

309. Dupressoir CAJ. A practical apparatus for measuring average exposure of operating theatre personnel to halothane. Anaesth Intensive Care 1975;3:345–347.

310. Choi-Lao AT. Trace anesthetic vapors in hospital operating-room environments. Nurs Res 1981;30:156–161.

311. Hunter L. An occupational health approach to anaesthetic air pollution. Med J Aust 1976;1:465–468.

312. Halliday MM, Carter KB. A chemical adsorption system for the sampling of gaseous organic pollutants in operating theatre atmospheres. Br J Anaesth 1978;50:1013–1018.

313. Bishop EC, Hossain MA. Field comparison between two nitrous oxide (N_2O) passive monitors and conventional sampling methods. Am Ind Hyg Assoc J 1984;45:812–816.

314. Cox PC, Brown RH. A personal sampling method for the determination of nitrous oxide exposure. Am Ind Hyg Assoc J 1984;45:345–350.

315. Ward BG. Development and application of a long dynamic range nitrous oxide monitoring system. An Ind Hyg Assoc J 1985;46:697–703.

316. Whitcher C. Clinical evaluation of two dosimeters for monitoring occupational exposure to N_2O. Anesthesiology 1984;61:A169.

317. Mcgill WA, Rivera O, Howard R. Time-weighted average for nitrous oxide: an automated method. Anesthesiology 1980;53:424–426.

318. Mehta S, Burton P, Simms JS. Monitoring of occupational exposure to nitrous oxide. Can Anaesth Soc J 1978;25:419–423.

319. Corbett TH. Retention of anesthetic agents following occupational exposure. Anesth Analg 1973; 52:614–618.

320. Anonymous. Workshop on anesthetic pollution. Anesthesiol Rev 1977;4:25–34.

321. Nikki P, Pfaffli P, Ahlman K. End-tidal and blood halothane and nitrous oxide in surgical personnel. Lancet 1972;2:490–491.

322. Salamonsen LA, Cole WJ, Salamonsen RF. Simultaneous trace analysis of nitrous oxide and halothane in air. Br J Anaesth 1978;50:221–227.

323. Hillman KM, Saloojee Y, Brett II, Cole PV. Nitrous oxide concentrations in dental surgery. Atmospheric and blood concentrations of personnel. Anaesthesia 1981;36:257–262.

324. Sonander H, Stenqvist O, Nilsson K. Exposure to trace amounts of nitrous oxide. Br J Anaesth 1983;55:1225–1229.

325. Sonander H, Stenqvist O, Nilsson K. Urinary N_2O as a measure of biologic exposure to nitrous oxide anaesthetic contamination. Ann Occup Hyg 1983;27:73–79.

326. Whitcher C. Correspondence. Anesthesiol Rev 1976;3:41–42.

327. Milliken RA. A plea for monitoring both haloge-

nated and non-halogenated anesthetic agents in the operating room. Anesthesiol Rev 1976;3:29–31.

328. Milliken RA. Correspondence. Anesthesiol Rev 1976;3:42, 51.

329. Gray WM. Occupational exposure to nitrous oxide in four hospitals. Anaesthesia 1989;44:511–514.

330. Draft report on anesthetic waste gas scavenging for Ministry of Health. Ontario, Canada, October 1977.

331. Geraci CL Jr. Operating room pollution: governmental perspectives and guidelines. Anesth Analg 1977;56:775–777.

332. Mazze RI. Waste anesthetic gases and the regulatory agencies. Anesthesiology 1980;52:248–256.

333. Anonymous: Scavenging systems to comply with "stiff laws" regulating trace gas exposure in OR described. Anesthesiol News, Aug 14, 1984.

334. Lambert-Jensen P, Christensen NE, Brynnum J. Laryngeal mask and anaesthetic waste gas exposure. Anaesthesia 1992;47:697–700.

335. Borm PJ, Kant I, Houben G, van Russen-Moll M, Henderson PT. Monitoring of nitrous oxide in operating rooms: identification of sources and estimation of occupational exposure. J Occup Med 1990;32:1112–1116.

336. Gardner RJ. Inhalation anaesthetics—exposure and control: a statistical comparison of personal exposures in operating theatres with and without anaesthetic gas scavenging. Ann Occup Hyg 1989;33:159–73.

337. Mondry GA. Medical-legal implications. In: Cohen EN, ed. Anesthetic exposure in the workplace. Littleton, MA: PSG, 1980:163-182.

338. Anonymous. OSHA inspections of hospital operating rooms. ASA Newslett 1980;(44):7.

Chapter 12

Hazards of the Anesthesia Machines and Breathing Systems

Happy is he who gains wisdom from another's mishaps.

Although enormous strides have been made in improving the safety of anesthesia apparatus, reports of problems continue to appear. Studies have shown that human error is more frequent than equipment failure (1–6).

This chapter will examine hazards of anesthesia machines and breathing systems from the perspective of their effect on the patient. Many examples are given, but this should not be considered a complete listing of all possible dangers. Many hazards involve older apparatus that may have been modified and is no longer sold or serviced by the manufacturer.

Hypoxia

HYPOXIC INSPIRED GAS MIXTURE

Incorrect Gas Supplied

Piping System

Cross-overs between oxygen and other gases may occur anywhere in a piped system. Most commonly the transposition is in the piping itself (7–10). Frequently the error is made during remodeling, repairs, or new construction. Following construction or repair, a pipeline may remain full of air or nitrogen rather than oxygen (11). Such a line must be purged thoroughly with oxygen before use.

It is possible for an incorrect gas to be installed at the central supply. Oxygen tanks have been reportedly filled with argon and nitrogen (12–15).

Inside the operating room, incorrect outlets may be installed (16–21). An incorrect connector may be placed on a hose (22–25) or the pipeline inlet of the anesthesia machine (19). Quick-connect fittings may be damaged or poorly designed so that an incorrect connection can be made (26). Finally, connections between piped gases can occur in peripheral equipment and result in the oxygen pipeline being contaminated with another gas (27–30). An air flowmeter may have an oxygen outlet connector (31,32).

If a cross-over or contamination has occurred, simply opening an oxygen cylinder on the anesthesia machine will not be effective because the pressure from the cylinder will be below that in the pipeline. The oxygen hose must be disconnected from the wall outlet.

Cylinders

It is possible for a cylinder labeled *oxygen* to contain another gas (33,34). A cylinder may be painted a color other than that normally used. Particular care should be taken with cylinders in other countries, because four different colors (green, white, blue, and black) are used around the world for oxygen (35). In a cylinder containing a mixture of two gases, incomplete mixing may result in a hypoxic mixture being delivered (36,37). Such a cylinder may require 45 min of rotating before mixing is complete.

Despite almost universal use of the Pin Index Safety System, reports of incorrect cylinders being connected to yokes continue to appear (38–44). An incorrect yoke block may be inserted (45,46).

Cross-overs in the Anesthesia Machine

Cross-overs between oxygen and other gases inside the anesthesia machine can occur (47,48). Whenever a new anesthesia machine or one that has been repaired or altered is used, it is particularly important to check for cross-overs using an oxygen analyzer calibrated on room air. The analyzer should read 100% oxygen when there is flow only through the oxygen flowmeter or oxygen flush.

Hypoxic Mixture Set

Flow Control Valve Malfunction

Damage to the oxygen flow control valve can result in low oxygen flow (49–51). Damage to the flow control valve for another gas may result in excessive flow of that gas relative to that of oxygen.

Incorrect Flowmeter Settings

Most anesthesia machines manufactured before 1979 do not have an oxygen-nitrous oxide interlock or proportioning system to prevent the user from dialing a hypoxic fresh gas flow. On these machines a hypoxic mixture can be caused by closing, partly or fully, the flow control valve for oxygen while allowing the nitrous oxide flow to continue (52–55). Machines manufactured after 1979 may have additional gases that are not incorporated into the interlock or proportioning system.

Oxygen flow can be inadvertently lowered (or flow of another gas increased) if the flow control knob is inadvertently rotated by an item on the surface below (56) or by a hose or wire allowed to drape around it. With some flowmeters, in and out movement of the flow control valve can change the flow significantly (57). Someone helping to move the machine could grab a flow control valve knob and change the flow (Fig. 12.1). Vari-

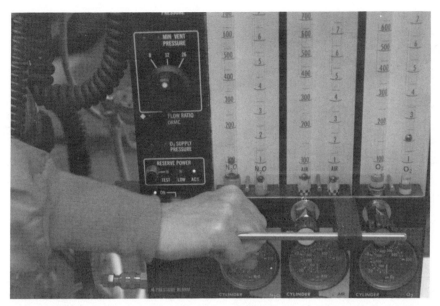

Figure 12.1. A dangerous practice. The flow control knob may look like a good thing to grab to someone moving an anesthesia machine. Flows may be altered in the process.

ous devices have been developed to protect the flow control valves (see Chapter 3).

Incorrect Flowmeter Reading

Observing the incorrect flowmeter scale is a possible cause of hypoxia. Accidental use of a low flow of oxygen when a high one is intended is a hazard whenever two oxygen flowmeter assemblies, one for low flows and one for high flows, are present.

On some older machines, the flowmeter indicator can disappear from view at the top of the tube when the flow of gas exceeds the maximum scale calibration. Such a flowmeter is very similar in appearance to one with the indicator resting at the bottom. If the flowmeter is for a gas other than oxygen, a hypoxic mixture may result.

If an air flowmeter is present on a machine, dialing air instead of oxygen can result in a hypoxic mixture (58). To prevent this, most modern anesthesia machines do not allow administration of air and nitrous oxide without oxygen flow (Fig. 12.2). A selector valve is one way to prevent this problem.

Inaccurate Flowmeter

Flowmeter inaccuracies are common and can occur in machines recently serviced. Causes include dirt, grease, or oil on the indicator or tube; a stuck or damaged indicator; misalignment of the tube; static electricity; improper calibration; the stop at the top of the tube falling down onto the indicator

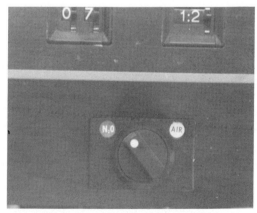

Figure 12.2. The valve prevents nitrous oxide and air from being administered together.

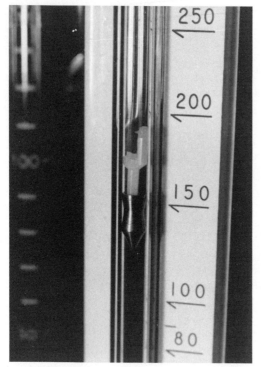

Figure 12.3. The stop at the top of the flowmeter tube has broken off and fallen onto the indicator. The flowmeter will read less than the actual flow.

(Fig. 12.3); and transposition of indicator, scale, or tube (59–63). This can sometimes be detected by an indicator not rotating or lying at an angle in the tube.

Increased Nitrous Oxide Supply Pressure

Once a flow control valve has been set, an increase in pressure upstream will result in increased flow (64). A pressure surge in the nitrous oxide pipeline can cause hypoxia by increasing the flow of nitrous oxide relative to oxygen flow (65).

Back Pressure on Flowmeters

Increased resistance to flow in the anesthesia machine can allow a preferential flow of nitrous oxide over oxygen if the pressure from the secondary nitrous oxide regulator is set higher than that from the oxygen regulator (66).

Loss of Oxygen to Atmosphere

If there is a leak at the top of the oxygen flowmeter tube, oxygen will be preferentially lost, even if the oxygen flowmeter is downstream of the other flowmeters (67–72) (see Fig. 3.26). The position of the flowmeter indicator may not be affected. Often the defect cannot be seen until the tube is disassembled.

Other leaks in the oxygen lines in the anesthesia machine can result in hypoxia, the magnitude of which will depend on the size of the leak and its location as well as the back pressure resulting from positive pressure ventilation, a direct-reading vaporizer in the fresh gas supply tube, or a defect in a vaporizer-mounting system (70–84). It is important to use a yoke plug in any yoke not containing a cylinder so that gas will not leak out in retrograde fashion if a flow control valve is left open.

Air Entrainment

If the pressure in the breathing system falls below atmospheric, air may be drawn into the system through a leak or disconnection and dilute the oxygen concentration. Subatmospheric pressure may be caused by the inspiratory effort of the patient, a ventilator with a hanging bellows, or a defect in the scavenging system (85–87).

In a ventilator powered by air, air may enter the system through a leak in the bellows. Air used to reduce the fogging of a lens on a bronchoscope may dilute the inspired oxygen (88).

A hypoxic mixture can be easily detected if a properly functioning and calibrated oxygen analyzer is used. Transposition of gases should be considered when a patient becomes cyanotic with 100% oxygen. If it is suspected that the pipeline oxygen system is delivering less than 100% oxygen, it is important to open an oxygen cylinder *and* to disconnect the oxygen pipeline hose. If the pipeline hose is not disconnected, gas from the piping system will still be delivered. If the cause of progressive cyanosis or a low oxygen concentration is not obvious and the situation is not corrected by disconnecting the oxygen pipeline hose and opening an oxygen cylinder, the patient should ventilated with room air.

HYPOXIA SECONDARY TO HYPOVENTILATION

Problems with equipment can result in less-than-adequate ventilation, with carbon dioxide retention and hypoxia.

Causes

Insufficient Gas in the Breathing System

Low Inflow. *Pipeline Problems.* Loss of pipeline oxygen pressure was discussed in Chapter 2. Causes include damage during construction, debris left in the line following installation, unannounced system shutdown, regulator malfunction, malfunction of the central supply system, disruption of the line between the central supply and the hospital, fires, and closure of an isolation valve (24,89–91). A station outlet may become blocked or not accept a quick-connect (92,93).

A hose may develop a leak (94–96), become blocked (97,98), or develop a kink that obstructs gas flow (99). The anesthesia machine may roll over a hose, occluding gas flow (100). The check valve in the pipeline inlet at the back of the machine may malfunction, blocking flow (101)

If piped oxygen pressure is lost, the oxygen failure safety valve should interrupt the flow of all gases. If that occurs, an oxygen cylinder should be opened and the pipeline hose disconnected from the wall to prevent flow from the cylinder into the pipeline. To minimize oxygen usage, the ventilator should be turned off and manual or spontaneous ventilation instituted and the fresh gas flow lowered.

If opening an oxygen cylinder does not repressurize the anesthesia machine, there is a problem in the intermediate pressure system

of the machine, unless the cylinder is empty or not connected properly (100). A resuscitation bag should be used to ventilate the patient until another machine can be obtained.

Cylinder Problems. A cylinder may be delivered empty or with an inoperable valve or blocked valve outlet (102,103).

Before a cylinder can be used it must be correctly installed on the machine. Frequently, the most inexperienced person in the operating room is told, without any instructions, to replace an empty cylinder. He or she may fail to crack the valve; install it without a washer, with a damaged washer, or with two washers; fail to remove the dust protection cap (Fig. 12.4); or fail to check to see that the cylinder is full. Another error is screwing the retaining screw of the yoke into the safety-relief device on the cylinder (104). It is sometimes possible to spot an incorrectly placed cylinder simply by looking at it. An improperly installed cylinder may hang at an angle instead of parallel to the machine (Fig. 12.5).

The fact that a full cylinder is present on an anesthesia machine does not mean that

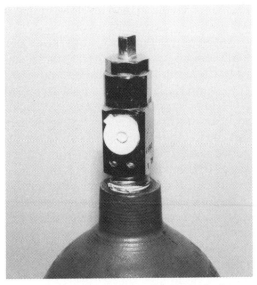

Figure 12.4. Failure to remove the dust protection cap from a cylinder before installing it on a machine caused a portion of the cap to be pushed into the cylinder valve port, and this blocked the exit of gas from the cylinder.

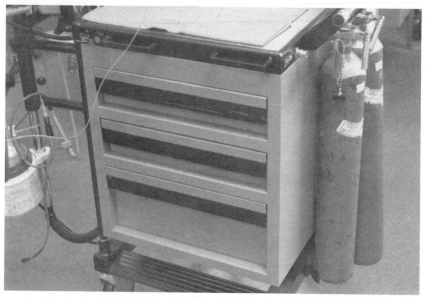

Figure 12.5.   A sure sign that a cylinder is not correctly fitted in its yoke is that it hangs at an angle to the machine rather than perpendicular to the floor.

there will be oxygen available when needed. First, there must be a means of opening the cylinder. Often a cylinder handle is borrowed for opening a portable cylinder or some other purpose and not returned. A good practice is to chain a handle to each machine so that it will always be there when needed.

Machine Problems. OBSTRUCTION. Obstruction to gas flow in the anesthesia machine caused by defects in the flush valve and flow control valve have been reported (105,106). Vaporizer connections, selector switches, interlocks, and mounting devices can cause obstruction (107,108). Other reported causes include the leaflet from a check valve (109) and a foreign body (110).

LEAKS.   If the check valve in the pipeline inlet of the anesthesia machine fails, gas may flow into the room (if the pipeline hose is disconnected) or into the piping system (if the hose is connected) (111,112). A leaking flowmeter tube or an open flow control valve with an opening to atmosphere upstream of the flowmeter can result in loss of gas.

Leaks may occur at a loose or defective vaporizer connection (113–127); at a loose, de-fective, or absent vaporizer filler cap or drain screw (128–130) (Fig. 12.6); or in the vaporizer itself (131). Some machines are designed so that when a vaporizer is removed, a manifold cap must be placed where the vaporizer was situated (Fig. 12.7). Failure to do so will result in a major leak.

Leaks downstream of the flowmeters and

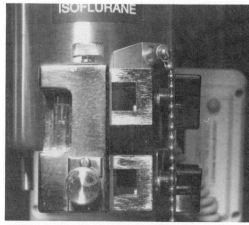

Figure 12.6.   When the block sitting on the filling block is missing there will be a leak when the vaporizer is turned on.

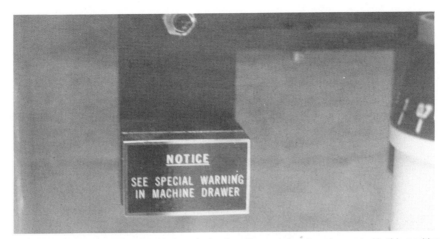

Figure 12.7. This manifold cap needs to be in place if a vaporizer is not mounted in this position.

vaporizers but upstream of the common gas outlet have been reported (132,133). The pressure relief device on the machine may vent fresh gas if resistance downstream causes the pressure to rise (134,135).

When a system designed to facilitate changing of vaporizers on the back bar is used, it is important that the machine be checked carefully after a vaporizer has been mounted. This includes sighting across the tops of the mounted and locked vaporizers to ensure that they are level and at the same height. An attempt should be made to lift each mounted and locked vaporizer off the manifold without unlocking it. If the vaporizer can be removed it is improperly positioned. Finally, the anesthesia machine should be checked for leaks with each vaporizer individually turned on and dialed to a concentration of 0% (136).

Problems with the Fresh Gas Supply.
The fresh gas supply hose, which goes from the anesthesia machine outlet to the breathing system, can become detached (86,137,138), occluded (139–145), or develop a leak (146). A component placed in the fresh gas line can develop a leak (147) or become disconnected (148). The inner tube of the Bain system, which carries the fresh gas flow, can become obstructed (99,149–152).

Excessive Outflow. *Breathing System Leaks.* Most breathing system leaks are too small to be of clinical significance, but some may be large enough that the patient cannot be ventilated adequately, especially if low fresh gas flows are used. Leaks also cause pollution of operating room air (see Chapter 11).

A common location for leaks in the circle system is the absorber. If the canisters do not fit together properly or the top and bottom do not seal well, large leaks can result. Accidental disengagement of the canister from the body of the absorber can occur (153,154). Humidifiers, breathing tubes, elbow adapters, bags, temperature probe sites, connectors for respiratory gas analyzer sensors, bag-ventilator selector valves, filters, heat and moisture exchangers, APL valves, and Y pieces have all been reported as sources of leaks (155–171) (Fig. 12.8). Breakage of a reservoir bag mount has been reported (172,173). A heated humidifier may burn a hole in a breathing tube (174,175).

The APL valve may fail to close (176–179). All new bag-ventilator selector valves cause the APL valve to be excluded from the system when switched to the automatic mode (see Chapter 7). On machines lacking this device, the user may forget to close the APL valve when switching to automatic ventilation.

Leaks may occur in a ventilator (180,181) or in its attachment to the breathing system (182–184). Loss of gas will occur if the pilot

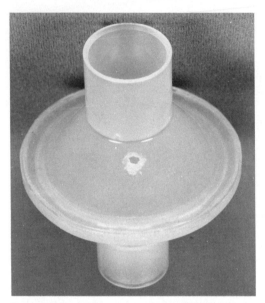

Figure 12.8. Various parts of the breathing system may have holes in them when they are received from the manufacturer.

line becomes disconnected or kinked during expiration, the spill valve ruptures or becomes stuck in the open position, or the exhaust valve malfunctions (185–189).

A defective nonrebreathing valve or misassembly of a manual resuscitator can result in part or all of the volume leaving the bag escaping to atmosphere (190–192).

Most leaks can be detected by checking before use. During a case, leaks may be detected by a low expired volume on a respirometer, an increase in end-tidal carbon dioxide or an increase in inspired nitrogen during spontaneous ventilation (193,194). With a standing bellows ventilator and especially with use of low fresh gas flows, the bellows may not return to its fully expanded position (195) and there may be a change in the sound of the ventilator. A low airway pressure monitor may detect a leak, but cannot be relied on.

When a leak is suspected, a systematic search of the anesthesia machine and breathing system should be made, following the route of gas travel. All components and connections should be examined, using leak detection fluid, soapy water, or a nitrous oxide trace gas analyzer if necessary.

Disconnections. A disconnection is an unintended separation of components in a breathing system. Studies show that disconnections are the most common type of preventable anesthetic mishap involving equipment (1,2,196,197). Most breathing system connectors are slip fittings that relay on friction to hold them together. They will come apart if sufficient tension is applied. Draping may make it difficult to see a disconnection (198).

Disconnections can occur anywhere in the breathing system. The most common site is between the breathing system and tracheal tube connector (1,199). Other common sites are between the common gas outlet and the fresh gas supply tube, at the end of the ventilator hose, and at the connection of the tubing to an airway pressure monitor or aspirating respiratory gas monitor.

Disconnections can be made less frequent by making secure connections. Connectors with lugs or other features that make them easy to grip may be easier to tighten. Wrung (push-and-twist) connections are much stronger than those made with a straight push and metal-to-metal or plastic-to-plastic joints are stronger than metal-to-plastic joints (200). Antidisconnect (locking) devices for use in breathing systems have been described (201–207) (Fig. 12.9). Many believe that they should not be used at the connection between the tracheal tube connector and the breathing system, reasoning that it is safer for such a joint to come apart under tension than for the tracheal tube to be pulled out of the patient (208). Also, it may be necessary to make a disconnection rapidly at this point for suctioning or to relieve a high pressure in the breathing system.

Adhesive tape is frequently used to prevent disconnections. Unfortunately, tape and adhesive residue can make reconnection more difficult.

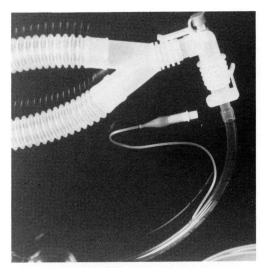

Figure 12.9. Antidisconnect devices are shown attached at the connection of the Y piece to the elbow adapter and between the elbow adapter and the tracheal tube connector. Use of such a device in the second location is controversial. Many believe that this increases the likelihood of inadvertent extubation.

Negative Pressure Applied to the Gas Flow Pathway. If the negative pressure inlet valve of a closed scavenging interface or the opening to atmosphere of an open interface becomes blocked, or the interface is omitted, a subatmospheric pressure may be transmitted across the APL valve to the breathing system (209–213).

If an enteric tube enters the trachea rather than the esophagus, respiratory gases will be removed from the lung and breathing system when suction is applied to the tube (214–216).

Improper Adjustment of the APL Valve. When manually controlled or assisted ventilation is used, gas is vented from the system during inspiration (unless a closed system technique is used). Part of the gas displaced from the bag goes to the patient and the rest is discharged from the breathing system. The person squeezing the bag may find it difficult to estimate how much gas is entering the patient and how much is escaping to atmosphere. Hypoventilation can occur if too much gas escapes through the valve.

Blockage of Inspiratory Pathway

Partial or complete blockage between the reservoir bag or ventilator and the patient can result in hypoventilation. Causes include manufacturing defects; water, blood, and/or secretions; and foreign bodies (166,217–230). Connecting a flow direction-sensitive component such as a PEEP valve or humidifier in the inspiratory limb of a breathing system in reverse will result in no flow to the patient (231). If the bag-ventilator selector valve is left in the wrong position, complete obstruction to gas flow will be the result.

Breathing tubes can become obstructed from kinking or twisting (232) (Fig. 12.10) as can the neck of the reservoir bag (Fig. 12.11). A heated humidifier may cause the inspiratory tubing to melt and become obstructed (233) (Fig. 12.12). Obstruction can result from the seals on a disposable absorbent

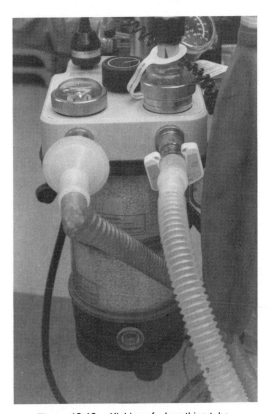

Figure 12.10. Kinking of a breathing tube.

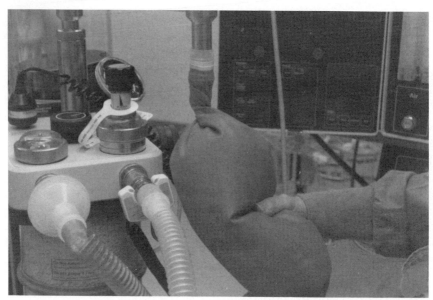

Figure 12.11. Twisting has caused this bag to become obstructed. Many bags have a guard in the neck to prevent this.

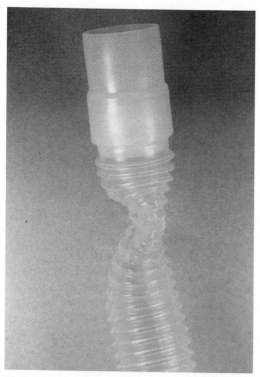

Figure 12.12. Contact with a heated humidifier can cause a breathing tube to melt and become obstructed.

package not being removed and from occlusions in the holes in the top and bottom panels (234–236) (Fig. 12.13).

With obstruction, the peak pressure recorded on the breathing system manometer may be increased. The travel of the ventilator bellows will be reduced, but not totally eliminated. An airway pressure monitor may alarm, depending on the location of the occlusion and the airway pressure sensor.

Ventilator Problems

Hypoventilation secondary to ventilator problems is discussed in Chapter 10. Causes include cycling failure, leaks of driving or breathing system gas, inaccurate settings, and the ventilator being turned off.

Wasted Ventilation

During controlled or assisted ventilation, not all of the gas discharged from a ventilator or reservoir bag enters the patient. Compression of gases and distension of components will tend to lower ventilation (see Chapter 5). These factors are particularly important when small patients are being ventilated.

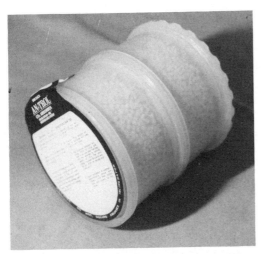

Figure 12.13. Prepacked absorbent container. Failure to remove the label from the top and/or bottom will result in obstruction to flow through the absorber.

Detection

Vigilance aids used to detect hypoventilation include airway pressure and carbon dioxide monitors and respirometers. They are discussed in Chapters 16 and 17. Because any single monitoring modality may fail to detect a problem (207,237–241), it is advisable to use all three. An oxygen analyzer may detect some disconnections (242, 243) but should not be relied on because it is effective in only a limited set of circumstances. Inadequate gas in the breathing system may be recognized by a ventilator bellows not returning to its fully expanded position at the end of expiration.

Response (244)

When inadequate ventilation is suspected, the operator should quickly check the breathing system pressure gauge, respirometer, capnometer, and the patient's chest movements and breath sounds. If ventilation appears to be inadequate, steps taken should include the following.

Check Ventilator Settings

A quick glance at the ventilator settings should be made to determine if they are correct.

Check Ventilator Bellows

Ventilator Bellows Does Not Move. Failure of the ventilator to cycle means that the driving gas supply has been shut off or that the ventilator electrical power has failed or been turned off. Manual ventilation should be resumed and the ventilator turned on or replaced.

Ventilator Bellows Fills but Fails to Compress Fully. If the bellows fills but fails to compress fully, there is obstruction to ventilation or a leak in the ventilator. The ventilator should be turned off and the bag-ventilator selector valve should be checked to make certain it is set for automatic ventilation. If it is, the user should disconnect the tracheal tube connector from the breathing system. If this results in an outrush of gas, there is an obstruction in the expiratory pathway. This should be checked quickly. A resuscitation bag should always be readily available in every operating room (Fig. 12.14). If the problem cannot be detected or corrected quickly, the tubing to the resuscitation bag should be connected to the common gas outlet on the anesthesia machine. This will supply oxygen and anesthetic agents for ventilation of the patient while the problem is corrected or a new breathing system is obtained.

If disconnection at the tracheal tube does not result in an outrushing of gas the user should attempt to blow down the tracheal tube. If the tube is obstructed, it should be replaced.

If there is no outrush of gas with disconnection and the tracheal tube is not blocked, there is an obstruction to inspiration. A switch should be made to manual ventilation. If the patient can now be ventilated, the problem is in the ventilator circuit, either an obstruction or a leak in the ventilator.

If the patient still cannot be ventilated a check should be made of the inspiratory pathway, starting with the reservoir bag and going through the system to the patient connection. If no problem is found, a resuscita-

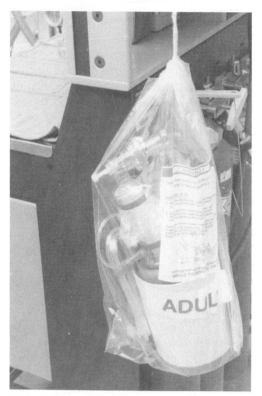

Figure 12.14. A resuscitation bag should be kept readily available in each operating room for use in emergencies.

tion bag with its supply tubing attached to the common gas outlet should be used to ventilate the patient and the breathing system replaced.

Ventilator Bellows Fails to Fill. If the bellows fails to fill, the flowmeters on the anesthesia machine should be checked. If low flows are being used, they should be increased. Often this will correct the problem. If the flowmeter indicators are at the bottom of their tubes, an oxygen cylinder should be turned on and the oxygen pipeline hose disconnected. If the indicators return to their normal positions, the problem is in the pipeline supply. If they do not return to their normal positions, there is a problem in the machine. A resuscitation bag should be used to ventilate with room air until a new machine

can be brought in. If an oxygen cylinder with an independent flowmeter can be quickly obtained, it can be used to supply oxygen to the resuscitation bag.

If the flowmeters are at their normal positions, the operator should perform a rapid visual scan for disconnections in the breathing system, starting with the patient connection and proceeding through the entire system. The cuff on the tracheal tube should be checked. If the problem is not found, a switch should immediately be made to manual ventilation. The reservoir bag should be filled with oxygen using the oxygen flush valve. If the bag fails to fill, the fresh gas supply hose should be checked for a leak, disconnection, or obstruction. A resuscitation bag or Mapleson D system with the fresh gas supply tube attached to the common gas outlet should be used to ventilate the patient and the breathing system replaced.

Reservoir Bag Stays Filled. If the bag fills as expected and the patient can be ventilated, the ventilator and its connections should be inspected. Common problems are a disconnection of the ventilator hose or a leak in the bellows.

Reservoir Bag Fails to Stay Filled. If the reservoir bag fills with use of the oxygen flush valve but does not stay filled when ventilation of the patient is attempted, there is excessive outflow from the breathing system. A systematic check should be made, starting with the fresh gas supply hose and moving around the entire system, looking for a leak, open APL valve, disconnection, or source of negative pressure. The tracheal tube should be disconnected from the breathing system and the patient connection port occluded. Applying positive pressure to the reservoir bag may make it possible to locate audibly the source of outflow. Equipment such as a humidifier that can be easily taken out of the system should be removed. This may eliminate the leak.

If the source of outflow cannot be found or easily corrected, a resuscitation bag with the fresh gas supply tube attached at the common gas outlet of the machine should be used to ventilate the patient. If the patient still cannot be ventilated, any enteric tube should be removed. If this does not help, the tracheal tube should be removed, and the patient should be ventilated using a mask and then reintubated.

HYPOXIA SECONDARY TO REBREATHING

As mentioned in Chapter 5, one of the consequences of rebreathing can be hypoxia. This will be discussed more fully in the section "Hypercapnia" (below).

INCORRECT PLACEMENT OF A PEEP VALVE

Low levels of PEEP may be beneficial in improving low arterial oxygen tension levels. If a bidirectional PEEP valve is incorrectly placed against the direction of flow or a unidirectional PEEP valve is placed in the inspiratory limb oriented with the flow, PEEP will not be applied to the patient's airway, although gas flow will not be obstructed.

Hypercapnia

HYPOVENTILATION

Causes of hypoventilation are discussed under hypoxia.

INADVERTENT ADMINISTRATION OF CARBON DIOXIDE (245)

In the United Kingdom and other countries, it is common to have a carbon dioxide cylinder and flowmeter on anesthesia machines. The flowmeter may be accidentally turned on and this not noticed, especially when the indicator is at the top of the tube (246).

In one reported case, a nitrous oxide hose was connected to the carbon dioxide station outlet (247). A cylinder may be mistakenly filled with carbon dioxide (248).

REBREATHING WITHOUT REMOVAL OF CARBON DIOXIDE

Absorbent Failure

Hypercarbia can occur if channeling allows gases to bypass the absorbent (249). Fluorescent lights in an operating room can deactivate the indicator around the outside of the canister so it does not change color when exhausted (250). Cases have been reported in which color change did not take place because the absorbent did not contain an indicator (251).

Bypassed Absorbent

Some older absorbers are fitted with a bypass that allows some or all of the gases to bypass the absorbent. Accidental activation of this bypass can lead to inadvertent hypercarbia. The danger is greater if low fresh gas flows are used. High fresh gas flows cause CO_2 to be washed out of the breathing system, so there is less dependence on the absorbent to remove the CO_2. As the fresh gas flow is lowered, the absorbent becomes more important for CO_2 removal.

The partial bypass on one older absorber is located opposite from where the user normally stands (Fig. 12.15). It is easy to miss seeing that the valve is in the bypass position unless a special effort is made to check it.

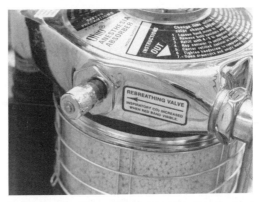

Figure 12.15. The partial bypass on this absorber is on the opposite side of the absorber from where anesthesia personnel normally stand and is not easily seen. A special effort should be made to check it.

The absorber may be defective so that gas flow is not directed through the absorbent (252).

Unidirectional Valve Problems

Correct movement of gases in a circle system depends on proper functioning of the unidirectional valves. If they do not close properly, the patient will rebreathe carbon dioxide (253–255). The disc or seat may become displaced, wet, sticky, or damaged so that the disc will not seat properly (255–262) (Fig. 12.16). Foreign material such as absorbent granules may prevent proper seating of the leaflet. A leaflet may be too large or small to function properly (257). A leaflet that has a projection to prevent its sticking to the top of the valve may leak if inserted with the projection downward (263). A disc may not be replaced after removal for cleaning or servicing.

Problems with Nonrebreathing Valves

Improper assembly or sticking of nonrebreathing valves can result in partial or total rebreathing. This is discussed more fully in Chapter 8.

Inadequate Fresh Gas Flow to a Mapleson System

In systems without carbon dioxide absorption a low fresh gas flow can result in

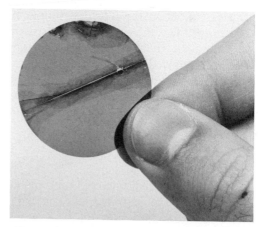

Figure 12.16. Damaged unidirectional valve leaflet.

dangerous rebreathing (see Chapter 6). Reported causes include the flow being set too low, a leak or obstruction in the machine, fresh gas supply line or a vaporizer, and an empty cylinder (109,162,264,265).

In Mapleson systems in which the fresh gases are delivered to the distal end of the system by an inner tube, rebreathing will occur if the inner tube is avulsed, damaged, kinked, or has a leak at the machine end; is omitted; or does not extend to the patient port (Fig. 12.17) (151,266–274).

Improper Assembly of Bain System

Cases of incorrect assembly of the Bain system have been reported (269,275). In one

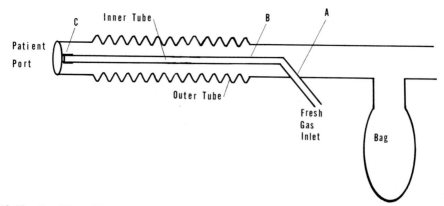

Figure 12.17. Possible problems with the inner tube of the Bain system that can result in hypercarbia. *A,* the fresh gas supply tube can become detached; *B,* the inner tube can become kinked or develop a leak; and *C,* the inner tube may not extend to the patient port.

case, the fresh gas supply tube was connected to the pressure manometer while the manometer was connected to the inflow orifice. In the other case, the system was assembled without the inner tube. In both cases the entire hose became dead space.

Excessive Dead Space

An increase in dead space will increase rebreathing, especially in small patients. One possible source is the heat and moisture exchanger. These come in a variety of sizes and if a large one is used on a patient with a small tidal volume, dangerous rebreathing may occur (276).

Leak in Inspiratory Limb

A leak in the inspiratory limb may allow exhaled gases to enter that limb and then be inhaled during the next inspiration (277). The amount of retrograde flow will be determined by the size and location of the leak.

Hypercarbia is best detected using capnometry. Inspired carbon dioxide will be zero if hypoventilation is the sole causes of hypercarbia. Inadvertent administration of carbon dioxide and rebreathing without carbon dioxide removal will result in an inspired concentration greater than zero. See Chapter 16 for a full discussion of CO_2 monitoring.

Hyperventilation

A hole or tear in the bellows can cause inadvertent hyperventilation (278–280). This can be detected by an increased oxygen concentration if oxygen is the driving gas (or a decreased concentration if air is used).

Increasing the fresh gas flow will increase the tidal volume during mechanically controlled ventilation (281). This is discussed more fully in Chapter 5.

Hyperventilation may be detected by increased volumes on a respirometer or a decrease in end-tidal CO_2.

Excessive Airway Pressure

In addition to interfering with ventilation, a high pressure can cause barotrauma and adverse effects on the cardiovascular system. Neurological changes and otorrhagia have been reported (282,283). A hyperinflated lung may interfere with surgery (284).

MODIFYING FACTORS

The rate and extent of the pressure rise are important and will be affected by a number of factors, including the reservoir bag, the volume and compliance of the system, the fresh gas flow, and use of a cuffed or uncuffed tube. The most important of these is the bag.

The pressure in the breathing system is normally limited to 50 cm H_2O by the reservoir bag. When an automatic ventilator is in use, the bellows buffers increase in pressure. Exclusion of the bag or ventilator bellows from the breathing system removes this buffering capacity so that dangerously high pressures may be attained rapidly when there is coincidental obstruction to the outflow of gases from, or high inflow into, the system. The most common cause of exclusion of the bag is obstruction of the expiratory limb upstream of the bag (see below). The bag may be obstructed by kinking at its neck (285) (see Fig. 12.11). Unfortunately, an anesthesiologist who finds a reservoir bag that is not filled may incorrectly assume that there is a leak in the system and operate the oxygen flush in an attempt to compensate for the leak (286).

Another factor that can affect the rate of pressure rise is an uncuffed tracheal tube or a tracheal tube whose cuff is not inflated to a high pressure. Adjusting cuff pressure to less than 34 cm H_2O will allow it to act as a safety valve for excessive pressure in the airway. Disconnection of components cannot be relied on to provide pressure relief because the pressures required for disconnection are far in excess of those that cause lung injury (200).

CAUSES

High Inflow

If the oxygen flush valve sticks in the on position, 35 to 75 liters/min will be delivered and excessive airway pressures can develop rapidly. On some older anesthesia machines, the oxygen flush valves could be locked in the flush position. Oxygen flush valves on newer machines are designed to close automatically, but can fail (287).

With some oxygen flush valves, it is possible for personnel accidentally to actuate them with their bodies. Other equipment may cause the flush valve to stick in the on position (288–290). A flush valve may stick in the open position (291).

Activation of the oxygen flush valve during the inspiratory phase of the ventilator cycle will cause a large volume of gas to be added to the inspired tidal volume. This will result in a greatly increased pressure in the lung (292,293).

Low Outflow

Buildup of pressure will occur when there is obstruction to the outflow of gases from the breathing system while inflow continues (286).

Obstruction in the Expiratory Limb

As noted above, exclusion of the bag from the breathing system results in loss of its buffering capacity. Thus obstruction of the expiratory limb is particularly hazardous if it occurs upstream of the reservoir bag.

Foreign Bodies. Various objects including ampules, coins, plastic wraps, discs, and caps have been found inside the expiratory limb (294–298).

Water. The expiratory pathway can become obstructed with condensed water (299,300).

Equipment Defects or Misassembly. Reported causes of obstruction to the flow of gases during expiration include defects in swivel ports, bacterial filters, ventilator hoses, heat and moisture exchangers, tub-

ings, and Y pieces (293,301–307). A PEEP valve may stick or become obstructed (308–310).

The expiratory breathing tube may be connected by mistake to the outlet of the APL valve (311–315), the ventilator spill valve (316), or the ventilator port of a bag-ventilator selector valve. A unidirectional PEEP valve placed backward in the expiratory limb (317,318) or attached in reverse to the expiratory port of a manual resuscitation bag (319) will cause complete obstruction to flow.

The expiratory limb of a T piece system can become obstructed by the user's finger, kinking, external compression, a misassembled scavenging valve, or adhesive (320–323). Cases have been reported in which the leaflet from a unidirectional valve was lost during servicing (324,325). It was later found obstructing the connection to the bag mount.

If a pediatric breathing system with an adapter that has the fresh gas inlet protruding near the end is used with a "low dead space" tracheal tube connector, the fresh gas supply tube may closely approximate or even press against the end of the connector, causing partial or complete obstruction of the exhalation pathway (326–329). The same problem has been reported with a bronchoscope (330).

Obstruction at the Ventilator

If the ventilator spill valve becomes stuck, the pressure in the breathing system will rise (187,300,331–333). Blockage of the exit of driving gas from the bellows housing may occur (334).

Obstruction at the APL Valve

Sticking, omission, malfunction, or blockage of an APL valve may occur (285,286,335). The user may fail to open the valve when switching from controlled to spontaneous ventilation (336). With some APL valves, subambient pressure from active scavenging will cause the valve to close, preventing gas from flowing out of the breathing system (337–340).

Obstruction in the Scavenging System

The scavenging system is essentially an extension of the breathing system. Obstruction between the APL valve in the breathing system or the spill valve in the ventilator and the interface will prevent gas from leaving the breathing system (339,341–343). The transfer tubing may be connected to an incorrect site, resulting in obstruction to flow (344–347).

Problems with Nonrebreathing Valves in Resuscitators

A sudden high inflow of gas or a quick squeeze or bump on the bag in a resuscitator may generate sufficient pressure to lock the nonrebreathing valve in the inspiratory position (348). Continuing inflow will cause a rise in pressure. Incorrect assembly or malfunction of a nonrebreathing valve may result in obstruction to exhalation (349–352).

Unintentional PEEP

An external PEEP valve may be left in the circuit and not removed or an integral PEEP valve may be left in the on position at the end of one case and not noticed by the next user (353). With older breathing systems, the airway pressure gauge is located on the absorber side of the unidirectional valves and PEEP cannot be observed on the gauge (318). With these systems, PEEP may be inadvertently set too high (284).

Misconnection of Oxygen Tubing

Misconnection of oxygen tubing directly to an indwelling tracheal or tracheostomy tube or laryngeal mask without provision for venting has occurred, often with disastrous results (354–358) (Fig. 12.18). Another cause is connection to a T piece with a closed expiratory limb (359,360).

Ventilator Malfunction

An anesthesia ventilator can stick in the inspiratory position (361).

DETECTION

When an automatic ventilator is used, it is essential that the chest wall motion, deflections on the breathing system pressure gauge, tidal and minute volumes registered on a respirometer, and breath sounds be monitored carefully. A ventilator that signals when it delivers a high pressure, changes sound with stacked breaths, and limits the maximum pressure should be used. A continuing or high airway pressure alarm may alert the operator of the hazard. Exhaled carbon dioxide monitoring may help to detect these problems. The waveform may show an ascending limb with a prolonged rise time and no plateau. Observation of the airway pressure waveform can also help to detect some problems.

RESPONSE

If there is a pressure buildup in the system, a disconnection should be made IMMEDIATELY at the tracheal tube connector. Ventilation can be carried on with a resuscitation bag until the problem is diagnosed and corrected. Time spent looking for the cause of the problem may result in ever increasing pressure.

Inhalation of a Foreign Substance

ABSORBENT DUST

Inhalation of absorbent dust can cause bronchospasm, laryngospasm, cough, decreased compliance, and burns of the patient's face (362,363). This can be avoided by placing a filter on the inspiratory side of the circle system, placing the reservoir bag on the inspiratory limb, releasing the pressure at the APL valve when checking for leaks (364), tapping each canister to remove dust before it is put into the absorber, and not overfilling canisters (365). Some absorbers have with a dust collector at the bottom (see Figs. 7.2 and 7.4).

Figure 12.18. **A,** The oxygen tubing is attached to the mask. **B,** The adapter has become detached from the mask and is attached to the tracheal tube connector. There is no way for the gas to escape.

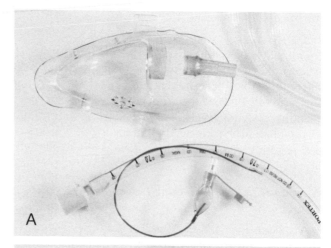

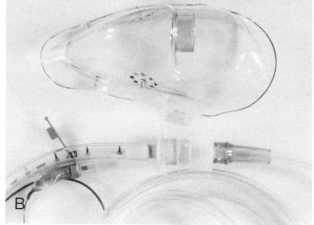

ETHYLENE OXIDE AND GLYCOL (SEE CHAPTER 19)

If equipment sterilized with ethylene oxide is not aerated adequately, residual ethylene oxide can diffuse into the breathing system and be inhaled. When nondisposable equipment is cleaned, water may remain. If wet equipment is sterilized with ethylene oxide, ethylene glycol (a toxic substance) will be formed and subsequently inhaled.

CONTAMINANTS IN MEDICAL GASES

Reported contaminants in medical gases include water (365), oil (366,367), hydrocarbons (21,102,368–371), higher oxides of nitrogen (372), and metallic fragments

(21,369). Bacteria may be found, especially in compressed air (373–376).

PARTS OF BREATHING SYSTEM COMPONENTS

Part of a breathing system component may become detached. Reported cases have involved parts of the sampling site for an aspirating respiratory gas monitor (377,378), an APL valve (379), an oxygen sensor (380), and HMEs (381,382). Some manufacturers plate the inside surfaces of components with materials that may flake off (383–385).

FOREIGN BODIES

A number of foreign bodies have been found in breathing systems, including a cap from a sampling port, a drug bottle top, an ampule cap, a coin, a spring from a humidifier, and part of a plastic bag (230,294,296–298,386). Often these enter the breathing system during cleaning. Part of a glove may be caught between two components (387).

Anesthetic Agent Overdosage

An overdose of anesthetic agent can result in severe cardiovascular depression. See Chapter 4 for a more complete discussion of overdosage caused by vaporizer malfunction.

TIPPING OF A VAPORIZER

If a vaporizer charged with liquid is tipped or agitated, a very high concentration may be delivered when the vaporizer is first turned on (388–390).

VAPORIZER INADVERTENTLY TURNED ON

Previous use of the machine by a colleague or servicing by a technician can result in the control dial being left in the on position (391,392). Someone helping to move the machine may grasp a control dial, inadvertently turning it on. Most newer vaporizers have locks to prevent a vaporizer from being turned on inadvertently.

INCORRECT AGENT

If an agent is incorrectly placed in a vaporizer designed for an agent with a lower vapor pressure and/or a higher MAC value, a hazardously high concentration may be delivered (393–395). Examples include placing isoflurane or halothane in a vaporizer designed for enflurane or placing halothane in a vaporizer designed for isoflurane.

IMPROPER VAPORIZER INSTALLATION

If a vaporizer is located in the fresh gas supply tube, there will be a higher-than-usual flow of gas through the vaporizer after the ox-

ygen flush is activated (396). If such a vaporizer is connected so that the flow runs in a reverse direction, the concentration of vapor coming from the vaporizer may be considerably higher than expected (397,398).

VAPORIZER CONTROL KNOB TURNED THE WRONG WAY

Clockwise rotation of the control on the top of modern vaporizers reduces the concentration of agent or turns it off. On some older vaporizers, this requires counterclockwise rotation. If both types of vaporizers are in the same department, an operator used to the turning motion of one vaporizer may accidentally turn the vaporizer to its maximum concentration while intending to turn the vaporizer off (399).

OVERFILLED VAPORIZER

Most vaporizers are designed so that they cannot be overfilled. Agent-specific filling devices prevent overfilling by connecting the air intake in the bottle to the inside of the vaporizing chamber. However, this safety feature can be overridden by slightly unscrewing the bottle adapter or turning the concentration dial on during filling.

INCORRECT CALCULATIONS

With measured-flow vaporizers it is necessary to make calculations to determine the settings that will give the desired delivered concentration. An error can result in anesthetic agent overdosage. Loss of diluent gas or an incorrect flowmeter reading may also result in overdosage.

When an overdose of anesthetic agent is suspected, the patient should be disconnected from the breathing system and ventilated using a resuscitation bag. If it is determined that the fresh gas flow does not contain anesthetic agent, a high flow of oxygen from the anesthesia machine can be used to ventilate the patient. Oxygen from the oxygen flush should not be contaminated with anesthetic agent. If anesthetic agent can be smelled in the fresh gas flow, the patient should be ventilated using room air or an independent oxygen source.

Inadequate Anesthetic Agent

Although not delivering enough anesthetic agent is usually not as serious as delivering too much, serious morbidity can result (400).

DECREASED NITROUS OXIDE FLOW

Loss of pipeline nitrous oxide caused by leaks, freezing of regulators, improper maintenance, depletion of a system too small to meet demand, and deliberate tampering have been reported (24,401–403). Cylinder supplies can also fail. An obstruction or leak in the anesthesia machine may decrease the nitrous oxide flow (404).

UNEXPECTEDLY HIGH OXYGEN CONCENTRATION

If a connection between the nitrous oxide and oxygen sources occurs, in either the pipeline system or the anesthesia machine, and the oxygen pressure is higher than that of nitrous oxide, oxygen will flow into the nitrous oxide line (405,406). An inward leak of oxygen downstream of the vaporizers will dilute volatile agents as well as nitrous oxide (407).

Accidental activation of the oxygen flush may occur (289,291,408–411). Repeated use of the oxygen flush to keep the reservoir bag filled can lead to patient awareness (137,412).

LEAK IN VAPORIZER

A leak in a vaporizer caused by a loose or absent filler cap or keyed filler block, or a defect in the inflow or outflow connections can cause a low concentration to be delivered (see Fig. 12.6). A vaporizer selector or interlock device can malfunction in such a way that no vapor is delivered, although the vaporizer appears to be situated normally (413).

EMPTY VAPORIZER

Another cause of underdosage is a vaporizer that runs empty (400). A vaporizer with a small vaporizing chamber may empty during a long case, especially if high fresh gas flows are used. Cases have been reported in which a fluid level was visible in the sight glass of a vaporizer when the vaporizer was empty (414).

INCORRECT AGENT IN VAPORIZER

If a vaporizer designed for use with a highly volatile agent is filled with one of low volatility, the patient will fail to receive the concentration expected (393,394). Examples include placing isoflurane or enflurane in a vaporizer designed for halothane and placing enflurane in a vaporizer designed for isoflurane.

INCORRECT VAPORIZER SETTING

An incorrect setting of a vaporizer control knob or flowmeter can be a cause of underdosage. It is important to check settings frequently during a case, as they can be altered without the operator's knowledge. It is not uncommon to forget to turn a vaporizer on after filling it during use.

INCORRECT VAPORIZER MOUNTING

Malfunction of a vaporizer mounting mechanism can result in a lower-than-expected vapor output (415–417).

INCORRECT CALCULATION

With a measured-flow vaporizer, incorrect calculations can result in a lower-than-expected delivered concentration.

AIR ENTRAINED INTO THE BREATHING SYSTEM

If a patient is breathing spontaneously, the negative pressure generated during inspiration may cause significant air entrainment through a leak or disconnection site. Negative pressure can also be caused by a ventilator that has a hanging bellows or a negative pressure phase (418) or by an active scavenging system (85).

DILUTION BY VENTILATOR DRIVING GAS

Driving gas (oxygen or air) can enter the breathing system if the bellows is improperly connected or has a hole (278,280,419–423).

AIR ADDED FROM LIGHT SOURCE

A stream of air used to reduce fogging of a lens may cause dilution of the inhaled anesthetic agents (88).

Inadvertent Exposure to Volatile Agents

It is possible that halothane-related hepatitis or malignant hyperthermia may be triggered by small amounts of agent present in a machine and breathing system even if the vaporizers are turned off (413,424–429).

When a patient with a history of one of these entities must be anesthetized, a machine should be prepared for use by removing all vaporizers (unless the machine isolates the vaporizers from the gas circuit when all vaporizers are in the off position), changing the absorbent, replacing the fresh gas supply hose, using a new disposable circle system, and flushing with oxygen at a rate of 12 liters/min for 6 min (430–433).

Should an episode of malignant hyperthermia occur during administration of anesthesia and the department has a machine from which vaporizers have been removed and that has been thoroughly flushed of volatile agents, it should be substituted for the machine in use. A fresh breathing system should be used. If the department does not have such a machine the following measures should be taken to reduce the inhaled concentration of volatile anesthetic (430,432):

1. Change the breathing system hoses and bag.
2. Change the fresh gas supply hose.
3. Change the absorbent.

4. Use very high flows of oxygen.
5. Insert a charcoal filter on the inspiratory port of the absorber.
6. Avoid using a contaminated ventilator.

Fires and Explosions

Flammable anesthetics have disappeared from operating rooms in the United States, but perioperative fires continue to occur. Most operating room fires ignite on or in the patient. These fires typically result in little damage to equipment, cause considerable injury to patients, and are a complete surprise to the staff (434). Tracheal tube fires during laser procedures will be discussed in Chapter 15.

FACTORS

Three things must be present for a fire to occur: a gas to support combustion, a source of ignition, and a flammable substance. Head and neck surgery offers a particularly good opportunity for all three to be present in close proximity.

Gas to Support Combustion

An oxygen-enriched atmosphere will cause materials that are flammable in air to ignite more easily and burn more vigorously and will lower the ignition threshold for some materials. Dilution of oxygen with nitrogen (air) and/or helium will reduce the potential for combustion.

Because oxygen is heavier than air, it collects in low-lying areas. Some materials such as some drape fabrics, absorb oxygen and retain it for some time.

Nitrous oxide supports combustion and in the process releases the energy of its formation, providing increased heat. Thus any mixture of oxygen and nitrous oxide will support combustion. Air will support combustion, since it contains oxygen.

Source of Ignition

A common source of ignition is the electrosurgical or electrocautery unit. Other reported sources include defibrillators, laser beams, resectascopes, operating room lights, heat lamps, fiberoptic light sources and cables, heated probes, drills and burs, argon beam coagulators, defective electrical equipment, and static electricity (94,434–441).

Another source of heat is adiabatic compression of a gas in a regulator. Rapid opening of a cylinder can result in temperatures up to 1700°F (434). Pieces of Teflon tape, chips from seal materials, latent hydrocarbon contaminants, and other materials may be ignited (442–445).

A Combustible Substance

A number of articles used in or near the patient can serve as the flammable material. These include (but are not limited to) tracheal and tracheostomy tubes, adhesive tape, oxygen cannulae and tubings, breathing tubes and bags, gauze pads and sponges, eye patches, masks, nasogastric tubes, lubricants and ointments, drapes, airways, paper products, blood pressure cuffs, tourniquets, gloves, stethoscope tubing, throat packs, egg crate foam mattresses, gowns, masks, hoods, and cleaning and prepping solutions and sprays (436,446–467). Disposable operating room drapes may be particularly difficult to extinguish because they are water repellent (460). Once ignited they burn rapidly (467).

MEASURES TO PREVENT FIRES

1. High-pressure oxygen equipment should not be contaminated with oil, grease, or other combustible materials. Such equipment should not be cleaned with a flammable agent such as alcohol.

2. A cylinder should always be opened slowly to allow dissipation of heat as the gas is recompressed.

3. Oxygen should be administered only when indicated and only in as high concentrations as are really needed. Use of air for insufflating under drapes should be considered. If oxygen must be used, a barrier should be established between the oxygen-enriched atmosphere and the surgical field, if possible. Tenting drapes around the patient's head will allow air to dilute the oxygen.

4. An attempt should be made to prevent oxygen and oxygen–nitrous oxide mixtures from being vented near a source of ignition or where they will be trapped under drapes. This can be accomplished by using a cuffed or tight-fitting tracheal tube and scavenging excess gases. If gases must be vented near the head or under the drapes, a local scavenging system will help to remove them from the vicinity of the surgery.

Electrosurgery, especially for cutting, should be avoided when the surgical field is adjacent to the oxygen source (468). When electrosurgery or electrocautery must be used while oxygen is being administered nearby (as during eye procedures done under local anesthesia), this should be anticipated by at least 1 min and oxygen administration discontinued.

When there must be an oxygen-rich environment near a heat source, it is advisable to put saline-soaked sponges around the surgical field to minimize the potential sources of fuel for combustion (469).

5. When diathermy is to be used in the oral cavity, the oxygen level should be minimized by using a cuffed tube (457). If an uncuffed tube must be used, a moist occlusive pharyngeal pack will reduce the leak of nitrous oxide and/or oxygen into the cavity (470). Gas that does leak into the cavity can be diluted by insufflating the cavity with a gas that does not support combustion. Gauze or packs to be used in the oral cavity should be moistened with a nonflammable liquid. A flammable liquid such as alcohol should not be used.

6. Water-based prep solutions should be used. If a flammable solution must be used, draping should be delayed until vapor dissipation has occurred.

7. Flammable liquids and sprays should be handled in such a way that pooling or saturation of drapes is avoided.

8. All aerosols should be considered flammable and the use of electrosurgery delayed

for several minutes following their application.

9. Hair near the operative site should be made nonflammable by coating it thoroughly with a water-soluble lubricating jelly or soaking it in saline (440).

10. The electrosurgical unit should function properly and have a proper dispersive (ground plate) circuit. This may shorten the required duty cycle and minimize extra heating of the tip. Use of bipolar rather than unipolar cautery will reduce the current density in the tissues surrounding the active electrode (470).

11. Electrical equipment should be kept in good condition.

12. Nitrogen or air rather than oxygen should be used for powering surgical tools.

13. Metal breathing system components should be used to prevent the spread of a fire (471).

14. Unnecessary foot switches should be removed to prevent accidental device activation.

PREPARATION FOR A FIRE (434,472)

Preparation for a fire will minimize the cost in dollars, lost time, emotional shock, and injury or death. Surgical teams should be trained in and practice drills for quickly stopping fires. Fire extinguishers should be located in convenient, easy-to-reach locations. These locations should be known by all OR staff, who should be well-trained in how to use the extinguishers.

ACTION IN CASE OF A FIRE

If a fire occurs the following steps should be taken (473).

1. Burning material on or in the patient should be removed and extinguished. A small area of burning can be patted out effectively and safely with a gloved hand. Larger areas can be smothered effectively with a blanket or wet towel. If the fire is under and in the drape and the drape material is water resistant, water and extinguishing materials poured on the drapes will be ineffective (474). The most effective method may be ripping the burning materials away from the patient.

If electrical equipment is involved, the power supply should be disconnected before using water to fight the fire, or a carbon dioxide or dry chemical extinguisher should be used (475).

2. The flow of oxygen, nitrous oxide, and air to any equipment involved should be turned off if this can be accomplished without injury to personnel. The zone valve to the operating room should be closed.

3. The immediately exposed patient(s) should be removed from the site of the fire if their hair or clothing are not burning.

In the event of a fire in an anesthetizing area while an operative procedure is in progress, it may be necessary to extinguish the fire before removing the patient from the room. It may be more hazardous to move the patient than to attempt to extinguish or contain the fire. The attending physician must determine which step would present the lesser hazard—hurriedly terminating an operative procedure or continuing the procedure and exposing the members of the operating team and the patient to the hazards stemming from the fire.

4. The fire alarm should be sounded.

5. The doors should be closed to contain the smoke and isolate the fire.

6. Whatever steps are necessary to protect or evacuate patients in adjacent areas should be taken.

7. Firefighters should be directed to the site of the fire.

Accident Investigation (476)

Whenever an adverse perioperative event occurs, one of the first concerns should be to determine the etiology. An often initially overlooked cause is the equipment used. The literature contains many unfortunate examples of two or more patients in succession suffering injury or death due to defective equipment continued to be used after an accident had occurred because the equipment was not suspected. Any time a patient has an unexplained problem, equipment malfunction or misuse should be suspected and the apparatus not used again until this has been disproved.

When there has been an injury to a patient, the hospital safety officer (risk manager) should be contacted at once to supervise investigation of the incident. This person should follow an established protocol so that all important areas are covered systematically. Such a protocol can ease the difficulties involved in gathering information about what may be emotionally charged details (476). All individuals involved in the incident should document their observations soon after the event, while details are still fresh in their minds. This should be a simple statement of facts, without judgments about causality or responsibility.

The following questions relating to equipment need to be asked:

1. What was the date and time of the problem?
2. In what area did the problem occur?
3. What monitors were being used?
4. On what values were the alarms set?
5. What was the first indication that there was a problem?
6. At what time did this occur?
7. Who first noted the problem?
8. What changes attracted attention? Were any alarms activated?
9. What signs or symptoms did the patient exhibit?
10. Had there been any recent modifications to the electrical system or gas pipelines in that area?
11. Was anything altered shortly before the incident?
12. Was this the first case performed in that area that day?
13. Were there any problems during previous cases performed in that area that day or the previous day?

14. Were there any unusual occurrences in other areas that day or the previous day?
15. Had any equipment been moved into that area recently? Were there any problems noted in the room where it was previously used?
16. What preuse checks were made of the anesthesia machine, breathing system, and ventilator?
17. Who last filled the vaporizers on the anesthesia machine?
18. If a vaporizer was recently attached to the machine, were precautions taken to prevent liquid from being spilled into the outflow tract?
19. After the initial indication of a problem, what was the sequence of events that occurred?

An important step involves construction of a time line, on which all events are listed in chronological order (476). This will help to sort out events and may lead to identification of missing data.

Numerous photographs should be taken of the area from various angles, with all equipment situated where it was at the time of the incident. Each piece of equipment should be photographed separately.

After pictures have been taken, all supplies and equipment associated with the case should be saved and sequestered in a secure location and labeled "DO NOT DISTURB" (477). Settings should not be changed. Relevant identifying information such as the manufacturer and lot and/or serial numbers should be recorded.

If, after all this has been done, it appears possible that equipment may be implicated in causing the problem, a thorough inspection of the equipment in the presence of the primary anesthesia personnel, insurance carrier, hospital safety officer, patient representative, and equipment manufacturers should be conducted. The investigation should consist of an in-depth examination of the equipment similar to the checking procedures described in Chapter 18. Vaporizers should be calibrated and checked to determine if vapor is delivered in the off position; an analysis should be made of the vaporizers' contents. Following the investigation, a report should be made, detailing all facts, analyses, and conclusions.

If a problem with the equipment is found, an attempt should be made to reconstruct the accident if this can be done without danger to anyone, and the equipment should again be locked up until any litigation is settled. If the investigation reveals no problems, the equipment can be returned to service with the consent of all parties.

The Safe Medical Devices Act of 1990 requires medical device user facilities to report incidents that reasonably suggest there is a probability that a medical device has caused or contributed to the death, serious injury, or serious illness of a patient (478). The report is due as soon as possible but no later than 10 working days after the user facility becomes aware of the incident.

Accident Prevention

SELECTION OF EQUIPMENT

Prevention of accidents associated with anesthesia equipment should start with proper selection. Reliability, safety, and cost should all be considered. Standardization of equipment, both within the anesthesia department and with other hospital areas, may help decrease mishaps.

REPLACEMENT OF OBSOLETE EQUIPMENT

Replacement of obsolete equipment is a necessary ongoing process. Apparatus that was the best available at one time may become unacceptable as improved models become available. There is no good answer as to when a particular piece of equipment needs to be replaced. Answers to the following questions can help determine this.

1. Can the equipment perform its functions within the manufacturer's specified tolerances?

2. Are the manufacturer's tolerances still satisfactory? Practice techniques change and may result in new demands being placed on the equipment. An example of this is the trend toward use of lower fresh gas flows. Vaporizers that are accurate at high but not low flows may be within the manufacturer's specifications but not suitable for this application.

3. What is the potential for human error? Most newer machines incorporate features designed to limit errors. Use of such equipment may prevent accidents. Examples include features to prevent dialing a hypoxic mixture on an anesthesia machine and a bag-ventilator selector valve that isolates the APL valve.

4. Can the equipment be upgraded? Although it may not be possible to upgrade equipment to meet new standards, there may be things that can be done to make it safer (479).

5. Can the equipment be serviced by qualified personnel? It is important that equipment be serviced by qualified people with proper components. In most cases this means the manufacturer's representative. If the manufacturer is no longer in existence or will no longer service the equipment, it will be necessary to replace it.

6. Will recent anesthesia trainees be able to use the equipment safely? Recent graduates of anesthesia training programs may not be acquainted with older equipment. This could lead to mistakes.

USE OF VIGILANCE AIDS

Use of vigilance aids (described in Chapters 16 and 17 and mentioned above) can provide warning of problems before the patient suffers harm.

EDUCATION AND COMMUNICATION

It is essential that all members of the department receive proper instruction in how to use new equipment properly. Manuals that come with equipment should be reviewed thoroughly.

Proper communication among members of the department is important. Information about equipment modifications or problems should be conveyed to each member. It is important that accidents and near accidents be discussed at department meetings, so that steps can be taken to prevent such occurrences in the future.

REFERENCES

1. Cooper JB, Newbower RS, Long CD, McPeek B. Preventable anesthesia mishaps: a study of human factors. Anesthesiology 1978;49:399–406.
2. Cooper JB, Newbower RS, Kitz RJ. An analysis of major errors and equipment failures in anesthesia management. Considerations for prevention and detection. Anesthesiology 1984;60:34–42.
3. Craig J, Wilson ME. A survey of anaesthetic misadventures. Anaesthesia 1981;36:933–936.
4. Currie M. A prospective survey of anaesthetic critical events in a teaching hospital. Anaesth Intensive Care 1989;17:403–411.
5. Desmonts JM. Role of equipment failure in the causation of anaesthetic morbidity and mortality: results from the French national survey and comparison with the Boston study. Eur J Anaesth 1987;4:200–203.
6. Kumar V, Barcellos WA, Mehta MP, Carter JG. Analysis of critical incidents in a teaching department for quality assurance. A survey of mishaps during anaesthesia. Anaesthesia 1988;43:879–883.
7. Anonymous. Emergency room mixup, deaths linked. Am Med News, August 8, 1971, p. 3.
8. Emmanuel ER, Teh JL. Dental anaesthetic emergency caused by medical gas pipeline installation error. Aust Dent J 1983;28:79–81.
9. LeBourdais E. Nine deaths linked to cross connection. Sudbury General Inquest makes hospital history. Dimens Health Serv 1974;51:10–12.
10. Sato T. Fatal pipeline accidents spur Japanese standards. APSF Newslett 1991;6:14.
11. Anonymous. Hospital death probe continues. Am Med News, August 15, 1977, p. 26.
12. Sprague DH, Archer GW. Intraoperative hypoxia from an erroneously filled liquid oxygen reservoir. Anesthesiology 1975;42:360–363.
13. Smith FP. Multiple deaths from argon contamination of hospital oxygen supply. J Forensic Sci 1987;32:1098–1102.
14. Holland R. Foreign correspondence: "wrong gas" disaster in Hong Kong. APSF Newslett 1989;4:26.
15. Anonymous. Puritan-Bennett quick connect valves for medical gases. Canadian medical devices alert warns of possible cracks. Biomed Safe Stand 1984;14:52–53.
16. Anonymous. Old-style Chemetron central gas outlets. Health Devices 1981;10(9):222–223.
17. Anonymous. Crossed connections in medical gas systems. Technol Anesth 1984;5:3.
18. Anonymous. Crossed N_2O & O_2 lines blamed for outpatient surgery death. Biomed Safe Stand 1992;22:14.
19. Downing JW. Safety of anaesthetic machines. South Afr Med J 1981;30:815.
20. Krenis LJ, Berkowitz DA. Errors in installation of a new gas delivery system found after certification. Anesthesiology 1985;62:677–678.
21. Tingay MG, Ilsley AH, Willis RJ, Thompson MJ, Chalmers AH, Cousins MJ. Gas identity hazards and major contamination of medical gas system of a new hospital. Anaesth Intensive Care 1978; 6:202–209.
22. Spurring PW, Shenolikar BK. Hazards in anaesthetic equipment. Br J Anaesth 1978;50:641–645.
23. Robinson JS. A continuing saga of piped medical gas supply. Anaesthesia 1979;34:66–70.
24. Feeley TW, Hedley-Whyte J. Bulk oxygen and nitrous oxide delivery systems: design and dangers. Anesthesiology 1976;44:301–305.
25. Anonymous. The Westminster inquiry. Lancet 1977;2:175–176.
26. Lane GA. Medical gas outlets—a hazard from interchangeable "quick connect" couplers. Anesthesiology 1980;52:86–87.
27. Carley RH, Houghton IT, Park GR. A near disaster from piped gases. Anaesthesia 1984;39:891–893.
28. Karmann U, Roth F. Prevention of accidents associated with air-oxygen mixers. Anaesthesia 1982;37:680–682.
29. Thorp JM, Railton R. Hypoxia due to air in the oxygen pipeline. Anaesthesia 1982;37:683–687.
30. Ziecheck HD. Faulty ventilator check valves cause pipeline gas contamination. Respir Care 1981; 26:1009–1010.
31. Anonymous. Patient receives air instead of oxygen: Canadian safety alert. Biomed Safe Stand 1991;21:97–98.
32. O'Connor CJ, Hobin KF. Bypassing the diameter-indexed safety system. Anesthesiology 1989; 71:318–319.
33. Boon PE. C-size cylinders. Anaesth Intensive Care 1990;18:586–587.
34. Jawan B, Lee JH. Cardiac arrest caused by an incorrectly filled oxygen cylinder. A case report. Br J Anaesth 1990;64:749–751.
35. Rendell-Baker L. Problems with anesthetic gas machines and their solutions. In: Rendell-Baker L,

ed. Problems with anesthetic and respiratory therapy equipment [Special issue]. Int Anesth Clin 1982;20(3):1–82.

36. Anonymous. Cylinders with unmixed helium/oxygen. Technol Anesth 1990;10:4.

37. Orr IA, Hamilton L. Entonox hazard. Anaesthesia 1985;40:496.

38. Sim P. Entonox hazard: a reply. Anaesthesia 1985;40:496.

39. Anonymous. Misconnection of oxygen regulator to nitrogen cylinder could cause death. Biomed Safe Stand 1988;18:90–91.

40. Anonymous. Nonstandard user modification of gas cylinder pin indexing. Technol Anesth 1989;10:2.

41. Goebel WM. Failure of nitrous oxide and oxygen pin-indexing. Anesth Prog 1980;27:188–191.

42. Jayasuriya JP. Another example of Murphy's law—mix up of pin index valves. Anaesthesia 1986;41:1164.

43. Mead P. Hazard with cylinder yoke. Anaesth Intensive Care 1981;9:79–80.

44. Saposnick AB. Maintenance and repair of gas, humidity, and aerosol equipment. Respir Care 1975;20:938–941.

45. MacMillan RR, Marshall MA. Failure of the pin index system on a Cape Waine ventilator. Anaesthesia 1981;36:334–335.

46. Fuller WR, Kelly R, Russell WJ. Pin-indexing failure. Anaesth Intensive Care 1985;13:440–441.

47. Spurring PW, Shenolikar BK. Hazards in anaesthetic equipment. Br J Anaesth 1978;50:641–645.

48. Bonsu AK, Stead AL. Accidental cross-connexion of oxygen and nitrous oxide in an anaesthetic machine. Anaesthesia 1983;38:767–769.

49. Beudoin MG. Oxygen needle valve obstruction. Anaesth Intensive Care 1988;16:130–131.

50. Khalil SN, Neuman J. Failure of an oxygen flow control valve. Anesthesiology 1990;73:355–356.

51. Rung GW, Schneider AJL. Oxygen flowmeter failure on the North American Drager Narkomed 2a anesthesia machine. Anesth Analg 1986;65:211–212.

52. Anonymous. Oxygen deprivation alleged in $2.5 million negligence suit. Biomed Safe Stand 1981;11:53.

53. McGarry PMF. Anaesthetic machine standard. Can Anaesth Soc J 1978;25:436.

54. Wyant GM. Some dangers in anaesthesia. Can Anaesth Soc J 1978;25:71–72.

55. Jenkins IR. A "too close to door" knob. Anaesth Intensive Care 1991;19:614.

56. Henling CE, Diaz JH. The cluttered anesthesia machine—a cause for hypoxia. Anesthesiology 1983;58:288–289.

57. Linton RAF, Foster CA, Spencer GT. A potential hazard of oxygen flowmeters. Anaesthesia 1982;37:606–607.

58. Russell WJ. The danger of air on anaesthetic machines. Anaesth Intensive Care 1988;16:499.

59. Battig CG. Unusual failure of an oxygen flowmeter. Anesthesiology 1972;37:561–562.

60. Chadwick DA. Transposition of rotameter tubes. Anesthesiology 1974;40:102.

61. Hodge EA. Accuracy of anaesthetic gas flowmeters. Br J Anaesth 1979;51:907.

62. Kelley JM, Gabel RA. The improperly calibrated flowmeter—another hazard. Anesthesiology 1970;33:467–468.

63. Thomas D. Interchangeable rotameter tubes. Anaesth Intensive Care 1983;11:385–386.

64. Hutton P, Boaden RW. Performance of needle valves. Br J Anaesth 1986;58:919–924.

65. Chi OZ. Another example of hypoxic gas mixture delivery. Anesthesiology 1985;62:543–544.

66. Riendl J. Hypoxic gas mixture delivery due to malfunctioning inlet port of a Select-a-Tec vaporizer manifold. Can J Anaesth 1987;34:431.

67. Chung DC, Jing QC, Prins L, Strupat J. Hypoxic gas mixtures delivered by anaesthetic machines equipped with a downstream oxygen flowmeter. Can Anaesth Soc J 1980;27:527–530.

68. Dudley M, Walsh E. Oxygen loss from rotameter. Br J Anaesth 1986;58:1201–1202.

69. Russell WJ. Hypoxia from a selective oxygen leak. Anaesth Intensive Care 1984;12:275–276.

70. McHale S. A critical incident with the Ohmeda Excel 410 machine. Anaesthesia 1991;46:150.

71. Powell J. Leak from an oxygen flow meter. Br J Anaesth 1981;53:671.

72. Wishaw K. Hypoxic gas mixture with Quantiflex monitored dial mixer and induction room safety. Anaesth Intensive Care 1991;19:127.

73. Hanning CD, Kruchek D, Chunara A. Preferential oxygen leak—an unusual case. Anaesthesia 1987;42:1329–1330.

74. Moore JK, Railton R. Hypoxia caused by a leaking rotameter—the value of an oxygen analyser. Anaesthesia 1984;39:380–381.

75. Julien RM. Potentially fatal machine fault. Anesthesiology 1983;58:584–585.

76. Cole AGH, Thompson JB, Fodor IM, Baker AB, Sear JW. Anaesthetic machine hazard from the selectatec block. Anaesthesia 1983;38:175–177.

77. Lenoir RJ, Easy WR. A hazard associated with removal of carbon dioxide cylinders. Anesthesiology 1988;43:892–893.

78. Russell WJ, Ward JB. Hypoxia with a third flowmeter tube on the anaesthetic machine. Anaesth Intensive Care 1978;6:355–357.

79. McQuillan PJ, Jackson IJB. Potential leaks from

anaesthetic machines. Anaesthesia 1987;42:1308–1312.

80. Williams AR, Hilton PJ. Selective oxygen leak. A potential cause of patient hypoxia. Anaesthesia 1986;41:1133–1134.

81. Wilson A. Dangerous leak. Anaesth Intensive Care 1990;18:575.

82. Katz D. Recurring cyanosis of intermittent mechanical origin in anesthetized patients. Anesth Analg 1968;47:233–237.

83. Bishop C, Levick CH, Hodbson C. A design fault in the Boyle apparatus. Br J Anaesth 1967;39:908.

84. Gupta BL, Varshneya AK. Anaesthetic accident caused by unusual leakage of rotameter. Br J Anaesth 1975;47:805.

85. Lanier WL. Intraoperative air entrainment with Ohio Modulus anesthesia machine. Anesthesiology 1986;64:266–268.

86. Ghanooni S, Wilks DH, Finestone SC. A case report of an unusual disconnection. Anesth Analg 1983;62:696–697.

87. Ditchik J, Herr GP. Can we do without O_2 analyzers? Anesthesiology 1984;61:629–630.

88. Mostello LA, Patel RI. Dilution of anesthetic gases by a new light source for bronchoscopy. Anesthesiology 1986;65:445.

89. Russell WG. Oxygen supply at risk. Anaesth Intensive Care 1985;13:216–217.

90. Johnson DL. Central oxygen supply versus mother nature. Respir Care 1975;20:1043–1044.

91. Newson AJ, Dyball LA. A visual monitor for piped oxygen supply systems to anaesthetic machines. Anaesth Intensive Care 1978;6:146–148.

92. Anderson B, Chamley D. Wall outlet oxygen failure. Anaesth Intensive Care 1987;15:468–469.

93. Chung DC, Hunter DJ. The quick-mount pipeline connector. Failure of a "fail-safe" device. Can Anaesth Soc J 1986;33:666–668.

94. Anderson EF. A potential ignition source in the operating room. Anesth Analg 1976;55:217–218.

95. Ewart IA. An unusual cause of gas pipeline failure. Anaesthesia 1990;45:498.

96. Lacoumenta S, Hall GM. A burst oxygen pipeline. Anaesthesia 1983;38:596–597.

97. Craig DB, Culligan J. Sudden interruption of gas flow through a Schrader oxygen coupler unit. Can Anaesth Soc J 1980;27:175–177.

98. Janis KM. Sudden failure of ceiling oxygen connector. Can Anaesth Soc J 1978;25:155.

99. Muir J, Davidson-Lamb R. Apparatus failure—cause for concern. Br J Anaesth 1980;52:705–706.

100. Anderson WR, Brock-Utne JG. Oxygen pipeline supply failure. A coping strategy. J Clin Monit 1991;7:39–41.

101. Varga DA, Guttery JS, Grundy BL. Intermittent oxygen delivery in an Ohmeda Unitrol anesthesia machine due to a faulty O-ring check valve assembly. Anesth Analg 1987;66:1200–1201.

102. Feeley TW, Bancroft ML, Brooks RA, Hedley-Whyte J. Potential hazards of compressed gas cylinders: a review. Anesthesiology 1978;48:72–74.

103. Blogg CE, Colvin MP. Apparently empty oxygen cylinders. Br J Anaesth 1977;49:87.

104. Milliken RA. An explosion hazard due to an imperfect design. Arch Surg 1972;105:125–127.

105. Fitzpatrick G, Moore KP. Malfunction in a needle valve. Anaesthesia 1988;43:164.

106. McMahon DJ, Holm R, Batra MS. Yet another machine fault. Anesthesiology 1983;58:586–587.

107. Boscoe MJ, Baxter RCH. Failure of anaesthetic gas supply. Anaesthesia 1983;38:997–998.

108. From R, George GP, Tinker JH. Foregger 705 malfunction resulting in loss of gas flow. Anesthesiology 1984;61:321–322.

109. Chang JL, Larson CE, Bedger RC, Bleyaert AL. An unusual malfunction of an anesthetic machine. Anesthesiology 1980;52:446–447.

110. Wan YL, Swan M. Exotic obstruction. Anaesth Intensive Care 1990;18:274.

111. Bamber PA. Possible safety hazard on anaesthetic machines. Anaesthesia 1987;42:782.

112. Heine JF, Adams PM. Another potential failure in an oxygen delivery system. Anesthesiology 1985;63:335–336.

113. Capan L, Ramanathan S, Chalon J, O'Meara JB, Turndorf H. A possible hazard with use of the Ohio Ethrane Vaporizer. Anesth Analg 1980;59:65–68.

114. Forrest T, Childs D. An unusual vaporiser leak. Anaesthesia 1982;37:1220–1221.

115. Eldrup-Jorgensen S, Sprissler GT. Gas leaks in anesthesia machines. Anesthesiology 1977;46:439.

116. Pyles ST, Kaplan RF, Munson ES. Gas loss from Ohio Modulus vaporizer selector-interlock valve. Anesth Analg 1983;62:1052.

117. Loughnan TE. Gas leak associated with a selectatec. Anaesth Intensive Care 1988;16:501.

118. Van Besouw JP, Thurlow AC. A hazard of free-standing vaporizers. Anaesthesia 1987;42:671.

119. Qadri AM. Unusual detection of an old problem. Anaesthesia 1988;43:611.

120. Berry PD, Ross DG. Missing O-ring causes unrecognised large gas leak. Anaesthesia 1992;47:359.

121. Patterson KW, Kean PK. Hazard with a Boyle Vaporizer. Anaesthesia 1991;46:152–153.

122. Wraight WJ. Another failure of Selectatec block. Anaesthesia 1990;45:795.

123. Hogan TS. Selectatec switch malfunction. Anaesthesia 1985;40:66–69.

124. Jove F, Milliken RA. Loss of anesthetic gases due to defective safety equipment. Anesth Analg 1983;62:369–370.

125. Jablonski J, Reynolds AC. A potential cause (and cure) of a major gas leak. Anesthesiology 1985;62:842–843.

126. Childres WF. Malfunction of Ohio Modulus anesthesia machine. Anesthesiology 1982;56:330.

127. Carter JA, McAtteer P. A serious hazard associated with the Fluotec Mark 4 vaporizer. Anaesthesia 1984;35:1257–1258.

128. Anonymous. Anesthesia unit vaporizers. Technol Anesth 1987;7:4.

129. Dolan PF. Vaporizer leak. Anesthesiology 1978;49:302.

130. Cooper PD. A hazard with a vaporizer. Anaesthesiology 1984;39:935.

131. Rosenberg M, Solod E, Bourke DL. Gas leak through a Fluotec Mark III Vaporizer. Anesth Analg 1979;58:239–240.

132. Comm G, Rendell-Baker L. Back pressure check valves a hazard. Anesthesiology 1982;56:327–328.

133. Dedrick DF, Mieras CD. Hazard associated with new Foretrend anesthesia machine. Anesthesiology 1979;51:483.

134. Beavis R. Boyles machine. Anaesth Intensive Care 1983;11:80.

135. Kataria B, Price P, Slack M. Delayed filling of the breathing bag due to a portable vaporizer. Anesth Analg 1987;66:1055.

136. Riddle RT. A potential cause (and cure) of a major gas leak. Anesthesiology 1985;62:842–843.

137. Longmuir J, Craig DB. Misadventure with a Boyle's gas machine. Can Anaesth Soc J 1976;23:671–673.

138. Okell RW:Chain of errors. Anaesthesia 1989;44:703–704.

139. Friesen RM. Safety of anaesthetic machines. Can J Anaesth 1989;36:364.

140. Dolan PF. Connections from anesthetic machine to circle system unsatisfactory. Anesthesiology 1979;51:277.

141. Goldman JM, Phelps RW. No flow anesthesia. Anesth Analg 1987;66:1339.

142. Mantia AM. A defective Washington T-piece. An example of inevitable failure and lessons to be learned. Anesthesiology 1983;59:167–168.

143. Milliken RA, Bizzarri DV. An unusual cause of failure of anesthetic gas delivery to a patient circuit. Anesth Analg 1984;63:1047–1048.

144. Anonymous. Anesthesia breathing circuits & fresh gas elbows recalled. Biomed Safe Stand 1989;19:19.

145. Bissonnette B, Roy WL: Obstruction of fresh gas flow in an Ayre's T-piece. Can Anaesth Soc J 1986;33:535–536.

146. Miguel R, Vila H. Machine wars. Another cause of pressure loss in the anesthesia machine. Anesthesiology 1992;77:398–399.

147. Nimocks JA, Modell JH, Perry PA. Carbon dioxide retention using a humidified "nonrebreathing" system. Anesth Analg 1975;54:271–273.

148. Tyler IL, Hammill M. Gas analyzer or anesthesia circuit malfunction? Let room air decide. Anesth Analg 1984;63:702–703.

149. Goresky GV. Bain circuit delivery tube obstructions. Can J Anaesth 1990;37:385.

150. Mansell WH. Bain circuit. The hazard of the hidden tube. Can Anaesth Soc J 1976;23:227.

151. Inglis MS. Torsion of the inner tube. Br J Anaesth 1980;52:705.

152. Forrest PR. Defective anaesthetic breathing circuit. Can J Anaesth 1987;34:541–542.

153. Anonymous. Anesthesia machine owners alerted to potential breathing circuit leak. Biomed Safe Stand 1989;19:122.

154. Birch AA, Fisher NA. Leak of soda lime seal after anesthesia machine check. J Clin Anesth 1989;1:474–476.

155. Brown MC, Burris WR, Hilley MD. Breathing circuit mishap resulting from Y-piece disintegration. Anesthesiology 1988;69:436–437.

156. Cottrell JE, Chalon J, Turndorf H. Faulty anesthesia circuits: a source of environmental pollution in the operating room. Anesth Analg 1977;56:359–362.

157. Colavita RD, Apfelbaum JL. An unusual source of leak in the anesthesia circuit. Anesthesiology 1985;62:208–209.

158. Cullingford D. Broken yoke. Anaesth Intensive Care 1985;13:442.

159. Cooper MG, Vouden J, Rigg D. Circuit leaks. Anaesth Intensive Care 1987;15:539–540.

160. Ferderbar PJ, Kettler RE, Jablonski J, Sportiello R. A cause of breathing system leak during closed circuit anesthesia. Anesthesiology 1986;65:661–663.

161. Kemen M, Desai K, Roizen MF, Jennnings J, Outly S. Over fifty percent of disposable circuits leak. Anesth Analg 1990;70:S194.

162. Lamarche Y. Anaesthetic breathing circuit leak from cracked oxygen analyzer sensor connector. Can Anaesth Soc J 1988;32:682–683.

163. Mantia AM. Faulty Y-piece. Anesth Analg 1981;60:121–122.

164. Lee O, Sommer RM. Pressure monitoring hose causes leak in anesthesia breathing circuit. Anesth Analg 1991;73:365.

165. Poulton TJ. Unusual corrugated tubing leak. Anesth Analg 1986;65:1365.

166. Prasad KK, Chen L. Complications related to the use of a heat and moisture exchanger. Anesthesiology 1990;72:958.

167. Patil AR. Melting of anesthesia circuit by humidifier. Anesth Prog 1989;36:63–65.

168. Raja SN, Geller H. Another potential source of a major gas leak. Anesthesiology 1986;64:297–298.

169. Sosis MB, Payne MN. Another cause for a leak in a disposable breathing circuit. Anesthesiology 1989;71:806.

170. Shampaine EL, Helfaer M. A modest proposal for improved humidifier design. Anesth Analg 1991;72:130–131.

171. Warren PR, Gintautas J. Problems with Dupaco ventilator valve assembly. Anesthesiology 1980; 53:524–525.

172. Stevenson PH, McLeskey CH. Breakage of a reservoir bag mount, an unusual anesthesia machine failure. Anesthesiology 1980;53:270–271.

173. Milliken RA. Bag mount detachment. A function of age? Anesthesiology 1982;56:154.

174. Wood D, Boyd M, Campbell C. Insulation of heated wire circuits. Anesth Analg 1992;74:471.

175. Mizutani AR, Ozaki G, Rusk R. Insulation of heated wire circuits. In response. Anesth Analg 1992;74:472.

176. Brown CQ, Canada ED, Graney WF. Failure of Bain circuit breathing system. Anesthesiology 1981;55:716–717.

177. Breen DP. Failure of a valve in a Bain system. A dangerous design? Anaesthesia 1990;45:417.

178. Miller DC, Collins JW, Wallace L. Failure of the expiratory valve on a Bain System. Anaesthesia 1990;45:992.

179. Nelson RA, Snowdon SL. Failure of an adjustable pressure limiting valve. Anaesthesia 1989;44:788–789.

180. Judkins KC, Safe M. Routine servicing of the Cape-Wane Ventilator. Anaesthesia 1983; 38:1102.

181. Ripp CH, Chapin JW. A bellow's leak in an Ohio anesthesia ventilator. Anesth Analg 1985; 64:942.

182. Hutchinson BR. An unusual leak. Anaesth Intensive Care 1987;15:355.

183. Rolbin S. An unusual cause of ventilator leak. Can Anaesth Soc J 1977;24:522–524.

184. Wolf S, Watson CB, Clark P. An unusual cause of leakage in an anesthesia system. Anesthesiology 1981;55:83–84.

185. Choi JJ, Guida J, Wu W. Hypoventilatory hazard of an anesthetic scavenging device. Anesthesiology 1986;65:126–127.

186. Eisenkraft JB, Sommer RM. Flapper valve malfunction. Anesth Analg 1988;66:1132.

187. Eisenkraft JB. Potential for barotrauma or hypoventilation with the Drager AV-E ventilator. J Clin Anesth 1989;1:452–456.

188. Sommer RM, Bhalla GS, Jackson JM, Cohen MI. Hypoventilation caused by ventilator valve rupture. Anesth Analg 1988;67:999–1001.

189. Khalil SN, Gholston TK, Binderman J, Antosh S.

Flapper valve malfunction in an Ohio closed scavenging system. Anesth Analg 1987;66:1334–1336.

190. Munford BJ, Wishaw KJ. Critical incidents with nonrebreathing valves. Anaesth Intensive Care 1990;18:560–563.

191. Oliver JJ, Pope R. Potential hazard with silicone resuscitators. Anaesthesia 1984;39:933–934.

192. Anonymous. Valve component on resuscitation kits may leak. Biomed Safe Stand 1989;19:35–36.

193. Jameson LC, Popic PM. Detection of anesthesia machine leaks during controlled ventilation in anesthetized dogs. Anesthesiology 1990; 73:A1063.

194. Jameson LC, Popic PM. Detection of anesthesia machine leaks with nitrogen, endtidal CO_2 and pulse oximetry during spontaneous ventilation in anesthetized dogs. Anesthesiology 1990;73:A1031.

195. Graham DH. Advantages of standing bellows ventilators and low-flow techniques. Anesthesiology 1983;58:486.

196. Vistica MF, Posner KL, Caplan RA, Cheney FW. Role of equipment failure and misuse in anesthetic-related malpractice claims. Anesthesiology 1990;73:A1007.

197. Heath ML. Accidents associated with equipment. Anaesthesia 1984;39:57–60.

198. Brahams D. Two locum anaesthetists convicted of manslaughter. Anaesthesia 1990;45:981–982.

199. Neufeld PD, Johnson DL. Results of the Canadian Anaesthetists' Society opinion survey on anaesthetic equipment. Can Anaesth Soc J 1983; 30:469–473.

200. Neufeld PD, Johnson DL, deVeth J. Safety of anaesthesia breathing circuit connectors. Can Anaesth Soc J 1983;30:646–652.

201. Condon HA. An antidisconnexion device. Anaesthesia 1982;37:103–104.

202. Dolan PF. A simple safety device. Br J Anaesth 1976;48:499.

203. Gilston A. Safety clip for Tunstall paediatric connections. Anaesthesia 1980;35:1119.

204. Knell PJW. Accidental disconnection of anaesthetic breathing systems. Anaesthesia 1980;35:825–826.

205. Malloy WF, Poznak AV, Artusio JF. Safety clip for endotracheal tubes. Anesthesiology 1979;50:353–354.

206. Star EG. A simple safety device. Br J Anaesth 1975;47:1034.

207. Spurring PW, Small LFG. Breathing system disconnexions and misconnexions. Anaesthesia 1983;38:683–688.

208. Janowski MJ. Feedback on ventilators. Am J Nurs 1984;84:1494.

209. Blackstock D, Forbes M. Analysis of an anaes-

thetic gas scavenging system hazard. Can J Anaesth 1989;36:204–208.

210. Morr ZF, Stein ED, Orkin LR. A possible hazard in the use of a scavenging system. Anesthesiology 1977;47:302–303.

211. Mostafa SM, Sutcliffe AJ. Antipollution expiratory valves. A potential hazard. Anaesthesia 1982;37:468–469.

212. Seymour A. The need for care in using electric warming blankets. Anaesthesia 1982;37:1218–1219.

213. Patel KD, Dalal FY. A potential hazard of the Drager scavenging interface for wall suction. Anesth Analg 1979;58:327–328.

214. Hodgson CA, Mostafa SM. Riddle of the persistent leak. Anaesthesia 1991;46:799.

215. Stirt JA, Lewenstein LN. Circle system failure induced by gastric suction. Anaesth Intensive Care 1981;9:161–162.

216. Lee T, Schrader MW, Wright BD. Pseudo-failure of mechanical ventilator caused by accidental endobronchial nasogastric tube insertion. Respir Care 1980;25:851–853.

217. Anonymous. Two firms near completion of class II recalls involving anesthesia face mask elbow connectors. Biomed Safe Stand 1985;15:98–99.

218. Anonymous. Breathing-circuit connectors blocked by plastic membrane. Biomed Safe Stand 1991;21:91.

219. Anonymous. Valves, positive end expiratory pressure. Technol Anesth 1991;12:11.

220. Anonymous. Videotape explains OR fires. Technol Anesth 1992;13:7.

221. Baker AJ, Hall R. Malfunction of Hudson electrochemical oxygen sensor. Anaesth Intensive Care 1989;17:516–517.

222. Cook WP, Gravenstein JS. Breathing circuit occlusion due to a defective paediatric face mask. Can J Anaesth 1988;35:205–206.

223. Daley H, Amoroso P. Dangerous repairs. Anaesthesia 1991;46:997.

224. Frankel DZN. Adhesive tape obstructing an anesthetic circuit. Anesthesiology 1983;59:256.

225. Gaines CY, Rees DI. Ventilator malfunction-another cause. Anesthesiology 1984;60:260–261.

226. Koga Y, Iwatsuki N, Takahashi M, Hashimoto Y. A hazardous defect in a humidifier. Anesth Analg 1990;71:712.

227. Prados W. A dangerous defect in a heat and moisture exchanger. Anesthesiology 1989;71:804.

228. Sabo BA, Olinder PJ, Smith RB. Obstruction of a breathing circuit. Anesth Rev 1983;10:28–30.

229. Springman SR, Malischke P. A potentially serious anesthesia system malfunction. Anesthesiology 1986;65:563.

230. Williams EL, Reede L. One cap too many. Anesth Analg 1987;66:1340–1341.

231. Cameron AE, Power I, Tierney B. Portex swivel connector hazard. Anaesthesia 1984;39:496.

232. Crowhurst P. Mishaps with the Mera-F circuit. Anaesth Intensive Care 1987;15:121–122.

233. Shroff PK, Skerman JH. Humidifier malfunction—a cause of anesthesia circuit occlusion. Anesth Analg 1988;67:710–711.

234. Feingold A. Carbon dioxide absorber packaging hazard. Anesthesiology 1976;45:260.

235. Anonymous. Sodasorb prepack CO_2 absorption cartridges. Health Devices 1988;17:35–36.

236. Anonymous. Sodasorb prepac safety advisory. Lexington, MA: WR Grace & Co., March 6, 1992.

237. Heath ML. Accidents associated with equipment. Anaesthesia 1984;39:57–60.

238. Levins RA, Francis RI, Burnley SR. Failure to detect disconnexion by capnography. Anaesthesia 1989;44:79.

239. Morrison AB. Failure to detect anesthetic circuit disconnections. Canadian "medical devices alert" issued by HPB. Biomed Safe Stand 1981;11:28.

240. Slee TA, Pavlin EG. Failure of low pressure alarm associated with the use of a humidifier. Anesthesiology 1988;69:791–793.

241. Wald A. Front panel cover for Frazer-Harlake ventilator. Anesth Analg 1983;62:619–620.

242. McGarrigle R, White S. Oxygen analyzers can detect disconnections. Anesth Analg 1984;63:464–465.

243. Meyer RM. A case for monitoring oxygen in the expiratory limb of the circle. Anesthesiology 1984;61:374.

244. Raphael DT, Weller RS, Doran DJ. A response alogrithm for the low-pressure alarm condition. Anesth Analg 1988;67:876–883.

245. Barry JES, Adams A. Inadvertent administration of carbon dioxide. Surv Anesth 1991;35:368–374.

246. Dinnick DP. Accidental severe hypercapnia during anaesthesia. Br J Anaesth 1968;40:36–45.

247. Klein SL, Lilburn JK. An unusual case of hypercarbia during general anaesthesia. 1980; Anesthesiology 53:248–250.

248. Holland R. Foreign correspondence. Another "wrong gas" incident in Hong Kong. APSF Newslett 1991;6:9.

249. Whitten MP, Wise CC. Design faults in commonly used carbon dioxide absorbers. Br J Anaesth 1972;44:535–537.

250. Andrews JJ, Johnston RV, Bee DE, Arens JF. Photodeactivation of ethyl violet. A potential hazard of sodasorb. Anesthesiology 1990;72:59–64.

251. Detmer MD, Chandra P, Cohen PJ. Occurrence of hypercarbia due to an unusual failure of anesthetic equipment. Anesthesiology 1980;52:278–279.

252. Loughman E. Defective soda lime canisters. Anaesth Intensive Care 1990;18:275.

253. Podraza AG, Salem MR, Joseph NJ, Brenchley JL.

Rebreathing due to incompetent unidirectional valves in the circle absorber system. Anesthesiology 1991;75:A422.

254. Parry TM, Jewkes DA, Smith M. A sticking flutter valve. Anaesthesia 1991;46:229.

255. Nunn BJ, Rosewarne FA. Expiratory valve failure. Anaesth Intensive Care 1990;18:273–274,

256. Anonymous. Anesthesia gas absorber check valves may "stick open." Biomed Safe Stand 1990;20:156.

257. Fogdall RP. Exacerbation of iatrogenic hypercarbia by PEEP. Anesthesiology 1979;51:173–175.

258. Pyles ST, Berman LS, Hodell JH. Expiratory valve dysfunction in a semiclosed circle anesthesia circuit—verification by analysis of carbon dioxide waveform. Anesth Analg 1984;63:536–537.

259. Kim JM, Kovac AL, Mathewson HS. Incompetency of unidirectional dome valves. A multi-hospital study. Anesth Analg 1985;64:237.

260. Rosewarne F, Wells D. Three cases of valve incompetence in a circle system. Anaesth Intensive Care 1988;16:376–377.

261. Whalley DG. Malfunctioning unidirectional valves of Ohmeda series 5 and 5A carbon dioxide absorbers. Can J Anaesth 1988;35:668–669.

262. Dzwonczyk D, Dahl MR, Steinhauser R. A defective unidirectional dome valve was not discovered during normal testing. J Clin Eng 1991;16:485–490.

263. Hornbein TF, Glauber DT. Inadvertent inspiration of carbon dioxide. Anesthesiology 1984;61:114.

264. Berner MS. Profound hypercapnia due to disconnection within an anaesthetic machine. Can J Anaesth 1987;34:622–626.

265. Dunn AJ. Empty tanks and Bain circuits. Can Anaesth Soc J 1978;25:337.

266. Breen M. Letter to the editor. Can Anaesth Soc J 1975;22:247.

267. Hannallah R, Rosales JK. A hazard connected with re-use of the Bain's circuit: a case report. Can Anaesth Soc J 1974;21:511–513.

268. Naqvi NH. Torsion of inner tube. Br J Anaesth 1981;53:193.

269. Peterson WC. Bain circuit. Can Anaesth Soc J 1978;25:532.

270. Mansell WH. Spontaneous breathing with the Bain circuit at low flow rates: a case report. Can Anaesth Soc J 1976;23:432–434.

271. Fukunaga AF. Torsion and disconnection of inner tube of coaxial breathing circuit. Br J Anaesth 1981;53:1106–1107.

272. Roberts PJ. Unattached inner coaxial tube. Anaesthesia 1987;42:1128.

273. Read PJH, Lukey R. Potential hazard of the Kendall "Bain" circuit. Anaesth Intensive Care 1989;17:510.

274. Wildsmith JAW, Grubb DJ. Defective and misused co-axial circuits. Anaesthesia 1977;32:293.

275. Paterson JG, Vanhooydonk V. A hazard associated with improper connection of the Bain breathing circuit. Can Anaesth Soc J 1975;22:373–377.

276. Raju R. Humidifier-induced hypercarbia. Anaesthesia 1987;42:672-673.

277. McNulty S, Barringer L, Browder J. Carbon dioxide associated with a humidifier defect. Can J Anaesth 1987;34:519–521.

278. Rigg D, Joseph M. Split ventilator bellows. Anaesth Intensive Care 1985;13:213.

279. Podraza A, Salem MR, Harris TL, Moritz H. Effects of bellows leaks on anesthesia ventilator function. Anesth Analg 1991;72:S215.

280. Waterman PM, Pautler S, Smith RB. Accidental ventilator-induced hyperventilation. Anesthesiology 1978;48:141.

281. Ghani GA. Fresh gas flow affects minute volume during mechanical ventilation. Anesth Analg 1984;63:619.

282. Dogu TS, Davis HS. Hazards of inadvertently opposed valves. Anesthesiology 1970;33:122–123.

283. Weaver LK, Fairfax WR, Greenway L. Bilateral otorrhagia associated with continuous positive airway pressure. Chest 1988;93:878–879.

284. Mayle LL, Reed SJ, Wyche MQ. Excessive airway pressures occurring concurrently with use of the Fraser Harlake PEEP valve. Anesthesiol Rev 1990;17:41–44.

285. Thompson PW. Prevention of the hazard of excessive airway pressure. Anaesthesia 1979;34:593.

286. Newton NI, Adams AQ. Excessive airway pressure during anesthesia. Anaesthesia 1978;33:689–699.

287. Bailey PL. Failed release of an activated oxygen flush valve. Anesthesiology 1983;59:480.

288. Anderson EC, Rendell-Baker L. Exposed O_2 flush hazard. Anesthesiology 56:328.1982

289. Cooper CMS. Capnography. Anaesthesia 1987;42:1238–1239.

290. Hanafiah Z, Sellers WFS. Nudging the emergency oxygen. Anaesthesia 1991;46:331.

291. Puttick N. Hazard from the oxygen flush control. Anaesthesia 1986;41:222–224.

292. Andrews JJ. Understanding anesthesia ventilators (ASA Refresher Course #242). Park Ridge, IL: ASA, 1990.

293. Anonymous. Barotrauma from anesthesia ventilators. Technol Anesth 1988;9:1–2.

294. Alston RP. Expiratory obstruction in a circle system. Anaesthesia 1987;42:1120.

295. Anonymous. Malfunction of anesthesia machine [The Malpractice Reporter]. Anesthesiology 1991;10:1.

296. Bishay EG, Echiverri E, Abu-Zaineh M, Lee C. An unusual cause for airway obstruction in a young healthy adult. Anesthesiology 1984;60:610–611.

297. Hindman BJ, Sperring SJ. Partial expiratory limb obstruction by a foreign body abutting upon an Ohio 5400 volume monitor sensor. Anesthesiology 1986;65:349–350.

298. Jack TM. An unusual cause of complete expiratory obstruction. Anaesthesia 1987;42:564.

299. Hilgenberg JC, Burke BC. Positive end-expiratory pressure produced by water in the condensation chamber. Anesth Analg 1985;64:541–543.

300. Hilton PJ, Clement JA. Surgical emphysema resulting from a ventilator malfunction. Anaesthesia 1983;38:342–345.

301. Anonymous. Dryden anesthesia breathing circuits. Technol Anesth 1988;8:4–5.

302. Escobar A, Aldrete A. Bacterial filters for anesthesia apparatus. Anesthesiol Rev 1977;4:25A–25B.

303. Grundy EM, Bennett EJ, Brennan T. Obstructed anesthetic circuits. Anesthesiol Rev 1976;3:35–36.

304. Loeser EA. Water-induced resistance in disposable respiratory-circuit bacterial filters. Anesth Analg 1978;57:269–271.

305. Mason J, Tackley R. An acute rise in expiratory resistance due to a blocked ventilator filter. Anaesthesia 1981;36:335.

306. Register SD. Detection of defective equipment by proper preanesthetic checks. Anesthesiology 1985;62:546–547.

307. Smith CE, Otworth JR, Kaluszyk P. Bilateral tension pneumothroax due to a defective anesthesia breathing circuit filter. J Clin Anesth 1991;3:229–234.

308. Anagnostou JM, Hults SL, Moorthy SS. PEEP valve barotrauma [Letter]. Anesth Analg 1990; 70:674–675.

309. Anonymous. Valves, positive end expiratory pressure. Technol Anesth 1991;11:11.

310. Kacmarek RM, Dimas S, Reynolds J, Shapiro BA. Technical aspects of positive end-expiratory pressure (PEEP). Part II. PEEP with positive-pressure ventilation. Respir Care 1982;27:1490–1504.

311. Flowerdew RMM. A hazard of scavenger port design. Can Anaesth Soc J 1891;28:481–483.

312. Holley HS, Eisenman TS. Hazards of an anesthetic scavenging device. Anesth Analg 1983;62:458–460.

313. Mann ES, Sprague DH. An easily overlooked malassembly. Anesthesiology 1982;56:413–414.

314. Stevens IM. Hazardous misconnection. Anaesth Intensive Care 1988;16:374–375.

315. Tavakoli M, Habeeb A. Two hazards of gas scavenging. Anesth Analg 1978;57:286–287.

316. Edwards ND. Another misconnection. Anesthesiology 1988;43:1066.

317. Anonymous. PEEP valves in anesthesia circuits. Health Devices 1983;13:24–25.

318. Cooper JB. Unidirectional PEEP valves can cause safety hazards. APSF Newslett 1990;5:28–29.

319. Arellano R, Ross D, Lee K. Inappropriate attachment of PEEP valve causing total obstruction of ventilation bag. Anesth Analg 1987;66:1050–1051.

320. Arens JF. A hazard in the use of an Ayre T-piece. Anesth Analg 1971;50:943–946.

321. Anonymous. Dupaco bag tail scavenging valves. Technol Anesth 1983;4(6):1–2.

322. Prince GD. Nichols BJ. Kinked breathing systems—again. Anaesthesia 1989;44:792.

323. Lynch CGM. The tail of a bag: a hazard. Anaesthesia 1976;31:803–804.

324. Anonymous. CO_2 absorber subject of class I recall; firm disputes FDA designation for anesthesia device component. Biomed Safe Stand 1983;13:98–99.

325. Dean HN, Parsons DE, Raphaely RC. Case report. Bilateral tension pneumothorax from mechanical failure of anesthesia machine due to misplaced expiratory valve. Anesth Analg 1971;50:195–198.

326. Goldsmith M. FDA issues pediatric respiratory device alert. JAMA 1983;250:2264.

327. Anonymous. Incompatability of Nellcor ADAP-PS gas sampling Tee and Dryden CPRAM breathing circuit. Technol Anesth 1986;10:6–8.

328. Branson R, Lam AM. Increased resistance to breathing: a potentially lethal hazard across a coaxial circuit-connector coupling. Can J Anaesth 1987;34:S90–S91.

329. Villforth JC. FDA safety alert. Breathing system connectors. Rockville, MD: U.S. Food and Drug Administration, September 2, 1983.

330. Sloan IA, Ironside NK. Internal mis-mating of breathing system components. Can Anaesth Soc J 1984;31:576–578.

331. Anonymous. Wrongful death suit dismissal overturned. Am Med News, November 13, 1981.

332. Anonymous. Pre-use testing prevents "helpful" reconnection of anesthesia components. Technol Anesth 1987;8:1–2.

333. Henzig D. Insidious PEEP from a defective ventilator gas evacuation outlet valve. Anesthesiology 1982;57:251–252.

334. Roth S, Tweedie E, Sommer RM. Excessive airway pressure due to a malfunctioning anesthesia ventilator. Anesthesiology 1986;65:532–534.

335. Burgess RW. Blockage of spill valve. Anaesth Intensive Care 1986;14:327–328.

336. Sellery GR. Hazards of artificial ventilation in the operating room. Can Med Assoc J 1972;107:421–423.

337. Sharrock ME, Leith DE. Potential pulmonary barotrauma when venting anesthetic gases to suction. Anesthesiology 1977;46:152–154.

338. Rendell-Baker L. Hazard of blocked scavenging valve. Can Anaesth Soc J 1982;29:182–183.

339. O'Conner DE, Daniels BW, Pfitzner J. Hazards of

anaesthetic scavenging: case reports and brief review. Anaesth Intensive Care 1982;10:15–19.

340. Malloy WF, Wrightman AE, O'Sullivan D, Goldiner PL. Bilateral pneumothorax from suction applied to a ventilator exhaust valve. Anesth Analg 1979;58:147–149.

341. Davies G, Tarnawsky M. Letters to the Editor. Can Anaesth Soc J 1976;23:228.

342. Hamilton RC, Byrne J. Another cause of gas-scavenging-line obstruction. Anesthesiology 1979;51:365–366.

343. Hagerdal M, Lecky JH. Anesthetic death of an experimental animal related to a scavenging system malfunction. Anesthesiology 1977;47:522–523.

344. Hayes C. An interesting misconnexion. Anaesthesia 1991;46:508–509.

345. Sainsbury DA. Scavenging misconnection. Anaesth Intensive Care 1985;13:215–216.

346. Phillips S. Scavenging hazard. Anaesth Intensive Care 1991;19:615.

347. Moon JRA. Expiratory obstruction from coincidence of sizing. Anaesthesia 1992;47:538–539.

348. Anonymous. Improperly cleaned resuscitator valves may stick & block airway. Biomed Safe Stand 1991;21:105–107.

349. Dolan PF, Shapiro S, Steinbach RB. Valve misassembly—manually operated resuscitation bag. Anesth Analg 1981;60:66–67.

350. Klick JM, Bushnell LS, Bancroft ML. Barotrauma, a potential hazard of manual resuscitators. Anesthesiology 1978;49:363–365.

351. Jumper A, Desai S, Liu P, Philip J. Pulmonary barotrauma resulting from a faulty Hope II resuscitation bag. Anesthesiology 1983;58:572–574.

352. Pauca AL, Jenkins TE. Airway obstruction by breakdown of a nonrebreathing valve. How foolproof is foolproof? Anesth Analg 1981;60:529–531.

353. Markovitz BP, Silverberg M, Godinez RI. Unusual cause of an absent capnogram. Anesthesiology 1990;71:992–993.

354. Katz L,Crosby JW. Accidental misconnections to endotracheal and tracheostomy tubes. Can Med Assoc J 1986;135:1149–1151.

355. Wasserberger J, Ordog GJ, Turner AF, et al. Iatrogenic pulmonary overpressure accident. Ann Emerg Med 1986;15:947–951.

356. Onsiong MK. Potential hazard of Hudson facemask. Anaesthesia 1988;43:907.

357. Newton NI. Supplementary oxygen—potential for disaster [Editorial]. Anaesthesia 1991;46:905–906.

358. Davies JR. A false compatibility. Anaesthesia 1991;46:991.

359. Arnold WP. Application of OSHA standard to waste anesthetic gases. ASA Newslett 1992; 56(8):23.

360. Giesecke AH, Skrivanek GD. Respiratory obstruction in the recovery room. Anesth Analg 1992;75:639.

361. Murray AW, Easton JC. Another problem with an expiratory valve. Anaesthesia 1988;43:891–892.

362. Davis R. Soda lime dust. Anaesth Intensive Care 1979;8:390.

363. Lauria JI. Soda-lime dust contamination of breathing circuits. Anesthesiology 1975;42:628–629.

364. Ribak B. Reducing the soda lime hazard. Anesthesiology 1975;43:277.

365. Goodie D, Stewart I. Ulco carbon dioxide absorber. Anaesth Intensive Care 1991;19:609–610.

365. Schiller DJ. Rusty water in an oxygen flowmeter. Anaesthesia 1986;41:1061.

366. Dinnick OP. Medical gases—pipeline problems. Eng Med 1979;8:243–247.

367. Anonymous. Oxygen cylinders recalled because of oil contamination. Biomed Safe Stand 1991;21:20.

368. Russell WJ. Industrial gas hazard. Anaesth Intensive Care 1985;13:106.

369. Eichorn JH, Bancroft ML, Laasberg LH, du Moulin GC, Saubermann AJ. Contamination of medical gas and water pipelines in a new hospital building. Anesthesiology 1977;46:286–289.

370. Gilmour IJ, McComb C, Palahniuk RJ. Contamination of a hospital oxygen supply. Anesth Analg 1990;71:302–304.

371. Coveler LA, Lester RC. Contaminated oxygen cylinder. Anesth Analg 1989;69:674–676.

372. Clutton-Brock J. Two cases of poisoning by contamination of nitrous oxide with higher oxides of nitrogen during anaesthesia. Br J Anaesth 1967;39:388–392.

373. Bjerring P, Oberg B. Bacterial contamination of compressed air for medical use. Anaesthesia 1986;41:148–150.

374. Bjerring P, Oberg B. Possible role of vacuum systems and compressed air generators in cross–infection in the ICU. Br J Anaesth 1987;59:648–650.

375. Oberg B, Bjerring P. Comparison of microbiological contents of compressed air in two Danish hospitals. Effect of oil and water reduction in air-generating units. Acta Anaesth Scand 1986;30:305–308.

376. Warren RE, Newsom SWB, Matthews JA, Arrowsmith LWM. Medical grade compressed air. Lancet 1986;1:1438.

377. Anonymous. Device safety alert. Anesthesia gas elbow component may separate. Biomed Safe Stand 1989;19:90.

378. Paulus DA. Drilling remnants in elbow adapters. Anesth Analg 1986;65:824.

379. Oh T. Bagging a foreign body. Anaesth Intensive Care 1978;6:89–91.

380. Ross A. Oxygen analyser hazard. Anaesth Intensive Care 1986;14:466–467.

381. Taylor BL, Rainbow C, Ford D. Debris in a breathing system. Anaesthesia 1989;44:702.

382. James PD, Gothard JWW. Possible hazard from the inserts of condenser humidifiers. Anaesthesia 1984;39:70.

383. Austin TR. Metallic flaking: a further hazard of anaesthetic apparatus. Anaesthesia 1972;27:92–93.

384. Gold MI. Defect in a T-fitting connection. Anesthesiology 1980;52:184.

385. Wald A, Mercurio A. Blistering of epoxy material of Narco Airshields ventilator Anesthesiology 1983;58:390.

386. Nimmagadda UR, Salem MR, Klowden AJ, Smith D, Saab S. An unusual foreign body in the left main bronchus after open heart surgery. Anesth Analg 1989;68:803–805.

387. Siler JN, Neumann G. Latex glove hazard. APSF Newslett 1992;7:11.

388. Munson WM. Cardiac arrest: a hazard of tipping a vaporizer. Anesthesiology 1965;26:235.

389. Long GJ, Marsh HM. A danger—insecure positioning of anaesthetic vaporizers. Med J Aust 1969;1:1108.

390. Scott DM. Performance of BOC Ohmeda Tec 3 and Tec 4 vaporizers following tipping. Anaesth Intensive Care 1991;19:441–443.

391. Riley RH, Hammond KA, Currie MS. "Hazards" of oxygen therapy during spinal anaesthesia. Anaesthesia 1991;46:421.

392. Williams L, Barton C, McVey JR, Smith JD. A visual warning device for improved safety. Anesth Analg 1986;65:1364.

393. Bruce DL, Linde HW. Vaporization of mixed anesthetic liquids. Anesthesiology 1984;342–346.

394. Chilcoat RT. Hazards of mis-filled vaporizers. Summary tables. Anesthesiology 1985;63:726–727.

395. Martin S. Hazards of agent-specific vaporizers. A case report of successful resuscitation after massive isoflurane overdose. Anesthesiology 1985;62:830–831.

396. Kelly DA. Free-standing vaporizers. Anaesthesia 1985;40:661–663.

397. Marks WE, Bullard JR. Another hazard of free-standing vaporizers, increased anesthetic concentration with reversed flow of vaporizing gas. Anesthesiology 1976;45:445–446.

398. Railton R, Inglis MD. High halothane concentrations from reversed flow in a vaporizer. Anaesthesia 1986;41:672–673.

399. Anonymous. Inquest told anesthetic killed young mother. Winnipeg Globe and Mail, January 8, 1986, p. A3.

400. Lewyn MJ. Patient wins damages for injury secondary to "light" anesthesia. Anesth Malprac Protector 1991;3:109–113.

401. Francis RN. Failure of nitrous oxide supply to the atre pipeline system. Anaesthesia 1990;45:880–882.

402. Yogananthan S. Failure of nitrous oxide supply. Anaesthesia 1990;45:897.

403. Paul DL. Pipeline failure. Anaesthesia 1989;44:523.

404. Comber REH. Penlon rotameter block failure. Anaesth Intensive Care 1990;18:141–142.

405. Craig DB, Longmuir J. An unusual failure of an oxygen fail-safe device. Can Anaesth Soc J 1971;18:576–577.

406. Puri GD, George MA, Singh H, Batra YK. Awareness under anaesthesia due to a defective gas-loaded regulator. Anaesthesia 1987;42:539–540.

407. Anonymous. Internal leakage from anesthesia unit flush valves. Health Devices 1981;10:172.

408. Brahams D. Anaesthesia and the law. Awareness and pain during anaesthesia. Anaesthesia 1989;44:352.

409. Judkins KC. BOC Boyle M anaesthetic machine—a modification. Anaesthesia 1983;38:387–388.

410. Paymaster NJ. Inadvertent administration of 100% oxygen during anaesthesia. Br J Anaesth 1978;50:1268.

411. Dodd KW. Inadvertent admisistration of 100% oxygen during anaesthesia. Br J Anaesth 1979;51:573.

412. Peters KR, Wingard DW. Anesthesia machine leakage due to misaligned vaporizers. Anesth Rev 1987;14:36–39.

413. Duncan JAT. Select-a-tec switch malfunction. Anaesthesia 1985;40:911–924.

414. Barcroft JP. Is there liquid in the vaporizer? Anaesthesia 1989;44:939.

415. Cudmore J, Keogh J. Another Selectatec switch malfunction. Anaesthesia 1990;45:754–756.

416. Lamberty JM, Lerman J. Intraoperative failure of a fluotec Mark II vapourizer. Can Anaesth Soc J 1984;31:687–689.

417. Maltby JR. Intraoperative failure of a Fluotec Mark II vapourizer. Can Anaesth Soc J 1985;32:200.

418. Bookallil MJ. Entrainment of air during mechanical ventilation. Br J Anaesth 1967;39:184.

419. Baraka A, Muallem M. Awareness during anaesthesia due to a ventilator malfunction. Anaesthesia 1979;34:678–679.

420. Longmuir J, Craig DB. Inadvertent increase in inspired oxygen concentration due to defect in ventilator bellows. Can Anaesth Soc J 1976;23:327–329.

421. Love JB. Misassembly of a Campbell ventilator causing leakage of the driving gas to a patient. Anaesth Intensive Care 1980;8:376–377.

422. Hillyer KW, Johnston RR. Unsuspected dilution of anesthetic gases detected by an oxygen analyzer. Anesth Analg 1978;57:491–492.

423. Marsland AR, Solomos J. Ventilator malfunction detected by O_2 analyser. Anaesth Intensive Care 1981;9:395.

424. Varma RR, Whitesell RC, Iskandarani MM. Halothane hepatitis without halothane. Role of inapparent circuit contamination and its prevention. Hepatology 1985;5:1159–1162.

425. Ellis FR, Clarks IMC, Modgill EM, Appleyard TN, Dinsdale RCW. New causes of malignant hyperpyrexia. 1975;Br Med J 1:575.

426. Bridges RT. Vaporizers—serviced and checked? Anaesthesia 1991;46:695–697.

427. Cook TL, Eger EI, Behl RS. Is your vaporizer off? Anesth Analg 1977;56:793–800.

428. Robinson JS, Thompson JM, Barratt RS. Inadvertent contamination of anaesthetic circuits with halothane. Br J Anaesth 1977;49:745–753.

429. Ritchie PA, Cheshire MA, Pearce NH. Decontamination of halothane from anaesthetic machines achieved by continuous flushing with oxygen. Br J Anaesth 1988;60:859–863.

430. Beebe JJ, Sessler KI. Preparation of anesthesia machines for patients susceptible to malignant hyperthermia. Anesthesiology 1988;69:395–400.

431. McGraw TT, Keon TP. Malignant hyperthermia and the clean machine. Can J Anaesth 1989;36:530–532.

432. Cooper JB, Philip JH. More on anesthesia machines and malignant hyperpyrexia. Anesthesiology 1989;70:561–562.

433. Samulksa HM, Ramaiah S, Noble WH. Unintended exposure to halothane in surgical patients. halothane washout studies. Can Anaesth Soc J 1972;19:35–41.

434. ECRI. Understanding the fire hazard. Technol Anesth 1992;12:1–6.

435. Miller PH. Potential fire hazard in defibrillation. JAMA 1972;221:192.

436. Rita L, Seleny F. Endotracheal tube ignition during laryngeal surgery with resectoscope. Anesthesiology 1982;56:60–61.

437. Anonymous. Hazard: unshielded radiant heat sources. Technol Anesth 1984;5:1–2.

438. Anonymous. Laser starts fire in OR. Technol Anesth 1988;8:3–4.

439. Willis MJ, Thomas E. The cold light source that was hot. Gastrointest Endosc 1984;30:117–118.

440. Epstein RH, Brummett RR Jr., Lask GP. Incendiary potential of the flash-lamp pumped 585-nm tunable dye laser. Anesth Analg 1990;71:171–175.

441. Wegrzynowicz ES, Jensen NF, Pearson KS, Wachtel RE, Scamman FL. Airway fire during jet ventilation for laser excision of vocal cord papillomata. Anesthesiology 1992;76:468–469.

442. Anonymous. Oxygen regulator fire caused by use of two yoke washers. Technol Anesth 1990;11:1–2.

443. Garfield JM, Allen GW, Silverstein P, Mendenhall MK. Flash fire in a reducing valve. Anesthesiology 1971;34:578–579.

444. Ito Y, Horikawa H, Ichiyanagi K. Fires and explosions with compressed gases. Br J Anaesth 1965;37:140–141.

445. Newton BE, Langford RK, Meyer GR. Promoted ignition of oxygen regulators In: Stoltzful JM, Benz FJ, Stradling JS, eds. Flammability and sensitivity of materials in oxygen-enriched atmospheres. Vol. 4. Philadelphia: ASTM, 1989:241–266.

446. Perel A, Mahler Y, Davidson JT. Combustion of a nasal catheter carrying oxygen. Anesthesiology 1976;45:666–667.

447. Anonymous. Infant dies after operating room flash fire. Biomed Safe Stand 1988;18:154.

448. Anonymous. Use of acetone & "eggcrate" mattress cited in operating room fire. Indiana hospitals advised to review internal policies. Biomed Safe Stand 1989;19:26.

449. Ashcraft KE, Golladay ES, Guinee WS. A surgical field flash fire during the separation of dicephalus dipus conjoined twins. Anesthesiology 1981; 55:457–458.

450. Anonymous. Fires during surgery of the head and neck area. Health Devices Alerts 1980;4:3–4.

451. Bowdle TA, Glenn M, Colston H, Eisele D. Fire following use of electrocautery during emergency percutaneous transtracheal ventilation. Anesthesiology 1987;66:697–698.

452. Collee GG. A fire in the mouth. Anaesthesia 1984;39:936.

453. Datta TD. Flash fire hazard with eye ointment. Anesth Analg 1984;63:700–701.

454. Gupte SR. Gauze fire in the oral cavity: a case report. Anesth Analg 1972;51:645–646.

455. Gibbs JM. Combustible plastic drape. Anaesth Intensive Care 1983;11:176.

456. Simpson JI, Wolf GL. Endotracheal tube fire ignited by pharyngeal electrocautery. Anesthesiology 1986;65:76–77.

457. Wong A, Macdonald M, Walker P, Fear D, Crysdale W. Diathermy-induced airway fire during tonsillectomy. Anesthesiology 1992;77:A1060.

458. Anonymous. Laser-ignited latex glove causes airway fire. Biomed Safe Stand 1992;22:51.

459. Magruder GB, Gruber D. Fire prevention during surgery. Arch Ophthalmol 1970;84:237.

460. Milliken RA, Bizzarri DV. Flammable surgical drapes—a patient and personnel hazard. Anesth Analg 1985;64:54–57.

461. Milliken RA, Bizzarri DV. Combustible plastic drape. Anaesth Intensive Care 1984;12:275.

462. Marsh B, Riley RH. Double-lumen tube fire during tracheostomy. Anesthesiology 1992;76:480–481.

463. Le Clair J, Gartner S, Halma G. Endotracheal tube cuff ignited by electrocautery during tracheostomy. Am Assoc Nur Anesth 1990;58:259–261.

464. Plumlee JE. Operating-room flash fire from use of cautery after aerosol spray: a case report. Anesth Analg 1973;52:202–203.

465. Schettler WH. Correspondence. Anesth Analg 1974;53:288–289.

466. Simpson JI, Wolf GL. Flammability of esophageal stethoscopes, nasogastric tubes, feeding tubes, and nasopharyngeal airways in oxygen- and nitrous oxide-enriched atmospheres. Anesth Analg 1988;67:1093–1095.

467. Ott AE. Disposable surgical drapes—a potential fire hazard. Obstet Gynecol 1983;61:667–668.

468. Bowdle TA, Glenn M, Colston H, Eisele D. Fire following use of electrocautery during emergency percutaneous transtracheal ventilation. Anesthesiology 1987;66:697–698.

469. Lake CH. From the literature. ECRI review explains, warns of OR fires. APSF Newslett 1991;6:46.

470. Sommer RM. Preventing endotracheal tube fire during pharyngeal surgery. Anesthesiology 1987;66:439.

471. Sosis M, Braverman B, Ivankovich AD. Metal anesthesia circuit components stop laser fires. Anesthesiology 1991;75:A396.

472. Moxon MA, Reading ME, Ward MB. Fire in the operating theatre. Evacuation pre-planning may save lives. Anaesthesia 1986;41:543–546.

473. National Fire Protection Association. Health care facilities. Suggested procedures in the event of a fire or explosion, anesthetizing locations (NFPA 99.1990). Quincey, MA: NFPA, 1990:182–184.

474. Bruner JMR. Fire in the operating room. ASA News 1990;54:22–25.

475. The Compressed Gas Association. Handbook of compressed gases. 3rd ed. New York: Van Nostrand Reinhold, 1990.

476. Armstrong JN, Davies JM. A systematic method for the investigation of anaesthetic incidents. Can J Anaesth 1991;38:1033–1035.

477. Anonymous. Impounding incident-related devices. Technol Anesth 1984;4(10):1.

478. Anonymous. FDA proposed rule on user facility and manufacturer reporting under the Safe Medical Devices Act of 1990. Biomed Safe Stand 1991;14(suppl):1–16.

479. Schneider AJL. Older anesthesia machines targeted for component replacement. APSF Newslett 1989;4:25–27.

Chapter 13

Face Masks and Airways

Face Masks

The face mask, or face piece, allows administration of gases from the breathing system without introducing any apparatus into the patient.

GENERAL DESCRIPTION (1)

A face mask may be constructed of rubber or plastic.

Mask Body

The mask body constitutes the main part of the mask. A transparent body allows observation of the patient for vomitus, secretions, blood, lip color, and condensation of exhaled moisture. It may be better accepted by a conscious patient.

Face Seal

The face seal (also called rim or flap) is the part of the mask that comes in contact with the face. Two general types of seals are used. One is a cushion (rim pad) that is inflated with air or filled with a material that will conform to the face when pressure is applied. The second type of seal is a flange that is an extension of the body.

Connector

The connector, or orifice, is at the opposite side from the face seal. It consists of a thickened fitting with an internal diameter of 15 or 22 mm. A hook ring may be placed around the connector.

SPECIFIC MASKS

A wide variety of masks is available. Some are shown in Figures 13.1 through 13.10. Most are available in a variety of sizes. An assortment of different face masks should be kept readily available, because none will fit every face well.

Anatomical Mask

The anatomical mask (Fig. 13.1) has a body is made of rubber that can be widened or narrowed to fit the face. It is available in a variety of sizes.

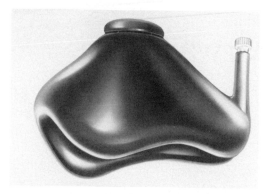

Figure 13.1. Anatomical mask (also known as Connell Mask or Form-It). Courtesy of Ohio Medical Products, a division of Airco, Inc.

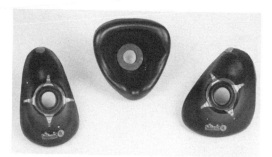

Figure 13.3. SCRAMs, or the selective contour retaining anatomical masks. Courtesy of Ohio Medical Products, a division of Airco, Inc.

Trimar Mask

The Trimar mask (Fig. 13.2) is similar to the anatomical mask but has a shallower body and less dead space.

SCRAM

The SCRAM, or selective contour retaining anatomical mask (Fig. 13.3), is designed for difficult-to-fit patients. The seal is a cushion filled with plastic. The entire mask body and seal can be molded.

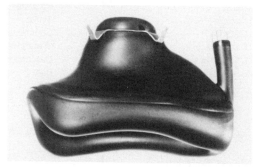

Figure 13.4. Bridgeless mask. Courtesy of Ohio Medical Products, a division of Airco, Inc.

Bridgeless Mask

The bridgeless mask (Fig. 13.4) is designed for a face with flat features or little or no nose bridge. It has an air-filled cushion. The nose notch is eliminated. The body is shallow and the curvature of the seal is flatter than that on the anatomical mask.

Ambu Transparent Mask

The Ambu transparent mask (Fig. 13.5) has a body of clear plastic. The seal is a pneumatic cuff. There is a thumb rest built into the body.

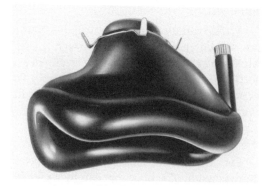

Figure 13.2. Trimar mask. Courtesy of Ohio Medical Products, a division of Airco, Inc.

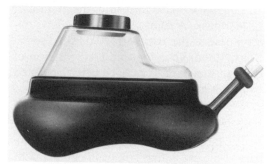

Figure 13.5. Ambu transparent mask. Courtesy of Ambu International.

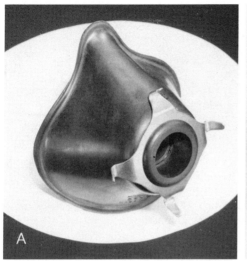
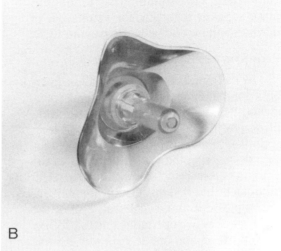

Figure 13.6. Rendell-Baker-Soucek masks. **A,** Black rubber version. **B,** Clear plastic version with pacifier. Courtesy of Ohio Medical Products, a division of Airco, Inc.

Rendell-Baker-Soucek Mask

The Rendell-Baker-Soucek (RBS) mask (Fig. 13.6) is designed to fit the pediatric patient. It has a solid triangular body made from rubber or clear plastic. It has a low dead space (2,3). Some of these masks are scented and may have a pacifier (Fig. 13.6*B*). This mask has been reported to be useful in ventilating postlaryngectomy patients (4,5).

Flotex Multifitting Mask (6)

The Flotex multifitting (antistatic) face mask (Fig. 13.7) has a rubber flange instead of a pneumatic cushion. The flange is extended so that it can be placed under the chin.

Laerdal Mask

The Laerdal mask (Fig. 13.8) is a soft one-piece silicone rubber mask with an inward-curving circular face seal. It can be boiled and

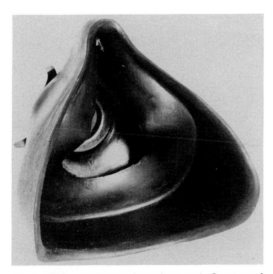

Figure 13.7. Flotex multifitting face mask. Courtesy of Harris-Lake, Inc.

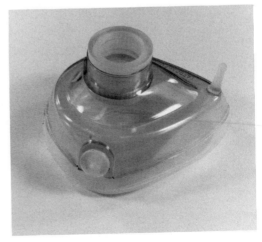

Figure 13.8. The Laerdal mask.

autoclaved. Two studies have found this mask superior to others for ventilation of newborn infants and pediatric patients (3,7).

Patil-Syracuse Endoscopic Mask (8,9)

The Patil mask is designed to allow fiberoptic intubation in a patient breathing spontaneously or receiving positive pressure ventilation by mask. The mask (Fig. 13.9) has an endoscopic port with a silicone diaphragm. A cap for covering the port is attached to the mask. A fiberscope with or without a tracheal tube can be inserted through the diaphragm, which provides an airtight seal. Use of the mask requires two operators: one to perform the intubation and one to maintain the airway, mask fit, and ventilation (10).

The diaphragm frequently ruptures as the tracheal tube cuff passes (11–14). Lubricating the tracheal tube or using an uncuffed tube will reduce this risk. Alternately, a rubber diaphragm can be fashioned and cut away and removed when the tracheal tube is advanced (12).

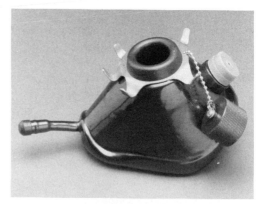

Figure 13.9. Patil-Syracuse endoscopic mask. Courtesy of Mercury Medical.

Clear Disposable Mask

A number of clear disposable masks are available from different manufacturers in various sizes. Two are shown in Figure 13.10.

MASK FIT

A good mask fit is essential, but it can be a difficult and vexing problem. Considerable

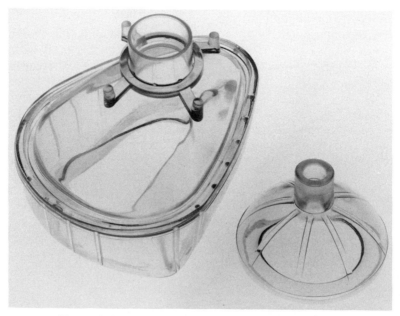

Figure 13.10.   Clear, disposable masks. Courtesy of Rusch Inc.

manual strength and dexterity may be necessary to achieve a tight seal and at the same time lift the jaw to prevent airway obstruction. A poor fit requires the anesthesia provider to maintain steady pressure. This may lead to cramped hands and tired forearms and limits the ability to do other tasks.

Failure to obtain a tight fit with spontaneous respirations will result in air dilution. This can be compensated for by increasing the fresh gas flow, but this is wasteful and contaminates the room with anesthetic gases. In addition, the reservoir bag no longer serves as a means of monitoring ventilation. With assisted or controlled respiration, development of adequate positive pressure to ventilate the patient will be impossible if the mask fit is poor.

Mask Selection

The best fit is obtained by selecting a mask and testing it before induction of anesthesia. The smallest mask that will do the job is the most desirable because it will cause the least increase in dead space, will usually be easiest to hold, and will be less likely to result in pressure on the eyes.

The Patient's Face

The mask rests on the skin over the nasal and maxillary bones above and the mandible below. The buccinator muscle forms out the cheeks and helps to create a seal in the area between the maxilla and the mandible.

A variety of face types will be encountered in clinical practice. These include fat, emaciated, and edentulous faces and those with prominent nares, burns, flat noses, receding jaws, beards, or drainage tubes in the mouth or nose.

The edentulous patient presents the most common problem. There is loss of bone of the alveolar ridge, causing a loss of distance between the points where the mask rests on the mandible and the nose. This makes a tight fit difficult. Inserting an oral airway will increase the distance by opening the mouth.

Furthermore, the buccinator muscle loses its tone in these patients. The cheeks sag, creating large gaps between them and the mask. Alveolar process resorption results in a shrinking of the corners of the mouth. Packing the cheek with gauze sponges may make up for the loss of bone structure and cheek tone. It may be desirable to leave the patient's dentures in place.

Holding the Mask

There are several methods of holding a mask to maintain an open airway and a tight seal. The method most commonly used is shown in Figure 13.11. The left hand grasps the mask. The thumb and index finger are placed on the body on opposite sides of the connector. These fingers push downward to hold the mask to the face and prevent leaks. Additional downward pressure can be exerted by the anesthesiologist's chin on the mask elbow. Three fingers are placed on the mandible. The middle finger is applied to the mentum and the ring and/or little finger to the angle of the mandible. It is important that there be no pressure applied to soft tissues of the patient's face or neck, as this may decrease patency of the airway.

A second method can be used to open any but the most difficult airway and obtain a

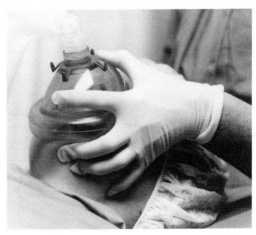

Figure 13.11.   Holding the mask with one hand.

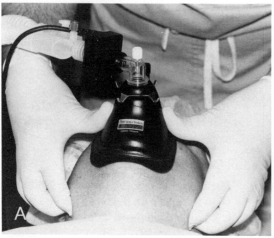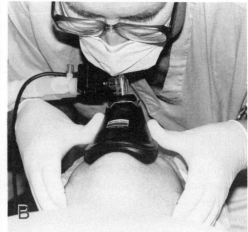

Figure 13.12.   A, Holding the mask with two hands. Also shown is the Esmarch-Heiberg maneuver, which involves dorsiflexion at the atlantooccipital joint and protrusion of the mandible anteriorly by exerting a forward thrust on the rami. **B,** The anesthesiologist's chin on the mask elbow helps create a better seal between the mask and the patient's face.

tight fit with the mask (Fig. 13.12). It is cumbersome in that it requires two hands so a second person is necessary for assisted or controlled respiration. The thumbs are placed on either side of the body of the mask. The index fingers are placed under the angle of the jaw. The mandible is lifted and the head extended. If a leak still occurs, downward pressure on the mask can be increased by the anesthesiologist's chin on the mask elbow (see Fig. 13.12*B*)

Another technique has been described that uses a triangular-shaped mask, such as the SCRAM or Trimar (15). The patient's mouth is opened and the horizontal border of the mask is placed between the gingiva of the maxilla and mandible. The mask is rotated onto the face so the superior angle of the mask conforms to the nose. The inferior margin of the mask is used as a fulcrum on which the mandible may be protruded.

DEAD SPACE

In any apparatus involving their use, the face mask and its adaptor contribute the major proportion of increased dead space, provided the fresh gas flow is adequate (16). This is of greatest significance in small patients. The entire volume of the face mask may not constitute dead space as channeling of air currents may reduce dead space (17). The dead space may be decreased by increasing the pressure on the mask, decreasing the volume of the cushion, using a smaller mask, extending the separation of the inspiratory and expiratory channels close to or into the mask, and blowing a jet of fresh gas into the mask.

MASK STRAPS

A mask strap (also called inhaler retainer, head strap, mask harness, mask retainer, headband, and head-restraining strap) serves to hold the mask firmly on the face. Its use may decrease leaks. A typical mask strap consists of thin rubber strips arranged in a circle with four or six projections (Fig. 13.13). The head rests in the circle and the straps attach around the mask connector.

The straps at the jaw may tend to pull the jaw posteriorly. Crossing the two lower straps under the chin may result in a better fit and counteract the pull of the upper straps so that there is less tendency for the mask to creep up above the bridge of the nose (18). Other suggestions are to insert a tongue depressor or

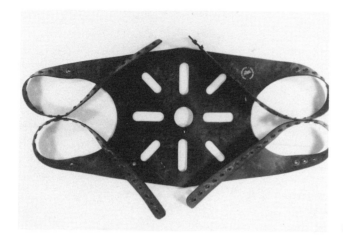

Figure 13.13.   Mask strap.

finger splint transversely under the strips below the jaw (19).

Care must be taken not to draw the straps too tight, because they can cause pressure damage from either the mask or the straps themselves. The straps should be kept as loose as is compatible with adequate ventilation and released periodically. Another danger of mask straps is that should vomiting or regurgitation occur, it takes longer to remove the mask.

COMPLICATIONS

Dermatitis

Dermatitis may occur if the patient is allergic to the material from which the mask is formed (20). Chemical or gas sterilization can leave a residue that can cause a dermatitis after contact with the skin (21,22). The pattern of the dermatitis follows the area of contact between the mask and skin.

Nerve Injury

Direct pressure from the mask or mask strap may cause injury to branches of the trigeminal or facial nerves. Forward displacement of the jaw may cause nerve injury from stretching. Fortunately, the sensory and motor dysfunctions reported have been transient (23–28).

If excessive pressure on the face or extreme forward displacement of the jaw must be exerted, intubation should be considered. The mask should be removed from the face periodically and readjusted to make certain that sustained pressure is not applied to one area.

Aspiration

A mask does not protect the tracheobronchial tree from aspiration of gastric contents (29). Ventilation with a mask may allow air to enter the stomach, increasing the risk of regurgitation and aspiration.

Injury to the Eye

Chemical disinfectants that gain access to the mask during cleaning and disinfection can run into the eye when the mask is applied to the face (30–32). Pressure on the medial angles of the eyes and supraorbital margins may result in edema of the eyelids, chemosis of the conjunctiva, pressure on the supraorbital or supratrochlear nerve, corneal injury, and possibly temporary blindness owing to acutely increased intraocular pressure (18). A corneal abrasion may be caused by a face mask placed inadvertently on an open eye (33).

Manufacturing Defects

A defective mask on which a plastic membrane occluded the connector portion of the mask was reported (34). Another mask had the end of a metal wire sticking out (35).

Movement of the Cervical Spine

Studies show that mask ventilation moves the cervical spine more than any commonly used method of tracheal intubation (36).

Latex Allergy

If rubber is a component of a face mask, anaphylactic reaction is a possible hazard (37,38).

Environmental Pollution

Studies show that use of a face mask is associated with greater environmental pollution with anesthetic gases and vapors than use of a tracheal tube or laryngeal mask (39–41). Pollution can be reduced by use of a close active scavenging device (42–44).

User Fatigue

Holding a mask securely onto the face and at the same time maintaining the correct position of the jaw can be difficult and may result in operator fatigue after a period of time. Failure to maintain the correct jaw position may result in loss of airway patency and air may be forced into the stomach.

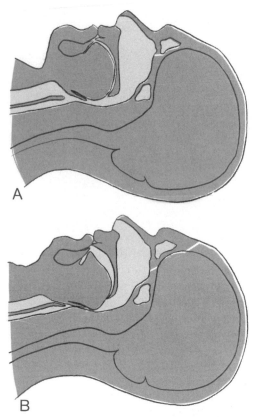

Figure 13.14. **A,** The normal airway. The tongue and other soft tissues are forward, allowing an unobstructed air passage. **B,** the obstructed airway. The tongue and epiglottis fall back to the posterior pharyngeal wall, occluding the airway. Courtesy of V. Robideaux, M.D.

Airways

PURPOSE (45,46)

A fundamental responsibility of the anesthesia provider is to maintain a patent airway. Failure to do so for more than a few minutes will result in brain damage or death.

Figure 13.14*A* shows the normal unobstructed airway in a supine patient. The air passage has a rigid posterior wall, supported by the cervical vertebrae, and a collapsible anterior wall, consisting of the tongue and epiglottis. Figure 13.14*B* shows the most common cause of airway obstruction. The muscles of the floor of the mouth and pharynx supporting the tongue relax, and the tongue and epiglottis fall back into the posterior pharynx, occluding the airway. When in place, an airway lifts the posterior aspect of the tongue and the epiglottis away from the posterior pharyngeal wall and prevents them from obstructing the space above the larynx.

Unlike other maneuvers to maintain a patent airway, including chin lift, jaw thrust, and tracheal intubation, insertion of an airway does not affect the stability of the cervical spine (47).

TYPES

Oropharyngeal Airways

Figure 13.15 shows an oropharyngeal (oral) airway in place. It extends from the lips to the pharynx, fitting between the lips and teeth and the tongue and posterior pharyn-

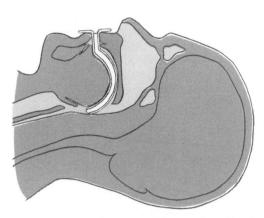

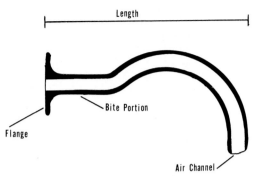

Figure 13.16. Oropharyngeal airway.

Figure 13.15. Oropharyngeal airway in place. The airway follows the curvature of the tongue, pulling it and the epiglottis away from the posterior pharyngeal wall and providing a channel for air passage. Courtesy of V. Robideaux, M.D.

geal wall. The pharyngeal end rests between the posterior wall of the oropharynx and the base of the tongue and, by pressure along the base of the tongue, pulls the epiglottis forward. The bite portion is between the teeth and the flange is outside the lips.

In addition to helping maintain an open airway, an oropharyngeal airway may be used to prevent a patient from biting and occluding a tracheal tube inserted through the mouth, protect the tongue during biting or seizure activity, facilitate suctioning, obtain a better mask fit, and/or provide a pathway for insertion of tubular devices into the esophagus or pharynx. Its use has not been associated with an increased incidence of sore throat or other symptoms (48,49).

General Description

An oropharyngeal airway is made of rubber or plastic (Fig. 13.16). It has a flange at the buccal end to prevent it from falling back into the mouth. It also may serve as a means to fix the airway in place. The flange may or may not rest on the patient's lips.

The bite portion is straight and fits between the teeth or gums. It must be firm enough that the patient cannot close the air channel by biting. The curved portion extends upward and backward to correspond to the shape of the tongue and palate.

The ANSI standard (50) on airways states that the size of an oropharyngeal airway shall be designated by a number that gives the nominal length in centimeters.

Specific Airways

Guedel Airway. The Guedel airway is perhaps the most frequently used type (Fig. 13.17). It has a large flange at the buccal end, a supported bite portion, and a gentle curve that follows the contour of the tongue. There is a tubular channel for air exchange and suction. A modification of this airway to aid flexible fiberoptic intubation in children has been described (51).

Berman Airway (52). The Berman airway has no enclosed air channel (see Figs. 13.15 and 13.16). There is a center support and the sides are open. This allows passage of tubular structures and provides air channels. The center support may have openings. There is a flange at the buccal end.

Patil-Syracuse Oral Airway. The Patil-Syracuse oral airway (or Patil endoscopic airway) was designed to aid in fiberoptic intubation (9). It has lateral suction channels and a groove in the center of the lingual surface to allow passage of a fiberscope and guide it in the midline. A slit in the distal end allows the fiberscope to be manipulated in the anteroposterior direction. Lateral manipulation is limited.

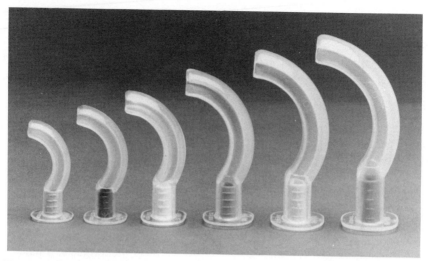

Figure 13.17.   Guedel airways. The bite portions are color coded to provide easy identification of size. Courtesy of Mercury Medical.

Williams Airway Intubator (53,54). The Williams airway intubator was originally designed for use in blind orotracheal intubations (55). It can also be used in fiberoptic intubations and as a conventional oral airway.

The airway is shown in Figure 13.18. It is plastic and available in two sizes, #9 and #10, which will admit up to an 8.0 or 8.5 tracheal tube, respectively. The proximal half is a cylindrical tunnel for placement of a fiberoptic scope and concentric tracheal tube, whereas the distal half is open on its lingual surface. The tracheal tube connector should be left off during intubation, because it will not pass through the airway.

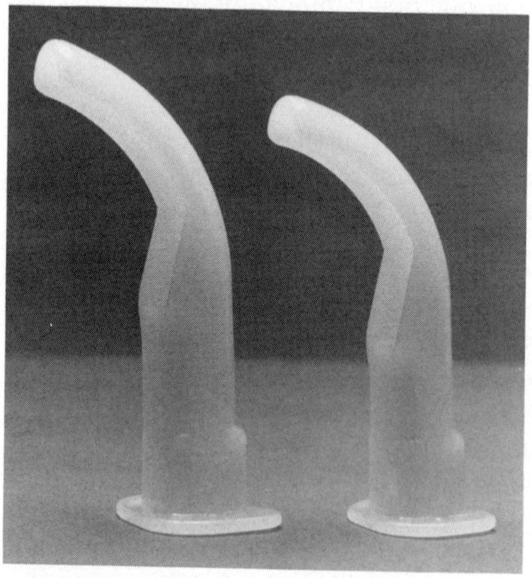

Ovassapian Fiberoptic Intubating Airway (56). The Ovassapian intubating airway is designed for use during fiberoptic intubation (Fig. 13.19). It has a flat, narrow lingual surface on the proximal end, which gradually widens at the distal end. At the buccal end are two vertical side walls. There are two pairs of curved guide walls between the side walls. The guide walls curve toward each other, leaving a space between them for a tracheal tube up to 9.0-mm ID. The guide walls are

Figure 13.18.   Williams airway intubators. Courtesy of Mercury Medical.

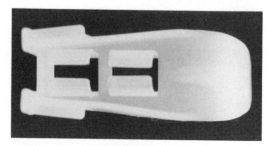

Figure 13.19.   Ovassapian fiberoptic intubating airway. Courtesy of A. Ovassapian, M.D.

flexible so that the airway may be removed from around the tracheal tube after intubation has been completed. The proximal half is tubular so that it can function as a bite block. The distal half of the airway has no posterior wall. This provides an open space in the oropharynx in which the distal end of the fiberscope can be maneuvered. It is not necessary to remove the tracheal tube connector when using this airway for fiberoptic intubation.

Tongue Retracting Airway. The tongue retracting airway is shown in Figure 13.20. The pharyngeal tip can be manipulated via a latching mechanism so that it moves the tongue to a more anterior position.

Computer Assisted Design Airway. The computer assisted design (CAD) airway (Fig. 13.21) is a modification of the Berman air-

way. It has a wide web with fenestrations. The lingual surface is tapered. The bite portion is elongated, especially on the lingual surface. The tip is slightly upturned. There is a ribbon slot near the buccal flange.

Berman Intubatation Pharyngeal Airway. The Berman intubation pharyngeal airway (Berman II) can be used the same way as a conventional airway or as an aid to blind orotracheal intubation or fiberoptic intubation via the oral route. This airway is tubular in its entire length to allow insertion of a lubricated tracheal tube (Fig. 13.22). The tip at the pharyngeal end fits into the vallecula, exerting a forward pull on the tongue. It is open on one side so that it can be split and removed, leaving the tracheal tube in place.

Insertion

Pharyngeal and laryngeal reflexes should be depressed before insertion is attempted. A smooth induction may be disturbed by a premature attempt to use an airway.

Selection of the correct size airway is important. Too small an airway may cause the tongue to kink and force the posterior part against the roof of the mouth, obstructing gas movement. Too large an airway may cause obstruction by displacing the epiglottis and may traumatize the larynx. The correct size can be estimated by holding the airway next to the patient's mouth. The tip should rest cephalad to the angle of the mandible.

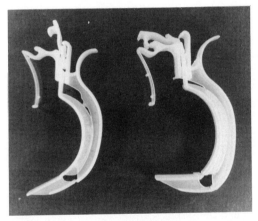

Figure 13.20. Tongue-retracting airways. The airway on the *right* is in the retracted position.

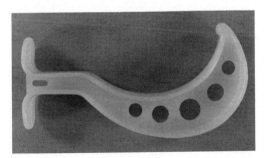

Figure 13.21. Computer assisted design (CAD) airway.

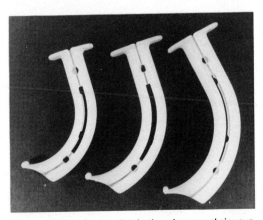

Figure 13.22. Berman intubation pharyngeal airways.

Wetting or lubricating the airway may facilitate insertion. The jaw is opened with the left hand. The teeth or gums are separated by pressing the thumb against the lower teeth or gum and the index or third finger against the upper teeth or gum. This crossed finger and thumb give the user increased leverage to open the mouth.

Oral airways may be inserted in two ways. One method is shown in Figure 13.23. The airway is inserted with its concave side toward the upper lip. When the tip has passed the uvula, the airway is rotated 180°, so that the tip lies posterior to the tongue.

An alternate method of insertion is shown in Figure 13.24. A tongue blade may be used to depress the tongue. The airway is held horizontal as the tip is inserted into the mouth. As the airway is advanced, it is rotated to a vertical position. This causes it to slide around behind the tongue.

The best criteria for proper size and position of the airway is unobstructed gas exchange.

Use with Fiberoptic Endoscopes

An adhesive transparent dressing can be used over an airway designed to aid in fiber-

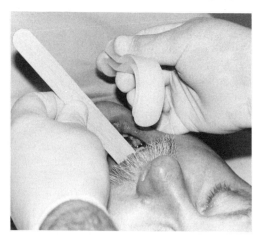

Figure 13.24.   Alternative method of inserting an oral airway. A tongue blade is used to displace the tongue forward.

optic intubation to provide a tight seal and allow for positive pressure ventilation (59).

Bite Block

A bite block (also called a gag or mouth prop) is placed between the teeth or gums to prevent them from occluding an oral tracheal tube or damaging a fiberscope and to keep the mouth open for suctioning. It also is used during electroconvulsive therapy and in unconscious individuals to prevent the patient from biting his or her tongue or lips. Because a bite block does not extend into the pharynx it is usually less irritating than an airway. Smaller bite blocks may be placed between the molar teeth.

A variety of bite blocks has been developed (Figs. 13.25 and 13.26). Some have channels for air passage. Many have an attached string that can be pinned to the patient's gown or taped to the side of the face so that it can be easily retrieved. A gauze sponge roll may serve as a bite block. A bite block may be part of a device used to secure a tracheal tube.

Nasopharyngeal Airways

A nasopharyngeal airway (also known as a nasal airway and nasal trumpet) is shown in position in Figure 13.27. It extends from the

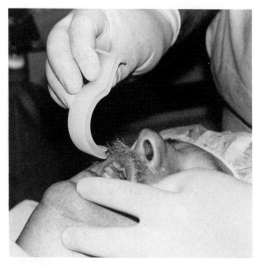

Figure 13.23.   Insertion of oral airway. Airway is turned 180° from the final resting position.

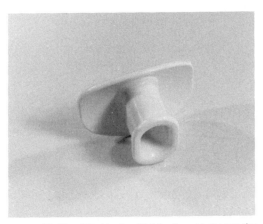

Figure 13.25. Bite block, which is placed between the teeth or gums (preferably in the molar area) to prevent occlusion of a tracheal tube or damage to a fiberoptic endoscope or to keep the mouth open for suctioning.

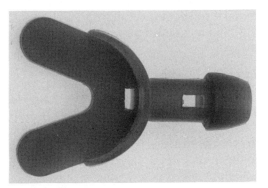

Figure 13.26. Oberto mouth prop, which is used for protecting the teeth during electroconvulsive therapy. Courtesy of Rusch Inc.

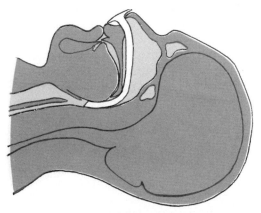

Figure 13.27. The nasopharyngeal airway in place. The airway passes through the nose and extends to just above the epiglottis. Courtesy of V. Robideaux, M.D.

nose to the pharynx, with the pharyngeal end above the epiglottis and below the base of the tongue with the flange just outside the nostril.

The nasopharyngeal airway offers an alternative to the oral airway. There are occasions when the mouth cannot be opened or an oral airway does not provide relief from obstruction. The nasal airway is better tolerated in the semiawake patient than is the oral airway and is less likely to be accidentally displaced or removed. A nasal airway may be preferable if the patient's teeth are loose or in poor condition, or there is trauma or pathology of the oral cavity (58). Nasopharyngeal airways have been used to aid in pharyngeal surgery, to apply continuous positive airway pressure, to facilitate suctioning, to reduce trauma when passing a flexible fiberoptic bronchoscope, and to help in the management of Pierre Robin syndrome (59) and singultus (hiccups).

Contraindications to the use of a nasopharyngeal airway include hemorrhagic disorders; use of anticoagulants; a basilar skull fracture; and pathology, sepsis, or deformity of the nose or nasopharynx. Special care should be exercised in children to avoid trauma to the adenoid tissues.

General Description

A nasopharyngeal airway resembles a shortened tracheal tube with a flanged end. It may be made of plastic or rubber. The ANSI standard (50) requires that the size of a nasopharyngeal airway be designated by a number expressing the inside diameter in millimeters.

Specific Airways

Bardex Airway. The Bardex (or Robertazzi) airway (Fig. 13.28) is made of rubber. The pharyngeal end has a bevel, and there is a large flange at the nasal end.

Rusch Airway. The Rusch nasal airway (see Fig. 13.28) is made of red rubber. It has an adjustable flange at the nasal end. The pharyngeal end has a short bevel.

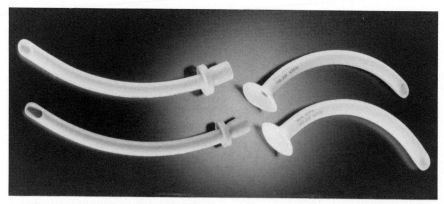

Figure 13.28. Nasopharyngeal airways. *Left,* Rusch. *Right,* Bardex (Robertazzi). Courtesy of Rusch Inc.

Linder Nasopharyngeal Airway (60).
The Linder nasopharyngeal airway is a clear plastic airway with a large flange (Fig. 13.29). The distal end is flat rather than beveled. The airway is supplied with an introducer, which has a balloon on its tip. The balloon can be inflated and deflated by attaching a Luer syringe to the one-way valve at the other end of the introducer.

Before insertion, the introducer is inserted into the airway until the tip of the balloon is just past the end. Air is injected through the one-way valve until the tip of the balloon is inflated to approximately the outside diameter of the tube. The complete assembly is inserted through the nostril. After it is in place, the balloon is deflated and the introducer removed.

Insertion

The length of airway needed for a patient can be estimated as the distance from the tragus of the ear to the tip of the nose plus 1 inch (61) or the distance from the tip of the nose to the meatus of the ear (62)

Before insertion, the nasal airway should be lubricated thoroughly along its entire length. Although the use of vasoconstrictors before insertion of the airway has been advocated, their use may not always be beneficial. Insertion should always be done gently to prevent epistaxis.

The nasopharyngeal airway should be inserted as shown in Figure 13.30*A*. The airway is held in the hand on the same side as it is to be inserted and pointed posteriorly. If resistance is encountered during insertion, the other nostril or a smaller airway should be used. Figure 13.30*B* shows an incorrect method for inserting the airway. The airway is being pushed into the turbinates and away from the nasopharynx.

The nasopharyngeal airway may be adjusted to fit the pharynx by sliding it in or out. If the tube is too long, laryngeal reflexes will

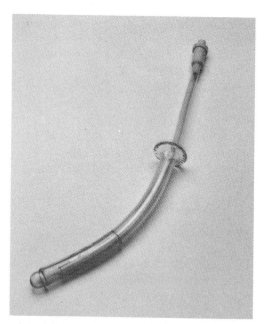

Figure 13.29. Linder nasopharyngeal airway. Courtesy of Polamedco, Inc.

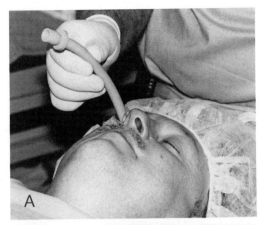

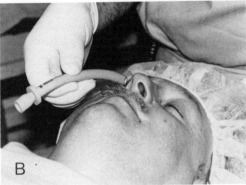

Figure 13.30. Insertion of a nasal airway. **A,** Correct method: the airway is inserted perpendicularly, in line with the nasal passage. **B,** Incorrect method: the airway is being pushed away from the air passage and into the turbinates.

be stimulated; if too short, airway obstruction will not be relieved.

Binasal Airway (63–65)

The binasal airway consists of two nasal airways joined together by a connection that

has an adaptor for attachment to the breathing system (Fig. 13.31). After the airway is inserted, the soft tissues often seal the hypopharynx, permitting assisted or controlled respirations. Excess gas will overflow through the mouth. These devices have been used as an alternative to intubation and to maintain ventilation during oral fiberoptic endoscopy (9).

COMPLICATIONS

Airway Obstruction

The tip of an airway can press the epiglottis against the posterior pharyngeal wall and cover the laryngeal aperture (66). If an oropharyngeal airway is incorrectly inserted or is too small it may push the tongue into the posterior pharynx (46). A foreign body may become lodged inside the air channel (67).

Epistaxis

Epistaxis can develop from the insertion of a nasal airway. This is usually self-limiting but can present a serious problem in patients with bleeding disorders or receiving anticoagulants.

Central Nervous System Trauma

Use of a nasal airway in a patient with a basilar skull fracture may result in trauma to the central nervous system.

Trauma to Uvula

A case of uvular edema apparently caused by entrapment of the uvula between the hard

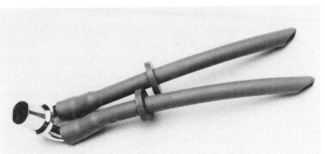

Figure 13.31. The binasal airway. Courtesy of Rusch, Inc.

palate and an oropharyngeal airway has been reported (68).

Dental Damage

Teeth can be cracked or avulsed if the patient bites an oral airway (69). Investigations into professional liability claims have shown that the oral airway was responsible for up to 55% of dental complications (70,71). Oral airways should be avoided if there is evidence of periodontal disease, teeth weakened by caries or restorations, crowns, fixed partial dentures, pronounced proclination (the front teeth having a forward inclination and overlapping the lower front teeth) or isolated teeth. With increasing age teeth become brittle and more likely to fracture. In these cases, use of a nasopharyngeal airway and/or a bite block between the back teeth may be preferable.

Damage to the Lip

When an oral airway is in place, the lip may be caught between the teeth and the airway. This may go unrecognized if a mask is in place.

Laryngospasm and Coughing

Insertion of an airway before establishment of adequate depth of anesthesia may cause coughing or laryngospasm, especially if it touches the epiglottis or vocal cords.

Ulceration and Necrosis

Ulceration of the nose or pharynx can occur if an airway remains in place for a long period of time. This is particularly a danger in infants with a strong sucking reflex who "tongue" the airway. Necrosis of the tongue when an oropharyngeal airway was left in place for an extended period of time has been reported (72).

Aspiration or Swallowing of the Airway

An oral or nasal airway may be aspirated into the pharynx or trachea (73–76) or swallowed (77).

Detachment of Esophageal Stethoscope Cuff

When an esophageal stethoscope was removed from a patient with a Berman airway in place the cuff became detached (78). It was postulated that the cuff got caught in the side grooves of the airway.

Equipment Failure

Airways made of rubber may fracture at the point of connection to the metal insert in the bite portion (79).

Cardiovascular Response

Studies have shown a significant increase in heart rate and blood pressure following insertion of an oral airway (80).

Latex Allergy

If an airway has rubber in it, a severe reaction may occur if the patient has an allergy to latex (37).

Laryngeal Mask

The laryngeal mask (LM), an alternative to both the face mask and tracheal tube, is designed to secure the airway by means of a low-pressure seal around the laryngeal inlet by use of an inflatable cuff (Fig. 13.32). The LM is also called the Brain mask, laryngeal mask airway (LMA), and Brain mask airway (BMA)

DESCRIPTION

The LM consists of a shallow silicone mask with a large-bore tube connected with its lumen at a 30° angle (Fig. 13.33). The tube portion may be made from a spiral reinforced tracheal tube (81). A black line runs the length of the tube so that twisting can be easily recognized. There are two vertical bars at the entry of the tube into the mask to prevent the epiglottis from obstructing the lumen. These act as a ramp up which the epiglottis slides during insertion. At the ma-

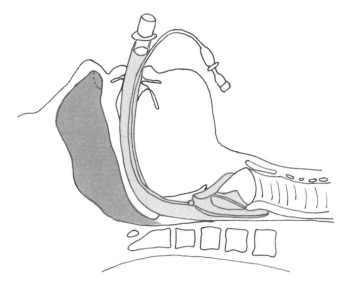

Figure 13.32. The laryngeal mask in place. The tip of the mask rests against the upper esophageal sphincter while the sides face the pyriform fossae.

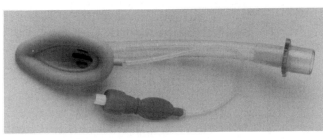

Figure 13.33. Laryngeal mask airway. Note the bars at the junction of the tube and the mask. Courtesy of Gensia Pharmaceuticals Inc.

chine end of the tube is a standard 15-mm tracheal tube connector. The mask is surrounded by an inflatable cuff that has an inflation tube with a pilot balloon and inflation valve.

The laryngeal mask is available in five sizes. Size 1 is designed for neonates and infants up to 6.5 kg but has been used in infants up to 10 kg (82). Size 2 is for patients between 6.5 and 20 kg. Size 2½ is for patients between 20 and 30 kg. Size 3 is for children over 30 kg and small adults. Size 4 is for normal-size and large adults.

USE

Inspection Before Use

Before insertion, the mask and tube should be examined carefully to make certain that they are free from blockage and do not contain any foreign material (83). The aperture bars should be gently probed to ensure they are not damaged.

The cuff should be inflated before insertion. The LM should be discarded if any discoloration, damage, or uneven bulging of the cuff is seen. The cuff should then be fully deflated to form a flat oval disc with the rim facing away from the aperture (Fig. 13.34). This is accomplished by pressing the hollow side down onto a flat surface with a finger pressing the tip. This is done so that during insertion the tip forms a smooth, thin, relatively stiff wedge capable of passing behind the epiglottis even when it is lying against the posterior pharyngeal wall (84). Slight downfolding of the epiglottis will cause little interference with the airway in normal use but may deflect a tracheal tube posteriorly, causing it to enter the esophagus. Complete downfolding of the epiglottis may result in airway obstruction.

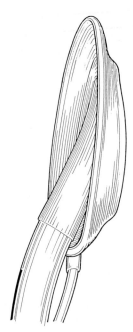

Figure 13.34. The laryngeal mask ready for insertion. The cuff should be deflated as tightly as possible with the rim facing away from the mask aperture. There should be no folds near the tip. Courtesy of Gensia Pharmaceuticals Inc.

If, after all the air has been removed, air leaks back into the cuff, the device should be discarded.

The tube should be bent back 180°. Kinking should not occur.

The back of the mask should be lubricated thoroughly. The anterior surface should be lubricated lightly or not at all. Globules of lubricant should not be present in the bowl of the mask or on the anterior surface of the cuff.

Insertion

Insertion of the LM requires a deeper level of anesthesia than is required for insertion of an oropharyngeal airway (85–87). Use of a neuromuscular-blocking drug may improve the success rate (88). It can be inserted in an awake patient following topical anesthesia (89–93).

After adequate general or topical anesthesia and/or complete muscle relaxation has been achieved, the head is extended and the neck flexed, as in rigid laryngoscopy. The LM can also be inserted without positioning in the classical intubating position (94). The mouth is propped open. The tube portion of the LM is grasped as if it were a pen; the index finger presses on the point where the tube adjoins the mask (Fig. 13.35). With the aperture facing anteriorly (and the black line facing the patient's upper lip), the tip of the mask is placed against the inner surface of the upper incisors or gums. If the user is inexperienced, an assistant should pull the jaw downward so that the user can see that the mask is not rolling over during insertion. The mask is pressed back against the hard palate to keep it flattened as it is advanced into the oral cavity. Some patients have a high, vaulted palate and in these individuals it may be easier to insert the mask from the side and then swing it into the midline after it has been flattened out. If the tip fails to stay flattened or the cuff begins to roll over, the mask should be removed and reinserted.

The mask is advanced, using the index finger at the junction of the mask and tube to push it upward against the palate. If resistance is felt, the tip may have folded over on itself or impacted on an irregularity or swelling in the posterior pharynx. A diagonal shift in direction is often helpful, or a gloved finger may be inserted behind the mask to lift it forward over the obstruction.

A change of direction can be sensed with the index finger as the mask tip encounters the posterior pharyngeal wall and follows it downward. The mask is inserted as deeply as possible. If cricoid pressure is being applied, it should be relaxed during final positioning. By withdrawing the other fingers as the index finger is advanced and slight pronation of the forearm it is often possible to insert the mask fully into position in a single movement (Fig. 13.36). If not, hand position is changed for the next movement. The tube is grasped with the other hand, straightened slightly, and then pressed down with a single, quick but gentle movement until resistance is felt (Fig. 13.37).

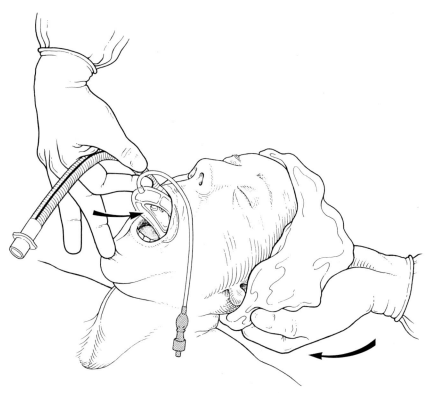

Figure 13.35.   Initial insertion of the laryngeal mask. Under direct vision, the mask tip is pressed upward against the hard palate. Using the index finger, the mask is pressed upward as it is advanced into the pharynx to ensure that the tip remains flattened and avoids the tongue. Courtesy of Gensia Pharmaceuticals Inc.

In pediatric patients, it may be better to insert the mask in reverse and turn it 180° on reaching the posterior pharyngeal wall (95,96).

If at any time during insertion the mask fails to stay flattened out or it starts to roll over as it is advanced, it should be withdrawn and reinserted.

The mask is now in place with the tip resting on the floor of the hypopharynx against the upper esophageal sphincter, the sides facing into the pyriform fossae and the upper border under the base of the tongue (Fig. 13.38 and see Fig. 13.32). The tip of the epiglottis may sit within or outside of the mask (97–99). In 10% to 15% of cases, the upper part of the esophagus lies within the rim of the mask.

The cuff should then be inflated without holding the tube, unless the position is obvi-ously unstable (as may be the case in elderly edentulous patients with slack tissues). For the size 1 mask, 2 to 5 ml should be injected; for the size 2 mask, 7 to 10 ml; for the size 2½ mask, up to 15 ml; for the size 3 mask, 15 to 20 ml; and for the size 4 mask, 25 to 30 ml. Insertion of greater than recommended volumes into the cuff will not improve the seal against the larynx, because it reduces the cuff's ability to conform to the shape of the laryngeal inlet. Inflation of the cuff usually causes slight upward movement (up to 1.5 cm) of the whole device. If placement is correct, it is common to see bulging of the front of the neck with cuff inflation (99). If the laryngeal mask is too large or the patient is too light, the mask may come out of the pharynx when the cuff is inflated.

After the cuff is inflated, a bite block or roll of gauze should be inserted into the mouth

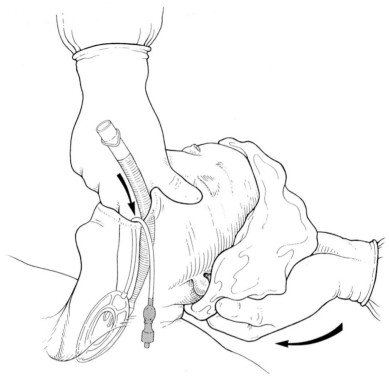

Figure 13.36. By withdrawing the other fingers and with a slight pronation of the forearm, it is usually possible to push the mask fully into position in one fluid movement. Note that the neck is kept flexed and the head extended. Courtesy of Gensia Pharmaceuticals Inc.

beside the tube. The tube should be secured with tape to prevent movement. This is done by affixing the tape first to the face, winding over the cephalad side of the tube, down around the caudal side to fix the tube and roll of gauze firmly to each other and back over the cephalad side before fixing to the opposite side of the face (84). The tube should never be bent upward, as this may cause rotation of the mask in the pharynx. It should be secured in a neutral position or down onto the chin.

A fiberscope can be inserted through the tube to confirm the position and rule out airway obstruction (100–102).

After the cuff is inflated, the tube should be connected to the breathing system. Airway patency and leaks are then assessed by squeezing the reservoir bag. Auscultation of normal breath sounds; observation of nor-

mal chest movement; the expired CO_2 waveform; normal excursions of the reservoir bag; and absence of stridor, tracheal tug, or out-of-phase respiratory movements of the chest and abdomen indicate correct positioning. An esophageal detector device can also be used (103).

If the airway is partially obstructed, it may be the result of incorrect positioning of the mask or downfolding of the epiglottis. In these cases, the obstruction can usually be eliminated by removing and reinserting the mask (104). However, the most common problem is inadequate depth of anesthesia. Manipulation of the jaw or repositioning of the head usually does not help to relieve airway obstruction.

The laryngeal mask tends to settle into place with time so that if there is a small air leak around the inflated rim, it may resolve

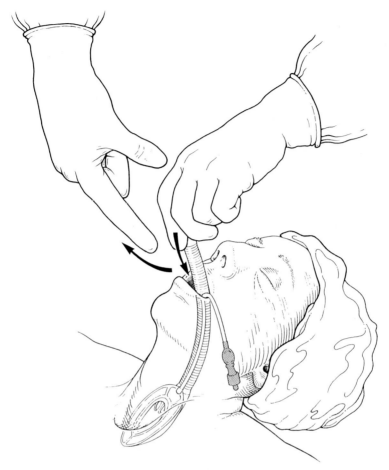

Figure 13.37. The laryngeal mask is grasped with the other hand and the index finger withdrawn from the pharynx. The hand holding the tube presses gently downward until the mask is fully inserted. Courtesy of Gensia Pharmaceuticals Inc.

spontaneously during the first few minutes (91,105,106). If it is large, and it is not the result of malposition or inadequate anesthesia, the device should be withdrawn and reinserted or a larger mask used.

Maintenance

During maintenance it is important that a depth of anesthesia adequate to prevent reaction to the surgical stimulus be maintained until the surgery is finished. If laryngospasm, coughing, straining, or breath holding occurs, the mask should not be removed. Instead the patient should be ventilated and anesthesia deepened. Patency of the airway and

the mask's correct orientation should be verified at regular intervals by confirming that the black line on the tube faces the upper lip.

The laryngeal mask can be used for controlled or spontaneous ventilation. If controlled ventilation is to be used, inspiratory pressure should be kept as low as is compatible with the desired end-tidal carbon dioxide concentration. Peak pressures usually need to be below 17 to 25 cm H_2O to avoid leakage of gas around the mask (86,87,106,107). With larger-size masks, it is sometimes possible to ventilate the lungs at pressures up to 30 cm H_2O (108). If higher pressures are required, leakage can sometimes be prevented

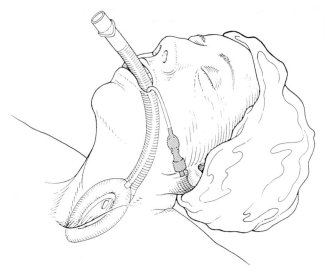

Figure 13.38. The laryngeal mask in place. Courtesy of Gensia Pharmaceuticals Inc.

by pressing on either side of the midline just above the thyroid cartilage (109,110).

Nitrous oxide can diffuse into the cuff so that partial cuff deflation may be necessary (111,112).

Patients can be positioned prone or laterally after the laryngeal mask is in place (110,113), but this should be attempted only after considerable experience with the device.

Tracheal Intubation

The LM can be used to intubate a patient who is difficult to intubate in the usual manner. It may be preferable to rigid laryngoscopy when there are fragile teeth or restorations. It may be desirable to intubate the patient when the laryngeal mask is in place if ventilation is unsatisfactory.

Blind

A 6.0-mm-ID cuffed tracheal tube is the largest that will fit through a size 3 or 4 LM. For a size 2 mask, a 4.5-mm-ID tube can be used, and for the size 1 mask, a 3.5-mm-ID tube (114). An LM that will allow passage of an 8.5-mm tracheal tube is being developed (115).

It is helpful to pass the tracheal tube through the same size LM outside the patient and note or mark the position on the tube shaft when the tracheal tube tip passes through the LM aperture.

The patient should be placed in the usual position for intubation with the neck flexed and the head extended. The tube should be well lubricated and rotated 90° to the left as it is passed down the mask tube, so that the bevel does not catch the bars at the junction of the tube and mask (116). Auscultation of the end of the tube during spontaneous breathing is useful. Flexion of the head may help avoid catching the tube tip on the anterior wall of the larynx. Application of cricoid pressure is usually not helpful and may lower the success rate (116–119). If it is being applied to prevent regurgitation, it may need to be released momentarily during intubation.

After positioning, the tracheal tube should be connected to the breathing system and a CO_2 monitor used to confirm intratracheal position. If the trachea is not entered initially, it is likely that the mask is not well situated over the laryngeal aperture or the aperture is blocked by the epiglottis. Adjustments in the patient's position should be made. If the tube still does not enter the trachea, it should be withdrawn until the bevel is just behind the aperture bars. The LM cuff is then deflated, and the LM is pushed a little farther into the hypopharynx. This maneuver causes elevation of the downfolded epiglottis. The tracheal tube is then pushed through the bars, and the cuff on the LM reinflated.

The laryngeal mask can also be used to guide a bougie into the trachea (92,120–124). Passage of the bougie may be easier if its angulated end is made to point anteriorly, followed by rotation through 180° as it clears the aperture of the LM, to bring the angulated end in line with the long axis of the trachea (120). Following removal of the LM, a tracheal tube is passed over the bougie.

Fiberoptic Guided (125,126)

Studies show that when fiberoptic-guided intubation is aided by use of a LM, the time taken to achieve intubation is significantly less and the success rate is higher (127,128). This may be a very useful method in children in whom it may be more difficult to intubate blindly or pass a guide through the LM (129).

The LM may be modified to aid in fiberoptic intubation by splitting the tube along its entire length and/or removing the pliable grates at the opening to the mask (127,128,130).

The LM is inserted. The fiberscope, with a tracheal tube threaded over its shaft, is placed in the tube. The fiberscope is passed into the trachea, and the tube railroaded over the scope into the trachea.

After intubation, the laryngeal mask may be left in place. The two connectors should be taped securely together (116). After the tracheal tube is removed, the mask can be left in place until it is appropriate to remove it.

If the LM must be removed after intubation, a fiberscope, jet stylet, or tube exchanger may be passed through the tube to facilitate reintubation should extubation accidentally occur during removal of the LM (131). The length of the tracheal tube can be extended by inserting a smaller or larger tracheal tube inside or over the existing tube (132). The LM is then removed from over the extended tube and the extender replaced by a standard connector.

Insertion of a Nasogastric Tube

It is preferable that a nasogastric tube be placed before the LM is inserted. It is, however, possible to pass it during anesthesia by slightly deflating the cuff and using a forceps to push the tube down behind the mask.

Use of a Fiberscope

The laryngeal mask can be used as a guide for fiberoptic laryngoscopy or bronchoscopy in both anesthetized and awake patients (89,101,121,133,134). Use of a connector incorporating a rubber seal will permit passage of a fiberscope without loss of seal.

Another technique is to insert a small tracheal tube through the LM, insert a bougie through the tube, remove the tracheal tube and LM, then thread a tracheal tube large enough to accommodate a fiberscope over the bougie (135).

Emergence

The laryngeal mask may be removed in either the operating room or the postanesthesia care unit (PACU). Use of the LM during transfer to the PACU will maintain a patent airway, while leaving the anesthesiologist's hands free for other tasks.

It has been recommended that the LM be left in position until full recovery of pharyngeal reflexes has occurred (136). Others have recommended that the LM be removed while the patient is under anesthesia (137). The incidence of airway complications is similar in awake and anesthetized patients (139). In a patient known to be difficult to intubate, the LM should be left in place and the cuff inflated until protective reflexes have recovered to the point at which the patient can maintain his or her airway unassisted. If the LM is left in position until full recovery of reflexes, the common practice of lightening anesthesia toward the end of the surgical procedures must be carried out later or avoided.

In the PACU, supplementary oxygen can be delivered with the LM in place, using a T piece (140). The patient should not be stimulated or turned onto his or her side, unless there is an important indication (such as regurgitation or vomiting), because this may cause premature rejection of the LM. The cuff should not be deflated until the patient can swallow or phonate and open the mouth on command. If the cuff is deflated before this, secretions in the upper pharynx may flood into the larynx, causing laryngospasm. Coughing should not necessarily be an indication for removal of the LM. The bite block or roll of gauze should be left in place until the LM is removed. Suctioning should not be performed before the LM is removed.

CARE OF THE LARYNGEAL MASK

The laryngeal mask is reusable, but should not be reused excessively because cuff herniation can become a problem (140). The inflation valve will eventually deteriorate with repeated autoclaving.

After use, the laryngeal mask should be cleaned with soap and water. Glutaraldehyde should not be used, as it can cause glottic edema. The mask can be autoclaved at temperatures up to 134°C (141). All air must be removed from the cuff and pilot tube immediately before autoclaving to prevent rupture of the cuff (115). This is important because any residual left in the cuff will expand. The valve will withstand repeated autoclaving, but will eventually deteriorate. The first sign is failure to maintain deflation of the cuff.

The LM will gradually discolor with age. Continued use is not recommended once obvious discoloration is present (141).

USEFUL SITUATIONS FOR THE LARYNGEAL MASK

The LM has been used for a wide variety of surgical procedures, but it is probably best suited to short procedures, especially while experience is being gained. It may be particularly useful in outpatient anesthesia, because it avoids the need for intubation or muscle relaxants.

It may also be useful in cases in which the

user would choose to administer anesthesia by face mask but elects not to because of the length of the procedure.

Use of a Face Mask Difficult

This includes patients with facial burns, those for whom it is difficult to obtain a good seal with the face mask, those undergoing laser treatment of the face, and patients in whom airway obstruction occurs when a face mask is used (93,142–145).

Failed Intubation

The LM may be useful in cases of failed intubation (146–152). Its use may avoid transtracheal ventilation.

Ocular Surgery

Three studies found that ocular pressure is lower during induction and emergence of the laryngeal mask than of the tracheal tube (153–155). Another study found that intraocular pressure was the same with both techniques (156). Reservations have been expressed about use of the LM in ocular surgery (157,158).

Abnormalities of the Trachea

The patient with tracheal stenosis may be difficult to manage. Minimal interference with airflow and avoidance of further tracheal damage is essential. Management of such a patient using the laryngeal mask has been described (159)

Head and Neck Surgery

Head and neck surgery is possible with the laryngeal mask. The head can be turned to either side without loss of airway, although extreme flexion can cause obstruction.

The laryngeal mask has been used in dental surgery and surgery on the tonsils (141,160,161). Correct placement of the mask should protect the larynx from blood and foreign matter from above.

The LM has also been used for surgery on the thyroid (162–164). Because damage to the recurrent laryngeal nerve is a complication of thyroid surgery, it may be desirable to stimulate that nerve during surgery and observe the motion of the vocal cords and to check motion of the cords following surgery. With the laryngeal mask in place, the motion of the vocal cords can be observed using a fiberscope. Possible problems with this technique include displacement of the mask and laryngospasm (164–166).

Pediatric Patients

The laryngeal mask can be used in children, although it is preferable that experience be gained in adults. Studies show more than 95% have a clear airway (167,168). Studies show fewer hypoxic episodes in children ventilated with the laryngeal mask than with a face mask (169). However, it should be used with caution in patients less than 6 months old (168).

Use of a Fiberscope in Children (134)

Children have small airways, and insertion of a fiberscope through a tracheal tube (which must be narrower than the patient's trachea) is limited. Because there is less airway resistance with a laryngeal mask than a tracheal tube, ventilation is easier.

MRI Imaging

Because there are no ferrous materials in the laryngeal mask, it can be used for magnetic imaging (170). Because some of the inflation valves contain metallic material, it may be necessary to remove such valves and knot the pilot tube (171). Special LMs with valves that do not contain ferrous material are available.

An Aid to Tracheal Suctioning

The laryngeal mask may have a role in intensive care in aiding oropharyngeal and tracheal suctioning without resorting to intubation or tracheostomy (172).

Professional Singers

The laryngeal mask may be especially useful for professional singers in whom laryn-

geal complications of intubation would be most serious (173).

Remote Anesthesia

Situations in which the anesthesiologist must be away from the patient can be managed using a laryngeal mask (104,170, 174,175).

COMPLICATIONS

Aspiration of Gastric Contents

The laryngeal mask cannot be relied on to protect the tracheobronchial tree from the contents of the gastrointestinal tract as reliably as a cuffed tracheal tube (87,91,107, 136,176–183). Although in some cases the distal part of the cuff will provide some protection by obstructing the upper esophagus, in others the esophagus communicates directly with the airway (101,184). The LM does not prevent passage of material into the larynx via the pyriform fossae. A reduction in lower esophageal sphincter barrier pressure may occur when a laryngeal mask is used (185). Studies show that up to 33% of patients anesthetized with a LM may regurgitate gastric contents (186,187). However, the chance of clinically significant aspiration has been estimated to be between 1 in 9,000 and 1 in 250,000 per insertion (188).

Gastric dilatation can occur with intermittent positive pressure breathing (108,189). This can be minimized by using the correct size mask size, careful positioning, good relaxation and low inflation pressures (190).

Cricoid pressure can be applied during use of the laryngeal mask and is effective in preventing reflux at intragastic pressures encountered clinically (191). However, tracheal intubation through the mask may be less likely to be successful if cricoid pressure is applied (116–119). In the event of a failed intubation in a patient for whom there is a significant risk of regurgitation and for whom ventilation can be maintained with a face mask while cricoid pressure is applied, it may be safer to continue with the face mask rather than try to insert a LM (118).

Foreign Body Aspiration

In one case, the inflation valve was found to be moving up and down inside the tube of a LM (192). It apparently entered during autoclaving, having been forced out of its housing as a result of high intracuff pressure after some air was inadvertently left in the cuff.

Airway Obstruction

There are a number of causes of complete or partial airway obstruction during use of a laryngeal mask, including malpositioning, backfolding of the distal cuff, downfolding of the epiglottis, forward displacement of the postcricoid area, cuff overinflation, increased cuff volume owing to warming or diffusion of nitrous oxide, kinking of the tube, presence of a foreign body, laryngospasm, and glottic closure (188). If the obstruction is of uncertain origin, patient reaction rather than mechanical obstruction should be assumed.

In a series of 50 infants, 12 developed complete or partial airway obstruction after a patent airway was secured initially. A total of 7 responded to minor adjustments of the jaw or LM, but in the remainder, the LMA had to be removed (82). Movement of the patient was often associated with deterioration of airway patency.

Glottis closure may occur following insertion if an inadequate induction dose is given, but this will last only 20 to 30 sec, provided the LM is not moved in the belief it is misplaced. The reported incidence of laryngospasm is 1% to 3% and has been noted during both induction and emergence (82,168,193–195).

In some cases, if the insertion technique is not carefully followed, the leading edge of the cuff folds backward against the posterior pharyngeal wall (99). If this occurs, the device must be withdrawn and reinserted. It may be a good idea to try a different size mask.

Overdistension of the cuff can cause obstruction (196,197). Overinflation of the cuff in an attempt to reduce leaks may have the effect of forcing the LM out of the hypopharynx and should be avoided (107). Cases of obstruction that occurred during use for which slight deflation of the cuff relieved the obstruction have been reported (112,198). It is thought that nitrous oxide diffused into the cuff and increased its volume so that it encroached on the laryngeal inlet.

Biting on the tube can cause obstruction. This can be avoided by using a bite block or gauze roll and leaving it in place until the LM is removed. Kinking of the tube also may occur (87,91,102,107,174,199–201). This can be avoided by proper preuse testing.

Airway obstruction may be caused by downfolding of the epiglottis across the laryngeal inlet or infolding of the aryepiglottic folds (86,99,101,202,208). The latter may be caused by the tip of the inflated cuff lying too high, so that it inflates against the arytenoids instead of the posterior surface of the cricoid cartilage. The epiglottis can become trapped in the mask portion of the LM, causing partial obstruction (204). This may occur more commonly in infants (82).

Airway obstruction may be caused by rotation of the LM, so that the inflated rim occludes the larynx (91). Rotation can be detected by checking for the black line, which should face the upper lip. The head can be turned to either side without loss of the airway. However, extreme flexion may cause obstruction, especially if the epiglottis is not completely clear of the mask apertures.

Airway Trauma

Use of the laryngeal mask may result in edema of the epiglottis or posterior pharyngeal wall (205). Edema of the epiglottis can occur if it becomes trapped in the grates over the opening of the tube into the mask (204). A hematoma above the vocal cords has been reported in a patient with a bleeding diathesis (206). Trauma to the uvula and tonsils have been reported (193,207,208). Transient swelling of the parotid glands has been reported (209).

Accidental Dislodgement

Once inserted, accidental dislodgement can occur during maintenance or emergence. Persistent difficulty in keeping the inflated LM in position may be solved by using a different size LM, reducing the cuff volume, elevating the mandible, or using a different head position (107). If the tube has come out only a short distance (2 to 3 cm), it can often be pushed back.

Damage to the LM

Disintegration of the tube has been reported (210,211). In one case, a patient bit through the LM during emergence (212).

Bacteremia

In one study 2 of 30 patients had bacteremia following introduction of a LM (213).

ADVANTAGES

1. The mask is easy to insert and use. Neither neuromuscular blockade nor a laryngoscope is required. Studies show a clean, unobstructed airway can be achieved in greater than 94% of cases (82,86,87,102, 104,167,169,193,194,214–216). The success rate increases with experience, and may exceed 99% (217). First-time insertion rates vary from 67% to 99% (169,188,194). People who are not skilled at intubation have a high success rate with the laryngeal mask (86,218–220).

Even in patients for whom airway maintenance might be expected to be difficult, such as the edentulous patient and the patient with an awkward jaw, it is possible to avoid leakage and obtain a satisfactory airway with the LM. Studies comparing the use of the LM with a face mask show fewer episodes of desaturation, less need to manipulate the airway, and reduced fatigue in the user with the LM (168,214). In the patient with a cervical collar, the LMA can be inserted more rapidly, more gently, and more reliably than a tracheal tube (94).

2. The LM may be useful in managing the patient with a difficult airway, either by using the LM alone or by using it to facilitate passage of a tracheal tube. In case of inability to intubate or ventilate the patient after induction of anesthesia, the LM may be life-saving (221–223).

The LM is useful in patients with airway distortion secondary to tumor, congenital problems, mandibular fracture, hematoma, burns involving the mouth and chin, poor mobility of the cervical spine, and presence of a cervical collar as well as in situations in which laryngoscopy and tracheal intubation are relatively contraindicated (instability of the cervical spine, use of muscle relaxants contraindicated) (94,107,109,114,123,124, 148,224–231). The patient who is incompletely reversed and whom it would be difficult to reintubate may be ventilated with a laryngeal mask (232).

3. The LM can facilitate tracheal intubation (90,114,116,233–236). The angle the tube enters the bowl was partly designed to allow blind tracheal intubation (237). One study found that 90% of patients could be intubated blindly through an LM (117). Another study found that it was as effective as an airway intubator for quickly directing the fiberscope to the vocal cords (238).

4. Insertion of the LM is possible with the patient's neck and head in any position, and with practice the operator can insert it from the side or from in front of the patient (221). It has been used in prehospital care when access to the patient was so limited that it was impossible to insert a tracheal tube (239).

5. The LM can be used with either spontaneous, manaully controlled, or artificial respiration.

6. The laryngeal mask can be left in place until protective reflexes have returned and the patient is able to swallow his or her secre-

tions. This makes suctioning before removal unnecessary in most cases.

7. There is less operating pollution with the laryngeal mask than with use of a face mask (106,240,241). Use of a close scavenging device will lower the levels of trace anesthetic gases so that they are similar to those associated with tracheal intubation.

8. The LM allows fiberoptic endoscopy to be performed while ventilation is maintained (89,133,242–244). This allows assessment of vocal cord function as well as visualization of the tracheobronchial tree.

9. The laryngeal mask offers less resistance to ventilation and requires less additional inspiratory work than a tracheal tube, especially if the tracheal tube is small (245).

10. Use of the LM avoids most of the complications of intubation. Because a laryngoscope is not used, dental damage should not occur. The incidence of sore throat following its use has been reported to be between 0% and 12% (86,87,110,156,193,194,246), which is lower than that following tracheal tube insertion. The incidence of bacteremia with insertion is low (214).

11. The use of the LM may be associated with less coughing, straining, breath holding, and an attenuated pressor response than use of a tracheal tube (86,155,156,247–251). A lesser anesthetic depth is needed (252).

12. Intraoperative airway manipulations and difficulty in maintaining a patent airway are less common with the LM than the face mask (214). Because there is no need to support the jaw or hold a face mask, the user's hands are free for other tasks. The problem of airway deterioration caused by the fatigue associated with manually maintaining correct jaw position is eliminated.

13. The LM avoids many of the complications associated with use of a face mask, including dermatitis and injury to the eye and nerves of the face.

14. The inability to generate high pressures with the LM protects the patient from barotrauma (107).

15. The LM is reusable and cost-effective

when used in place of disposable single-use tracheal tubes. It is manufactured to withstand repeated autoclavings, and with care can be reused up to 200 times.

DISADVANTAGES

1. The LM is not suitable for certain patients and situations. Because the laryngeal mask does not protect from aspiration, it should not be used in a patient with a high risk of aspiration. This includes the patient with a hiatus hernia, the grossly obese patient, the diabetic patient with autonomic neuropathies, the pregnant patient, the trauma patient, the patient receiving opiate medications, and the patient with an acute abdomen. Its use in such a patient might be justified only if, after induction of anesthesia, intubation is impossible (87,148). Most authors believe this device should not be used for a cholecystectomy because of the high incidence of regurgitation of bile (253–257)

Many authors do not recommend the use of the LM in obstetrical patients (87,259), although it has been used in pregnant patients up to the 14th week (141). It can be life-saving in obstetrical situations in which intubation and manual ventilation with a face mask are not possible (146,150,229). For this reason, keeping the larygeal mask in the obstetric OR should be considered (115).

The LM is not suitable for patients who require high inflation pressures (87,91). Insertion may be difficult or impossible if the patient has a small mouth or is unable to flex the neck (87,222). It is not suitable in the patient with laryngeal injury or edema.

Presence of a bleeding disorder is considered a relative contraindication to use of a LM (206,259,260). Extreme care should be exercised to insert the LM slowly and gently in these patients.

2. A fairly deep level of anesthesia is required both during insertion of the LM and maintenance of anesthesia to prevent patient reaction to surgical stimuli (222). Coughing, gaging, vomiting, biting, laryngospasm, and bronchospasm can occur in inadequately

anesthetized patients (86,104,261). These may be more of a problem in patients with asthma or chronic obstructive airway disease and heavy smokers (262). Superior laryngeal nerve block may help to prevent these problems (261).

3. Insertion of the LM causes cardiovascular stimulation (107,247,248,263). Although most studies show an attenuated pressor response associated with laryngeal mask insertion compared with conventional laryngoscopy and tracheal intubation (154, 247,251,253), one study found similar responses (263). Another study found that the cardiovascular stimulation with the laryngeal mask was about equal to that of insertion of an oral airway (248).

4. Leakage of the LM may result in significant pollution of the operating room air with anesthetic agents (264).

5. Although LM placement is an easier technique to learn than tracheal intubation, skill and confidence in its use requires instruction and practice. It would be unwise to use an LM in an emergency without first having become proficient in its use for routine cases (218). Inexperienced personnel may have more success ventilating patients using a face mask than a LM (266).

6. Personnel caring for the patient in the postanesthesia care unit must be educated on how to care for a patient with the laryngeal mask in place and when to remove it.

REFERENCES

1. American Society for Testing and Materials. Standard specification for minimum performance and safety requirements for resuscitators for use with humans (F920-85). Philadelphia: ASTM, 1985.
2. Rendell-Baker L, Soucek DH. New paediatric face masks and anaesthetic equipment. Br Med J 1962;1:1690.
3. Palmer C, Nystrom B, Tunell R. An evaluation of the efficiency of face masks in the resuscitation of newborn infants. Lancet 1985;1:207–210.
4. Aghdami A, Ellis R, Rah KH. A pediatric face mask can be a useful aid in lung ventilation on postlaryngectomy patients. Anesthesiology 1985;63:335.
5. Northwood D, Wade MJ. Novel use of the Rendell-Baker Soucek mask. Anaesthesia 1991;46:319.
6. Binning R. The development of a new face mask. Anaesthesia 1965;20:491–493.
7. Yamashita M, Motokawa K. Mask for child resuscitation. Anaesthesia 1986;41:557.
8. Mallios C. A modification of the Laerdal anesthesia mask for nasotracheal intubation with the fiberoptic laryngoscope. Anaesthesia 1980;35:599–600.
9. Patil V, Stehling LC, Zauder HL, Koch JP. Mechanical aids for fiberoptic endoscopy. Anesthesiology 1982;57:69–70.
10. Rogers SN, Bunumof JL. New and easy techniques for fiberoptic endoscopy-aided tracheal intubation. Anesthesiology 1983;59:569–572.
11. Waring PH, Vinik HR. A potential complication of the Patil-Syracuse endoscopy mask. Anesth Analg 1991;73:668–669.
12. Davis K. Alterations to the Patil-Syracuse mask for fiberoptic intubation. Anesth Analg 1992;74:472–473.
13. Williams L, Teague PD, Nagia AH. Foreign body from a Patil-Syracuse mask. Anesth Analg 1991;73:359–360.
14. Zornow MH, Mitchell MM. Foreign body aspiration during fiberoptic assisted intubation. Anesthesiology 1986;64:303.
15. Lanier WL. Improving anesthesia mask fit in edentulous patients. Anesth Analg 1987;66:1053.
16. Harrison GG, Ozinsky J, Jones CS. Choice of an anaesthetic facepiece. Br J Anaesth 1959;31:269–273.
17. Clarke AD. Potential deadspace in an anaesthetic mask and connectors. Br J Anaesth 1958;30:176–181.
18. Chandler S. A new head strap. Anesth Analg 1980;59:457–458.
19. Jeal DE. Head strap modification. Anesth Analg 1980;59:809–810.
20. Begenau VG. Allergic dermatitis due to rubber: report of a case. Anesthesiology 1951;12:771–772.
21. Anonymous. The physician and the law. Anesth Analg 1970;49:889.
22. Potgieter SV, Mostert JW. A hazard associated with the use of a face mask: case report. S Afr Med J 1959;33:989–990.
23. Azar I, Lear E. Lower lip numbness following anesthesia. Anesthesiology 1986;65:450–451.
24. Ananthanarayan C, Rolbin SH, Hew E. Facial nerve paralysis following mask anaesthesia. Can J Anaesth 1988;35:102–103.
25. Glauber DT. Facial paralysis after general anesthesia. Anesthesiology 1986;65:516–517.
26. Barron DW. Supra-orbital neurapraxia. Anaesthesia 1955;10:374.

27. Keats AS. Post-anaesthetic cephalagia. Anaesthesia 1956;11:341–343.

28. James FM. Hypesthesia of the tongue. Anesthesiology 1975;42:359–360.

29. Blitt CD, Gutman HL, Cohen DD, Weisman H, Dillon JB. Silent regurgitation and aspiration during general anesthesia. Anesth Analg 1970; 49:708–712.

30. Anonymous. Allegedly defective anesthetic mask blamed in eye injury suit. Biomed Safe Stand 1985;15:109.

31. Durkan W, Fleming N. Potential eye damage from reusable masks. Anesthesiology 1987;67:444.

32. Murray WJ, Ruddy MP. Toxic eye injury during induction of anesthesia. South Med J 1985;78:1012–1013.

33. Snow JC, Kripke BJ, Norton ML, Chandra P, Woodcome HA. Corneal injuries during general anesthesia. Anesth Analg 1975;54:465–467.

34. Cook WP, Gravenstein JS. Breathing circuit occlusion due to a defective paediatric face mask. Can J Anaesth 1988;35:205–206.

35. Gordon HL, Tweedie IE. Facemask hazard. 1989;Anaesthesia 44:84.

36. Hauswald M, Sklar DR, Tandberg D, Garcia JF. Cervical spine movement during airway management. Cinefluoroscopic appraisal in human cadavers. Am J Emerg Med 1991;9:535–538.

37. Parisian S. Latex allergies causing more anesthesia problems. APSF Newslett 1992;7:1.

38. McKinstry LJ, Fenton WJ, Barrett P. Anaesthesia and the patient with latex allergy. Can J Anaesth 1992;39:587–589.

39. Sarma VJ, Leman J. Laryngeal mask and anaesthetic waste gas concentrations. Anaesthesia 1990;45:791–792.

40. Barnett R, Gallant B, Fossey S, Finegan B. Nitrous oxide environmental pollution. A comparison between face mask, laryngeal mask, and endotracheal intubation. Can J Anaesth 1992;39:A151.

41. Lambert-Jensen P, Christensen NE, Brynnum J. Laryngeal mask and anaesthetic waste gas exposure. Anaesthesia 1992;47:697–700.

42. Carlsson P, Ljungqvist B, Hallen B. The effect of local scavenging on occupational exposure to nitrous oxide. Acta Anaesth Scand 1983;27:470–475.

43. Nilsson K, Stenquist O, Lindberg B, Kjelltoft B. Close scavenging. Experimental and preliminary clinical studies of a method of reducing anaesthetic gas contamination. Acta Anaesth Scand 1980; 24:475–481.

44. Sik MJ, Lewis RB, Eveleigh DJ. Assessment of a scavenging device for use in paediatric anaestheisa. Br J Anaesth 1990;64:117–123.

45. Boidin MP. Airway patency in the unconscious patient. Br J Anaesth 1985;57:306–310.

46. Marsh AM, Nunn JF, Taylor SJ, Charlesworth CH. Airway obstruction associated with the use of the Guedel airway. Br J Anaesth 1991;67:517–523.

47. Aprahamian C, Thompson B, Finger WA, et al. Experimental cervical spine injury model. Evaluation of airway management and splinting techniques. Ann Emerg Med 1984;13:584–587.

48. Browne B, Adams CN. Postoperative sore throat related to the use of a Guedel airway. Anaesthesia 1988;43:590–591.

49. Monroe MC, Gravenstein N, Saga-Rumley S. Postoperative sore throat. Effect of oropharyngeal airway in orotracheally intubated patients. Anesth Analg 1990;70:512–516.

50. American National Standards Institute. Oropharyngeal and nasopharyngeal airways (ANSI Z39.3-1983). New York: ANSI, 1983.

51. Wilton NCT. Aids for fiberoptically guided intubation in children. Anesthesiology 1991;75:549–550.

52. Berman RA, Lilienfeld SM. Correspondence. Anesthesiology 1950;11:136–137.

53. Palazzo MGA, Soltice NJ. A new aid to fiberoptic bronchoscopy. Anaesth Intensive Care 1983; 11:388–389.

54. Williams RT. Comments from an experienced user of the airway intubator. Anesthesiology 1984;61:108–109.

55. Williams RT, Harrison RE. Prone tracheal intubation simplified using an airway intubator. Can Anaesth Soc J 1981;28:288–289.

56. Ovassapian A, Dykes HM. The role of fiber-optic endoscopy in airway management. Semin Anesth 1987;6:93–104.

57. McAlpine G, Williams RT. Fiberoptic assisted tracheal intubation under general anesthesia with IPPV. Anesthesiology 1987;66:853.

58. Long TMW. Atraumatic nasopharyngeal intubation for upper airway obstruction. Anaesthesia 1988;43:510–511.

59. Heaf DP, Helms PJ, Dinwiddie R, Matthew DJ. Nasopharyngeal airways in Pierre Robin syndrome. J Pediatr 1982;100:698–703.

60. Gallagher WJ, Pearce AC, Power SJ. Assessment of a new nasopharyngeal airway. Br J Anaesth 1988;60:112–115.

61. Collins VJ. Principles of anesthesiology. Philadelphia: Lea & Febiger, 1966:245–249.

62. Monheim LM. General anesthesia in dental practice. 3rd ed. St. Louis: CV Mosby, 1968.

63. Elam JO, Titel JH, Feingold A, Weisman H, Bauer RO. Simplified airway management during anesthesia or resuscitation: a binasal pharyngeal system. Anesth Analg 1969;48:307–316.

64. Weisman H, Bauer RO, Huddy RA, Elam JO. An improved binasopharyngeal airway system for anesthesia. Anesth Analg 1972;51:11–13.

65. Weisman H, Weis TW, Elam JO. Use of double

nasopharyngeal airways in anesthesia. Anesth Analg 1969;48:356–361.

66. Brown TCK. The airway in mucopolysaccharidoses. Anesth Intensive Care 1992;12:178.

67. McNicol LR. Unusual cause of obstructed airway in a child. Anaesthesia 1986;41:668–669.

68. Shulman MS. Uvular edema without endotracheal intubation. Anesthesiology 1981;55:82–83.

69. Pollard BJ, O'Leary J. Guedel airway and tooth damage. Anaesth Intensive Care 1981;9:395.

70. Burton JF, Baker AB. Dental damage during anaesthesia and surgery. Anaesth Intensive Care 1987;15:262–268.

71. Solazzi RW, Ward RJ. The spectrum of medical liability cases. Int Anesthesiol Clin 1984;22:43–59.

72. Moore MW, Rauscher L. A complication of oropharyngeal airway placement. Anesthesiology 1977;47:526.

73. Howat DDC. Disposable nasopharyngeal airways—a potential hazard. Anaesthesia 1982; 37:101.

74. Hayes JD, Lockrem JD. Aspiration of a nasal airway. a case report and principles of management. Anesthesiology 1985;62:534–535.

75. Daly SM, Weinberg B, Murphy RJC, Shugar JMA, Rose JS. Unrecognized aspiration of an oropharyngeal airway. Pediatr Radiol 1983;13:227–228.

76. Milam MG, Miller KS. Aspiration of an artificial nasopharyngeal airway. Chest 1988;93:223–224.

77. Zaltzman J, Ferman A. An acute life-threatening complication caused by a Guedel airway. Crit Care Med 1987;15:1074.

78. Gandhi S, Dhamee MS. Detachment of an esophageal stethoscope cuff-possible role of an oral airway. Anesthesiology 1983;58:202.

79. Lloyd-Williams R. Fractured airways. Anaesth Intensive Care 1985;13:335–336.

80. Hickey S, Cameron AE, Asbury AJ. Cardiovascular response to insertion of Brain's laryngeal mask. Anaesthesia 1990;45:629–633.

81. Goodwin APL, Ogg TW. An armored laryngeal mask airway. Anesthesiology 1992;76:150.

82. Mizushima A, Wardall GJ, Simpson DL. The laryngeal mask airway in infants. Anaesthesia 1992;47:849–851.

83. Goldberg AAJ. Foreign body in a laryngeal mask airway. Anaesthesia 1991;46:700.

84. White A, Sinclair M, Pillai R. Laryngeal mask airway for coronary artery bypass grafting. Anaesthesia 1991;46:1083.

85. Brain AIJ. The laryngeal mask—a new concept in airway management. Br J Anaesth 1983;55:801–804.

86. Brodrick PM, Webster NR, Nunn JF. The laryngeal mask airway. Anaesthesia 1989;44:238–241.

87. Maltby JR, Loken RG, Watson NC. The laryngeal mask airway. Clinical appraisal in 250 patients. Can J Anaesth 1990;37:509–513.

88. Yaddanapudi LN, Kashyap L, Mallick A. Hypoxaemia and insertion of the laryngeal mask airway. Br J Anaesth 1992;69:661.

89. Brimacombe JR. LMA in awake fibreoptic bronchoscopy. Anaesth Intensive Care 1991;19:472.

90. Sellers WFS, Edwards RJ. Awake intubation with Brain laryngeal airway. Anaesth Intensive Care 1991;19:473.

91. Maltby JR. The laryngeal mask airway. Anesth Rev 1991;18:55–57.

92. McCrirrick A, Pracilio JA. Awake intubation: a new technique. Anaesthesia 1991;46:661–663.

93. Markakis DA, Sayson SC, Schreiner MS. Insertion of the laryngeal mask airway in awake infants with the Robin sequence. Anesth Analg 1992;75:822–824.

94. Pennant JH, Pace NA, Gajraj NM. Use of the laryngeal mask airway in the immobilized cervical spine. Anesthesiology 1992;77:A1063.

95. McNicol RL. Insertion of laryngeal mask airway in children. Anaesthesia 1991;46:330.

96. Chow BFM, Lewis M, Jones SEF. Laryngeal mask airway in children: insertion technique. Anaesthesia 1991;46:590–591.

97. Brain A. Proper technique for insertion of the laryngeal mask. Anesthesiology 1990;73:1053.

98. Grebenik CR, Ferguson C. In reply. Anesthesiology 1990;73:1054.

99. Nandi PR, Nunn JF, Charlesworth CH, Taylor SJ. Radiological study of the laryngeal mask. Eur J Anaesth 1991;4(suppl):33–39.

100. Monso E, Carreras A, Bassons J, Gonzalez-Tadeo M. Fibreoptic laryngoscopy as a method of assessing the risk of airway obstruction following laryngeal mask airway insertion. Anaesthesia 1992;47:631–632.

101. Payne J. The use of the fiberoptic laryngoscope to confirm the position of the laryngeal mask. Anaesthesia 1989;44:865.

102. Rowbottem SJ, Simpson DL, Grubb D. The laryngeal mask airway in children. A fiberoptic assessment of positioning. Anaesthesia 1991;46:489–491.

103. Ainsworth QP, Calder I. The oesophageal detector device and the laryngeal mask. Anaesthesia 1990;45:794.

104. Grebenik CR, Ferguson C, White A. The laryngeal mask airway in pediatric radiotherapy. Anesthesiology 1990;72:474–477.

105. Alexander CA, Leach AB, Thompson AR, Lister JB. Use your Brain. Anaesthesia 1988;43:893–894.

106. Lambert-Jensen P, Christensen NE, Brynnum J. Laryngeal mask and anaesthetic waste gas exposure. Anaesthesia 1992;47:697–700.

107. Leach AB, Alexander CA. The laryngeal mask—an overview. Eur J Anaesth 1991;4(suppl):19–31.

108. Brain AIJ. Further developments of the laryngeal mask. Anaesthesia 1989;44:530.
109. Brain AIJ. Three cases of difficult intubation overcome by the laryngeal mask airway. Anaesthesia 1985;40:353–355.
110. Brain AIJ, McGhee TD, McAteer EJ, Thomas A, Abu-Saad MAW, Bushman JA. The laryngeal mask airway. Development and preliminary trials of a new type of airway. Anaesthesia 1985;40:356–361.
111. Lumb AB, Wrigley MW. The effect of nitrous oxide on laryngeal mask cuff pressure. Anaesthesia 1992;47:320–323.
112. Wright ES, Filshie J, Dark CH. Laryngeal mask cuff pressure and nitrous oxide. Anaesthesia 1992;47:713–714.
113. Nagan Kee WD. Laryngeal mask airway for radiotherapy in the prone position. Anaesthesia 1992;47:446–447.
114. Benumof JL. Use of the laryngeal mask airway to facilitate fiberscope-aided tracheal intubation. Anesth Analg 1992;74:313–315.
115. McEwan AI, Mason DG. The laryngeal mask airway. J Clin Anesth 1992;4:252–257.
116. Heath ML. Endotracheal intubation through the laryngeal mask—helpful when laryngoscopy is difficult or dangerous. European J Anaesth Suppl 1991;4:41–45.
117. Heath ML, Allagain J. Intubation through the laryngeal mask. A technique for unexpected difficult intubation. Anaesthesia 1991;46:545–548.
118. Ansermino JM, Blogg CE. Cricoid pressure may prevent insertion of the laryngeal mask airway. Br J Anaesth 1992;69:465–467.
119. Brimacombe J. Cricoid pressure in the laryngeal mask airway. Anaesthesia 1991;46:986–987.
120. Allison A, McCrory J. Tracheal placement of a gum elastic bougie using the laryngeal mask airway. Anaesthesia 1990;45:419–420.
121. Brimacombe J, Newell S, Swainston T, Thompson J. A possible new technique for awake diagnostic bronchoscopy. Med J Aust 1992;156:876–877.
122. Chadd GD, Ackers JWL, Bailey PM. Difficult intubation aided by the laryngeal mask airway. Anaesthesia 1989;44:1015.
123. Chadd GD, Crane DL, Phillips RM, Tunell WP. Extubation and reintubation guided by the laryngeal mask airway in a child with the Pierre-Robin syndrome. Anesthesiology 1992;76:640–641.
124. Silk JM, Hill HM, Calder I. Difficult intubation and the laryngeal mask. Eur J Anaesth 1991;4(suppl):47–51.
125. Kadota Y, Oda T, Yoshimura N. Application of a laryngeal mask to a fiberoptic bronchoscope-aided tracheal intubation. J Clin Anesth 1992;4:503–504.
126. Asai T. Use of the laryngeal mask for tracheal intubation in patients at increased risk of aspiration of gastric contents. Anesthesiology 1992;77:1029–1030.
127. Maroof M, Khan RM, Siddique MSK, Bhattie TH, Hussain A. Fiber-optic intubation through a modified laryngeal mask. Anesthesiology 1992;77:A510.
128. Maroof M, Khan RM, Khan H, Stewart J, Mroze C. Evaluation of modified laryngeal mask airway as an aid to fiber optic intubation. Anesthesiology 1992;77:A1062.
129. Denman WT, Gouldsouzian NG. Position of the laryngeal mask airway. Anesthesiology 1992;77:401–402.
130. Brimacombe J, Johns K. Modified Intravent LMA. Anaesth Intensive Care 1991;19:607.
131. Loken RG, Moir CL. The laryngeal mask as an aid to blind orotracheal intubation. Can J Anaesth 1992;39:518.
132. Chadd GD, Walford AJ, Crane DL. The 3.5/4.5 modification for fiberscope-guided tracheal intubation using the laryngeal mask airway. Anesth Analg 1992;75:307–308.
133. Tuck M, Phillips R, Corbett J. LMA for fiberoptic bronchoscopy. Anaesth Intensive Care 1991;19:472–473.
134. Walker RWM, Murrell D. Yet another use for the laryngeal mask. Anaesthesia 1991;46:591.
135. Thomas DI. Another approach with the laryngeal mask airway. Anesth Analg 1992;75:156.
136. Brain AIJ. The laryngeal mask and the oesophagus. Anaesthesia 1991;46:701–702.
137. Erskine RJ, Rabey PG. The laryngeal mask airway in recovery. Anaesthesia 1992;47:354.
138. Laffon M, Plaud B, Hajhmida RB, Dubousset A-M, Ecoffey C. Removal of laryngeal mask: airway complications in children, anesthetized versus awake. Anesthesiology 1992;77:A1176.
139. Goodwin APL. Postoperative oxygen via the laryngeal mask airway. Anaesthesia 1991;46:700.
140. Brain AIJ. Studies on the laryngeal mask: first, learn the art. Anaesthesia 1991;46:417.
141. Brain AIJ. The intavent laryngeal mask instruction manual. Gensia Pharmaceuticals, Inc. 1992.
142. Garbin GS, Bogetz MS, Grekin RC, Frieden IJ. The laryngeal mask as an airway during laser treatment of port wine stains. Anesthesiology 1991;75:A953.
143. Michel MZ, Stubbing JF. Laryngeal mask airway and laryngeal spasm. Anaesthesia 1991;46:71.
144. Smith I, White PF. Comparison of laryngeal mask and face mask during ambulatory anesthesia. Anesthesiology 1992;77:A520.
145. Smith TGC, Whittet H, Heyworth T. Laryngomalacia—a specific indication for the laryngeal mask. Anaesthesia 1992;47:910.
146. Chadwick IS, Vohra A. Anaesthesia for emergency

caesarean section using the Brain laryngeal airway. Anaesthesia 1989;44:261–262.

147. Cork R, Monk JE. Management of a suspected and unsuspected difficult laryngoscopy with the laryngeal mask airway. J Clin Anesth 1992;4:230–234.

148. de Mello WF, Kocan M. The laryngeal mask in failed intubation. Anaesthesia 1990;45:689.

149. Dalrymple G, Lloyd E. Laryngeal mask: a more secure airway than intubation. Anaesthesia 1992;47:712–713.

150. McClune S, Regan M, Moore J. Laryngeal mask airway for caesarean section. Anesthesia 1990;45:227–228.

151. Priscu V, Priscu L, Soroker D. Laryngeal mask for failed intubation in emergency caesarean section. Can J Anaesth 1992;39:893.

152. White A, Sinclair M, Pillai R. Laryngeal mask airway for coronary artery bypass grafting. Anaesthesia 1991;46:234.

153. Watcha MF, White PF, Tychsen L, Stevens JL. Comparative effects of laryngeal mask airway and endotracheal tube insertion on intraocular pressure in children. Anesth Analg 1992;75:355–360.

154. Holden R, Morsman CDG, Butler J, Clark GS, Hughes DS, Bacon PJ. Intra-ocular pressure changes using the laryngeal mask airway and tracheal tube. Anaesthesia 1991;46:922–924.

155. Lamb K, James MFM, Janicki PK. The laryngeal mask airway for intraocular surgery: effects on intraocular pressure and stress responses. Br J Anaesth 1992;69:143–147.

156. Akhtar TM, McMurray P, Kerr WJ, Kenny GNC. A comparison of laryngeal mask airway with tracheal tube for intra-ocular ophthalmic surgery. Anaesthesia 1992;47:668–671.

157. McCartney CA, Wilkinson DJ. The laryngeal mask airway and intra-ocular surgery. Anaesthesia 1992;47:445.

158. Rabey PG, Murphy PJ. The laryngeal mask airway and intra-ocular surgery. Reply. Anaesthesia 1992;47:445–446.

159. Asai T, Fujise K, Uchida M. Use of the laryngeal mask in a child with tracheal stenosis. Anesthesiology 1991;75:903–904.

160. Allen JG, Flower EA. The Brain layrngeal mask. An alternative to difficult intubation. Br Dent J 1990;168:202–204.

161. Noble H, Wooller DJ. Laryngeal masks and chair dental anaesthesia. Anaesthesia 1991;46:591.

162. Akhtar TM. Laryngeal mask airways and visualization of vocal cords during thyroid surgery. Can J Anaesth 1991;38:140.

163. Maroof M, Siddique M, Khan RM. Post-thyroidectomy vocal cord examination by fiberoscopy aided by the laryngeal mask airway. Anaesthesia 1992;47:445.

164. Tanigawa K Inoue Y, Iwata S. Protection of recurrent laryngeal nerve during neck surgery. A new combination of neutracer, laryngeal mask airway, and fiberoptic bronchoscope [Letter]. Anesthesiology 1991;74:966–967.

165. Charters P, Cave-Bigley D, Roysam CS. Should a laryngeal mask be routinely used in patients undergoing thyroid surgery? Anesthesiology 1991; 75:918–919.

166. Tanigawa K, Inoue Y, Iwata S. In reply. Anesthesiology 1991;75:919.

167. Mason DG, Bingham RM. The laryngeal mask airway in children. Anaesthesia 1990;45:760–763.

168. Fawcett WJ, Ravilia A, Radford P. The laryngeal mask airway in children. Can J Anaesth 1991;38:685–686.

169. Johnston DF, Wrigley SR, Robb PJ, Jones HE. The laryngeal mask airway in paediatric anaesthesia. Anaesthesia 1990;45:924–927.

170. Rafferty C, Burke AM, Cossar DF, Farling PA. Laryngeal mask and magnetic resonance imaging. Anaesthesia 1990;45:590–591.

171. Langton JA, Wilson I, Fell D. Use of the laryngeal mask airway during magnetic resonance imaging. Anaesthesia 1992;47:532–533.

172. Lim W. Yet another use for the laryngeal mask. Anaesthesia 1992;47:175–176.

173. Harris TM, Johnston DF, Collins SRC, Heath ML. A new general anaesthetic technique for use in singers. The Brain laryngeal mask airway versus endotracheal intubtion. J Voice 1990;4:81–85.

174. Taylor DH, Child CSB. The laryngeal mask for radiotherapy in children. Anaesthesia 1990;45:690.

175. Waite K, Filshie J. The usc of a laryngeal mask airway for CT radiotherapy planning and daily radiotherapy. Anaesthesia 1990;45:894.

176. Boyce JR, Peters G. Vessel dilator cricothyrotomy for transtracheal jet ventilation. Can J Anaesth 1989;36:350–353.

177. Brain AIJ. The laryngeal mask in patients with chronic respiratory disease. Anaesthesia 1989; 44:790–791.

178. Cyna AM, MacLeod DM. The laryngeal mask: cautionary tales. A reply. Anaesthesia 1990; 45:167.

179. Campbell JR. The laryngeal mask: cautionary tales. A reply. Anaesthesia 1990;45:167–168.

180. Criswell J, John R. The laryngeal mask: cautionary tales. A reply. Anaesthesia 1990;45:168.

181. Griffin RM, Hatcher IS. Aspiration pneumonia and the laryngeal mask airway. Anaesthesia 1990;45:1039–1040.

182. Koehli N. Aspiration and the laryngeal mask airway. Anaesthesia 1991;46:419.

183. Nanji GM, Malt JR. Vomiting and aspiration pneumonitis with the laryngeal mask airway. Can J Anaesth 1992;39:69–70.

184. John RE, Hill S, Hughes TJ. Airway protection by

the laryngeal mask. A barrier to dye placed in the pharynx. Anaesthesia 1991;46:366–367.

185. Rabey PG, Murphy PJ, Langton JA, Barker P, Rowbothan DJ. Effect of the laryngeal mask airway on the lower oesophageal sphincter pressure in patients during general anaesthesia. Br J Anaesth 1992;69:346–348.

186. Barker P, Langton JA, Murphy PJ, Rowbotham DJ. Regulation of gastric contents during general anaesthesia using the laryngeal mask airway. Br J Anaesth 1992;69:314–315.

187. Barker P, Murphy P, Langton JA, Rowbotham DJ. Regurgitation of gastric contents during general anaesthesia using the laryngeal mask airway. Br J Anaesth 1990;67:660P.

188. Brimacombe JR. The laryngeal mask airway. A review for the nurse anesthetist. J Am Assoc Nurse Anesth 1992;60:490–499.

189. Wittmann PH, Whittmann FW. Laryngeal mask and gastric dilitation. Anaesthesia 1991;46:1083.

190. Hammond JE. Controlled ventilation and the laryngeal mask. Anaesthesia 1989;44:616–617.

191. Strang TI. Does the laryngeal mask airway compromise cricoid pressure? Anaesthesia 1992;47:829–831.

192. Conacher ID. Foreign body in a laryngeal mask airway. Anaesthesia 1991;46:164.

193. McCrirrick A, Ramage DTO, Pracilio JA, Hickman JA. Experience with the laryngeal mask airway in two hundred patients. Anaesth Intensive Care 199119:256–260.

194. Sarma VJ. The use of a laryngeal mask airway in spontaneously breathing patients. Acta Anaesthesiol Scand 1990;34:669–672.

195. Wilkinson PA. The laryngeal mask: cautionary tales. Anaesthesia 1990;45:167.

196. Welsh BE. Will we ever learn? Anaesthesia 1990;45:892.

197. Martin DW. Will we ever learn? A reply. Anaesthesia 1990;45:892.

198. Collier C. A hazard with the laryngeal mask airway. Anaesth Intensive Care 1991;19:301.

199. Goldberg PL, Evans PF, Filshie J. Kinking of the laryngeal mask airway in two children. Anaesthesia 1990;45:487–488.

200. Herrick NJ, Kennedy DJ. Airway obstruction and the laryngeal mask airway in paediatric radiotherapy. Anaesthesia 1992;47:910.

201. Rowbottom SJ, Simpson DL. Partial obstruction of the laryngeal mask airway. Anaesthesia 1990;45:892–893.

202. Dubreuil M, Janvier G, Dugrais, Berthoud MC. Uncommon laryngeal mask obstruction. Can J Anaesth 1992;39:517–518.

203. Young TM. The laryngeal mask in dental anaesthesia. Eur J Anaesth 1991;4(suppl):53–59.

204. Miller AC, Bickler P. The laryngeal mask airway. Anaesthesia 1991;46:659–660.

205. Marjot R. Trauma to the posterior pharyngeal wall caused by a laryngeal mask airway. Anaesthesia 1991;46:589–590.

206. Thompsett C, Cundy JM. Use of the laryngeal mask airway in the presence of a bleeding diathesis. Anaesthesia 1992;47:530–531.

207. van Heerden PV, Kirrage D. Large tonsils and the laryngeal mask airway. Anaesthesia 1989;44:703.

208. Lee JJ. Laryngeal mask and trauma to uvula. Anaesthesia 1989;44:1014.

209. Harada M. Transient swelling of the parotid glands following laryngeal mask airway. Can J Anaesth 1992;39:745–746.

210. Crawford M, Davidson G. A problem with a laryngeal mask airway. Anaesthesia 1992;47:76.

211. Squires SJ. Fragmented laryngeal mask airway. Anaesthesia 1992;47:274.

212. Kramer-Kilper OT. Removal of laryngeal mask airway during light anesthesia. Anesthesia 1992;47:816.

213. Stone JM, Karalliedde LD, Carter ML, Cumberland NS. Bacteremia and insertion of laryngeal mask airways. Anaesthesia 1992;47:77.

214. Smith I, White PF. Use of the laryngeal mask airway as an alternative to a face mask during outpatient arthroscopy. Anesthesiology 1992;77:850–855.

215. Ravalia A, Fawcett W, Radford P. The Brain laryngeal mask airway in paediatric anaesthesia. Anesth Analg 1991;72:S220.

216. Haynes SR, Allsop JR, Gillies GWA. Arterial oxygen saturation during induction of anaesthesia and laryngeal mask insertion. Prospective evaluation of four techniques. Br J Anaesth 1992;68:519–522.

217. Brain AJ. Personal communication, 1992.

218. Davies PRF, Tighe SQM, Greenslade GL, et al. Laryngeal mask airway and tracheal tube insertion by unskilled personnel. Lancet 1990;2:977–979.

219. de Mello WF, Ward P. The use of the laryngeal mask airway in primary anaesthesia. Anaesthesia 1990;45:793–794.

220. Pennant JH, Walker MB. Comparison of the endotracheal tube and laryngeal mask in airway management by paramedical personnel. Anesth Analg 1992;74:531–534.

221. Riley RH, Swan HD. Value of the laryngeal mask airway during thoracotomy. Anesthesiology 1992;77:1051.

222. Fisher JA, Ananthanarayan C, Edelist G. Role of the laryngeal mask in airway management. Can J Anaesth 1992;39:1–3.

223. Calder I, Ordman AJ, Jackowski A, Crockard HA. The Brain laryngeal mask airway. Anaesthesia 1990;45:137–139.

224. Beveridge ME. Laryngeal mask anaesthesia for repair of cleft palate. Anaesthesia 1989;44:656–657.

225. Bailey C, Chung R. Use of the laryngeal mask air-

way in a patient with Edward's syndrome. Anaesthesia 1992;47:713.

226. Brimacombe J. The laryngeal mask airway: use in the management of stridor. Anaesth Intensive Care 1992;20:117–118.

227. Denny NM, Desilva KD, Webber PA. Laryngeal mask airway for emergency tracheostomy in a neonate. Anaesthesia 1990;45:895.

228. Logan A. Use of the laryngeal mask in a patient with an unstable fracture of the cervical spine. Anaesthesia 1991;46:987.

229. McClune S, Moore JA. The laryngeal mask in failed intubation: a reply. Anaesthesia 1990;45:689.

230. Russell R, Judkins KC. The laryngeal mask airway and facial burns. Anaesthesia 1990;45:894.

231. Ravalia A, Goddard JM. The laryngeal mask and difficult tracheal intubation. Anaesthesia 1990;45:168.

232. Kumar CM. Laryngeal mask airway for inadequate reversal. Anaesthesia 1990;45:792.

233. Brain AIJ. The laryngeal mask airway—a possible new solution to airway problems in the emergency situation. Arch Emerg Med 1984;1:229–232.

234. Heath ML, Allagain J. The Brain laryngeal mask airway as an aid to intubation. Br J Anaesth 1990;64:382P–383P.

235. Smith JE, Sherwood NA. Combined use of a laryngeal mask airway and fiberoptic laryngoscope in difficult intubation. Anaesth Intensive Care 1991;19:471–472.

236. Thompson KD, Ordman AJ, Parkhouse N, Morgan BDG. Use of the Brain laryngeal mask airway in anticipation of difficult tracheal intubation. Br J Plast Surg 1989;42:478–480.

237. Brain AIJ. The development of the laryngeal mask—a brief history of the invention, early clinical studies and experimental work from which the laryngeal mask evolved. Eur J Anaesth 1991;4(suppl):5–17.

238. Crichlow A, Locken R, Todesco J. The laryngeal mask airway and fibreoptic laryngoscopy. Can J Anaesth 1992;39:742–744.

239. Greene MK, Roden R, Hinchley G. The laryngeal mask airway. Two cases of prehospital trauma care. Anaesthesia 1992;47:688–689.

240. Barnett R, Gallant B, Fossey S, Finegan B. Nitrous oxide environmental pollution. A comparison between face mask, laryngeal mask, and endotracheal intubation. Can J Anaesth 1992;39:A151.

241. Sarma VJ, Leman J. Laryngeal mask and anaesthetic waste gas concentrations. Anaesthesia 1990;45:791–792.

242. McNamee CJ, Meyns B, Pagliero KM. Flexible bronchoscopy via the laryngeal mask: a new technique. Thorax 1991;46:141–142.

243. Maekawa N, Mikawa K, Tanaka O, Goto R, Obara H. The laryngeal mask may be a useful device for fiberoptic airway endoscopy in pediatric anesthesia. Anesthesiology 1991;75:169–170.

244. Tuck M, Phillips R, Corbett J. LMA for fibreoptic bronchoscopy. Anaesth Intensive Care 1991;19:472–473.

245. Bhatt SB, Kendall AP, Lin ES, Oh TE. Resistance and additional inspiratory work imposed by the laryngeal mask airway. Anaesthesia 1992;47:343–347.

246. Alexander CA, Leach AB. Incidence of sore throats with the laryngeal mask. Anaesthesia 1989;44:791.

247. Braude N, Clements EAF, Hodges UM, Andrews BP. The pressor response and laryngeal mask insertion. Anaesthesia 1989;44:551–554.

248. Hickey S, Cameron AE, Asbury AJ. Cardiovascular response to insertion of Brain's laryngeal mask. Anaesthesia 1990;45:629–633.

249. Wilkins CJ, Cramp PGW, Staples J, Stevens WC. Comparison of the anesthetic requirement for tolerance of laryngeal mask airway and endotracheal tube. Anesth Analg 1992;75:794–797.

250. Wood MLB, Forrest ETS. Haemodynamic response to insertion of the laryngeal mask. Anaesthesia 1989;44:938.

251. Wilson IG, Fell D, Robinson SL, Smith G. Cardiovascular responses to insertion of the laryngeal mask. Anaesthesia 1992;47:300–302.

252. Wilkins CJ, Cramp PGW, Staples J, Stevens WC. Less anesthetic is required to tolerate a laryngeal mask airway than an endotracheal tube. Anesth Analg 1992;74:S349.

253. Braude N, Clements EAF, Hodges UM, Andrews BP. The pressor response and laryngeal mask insertion. A comparison with tracheal intubation. Anaesthesia 1989;44:551–554.

254. Griffin RM, Hatcher IS. Aspiration pneumonia and the laryngeal mask airway. Anaesthesia 1991;46:419.

255. Krapez JR. Aspiration pneumonia and the laryngeal mask airway. Anaesthesia 1991;46:418–419.

256. Philpott B. Aspiration pneumonia and the laryngeal mask airway. Anaesthesia 1991;46:418.

257. Riddell PL. Aspiration and the laryngeal mask airway. Anaesthesia 1991;46:18.

258. Freeman R, Baxendale B. Laryngeal mask airway for caesarean section. Anaesthesia 1990;45:1094.

259. Brimacombe J. Laryngeal mask and bleeding diathesis. Anaesthesia 1992;47:1004–1005.

260. Brain AIJ. Laryngeal mask misplacement—causes, consequences and solutions. Anaesthesia 1992;47:531–532.

261. Dasey N, Mansour N. Coughing and laryngospasm with the laryngeal mask. Anaesthesia 1989;44:865.

262. Gunawardene RD. Laryngeal mask and patients with chronic respiratory disease. Anaestheisa 1989;44:531.

263. Griffin RM, Dodd P, Buckoke PC, Tosh GC, Day SJ. Cardiovascular responses to insertion of the Brain laryngeal mask. Br J Anaesth 1989;63:624P–625P.

264. Fullekrug B, Pothmann W, Esch JS. The laryngeal mask. Fiberoptic detection of positioning and measurements of anesthetic gas leakage. Anesth Analg 1992;74:S101.

265. Davies PRF, Tighe SQM, Greenslade GL, Evans GH. Laryngeal mask airway and tracheal tube insertion by unskilled personnel. Lancet 1990;(336):977–979.

266. Tolley PM, Watts ADJ, Hickman JA. Comparison of the use of the laryngeal mask and face mask by inexperienced personnel. Br J Anaesth 1992;69:320–321.

Laryngoscopes

A laryngoscope is used to view the larynx and adjacent structures, most commonly for the purpose of inserting a tube into the tracheobronchial tree.

The Rigid Laryngoscope

Most laryngoscopes in use today are manufactured as detachable blade and handle units on which the light source is energized when the blade and handle are locked in the operating position.

DESCRIPTION

Standards for the connection between the handle and the blade include ASTM standard F965-85 and ISO 7376/1, which cover fittings that have the lamp in the blade (1,2). Among other things, they specify critical dimensions for the hook-on fittings to ensure interchangeability of different manufacturers' blades and handles. ASTM standard F1195-88 covers blades and handles that are fiberoptic illuminated (3). It provides methods of identifying compatible blades and handles by color.

Handle

The handle is held in the hand during use. It may have a rough surface for traction. It provides the power source for the light. Most often this is from disposable batteries. Handles with rechargeable batteries are available. Fiberoptic-illuminated laryngoscopes may use a remote light source (4), and their handles are required by the ASTM (3) standard to have a circumferential band of color, distinct from the handle, located between the hook-on fitting and the midpoint of the handle. The critical dimensions of the fittings for each color system are also specified in the standard.

A hook-on connection between the handle and blade is most commonly used. One end of the handle is fitted with a hinge pin that fits a slot on the base of the blade. This allows for quick-and-easy attachment and detachment.

Handles designed to accept blades that have a light bulb have a metallic contact, which completes an electrical circuit when the handle and blade are engaged in the operating position. Handles containing batteries and using fiberoptic illumination contain a halogen lamp bulb. When the handle and blade are locked in the operating position, an activator switch is depressed. This provides a connection between the bulb and the batteries. A halogen lamp bulb has a useful life three times that of light bulbs used in other laryngoscopes.

Handles are available in several sizes. A narrow handle may be advantageous when intubating a small patient. Short handles may be advantageous for patients in whom the chest and/or breasts contact the handle during use, when cricoid pressure is being applied or when the patient is in a body cast (5). Other techniques for handling this situation include inserting the blade laterally into the mouth, advancing it halfway into the mouth and gradually rotating it back to the normal position (6,7), and inserting a detached blade into the mouth and then attaching the handle (8,9).

Although most blades form a right angle with the handle when ready for use, the angle may also be acute or obtuse. An adaptor may be fitted between the handle and the blade to allow the angle to be altered (10–12) (Fig. 14.1). The Patil-Syracuse handle (Fig. 14.2) can be positioned and locked in four different positions (13).

Most handles are designed to accept either nonfiberoptic-illuminated or fiberoptic-illuminated blades, but handles that can engage either have been developed.

Blade

The blade is the rigid component that is inserted into the mouth. When a blade is

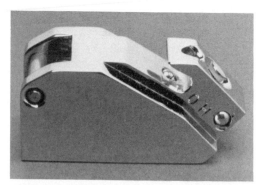

Figure 14.1.   Howland lock. The Howland lock fits between the handle and the blade by means of hook-on connections on both parts. It changes the angle between the handle and the blade. Courtesy of Mercury Medical.

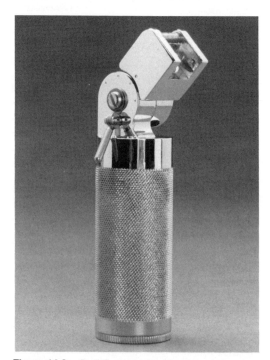

Figure 14.2.   Patil-Syracuse handle. With this handle, the blade can be adjusted and locked in four different positions (180°, 135°, 90°, or 45°). Courtesy of Mercury Medical.

available in more than one size, the blades are numbered, with the number increasing with size. Disposable blades are available for attachment to a regular or disposable handle (Fig. 14.3). The blade is composed of several

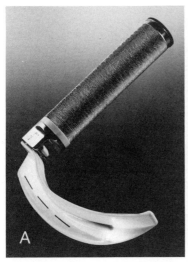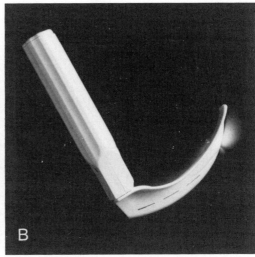

Figure 14.3. **A,** Disposable blade attached to reusable handle. **B,** Disposable handle and blade. Courtesy of Vital Signs.

parts, including the base, heel, tongue, flange, web, tip, and light source (Fig. 14.4).

The base is the part that attaches to the handle. It has a slot for engaging the hinge pin of the handle. The proximal end of the base is called the heel.

The tongue (spatula) is the main shaft. It serves to compress and manipulate the soft tissues (especially the tongue) and lower jaw so that a direct line of vision to the larynx is achieved. The long axis of the tongue may be straight or curved in part or all of its length. Blades are commonly referred to as curved or straight, depending on the predominant shape of the tongue.

The flange is parallel to the tongue and connected to it by the web. It serves to guide instrumentation and deflect interfering tissues. The flange determines the cross-sectional shape of the blade.

The tip (beak) contacts either the epiglottis or the vallecula and directly or indirectly elevates the epiglottis. It is usually blunt and thickened to decrease trauma.

The blade may have a lamp (bulb) (Fig. 14.5) or a fiberoptic bundle that transmits light from a source in the handle (Fig. 14.6). The lamp screws into a socket that has a me-

tallic contact. On most blades the socket is located near the tip. On some blades it is in the base of the blade. When the blade is snapped into place, electrical contact with the batteries in the handle is made. The socket area is subject to soiling by fluids that can affect the electrical contacts, causing the light to fail.

A fiberoptic-illuminated blade has an encased fiberoptic bundle that transmits light from a source in the handle or base of the blade. This provides a light intensity greater than that obtained with a regular light bulb in the blade (14). Because there is no bulb or electrical contact in the blade, cleaning and sterilization are easier and the laryngoscope is more reliable. Even if the light is left on for an extended period of time, the blade stays cool. The ASTM (3) standard requires fiberoptic-illuminated blades to be color coded by means of a mark on the heel.

In most cases, use of a laryngoscope presents little or no difficulty to the experienced operator, and skill is of more importance than the type of blade employed. There are, however, situations in which a certain blade is particularly advantageous (15). This has led to the development of a number of blades. The blades discussed here are avail-

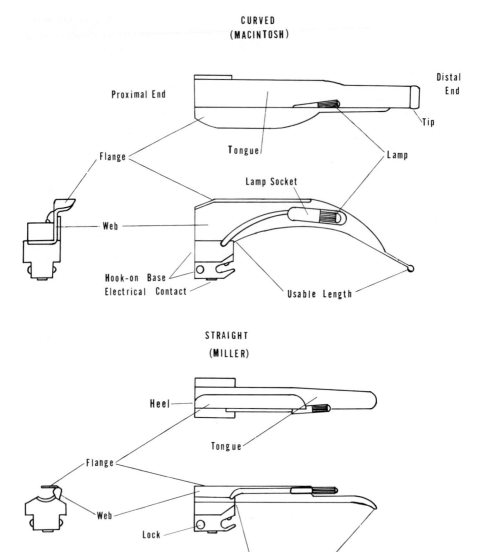

CURVED
(MACINTOSH)

Proximal End

Distal
End

Tip

Flange

Tongue

Lamp

Lamp Socket

Web

Hook-on Base
Electrical Contact

Usable Length

STRAIGHT
(MILLER)

Heel

Tongue

Flange

Web

Lock

Usable Length

Figure 14.4. The parts of the Macintosh (**top**) and the Miller (**bottom**) blades are illustrated. The tip is the distal end of the blade intended for insertion into the patient. The proximal end is the part closest to the handle. Redrawn from a drawing in Committee, American National Standards Institute. Draft standard, laryngoscopes for tracheal intubation (Z-79). Philadelphia: ASTM.

Figure 14.5. Left-handed Macintosh blade. Courtesy of Penlon Ltd.

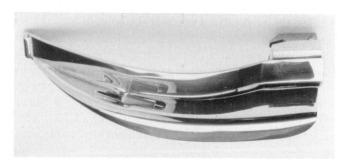

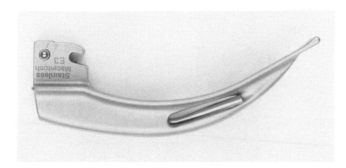

Figure 14.6. English Macintosh blade. Courtesy of Welch Allyn, Inc.

able commercially in the United States. A number of other blades have been described in the literature.

Macintosh Blade (16,17)

The Macintosh blade (Figs. 14.4 and 14.7) is one of the most popular. The tongue has a smooth, gentle curve that extends from the base to the tip. There is a flange at the left to push the tongue out of the way. In cross-section, the tongue, web, and flange form a reverse *Z*. Numerous modifications have been made (18–24).

Left-Handed Macintosh Blade (25)

The left-handed Macintosh blade (see Fig. 14.5) has the flange on the opposite side from the usual Macintosh blade. This blade may be useful for abnormalities of the right side of the face or oropharynx, left-handed persons, intubating in the right lateral position, and positioning a tracheal tube directly on the left side of the mouth (26,27).

Polio Blade

The polio blade (see Fig. 14.7) is also a modification of the Macintosh. The blade is offset from the handle at an obtuse angle to allow intubation of patients in iron lung respirators or body jackets; after the anesthesia screen is in place; and of patients with obesity, breast hypertrophy, kyphosis with severe barrel chest deformity, a short neck, or restricted neck mobility (28,29). Disadvantages of this blade are that little force can be applied and control is minimal (8).

Improved Vision Macintosh Blade (30)

The improved vision (I.V.) Macintosh blade (Fig. 14.8) is similar to the standard version except that the midportion of the tongue is concave to allow greater visualization of the larynx.

Oxiport Macintosh (Mac/Port)

The oxiport Macintosh blade (Fig. 14.9) is a conventional Macintosh blade with a tube added to deliver oxygen.

English Macintosh

The English Macintosh (see Fig. 14.6) is similar to the conventional Macintosh except the flange is curved and lower at the handle end.

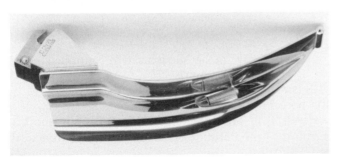

Figure 14.7. The polio blade. Courtesy of Penlon Ltd.

Figure 14.8. A, The improved vision (I.V.) Macintosh blade (**left**) and the conventional Macintosh blade (**right**). Note the improved vision when the blade is viewed from the proximal end. **B,** Conventional Macintosh blade (**top**) and the I.V. Macintosh blade (**bottom**). On the I.V. Macintosh, the midportion of the spatula is concave. Courtesy of Gabor B. Racz, M.D.

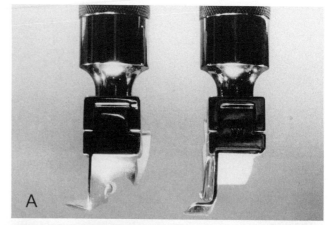

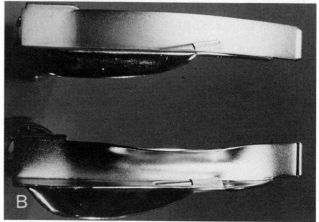

Figure 14.9. The oxiport Macintosh blade. Courtesy of Mercury Medical.

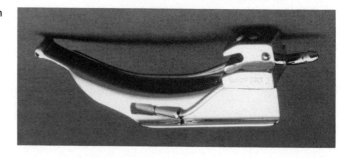

Tull Macintosh

The Tull (suction) blade (Fig. 14.10) is a modified Macintosh that has a suction port near the tip. The suction channel extends next to the handle and has a finger-controlled valve so that suction can be controlled by the laryngoscopist.

Fink Blade

The Fink blade (Fig. 14.11) is another modification of the Macintosh. The tongue is

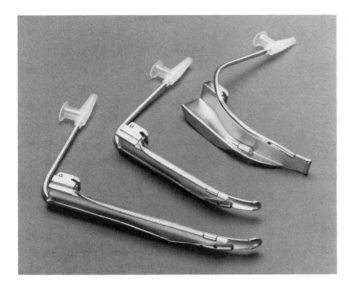

Figure 14.10. Tull (suction) Macintosh and Miller blades. The finger-controlled valve allows suction to be regulated by the laryngoscopist. Courtesy of Mercury Medical.

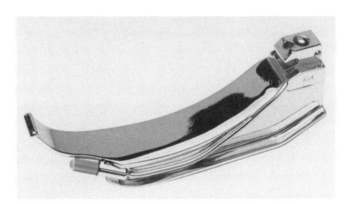

Figure 14.11. The Fink blade. Note that the tongue is more curved at the tip and the flange is reduced at the proximal end compared with the Macintosh blade. The light bulb is placed nearer the distal end. Courtesy of Puritan-Bennett Corp.

wider and has a sharper curve at the distal end. The height of the flange is reduced, especially at the proximal end. The light bulb is placed farther forward than on the Macintosh.

Bizarri-Guiffrida Blade (31)

The Bizarri-Guiffrida blade (Fig. 14.12) is a modified Macintosh. The flange is removed, except for a small part that encases the light bulb. This was done to attempt to limit damage to the upper teeth. The blade is designed particularly for patients with a limited mouth opening, prominent incisors, receding mandible, short thick neck, or anterior larynx.

Miller Blade (32)

The Miller blade is one of the most popular blades (Figs. 14.4 and 14.13). The tongue is straight with a slight upward curve near the tip. In cross-section the flange, web, and tongue form a *C* with the top fattened. Some commercial versions of the blade have the lamp socket on the tongue, whereas other versions have it on the web. The lamp may be either on the right or left side of the blade. Several modifications have been described in the literature (33,34).

Oxiport Miller Blade (35-38)

The oxiport Miller (also called Mil/port and oxyscope) blade has a built-in tube that

Figure 14.12. The Bizarri-Guiffrida blade. Courtesy of Puritan-Bennett Corp.

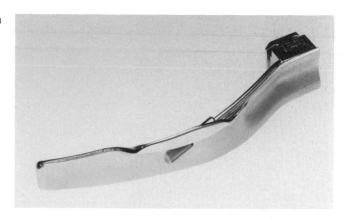

Figure 14.13. The Miller blade. Courtesy of Penlon Ltd.

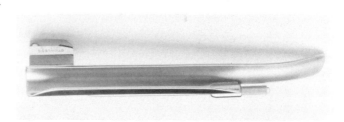

Figure 14.14. The oxiport Miller blade. Courtesy of Mercury Medical.

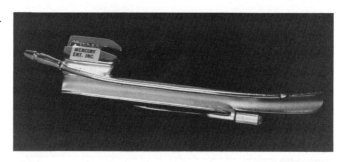

allows delivery of oxygen or other gases during intubation (Fig. 14.14). The tube also may be used for suction. Insufflation of oxygen during intubation using this blade has been found to decrease oxygen desaturation in spontaneously breathing anesthetized patients (39,40).

Tull Miller Blade

The Tull (suction) Miller blade is a standard Miller blade with a suction tube whose port ends near the tip of the blade (see Fig. 14.10). Near the handle is a finger-controlled

port that allows control of suction with a finger.

Mathews Blade

The Mathews blade is a straight blade with a wide and flattened petalloid configuration tip (Fig. 14.15). It is designed for difficult nasotracheal intubations.

Wisconsin Blade

Unlike the Miller blade, the Wisconsin blade's tongue has no curve (Fig. 14.16). The

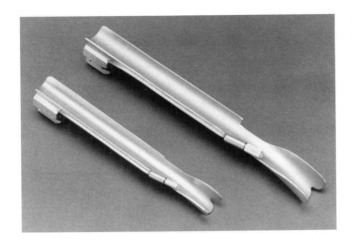

Figure 14.15. The Mathews blade. Courtesy of Mercury Medical.

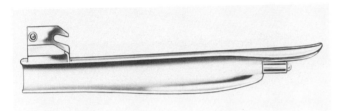

Figure 14.16. The Wisconsin blade. Courtesy of Ohio Medical Products, a division of Airco, Inc.

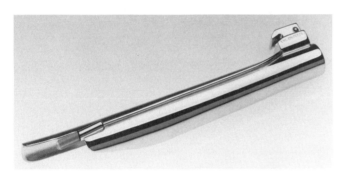

Figure 14.17. The Wis-Foregger blade. Courtesy of Puritan-Bennett Corp.

flange is curved to form two-thirds of a circle in cross-section. The depth of the flange is small at the proximal end and widened in the distal portion.

Wis-Foregger Blade (41)

The Wis-Foregger is a modification of the Wisconsin blade with a straight tongue and a flange that expands slightly toward the distal end (Fig. 14.17). The distal portion of the blade is wider and formed slightly to the right.

Wis-Hipple Blade

The Wis-Hipple also is a modified Wisconsin blade (Fig. 14.18). The tongue is straight, and the flange is large and circular. Compared with the Wisconsin blade, the flange is straighter and runs parallel to the tongue and the tip is wider. It is designed primarily for use in infants.

Figure 14.18. The Wis-Hipple blade Courtesy of Puritan-Bennett Corp.

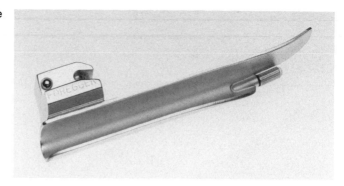

Figure 14.19. The Schapira blade Courtesy of Puritan-Bennett Corp.

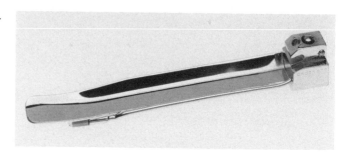

Figure 14.20. The Alberts (**top**) and Michaels (**bottom**) blades. The Alberts blade offers a sharp 67° angle, whereas the Michaels blade has a slight 93° angle. Courtesy of North American Drager.

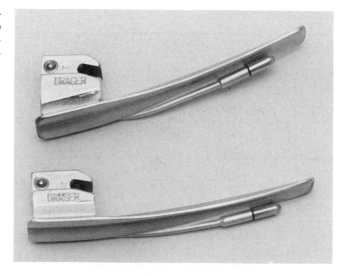

Figure 14.21. The Soper blade. Courtesy of Penlon Ltd.

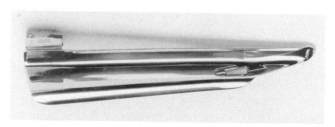

Schapira Blade (42)

The Schapira blade is a straight blade with a tip that curves upward (Fig. 14.19). There is no vertical component. The blade's curvature is designed to facilitate intubation by cradling the tongue and pushing it to the left side of the mouth.

Alberts Blade

The Alberts blade combines characteristics of the Miller and Wis-Hipple blades with a cut-away flange to increase visibility (Fig. 14.20). There is a recess to facilitate insertion of a tracheal tube. The blade forms a 67° angle with the handle. It is used for pediatric patients.

Michaels Blade

The Michaels blade differs from the Alberts blade only in that it forms a 93° angle with the handle (see Fig. 14.20).

Soper Blade (43)

The Soper blade combines the Z shape of the Macintosh blade with a straight blade (Fig. 14.21).

Heine Blade

The Heine, or Propper, blade is straight with a slight upward curve at the tip (Fig.

14.22). The flat flange is curved away from the blade. It is useful for children with large tongues.

Snow Blade (44)

The Snow blade is a hybrid blade consisting of a Miller tongue and a Wis-Foregger flange (Fig. 14.23).

Flagg Blade (45)

The Flagg blade has a straight tongue (Fig. 14.24). The flange has a C shape that gradually decreases in size as it approaches the distal end.

Guedel Blade

The Guedel blade is a straight blade on which the tongue is set at a 72° angle to the handle (Fig. 14.25). The flange has the shape of a U on its side. The light is close to the tip, which has an uptilt of 10°.

Bennett Blade

The Bennett blade is a modification of the Guedel blade (Fig. 14.26). It also forms an acute angle with the handle. The upper part of the flange has been omitted.

Eversole Blade

The Eversole blade has a straight tongue (Fig. 14.27). The flange forms a C with the

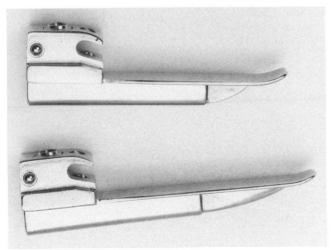

Figure 14.22. Heine blades. Courtesy of Propper Manufacturing Co., Inc.

Figure 14.23. The Snow blade. Courtesy of Air Products and Chemicals, Inc.

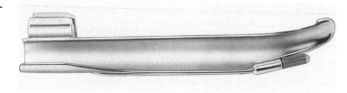

Figure 14.24. The Flagg blade. Courtesy of Ohio Medical Products, a division of Airco, Inc.

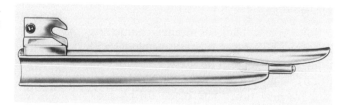

Figure 14.25. The Guedel blade. Courtesy of Penlon Ltd.

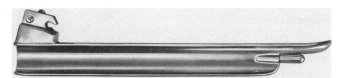

Figure 14.26. The Bennett blade. Courtesy of Puritan-Bennett Corp.

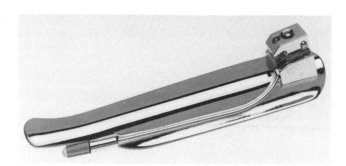

Figure 14.27. The Eversole blade. Courtesy Puritan-Bennett Corp.

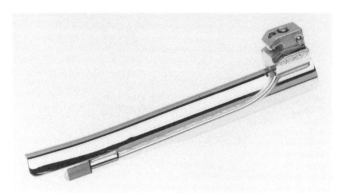

tongue and web near the proximal end. Midway to the tip the upper flange tapers.

Seward Blade (46)

The Seward blade has a straight tongue with a curve near the tip (Fig. 14.28). It has a small reverse Z-shaped flange. The blade is useful for nasotracheal intubation because its shape allows a Magill forceps to be introduced with minimum loss of view (47).

Phillips Blade (48)

The Phillips blade is straight with a low flange and a curved tip similar to a Miller blade (Fig. 14.29). The light bulb is placed along the left side of the blade.

Racz-Allen Blade (49)

The Racz-Allen blade is straight with a curved tip. The proximal portion of the blade flexes to relieve pressure on the teeth. The vertical portion is hinged and held in position by a spring. The spring allows lateral deflection of the vertical portion without occluding the view. Exposure is improved by tilting the handle of the laryngoscope to the left. The hinged portion is concave along its length. The tongue surface is rough and unpolished to reduce slipping.

Robertshaw Blade (50)

The Robertshaw blade has a straight tongue with a gentle curve near the tip (Fig. 14.30). It is designed to lift the epiglottis indirectly. The flange is extended to the left. The blade was designed for infants and children. It has been found to be useful for nasotracheal intubation because it allows a Magill forceps to be introduced with a minimum loss of view (47).

Oxford Infant Blade (51)

The Oxford infant blade has a straight tongue that curves up slightly at the tip (Fig. 14.31). It has a U shape at the proximal end with the bottom limb of the U decreasing toward the tip so that the distal part is open. It tapers from a maximum width at the proximal end to the tip. Although intended primarily for newborns, it can be used for children up to the age of 4.

Bainton Laryngoscope Blade (52)

The Bainton blade has a straight tongue (Fig. 14.32). The distal 7-cm section is tubular and has an intraluminal light source so that it is protected from obstruction by edematous tissue, blood, secretions, intraoral masses, and scar tissue. The tip is beveled at

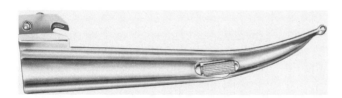

Figure 14.28. The Seward blade. Courtesy of Penlon Ltd.

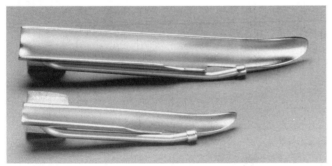

Figure 14.29. Phillips blades. Courtesy of Mercury Medical.

Figure 14.30. The Robertshaw blade. Courtesy of Penlon Ltd.

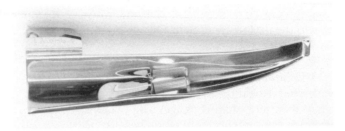

Figure 14.31. The Oxford infant blade. Courtesy of Penlon Ltd.

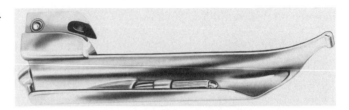

Figure 14.32. The Bainton blade. Note the distal tubular section. Courtesy of Mercury Medical.

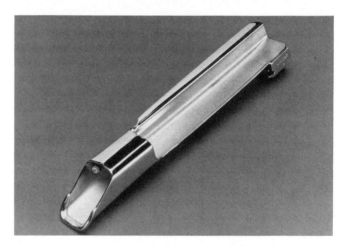

a 60° angle to create an oval opening at the distal end of the tube. A tracheal tube of 8 mm or less can be inserted through the tubular lumen without significantly obstructing vision.

A modified two-piece tubular pharyngolaryngoscope is also available. The two parts of the blade are held together by a screw during intubation. A tracheal tube is placed intraluminally into the glottis, then the two pieces are dismantled for removal from around the tube.

Double-Angle Blade (53,54)

The spatula of the double-angle blade (also called the Choi blade) has two incre-mental angulations, 20° and 30°, to improve lifting of the epiglottis and reduce the need to tilt the blade posteriorly (Fig. 14.33). The spatula and tip form a wide, flat surface. The bulb is located on the left edge of the blade between the two curvatures. The flange has been eliminated. The blade may be especially useful for the patient with an anterior larynx. Because there is no flange, there is more room to pass the tracheal tube than there is with a straight blade.

Blechman Blade

The Blechman blade is a modification of the Macintosh-style blade, with the tip an-

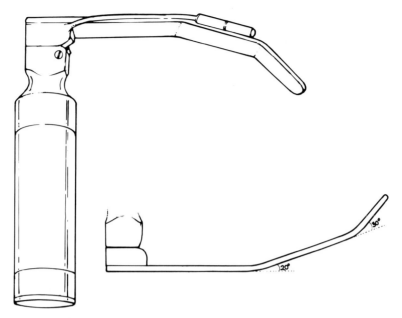

Figure 14.33. The double-angle blade. Courtesy of Jay J. Choi, M.D.

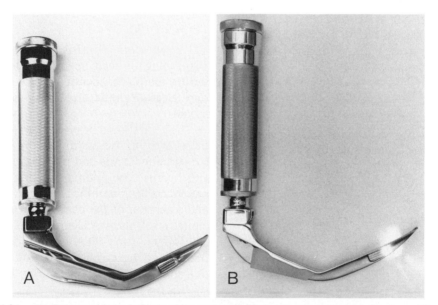

Figure 14.34. The Belscope blade. **A,** Blade without prism. **B,** Blade with prism attached. Courtesy of Dr. Paul Bellhouse.

gled sharply. The flange has been removed near the handle end of the blade.

Belscope Blade (55,56)

The Belscope blade is a straight blade that has been modified by bending it forward through 45° at the midpoint so that from the side the blade has a broad *V* shape (Fig. 14.34). The angulation makes this blade useful when there is poor dentition, because the proximal part remains well away from the upper teeth. The horizontal spatula has a small horizontal step and a low vertical component, so that the blade has the shape of an inverted *L* in cross-section. The tip is beaded on the underside. The blade is used like a straight blade, with the tip lifting the epiglottis.

For the occasional situation in which a satisfactory view of the larynx cannot be obtained, a prism cut from a transparent acrylic material can be attached to the blade just proximal to the angle (see Fig. 14.34*B*). To prevent fogging an antifog preparation may be applied to the leading and trailing surfaces of the prism or the prism may be warmed before use.

This blade feels different from other blades, so practice is essential to develop skill with this blade (54). Fogging of the prism can be a problem.

Cranwall Blade

The Cranwall blade has a curved tip like a Miller blade (Fig. 14.35). There is a reduced flange to decrease the potential for damage to the upper teeth.

Whitehead Blade

The Whitehead blade is a modification of the Wis-Foregger blade. The flange is reduced in height and open proximally and distally (see Fig. 14.35).

Accessories

Huffman Prism and Prism Laryngoscope Blade (57–59)

The Huffman prism and prism laryngoscope blade are designed to provide an indirect view of the larynx in patients in whom direct exposure is difficult. The prism is a block of Plexiglas shaped to fit on the proximal end of a No. 3 Macintosh blade (Fig. 14.36). The ends are polished to produce optically flat surfaces. A refraction of 30° in the line of sight is provided, thereby bringing into view structures within a few millimeters of the tip of the blade. The image is right side up. It is necessary to warm the prism before use to prevent condensation.

The prism laryngoscope blade has the prism built into the blade. An additional 20° refraction from right to left is added, because the prism is to the left of the midline. The prism laryngoscope blade allows either conventional direct exposure of the larynx or indirect exposure through the prism. It allows more space for insertion of a tracheal tube than does the prism attached to a Macintosh blade.

TECHNIQUES OF USE

Laryngoscopy consists of several steps: positioning the head, opening the mouth, inserting the blade, identifying the epiglottis, raising the epiglottis, and finally viewing the larynx.

The head should be positioned so that the passageway to the larynx is brought into a straight line for the best possible view of the vocal cords. The optimal position for most patients is flexion of the lower cervical spine and extension of the head at the atlantooccipital level, the so-called sniffing position. The lower portion of the cervical spine can be maintained in a position of flexion by means of a small pillow under the head. Extension

Figure 14.35.   Cranwall (**top**) and Whitehead (**bottom**) blades. Blades courtesy of Bay Medical, Inc.

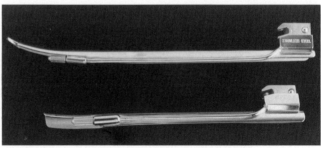

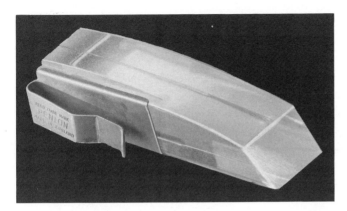

Figure 14.36. The Huffman prism. Courtesy of Penlon Ltd.

of the atlantooccipital joint is achieved by pressure on the top of the head and/or upward traction on the upper teeth or gums by the laryngoscopist's hand (60). In children, it may be unnecessary to flex the lower cervical vertebrae, and in neonates it may be necessary to elevate the shoulders.

The laryngoscope handle is held in the left hand unless the operator is left-handed. Many left-handed people also hold the scope in the left hand, because most blades are designed for insertion on the right side of the mouth. Moistening or lubricating the blade will facilitate insertion if the mouth is dry. In some situations the chest will impinge on the handle, making insertion of the blade difficult. In these cases, a short handle may be used, the blade may be inserted sideways (6,7), or the blade may be inserted and then attached to the handle (8,9).

The fingers of the right hand are used to open the mouth and spread the lips apart. In patients with dentition, the optimum opening of the mouth is often with a thumb-over-index-finger approach, with the index finger on the maxillary dentition as far to the right as possible and the thumb placed on the lower dentition (61).

The blade is inserted at the right side of the mouth. This reduces the likelihood that the incisor teeth will be damaged and helps push the tongue to the left. The blade is advanced on the side of the tongue toward the right tonsillar fossa, so that the tongue lies on the left side of the blade. The right hand keeps the lips from getting caught between the teeth or gums and the blade. If the tongue is slippery, placement of tape on the lingual surface of the blade may be helpful (62). When the right tonsillar fossa is visualized, the tip of the blade is moved toward the midline. The blade is then advanced behind the base of the tongue, elevating it, until the epiglottis comes into view.

There are two methods for elevating the epiglottis, depending on whether a straight or curved blade is being used.

Straight Blade

The straight blade is shown in position for intubation in Figure 14.37*A*. The tip is alternately advanced and the handle rotated backward until the epiglottis is exposed. The blade is then made to scoop under the epiglottis and lift it anteriorly. The vocal cords should be identified. If they are not seen, an assistant should be asked to push gently downward on the larynx.

If the blade is advanced too far, it will result in elevation of the larynx as a whole rather than exposure of the vocal cords. Occasionally, the blade will expose the esophagus. It should then be withdrawn slowly. If it is then withdrawn too far, the tip of the epiglottis will be released and will flip over the glottis.

The straight blade can also be inserted into the vallecula (the angle made by the epiglottis with the base of the tongue) and used in the same manner as a curved blade.

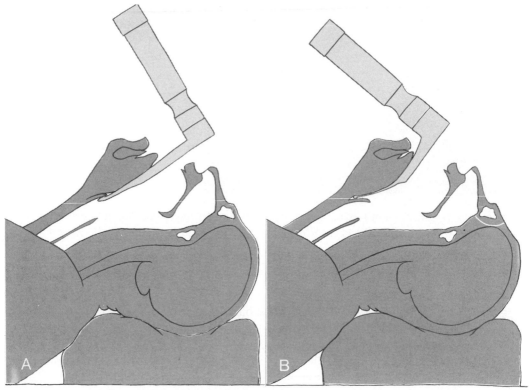

Figure 14.37. **A,** Intubation with a straight laryngoscope blade. The tip of the blade picks up the epiglottis. **B,** Intubation with the curved laryngoscope blade. The epiglottis is below the tip of the blade. A small pillow under the head allows better visualization on the larynx. Courtesy of Vance Robideaux.

Curved Blade

Figure 14.37*B* shows the curved blade in position for intubation. After the epiglottis is seen, the blade is advanced until the tip fits into the vallecula. Traction is then applied along the handle, at right angles to the blade to carry the base of the tongue and the epiglottis forward. The glottis should come into view. If it is not seen, external pressure on the larynx may be helpful. It is important that the handle not be pulled backward. This will cause the tip to push the larynx upward and out of sight and could cause damage to the teeth or gums. A curved blade can be used as a straight blade, lifting the epiglottis directly, if it is long enough (63).

Use of laryngoscopes during magnetic resonance imaging (MRI) creates special problems (64). Plastic laryngoscopes are available, but the batteries in the handle still cause a pull from the magnetic field. Laryngoscopes have been modified to operate from a DC source connected to the MRI machine (65). A special cable with nonmagnetic connectors is used to connect the laryngoscope to the power source.

Flexible Fiberoptic Endoscope (66,67)

Compared with a rigid laryngoscope, the flexible fiberoptic endoscope (also called fiberscope) is more expensive, fragile, and difficult to use and clean. Fiberoptic techniques require more time than conventional intubation, and an assistant is often needed to help with the procedure. However, the fiber-

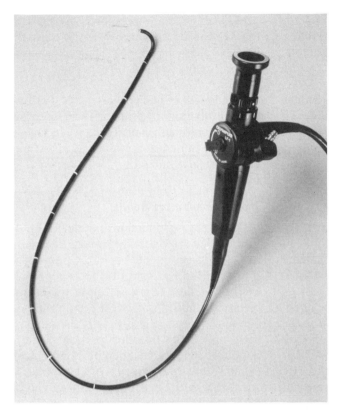

Figure 14.38. Flexible fiberoptic laryngoscope. Light is supplied from a separate source. The lever on the handle controls deflection of the tip in two directions. Two ports attach to the working channel. One is for insufflation or injection and one for suctioning. Courtesy of Olympus Corp.

scope can be used to intubate patients who are difficult or impossible to intubate with a rigid laryngoscope (68–78), to assess tracheal or bronchial tube placement (66,79,80), to change tracheal tubes (66,81,82), to locate and remove secretions, to examine the airway, and to place and evaluate the position of a nasogastric tube (83). The only major impediment to its successful use in a properly prepared patient is the presence of significant amounts of blood and/or secretions (54).

DESCRIPTION (66,67,84)

The fiberscope is composed of several parts, including the light source, handle, and flexible insertion portion (Fig. 14.38).

Light Source

Light may be provided by a handle with batteries or a high-intensity source with a fiberoptic cable (light cord) that connects to the handle. If the fiberscope has sustained

damage and part of the light-carrying fibers are broken, a more powerful light source will usually be needed.

Handle with Batteries

A handle with batteries that uses a low-power halogen light bulb is compact, convenient, and inexpensive. However, the illumination will be weaker than that from other sources.

Halogen Light Source

The halogen light source is contained in a separate box and is connected to the scope by a fiberoptic cable (light cord, tube, or transmission cord). This produces a bright light without much heat.

Xenon Light Source

Xenon is the brightest available light source and is needed for videotaping. It also is quite hot, and the connector to the handle can cause a burn if it contacts the skin of the patient or the endoscopist. This is the most expensive light source.

Handle

The handle, or body, is the part held in the hand during use. It houses the batteries, if they are used as the power source, or there may be an adapter to a high-intensity remote light source. Other parts of the handle include the eyepiece, focusing ring, working channel port, and the tip control lever or knob. The eyepiece is at the proximal end. By rotating the focusing (adjusting) ring the image just in front of the tip of the scope can be brought into focus. Often a camera adapter or teaching attachment can be fitted to the eyepiece.

The tip control (also called bending or angulation control) lever or knob may be on the side of the body, but a thumb-controlled lever system on the back section of the handle is considered superior by many (66). By turning this, the tip of the flexible portion can be flexed or extended. A full range of motion can be attained by rotating the entire instrument. The connection of the handle to the insertion portion is usually tapered to hold the tracheal tube.

Insertion Portion

The insertion portion (also called insertion cord or tube) is inserted into the patient, and a tracheal tube is passed over it during fiberoptic intubation. It contains one image-transmitting bundle, one or two light-conducting bundles, angulation wires, and may contain a working channel. These are surrounded by a protective wire mesh and covering. This portion is fully submersible, which facilitates cleaning.

Its thickness is of some importance, as this determines the size of the smallest tracheal tube that can be used. In general, the inside diameter of the tracheal tube should be at least 1 mm larger than the diameter of the insertion cord. If the tube is passed through the nose, a difference of 2 mm is appropriate (85). Fiberscopes as narrow as 2.0 mm OD have been developed (86). These allow intubation with a tracheal tube as small as 3.0 mm ID (72,87).

The length of this portion varies. For tracheal intubation in adults, a 50-cm insertion cord is usually sufficient. To allow placement of double-lumen endobronchial tubes and nasotracheal intubation, 55 to 60 cm are needed.

Image-Conducting Bundle

The image-conducting bundle is sometimes called the optic fiber, image transmission, or image guide bundle. Optic fibers transmit the image in front of the scope to the eyepiece. These fibers are quite small and precisely grouped so that the relationship of one fiber to the other is exactly the same at each end of the insertion portion. Such a bundle of organized filaments is called *coherent* and allows transmission of a clear image. An objective lens is placed at the distal end to focus the image being transmitted by the fibers. Except at the ends where the fibers are fused for strength, the bundle is flexible. However, the fibers are delicate and breakage may occur. When broken, a fiber will no longer pass its image and the viewer will see a black dot in that fiber's location.

Light-Conducting Fiber Bundle(s)

The light-conducting fiber bundle also is called the light guide or light transmission bundle. Flexible glass fibers are very efficient light conductors and can transmit light from a powerful source without producing dangerous heating. Unlike the image-conducting bundle, the fibers are not arranged in a precise manner. This is known as an *incoherent* bundle.

Working Channel

Although the working channel is optional, most scopes have one, extending from the tip to the body. This can be used for suctioning, injection of water or medications, insufflation of gases, and passage of other instruments (such as forceps or a guide wire).

Tip Flexion Cables

The tip flexion cables are also known as angulation wires and tip-bending control wires. Cables connecting the tip to the bending knob on the handle are placed along two sides of the insertion portion. Flexion and extension can be performed in only one plane. When the handle is rotated, the insertion portion also rotates, because it is semirigid. Thus the tip can be manipulated in any direction by a combination of rotation and bending.

Endoscopic Accessories

Accessory devices to protect the fiberscope from the teeth and to keep it in the midline and carry it forward to the vicinity of the larynx are often used. These are discussed in Chapter 13.

TECHNIQUES OF USE

Use of the fiberscope is an indispensable skill for anesthesia personnel confronted with anatomic or physiologic abnormalities of the upper airway. Many users become disenchanted when they attempt to use it for the first time for a difficult intubation and do not meet with success. Frequently, it is used only after multiple unsuccessful attempts with a rigid laryngoscope. After the airway is filled with secretions or blood and compromised by edema, a high failure rate is not surprising.

A full discussion of fiberoptic techniques is beyond the scope of this book. The reader is referred to two excellent textbooks and a number of review articles (66,67,83,88–90). Only the basics will be mentioned here.

It can be inserted either nasally or orally, in awake or anesthetized patients who are either breathing spontaneously or paralyzed. If the patient is anesthetized, the pharynx may collapse, leaving little or no air space to see

through (91). For this reason, most authors recommend that when a difficult intubation is expected, that it be carried out in the awake patient using sedation and topical anesthesia. Transtracheal ventilation through a catheter passed through the cricothyroid membrane may be useful, especially when there are abnormalities of the upper airway (92,93). Other methods of ventilation during use of a fiberscope have been described (66,67,94–97).

Practice is needed to learn to manipulate the tip control while advancing the scope. Furthermore, the anatomy appears different from that viewed with a rigid laryngoscope. Nevertheless, facility with this instrument can be achieved without an inordinate expenditure of time or effort. As experience is gained, the average time required for intubation will decrease.

Rather than making first attempts with a difficult intubation, facility should be developed first with an intubation mannequin or animal model then with awake, spontaneously breathing patients in whom no difficulty with intubation is anticipated.

Because this instrument is expensive and delicate, great care must be taken not to damage it. A minor blow can break glass fibers. Care must be taken not to put excessive pressure on the bending lever, as this will result in breakage of the tip flexion cables. A blow to the distal end may crack the objective lens. The flexible insertion portion should not be squeezed, bent, or twisted by hand or forced into a tracheal tube that is too small. The insertion portion must not be withdrawn or advanced with the distal tip angulated.

Before use, the light and suction source should be tested. The tip should be treated with antifogging solution or placed in warm water (not saline) for several minutes before use. The light source should be connected and tested. The focusing ring should be adjusted by viewing some small print at a distance of 2 to 3 cm. The outside of the flexible portion should be coated with a lubricating gel, but the lubricant should not contact the lens.

There are several basic techniques. The first is to thread a tracheal or double-lumen tube over the fiberscope until it abuts the handle, advance the flexible portion until the tip enters the larynx, then thread the tube over the flexible portion. A flexometallic tube may be easier to pass through the glottis than one with a preformed curve (98). With the second technique, the tracheal tube is first advanced into the pharynx so that it acts as a guide to bring the tip of the scope close to the entrance of the larynx. The fiberscope is passed through the tube and into the trachea, then the tube is threaded over the flexible portion. A third technique is to use the fiberscope to place a guide (bougie) into the trachea under direct vision (71,78,99,100). The fiberscope is withdrawn and the tracheal tube slipped over the guide into the trachea. Another approach is to position the fiberscope near the laryngeal entrance, then separately advance the tracheal tube until it can be visualized through the fiberscope. The tube is then advanced under direct fiberoptic vision.

The handle is held close to the eye with one hand, and the index finger or thumb can be used to turn the tip control. The other finger may be used to intermittently occlude the external suction. The other hand manipulates the insertion cord or tracheal tube.

Because the flexion cables are not strong enough to lift, part, or dislodge tissues, it is important to have an air space at the end of the tip. In the anesthetized patient visualization is often difficult or impossible unless some means to expand the pharynx is used. This may be accomplished by having a second person pull the tongue anteriorly or elevate the jaw. Occasionally, it may be necessary to lift the larynx by grasping it externally between the thumb and fingers. Alternately, a modified surgical tongue retractor or a conventional rigid laryngoscope can be used to push the tongue forward (91,101). The awake patient can be asked to stick out his or her tongue, which is then held gently between gauze by an assistant.

Oral Intubation

Optimal positioning for fiberoptic laryngoscopy by the oral route includes extension of the cervical spine rather than flexion as recommended for direct laryngoscopy (102,103). Oral intubation will usually be easier if used with an accessory that will protect the instrument from the patient's teeth, guide it into the midline, and keep the tongue from falling backward. Such accessories are discussed in Chapter 13. A rigid laryngoscope may be used to direct the fiberscope near the glottis (104).

The fiberscope is placed in the midline and advanced under direct vision, curving downward at the posterior pharyngeal wall, seeking the epiglottis. It is important that the laryngoscope be kept in the midline as it is advanced.

Disorientation in the airway is best resolved by withdrawing the tip a bit and examining the area with gentle up and down tip deflection, by rotating the scope, or by alternately advancing the tip and withdrawing it slightly. If the view is consistently foggy or hazy, irrigation with saline and suction will usually resolve this problem. Adherent secretions may require withdrawal of the entire instrument and mechanical cleaning of the tip with a moist gauze. Insufflation of oxygen serves the dual purpose of maintaining the distal lens clear from secretions and increasing the oxygen concentration at the end of the fiberscope.

When the epiglottis has been located, the fiberscope tip is rotated downward so that it passes beneath the epiglottis and is then turned upward until the vocal cords are seen. The tip is then passed between the cords and advanced several centimeters into the trachea. For endobronchial intubation, the tip is advanced to view the carina, then into the desired mainstem bronchus.

With the tip of the fiberscope in the neutral position, the tube is advanced into the trachea or bronchus using a gentle twisting motion. If an obstruction is encountered, the tracheal tube should be rotated counterclockwise 90°, then again advanced (105,106). If the tube does not advance smoothly, the tongue and epiglottis should be elevated by pushing or pulling the mandible forward, pulling the tongue forward, or using a tongue retractor or rigid laryngoscope (107). Application of external pressure to the larynx also may assist tube advancement (108). The fiberscope should be used to verify that the tip of the tube is correctly positioned, then withdrawn, leaving the tube in place.

A technique for pediatric patients involves threading a tracheal tube of a size larger than can be accommodated by the trachea over the fiberscope until it impacts in the larynx (109). The fiberscope is then removed and a tube changer slipped through the tube and into the trachea. The tracheal tube is then removed and a smaller tracheal tube threaded over the tube changer into the trachea.

The fiberoptic endoscope can be used in a manner similar to a light wand (110,111).

Nasal Intubation

Despite the potential for bleeding, nasotracheal intubation is usually easier than orotracheal intubation. It is important to pass the fiberscope through the most patent nares. The tracheal tube must be large enough to pass over the laryngoscope but not too large to pass through the nose. Some tubes are compressed in the nose so that they will not accommodate the laryngoscope, even when the tube lumen would otherwise be adequate. In some patients, narrow nasal passages will not allow passage of either the tracheal tube or the endoscope. Unrecognized pathology in the pharynx may prevent the fiberscope from advancing into the trachea.

It may be helpful to pass the fiberscope through a soft well-lubricated nasal airway that is split lengthwise (89). Once the insertion portion of the fiberscope is advanced into the trachea, the airway is removed and the tracheal tube threaded over the fiberscope.

Difficulty in advancing the tube over the fiberscope is usually the result of the tip hanging up on the epiglottis (106). The tube should be withdrawn, rotated 180°, then advanced. If it still does not advance smoothly, the epiglottis should be moved anteriorly by elevating the mandible or applying external pressure on the larynx.

For patients who require a tube too small to allow a fiberscope, the fiberscope can be passed through one nostril for visualization of the larynx and the tracheal tube passed through the other nostril. The scope is used to visualize the tube and larynx and allow the tube to be manipulated into the larynx under direct vision (112,113).

Tracheal Tube Exchange (81)

To exchange a tracheal tube, the new tube is threaded over the fiberscope. In one technique, the insertion portion of the fiberscope is advanced into the tube to be replaced (114). As the old tube is pulled out, it is cut and removed from around the fiberscope. The new tube is then advanced into place over the fiberscope. In an alternative technique, the malfunctioning tube is visualized in the pharynx using the fiberscope and followed down to the level of the vocal cords (81,115). It may be advisable to insert a jet stylet catheter through the old tracheal tube before removing it to allow for ventilation or reintubation over it if the new tracheal tube cannot be passed into the trachea (116). The cuff on the malfunctioning tube is then deflated and the fiberscope advanced through the space around the tube past the cords. The old tube is gently removed and the new one advanced over the fiberscope into position.

Stylet Laryngoscope (117)

DESCRIPTION

The stylet laryngoscope also is called the optical stylet, malleable fiberoptic laryngo-

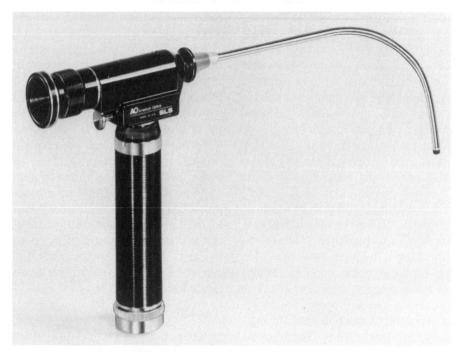

Figure 14.39.   Fiberoptic stylet laryngoscope. Courtesy of American Optical.

scope, and malleable fiberoptic stylet and is composed of a handle, body, and stylet (Fig. 14.39). The body has an eyepiece for viewing at the end of the stylet. The stylet portion has fiberoptic bundles for transmitting light to the tip and an image from the tip to the eyepiece. Power may be furnished by batteries or an external light source. The distal portion of the stylet is malleable.

TECHNIQUES OF USE

The stylet laryngoscope is restricted to oral use. It is recommended particularly where movement of the mouth, jaw, head, or neck is limited, because it can be adjusted to the patient's position or abnormal anatomy.

Before use, the light should be checked for brightness and the curve of the distal malleable portion should be shaped as deemed appropriate to fit the patient's oropharynx. The tip of the scope is immersed in warm water to prevent fogging. The stylet is lubricated with a water-based lubricant and the tracheal tube (without a connector) is threaded over it.

The laryngoscopist stands behind the patient or in front and to the side. Intubation in the sitting position has been described (118). The neck is not extended or flexed. The laryngoscope and tube are inserted together under direct vision in the midline of the mouth until the tips of both can no longer be seen. The laryngoscopist then directs the advance by looking through the eyepiece. The stylet is advanced behind the epiglottis to visualize the vocal cords. The tube is slid off the laryngoscope and into the trachea. The tip of the stylet should not pass beyond the vocal cords.

Lighted Intubation Stylet

The lighted intubation stylet is sometimes called the lightwand, (flexible) lighted stylet, and illuminating intubating stylet. It uses transillumination of the neck tissues to guide the placement of a tracheal tube. The larynx is not visualized.

DESCRIPTION

The lighted intubation stylet has a handle and a malleable stylet with a light at the end (Fig. 14.40). Some have a light bulb at the tip. Later models have the shaft and bulb encased in a plastic covering to prevent detachment of the bulb from the wire (119). Some models have a fiberoptic lighting system. One model has a retractable inner trocar that can be removed to make the stylet more flexible (and more suitable for nasal intubation) and a side clip to secure the tube to the stylet (120,121).

TECHNIQUES OF USE (122–127)

Intubation with a lighted stylet can be performed under general anesthesia or in an awake patient who has had topical anesthesia of the airway. A lubricated light wand is passed through a transparent tracheal tube whose connector has been removed so that the light is just short of the end of the tube. For nasal intubation a more flexible and longer lighted stylet should be used (128). The tube-stylet is bent to the desired shape. For oral intubation a hockey stick bend is placed in the distal portion beginning just proximal to the proximal end of the tube cuff

(54,128). Care should be taken not to bend the stylet at the point at which the bulb meets the shaft (127). It may be useful to measure the mandibular-hyoid distance by placing the index, middle, and ring fingers if necessary between the submental area of the mandible and the hyoid bone (129). The index finger is then placed at the junction of the light bulb and stylet, and the bend is made at the finger corresponding to the previous measurement.

The head may be in a neutral position, elevated slightly, or put in the traditional "sniffing" position (129,130). The mouth is opened and the tongue pulled forward. A bite block may be inserted to prevent the patient from biting the tube-stylet. The stylet is illuminated, the room lights are dimmed, and the tube-stylet is inserted in the midline of the oral cavity or nares and advanced into the hypopharynx. A Williams airway intubator (see Chapter 13) may be used to keep the stylet in the midline (130).

As the tube-stylet is advanced, transillumination will appear suddenly as it passes the bulk of the tongue and epiglottis, just superior to the thyroid cartilage. As the stylet is advanced farther, its position can be dis-

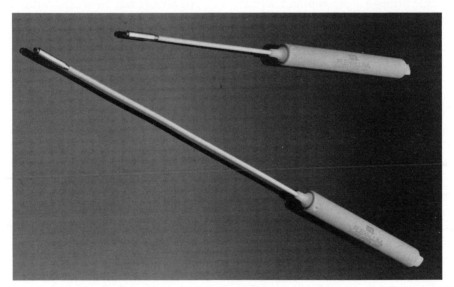

Figure 14.40. Lighted intubation stylets. There is a light bulb at the tip of the malleable stylet. Courtesy of Concept Inc.

cerned by observing the transillumination of the soft tissues of the neck. The intensity of the illumination may be increased by applying cricoid pressure. A bright area of illumination in the midline at the thyroid prominence indicates entry into the trachea. The trocar, if present, should be pulled back several centimeters and the tube-stylet advanced so that the glow rests at the level of the sternal notch (131). The tube is held in place, and the stylet is removed.

If the esophagus is entered, the transillumination will disappear (55,119). This can be corrected by lifting the stylet to bring the tip more anterior in the neck (129). With placement in the pyriform fossa, transillumination will appear lateral to the midline. A bright glow in the submental area indicates the tip is in the vallecula, and it may be necessary to flex the neck to allow the tube to enter the trachea.

A digital technique can also be used. Gloved fingers are inserted into the mouth and the tongue and jaw pulled forward (127). The tube and stylet are slid along the tongue and guided into the trachea. The patient with a clenched jaw can be intubated by retracting the cheek and inserting the lightwand from the right side through a gap behind the rearmost teeth (132).

HAZARDS

Detachment of the bulb or lens has been reported (124,127,130,133,134).

ADVANTAGES

Advantages of this technique include rapidity of intubation and ability to intubate without movement of the head or neck (which may make it useful when a cervical spine injury may be present and/or neck mobility is limited). The technique is easily learned, permits cricoid pressure to be used, is effective when blood or secretions are present, and can be used in intoxicated or uncooperative patients (135). It may be especially useful when anatomical abnormalities preclude insertion of a conventional laryngoscope or extension of the head and in pa-

tients with extensive or expensive dental work or poor teeth (136,137). It has been used successfully with rapid sequence induction and in patients who are difficult to intubate with conventional direct laryngoscopy (121,138,139). Because the method does not require that the user crouch down or be at the patient's head, the technique can be used in cramped quarters such as hallways and helicopters (127). It will rapidly and reliably distinguish intratracheal from inadvertent esophageal placement (119). It can be used in pediatric patients (137,140,141). The equipment is simple, inexpensive, reusable, reliable, compact, easily cleaned, portable, and reasonably durable.

No significant problems with this method have been noted when it was compared with the conventional laryngoscopic methods (124,129,142,143), although more attempts before successful intubation may be required than with conventional rigid laryngoscopy (129). Use of the lighted intubation stylet has been found to be superior to blind techniques for both oral and nasal intubations (125,144).

DISADVANTAGES

Anything that interferes with transmission of the light from the neck such as anterior neck scarring, flexion contractions, excessive cervical adipose tissue, midline neck tumors or swellings, covering of the bulb with blood and/or secretions, and inability to darken the room lights will decrease the effectiveness of the technique (54,55). Experience and practice in routine cases is needed for successful use in the occasional difficult case.

The Bullard Laryngoscope (145,146)

DESCRIPTION

The Bullard laryngoscope combines an anatomically shaped rigid blade with a fiberoptic bundle on its posterior aspect. Adult

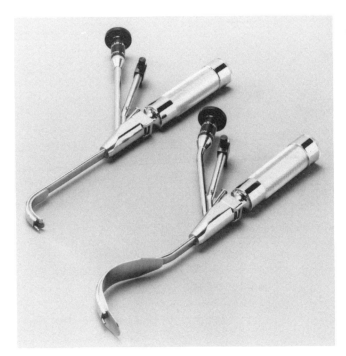

Figure 14.41. Bullard laryngoscopes. **Top,** Pediatric version. **Bottom,** Adult version. The handle contains batteries that power a halogen light bulb. The viewing arm with eyepiece extends at a 45° angle from the handle. Between the handle and the viewing arm are two working channels. The one nearest the viewing arm is for the intubating forceps, which protrudes from the distal end. The other is for insufflation, injection, or suctioning. Courtesy of Circon ACMI, a division of Circon Corp.

and pediatric versions are available (Figs. 14.41 and 14.42). The pediatric version is *L*-shaped with a short blade and is recommended for use in patients up to 8 to 10 years of age. The blade on the adult version has a deeper curve and resembles an inverted question mark.

A handle with batteries and a halogen bulb may provide the light. Alternately, a handle with an adaptor for a cord from a high-intensity light source may be used. A viewing arm with eyepiece extends at a 45° angle from the handle. A teaching attachment with an additional eyepiece is available and video cameras from several manufacturers fit the eyepiece.

Fiberoptic bundles for illumination and operator viewing are housed in a rigid sheath that follows the curve of the blade. The sheath is sealed at its distal end to protect the bundles and allow the blade to be immersed for cleaning.

In the older version between the handle and the viewing arm are two ports, both of which connect to the working channel that is in the same sheath as the fiberoptic bundles (see Fig. 14.41). The smaller port has a Luer-lock connection for oxygen insufflation, injection of fluid, or suctioning. The larger port accepts the nonmalleable intubating forceps, which has a thumb-activated lever. It allows the operator both to advance the forceps (with attached tracheal tube) into the larynx and to release the tube when it is properly positioned. If the intubating forceps is not in place, the larger port must be plugged if the small port is to be used for suctioning or oxygen administration.

On later models there is only one port, which can be used for administration of oxygen or local anesthetics or suctioning (Fig. 14.43 and see Fig. 14.42). In place of the larger port is a connection for a detachable stylet, which is used instead of the intubating forceps. A tip extender is available. This is used when the blade is not long enough to lift the epiglottis. Studies indicate that the new intubating stylet results in fewer attempts at intubation, less time to intubate, and less trauma (54,147).

TECHNIQUES OF USE (145,146,148)

Designed for the difficult-to-intubate patient, the Bullard laryngoscope can be used

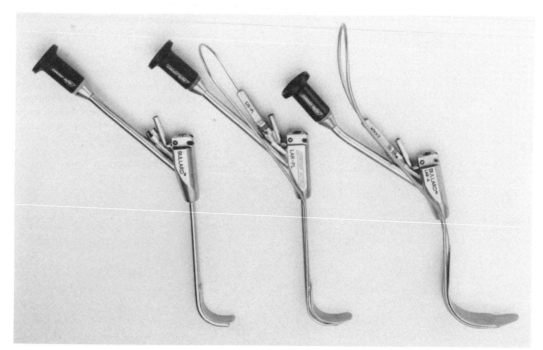

Figure 14.42.   Bullard laryngoscope with intubation forceps, later version. **Left,** Pediatric version without stylet. **Middle,** Pediatric version with stylet in place. **Right,** Adult version with stylet in place. Courtesy of Circon ACMI, a division of Circon Corp.

routinely in patients with normal airways. It can be used in awake or anesthetized patients either paralyzed or breathing spontaneously and can be used for nasal intubation.

Before use, the image bundle window at the distal end of the sheath should be treated with an antifog solution. The laryngoscopist is positioned at patient's head, and the scope is held with the handle horizontal. The patient's head is kept in the neutral position. The blade is inserted midline in the oral cavity, much like an oral airway. As the blade is advanced, the handle is rotated to the vertical position so that the blade slides over the tongue. Once the blade has been rotated around the tongue, upward movement along the axis of the handle is exerted to visualize the larynx. Either the epiglottis or the glottis should come into view. The tip of the blade can be used to lift the epiglottis directly or indirectly.

Older Version

Intubation can be accomplished with a styleted tracheal tube, a tracheal tube with a directional tip, or the Bullard intubating forceps. If the intubating forceps is used, a tracheal tube with a Murphy eye is required. Before use, the forceps is inserted through the channel in the scope and made to grasp the tracheal tube by its Murphy eye. After the larynx is visualized, the scope should be angled to the right so that the tube tip and forceps, which advance from the left of the field of view, point at the vocal cords. Pressure on the thumb lever advances the tube into the larynx. Additional pressure causes the forceps jaw to open, releasing the tube, which is then advanced to the appropriate intratracheal position. The thumb lever is then retracted fully, closing the jaws and retracting the forceps. After placement of the tracheal

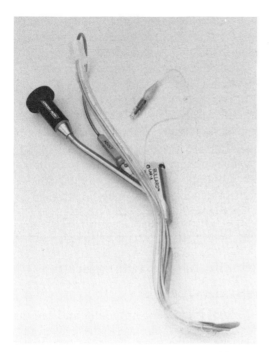

Figure 14.43. Later version of adult Bullard laryngoscope with tracheal tube in place over stylet. Note that the stylet comes out through the Murphy eye. Courtesy of Circon ACMI, a division of Circon Corp.

tube is confirmed visually, the laryngoscope and forceps are removed.

If the intubating forceps is not used, a styleted tube that mimics the shape of the laryngoscope blade or a tracheal tube with a directional tip should be used. After the larynx has been visualized, the tip of the tracheal tube is introduced into the mouth next to the blade on either side. It is then advanced in a fashion similar to that of the blade and manipulated until it comes into the field of vision. It is then inserted into the larynx as with conventional direct laryngoscopy.

Another technique is to use a stylet designed especially for use with this laryngoscope (149). The stylet attaches to the laryngoscope at the same site as the forceps and is designed to hold the tracheal tube close to the underside of the blade. A well-lubricated tube is loaded onto the stylet. The tip of the stylet may be allowed to protrude through the Murphy eye or may be inside the tube. If

the stylet is inside the tube, the tube should be rotated so that the long part of the bevel is in view (149). The entire apparatus is advanced into the pharynx. When the tip of the tube or stylet is seen in proximity to the glottis, the tube is slipped off the stylet into the larynx.

Alternately, a flexible wire or bougie may be placed into the trachea through the forceps port, the laryngoscope removed, and a tracheal tube passed over the wire (150,151).

Newer Version

A tracheal tube is placed over the stylet and the stylet is advanced through the Murphy eye. After the vocal cords are visualized, the tip of the stylet is manipulated until it points between the cords. The tube is then advanced off the stylet and into the trachea. If the tube does not enter the larynx, the tube and stylet must be withdrawn and the tube again placed over the stylet with the tip of the stylet projecting through the Murphy eye before another attempt at intubation is made.

For nasotracheal intubation, the larynx is visualized using the Bullard laryngoscope; the patient's head position and the thyroid cartilage are manipulated to allow the tube to be advanced between the vocal cords (152). A directional tip tracheal tube may be especially useful in this situation.

Reported advantages of the Bullard laryngoscope include rapidity of intubation, low risk of failed intubation and trauma to lips and teeth, less discomfort in the awake patient than direct laryngoscopy, and no need for neck flexion or extension or anterior displacement of the tongue (149,153,154). Minimal mouth opening is required.

Disadvantages include the fact that practice is needed to achieve proficiency. The forceps teeth may lacerate the tracheal tube cuff and could cause trauma if they are allowed to close on tissue or if the forceps is not fully retracted before laryngoscope removal. The equipment is expensive. Cleaning is somewhat involved. The large number of individual parts require careful handling and storage to prevent loss. It may not be suitable for intubation of adults with necks that are significantly longer than average (149).

A study comparing ease of learning to use the Bullard laryngoscope with the flexible fiberoptic laryngoscope found that both devices require a similar amount of practice (150). Passage of the tracheal tube took longer with the Bullard.

Tooth Protector

Tooth protectors (mouth guards, mouth protectors, or dentguards) are placed over the upper teeth to protect them from damage by contact with the flange of the laryngoscope blade. They can also be used to prevent the laryngoscope blade from getting caught in a gap between teeth. Use of a protector does not guarantee avoidance of dental trauma (155). Although it will prevent direct trauma to the surface of the teeth, it cannot prevent transmission of pressure to the roots.

Tooth protectors are available in different designs (Fig. 14.44). They may by fashioned by the user from various materials, including rubber, adhesive tape, gauze, silicone elastomers, lead foil, cellulose acetate, or orahesive (156–158).

These devices may make it harder to visualize the larynx and may inhibit insertion of the tracheal tube because of lack of space (155). Cutting off part of the right side of the protector or using a transparent protector may decrease these problems (155,159). It may be necessary to remove the protector before intubation can be accomplished. A tooth protection device may be attached to the laryngoscope blade (160–163).

Complications of Laryngoscopy

DENTAL INJURY

One of the most common complications of laryngoscopy is damage to the teeth, gums, or dental prostheses. There not only may be cosmetic disfigurement and discomfort but also may be serious pulmonary complications if a dislodged tooth or fragment is aspirated.

A tooth or prosthetic device may be chipped, broken, loosened or avulsed. The

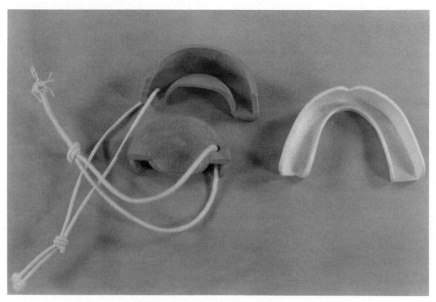

Figure 14.44. Tooth protectors.

teeth most likely to be damaged are those that have been restored or weakened through periodontal disease (164). The upper incisors are most frequently involved (165). This usually is caused by using the teeth as a fulcrum point for the laryngoscope while elevating the epiglottis.

The condition of each patient's teeth should be carefully assessed preoperatively to identify possible problems. Inquiry should be made concerning vulnerable dental repair work or loose or carious teeth. Anatomical variations of the mouth and pharynx that can cause difficulty in exposing the larynx should be noted. The patient should be advised beforehand if there is likely to be a problem.

In patients 4 to 11 years old, the deciduous teeth may be easily dislodged. Removal of such teeth before or during anesthesia may be indicated if they are loose. A suture may be placed around a loose tooth to prevent it from entering the airway should it become dislodged.

When there are gaps between the upper front teeth, a portion of a tracheal tube or other device may be used to bridge the gap (166,167) or a tooth protector may be used. Keeping partial upper dentures in place may prevent the laryngoscope from slipping into gaps between teeth.

If a tooth, fragment or dental appliance is dislodged, prevention of foreign body aspiration should be of major concern. An immediate search should be conducted, starting with an examination of the oral cavity and the area surrounding the patient's head. X-rays of the chest and neck must be taken if the fragment is not found (168).

Different types of tooth damage may occur (169). These require different treatments. A qualified dentist or oral surgeon should be consulted.

DAMAGE TO SOFT TISSUES AND NERVES

Damage to all areas of the upper airway have been reported, including abrasion, he-matoma, and laceration of the lips, tongue, palate, pharynx, hypopharynx, larynx, and esophagus (127,170–76). The lingual nerve may be injured (177–180).

INJURY TO CERVICAL SPINAL CORD

Aggressive positioning of the head for intubation, especially extension of the head or neck can aggravate a preexisting cervical spine injury (181–184). Cervical cord damage may be especially likely in patients with fractures, dislocations of cervical vertebrae, congenital weaknesses or malformations, or other pathologic fragility such as that seen with osteoporosis, connective tissue diseases, and lytic bone tumors (185). Although there are no good data to define whether the small amounts of movement that result from carefully executed airway maneuvers increase the risk of a secondary injury, clinical experience suggests they do not (186–188). There are also no data to suggest that any mode of airway intervention is superior to another in decreasing secondary injury or improving outcome (186,189–192). However, studies show that mask ventilation moves the cervical spine more than any commonly used method of tracheal intubation. There is good evidence that in-line immobilization reduces spinal movement and the likelihood of secondary injury (187,190,192).

ESOPHAGEAL INTUBATION WITH FIBEROPTIC SCOPE

A case has been reported in which a tracheal tube threaded over a flexible fiberoptic endoscope repeatedly entered the esophagus despite placement of the end of the endo-scope in the trachea (193). Use of a stiffer fiberscope may avoid this problem (194).

ADVANCEMENT OF FIBERSCOPE THROUGH MURPHY EYE

If the tip of the fiberscope protrudes through the Murphy eye of the tracheal tube, it may not be possible to slip the tracheal tube off the endoscope or to withdraw the fiberscope from the tracheal tube (195,196,197). The fiberscope and tracheal tube should be withdrawn together as a unit.

To avoid this problem, the tracheal tube should be threaded onto the fiberscope before endoscopy or the fiberscope should be advanced through the tube under direct vision, identifying both the side and distal openings and taking care to pass the fiberscope through the distal one. The tip of the endoscope should be in the neutral position as the tracheal tube is advanced and the fiberscope is withdrawn.

CIRCULATORY CHANGES

Laryngoscopy can result in significant hemodynamic changes. Many studies pertaining to the effect of laryngoscopy on heart rate and blood pressure have been carried out in both awake and anesthetized patients. In awake patients who have received i.v. sedation and topical anesthesia, neither fiberoptic nor rigid laryngoscopy caused a significant increase in heart rate, although rigid laryngoscopy produced an increase in blood pressure (198).

In anesthetized patients, the results are somewhat confusing. Some studies show similar increases in blood pressure and heart rates with fiberoptic and rigid laryngoscopy (199,200). Another study found lower pressures but higher heart rates in the fiberoptic group (201). Another study found similar pressures but higher heart rates in the fiberoptic group (202). Other studies have found that both pressures and heart rates were significantly greater and more prolonged in fiberoptic patients than rigid laryngoscopy patients (203–205).

Two studies comparing the use of the light stylet with direct rigid laryngoscopy found no differences in the postintubation heart rates and blood pressures (142,143).

Studies comparing a curved blade and a straight blade either with the tip in the vallecula or used to lift the epiglottis have found no differences in heart rate and blood pressure responses (206,207).

SWALLOWING OR ASPIRATION OF A FOREIGN BODY

Cases have been reported in which the bulb from a laryngoscope was aspirated during intubation (124,127,130,133,134,208, 209). A portion of the diaphragm of a Patil-Syracuse mask may enter the airway (210–212).

It is important to make every effort to find these foreign bodies. If they cannot be found in the oral cavity or around the patient's head, x-rays of the chest and neck should be taken.

SHOCK AND/OR BURN

A case has been reported where a laryngoscope light was left on and contacted the patient's skin, resulting in a burn (213). Malpositioning of a blade on the handle can produce a short circuit, which leads to rapid heating of the handle (214). The tip of a fiberscope connected to a powerful light source may be hot enough to produce a burn (215). Interference on an ECG tracing from a flexible fiberscope has been reported (216).

LARYNGOSCOPE MALFUNCTION (217)

The most common malfunction of the laryngoscope is failure of the light to illuminate. This may be the result of a defective power source, defective lamp, faulty socket, or poor contact between the blade and handle. Fiberoptic laryngoscopes are more reliable, because the useful light of a halogen lamp is longer than an ordinary light bulb and the lamp is usually in the handle rather than the blade. Breakage of the blade (218,219) and handle (217,220,221) have been reported.

A preuse check will detect most malfunctions. An extra handle and blade should always be immediately available. Neglecting to observe these precautions could spell disaster, especially when a rapid sequence induction is being performed.

DIFFICULTIES IN CLEANING AND STERILIZATION

Flexible fiberoptic instruments have nooks and crannies that make it difficult to clean and sterilize them effectively between patients. Ineffective reprocessing may result in the introduction of infectious debris from one patient into a subsequent patient, growth of opportunistic pathogens in the scopes and their introduction into subsequent patients, and introduction of chemical agents used in reprocessing equipment into subsequent patients (222).

TMJ DYSFUNCTION

Patients with TMJ derangements sometimes report that the problem began following general anesthesia (223).

REFERENCES

1. American Society for Testing and Materials. Standard specification for rigid laryngoscopes for tracheal intubation. Hook-on fittings for laryngoscope handles and blades with lamps (F965-85). Philadelphia: ASTM, 1985.
2. International Standards Organization. Laryngoscopic fittings. Part 1. Hook-on type handle—blade fittings (ISO 7376/1). Geneva Switzerland: ISO, 1984
3. American Society for Testing and Materials. Standard specification for rigid laryngoscopes for tracheal intubation. Hook-on fittings for fiberilluminated blades and handles (F1195-88). Philadelphia: ASTM, 1988.
4. Greenblatt GM. Fiberoptic illuminating laryngoscope with remote light source—further development. Anesth Analg 1981;60:841–842.
5. Datta S, Briwa J. Modified laryngoscope for endotracheal intubation of obese patients. Anesth Analg 1981;60:120–121.
6. King H, Wang L, Khan AK. A modification of laryngoscopy technique. Anesthesiology 1986; 65:566.
7. Thomas DV. Difficult tracheal intubation in obstetrics. Anaesthesia 1985;40:307.
8. Bourke DL, Lawrence J. Another way to insert a Macintosh blade. Anesthesiology 1983;59:80.
9. Gandhi SK, Burgos L. A technique of laryngoscopy for difficult intubation. Anesthesiology 1986;64:528–529.
10. Dhara SS, Cheong TW. An adjustable multiple angle laryngoscope adaptor. Anaesth Intensive Care 1991;19:243–245.
11. Jellicoe JA, Harris NR. A modification of a standard laryngoscope for difficult tracheal intubation in obstetric cases. Anaesthesia 1984;39:800–802.
12. Yentis SM. A laryngoscope adaptor for difficult intubation. Anaesthesia 1987;42:764–766.
13. Patil VU, Stehling LC, Zauder HL. An adjustable laryngoscope handle for difficult intubations. Anesthesiology 1984;60:609.
14. Lewis JJ. Autoclavable Macintosh laryngoscope with high-intensity fiberoptic illumination for routine anesthetic use. Anesthesiology 1975;43:573–574.
15. McIntyre JWR. Laryngoscope design and the difficult adult tracheal intubation. Can J Anaesth 1989;36:94–98.
16. Macintosh RR. A new laryngoscope. Lancet 1943;1:205.
17. Jephcott A. The Macintosh laryngoscope. A historical note on its clinical and commercial development. Anaesthesia 1984;39:474–479.
18. Campbell NN, Millar R. Modification of laryngoscope for nasogastric intubation. Anaesthesia 1985;40:703–704.
19. Callander CC, Thomas J. Modification of Macintosh laryngoscope for difficult intubation. Anaesthesia 1987;42:671–672.
20. Gabrielczyk MR. A new integrated suction laryngoscope. Anaesthesia 1986;41:970–971.
21. Ibler M. Modification of Macintosh laryngoscope blade. Anesthesiology 1983;58:200.
22. Kessell J. A laryngoscope for obstetrical use. An obstetrical laryngoscope. Anaesth Intensive Care 1977;5:265–266.
23. Mazumder JK. Laryngoscope blade with suction unit. Can Anaesth Soc J 1979;26:513–514.
24. McWhinnie F. Modification of laryngoscope for nasogastric intubation. Anaesthesia 1986;41:218–219.
25. Pope ES. Left handed laryngoscope. Anaesthesia 1960;15:326–328.
26. McComish PB. Left sided laryngoscopes. Anaesthesia 1965;20:372.
27. Lagade MRG, Poppers PJ. Use of the left-entry laryngoscope blade in patients with right-sided orofacial lesions. Anesthesiology 1983;58:300.
28. Legade MRG, Poppers PJ. Revival of the polio laryngoscope blade. Anesthesiology 1982;57:545.
29. Weeks DB. A new use of an old blade. Anesthesiology 1974;10:200–201.
30. Racz GB. Improved vision modification of

the Macintosh laryngoscope. Anaesthesia 1984; 39:1249–1250.

31. Bizarri DV, Guffrida JG. Improved laryngoscope blade designed for ease of manipulation and reduction of trauma. Anesth Analg 1958;37:231–232.

32. Miller RA. A new laryngoscope. Anesthesiology 1941;2:317–320.

33. Jones RDM. Lamp placement and the Miller I laryngoscope blade. Anesthesiology 1985;62:207.

34. Rokowski WJ, Gurmarnik S. Laryngoscope blades modified for neonates and infants. Anesth Analg 1983;62:241–2.

35. Cork RC, Woods W, Vaughn RW, Harris T. Oxygen supplementation during endotracheal intubation of infants. Anesthesiology 1979;51:186.

36. Diaz JH. Further modifications of the Miller blade for difficult pediatric laryngoscopy. Anesthesiology 1984;60:612–613.

37. Wung J, Stark RI, Indyk L, Driscoll JM. Oxygen supplement during endotracheal intubation of the infant. Pediatrics 1977;59:1046–1048.

38. Hencz P. Modified laryngoscope for endotracheal intubation of neonates. Anesthesiology 1980; 53:84.

39. Ledbetter JL, Rasch DK, Pollard TG, Helsel P, Smith RB. Reducing the risks of laryngoscopy in anaesthetised infants. Anaesthesia 1988;43:151–153.

40. Todres ID, Crone RK. Experience with a modified laryngoscope in sick infants. Crit Care Med 1981;9:544–545.

41. Portzer M, Wasmuth CE. Endotracheal anesthesia using a modified Wis-Foregger laryngoscope blade. Cleve Clin Q 1959;26:140–143.

42. Schapira M. A modified straight laryngoscope blade designed to facilitate endotracheal intubation. Anesth Analg 1973;52:553–554.

43. Soper RL. A new laryngoscope for anaesthetists. Br Med J 1947;1:265.

44. Snow JC. Modification of laryngoscope blade. Anesthesiology 1962;23:394.

45. Flagg P. Exposure and illumination of the pharynx and larynx by the general practitioner. A new laryngoscope designed to simplify the technique. Arch Laryngol 1928;8:716–717.

46. Seward EH. Laryngoscope for resuscitation of the newborn. Lancet 1957;2:1041.

47. Hatch DJ. Paediatric anaesthetic equipment. Br J Anaesth 1985;57:672–684.

48. Phillips OC, Duerksen RL. Endotracheal intubation. A new blade for direct laryngoscopy. Anesth Analg 1973;52:691–698.

49. Racz GB, Allen FB. A new pressure-sensitive laryngoscope. Anesthesiology 1985;62:356–358.

50. Robertshaw FL. A new laryngoscope for infants and children. Lancet 1962;2:1034.

51. Bryce-Smith R. A laryngoscope blade for infants. Br Med J 1952;1:217.

52. Bainton CR. A new laryngoscope blade to overcome pharyngeal obstruction. Anesthesiology 1987;67:767–770.

53. Choi JJ. A new double-angle blade for direct laryngoscopy. Anesthesiology 1990;72:576.

54. Benumof JL. Management of the difficult adult airway. Anesthesiology 1991;75:1087–1110.

55. Mayall RM. The Belscope for management of the difficult airway. Anesthesiology 1992;76:1059–1060.

56. Bellhouse CP. An angulated laryngoscope for routine and difficult tracheal intubation. Anesthesiology 1988;69:126–129.

57. Huffman J. The application of prisms to curved laryngoscopes: a preliminary study. J Am Assoc Nurse Anesth 1968;35:138–139.

58. Huffman J, Elam JO. Prisms and fiber optics for laryngoscopy. Anesth Analg 1971;50:64–67.

59. Huffman J. The development of optical prism instruments to view and study the human larynx. J Am Assoc Nurse Anesth 1970;38:197–202.

60. Murrin KR. Intubation procedure and causes of difficult intubation. In: Latto IP, Rosen M, eds. Difficulties in tracheal intubation. London: Bailliere Tindall, 1985:75–89.

61. Brown A, Norton ML. Instrumentation and equipment for management of the difficult airway. In: Norton ML, Brown ACD, eds. Atlas of the difficult airway. A source book. St. Louis: Mosby Year Book, 1991:24–32.

62. Moynihan P. Modification of pediatric laryngoscope. Anesthesiology 1982;56:330.

63. Eldor J, Gozal Y. The length of the blade is more important than its design in difficult tracheal intubation. Can J Anaesth 1990;37:268.

64. Patteson SK, Chesney JT. Anesthetic management for magnetic resonance imaging: problems and solutions. Anesth Analg 1992;74:121–128.

65. Karlik SJ, Heatherley T, Pavan F, Stein J, Lebron F, Rutt B. Patient anesthesia and monitoring at a 1,5-T MRI installation. Magn Reson Med 1988;7:210–221.

66. Ovassapian A. Fiberoptic airway endoscopy in anesthesia and critical care. New York: Raven Press, 1990.

67. Patil VU, Stehling NC, Zauder HL. Fiberoptic endoscopy in anesthesia. Chicago: Year Book Medical Publishers, 1983.

68. Daum REO, Jones DJ. Fiberoptic intubation in Klippel-Feil syndrome. Anaesthesia 1988;43:18–21.

69. Divatia JV, Upadhye SM, Sareen R. Fiberoptic intubation in cicatricial membranes of the pharynx. Anaesthesia 1992;47:486–489.

70. Hemmer D, Lee T, Wright BD. Intubation of a

child with a cervical spine injury with the aid of a fiberoptic bronchoscope. Anaesth Intensive Care 1982;10:163–165.

71. Howardy-Hansen P, Berthelsen P. Fiberoptic bronchoscopic nasotracheal intubation of a neonate with Pierre-Robin syndrome. Anaesthesia 1988;43:121–122.

72. Kleeman P, Jantzen JAH, Bonfils P. The ultra-thin bronchoscope in management of the difficult paediatric airway. Can J Anaesth 1987;34:606–608.

73. Keenan MA, Stiles CM, Kaufman RL. Acquired laryngeal deviation associated with cervical spine disease in erosive polyarticular arthritis. Use of fiberoptic bronchoscope in rheumatoid disease. Anesthesiology 1983;58:441–448.

74. Ovassapian A, Land P, Schaffer MF, Cerullo L, Zalkind MS. Anesthetic management for surgical corrections of severe flexion deformity of the cervical spine. Anesthesiology 1983;58:370–372.

75. Ovassapian A, Doka JC, Romsa DE. Acromegaly; use of fiberoptic laryngoscopy to avoid tracheostomy. Anesthesiology 1984;43:429–430.

76. Rashid J, Warltier B. Awake fiberoptic intubation for a rare cause of upper airway obstruction: an infected laryngocoel. Anaesthesia 1989;44:834–836.

77. Stella JP, Kageler WV, Epker BN. Fiberoptic endotracheal intubation in oral and maxillofacial surgery. J Oral Maxillofac Surg 1986;44:923–925.

78. Scheller JG, Schulman SR. Fiber-optic bronchoscopic guidance for intubating a neonate with Pierre-Robin syndrome. J Clin Anesth 1991;3:45–47.

79. Ovassapian A, Schrader C. Fiber-optic-aided bronchial intubation. Semin Anesth 1987;6:133–142.

80. Slinger PD. Fiberoptic bronchoscopic positioning of double-lumen tubes. J Cardiothorac Anesth 1989;3:486–496.

81. Rosenbaum SH, Rosenbaum LM, Cole RP, Askanazi J, Hyman AI. Use of the flexible fiberoptic bronchoscope to change endotracheal tubes in critically ill patients. Anesthesiology 1981;54:169–170.

82. Watson CB. Use of fiberoptic bronchoscope to change endotracheal tube endorsed. Anesthesiology 1981;55:476–477.

83. Ovassapian A, Dykes HM. The role of fiber-optic endoscopy in airway management. Semin Anesth 1987;6:93–104.

84. Dierdorf SF. Types and physics of fiberscopes. In: Roberts JT, ed. Fiberoptics in anesthesia [Special issue]. Anesth Clin North Am 1991;9:19–42.

85. Wang JF, Reves JG, Corssen G. Use of the fiberoptic laryngoscope for difficult tracheal intubation. Ala J Med Sci 1976;13:247–251.

86. Bloch EC, Filston HC. A thin fiberoptic bronchoscope as an aid to occlusion of the fistula in infants with tracheoesophageal fistula. Anesth Analg 1988;67:791–793.

87. Laravuso RB, Perloff WH. Difficult pediatric intubation. Anesthesiology 1986;64:668–669.

88. Boysen PG. Fiberoptic intervention of the airway (ASA Refresher Course 116). Park Ridge, IL: ASA, 1991.

89. Patil VU. Oral and nasal fiberoptic intubation with a single lumen tube in fiberoptics in anesthesia. In: Roberts JT, ed. Fiberoptics in anesthesia [Special issue]. Anesth Clin North Am 1991;9:83–96.

90. Stehling L. The difficult intubation and fiberoptic endoscopy (ASA Refresher Course 262). Park Ridge, IL: ASA, 1989.

91. Childress WF. New method for fiberoptic endotracheal intubation of anesthetized patients. Anesthesiology 1981;55:595–596.

92. Cooper DW, Long GT. Difficult fiberoptic intubation in an intellectually handicapped patient. Anaesth Intensive Care 1992;20:227–229.

93. Baraka A. Transtracheal jet ventilation during fiberoptic intubation under general anesthesia. Anesth Analg 1986;65:1091–1092.

94. Lu GP, Frost EAM, Goldiner PL. Another approach to the problem airway. Anesthesiology 1986;65:101–102.

95. Patil V, Stehling LC, Zauder HL, Koch JP. Mechanical aids for fiberoptic endoscopy. Anesthesiology 1982;57:69–70.

96. Rogers SN, Benumof JL. New and easy techniques for fiberoptic endoscopy-aided tracheal intubation. Anesthesiology 1983;59:569–572.

97. Wangler MA, Weaver JM. A method to facilitate fiberoptic laryngoscopy. Anesthesiology 1984;61:111.

98. Calder I. When the endotracheal tube will not pass over the flexible fiberoptic bronchoscope. Anesthesiology 1992;77:398.

99. Gerrish SP, Weston GA. The use of a biopsy brush wire as a bronchoscope guide. Anaesthesia 1986;41:444.

100. Suriani RJ, Kayne RD. Fiberoptic bronchoscopic guidance for intubating a child with Pierre-Robin Syndrome. J Clin Anesth 1992;4:258.

101. Johnson C, Hunter J, Ho E, Bruff C. Fiberoptic intubation facilitated by a rigid laryngoscope. Anesth Analg 1991;72:714.

102. Shorten GD, Ali HH, Roberts JT. Assessment of patient position for fiberoptic intubation using videolaryngoscopy. Anesth Analg 1991;72:S253.

103. Roberts JT, Ali HH, Shorten GD, Gorback MS. Why cervical flexion facilitates laryngoscopy with a Macintosh laryngoscope, but hinders it with a flexible fiberscope. Anesthesiology 1990;73:A1012.

104. Ross DG. Fiberoptic intubation and double-lumen tubes. Anaesthesia 1990;45:895.

105. Schwartz D, Johnson C, Roberts J. A maneuver to facilitate flexible fiberoptic intubation. Anesthesiology 1989;71:470–471.

106. Katsnelson T, Frost EAM, Farcon E, Goldiner PL. When the endotracheal tube will not pass over the flexible fiberoptic bronchoscope. Anesthesiology 1992;76:151–152.

107. Couture P, Perreault C, Girard D. Fiberoptic bronchoscopic intubation after induction of general anaesthesia: another approach. Can J Anaesth 1992;39:99.

108. Bond A. Assisting fiberoptic intubation. Anaesth Intensive Care 1992;20:247–248.

109. Berthelsen P, Prytz S, Jacobsen E. Two-stage fiberoptic nasotracheal intubation in infants: a new approach to difficult pediatric intubation. Anesthesiology 1985;63:457–458.

110. Foster CA. An aid to blind nasal intubation in children. Anaesthesia 1977;32:1038.

111. Stone DJ. Another use for the fiberoptic bronchoscope. Anesthesiology 1987;67:608.

112. Skinner AC. Glottic illumination by fibrescope. Anaesthesia 1983;38:1100–1101.

113. Alfery DD, Ward CF, Harwood IR, Mannino FL. Airway management for a neonate with congenital fusion of the jaws. Anesthesiology 1979;51:340–342.

114. Hudes ET, Fisher JA, Guslitz B. Difficult endotracheal reintubations. A simple technique. Anesthesiology 1986;64:515–517.

115. Halebian P, Shires T. A method of replacement of the endotracheal tube with continuous control of the airway. Surg Gynecol Obstet 1985;161:285–286.

116. Benumof JL. Additional safety measures when changing endotracheal tubes. Anesthesiology 1991;75:921–922.

117. Kraft M. Stylet laryngoscopy for oral tracheal intubation. Anesthesiol Rev 1982;9:35–37.

118. Shapiro HM, Sanford TJ, Schaldah AL. Fiberoptic stylet laryngoscope and sitting position for tracheal intubation in acute superior vena caval syndrome. Anesth Analg 1984;63:161–162.

119. Stewart RD, LaRosee A, Stoy WA, Heller MB. Use of a lighted stylet to confirm correct endotracheal tube placement. Chest 1987;92:900–903.

120. Stevens SC, Hung OR. A new device for oral and nasotracheal light-guided intubation. Can J Anaesth 1992;39:A86.

121. Hung OR, Stevens SC, Hawboldt G. Light-guided vs. laryngoscope intubation in surgical patients. Clinical trial of a new lightwand device. Can J Anaesth 1992;39:A147.

122. Ainsworth QP, Howells TH. Transilluminated tracheal intubation. Br J Anaesth 1989;62:494–497.

123. Ducrow M. Throwing light on blind intubation. Anaesthesia 1978;33:827–829.

124. Ellis DG, Jakymec A, Kaplan RM, et al. Guided orotracheal intubation in the operating room using a lighted stylet. A comparison with direct laryngoscopic technique. Anesthesiology 1986;64:823–826.

125. Fox DJ, Castro T, Rastrelli AJ. Comparison of intubation techniques in the awake patient. The Flexi-lum surgical light (lightwand) versus blind nasal approach. Anesthesiology 1987;66:69–71.

126. Mehta S. Transtracheal illumination for optimal tracheal tube placement. A clinical study. Anaesthesia 1989;44:970–972.

127. Vollmer TP, Stewart RD, Paris PM, Ellis D, Berkebile PE. Use of a lighted stylet for guided orotracheal intubation in the prehospital setting. Ann Emerg Med 1985;14:324–328.

128. Weiss FR, Hatton MN. Intubation by use of the lightwand: experience in 253 patients. J Oral Maxillofac Surg 1989;47:577–580.

129. Ellis DG, Stewart RD, Kaplan RM, Jakymec A, Freeman JA, Bleyaert A. Success rates of blind orotracheal intubation using a transillumination technique with a lighted stylet. Ann Emerg Med 1986;15:138–142.

130. Williand RT, Stewart RD. Transillumination of the trachea with a lighted stylet. Anesth Analg 1986;65:542–543.

131. Stewart RD, LaRosee A, Kaplan RM, Ilkhanipour K. Correct positioning of an endotracheal tube using a flexible lighted stylet. Crit Care Med 1990;18:97–99.

132. Hartman RA, Castro T, Matson M, Fox DJ. Rapid orotracheal intubation in the clenched-jaw patient. A modification of the lightwand technique. J Clin Anaesth 1992;4:245–246.

133. Stone DJ, Stirt JA, Kaplan MJ, McLean WC. A complication of lightwand-guided nasotracheal intubation. Anesthesiology 1984;61:780–781.

134. Dowson S, Greenwald KM. A potential complication of lightwand-guided intubation. Anesth Analg 1992;74:169.

135. Weis FR. Light-wand intubation for cervical spine injuries. Anesth Analg 1992;74:622.

136. Graham DH, Doll WA, Robinson AD, Warriner CB. Intubation with lighted stylet. Can J Anaesth 1991;38:261–262.

137. Rayburn RL. Light wand intubation. Anaesthesia 1979;34:677–678.

138. Culling RD, Mongan P, Castro T. Lightwand guided rapid sequence orotracheal intubation. Anesthesiology 1989;71:A994.

139. Robelen GT, Shulman MS. Use of the lighted stylet for difficult intubation in adult patients. Anesthesiology 1989;71:A438.

140. Holzman RS, Nargozian CD, Florence B. Lightwand intubation in children with abnormal upper airways. Anesthesiology 1988;69:784–787.

141. Fox DJ, Matson MD. Management of the difficult pediatric airway in an austere environment using the lightwand. J Clin Anesth 1990;2:123–125.

142. Knight RG, Castro T, Rastrelli AJ, Maschke S, Scavone JA. Arterial blood pressure and heart rate response to lighted stylet or direct laryngoscopy for endotracheal intubation. Anesthesiology 1988; 69:269–272.

143. Kashin BA, Wynands JE. A comparison of haemodynamic changes during lighted stylet or directed laryngoscopy for endotracheal intubation. Can J Anaesth 1989;36:S72–S73.

144. Verdile VP, Chang JL, Bedger RM, Stewart RD, Kaplan R, Paris PM. Nasotracheal intubation using a flexible lighted stylet. Ann Emerg Med 1988;17:410.

145. Borland LM, Casselbrant M. The Bullard laryngoscope. A new indirect oral laryngoscope (pediatric version). Anesth Analg 1990;70:105–108.

146. Bjoraker DG. The Bullard intubation laryngoscopes. Anesthesiol Rev 1990;17:64–70.

147. Gaughan SD, Benumof JL Ozaki GT. Evaluation of the Bullard laryngoscope with the new intubating stylet. Anesthesiology 1992;77:A512.

148. Gaughan SD. Clinical experiences with the difficult airway using the Bullard laryngoscope. ASA exhibit presentation. San Francisco, October 28, 1991.

149. Gorback MS. Management of the challenging airway with the Bullard larygnoscope. J Clin Anesth 1991;3:473–477.

150. Dyson A, Harris J, Bhatia K. Rapidity and accuracy of tracheal intubation in a mannequin. Comparison of the fibreoptic with the Bullard laryngoscope. Br J Anaesth 1990;65:268–270.

151. Baraka A, Muallem M, Sibai AN, Louis A. Bullard laryngoscopy for tracheal intubation of patients with cervical spine pathology. Can J Anaesth 1992;39:513–514.

152. Shigematsu T, Miyazawa N, Yorozu T. Nasotracheal intubation using Bullard laryngoscope. Can J Anaesth 1991;38:798.

153. Saunders PR, Geisecke AH. Clinical assessment of the adult Bullard laryngoscope. Can J Anaesth 1989;36:S118–S119.

154. Abrams KJ, Desai N, Katsnelson T. Dullard laryngoscopy for trauma airway management in suspected cervical spine injuries. Anesth Analg 1992;74:623.

155. Aromaa U, Pesonen P, Linko K, Tammisto T. Difficulties with tooth protectors in endotracheal intubation. Acta Anaesthesiol Scand 1988;32:304–307.

156. Davis FO, DeFreece AB, Shroff PF. Custom-made plastic guards for tooth protection during endoscopy and orotracheal intubation. Anesth Analg 1971;50:203–206.

157. Evers W, Racz GB, Glazer J, Dobkin AB. Orahesive as a protection for the teeth during general anaesthesia and endoscopy. Can Anaes Soc J 1967;14:123–128.

158. Rosenberg M, Bolgla J. Protection of teeth and gums during endotracheal intubation. Anesth Analg 1968;47:34–36.

159. Beneby G. The use of a transparent mouthguard at induction. Anaesthesia 1989;44:705.

160. Haddy S. Protecting teeth during endotracheal intubation. Anesthesiology 1989;71:810–811.

161. Hohmann JE. Practice gems. Welcome Trends Anesthesiol 1992;10:10.

162. Lisman SR, Shepherd NJ, Rosenberg M. A modified laryngoscope blade for dental protection. Anesthesiology 1981;55:190.

163. Nique TA, Bennett CR, Altop H. Laryngoscope modification to avoid trauma due to laryngoscopy. Anesth Prog 1982;29:47–49.

164. Burton JF, Baker AB. Dental damage during anaesthesia and surgery. Anaesth Intensive Care 1987;15:262–268.

165. Lockhart PB, Feldbau EV, Gabel RA, Connolly SF, Silversin JB. Dental complications during and after tracheal intubation. J Am Dent Assoc 1986;112:480–483.

166. Fry ENS. A lead tooth-bridge. Br J Anaesth 1974;46:543.

167. Sniper W. Filling a gap. Br J Anaesth 1984;56:313–314.

168. Siek GW, Bjorkman LL. Missed pharyngeal foreign body. JAMA 1978;239:722.

169. Clokie C, Metcalf I, Holland A. Dental trauma in anaesthesia. Can J Anaesth 1989;36:675–680.

170. Hawkins DB, Seltzer DC, Barnett TE, Stoneman GB. Endotracheal tube perforation of the hypopharynx. West J Med 1974;120:282–286.

171. Hirsch IA, Reagan JO, Sullivan N. Complications of direct laryngoscopy. Anesthesiol Rev 1990; 17:34–40.

172. Hawkins DB, House JW. Postoperative pneumothorax secondary to hypopharyngeal perforation during anesthetic intubation. Ann Otol 1974; 93:556–557.

173. McGoldrick KE, Donlon JV. Sublingual hematoma following difficult laryngoscopy. Anesth Analg 1979;58:343–344.

174. Roberts J. Fundamentals of tracheal intubation. New York: Grune & Stratton, 1983.

175. Stauffer JL, Petty TL. Accidental intubation of the pyriform sinus. A complication of "roadside" resuscitation. JAMA 1977;237:2324–2325.

176. Wolf AP, Kuhn FA, Ogura JH. Pharyngeal-esophageal perforations associated with rapid oral endotracheal intubation. Ann Otol 1972;81:258–261.

177. Teichner RL. Lingual nerve injury: a complication

of orotracheal intubation. Br J Anaesth 1971; 43:413–414.

178. Jones BC. Lingual nerve injury: a complication of intubation. Br J Anaesth 1971;43:730.

179. Loughman E. Lingual nerve injury following tracheal intubation. Anaesth Intensive Care 1983;11:171.

180. Silva DA, Colingo KA, Miller R. Lingual nerve injury following laryngoscopy. Anesthesiology 1992;76:650–651.

181. Blanc VF, Tremblay NAG. The complications of tracheal intubation. A new classification with a review of the literature. Anesth Analg 1974;53:202–213.

182. Aprahamian C, Thompson B, Finger WA, et al. Experimental cervical spine injury model. Evaluation of airway management and splinting techniques. Ann Emerg Med 1984;13:584–587.

183. Doolan LA, O'Brian JF. Safe intubation in cervical spine injury. Anaesth Intensive Care 1985;13:319–324.

184. Hastings RH, Marks JD. Airway management for trauma patients with potential cervical spine injuries. Anesth Analg 1992;73:471–482.

185. Stout DM, Bishop MJ. Perioperative laryngeal and tracheal complications of intubation. Probl Anesth 1988;2:225–234.

186. Crosby ET. Tracheal intubation in the cervical spine-injured patient. Can J Anaesth 1992; 39:105–109.

187. Grande CM, Barton CR, Stene JK. Appropriate technique for airway management of emergency patients with suspected spinal cord injury. Anesth Analg 1988;67:714–715.

188. Stewart RD, LaRosee A, Stoy A, Heller MB. Use of a lighted stylet to confirm tube placement. Chest 1987;92:900.

189. Suderman VS, Crosby ET, Lui A. Elective oral tracheal intubation in cervical spine-injured adults. Can J Anaesth 1991;38:785–789.

190. Majernick TG, Bieniek R, Houston JB, Hughes HG. Cervical spine movement during orotracheal intubation. Ann Emerg Med 1986;15:417–420.

191. Majernick TG, Bieniek R, Houston JB, Hughes HG. Cervical spine movement during orotracheal intubation. Ann Emerg Med 1986;15:417–420.

192. Hastings RH, Marks JD. Airway management for trauma patients with potential cervical spine injuries. Anesth Analg 1991;73:471–482.

193. Moorthy SS, Dierdorf SF. An unusual difficulty in fiberoptic intubation. Anesthesiology 1985; 63:229.

194. Green CG. Improved technique for fiberoptic intubation. Anesthesiology 1986;64:835.

195. Ovassapian A. Failure to withdraw flexible fiberoptic laryngoscope after nasotracheal intubation. Anesthesiology 1985;63:124–125.

196. MacGillivray RG, Odell JA. Eye to eye with Murphy's Law. Anaesthesia 1986;41:334.

197. Nichols KP, Zornow MH. A potential complication of fiberoptic intubation. Anesthesiology 1989;70:562–563.

198. Schrader S, Ovassapian A, Dykes MH, Avram M. Cardiovascular changes during awake rigid and fiberoptic laryngoscopy. Anesthesiology 1987; 67:A28.

199. Saddler JM, Finfer SR, MacKenzie SIP, Watkins TGL. Fiberoptic technique does not diminish pressor response to intubation. Anesthesiology 1988;69:A144.

200. Schaefer H-G, Marsch SCU. Comparison of orthodox with fibreoptic orotracheal intubation under total IV anaesthesia. Br J Anaesth 1991;66:608–610.

201. Smith JE, Mackenzie AA, Sanghera SS, Scott-Knight VCE. Cardiovascular effects of fiberscope-guided nasotracheal intubation. Anaesthesia 1989;44:907–910.

202. Finfer SR, MacKenzie SIP, Saddler JM, Watkins TGL. Cardiovascular responses to tracheal intubation. A comparison of direct laryngeal and fiberoptic intubation. Anaesth Intensive Care 1989;17:44–48.

203. Smith JE. Heart rate and arterial pressure changes during fibreoptic tracheal intubation under general anaesthesia. Anaesthesia 1988;43:629–632.

204. Smith JE, Mackenzie AA, Scott-Knight VCE. Comparison of two methods of fiberscope-guided tracheal intubation. Br J Anaesth 1991;66:546–550.

205. Hawkyard SJ, Morrison A, Doyle LA, Croton RS, Wake PN. Attenuating the hypertensive response to laryngoscopy and endotracheal intubation using awake fibreoptic intubation. Acta Anaesthesiol Scand 1992;36:1–4.

206. Norris TJ, Baysinger CL. Heart rate and blood pressure response to laryngoscopy. The influence of laryngoscopic technique. Anesthesiology 1985;63:560.

207. Cozanitis DA, Nuuttila K, Merrett JD, Kala R. Influence of laryngoscope design on heart rate and rhythm changes during intubation. Can Anaesth Soc J 1984;31:155–159.

208. Johnson JD, Love JD. Lights out! A preventable complication of endotracheal intubation. Chest 1985;87:701–702.

209. Perel A, Katz E, Davidson JT. Fiberbronchoscopic retrieval of an aspirated laryngoscope bulb. Intensive Care Med 1981;7:143–144.

210. William L, Teague PO, Nagia AH. Foreign body from a Patil-Syracuse mask. Anesth Analg 1991;73:359–360.

211. Waring PH, Vinik HR. A potential complication of the Patil-Syracuse endoscopy mask. Anesth Analg 1991;73:668–669.

212. Zornow MH, Mitchell MM. Foreign body aspiration during fiberoptic–assisted intubation. Anesthesiology 1986;64:303.

213. Toung TJK, Donham RT, Shipley R. Thermal burn caused by a laryngoscope. Anesthesiology 1981;55:184–185.

214. Siegel LC, Garman JK. Too hot to handle. A laryngoscope malfunction. Anesthesiology 1990; 72:1088–1089.

215. Willis MJ, Thomas E. The cold light-source that was hot. Gastrointest Endosc 1984;30:117–118.

216. Anonymous. Bronchoscopes, flexible. Technol Anesth 1986;6:3–4.

217. Daley H, Amoroso P. Dangerous repairs. Anaesthesia 1991;46:997.

218. Desmeules H, Tremblay P. Laryngoscope blade breakage during intubation. Can J Anaesth 1988;35:202–203.

219. Smith MB, Camp P. Broken laryngoscope. Anaesthesia 1989;44:179.

220. Rocco M, Chatwani A, Shupak R. Laryngoscope handle malfunction. Anesthesiology 1986;65:107.

221. Vernon JM. A broken laryngoscope. Anaesthesia 1990;43:697.

222. Anonymous. Flexible fiberoptic endoscopes. ASTM Standard News 1991;19:40–43.

223. Upton LG. Oral and maxillofacial surgical considerations in the difficult airway. In: Norton, ML, Brown ACD, eds. Atlas of the difficult airway. A source book. St. Louis: Mosby Year Book, 1991:129–144.

Chapter 15

Tracheal Tubes

The tracheal tube (also called the endotracheal tube, intratracheal tube, and catheter) is inserted into the trachea and is used to conduct gases and vapors to and from the lungs. An orotracheal tube is designed to be inserted through the mouth, and a nasotracheal tube is designed to be inserted through the nose. Most disposable tracheal tubes are designated "oral/nasal," indicating that they can be inserted either orally or nasally.

General Principles

RESISTANCE AND WORK OF BREATHING

A tracheal tube places a mechanical burden on the spontaneously breathing patient

(1–6). It is the source of more resistance and is a more important factor in determining the work of breathing than the breathing system components (7,8). Work of breathing may be a more relevant parameter than resistance (9). Pressure-support ventilation can be used to compensate for the additional work of breathing during inspiration (3,10,11).

Several factors help to determine the resistance to gas flow imposed by a tracheal tube.

Internal Diameter

The single most important factor is the internal diameter of the tube and its connector. A tube with a thick wall will offer more resistance than a thin-walled tube with the same outer diameter (12,13). The wall thick-

439

ness:tube diameter ratio is greater in small tubes, leading to a relatively higher increase in airway resistance after intubation in children (14). Resistance will be increased if a suction catheter or fiberscope is passed through the tube, because this decreases the size of the lumen (15,16).

To minimize the work of breathing, one should use the widest tracheal tube that will fit the larynx. It should, however, be kept in mind that use of too large a tube can increase laryngeal damage. It is also important to use a thin-walled tube. If the wall is too thin, it may be prone to kinking, which increases resistance. Furthermore, try to use as large a connector as will fit in the tube.

Length

Decreasing tube length lowers its resistance, but the decrease is much less than could be accomplished by increasing the internal diameter (6,12,17). Disposable tubes are usually supplied longer than needed and may be cut to a suitable length to reduce resistance.

Configuration

Abrupt changes in direction and diameter increase resistance (17–19). A RAE tube offers more resistance than a tube with gentler curves (14). Kinking increases resistance.

Curved connectors offer more resistance than straight ones (20). A gently curved connector offers less resistance than a right-angled one. The resistance of swivel connectors is similar to that of curved connectors (21).

Gas Density

Decreasing the density of the gas flowing through the tube (by including helium in the inspired gases) will reduce resistance (6,12,15).

DEAD SPACE

The tracheal tube and connector constitute mechanical dead space, which was discussed in Chapter 5. Because the volume of a tracheal tube and its connector is usually less than that of the natural passages, dead space is normally reduced by intubation. In pediatrics, however, long tubes and connectors may increase the dead space beyond that generally present. Special low-volume pediatric connectors are available.

Tracheal Tubes

MATERIALS OF CONSTRUCTION (22–24)

The material from which a tracheal tube is manufactured should have the following characteristics:

1. Low cost.
2. Lack of tissue toxicity.
3. Transparency.
4. Ease of sterilization and durability with repeated sterilizations (unless disposable).
5. Nonflammability.
6. A slippery, smooth, nonwettable surface inside and outside to prevent secretion buildup, allow easy passage of a suction catheter or bronchoscope, and prevent trauma.
7. Sufficient body to maintain its shape during insertion and prevent occlusion by torsion, kinking, or compression by the cuff or external pressure.
8. Sufficient strength to allow thin wall construction.
9. Thermoplasticity to conform to the patient's anatomy without kinking when in place.
10. Nonreactivity with lubricants and anesthetic agents.

To date no substance has been found that will meet all of the above requirements. This section will describe some of the substances that have been used for tracheal tubes and some of the problems encountered.

For many years, tracheal tubes were made from rubber. Rubber tubes can be cleaned, sterilized, and reused multiple times. However, they harden with age, become sticky, have poor resistance to kinking, become clogged by inspissated secretions more easily than plastic tubes, and do not soften appreciably at body temperature. Their lack of transparency is another disadvantage. Latex allergy is another possible problem (25).

In the late 1960s disposable tubes made from plastics began to appear. At present, polyvinyl chloride (PVC) is the most widely used plastic in disposable tracheal tubes. It is relatively inexpensive and compatible with tissues. Tubes made from PVC have less tendency to kink than rubber tubes. They are stiff enough for intubation at room temperature but soften at body temperature, so that the tubes tend to conform to the anatomy of the patient's upper airway, reducing pressure at points of contact. They present a smooth surface that facilitates passage of a suction catheter or bronchoscope. Their transparency permits observation of the tidal movement of respiratory moisture as well as objects or materials in the lumen.

Silicone is used in the manufacture of some tracheal tubes. Although more expensive than PVC, many products made from it can be sterilized and reused.

Some materials used in the manufacture of tracheal tubes in the past have shown evidence of tissue toxicity. To meet the ASTM (24) standard, materials must pass a USP implantation test in which the material to be tested is implanted in the paravertebral muscle of a rabbit. Tissue reaction is then compared with a control. Other test methods, including cell cultures, may be used, provided they yield equivalent results. The marking *F-29* or *I.T.* on a tube is proof that the tube material has been tested and no evidence of toxicity was found.

TUBE DESIGN (22)

An ASTM (24) standard contains requirements and recommendations for tracheal tubes, including the material from which the tube is constructed, the inside diameter, length, inflation system, cuff, radius of curvature, markings, Murphy eye, packaging, and labeling.

A typical tracheal tube is shown in Figure 15.1. The ASTM (24) standard specifies a ra-

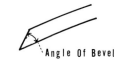

Angle Of Bevel

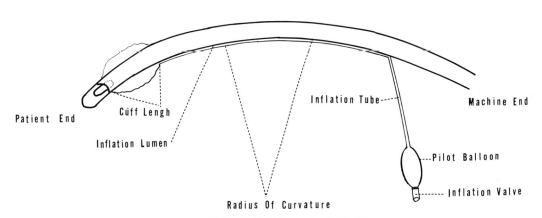

Patient End

Cuff Lengh

Inflation Lumen

Inflation Tube

Machine End

Pilot Balloon

Inflation Valve

Radius Of Curvature

Figure 15.1. Cuffed Murphy tracheal tube.

dius of curvature from 12 to 16 cm. In cross-section, the tube's internal and external walls should be circular. A tube whose lumen is oval or elliptical in shape is more prone to kinking than one that is round.

The machine (proximal) end receives the connector and projects from the patient. It should be possible (and is often necessary when received from the manufacturer) to shorten this end to adjust the tube length. The patient (tracheal or distal) end is inserted into the trachea. It usually has a slanted portion called the bevel. The angle of the bevel is the acute angle between the bevel and the longitudinal axis of the tracheal tube. The tracheal tube standard specifies a bevel angle of 38 ± 8 degrees (24). The opening of the bevel faces left when viewing the tube from its concave aspect. This is because most often the tube is introduced from the right. Having the bevel facing left facilitates visualization of the larynx as the tube is being inserted.

The tip should be rounded with no sharp points or edges. Figure 15.1 shows a hole through the tube wall on the side opposite to the bevel. This is known as a Murphy eye, and a tube with this eye is called a Murphy or Murphy-type tube (26). The purpose of the eye is to provide an alternate pathway for gas flow if the bevel is occluded (27). Some authors think that the hole is a disadvantage, because secretions tend to accumulate there (28). The tracheal tube standard specifies that the area of a Murphy eye must not be less than 80% of the cross-sectional area of the tube lumen. Forceps, tube changers, and fiberscopes have been inadvertently advanced through a Murphy eye (29–32). Some tubes have a second eye on the bevel side. This may provide a measure of safety should the tube be accidentally advanced into the right main-stem bronchus. Tracheal tubes lacking the Murphy eye are known as Magill or Magill-type tubes (Fig. 15.2A). Absence of a Murphy eye allows the cuff to be placed close to the tip. This may decrease the chances of inadvertent bronchial intubation and may reduce injury to the trachea (33).

Frequently, a radiopaque marker is placed at the tip or along the entire length of the tube to aid in determination of tube position after intubation. A barium sulfate stripe significantly lowers the temperature at which ignition of the tube occurs and thus increases the risk of fire (34).

SPECIAL TUBES

There are many tubes available. Most are familiar to the majority of anesthesiologists and do not require any special descriptions. A few have particular characteristics or purposes that deserve mention.

Cole Tube (35)

The Cole tube is shown in Figure 15.3. It was designed for pediatric patients. The patient end is smaller in diameter than the rest of the tube. Cole tubes are sized according to the internal diameter of the tracheal portion.

The shoulder, the portion at which the transition from the oral portion to the laryngo-tracheal portion occurs, provides some protection against inadvertent bronchial intubation. The tube should not, however, be inserted so far that the widened portion contacts the larynx, because this will result in pressure on, and possibly dilatation of, the larynx (36).

Some studies have found that the resistance offered by the Cole tube is less than that of comparable tubes of constant lumen (20, 37). Others have found that resistance is higher with Cole tubes (19). The wide bore section increases dead space slightly, but this is believed to be insignificant (37).

A disadvantage of this tube is that it cannot be used nasally because the larger segment will not pass through an infant's nares.

RAE Preformed Tracheal Tube (38,39)

RAE tracheal tubes are plastic tubes that are longer than most other tubes (Fig. 15.4). Nasal and oral versions are available. There is a preformed bend in the tube that may be temporarily straightened to allow passage of a suction catheter.

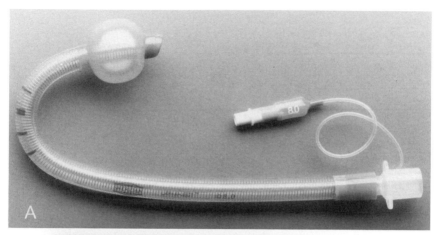

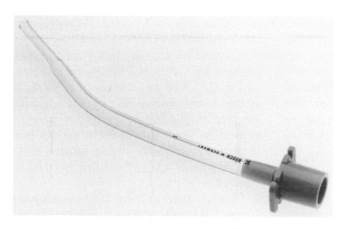

Figure 15.2. Laryngectomy tubes. **A,** This spiral-wound steel wire tube has a short Magill-type tip. Courtesy of Sheridan Catheter Corp. **B,** Another version with a Murphy eye. Courtesy of Mallinckrodt Anesthesia Division, Mallinckrodt Medical, Inc.

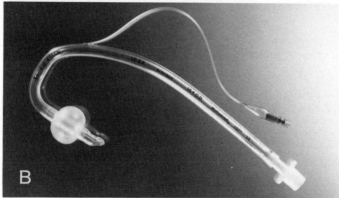

Figure 15.3. Cole tracheal tube. These tubes are sized according to the intratracheal portion. Note that the tube's size is designated by the French scale. Courtesy of Rusch, Inc.

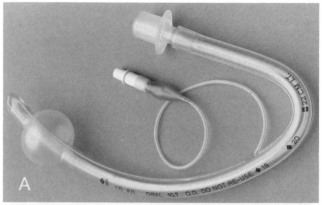

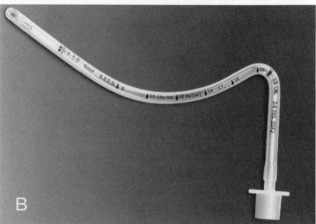

Figure 15.4. RAE tubes. Note the rectangular mark at the center of the sharp bend on each tube. **A**, Oral tube. The one shown is the adult version fitted with a low-pressure cuff. The rectangular mark should be placed at the teeth. **B**, Nasal tube. The one shown is the uncuffed version with two ports at the tip, one on the bevel side and one on the opposite side. Note that both the internal and external diameters are marked. Courtesy of Mallinckrodt Anesthesia Division, Mallinckrodt Medical, Inc.

Cuffed and uncuffed versions are available. Uncuffed versions have two ports near the tip. These tubes come in various sizes. As the diameter increases, the length and distance from the distal tip to the curve also increases. Each tube has a rectangular mark at the center of the bend. The distance from this mark to the distal tip is printed on each tube. In the majority of cases when this mark is at the teeth or naris, the cuff will be satisfactorily positioned in the trachea, if the proper diameter tube for the patient was selected. This is only a guide and should not be used as the sole criterion for judging correct positioning of the tube.

The nasal RAE has a curve opposite to the curvature of the oral tube, so that when in place the outer portion of the tube is directed over the patient's forehead. This helps to reduce pressure on the nares. This tube may be useful for oral intubation of patients who are to be in the prone position (40).

The oral RAE tubes are shorter than the nasal ones. The external portion is bent at an acute angle toward the concavity of curvature of the tube, so that when in place it rests on the patient's chin.

These tubes are easy to secure and their use may reduce the risk of unintended extubation (14). The curve allows the breathing system connection to be placed away from the surgical field during operations in the region of the head without use of special connectors and helps to protect against kinks that may occur when other tubes are used for these applications.

Disadvantages of RAE tubes include the fact that it is difficult to pass a suction catheter down them. RAE tubes offer more resistance than comparably sized conventional tubes (14,41). Since they are designed to fit the average patient, a tube may be either too long or too short for a given patient (42,43). When selecting tube size, reference to height and weight may be more useful than age in years, and the user should always be alert to the possibility of bronchial intubation or accidental extubation (44).

Spiral Embedded Tubes

The spiral embedded tube is also called the flexometallic, armored, reinforced, anode, metal spiral, and woven tube. These tubes have a metal or nylon spiral-wound reinforcing wire covered both internally and externally by rubber, latex, PVC, or silicone (Fig. 15.5; see also Fig. 15.2A). The spiral

does not extend into the distal and proximal ends. A forceps and/or a stylet will often be needed for intubation.

Spiral embedded tubes are especially useful in situations in which bending or compression of the tube is likely to occur, as in neurosurgery and head and neck surgery. Another use is in surgery on the trachea. A sterile spiral embedded tube can be placed in the trachea by the surgeon.

The primary advantage of these tubes is resistance to kinking and compression (45). The portion of the tube outside the patient can be easily angled away from the surgical field without causing kinking (46). This may make them useful in patients with tracheostomies. In one study, use of a spiral embedded silicone tube resulted in less pressure on the larynx than any other type of tube tested

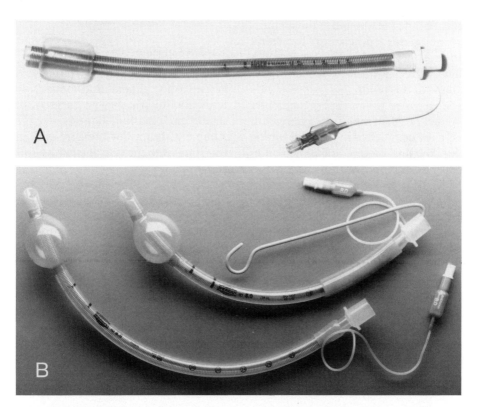

Figure 15.5.   Spiral embedded tracheal tubes. **A**, This disposable tube is fitted with a high-volume, low-pressure cuff. Courtesy of Rusch, Inc. **B**, These tubes have a reinforcing covering over the bite area. Note the marks near the patient end of the tubes to aid in positioning with respect to the vocal cords. Courtesy of Sheridan Catheter Corp.

(47). A spiral embedded tube may pass more easily over a fiberscope than a tube with a preformed curve (48).

There are a number of problems with spiral embedded tubes. The tube may rotate on the stylet during insertion. Insertion through the nose is difficult and sometimes impossible. Because of the spiral, these tubes cannot be shortened. Secure fixation is more difficult than with other tubes.

There are numerous reports of respiratory obstruction with spiral embedded tubes (49–66). Most have been with tubes that have been resterilized. For this reason, it is recommended that these tubes not be reused.

Cases have been reported in which patients bit the tube, causing it to be permanently deformed and resulting in obstruction (67–72). Some spiral embedded tubes have an external covering over the bite area (see Fig. 15.5B). On some older tubes, kinking could occur at the patient end if the connector were not pushed down into the spiral (51). On most newer tubes the connector is permanently sealed against the spirals to prevent kinking at this point.

Cuff deflation occurs relatively frequently (65). Another problem is failure of the cuff to deflate as a result of debris in the pilot tubing or double layering of the cuff (73,65). On some older tubes, the inflation tube passes outside distal to the point where the spiral ends. If the connector is pushed into the spiral to prevent kinking, it may pinch off the inflation tube so that the cuff can be neither inflated nor deflated, although the pilot balloon will inflate and deflate (59,74,75). This problem can be avoided by making a small notch in the connector at the point where the inflation tube passes outside (76). On most newer tubes, the inflation tube is attached outside the wall of the tube or the connector is permanently sealed against the coils to prevent this problem.

Carden Bronchoscopy Tube

The Carden bronchoscopy tube (Fig. 15.6) is specially designed for fiberoptic bronchoscopy. The machine end is wider than the patient end. The tube is sized by the internal diameter at the patient end. The larger diameter of the machine end decreases the increase in resistance caused by passage of the bronchoscope. The tube is made of silastic and can be sterilized and reused. A swivel adapter with a port for a bronchoscope is supplied with each tube.

Carden Laryngoscopy Tube (77,78)

The Carden laryngoscopy tube (Fig. 15.7) is used when general anesthesia is administered for microlaryngeal surgery. It is less than 7 cm long. It is manufactured from silicone and has a low-pressure cuff and a jet tube built into the side. It can be sterilized for reuse.

This tube is difficult to insert below the vocal cords. Various methods have been described (77–82). After insertion, the cuff is inflated to hold it in position. Intermittently jetting gases into the tube causes intermittent

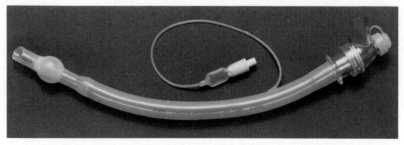

Figure 15.6.   Carden bronchoscopy tube. The larger diameter of the part of tube that lies outside the larynx and trachea reduces resistance to gas flow. Courtesy of Xomed-Trease.

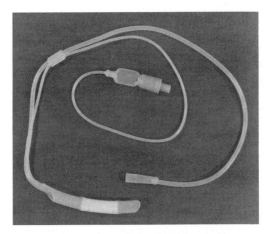

Figure 15.7. Carden laryngoscopy tube.

inflation of the patient's lungs. During the noninflation phases, the patient can passively exhale through the tube and the cords. To remove the tube, the cuff is first deflated, and then the jet is activated. This causes the tube to be blown from the trachea (83).

Use of this tube with a jetting device usually results in a good operating field for the surgeon. The gas passing out through the cords during both inflation and exhalation tends to blow blood and debris out of the operating area and away from the lungs. Work below the level of the cords can be performed by placing the tube below the lesion in the trachea (78). Because the jet is mounted in the tube, there is little or no Venturi effect (78).

Problems include accidental dislodgement, cephalad movement, and difficulty with removal (84). Respiratory obstruction can occur before the surgeon places the scope and maintains a clear airway or if the cords are allowed to close (82,85). Obstruction will prevent gas from exiting the lung and can result in high pressures in the lower airway.

Injectoflex

The injectoflex also is used for laryngeal microsurgery (Fig. 15.8). It is a short-cuffed silicone tube designed to be placed below the vocal cords. The tube has an embedded wire spiral to prevent kinking and compression. The cuff inflation lumen and the gas jet lumen are integrally joined in a sheath with a

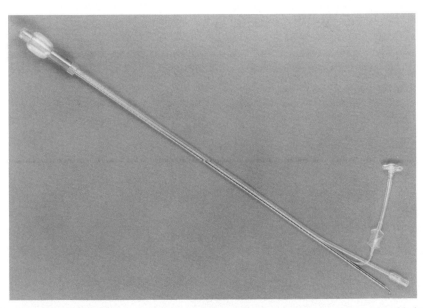

Figure 15.8. Injectoflex tube, which is used for procedures on the larynx. The tube has an embedded metal spiral and low-pressure cuff. The insufflation lumen and cuff inflation tube are combined in one sheath with the malleable introducer. Courtesy of Rusch, Inc.

malleable introducer. The introducer remains in place during the procedure.

Microlaryngeal Tracheal Surgery Tube

The microlaryngeal tracheal surgery tube (also called LTS or MLT tracheal tube) is available with an ID of 4, 5, or 6 mm, each of which has the same length and cuff diameter as a standard 8-mm-ID tube (Fig. 15.9). One version has a yellow-colored cuff.

This tube is designed for microlaryngeal tracheal surgery or for patients whose airway has been narrowed to such an extent that a normal-size tracheal tube cannot be inserted. The small diameter provides better visibility and access to the surgical field. Problems with a tube having such a small bore include the dangers of incomplete exhalation and occlusion. These tubes are not safe for use with lasers.

Laryngectomy Tube (86)

Laryngectomy tubes are designed for insertion into a tracheostomy site. The tube is preformed in a *J* configuration (see Fig. 15.2*A*). This allows the part of the tube external to the patient to be directed away from the surgical field. The tip may be short and/ or without a bevel to avoid inadvertent advancement into a bronchus.

The curve may need to be straightened to facilitate insertion. The tube can be secured by suturing during intraoperative tracheostomies or by taping to the chest wall in patients with preexisting tracheostomies (86).

Endotrol Tracheal Tube

The endotrol tracheal tube is disposable (Fig. 15.10) and provides a means to control the direction of the tip via a ring loop. Pulling on the ring decreases the radius of distal end of the tube via a cable-like mechanism so that the tip moves anteriorly. This may make the tube useful during certain difficult intubations (87).

In one reported case, obstruction to gas flow was noted after the tube had been inserted nasally (88). The pull ring was exerting tension on the pull wire, causing the tip of the tube to abut against the tracheal wall. Cutting the pull ring alleviated the tension and the airway obstruction.

Tubes with Monitoring Lumen(s)

Tubes are available with one or more separate lumens terminating near the tip. Two are shown in Figure 15.11. They are useful for respiratory gas sampling, pressure monitoring, and injection of fluids and drugs.

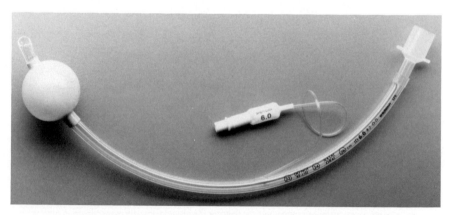

Figure 15.9. Tube for microlaryngeal tracheal surgery. The small diameter tube allows greater access to the surgical field. The cuff on this tube is colored yellow for greater visibility. Courtesy of Sheridan Catheter Corp.

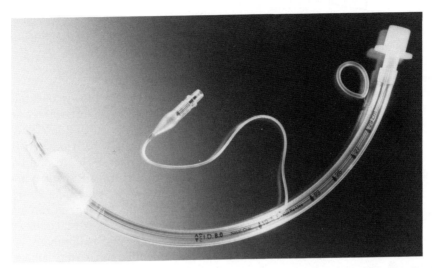

Figure 15.10.   Endotrol tracheal tube. The ring is attached to the tip by a cable-like mechanism that allows the tip to be maneuvered. Courtesy of Mallinckrodt Anesthesiology Division, Mallinckrodt Medical, Inc.

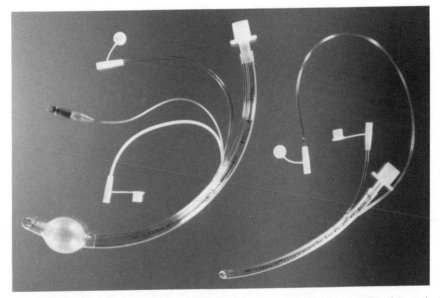

Figure 15.11.   Tubes with monitoring lumen(s). These tubes have a main lumen for ventilation of the patient and one or more additional lumens for monitoring or irrigation. On the adult version, the clear lumen is used for jet ventilation and administration of oxygen during suctioning and bronchoscopy. The opaque lumen can be used for irrigation and sampling of gases from the trachea. This type of tube has been used for high-frequency ventilation. Courtesy of Mallinckrodt Anesthesiology Division, Mallinckrodt Medical, Inc.

In patients weighing less than 8 kg, gas aspirated from the lumen of such a tube may provide end-tidal concentrations that correlate better with arterial concentrations than samples taken farther from the patient (89).

A number of problems are associated with these tubes (90). Good stabilization of the sampling tube is necessary to minimize tension on the tube and avoid kinking or accidental extubation. The port of the monitoring lumen can easily become obstructed by mucus, blood, etc. Many tubes with a monitoring lumen do not have a Murphy eye, and this may increase the risk of obstruction.

Laser-Shield II Tracheal Tube

The Laser-Shield II (Fig. 15.12) is the successor to the Laser-Shield tube, which is no longer manufactured. It is designed for use with CO_2 and KTP lasers. This tube is made from silicone with an overlapping spiral aluminum wrap and a smooth Teflon outer wrap. There is 1 cm of unprotected silicone tubing proximal to the cuff. The part of the tube distal to the cuff also is unprotected. The cuff contains methylene blue crystals. Cottonoids for wrapping around the cuff are supplied with each tube. These must be moistened and kept moist during the entire procedure.

Studies have shown that the wrapped portion of the shaft is not penetrated by a CO_2 or Nd-YAG laser, but the overlying Teflon may be vaporized (91,92). Exposure of the unprotected parts of the tube proximal and distal to the cuff can result in rapid combustion. Blood on the outside of the tube does not affect the protection from combustion with the CO_2 laser (93).

Laser-Flex Tracheal Tube

The Laser-Flex tube is a flexible stainless-steel tube with a smooth surface designed for use with CO_2 and KTP lasers (Fig. 15.13). The wall of the tube is thicker than that of most other tubes (94). The adult version has two PVC cuffs and a PVC tip with a Murphy eye. The two cuffs are inflated by two separate inflation tubes, which run along the inside of the tube. The distal cuff can be used if the proximal one is damaged by the laser. Small uncuffed tubes are available.

The cuffs should be filled with saline. The distal cuff should be filled first until sealing occurs, then the proximal cuff is filled with saline colored with methylene blue (95).

Studies show that the shaft holds up well when exposed to a CO_2 or KTP laser but not the Nd-YAG laser (94,96–100). Blood on the outside of the tube renders it less resistant to combustion with the CO_2 laser (93). The cuff and distal tip are vulnerable to all lasers.

In a study of damage from reflected CO_2 laser beams from laser-resistant and foil-wrapped tubes, it was found that the danger was least with this tube (101).

Reported problems with the Laser-Flex tube include stiffness and roughness (100). It

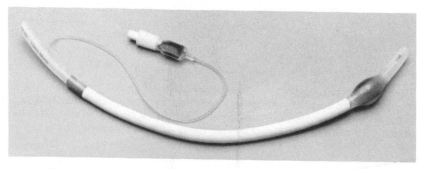

Figure 15.12.   Laser-shield II tracheal tube. Courtesy of Xomed-Trease.

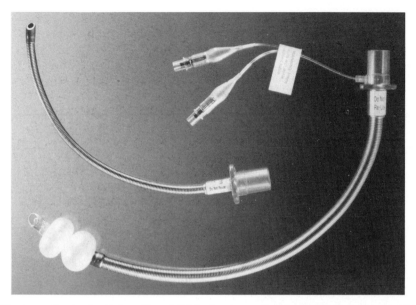

Figure 15.13.   Laser-flex tracheal tubes. The adult tube has two cuffs. The distal cuff can be used if the proximal one is damaged. Courtesy of Mallinckrodt Anesthesiology Division, Mallinckrodt Medical, Inc.

cannot be trimmed, but it can be bent and will hold its shape. The double cuff adds to the time of intubation and extubation. The large external diameter can be a problem in small patients (94). In one reported case, great difficulty was experienced in removing the cuffed tube because of a subglottic mass (102).

Sheridan YAG Tracheal Tube

The Sheridan YAG tracheal tube is a clear PVC tube with a Murphy eye designed for use with the Nd-YAG laser. The tube itself has no markings; tube size is indicated on the pilot balloon. One study found that this tube ignited under typical clinical conditions (100). Another study found that the tube itself was resistant to the Nd-YAG laser, but it was ignited when drops of blood or saline or mucus were applied to the outside of the tube (103).

Norton Tube (104)

The Norton tube is a reusable, flexible, spiral-wound metal tube with a stainless-steel connector designed for laser surgery. It has thick walls. The exterior of the tube has a matt finish to decrease reflection of the laser beam. The finish is obtained by creating microscopic pits from which the laser beam is deflected in all directions. It has no cuff. However, a separate cuff may be placed over the distal tip or packing can be used to achieve a seal. Studies show this tube is acceptable for use with KTP, Nd-YAG, and, CO_2 lasers (100).

There are a number of problems with the Norton tube. Its flexible coils are not airtight and angulation can result in a large leak (105). The tube's exterior is somewhat rough and may have sharp edges that could cause tissue damage (106). The large external diameter and stiffness may make surgical exposure and positioning of an operating laryngoscope difficult (107). The tube tends to twist on the stylet during intubation (100). It requires special ventilating techniques when it is used cuffless. If it is used with a separate cuff, the cuff and its inflating tube can be ignited and may or may not remain attached to the tube.

Bivona Fome-Cuf Laser Tube

The Bivona Fome-Cuf laser tube has an aluminum and silicone spiral with a silicone covering (Fig. 15.14). It is marketed for use with the CO_2 laser. It has a self-inflating cuff that consists of a polyurethane foam sponge with a silicone envelope. The cuff must be deflated before intubation or extubation (108). The cuff should be filled with saline during use. The cuff retains its shape and keeps a seal when it is punctured (100). The inflation tube runs along the exterior of the tube and is colored black so that it can be positioned away from areas where the laser will be used.

Studies show that a fire can result when the CO_2 laser operating at high power is applied to this tube (97). Damage also occurs when it is exposed to a Nd-YAG or KTP laser (96,98,100). When burned, the silicone covering forms an ash that sloughs off and is left in the trachea, but most of the tube stays intact (100).

A high incidence of sore throats has been noted with this cuff (109). If the inflation tube is severed or the cuff punctured, the cuff cannot be deflated.

Combitube

The Combitube is a double-lumen tube designed to provide a patent airway during difficult and emergency intubation (Fig. 15.15). It has two cuffs. The large pharyngeal cuff is inflated with 100 ml of air. The distal cuff requires only 15 ml. There are eight ventilating eyes between the cuffs.

Blind placement of the tube usually results in esophageal placement (Fig. 15.16). In this case, the anesthesia breathing system is connected to the No. 1 lumen. Air is blocked from entering the stomach by the distal cuff and from escaping out through the mouth and nose, so it goes into the trachea. Should the tube enter the trachea, the breathing system is moved to the No. 2 extension, and the tube is used as a standard tracheal tube.

TUBE SIZE

Three methods have been used for sizing tracheal tubes. The oldest is the Magill scale by which tubes went from size 0 (infant) to 10 (large adult). The French scale, which multiplied the external diameter, in millimeters, by 3, was commonly used for many years. Current standards designate tracheal tube

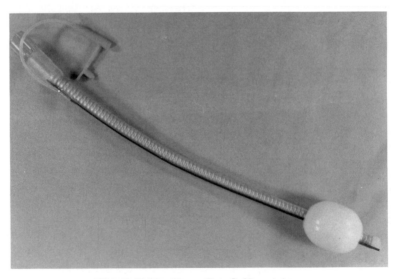

Figure 15.14.   Bivona Fom-Cuf laser tube.

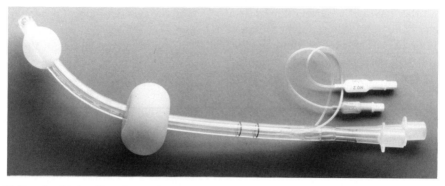

Figure 15.15. Combitube. Note the ventilating eyes between the two cuffs. Courtesy of Sheridan Catheter Corp.

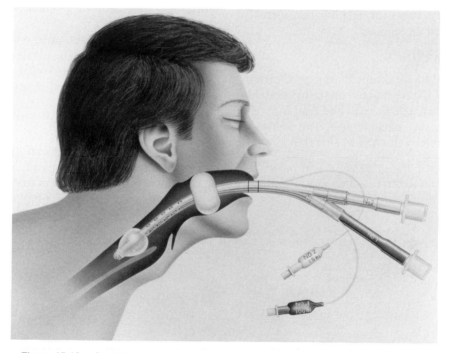

Figure 15.16. Combitube in place in the esophagus. Courtesy of Sheridan Catheter Corp.

size by the internal diameter in millimeters (24). The French scale size may still be listed in catalogs and on packages for those not accustomed to using the internal diameter and is still used on some tubes (see Fig. 15.3).

The ASTM (24) standard requires tube size to be indicated between the cuff and the take-off point for the inflation tube for cuffed tubes (see Fig. 15.4A). For uncuffed tubes, the size marking should be toward the patient end (see Fig. 15.3). Some manufacturers also put the tube size on the pilot balloon so the size can be determined when the tube is in the patient. Because of variations in wall thickness, tubes having the same internal diameter may have quite different external diameters (110,111). The outside diameter is important, especially in children, because this is what must pass through the larynx. Accordingly, the tracheal tube standard specifies that tubes size 6.0 and smaller show the external diameter in millimeters (see Figs. 15.3*B* and 15.8). Many manufacturers also mark this on larger tubes (see Fig. 15.3*A*).

TUBE LENGTH

The ASTM (24) standard specifies the minimum tube length, which increases as internal diameter increases. Most manufacturers supply tubes in lengths considerably longer than the standard.

TUBE MARKINGS

Typical tracheal tube markings, shown in Figure 15.5*B*, are situated on the beveled side of the tube above the cuff and read from the patient to the machine end. The following are required by the ASTM (24) standard:

1. The word *oral* or *nasal* or *oral/nasal.*
2. Tube size in internal diameter (ID) in millimeters.

3. The outside diameter (OD) for size 6 and smaller.
4. The name or trademark of the manufacturer or supplier.
5. The notation *F-29* or *Z-79* or *IT,* which indicates that the tube has passed the tissue toxicity test.
6. Length (depth) markings in centimeters measured from the patient end.
7. A cautionary note such as "Do not reuse" or "Single use only," if the tube is disposable.
8. A radiopaque marker at the patient end or along the full length.

Other markings not in conflict with the above may be applied.

Many tubes have black lines or rings to help position the tube with respect to the vocal cords (Fig. 15.17; see also Fig. 15.5*B*). The distal portion of some pediatric tubes are colored to aid in positioning.

CUFF SYSTEMS

A cuff system includes the cuff itself plus an inflation system, which typically includes an inflation lumen in the wall of the tube, an external inflation tube, a pilot balloon, and

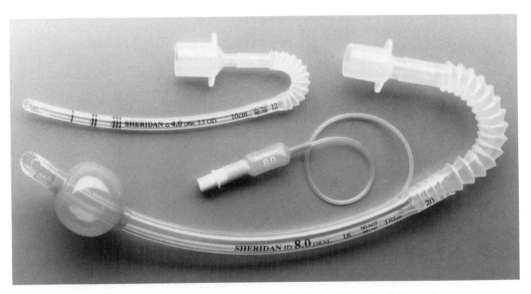

Figure 15.17. Tubes with flexible connectors. Courtesy of Sheridan Catheter Corp.

an inflation valve (see Fig. 15.1). The purpose of the cuff system is to provide a seal between the tube and the tracheal wall to prevent aspiration of pharyngeal contents into the trachea and ensure that no gas leaks past the cuff during positive pressure ventilation. The cuff also serves to center the tube in the trachea so that its tip is less likely to traumatize the mucosa.

Cuff

The cuff is an inflatable sleeve near the patient end of the tracheal tube. The cuff material should be strong and tear resistant but thin, soft, and pliable. Cuffs are usually made of the same material as the tracheal tube. Cuff materials are subject to the same tissue-testing requirements as the tube itself.

The ASTM (24) standard specifies the maximum distance from the tip of the tube to the machine end of the cuff. This varies with tube size. If the distance from the machine end of the cuff to the tip of the tube were too great, the tip of the tube could rest on the carina while the cuff impinged on the vocal cords. The standard (24) also requires that the bonded edge of the cuff not encroach on the Murphy eye, if present. Other requirements are that the cuff must not herniate over the tube tip under normal conditions of use and must inflate symmetrically.

Cuff Pressures

Intracuff Pressure and Pressure on the Tracheal Wall. Many of the complications associated with tracheal tubes are the result of excessive pressure exerted on the tracheal wall by the cuff. It is desirable that the cuff seal the airway without exerting so much pressure on the trachea that its circulation is compromised or the trachea is dilated. A high cuff pressure prevents aspiration and ventilatory leaks and prevents eccentric positioning of the tube in the trachea, but it can result in tracheal damage secondary to ischemia. A low cuff pressure minimizes tracheal damage secondary to ischemia and can act to relieve excessive airway pressure, but it may result in aspiration, leaks, and eccentric positioning of the tube in the trachea.

Most authors recommend that the pressure on the lateral tracheal wall measured at end expiration be kept between 25 and 34 cm H_2O (112,113). Studies show impaired tracheal blood flow at 30 cm H_2O (114). If the pressure exceeds 25 cm H_2O, aspiration should not occur, provided the density of the material above the cuff is similar to that of water (112,115).

Intracuff Pressure and Use of Nitrous Oxide. Studies show that the resting intracuff pressure and volume of a cuff inflated with air rise during nitrous oxide anesthesia (109,116–124). The increase in pressure varies directly with the partial pressure of the nitrous oxide and time, and inversely with cuff thickness. The increase in pressure may result in ischemia of the tracheal mucosa or compression of the tube, and the increase in volume may lead to cuff herniation. Several methods have been suggested to modify or avoid this increase (125).

1. Filling the cuff with the gas mixture to be used for anesthesia (120,121,124–128). This is somewhat awkward to perform. A cuff that is at just the correct volume will lose volume and may allow a leak of gas when nitrous oxide administration is discontinued or during extracorporeal circulation (129–130,131).
2. Filling the cuff with saline (132,133).
3. Fitting the cuff system with a pressure relief valve or pressure-regulating device (see below).
4. Use of special systems. Special cuff systems are incorporated in the Brandt tube (134), a tube with a Lanz Pressure-Regulating Valve (135), and a tube with a sponge cuff (118). All three are discussed below.
5. Monitoring cuff pressure and inflating or deflating the cuff as needed (116,124,130).

Low-Volume, High-Pressure Cuff

The low-volume, high-pressure cuff is referred to by a number of terms: small resting diameter cuff, low residual volume cuff, low-volume cuff, small cuff, standard or conventional cuff, and low-compliance, high-pressure cuff.

Characteristics. A high-pressure cuff has a small diameter at rest and a low residual volume (the amount of air that can be withdrawn from the cuff after it has been allowed to assume its normal shape) in the natural intratracheal position, with the inflation tube exposed to atmospheric pressure (136). It requires a high intracuff pressure to achieve a seal with the trachea. It has a small area of contact with the trachea and distends and deforms the trachea to a circular shape (Fig. 15.18).

Intracuff Pressure and Pressure on the Tracheal Wall. With a high-pressure cuff most of the pressure inside the cuff is used to overcome cuff wall compliance so that the pressure exerted laterally on the tracheal wall will be less than the intracuff pressure. The intracuff pressure does not change when the tracheal wall is contacted and does not bear a consistent relationship to the tracheal wall pressure.

The pressure of the tracheal wall exerted by such a cuff is difficult to ascertain but will

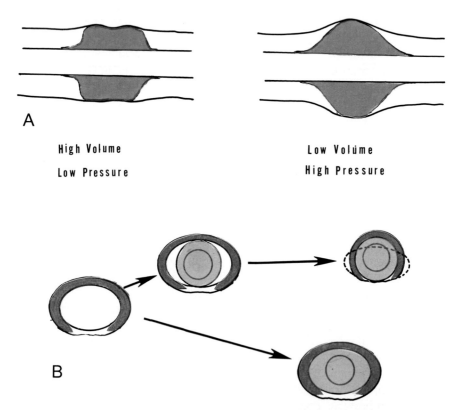

Figure 15.18. Relation of different types of cuffs to the trachea. **A,** side view. *Left,* The high-volume, low-pressure cuff has a large area of contact with the trachea. The cuff adapts itself to the irregular tracheal wall. *Right,* The low-volume, high-pressure cuff has a small area of contact with the trachea. It distends the trachea and distorts it to a circular shape. **B,** Cross-sectional view. At the *left* is the normal trachea. At the *top,* the low-volume, high-pressure cuff distorts the trachea and makes the tracheal contour the same as the shape of the cuff. At the *bottom,* the soft high-volume, low-pressure cuff conforms to the normal tracheal lumen.

be well above mucosal perfusion pressure (112,137,138). Ischemic damage to the tracheal mucosa can be expected to result from its prolonged use.

With this type of cuff, intracuff pressure and the lateral pressure on the tracheal wall increase sharply as increments of air are added to the cuff (139). For this reason, use of the largest intratracheal tube possible has been advocated, so the cuff will be minimally inflated when a seal is created (139).

Evaluation. These cuffs offer some advantages over low-pressure cuffs. Because they can usually be reused, they are less expensive. They offer better protection against aspiration and better visibility during intubation than low-pressure cuffs. Several investigators have reported a lower incidence of sore throat with their use than with use of high-volume, low-pressure cuffs (109,140–142).

The most serious risk associated with high-pressure cuffs is ischemic damage to the trachea following prolonged use. Therefore, these cuffs should not be used for long-term intubation. The question of whether they should be used for short periods of general anesthesia is more controversial. The authors of this text feel that at the present time there is no convincing evidence that high-pressure cuffs are less desirable than low-pressure cuffs for short-term intraoperative procedures. However, if a tube with a high-pressure cuff is used intraoperatively and for some reason the tube must be left in place following surgery or if the surgery is expected to last more than a few hours, it should be replaced with a tube with a low-pressure cuff.

High-Volume, Low-Pressure Cuff

High-volume, low-pressure cuffs also are called large resting diameter cuffs; large residual volume cuffs; large cuffs; high-volume cuffs; high-compliance, low-pressure cuffs; floppy cuffs; and low-pressure cuffs.

Characteristics. A high-volume, low-pressure cuff has a large resting volume and diameter, and a thin compliant wall that en-

ables a seal with the trachea to be achieved without stretching of its wall. This type of cuff is floppy and easily deformed. As it is inflated, it first touches the trachea at its narrowest point at that level. As cuff inflation continues, the area of contact becomes larger and the cuff adapts itself to the irregular tracheal surface (139) (see Fig. 15.18). If cuff inflation is continued, the areas in contact will be subject to increasing pressure, and the trachea will be distorted to a circular cross-section, similar to a high-pressure cuff (143).

Different shapes have been used for the low-pressure cuff (144,145). A cuff with a short tracheal contact area may have fewer folds and wrinkles when inflated and may be associated with a lower incidence of postoperative sore throat (146). When high airway pressures must be used, such a cuff requires higher intracuff pressures than a cuff with a larger volume, which provides a greater reservoir of gas within the cuff, allowing additional gas to be "milked" into the proximal end of the cuff without increasing the resting cuff pressure (144).

Intracuff Pressure and Pressure on the Tracheal Wall. A significant advantage of these cuffs is that provided the cuff wall is not stretched the intracuff pressure closely approximates that on the wall of the trachea (147–150). Thus with this type of cuff it is possible to measure and regulate the pressure exerted by the cuff on the tracheal mucosa.

The intracuff pressure varies during the ventilatory cycle (143,144). During spontaneous breathing, airway (and cuff) pressure will be negative during inspiration and positive during exhalation (143). If the cuff is located above the thoracic inlet, the intracuff pressure may rise during inspiration (18). With controlled ventilation, when airway pressure exceeds intracuff pressure, a positive pressure will be applied to the lower face of the cuff. If the cuff wall is pliable, it will be unable to resist this pressure and will be deformed into a cone shape as the distal portion is compressed and the proximal portion is distended (144). The air in the cuff will be compressed until intracuff pressure equals airway pressure. During exhalation, the intracuff pressure will decrease until its resting pressure is reached. By increasing its intracuff pressure the cuff automatically compensates for the increase in airway pressure without additional inflation (self-sealing action). A leak will develop if the diameter of the expanded trachea becomes greater than the diameter of the proximal end of the cuff. At that point, more gas must be added to the cuff to abolish the leak. Unfortunately, this additional cuff inflation will elevate the baseline cuff inflation pressure.

It is desirable that cuff circumference at residual volume be at least equal to the circumference of the trachea (125,148,151). If the cuff is smaller, it must be stretched beyond its residual volume to create a seal. At this point it will act like a high-pressure cuff (144). On the other hand, if the residual diameter of the cuff is much greater than the diameter of the trachea, cuff infolding may occur, with the possibility of aspiration along the folds.

Evaluation. The main advantage of high-volume, low-pressure cuffs is that the frequency of significant cuff-induced complications following prolonged intubation is reduced with their use (145,152,153). However, tracheal injury can occur even when these cuffs are used properly (154,155). During hypotension the mucosal contact pressure that will produce ischemia is reduced (156). A tendency toward tracheal dilatation has been reported (157).

Tubes with these cuffs may be more difficult to insert, as the cuff may obscure the view of the tube tip and larynx so that trauma to the airway may be more common (158,159). The cuff is more friable and thus more likely to be torn during intubation, especially if forceps are used (160).

The incidence of sore throat has been found to be greater than with high-pressure cuffs, unless the cuff is specially designed so that the tracheal contact area is small (109,140–142,146). Severe postextubation stridor has been reported with their use (159).

Aspiration past low-pressure cuffs has been reported (112,161–164). This may be caused by folds or wrinkles in an oversize cuff. Another cause is spontaneous respiration. The dilatation of the trachea and negative pressure applied to the cuff during inspiration may allow passage of fluids around the cuff.

It is relatively easy to pass devices such as esophageal stethoscopes, temperature probes, and nasoenteric tubes around low-pressure cuffs (165–171).

There may be a greater likelihood of dislodgement (including extubation) with these cuffs, especially with oral intubation and positive pressure ventilation (62).

One of the biggest problems with use of low pressure cuffs stems from a lack of understanding by the user. There is widespread belief that simply using this type of cuff will prevent high pressures from being exerted on the wall of the trachea. Any cuff, even a so-called low-pressure cuff, can be overfilled or the volume and pressure can increase during nitrous oxide anesthesia, resulting in high intracuff and tracheal wall pressures (114,172). The volume of gas necessary to raise the cuff pressure from the point of seal to an unsafe pressure is only 2 to 3 ml (145).

Foam Cuff

The foam cuff is also known as the sponge, Fome, and Kamen-Wilkinson cuff.

Characteristics. The foam cuff has a large diameter, residual volume, and surface area (Fig. 15.19). It is filled with polyurethane foam covered with a sheath. Applying suction to the inflation tube causes the foam to contract. When the negative pressure is released, the cuff expands.

The tube was originally designed to be used with the inflation tube open to atmosphere (108). Later, the tube was supplied with a T piece to fit between the connector and the breathing system (Fig. 15.20). When the inflation tube is connected to this T piece, the pressure inside the cuff will follow proximal airway pressure during the ventilatory cycle (118,173).

Before extubation the cuff should be col-

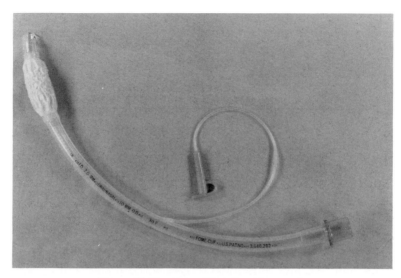

Figure 15.19.   Tube with deflated foam cuff.

lapsed by aspirating with a syringe and clamping the inflation tube. Several investigators have found no harmful effects from the gentle removal of the tube without prior removal of air from the cuff. This technique permits removal of secretions that have accumulated above the cuff (174). However, it is possible that if the tube must be removed quickly, damage to the vocal cords could occur.

Intracuff Pressure and Pressure on the Tracheal Wall.   When in place in the trachea, the degree of expansion of the foam determines the resting pressure exerted laterally on the tracheal wall (157). The more the foam is expanded, the lower the pressure

(173). Thus the pressure on the tracheal wall depends on the relationship between cuff diameter at residual volume and the diameter of the trachea. If too large a cuff is used, the cuff:tracheal wall pressure ratio will be high. If too small a cuff is used, there is risk of aspiration and leaks during positive pressure ventilation.

Diffusion of anesthetic agents into the cuff can occur but will not cause an increase in pressure (116,118).

Evaluation.   Use of this cuff obviates the need for measurement of cuff pressure or use of a pressure-regulating device. One study found this cuff to be an effective barrier to aspiration (173). However, if a small tube is

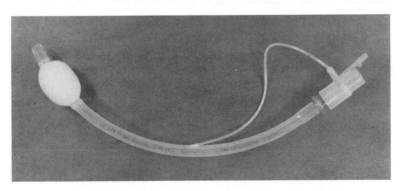

Figure 15.20.   Tube with inflated foam cuff and a T piece.

used, the lateral wall pressure may be less than that required to prevent aspiration.

It provides a seal at a low tracheal wall pressure, provided the relationship between the cuff and tracheal diameters is optimal (108,173,175). A reduced incidence of tracheal dilatation has been reported with its use (157). It has been reported that the foam may change shape with time, allowing an air leak to occur after 18 to 36 hr of intubation (152). However, this was with the inflation tube open to atmosphere.

One study found a high incidence of sore throat associated with its use (109). In two reported cases, the inflation tube was accidentally pulled out at the point of insertion on the tube, making cuff deflation impossible (176,177). It has been suggested that the cuff can be removed without deflation without untoward effects (174).

Inflation System

See Figure 15.1.

Inflation Lumen

The inflation lumen, which connects the inflation tube to the cuff, is located within the wall of the tracheal tube. The ASTM (24) standards requires that it not encroach on the lumen of the tube and recommends that it not bulge outward.

External Inflation Tube

The external inflation tube (cuff tube, pilot tube or line, pilot balloon line, inflating tube, or tail) is external to the tube. The ASTM (24) standard requires that its external diameter not exceed 2.5 mm and recommends that it be attached to the tube at a small angle. The standard also specifies the distance from the tube tip to the point where the external inflation tube is attached and requires that the tube extend at least 3 cm beyond the machine end of the tube before a pilot balloon or inflation valve is incorporated.

The inflation tube can become obstructed by kinking or by crushing from a clamp. On spiral embedded tubes, the inflating tube may connect to the inflation lumen above the first spiral ring. If the connector is inserted into the tube far enough to contact the first spiral to prevent kinking at that spot, it may cause the inflation tube to be blocked (75,76,178). This can be remedied by cutting a small V in the connector and inserting the connector so that the inflation tube passes through the V. Most spiral embedded tubes presently available have the inflation tube outside the spirals to prevent this problem.

Pilot Balloon

The pilot balloon (bulb, external reservoir, or external balloon) may be located near the midpoint of the inflating tube or adjacent to the inflation valve. Its function is to give an indication of inflation or deflation of the cuff.

Inflation Valve

The ASTM (24) standard requires that the external inflation tube either be fitted with an inflation valve with an inlet that will mate with a male Luer's syringe tip or have a female end capable of accepting a standard Luer's syringe.

The inflation valve is designed so that when a syringe with a standard Luer's tip is inserted into it, a plunger is displaced from its seat and gas can be injected into the cuff. Upon removal of the syringe, the valve seals and gas cannot escape from the cuff unless a syringe is reinserted and the gas deliberately removed.

Some tubes, such as red rubber ones, may lack an inflation valve. Cuff inflation is maintained by application of a clamp to the external inflation tube or by placing a plug in its free end.

DEVICES TO MEASURE CUFF PRESSURE

Monitoring of cuff pressure is desirable so that the pressure can then be adjusted to a safe level. Several methods have been used to monitor intracuff pressures either continuously or intermittently (113,179–181). Devices for this purpose are available commercially (Fig. 15.21). If the pressure is measured intermittently, the cuff and manometer should be inflated simultaneously (182).

DEVICES TO LIMIT CUFF PRESSURE

Devices that will bleed the cuff when the intracuff pressure rises above a set value have been developed.

Lanz Pressure-Regulating Valve (183,184)

The Lanz pressure-regulating valve (or McGinnis balloon system) on the Lanz tube consists of a very compliant latex pilot balloon inside a transparent plastic sheath with an automatic pressure-regulating valve between it and the cuff (Fig. 15.22). The pilot

balloon has three functions: (*i*) an indication of cuff inflation, (*ii*) an external reservoir for the cuff, and (*iii*) a pressure-limiting device. It is designed to maintain an intracuff pressure of 20 to 25 torr at end expiration while preventing overinflation of the cuff.

The pressure-regulating valve permits rapid gas flow from the balloon to the cuff but only slow gas flow from the cuff to the balloon. This prevents gas from being squeezed back into the balloon when the airway pressure rises rapidly, so there is no leakage of gas around the cuff during positive pressure ventilation. It also prevents increases in cuff volume and pressure caused by diffusion of nitrous oxide and other gases into the cuff.

As air is injected, the cuff and balloon are

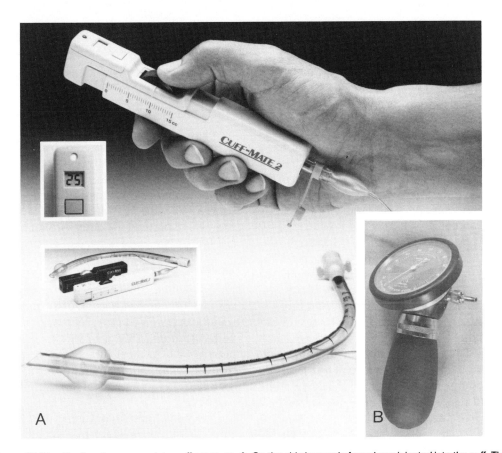

Figure 15.21. Devices to measure intracuff pressure. **A,** On the side is a scale for volume injected into the cuff. This is increased by turning the wheel. A window on the top shows the intracuff pressure in cm H$_2$O. Courtesy of Diemolding Heathcare Division.

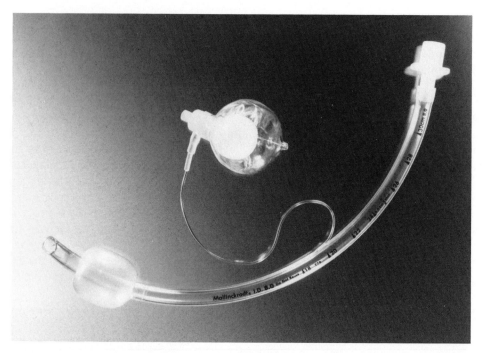

Figure 15.22.   Lanz pressure-regulating valve. The pilot balloon is confined inside a transparent plastic sheath. There is a pressure-regulating valve between the pilot balloon and the cuff. Air should be injected into the cuff until the pilot balloon is stretched, but it should be smaller than the confining sheath.

inflated in parallel. When the balloon has a stretched appearance, a pressure of approximately 26 to 33 cm H_2O will be present in the cuff. As injection continues, the pilot balloon fills preferentially. The intraballoon pressure remains constant and will not increase until it strikes the confining sheath. Should the trachea expand, air will slowly flow from the balloon into the cuff. The pressure-regulating valve protects against rapid loss of cuff volume into the balloon during inspiration.

This valve has been found by several investigators to be effective in keeping lateral tracheal wall pressure low and preventing increases in pressure as a result of nitrous oxide diffusion (116,135,145,185–187). One study found that to go from the point of tracheal occlusion to an unsafe cuff pressure required 45 ml of air (145). Use of it eliminates the need to measure cuff pressure.

If the patient happens to lie on the balloon

or the balloon is compressed or overinflated, the intracuff pressure will rise (188).

In patients with mean airway pressures above 33 cm H_2O, this system may fail to form a seal with the trachea (113). The cuff may leak, particularly after prolonged use (189).

Brandt Tube (190)

The Brandt tube is specially designed to compensate for the diffusion of nitrous oxide into the cuff by means of a large pilot balloon with a thin cuff (Fig. 15.23). Nitrous oxide entering the tracheal tube cuff will migrate through the inflation tube into the pilot balloon and then diffuse through it into the atmosphere.

One study found that when exposed to nitrous oxide the pressure in the cuff of the Brandt tube stayed within 14% of its initial value, whereas that of another cuff increases

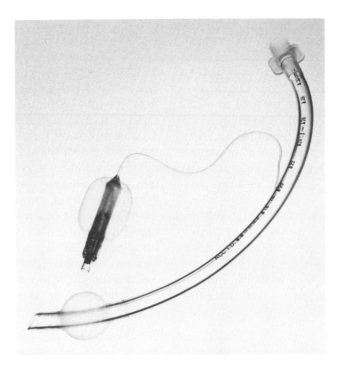

Figure 15.23.   Brandt tube. Nitrous oxide entering the tracheal tube cuff will migrate through the inflation tube to the large pilot balloon, which has a thin cuff, and diffuse through it to the atmosphere. Courtesy of Mallinckrodt Medical, Inc.

232% over the course of 1 hr (191). Another study showed that the incidence of sore throat after intubation could be reduced using this tube (192).

Others (113)

Other mechanisms of automatic cuff pressure control have included a modified epidural syringe (193,194), pneumatic devices (113,195), a water column (196,197), and electropneumatic devices (180,198–200). Several of these devices are available commercially, but variability may limit their usefulness (201).

TRACHEAL TUBE CONNECTORS

The tracheal tube connector (union) serves to attach the tube to the breathing system. It may be made of plastic or metal. The basic taper dimensions of the connector are set by an ASTM (202) standard.

The end that fits into the tube is called the patient (distal) end, and the size of the connector is designated by the internal diameter of this end in millimeters. The end that connects to the breathing system is called the machine (proximal) end and has a 15-mm male (OD) fitting.

The connector may have protrusions, lugs, or other features to which elastic bands or other devices may be attached to prevent accidental disconnection from the breathing system (see Figure 12.9), but there is controversy as to their desirability. Some connectors have a side port for respiratory gas sampling.

Special connectors with low dead space are available for pediatric use. A hazard is associated with their use (203,204). When used in association with a breathing system adaptor that has a fresh gas inlet tube that protrudes into the lumen of the adaptor, the inlet tube may press against the end of the connector. This can cause partial or complete obstruction of the exhalation pathway and result in barotrauma.

The connector should be the same size as the tube with which it is intended to mate. This will result in minimal reduction of the lumen and make separation unlikely. There should be no shoulder within the lumen, and transitions in the internal diameter should be tapered to facilitate passage of a suction catheter (202).

The most commonly used connectors are the straight and 90° curved (right angle). Acute angle connectors with less than a 90° curve (Fig. 15.24) and flexible connectors (205) (see Fig. 15.17) are available. For operations around the face, a curved connector may facilitate positioning of the breathing system away from the surgical field. Curved and flexible connectors have two disadvantages: (*i*) they increase resistance (20,206,207) and (*ii*) they must be removed from the tube when it is desired to insert a stylet or suction catheter.

Most disposable tracheal tubes come with the connector only partly inserted into the tube. Before use, the connector should be fully inserted. Removing it from the tube and wiping the distal end with alcohol will facilitate insertion into the tube and cause bonding with the tube. Removal of a connector from the tracheal tube may be facilitated by use of a towel clip (208).

Occasionally, when a tube is cut fairly short and the connector firmly seated, the

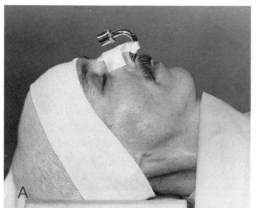

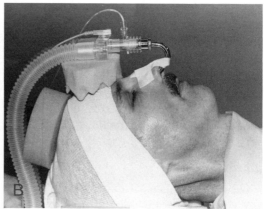

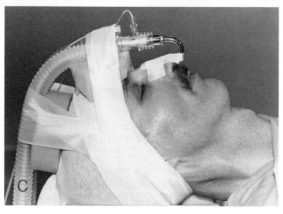

Figure 15.24. Method of securing a nasotracheal tube. **A**, A skull cap is placed around the head. An acute-angle connector is used and taped so that it does not exert pressure on the nasal ala. **B**, Foam padding is used to keep the breathing system from exerting pull on the tracheal tube. **C**, Tape is added to keep the breathing system firmly in place.

pilot tube to the cuff may be occluded, making inflation or deflation of the cuff impossible (209).

LASER-RESISTANT WRAPS FOR TRACHEAL TUBES

Products

In an effort to protect the shafts of combustible tracheal tubes from laser beams, tubes have been wrapped with various materials, including aluminum foil, aluminum tape, copper tape, and moist cotton (92,97,100,210–215). Copper foil (Venture) has been found to protect tubes from CO_2, Nd-YAG, and KTP lasers (96,97,100,210,216,217). 3M 425 aluminum tape has been shown to provide adequate protection from the CO_2 laser in several studies (92,96,97,216,217). Although most studies have shown it offers protection against the Nd-YAG laser (92,100,210), one study found it did not protect PVC tubes from this laser (100). Blood on the outside of aluminum- or copper-wrapped tubes can compromise the protection from combustion (93).

The possibility of changes in the composition of any tape requires that every batch be evaluated for its incendiary characteristics. Thus every foil- or tape-wrapped tube should be tested with the laser before use (218,219).

The only product approved by the FDA for this purpose is a two-layered sheet of synthetic surgical sponge and adhesive-backed corrugated silver foil (Merocel Laser Guard), which is available in several sizes. It can be applied more quickly to the tracheal tube than can foil tapes (211). Before intubation, the tube with wrap is saturated with water or saline. When wet, the sponge and reflective foil act as a heat sink and disperse argon, CO_2, Nd-YAG, and KTP lasers (100,220,221). There is less likelihood of a reflected laser beam causing damage with this product than with foil-wrapped tubes

(101). Blood on the coating does not reduce its protective effect (93).

Wrapping Procedure with Tapes (100,211,219)

Some investigators believe that only red rubber tubes should be used for wrapping (100). A burned silicone tube loses its structural integrity, and combustion of a PVC tube will produce toxic gases.

The tube should be cleaned with alcohol to remove any residue that would prevent the tape from adhering to it. The tube should be thoroughly dry before wrapping. Painting the tube with tincture of benzoin may strengthen the adhesion of some tapes. The tape should be wrapped in an overlapping spiral starting from just above the cuff and proceeding toward the machine end. The inflation tube should be placed against the tube and wrapped together with it. The cuff should not be wrapped. In the case of an uncuffed tube, the wrapping should extend far enough toward the tip that it will be at least 1 cm below the vocal cords (214,222). The spiral should overlap by one-third to one-half of the tape width. This allows the tube to be flexed without exposing the underlying tube or breaking or kinking the tape. Applying tension on the tape as it is wrapped around the tube will help it conform to the tube and eliminate kinks, bumps, and wrinkles. The tube should be allowed to retain its manufactured shape.

An alcohol wipe of the wrapped tube will provide a minimal level of disinfection without damaging the tube or tape. Foil-wrapped tubes can be gas sterilized before use without affecting their combustibility (211,217).

The tube should be inspected for gaps or holes in the wrap before use. Tubes that are not fully protected or that have bumps or wrinkles should not be used.

Disadvantages

Wrapping reduces tube flexibility, can predispose to tube occlusion, and may create a rough surface (213,223). The outer diameter of the tube is increased. Reflection of the laser beam from metallic tape could cause damage to nontargeted tissues (101). The wrapping material may come off and obstruct the airway (224). Errors in wrapping may expose the tube to the laser beam.

The cuff remains vulnerable to penetration and ignition of the tube distal to the cuff may occur (100,222,225). Wet cottonoids should be used to protect the cuff, which should be filled with colored saline (225,226). A slight separation or tear in the tapes will make the tube vulnerable to ignition. The interior of a tube can be ignited by flaming pieces of tissue either in close proximity to or inhaled into the tip of the tube (227,228).

Wrappings with cotton or sponge material must be kept moist and may ignite if allowed to dry out. A catheter irrigation system has been described (229).

A medicolegal problem is possible if tapes not approved for medical use are used (100). In addition, most manufacturers of standard tracheal tubes state that their tube should not be used with a laser.

It has been recommended that tapes on tracheal tubes be used only as a last resort when other methods of providing laser resistance (laser-resistant tracheal tubes or Merocel wrap or techniques not using a tracheal tube) are unavailable or cannot be used, such as laser surgery on small patients (100).

Use of the Tracheal Tube

CHOOSING THE TUBE

Cuffed Versus Uncuffed

It has been common practice to avoid cuffed tracheal tubes in young children for fear of the patient developing postintubation stridor (230). Some studies indicate that their use is not associated with increased problems (231). Advantages of cuffed tubes include improved monitoring, absence of leaks during ventilation, and the ability to use PEEP. A drawback is the need to choose a slightly smaller tube, which makes suction more difficult and increases resistance. Use of uncuffed tubes can result in a high incidence of silent aspiration (232).

Size

Choosing the correct size tube before intubation is attempted will avoid trauma from trying to insert too large a tube or reintubation if the tube is too small. The choice of tube size involves many considerations.

Smaller-diameter tubes are easier to insert and require a smaller reshaping force to adapt to the patient's anatomical airway (233), but they are associated with higher resistance, difficulty in providing adequate tracheobronchial toilet, leaks with positive pressure ventilation, and increased risk of occlusion and kinking. Passage of a fiberscope may not be possible if the tube is too small. In general, the inside diameter of the tracheal tube should be at least 1 mm larger than the outside diameter of the fiberscope. For best results, and especially if the tube is inserted nasally, a difference of 2 mm is needed.

Larger tubes are associated with less risk of occlusion and lower resistance but may predispose to laryngotracheal injury.

Because no system of choosing the correct size tube is foolproof, the user should always have readily available tubes one size larger and one size smaller than the one chosen. If a difficult intubation is anticipated, a small tube should be used. A tube changer can be used later to insert a larger tube.

Cuffed Tubes

In adults and larger pediatric patients, the circumference of the cuff, not internal tube diameter, should be used to determine the best fit. If the tube size results in the cuff being too small for the trachea, then a higher cuff pressure will be required to effect a seal, converting the low-pressure cuff into a high-pressure one. If the cuff is too large in relation to the tracheal lumen, it will have folds when it is inflated to occlusion. Aspiration may occur along those folds (234).

Ideally, the cuff circumference should equal diameter of the tracheal lumen (151). Based on this, one study found that the ideal tube in the average adult would be a 7.5-mm-ID tube for females and a 8.5-mm-ID tube for males (235). However, there is great variation in sizes and shapes of tracheas in adults (234,236–238). The transverse dimensions increase with age, but in general, the correlation between age, race, height, weight, body surface area, and tracheal shape or size is poor (234,236). There is some variation in the cuff circumference of tubes.

Uncuffed Tubes

In small children, an airtight seal is often achieved not by means of a cuff but by selection of the correct size of an uncuffed tube to fit the cricoid ring. There is considerable variation in subglottic size in children.

For prolonged intubation in children, many think that there should be a small leak of gas between the tube and the trachea head using a stethoscope with the head in the neutral position at a peak pressure of 20 to 40 cm H_2O. Reintubation with a smaller tube should be considered if the leak pressure approaches 40 cm H_2O (239–241).

The following have been used as general guidelines for selection of a tube size in children.

1. 1 to 6 months — 3.0 to 4.0 mm ID
   6 months to 1 year — 3.5 to 4.5 mm ID
   older than 1 year — ID in mm = (16 + age in years) ÷ 4 (233,242)
2. Premature — gestational age in weeks ÷ 10 + 0.5 = ID in mm (243)

younger than 6.5 years — 3.5 + age in years ÷ 3 = ID in mm

older than 6.5 years — 4.5 + age in years ÷ 4 = ID in mm (244)

3. infant below 1 kg — 2.5 mm
   infant between 1 and 2 kg — 3.0 mm
   infant between 2 and 3 kg — 3.5 mm
   infant over 3 kg — 4.0 mm (245)
4. Choosing a tube whose external diameter is the same width as the patient's distal little finger (246,247).
5. Use of a tape measure based on body length (248,249).

It has been recommended that a smaller tube be used for children with a history of croup or asthma presenting for routine surgery and also for patients with upper airway obstruction caused by larygotracheobronchitis or epiglottis (250–252).

CHECKING THE TUBE

Before insertion, the tube should be examined carefully for defects such as splitting, holes, and missing sections (253–255). The cuff, if present, should be inflated and the syringe removed to check the functioning of the inflation valve. If the syringe is left in the valve, the valve housing may crack and leak (256). The cuff should be inspected to make certain it inflates evenly and does not cause the tube lumen to be reduced. It should be left inflated for at least 1 min to check for a slow leak.

If the tube has a sponge cuff, all the air should be removed by aspiration. The inflation tube should then be closed or clamped off. The cuff should remain collapsed. If it fills, there is a leak, and the tube should be discarded.

The tube should be checked for obstructions. With transparent tubes, simple observation will suffice. With other tubes, the user should look into both ends and/or insert a stylet.

PREPARING THE TUBE

After the sterile wrapper is opened, the tube should be handled only at the connector end. The connector should be inserted as far as possible. Removing it from the tube and wiping the distal end with alcohol will make insertion into the tube easier and cause bonding with the tube.

Lubricants have been used on tracheal tubes for many years, although their value has been questioned. It has been suggested that use of a lubricant jelly on a low-pressure, high-volume cuff may decrease aspiration by filling in the folds (164). Only a sterile water-soluble lubricant should be used (257). For oral intubation, only the distal end of the tube should be lubricated. If nasal intubation is planned, lubricant should be placed along the entire length of the tube.

The curvature of the tube can be increased by inserting the tip of the tube into the connector (258). This may facilitate insertion in a patient with an anterior larynx.

INSERTING THE TUBE

Techniques

Oral Intubation

Oral intubation is generally preferred for general anesthesia and in emergencies because it can be performed more quickly than nasal intubation. It allows passage of a larger and shorter tube with a larger radius of curvature than nasal intubation. This facilitates flexible bronchoscopy and suctioning and lowers resistance to airflow.

Studies comparing orotracheal and nasotracheal intubation in patients requiring ventilatory assistance have found little difference, except that the ease of initial intubation was greater with orotracheal intubation (259,260). There is less movement of the tube within the trachea with changes in head position with oral intubation (261).

Disadvantages include the possibility of dental and oropharyngeal complications.

Oral intubation is usually not well-tolerated by the conscious patient. The patient with an oral tube has difficulty swallowing secretions. Prolonged oral intubation in the infant has been found to be associated with damage to unerupted teeth and the palate (262–265).

Insertion of the tube is usually easy once the vocal cords are exposed. The tube should be introduced into the right corner of the mouth and directed toward the glottis with the bevel parallel to the cords. If there is movement of the cords, the tube should be inserted between them during the moment of greatest abduction.

A bite block, rolled gauze, or oral airway may be placed between the teeth to prevent the patient from biting down and occluding the lumen.

Nasal Intubation

The nasal route is often used for surgical procedures involving the oral cavity, oropharynx, and face, when an oral tube would hinder the surgeon's access to the operative field. Other indications may include a fractured mandible, limitation of movement at the temporomandibular joints, and an obstructing mass in the mouth or oropharynx. It may be preferable when the patient is awake or combative, has a neck injury, or has a mechanical obstruction to orotracheal intubation.

Intubation by the nasal route has many advantages. Fixation of the tube is easier and there may be less tendency for inadvertent extubation (62,266), although a study of long-term intubation found no significant differences between patients who received oral intubation and those who received nasal intubation (267). During long-term intubation, oral feedings and improved oral hygiene are possible. Use of the nasal route eliminates the possibility of tube occlusion by biting.

Disadvantages of this route include the possibility of cosmetic nasal deformities and meteorism with long-term intubation. The chances of cuff damage during intubation are increased. Smaller tubes must be used, resulting in increased resistance, difficulty in suctioning, and difficulty in using a fiberscope. The time for tube placement is longer. Nasal bleeding may occur in a large number of patients.

Nasal intubation has been shown to result in a high incidence of bacteremia (268–271). For this reason, it may be prudent to administer prophylactic antibiotics to susceptible patients. A high incidence of sinusitis and otitis during and following nasotracheal intubation has been reported (266,272–286). Sinusitis may lead to severe complications such as meningitis, pneumonia, and septicemia. Nasotracheal tubes should not be used in patients with a head injury, because a cerebrospinal fluid leak into the nose could become a route of infection (287).

Contraindications to nasotracheal intubation include coagulopathy; basilar skull fracture; and any mechanical impediment of the nasotracheal route, including polyps, abscesses, foreign bodies, and possibly epiglottitis (288). Relative contraindications include patients who have undergone nasal surgery or have nasal pathology.

Before insertion of a nasotracheal tube, there should be local application of a vasoconstrictor. The patency of each nasal cavity should be assessed by having the patient inhale through each nostril separately. Often a tube one size smaller than would be considered optimal for oral intubation is selected to minimize epistaxis. It should be thoroughly lubricated along its entire length with a water-soluble lubricant (257). The tube can be softened by placing it in an oven at 50°C for 15 min before expected intubation time (289).

The patient's head should be put in the usual position for laryngoscopy (see Chapter 12). The tube should be inserted into the larger or more patent nasal cavity. Inserting progressively larger lubricated nasal airways will serve to test the patency of the nostril and dilate it (290,291).

When the tracheal tube is inserted, its bevel should face laterally, so as to direct its leading edge away from the turbinates (289,292). Then, before it is advanced, it should be pulled cephalad so that its bevel is directed along the floor of the nasal cavity and below the inferior turbinate (292). The tube should be directed gently posteriorly until it contacts the posterior pharyngeal wall. Here the natural curve of the tube and the anterior body of the cervical spine will usually direct it anteriorly. When it is judged that the tip has passed the uvula, the tube should be rotated 180°, then advanced toward the larynx.

Resistance to passage of the tube may be met at various points along its course. Only moderate pressure should be used. If excessive resistance is encountered, the other nostril or a smaller tube should be tried. Sometimes the tube will impact against the posterior pharyngeal wall and resist attempts to advance it farther. The tube should be pulled back a short distance, and the patient's head extended to facilitate passage beyond this point. It may be useful to withdraw the tube and place a stylet in it, making an acute bend in the distal 1.5 cm of the tube. The tube is inserted until it passes the posterior nasopharynx, then the stylet is withdrawn. Another technique is to pass a small suction catheter through the tube and into the oropharynx (223,293). The tube can usually be threaded over the catheter, or the tip of the catheter can be picked up and brought out of the mouth. A forward pull on the catheter will usually bring the tip of the tracheal tube forward.

Direct Laryngoscopy.   After the tube is in the pharynx, the larynx is exposed using a laryngoscope. The tube tip can usually be directed laterally by twisting. The position of the larynx relative to the tube tip may be altered by flexing or extending the neck and/or external pressure on the larynx. If these manipulations do not line up the tube and laryngeal opening, forceps can be used to grasp the tip and direct it through the vocal cords. The cuff should not be grasped, as it may be damaged by the forceps.

If the tip passes through the vocal cords but then encounters resistance, it is most likely because the curve of the tube is directing the tip into the anterior wall of the larynx. Withdrawing the tube slightly and flexing the neck will usually allow advancement. Other techniques include rotating the tube 180° before pushing it forward, passing a suction catheter through the tube into the larynx as a guide (294), and inserting a stylet with an anterior bend near the tip (295,296).

Flexible Fiberoptic Laryngoscopy. Flexible fiberoptic laryngoscopy is the preferred method if a conventional rigid laryngoscope cannot be used because of inability to move the patient's neck or open the mouth. Blind nasal intubation may stir up bleeding and ruin the chance to view the larynx through the fiberscope. The technique is described in Chapter 14.

Blind (297,298). The blind technique may be useful when direct laryngoscopy or use of a fiberscope would be difficult. It may be associated with more trauma than intubation under direct vision or using a fiberscope.

It may be performed under general or local anesthesia. The classical technique of blind nasal intubation requires a spontaneously breathing patient and uses breath sounds as a guide to placement. The patient is placed in the classical intubation position with the neck flexed and the head extended. After the tube is inserted through the nostril, it is advanced blindly. If the patient is breathing spontaneously, breath sounds can be heard as the tip approaches the larynx. When the sounds are at maximal intensity, the tube is gently but swiftly advanced during early to end inspiration. If the sounds suddenly cease but the patient continues to breathe, the tube has passed into a location other than the trachea. Flexion or extension of the head or manipulation of the larynx by external pressure may line up the tube and larynx. The tube tip may be rotated by twisting the tube at the connector end (299). Insertion of a preformed stylet with an anterior curve may help to advance the tip through the vocal cords (295).

A technique for blind intubation if the patient is not breathing has been described (297). Certain landmarks on the front of the neck (hyoid bone, notch of the thyroid cartilage, and the cricoid cartilage) are observed. As the tube moves anteriorly, the landmarks are moved by the tip of the tube. The object is to move the tip to the midline at the thyroid angle, where it should enter the larynx. If the tip is above the thyroid cartilage, flexion of the head will move the tip more caudad. If the tip is below the thyroid cartilage, extension of the neck will move it cephalad. If the tip is observed resting laterally, the tube should be withdrawn and twisted to direct it toward the midline. If the tube tip passes the laryngeal inlet but impinges on the anterior trachea, increasing cervical flexion or rotating the tube through 180° may allow it to pass into the trachea.

For difficult intubations when the above techniques do not work, a retrograde intubation technique may be used (300). This may be performed in cases of suspected cervical spine injury or when a difficult intubation is anticipated. The procedure begins with puncture of the cricothyroid membrane and insertion of a wire (Seldinger technique) or an epidural catheter in a cephalad direction. It is retrieved through the oropharynx. If the patient has a large amount of blood or secretions in the mouth, a catheter is best used, because air can be injected through it to facilitate visualization of the tip. Once the line is retrieved, it is used to guide a tracheal tube into the airway.

Depth of Insertion

The tube should be passed until the cuff is 2.25 to 2.5 cm below the vocal cords (301). If no cuff is present, the tube tip should be inserted not more than 1 cm past the cords in children under 6 months, not more than 2 cm past the cords for patients up to 1 year, and not more than 3 to 4 cm past the cords in larger patients. In children, it is possible to pass a tube through the cords but have its passage blocked just below this level. The tube should not be forced, but a smaller tube used instead.

In average-size adult patients, securing the tube at the anterior incisors at 23 cm in males and 21 cm in females will usually avoid endobronchial intubation (302). For nasal intubations, 3 cm should be added to these lengths for positioning at the nares.

In children, the optimal depth to which the tracheal tube should be inserted nasally can be estimated by the following formula:

$$L = (3 \times S) + 2$$

where S is the internal diameter of the tube in millimeters and L, the length in centimeters (303).

CHECKING THE POSITION

After the tube has been inserted, its position should be checked: first to be sure that it is in the tracheobronchial tree and not the esophagus, and second, to make sure that it is neither too deep nor too shallow in that tree. Methods to detect intubation of a bronchus or the esophagus are discussed in "Perioperative Complications." After confirmation of correct placement, the portion external to the patient may be shortened to prevent kinking.

INFLATING THE CUFF

Low-Volume, High-Pressure Cuff

If the tube has a high-pressure cuff, the cuff should be inflated with the minimal amount of gas that will cause it to seal against the trachea at peak inspiratory pressure. Listening with the unaided ear will often miss small leaks. These can be detected by palpation or auscultation of the suprasternal pretracheal area (304,305). Inflating until the pilot balloon is tense and/or inflating beyond seal will result in unnecessarily high cuff volume and tracheal wall pressure.

Low-Pressure, High-Volume Cuff

With a low-pressure, high-volume cuff, measurement of cuff pressure is necessary to prevent overinflation or underinflation. If a low-pressure cuff is adjusted to the point of just abolishing audible leakage at peak inspiratory pressure, the resulting intracuff pressure may not be high enough to prevent aspiration (306).

The cuff should be inflated to a pressure of 25 to 34 cm H_2O (112,113). The pressure should be measured and adjusted approximately 10 min after the tube has been inserted (307). This delay is necessary to allow for softening of the cuff material at body temperature and for the patient to become settled, because the volume necessary for occlusion will vary with muscle tone.

After cuff pressure has been adjusted, a check should be made to make sure there is no leak at peak airway pressure. If there is a leak, and peak airway pressure does not exceed intracuff pressure, the cuff is probably too small for the trachea, and a tube with a larger cuff should be used (172).

Cuff pressure should be measured and readjusted frequently. Changes in muscle tone in the trachea and diffusion of gases across the cuff may result in large changes in cuff pressure.

When a tracheal tube with a Lanz pressure-regulating valve is used, the cuff should be inflated until a seal is achieved during peak inspiration. The pilot balloon should be distended but should be smaller than the confining sheath.

Sponge Cuff

After intubation, the inflation tube should be opened to atmosphere and the cuff be allowed to fill with air. The amount of air in the cuff should be ascertained by withdrawal with a syringe. The ability to remove 2 to 3 ml from the smallest cuff or 5 to 6 ml or more from the largest cuff usually signifies that a cuff:tracheal wall pressure ratio will allow adequate mucosal perfusion. If little or no air can be aspirated, the cuff may be too large.

If a leak is present after the cuff has been allowed to refill, wrinkles in the cuff may be present and may be straightened out by injecting 2 or 3 ml of air into the cuff then allowing it to deflate. If the leak persists, consideration should be given to using a larger tube. Alternatively, the inflating tube can be capped at the end of exhalation. If this is not effective, the minimum amount of air required to stop the leak should be injected and the inflation tube should be clamped.

SECURING THE TUBE

A well-secured tracheal tube is essential for safe anesthesia, particularly in pediatric patients in whom the distance from the mid-trachea to the cords or carina is short. If the tube is not well-fixed there is danger of either unplanned extubation or advancement of the tube deeper into the trachea or into one of the mainstem bronchi. Lesions of the airway owing to friction may be increased if the tube is not well-secured. The securement technique must be appropriate for the nature of the surgery and accessibility of the tube.

Adhesive tape is most commonly used to maintain the tube in the desired position. The part of the tube to which the tape is to be applied should be thoroughly dried. All tapes do not adhere to all tracheal tubes equally well (308), so it is advisable to test available tapes to determine which works best for the chosen tube. Cohesion can be improved by wrapping the tube with a transparent adhesive dressing (308–310). Use of an adhesive such as tincture of benzoin on the tube and skin may make the tape stick better.

The tube may be secured by having the tape completely encircle the head (311). Fixation to the lower lip may be safer than fixation to the upper lip (312).

Use of adhesive tape has the following disadvantages:

1. Some patients have skin conditions that are aggravated by contact with adhesives or adhesive tape. Others may have allergic responses. Tape can damage the skin of burn patients.
2. It may interfere with preparation of the head and neck.
3. Many male patients have beards or mus-

taches, making it difficult to attach the tape.
4. Secretions from the mouth, sweat, or prep solutions may make the tape slippery and ineffective.

For these reasons other materials such as umbilical tape or surgical suture may be used to anchor the tube (313–315). The suture may be passed either around a ring of adhesive tape on the tube or through the wall of the tube and may be anchored by passing it through the gum or around a tooth or by taping it to the skin. Placing a safety pin through the wall of the tube may be helpful. The tube may be sutured to the tongue (316).

Because the hair is an insecure medium for fixing a tube, a close-fitting skull cap, elastic net or a towel taped around the head may be used to provide a firm structure to which to attach tape or ties (Fig. 15.24) (317,318).

Other methods used to secure the tube include circumpalatal fixation (319), use of liquid silicone foam to form a cast around the tube (320), and use of an umbilical cord clamp to snap around the tube (321). Special devices for securing tracheal tubes without use of adhesives or ties are available commercially. A tube holder may be combined with a bite block and/or nasogastric tube holder.

With nasal intubation, padding around the tube may help to prevent pressure necrosis (321). Fixation in the direction of the mouth rather than cephalad may decrease the risk of damage to the nasal alae with prolonged intubation (322).

Equally important to fixing the tube properly is making sure there is no pull on it. Use of a lightweight extension between the tracheal tube connector and the breathing system and/or a tube support may be helpful. Figure 15.24 shows a method of securing the breathing system so that it does not exert pull on a tracheal tube inserted nasally.

CHANGING THE TUBE (323–326)

There are three general techniques available for changing a tracheal tube: use of a fiberscope; direct laryngoscopy; and use of a tube changer (discussed later in this chapter). Exchange of a tracheal tube using a fiberscope is discussed in Chapter 14.

Direct laryngoscopy can be used for changing an orotracheal or nasotracheal tube or substituting one for the other. A laryngoscope blade is placed into the mouth and positioned in the hypopharynx. The existing tube is visualized entering the glottis. The replacement tracheal tube is positioned as near to the glottis as possible, the existing tracheal tube pulled out, and the replacement tube is inserted. Passage of a jet-stylet tube exchanger through the existing tube and leaving it in place will allow jet ventilation until the new tube enters the trachea (325).

When changing a tracheal tube using a tube exchanger, the lubricated exchanger is inserted into the tube and advanced until it has passed the end of the tube. Most tracheal tube changers have depth marks printed on their sides to aid in precise placement. While the tube changer is held firmly in place, the existing tube is withdrawn. Care must be taken not to alter the position of the changer. The new tracheal tube is then threaded over the tube changer and advanced until it is at the proper depth. The tube changer is then withdrawn.

Use of a jet stylet tube changer allows administration of oxygen, suctioning, and ventilation while the changer is in place (324).

REMOVING THE TUBE

When it is time for extubation, the mouth and pharynx should be suctioned and the tape or other fixation device removed. Withdrawing the tube until resistance is met before deflating the cuff may push material that has accumulated above the cuff into the pharynx where it can be removed by suctioning. The patient should be given a large sustained inflation or the APL valve should be closed and airway pressure allowed to rise to 5 to 10 cm H_2O. While the lung is near total capacity, the cuff should be deflated and the tube removed during inspiration (327,328). This will blow secretions collected above the

cuff into the mouth and pharynx, which should then be suctioned.

If the tube cannot be removed easily, the inflating tube should be checked for obstruction distal to the pilot balloon, especially at the point where tape was used to hold the tube in place. If the surgery has involved the mouth or thorax, a suture may be around or through the tube or cuff. If the tube is forceably removed in these circumstances, disastrous consequences may result.

Extubation of a patient with a possible difficult airway is best carried out over a jet stylet (329). After the tracheal tube is withdrawn, the small hollow catheter may then be used as a means of ventilation and/or a guide for reintubation. The jet function may allow additional time to assess the need for reintubation. After the tracheal tube has been passed over the jet stylet, the intratracheal location of the jet stylet may be maintained while confirming intratracheal placement of the reintubation tracheal tube by passing the tube exchanger through the self-sealing diaphragm of a fiberoptic elbow adapter. Positive pressure ventilation and carbon dioxide sampling can be done around the tube exchanger.

If the tracheal tube is to stay in place and nitrous oxide has been in use, the cuff should be evacuated and filled with air to avoid a leak in the postoperative period (131).

Perioperative Complications

Complications associated with short-term intubation are usually mild in nature. As the length of intubation increases, so do the incidence and severity of complications.

AT THE TIME OF INTUBATION

Trauma During Insertion

Intubation is inevitably associated with some incidence of trauma. A delicate epithelium plus a small lumen place infants and children at greater risk. Elderly and emphysematous patients have a thin, friable, less-elastic trachea so that perforation is a greater hazard. Trauma is often associated with use of excessive force or repeated attempts at intubation. It varies with the skill of the operator, the difficulty of the intubation, and the quality of muscle relaxation. Damage may be increased with use of a stylet protruding beyond the end of the tube or through the Murphy eye. Mucosa can be torn when a metal or foil-wrapped tube is used (106,223). A defective tube may have a barb (295). Plastic tubes become stiffer when cold and this may increase the likelihood of trauma on insertion.

Trauma to the lips, tongue, teeth, nose, pharynx, larynx, trachea, or bronchus may occur. Injuries ranging from simple abrasion to severe laceration and perforation have been reported.

Reported injuries to the larynx include hematomas, contusions, lacerations, puncture wounds, cord avulsions, and fractures (330–333). Recovery is generally prompt with conservative management. Arytenoid cartilage dislocation is an uncommon complication (334–336). The left arytenoid is usually the one dislocated (337,338). Bilateral dislocation resulting in severe upper airway obstruction has been reported (339,340). Problems associated with arytenoid dislocation or subluxation include alterations in phonation, increased resistance to breathing, aspiration, dyspnea, impaired cough, and pain on swallowing.

With nasotracheal intubation, abrasion or laceration of the mucosa is common (341,342). The nasal septum may be dislocated or perforated. Fragments of adenoid tissue, nasal polyps, or tubinates may be dislodged (343–348). Retropharyngeal passage of a tube has been reported (349,350). This may progress to formation of an abscess or even mediastinitis.

Cases of tracheal, bronchial, esophageal, pharyngeal, hypopharyngeal, and laryngeal perforation have been reported, sometimes with fatal consequences (341,351–379). Consequences of perforation include hema-

toma, upper airway obstruction, pneumomediastinum, pneumothorax, subcutaneous emphysema, mediastinitis, aspiration pneumonia, hydrothorax, pneumoretroperitoneum, and pyopneumothorax. An abscess, fistula, or cellulitis may develop (380–382). Bronchial rupture has been associated with use of a tube changer (383).

The best way to avoid trauma is never use more than gentle pressure during intubation. Muscle relaxants should be used to avoid patient movement. Stylets should be flexible and never extend beyond the tip of the tube.

Use of vasoconstrictors on the nasal mucosa before intubation, warming the tube, and sequential dilatation (inserting progressively larger, lubricated nasal airways) will reduce the trauma associated with nasal intubation (289–291,384). Tubes used for nasal intubation should be smaller than considered optimal for oral intubation and should be well-lubricated along their entire length.

Failure to Achieve Satisfactory Seal

A leaking cuff or tube may make maintenance of adequate ventilation difficult, fail to protect against aspiration, and make surgery involving the oral cavity extremely difficult.

If the cuff protrudes above the cords, there may be a leak despite a large amount of air being injected into the cuff. Further inflation may seal the leak, but it will gradually return.

During insertion, the cuff, inflation tube, or the tube itself may be torn by a tooth or turbinate, the laryngoscope blade, forceps, or the sharp edge of a stylet (385). High-volume, low-pressure cuffs are more liable to be torn than low-volume, high-pressure ones. A kink in the inflation tube where it joins the tube can prevent the cuff from being inflated (386). A defect in the tube or eccentric cuff inflation can cause a leak (254,387). If the compliance of the pilot balloon is greater than that of the cuff, the cuff may empty into it (388). Leaving the inflating syringe attached to the valve assembly may cause a crack in the valve housing so that it leaks when air is injected (256). A problem with the syringe used to inflate the cuff may make it impossible to inflate the cuff (389,390). Failure to establish a seal may result from inserting a small tube into a patient with large or highly compliant airways or tracheomalacia.

When a leak is present, laryngoscopy should be performed to determine if the cuff is above the cords. If so, the cuff should be deflated, the tube advanced and the cuff reinflated. If this fails to solve the problem, the tube should be replaced. If intubation was difficult, consideration should be given to using a tube exchanger or fiberscope for replacing the tube.

Intubation of the Esophagus

Esophageal intubation is a potentially disastrous complication that can occur even with an experienced anesthesia provider (391–396). In addition to hypoxia and brain injury, consequences include ruptured stomach and pneumoperitoneum (395,397). Distension of the stomach can predispose to regurgitation and aspiration. The tracheal tube may be lost into the stomach (398).

Recognition that this has occurred and prompt correction are necessary to prevent dire consequences. The tube should be checked immediately after intubation to determine if it is in the tracheobronchial tree.

In most patients, distinguishing between esophageal and tracheal intubation is not difficult. In a small number, however, some signs can so closely resemble tracheal placement that they can deceive even a careful, experienced individual. In many of the reported incidents involving esophageal intubation, one or more of the following tests have been performed and were misleading.

1. Visualization of the tube passing between the vocal cords is one of the most reliable signs. Unfortunately, the glottis frequently cannot be visualized. In these cases, posterior displacement of the tracheal tube with the laryngoscope blade still in the mouth will usually bring the tube and vocal cords into view (399). However, even if a direct view is achieved, the tube may be displaced before or during securement.

2. The characteristic feel of the reservoir bag associated with normal lung compliance is another method. Decreased compliance and expiratory time may be seen with esophageal intubation (400). Unfortunately, this test is unreliable (396,401–405).

A related test is movement of the reservoir bag and measurable tidal volumes in time with the patient's spontaneous respiratory efforts. However, tidal volumes have been noted through a tube in the esophagus (396,401,402,404,406,407).

Another test is assessment of bag refilling with the bag full but with no flow from the machine (408). The bag is squeezed three to five times, and if the tube is correctly placed, the bag will refill each time. If the tube is in the esophagus, significant refilling will not occur.

3. Some users rely on visual and/or manual confirmation of chest wall movement on inflation. Unfortunately, movement of the chest wall simulating ventilation of the lungs can occur with the tube in the esophagus, especially in patients whose respiration is primarily abdominal (401–404,409–413). Low lung or chest wall compliance may result in poor chest movement, even when the tube is in the trachea (396).

4. Hearing normal breath sounds on auscultation of the chest is another sign. Auscultation should be performed in the mid-axillary areas bilaterally, not just the anterior chest. The quality of the sounds is important. A gurgling sound in the tube (the death rattle) suggests esophageal placement. This test is not totally reliable, because there are cases documented in the literature for which apparently normal and symmetrical breath sounds were heard with esophageal intubation (396,401,404,407,409,412–414). With a large intrathoracic hiatal hernia, a gastric pullup, or intrathoracic esophagogastrostomy, sounds that mimic normal breath sounds may be heard (402).

5. With the cuff deflated, the high-pitched

sounds of air escaping around a tracheal tube, compared with the more guttural sounds of leakage around a tube in the esophagus, have been used as a distinguishing feature (396). However, if the cuff of the tube is near the cricoid cartilage, the distinction in sound may not be present (404).

6. Epigastic auscultation and observation for air movement into the stomach have also been used. Auscultation of the upper abdomen as well as the lungs has been found more reliable than auscultation of the lungs alone (409). Yet such sounds may be confused with breath sounds often heard in the epigastric area in thin individuals and pediatric patients (396,407).

7. Some users observe the epigastrium for lack of gastric distension. Unfortunately, the abdomen does not always distend with intermittent gastric inflation and the presence of gastric distension can be the result of mask ventilation before attempted intubation (403,404,411). The presence of a hiatal hernia or intrathoracic gastrointestinal contents may result in the absence of abdominal distension with esophageal intubation (402).

8. Appearance of moisture in a transparent tracheal tube (400) is not necessarily reliable. Moisture can appear with esophageal intubation (396,409,415).

9. Absence of changes in blood pressure or heart rate is another test. Unfortunately neither blood pressure nor heart rate is a reliable indication of hypoxia or hypercarbia (317,318). The electrocardiogram also cannot be relied on.

10. Persistence of good patient color or satisfactory pulse oximeter readings has been used. However, color changes will be delayed a number of minutes with esophageal intubation if preoxygenation has been performed, and at that time a number of other causes for the hypoxemia must be ruled out (396,416). If oxygen saturation improves after intubation, it is likely that the tube is in the tracheobronchial tree (417).

11. Listening through the open end of the tracheal tube while the sternum is abruptly depressed can be misleading for a variety of reasons (396,404).

12. Obtaining a chest x-ray is time-consuming and expensive and may not be definitive in determining if the tube is in the esophagus without a lateral view, unless the tip is seen below the carina or gastric dilation is present (396,418,419).

13. Palpation of the cuff in the suprasternal notch has been used. With this test, the pilot balloon is rapidly and intermittently squeezed while the other hand palpates the neck suprasternally (420). This test is not reliable in detecting esophageal replacement (396,406,415,421).

14. Another test is to note the requirement for excessive air to cause the cuff to seal in the trachea with a tube appropriately sized for the patient. However, placement of the cuff at or just above the vocal cords, a tear in the cuff, or failure of the cuff to expand uniformly can also result in the need for high volumes in the cuff.

15. Some users visualize the tracheal rings, using a fiberscope. A special adapter with a port will allow ventilation while the examination is carried out (Fig. 15.25). This is a reliable method verifying tracheal placement but requires special instruments and skill, takes time, and cannot be used with small tubes.

16. The presence of gastric fluid in the tube lumen may indicate misplacement. However, gastric fluid may not appear with esophageal placement and may be difficult to distinguish from secretions in the lungs (396).

17. Intraoral tactile tests (422,423) involve placing one hand inside the patient's mouth and the other hand on the patient's neck and confirming that the tube lies immediately anterior to the interarytenoid groove.

18. The esophageal detector device has been used. A 60-ml syringe or compressible bulb is attached to the tracheal tube connector using an adaptor, and the plunger is withdrawn or the compressed bulb is released (424,425). If the tube is in the trachea and an

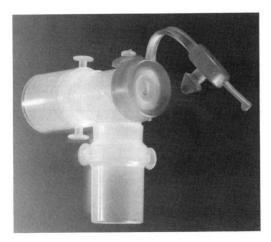

Figure 15.25. Adaptor for use of fiberscope. Courtesy of Mallinckrodt Medical, Inc.

airtight seal has been achieved, withdrawal of the plunger of the syringe or release of the bulb will aspirate gas from the patient's lungs without resistance. However, if the tube is in the esophagus, apposition of the walls of the esophagus around the tube will occur. This will occlude the lumen and cause a negative pressure or resistance when the plunger is pulled back or the bulb released. Deflation of the cuff helps to distinguish between the two sites (426). As a confirmatory test, the device can be used to inject a bolus of air into the tube while listening over the epigastrium for gas bubbling in the stomach. This test will also detect a blocked tracheal tube (425).

This test has a high degree of accuracy (425,427–431), but false negatives may occur (425,429,432). The presence of a nasogastric tube does not limit the efficacy of this test (429).

19. Intentional bronchial intubation (433) is another test. The tube is advanced sufficiently far for the tube to enter a bronchus. The chest is then auscultated during positive pressure ventilation. If breath sounds can be heard on only one side, bronchial intubation has been achieved. With esophageal intubation, the breath sounds are either equal in intensity bilaterally or equally diminished or absent on both sides of the chest. This test is not foolproof (433).

20. An introducer can be passed down the tracheal tube (396,434). With the tracheal tube in the esophagus, the introducer will pass unopposed to the distal esophagus or stomach. If the tracheal tube is in the trachea, the tube will meet the carina at approximately 26 to 32 cm in adults. Other criteria indicating placement in the trachea include resistance to further insertion, the ability to maintain air entrainment through the open end of the tracheal tube while suction is applied to the tube, the ease of withdrawal of the tube with suction, and the absence of bile or gastric contents in the aspirate.

21. Tracheal palpation during insertion is another method. During attempted intubation with gentle palpation of the trachea in the sternal notch or application of cricoid pressure, a washboard-like sensation can be appreciated as the tube passes over the tracheal rings (435). This sensation may not be present when the intubation is performed with a relatively small-diameter tube compared with the trachea.

22. Presence of carbon dioxide in the exhaled gases (396,403,436,437) is one of the best available methods. It allows reliable and rapid detection of esophageal intubation. Both qualitative and quantitative carbon dioxide monitors are available (see Chapter 16). Tube placement can be reliably checked on the first few breaths with either spontaneous or controlled ventilation. It can be used when the vocal cords cannot be visualized, breath sounds are difficult to hear, and access to the patient is limited.

There are some special circumstances in which carbon dioxide may be detected if the tube is in the esophagus (438). Exhaled gases may be forced into the stomach during mask ventilation before intubation. Carbon dioxide can be in the stomach as a byproduct of magnesium trisilicate or sodium bicarbonate that has reacted with gastric acid and from ingestion of carbonated beverages. In these cases, the end-tidal CO_2 will be low, the wave pattern will be irregular, and CO_2 levels will rapidly diminish with repeated ventilation.

The capnogram will not be normal in configuration. Carbon dioxide may not appear despite correct placement with severe bronchospasm or if there is no pulmonary blood flow (405,435).

If there is the slightest doubt as to where the tube has been placed and the patient's condition permits, a check of tube position by direct laryngoscopy should be made. Posterior displacement of the tracheal tube may help to bring the tube and vocal cords into direct view (399). Alternately, the patient can be ventilated using a mask placed over the open tube and mouth. Cyanosis relieved by this maneuver is evidence of tube misplacement (401). If the patient's condition is deteriorating and these maneuvers are not helpful or cannot be performed for some reason, the tube should be removed. "When in doubt, take it out" is a good rule to follow.

Swallowed Tracheal Tube

There are a number of case reports of a tracheal tube being lost in the esophagus (398,439–451). The majority of these occurred during newborn resuscitation. The tubes were removed and no permanent sequelae occurred.

This complication can be prevented by using a connector that fits firmly into the tube. Bonding between the connector and the tube will be increased if the connector is wiped with alcohol before insertion into the tube. The tube should be long enough that it protrudes from the mouth when correctly placed. It should be firmly secured.

If this complication does occur, removal of the tube need not be immediate. Resuscitation should continue and the patient's condition stabilized.

Inadvertent Bronchial Intubation

Insertion of a tracheal tube into a mainstem bronchus is a relatively common and sometimes fatal complication. If not rectified, it leads to atelectasis and intrapulmonary shunting in the nonventilated lung.

Other possible consequences include alveolar rupture, interstitial emphysema, and pneumothorax on the side where the tube is placed. A tube inserted into the right main bronchus may occlude the bronchus to the right upper lobe (452). If the tip impinges on the carina, persistent coughing and bucking may occur.

The adverse effects can be slow in onset and this may delay the diagnosis. Because the clinical features vary considerably, a high index of suspicion should be maintained in every intubated patient.

Inadvertent bronchial intubation has been found to occur more frequently during emergency intubations (453,453a) and in pediatric patients (453b,453c). A short trachea is associated with a number of pediatric syndromes (453d). One study showed that RAE tubes were too long in 32% of children and bronchial intubation occurred in 20% (42).

Intubation of a bronchus can occur either at the time of initial insertion or subsequently. If not firmly anchored, the tube may descend into a bronchus as a result of the weight of the attachments or from suctioning or other maneuvers. The tube will move caudad with neck flexion, opening of the mouth, movement of the head from the side to the center, and going from an erect to a recumbent position (453e–453k). Trendelenburg or lithotomy position, placement of upper abdominal packs, and compression of the abdomen will move the carina upward (454).

After intubation, an effort should be made to detect bronchial intubation. This should be repeated at intervals, whenever changes in the patient's position are made, and whenever there is any indication of hypoxia. If a patient fails to settle down and continues to cough, it should be suspected that the tube may be irritating the carina.

There are several methods used to detect bronchial intubation.

1. Auscultation for Bilateral Breath Sounds

The commonly used method of auscultating the lower and upper peripheral lung fields bilaterally may be misleading as breath sounds can be transmitted to the opposite side of the chest in the presence of endobronchial intubation, unless the tube is wedged firmly in a main bronchus (454,455).

2. Visualization of Symmetrical Chest Expansion.

Visualization is easily performed but is not reliable.

3. Chest X-Rays (455)

Chest x-rays are highly reliable if performed correctly but are time-consuming and expensive. Most workers believe that the tip of the tube should be in the middle third of the trachea with the head in a neutral position (midway between full extension and full flexion) (453f,453j,456). If the neck is flexed, the tube will appear to be too deep in the trachea. If the head is extended it will appear to be too near the cords.

Appropriate tube position can also be assessed by noting which vertebral body the tip overlies. A safe level is over the second to fourth thoracic vertebrae (405,453f,457).

The distance between the tube tip and carina can also be used. In the neonate, infant, and young child the tip should be 2 cm above the carina with the neck in the neutral position (453c,458). In children approaching 5 to 6 years of age, this distance should be increased to 3.0 cm (458). In adults, the ideal distance is 3, 5, or 7 cm with the neck flexed, neutral, or extended, respectively (453f,457,459).

A pitfall in the interpretation of a chest x-ray for tube placement is that not all tubes contain radiopaque lines extending to the tip (460). In this case, the tube may be reported to be correctly positioned when it is in fact too deep.

4. Tube Position at the Lips/Nostril

Adult Patients. It is recommended that oral tubes be positioned 21 cm at the teeth (or upper anterior gums in edentulous patients) in normal-size females and 23 cm in normal-size males (302,435). Studies show this is a better method of preventing endobronchial intubation than auscultation of the chest. However, it may result in high placement in some patients, with the danger of accidental extubation (461). For nasal intubation 3 cm should be added to these lengths for positioning at the nares.

For patients whose body lengths lie outside the normal range, the tube can be placed alongside the patient's face and neck with the tip lying at the suprasternal notch. The tube is aligned to conform externally to the position of a nasal or oral tracheal tube. The centimeter markings at which the tube intersects with the teeth or gums (oral intubation) or the nares (nasal intubation) are noted, and the tube is secured in that position after intubation. One study determined that the maximum safe tube length at the naris was best determined by measuring the distance between the upper border of the cricoid cartilage and the tip of the xiphoid process (462).

Pediatric Patients. The margin of safety in children is less than that in adults because of a shortened trachea. A number of formulas and tables based on body size and gestation age have been developed, including the following:

Oral Intubation

1. Length in centimeters = age $\div$ 2 + 12 cm (453,463).
2. Length in centimeters = weight in kilograms $\div$ 5 + 12 cm (463).
3. Length in centimeters = height in centimeters $\div$ 10 + 5 cm (464).
4. Rule of 7-8-9: infants weighing 1 kg are intubated to a depth of 7 cm at the lips; 2-kg infants, to a depth of 8 cm; and 3-kg infants, to a length of 9 cm (465).

Nasotracheal Intubation

1. $L = (S \times 3) + 2$, where L is the length in centimeters and S is the internal diameter of the tube in millimeters (303).

2. Multiplying crown-heel length by 0.21 (466).
3. For total tube length, 0.16 × height in centimeters + 4.5 cm, then leave 2 cm of tube outside the nostril of an infant and 3 cm outside for an older child (467).

While use of special formulas will decrease the incidence of this complication, such formulas are based on averages and should not be considered totally reliable (454). Furthermore, tube length markings are not always accurate (468).

5. Guide Marks on the Tracheal Tube (301,469,470)

Many tubes have lines or rings to help position the tube with respect to the vocal cords (see Figs. 15.4B and 15.17), and the distal portion of some pediatric tubes are colored.

6. Breath Sounds

Advance the tube until unilateral breath sounds and chest rise are observed. Then slowly withdraw the tube, noting the tube length at nares or gum at which symmetrical breath sounds and chest movement return. Withdraw the tube an additional 2 cm, and secure it (458,471).

7. Fiberscope Through the Tube (472)

Passing a fiberscope through the tube is equal in accuracy to chest x-ray for determining tube position relative to the carina in both adults and pediatric patients (472–474). Furthermore, it is considerably faster than x-rays. The ready availability of fiberscopes in most operating room suites makes this a practical method of checking tube position.

8. Inflation and Deflation of Cuff While Palpating

Another method is inflation and deflation of the cuff while palpating the anterior neck (475–477). The lower border of the cuff should be felt just above the suprasternal notch. This method may not be useful in obese patients and with high-volume, low-pressure cuffs (478,479). A better method may be to palpate the trachea downward from below the cricoid cartilage while applying constant pressure to the filled pilot balloon (479). When the region of the trachea with the inflated cuff is palpated, an increase in pressure should be detected in the balloon. With uncuffed tubes, the tip of the tube is palpated during insertion and advancement is stopped when the tip has just passed the suprasternal notch (453b).

9. Fluid in Cuff (480)

Injection of fluid into the cuff, followed by gentle compression of the pilot balloon while auscultating over the suprasternal notch is another method. The characteristic gurgling sound produced is not heard if the tip is in a mainstem bronchus or near the carina.

10. Magnetically Detectable Metallic Element (481,482)

A portable locator is used to detect a metallic element that has been placed near the tip of the tube. This method reduces the rate of malpositioning of tubes, but does not eliminate it (481).

A thin foil band wrapped around a tracheal tube and detectable by a electronic sensor has also been used to position the tube tip in the midtrachea (478).

11. Monitoring Expired Carbon Dioxide

Monitoring of expired carbon dioxide may lead to the discovery of endobronchial intubation (483–486), but it is not a reliable means to detect this problem. Either an increase or decrease in end-tidal CO_2 may be seen.

12. Lighted Intubation Stylet

One study showed that by inserting a lighted intubation stylet so that the light is at the tip of the tube and positioning the tube so that the maximum transilluminated glow is at the sternal notch, the tip can be consistently placed at a satisfactory level (487).

13. Illumination by a Fiberoptic Strand

Tracheal tubes in which the tip is illuminated by a fiberoptic strand that is incorporated into the tube wall and terminates just proximal to the cuff, or near the tip on uncuffed tubes have been used (488,489). When a light source is connected, a bright transillumination appears distal to the cricoid cartilage.

14. Transcutaneous Oxygen Monitor or Pulse Oximeter

Sudden and immediate falls in arterial and transcutaneous oxygen can occur with bronchial intubation (490). Pulse oximetry is somewhat less sensitive. However, desaturation does not necessarily occur with endobronchial intubation even in the presence of massive atelectasis (435,491).

When a tracheal tube is believed to be in a bronchus, the cuff should be deflated, the tube withdrawn several centimeters, the cuff reinflated, and the position rechecked. If reintubation would be difficult because of the patient's position or because the initial intubation was difficult, consideration should be given to advancing a fiberscope or bougie into the tube before withdrawing it. Even if extubation should occur, the tracheal tube can be quickly reinserted. The lungs should then be hyperinflated sufficiently to expand atelectatic segments. For long-standing atelectasis, bronchoscopy may be required to remove mucous plugs.

Bronchial Obstruction

Bronchial obstruction secondary to bronchial intubation was discussed above. Bronchial obstruction also can occur as a result of an anomalous tracheal bronchus (269). Such bronchi are nearly always on the right side, usually supplying the right upper lobe.

Foreign Body Aspiration

During intubation a variety of materials can be aspirated into the trachea and can cause blockage or check valve obstruction to part of the lungs. In some reported cases, serious, life-threatening airway obstruction has occurred.

A tracheal tube may dislodge fragments of tumors of the oral cavity, pharynx, or larynx. A tube inserted nasally may dislodge a fragment of adenoid or nasal tissue during its passage (492). Obstruction of a bronchus by a blood clot following a traumatic intubation has been reported (493).

It is possible for a tracheal tube to become separated from its connector and lost in the trachea or pharynx (494–496).

A tracheal tube may have the punched-out area forming the Murphy eye still in situ (497–499), and this may be aspirated. A portion of a ruptured cuff may fall into a bronchus (500–502).

The coating of a stylet may be scraped off as it is removed (503–505). Other foreign bodies have included a cottonoid used to protect the cuff from a laser beam (215), the distal portion of a tracheal tube (506,507), pieces of aluminum used to protect the tube from ignition by a laser beam (224), parts of defective connectors (508,509), a cap liner from a tube of lidocaine ointment (510), and parts of sprays and atomizers (511–513). Aspiration of teeth, dentures, and parts of laryngoscopes have all been reported.

Careful inspection of connectors, tubes, and stylets before use will help to avoid introduction of foreign bodies. The connector should fit firmly in the tracheal tube and the tape or securing device should be attached to the tube, not the connector. Whenever a cuff leaks, it should be carefully examined for missing portions after removal from the patient.

Foreign body aspiration should always be

suspected whenever obstructive signs or symptoms appear, and an immediate search should be made of the patient's air passages. This should include bronchoscopy if examination above the level of the larynx proves fruitless.

WHILE THE TRACHEAL TUBE IS IN PLACE

Unsatisfactory Seal

The cuff can rupture or become separated from the tube while in place (502,514). Application of lubricant or local anesthetic spray has been associated with cuff leaks (515–517). The inflation system may have a defect (518–520). Puncture of a cuff may occur during internal jugular or subclavian intravenous cannulation (521,522). A laser beam can perforate the cuff and cause a leak (215). If a device to monitor cuff pressure is left attached to the inflation valve, the valve housing may crack (256). The connector may leak or separate from the tube (523–525).

When the tube is adjacent to the site of surgery, as during thoracic or intraoral surgery, tube damage can occur (324,526–536). The patient may chew a hole in a tube (68,537,538).

When a leak occurs, laryngoscopy should be performed to check the position of the cuff. If it is not completely below the vocal cords, the cuff should be deflated, the tube advanced, then the cuff reinflated. If the problem is in the inflation system, it may be possible to repair the damage or the leak can be bypassed using a three-way stopcock or a needle inserted into the line below the defect (539–542).

If the tube is cut, it may be possible to pass a small uncuffed tube past the cut (534). The small tube can then be used to ventilate the patient until the tube can be changed. In some cases, it may be possible to approximate the ends of the tube and seal the leak (530).

If the cuff is leaking, several alternatives are available:

1. Do nothing (if the leak is small and the patient is not in danger of aspiration).
2. Fill the cuff with a mixture of lidocaine jelly and saline (543,544).
3. Attach a mechanism for maintaining a continuous infusion of air into the inflation tube. Methods described include an intravenous tubing connected to an air-filled plastic container to which constant external pressure is applied (531), a flowmeter (545,546), and a system for maintenance of intraocular pressure (547).
4. Increase the fresh gas flow to compensate for the leak.
5. Reintubation. If this is elected, consideration should be given to use of a tube exchanger or fiberscope.
6. Put a mask over the patient's face and the tube and ventilate.
7. Remove the tube and ventilate with a mask.
8. Use pharyngeal packing to control the leak.
9. Establish an acceptable airway in another fashion (tracheostomy or cricothyroid membrane puncture.)

When a tube with a leaking cuff is removed, the damaged cuff should be carefully examined for missing portions.

Airway Perforation

Tracheal or bronchial perforation is a rare but serious complication of intubation (372,548–552). It is usually associated with preexisting pathology of the airway, use of a stiff tracheal tube, hyperextension of the neck, violent movements of the head and neck, traction on the trachea, or overinflation of the cuff (333). In one case, the trachea was ruptured because the cuff was connected to a jet ventilation device (553). If airway rupture is suspected, it is essential to establish a diagnosis by bronchoscopy.

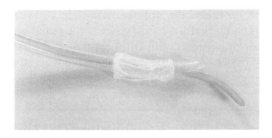

Figure 15.26. The tube changer has become caught in the Murphy eye.

Murphy Eye Complications

Anything passed down the tracheal tube such as a suction catheter, tube exchanger, or fiberscope can pass through a Murphy eye and become caught (Fig. 15.26). It may be impossible to remove the device without also removing the tracheal tube (554).

Laser-Induced Tracheal Tube Fire

A tracheal tube fire is one of the most serious hazards of laser surgery (222,228,555–559).

Physics of Lasers (560,561)

A laser (light amplification by stimulated emission of radiation) is a source of coherent light, a form of electromagnetic radiation. Coherent light results from the stimulation of atoms, ions, or molecules (the laser medium) by electrical, optical, or thermal energy. The stimulated laser medium spontaneously gives off energy in the form of light, which is then amplified and emitted as the laser beam. Coherent radiation has three important characteristics that account for specific interaction between laser light and tissues: coherence (all waves are in phase in both time and space); collimation (all waves are traveling in parallel directions); and monochromaticity (all waves are of the same wavelength).

Laser devices have three components: a laser medium, an optical cavity, and a pumping source.

1. Laser Medium. The name of the laser refers to the type of material used within the optical cavity as the laser medium, which may be a solid, liquid, or gas. The laser medium determines the wavelength of the emitted radiation.

2. The Optical Cavity. The optical or resonator cavity provides the controlled environment in which the laser medium is confined. Energy released from the medium travels in all directions. Mirrors are used to reflect the atoms liberated and to increase the energy of the stimulated emission.

3. Pumping Source. The pumping source supplies electrons to the laser medium, liberating energy.

Types (211,560)

Carbon Dioxide Laser. Since its introduction in the early 1970s, the carbon dioxide laser has been widely used for surgery in the upper airway. The CO_2 laser beam is invisible and so must be used with a helium-neon aiming beam as a marker. It cannot be transmitted using fiberoptic instruments.

Nd-YAG Laser. Nd-YAG is short for neodymium-yttrium aluminum-garnet laser. It is used for palliative procedures in the trachea and bronchi. Its short wavelength allows the beam to be transmitted by fiberoptic fibers. It is useful for surgery on the distal tracheobronchial tree and the retina. Because it is taken up by pigment, colored markings on tracheal tubes are more likely to be damaged than clear portions (95). Blood or debris on or in the tracheal tube make it more laser sensitive. Fires from a Nd-YAG laser passed through a channel of a flexible bronchoscope have been reported (562–564).

KTP Laser. The KTP laser is the potassium-titanylphosphate laser. It can be transmitted by fiberoptic bundles. It has been used for neurosurgical and otolaryngological procedures.

Argon Laser. The argon laser has been used during neurosurgery, retinal and otolaryngological surgery, and treatment of cutaneous lesions. It can be transmitted by fiberoptic bundles. Prolonged exposure of PVC or red rubber tubes to the argon laser causes minimal damage (565).

Minimizing Risk

The tube may be exposed to either the direct or reflected laser beam. Flaming tissue in close proximity to the tube may ignite it (228). The interior surface of a tube can be ignited by burning pieces of tissue inhaled into the tube.

Low Inspired Oxygen Concentrations (566,567). Nitrogen, air, or helium should be used to reduce the oxygen concentration to the lowest level that will provide satisfactory patient oxygenation, because some tubes that will ignite at high oxygen concentrations are safe at low concentrations. Helium may be preferable to nitrogen (34,568–570). Nitrous oxide supports combustion and should not be used as the diluent gas (34,571–547).

Although using low inspired oxygen concentrations will make ignition less likely to occur, it will not totally prevent it. If there is a significant leak, the anesthesiologist may fill the reservoir bag by pushing the oxygen flush valve (566). This will result in an elevated oxygen concentration. If there is a leak, a more appropriate response would be to increase the gas flow while maintaining the same inspired oxygen concentration or to replace the tracheal tube with one that has a competent cuff.

Limiting Laser Power Density and Duration (566,569,575). Lasers should always be kept in the standby mode except when ready to fire, so that inadvertent activation does not occur.

Filling the Cuff with Saline. The cuff is not laser resistant. If a beam penetrates an air-filled cuff, airway gas can leak into the operative field and, if the oxygen or nitrous oxide content is high, increase the risk of fire. Fluid in a cuff acts as a heat sink, which

prevents heat buildup and makes the cuff less likely to perforate (576,577). If the cuff does perforate, a jet of fluid may extinguish the fire (578). Addition of methylene blue or any other biocompatible and highly visible dye to the saline will help the surgeon to recognize a perforated cuff.

Care must be taken to flush all air from the cuff, because any remaining air will settle in the most superior part of the cuff, which is the part most likely to be hit by the laser beam (95). As a further precaution, cottonoids or pledgets, which must be kept wet, should be placed on the cuff (579). It is important that they be kept moist. Continuous insult from the laser beam may dry them, so that they lose their protective properties. Further hits can then cause combustion of the cottonoids and/or the cuff (225). The cottonoids must be carefully retrieved after surgery.

Use of a Technique Not Requiring Intubation (94,580,581). A tube in the airway can be avoided by using jet (Venturi) ventilation, insufflation, or by removing the tracheal tube during treatment. Possible complications of these techniques include barotrauma and aspiration.

If jet ventilation is being used and an errant laser strikes an object outside the oropharynx, the resultant burning vapors may be entrained into the airway and exhaled, possibly causing facial burns (582).

Use of Protective Wrappings. The tube can be covered with a protective wrapping. These were discussed earlier in this chapter.

Use of Special Tubes. Use of special tubes was discussed above. No one tube is completely safe for all lasers (100,579). Tubes sold for laser use should indicate the type of laser for which they are suited as well as the conditions (power, power density, spot size, and/or oxygen concentration) under which the tube is supposedly free from the hazard of ignition. A metal bronchoscope for pulmonary Nd-YAG laser surgery also can be used (583,584).

Action in Case of Fire (100,211,585)

Because a completely safe anesthetic technique has not yet been devised, the entire OR team should be well-rehearsed in a protocol to follow if an airway fire occurs. The surgical team should be vigilant whenever the laser is in or near the airway. A flash, pop, or snap or the sight or smell of smoke may signal an airway fire. The tube should be loosely fixed to the patient so that it can be removed rapidly if necessary (569,562). The patient should not be excessively draped. A container of water should be available to douse any flames.

If a fire occurs, the flow of all gases, including oxygen, should be stopped and the pilot tube cut. Stopping the gas flow will reduce the intensity of the fire or allow it to go out. In addition, it will prevent setting fire to drapes or other materials around the patient. Cutting the pilot tube will deflate the cuff and facilitate extubation. The tube and cuff protective devices should be removed immediately (100). The fire should be extinguished with water or saline or by smothering it with a wet towel. Alcohol or other flammable fluids should not be used.

The airway should be reestablished and the patient ventilated with air until it is certain that nothing remains burning in the throat, then 100% oxygen should be used. A search for burning fragments that remain in the trachea and assessment of damage to the larynx and tracheobronchial tree should be made.

Tracheal Tube Obstruction

One of the reasons for insertion of a tracheal tube is to provide a patent airway. Unfortunately, the tube itself may become the cause of obstruction. This can occur anytime. In infants and children, serious tracheal tube obstruction occurs in 4% to 5% of intubations (586).

The obstruction can be partial or complete. It is possible to have a ball valve obstruction so that inspiration is unimpeded, but resistance to expiration is increased (54,587–590).

An obstruction of slow onset may present as a decrease in compliance and high inspiratory pressures with controlled ventilation coupled with wheezing resembling bronchospasm, for which bronchodilators are often given in error (591). Paradoxical movements may be seen in spontaneously breathing patients (333). Acute complete obstruction is much less ambiguous in its presentation, while a problem that permits inhalation but prevents exhalation may present as circulatory collapse (589).

Causes

Biting. Unless protection in the form of an airway or bite block is provided, the patient may bite the tube (67–70,72,592,593). Most of the reported cases involved spiral embedded tubes that were permanently deformed after the bite was released. Care should be taken to prevent the tube from slipping between the molar teeth where occlusion may occur in spite of an airway or bite block.

Kinking. Kinking, formerly a common occurrence with reusable tubes that had become old and weakened, still may be a cause of tracheal tube obstruction. Spiral embedded tubes have been used to overcome this problem, but kinking can still occur at the patient end if the connector is not inserted inside the spirals (51).

Kinking sometimes occurs when the position of the patient's head is changed, especially when the neck is flexed (594–598). It also can occur when a tube inserted from the right side of the mouth is transferred to the left side without ensuring that the entire tube has been moved to the left of the tongue (361).

Tubes vary in their resistance to kinking. Smaller tubes kink more readily than larger ones. This can be remedied by placing a larger tube over the small one (599,600). If a larger tube kinks, a smaller tube may be passed through it (597). A structural fault in the tube such as at the point where the inflating tube enters the wall of the tube can predispose to kinking (601).

When tubes are wrapped for laser microlaryngeal surgery, they may become occluded as a result of compression by the foil as the tube accommodates to the curvature of the posterior pharynx (214).

When placing a tracheal tube in the trachea through a tracheostomy stoma, care must be taken that the tube does not bend back on itself (602). Obstruction of a tracheal tube from a peritonsillar abscess has been reported (45). The problem did not recur when an armored tube was used.

Obstruction by Material in the Lumen of the Tube. A tracheal tube may be obstructed by dried secretions, blood, pus, debris, or tissue (529,590,603–609). Nasal conchae, turbinates, and adenoid material may be found in a tube after intubation (347,610–612).

Foreign bodies reported in occluded tracheal tubes have included foam rubber from a mask (613), an inflation valve (614), a cleaning brush (615), an adaptor from an intravenous set (616), an intravenous needle (617), a stop from a stylet (618), a cork (619), a glass ampule (620), pieces of plastic (589,621–623), part of a nasogastric tube (623), an oral medication tablet (630), a smaller tracheal tube (631), part of a paper towel (632), and dead organisms (633,634).

Defective Spiral Embedded Tubes. Overuse and repeated sterilization of spiral embedded tubes can predispose to problems. In one case, insertion of a connector caused the inside of the tube to pucker up and occlude the lumen (61). The inner wall may become detached (55,635).

During manufacture, air bubbles may form between the layers. If these tubes are gas-sterilized or steam auto-claved with vacuum, blebs may form (63). During anesthesia, nitrous oxide may diffuse into the blebs and cause swelling or gas from the cuff can enter the space between layers. Herniation into the tube lumen will cause obstruction (52,54,58,60,61,635–638).

Bevel Abutting Against the Tracheal Wall. The bevel may impinge against the wall of the trachea (Figs. 15.27 and 15.28) (51,587,639–643). In many of these cases, the cuff inflated eccentrically (see Fig. 15.28). If the tube has a Murphy eye, ventilation may continue through it but passage of a suction catheter or bougie may be impossible (27).

An unusual cause of obstruction involved the endotrol tube (88). When it was inserted nasally, the loop on the pull cord abutted against the nares, causing the tip of the tube to bend and obstruct against the tracheal wall. The problem was solved by cutting the pull cord.

In infants when the tube orifice faces in one direction and the infant's head is turned to the other, the orifice may abut against the tracheal wall (644). This occurs more readily with higher tube positions and/or neck flexion. Displacement of the trachea by part of the aortic arch may cause the bevel to lie against the tracheal wall (645–647).

Obstruction by the Cuff. It is possible for an overinflated cuff to balloon over the tip of the tube (57,648–651) (see Fig. 15.27). Distension of the cuff may cause compression of the tube lumen (Fig. 15.29) (66,652–662).

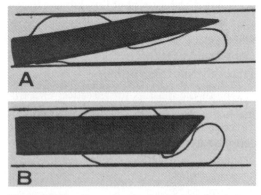

Figure 15.27. Two causes of tracheal tube obstruction. **A,** The bevel is pushed against the wall of the trachea by an eccentrically inflated cuff. **B,** The cuff has ballooned over the end of the tube.

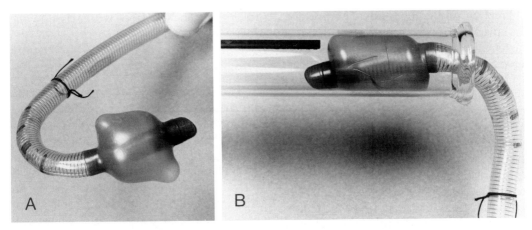

Figure 15.28.   Tracheal tube obstruction secondary to eccentric cuff inflation. **A**, The cuff as removed from the patient. **B**, When placed in a glass tube, the inflated cuff pushes the bevel toward the wall of the tube.

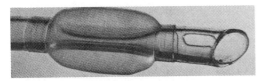

Figure 15.29.   Reduction of tube lumen by cuff. Inflation of the cuff caused narrowing of the tube lumen.

Obstruction from these causes may not occur for some time after initial cuff inflation; as the cuff softens with increased temperature, nitrous oxide diffuses into it.

Cases have been reported for which a feeding tube was connected to the cuff inflation system (648,663,664). This caused the cuff to overdistend and obstruct the tube.

External Compression.   A case has been reported in which a tube was forced through an obstruction in the nose. This caused lateral compression of the tube (665). Another case of compression occurred when a suction catheter became knotted around a tracheal tube (666).

Defective Connector.   If the connector is defective or damaged on insertion, it can partially or completely obstruct the lumen (509,667–672).

Prevention

Prevention of tracheal tube obstruction starts with the choice of tube. Spiral embedded tubes should not be reused. Transparent tubes facilitate identification of material or objects blocking the lumen. Use of a fenestrated (Murphy) tube may avoid some cases of obstruction. A spiral embedded tube may be advisable if an operation involves turning the head or other maneuvers that may induce kinking.

The tracheal tube should be examined carefully before use and the patency of the lumen verified. Foreign bodies inside the lumen can be detected by inserting a stylet. The cuff should be examined to make certain that it is securely attached and inflates symmetrically. The lumen should not be reduced nor should the cuff balloon over the end of the tube when it is inflated. It may be necessary to rotate and examine the tube from several angles to detect obstruction (653). After insertion, the cuff should be inflated as described in "Use of the Tracheal Tube," above. Cuff pressure should be readjusted frequently, especially if nitrous oxide is used. When an x-ray is taken, the position of the orifice and the configuration of the cuff should be examined.

Biting of the tube may be prevented by using an oral airway or a bite block, maintaining an adequate level of anesthesia and securing the tracheal tube at the center of the mouth.

Traction on the tube should be avoided. Kinking of the tube outside the mouth can be prevented by covering the tube with a short piece of a larger tracheal tube (600).

Once inserted, the tube should not be withdrawn while the cuff is inflated, as this may cause the cuff to balloon over the end of the tube.

When secretions are heard, they should be removed with a suction catheter. Humidifying the inspired gases will prevent drying of secretions. This is especially important with long intubations and small tubes. Secretions that cannot be removed in this way may be removed using an embolectomy or Foley catheter (673,674).

Treatment

The occurrence of "bronchospasm" in the middle of an anesthetic should always raise the suspicion of a mechanical problem such as obstruction of the tube. Immediate steps must be taken to reestablish airway patency. If tube patency cannot be reestablished quickly, the tube should be removed.

If there is time, the tube should be checked for kinking, either by feeling with a gloved finger or by direct vision with a laryngoscope. Digital pressure on the site of a kink may relieve the obstruction (674). Alteration of the patient's head position may also help. If these simple maneuvers are unsuccessful, the cuff should be deflated. If the obstruction is still not relieved, the tube should be rotated and the patient's head position adjusted. Passing a fiberscope down the tube will facilitate diagnosis, but complete removal of the tube with replacement is usually warranted as a quicker option. Passage of a suction catheter down the tube is usually not helpful (676).

Aspiration of Gastric Contents

Although it is generally assumed that a tracheal tube will protect the lungs from the entry of foreign material, aspiration to some extent has been found to be a common occurrence in patients with artificial airways (677,678). The incidence is increased by the following factors.

Use of Low-Pressure Cuffs (164,678)

The baseline intracuff pressure at occlusion is significantly lower in high-volume, low-pressure cuffs than low-volume, high-pressure cuffs. Many low-pressure cuffs wrinkle despite proper inflation. Fluid can pass through channels formed along the folds of the cuff. Infolding can be decreased by increasing the pressure in the cuff, using a thin-walled cuff, and using a tube whose cuff diameter at residual volume approximates the internal diameter of the trachea (112,151,161,164). It has been suggested that lubricant jelly applied to the cuff may fill in the folds (164).

Spontaneous Ventilation

Aspiration past high-volume cuffs has been reported in spontaneously breathing patients (161,163,679). With thin-walled cuffs, a negative airway pressure will be transmitted to the cuff during inspiration. In addition, the tracheal tends to dilate during spontaneous inspiration.

Accumulation of Fluid above the Cuff

Frequent suctioning to maintain a clear oropharynx will decrease the pressure exerted by fluid above the cuff. It has been suggested that the cuff be placed just below the vocal cords, reasoning that the shorter the distance between the top of the cuff and the vocal cords, the smaller the volume of fluid that cannot be removed by suctioning. If the cuff is just below the cords, however, movement of the head may cause the tube to move upward, causing the cuff to exert pressure on the cords and increasing the risk of inadvertent extubation. Furthermore, a cuff placed just below the cords may compress nerve endings against the thyroid cartilage, resulting in vocal cord paralysis.

Head-Up Position

If the pharynx is filled with fluid when the patient is in a head-up position, the hydrostatic pressure exerted on the cuff will be higher than if the patient is supine.

Use of Uncuffed Tubes (232)

The incidence of aspiration can be lowered by using PEEP (679).

Misplacement of Other Equipment into the Trachea

A tracheal tube keeps the glottis open, making it easier to pass other equipment into the tracheobronchial tree (165–167,169–171,529,680). Misplaced items have included nasogastric tubes, esophageal stethoscopes, ECG leads, and temperature probes. Connection of the nasogastric tube to suction will cause rapid emptying of the breathing system if the tip is in the trachea. Water should not be used to test the location of a nasogastric tube.

A case has been reported in which a nasogastric tube previously in the stomach was found in the lung after a tracheal tube was changed (681). It was surmised that the nasogastric tube was pulled out of the stomach during the tube change and entered the trachea beside the tracheal tube.

CT Scan Artifact

Artifacts may be seen on a CT scan when radiopaque markers are present on tracheal tubes. Tubes without these markers are available and should be used for this application (682,683).

Accidental Extubation

Accidental dislocation of a tracheal tube from the trachea into the pharynx is at best a nuisance and at worst a life-threatening emergency. It occurs more commonly in smaller patients (684).

Extension or lateral rotation of the neck can cause cephalad movement of the tube and may result in extubation (312,453f,453g,453k,454). The cephalad movement is increased with nasal intubation (261). Certain positions create pull on the tube.

Another cause is improper tube fixation. Secretions, skin oils, and prep solutions can cause the tape to loosen. Securement techniques appropriate to the nature of the surgery or accessibility of the tube are needed to prevent accidental dislodgement. Adhesive tape, benzoin, and stainless-steel wire to secure the tube to the teeth are all tools that may be considered.

Another cause is positioning the cuff between or just below the cords. Distension of the cuff as a result of overinflation or diffusion of nitrous oxide may cause it to herniate upward. This may result in failure to achieve a seal. A likely response is to inject more air into the cuff. If the cuff is at or just above the vocal cords, more air in the cuff may push the tube farther out of the trachea.

Use of antidisconnect devices may increase the danger of inadvertent extubation. It may be preferable for the connection between the tube and the breathing system to give way under strain than to permit the tube to be pulled out.

During insertion, a nasogastric tube may form a loose knot around the tracheal tube, and the tracheal tube may be removed with the nasogastric tube (685). If a mouth gag that has a groove for a tube is used, the tube can become wedged into this groove (657). It may not be possible to remove the gag without removing the tracheal tube.

Prevention of dislodgement begins with the realization that it is a possibility. The tube should be positioned with the tip in the middle third of the trachea with the neck in a neutral position. It has been suggested that manufacturers place a marking 2 to 4 cm from the proximal end of the cuff for positioning at the level of the vocal cords to ensure placement in the middle third of the trachea (301).

Once properly positioned, the tube should be well-secured to avoid subsequent slippage. Fixation to the lower lip may be safer than fixation at the upper lip (312). Pull on the tube should be avoided.

Great care should be taken to avoid accidental extubation during procedures that involve repositioning of the head or neck. Careful observation should be made for air leakage, indicating that the cuff may be located at the level of the vocal cords. A cuff that requires frequent inflation should suggest that it may be situated between instead of below the level of the cords.

Use of an RAE tube may decrease the incidence of accidental extubation (14).

DURING EXTUBATION

Difficulty in Extubation

Difficulty in removing a tracheal tube is a rare yet dangerous problem. The most common cause is inability to deflate the cuff. This is most often due to obstruction of the inflation tube. If the obstruction is distal to the pilot balloon, the balloon will offer no clue that the cuff has not deflated (686). One case has been reported in which heat from a drill melted the inflating tube, occluding both distal and proximal parts (528). Biting by the patient may cause the inflating tube to be occluded (176). Some users pull the pilot balloon and inflation valve from the inflation tube to deflate the cuff. This can cause the inflation tube to seal (687,688).

With a sponge cuff, deflation will be difficult if the inflation tube is cut or detached (176,177). With a spiral embedded tube, air from the cuff may pass into the wall between layers. When the cuff is deflated, air will be trapped in the wall of the tube (73).

The connector may occlude the inflation tube if it fits below the point where the tube leaves the wall of the tracheal tube (74,75,209).

The pilot tube may be kinked by a retaining bandage (689,690). Cases of difficult extubation have been reported in which the inflating tube became twisted around a nasogastric tube or turbinate (691,692). A fold or flange in the cuff may impede extubation (693–698).

Another cause of difficult extubation is surgical transfixion of the tube to adjacent tissue (699–703). In this case, forceably removing the tube could lead to fatal consequences. If a partial cut is made in the tube during maxillofacial surgery, the cut edge can form a barb that makes extubation difficult (535).

In cases in which it is impossible to deflate the cuff, the inflation tube should be cut as close to the tube as possible. If the cuff still remains inflated, the tube should be pulled until the cuff is close to the surface of the vocal cords. A needle can then be inserted through the cricothyroid membrane, puncturing the cuff (704). Alternately, the tube can be withdrawn so that the cuff is seen below the cords and the cuff punctured with a spinal needle (705). Removal may be aided by relaxing the vocal cords and/or rotation of the tube (402,706).

Difficulty in extubation may be the result of a subglottic mass that causes the cuff to hang up (102).

Aspiration at Extubation

Fluid can accumulate in the trachea above the cuff. Pharyngeal suction may not remove all this fluid and it can find its way into the lungs when the cuff is deflated before extubation. To reduce this, it has been recommended that the inflated cuff be withdrawn until it is impinging on the lower surface of the vocal cords (707).

Aspiration can be minimized by placing the patient in a head down and lateral position before cuff deflation and deflating the cuff during the application of positive airway pressure to blow material collected above the cuff into the pharynx where it can be removed by suctioning (see "Removing the Tube," above).

AFTER INTUBATION

Sore Throat

Sore throat is common after intubation. It usually abates within 24 to 48 hr without any special treatment. Persistent symptoms deserve further investigation, which can include laryngoscopy. The reported incidence varies from 6% to 90% of intubations (142,146,341,708–712). It has also been reported in 10% to 22% of nonintubated patients (141,142,146,711). The use of a nasogastric tube is very likely to produce a sore throat (713).

It is more common in females (140,141,535,714), when blood is found in the airway (715), and after operations involving the head and neck or when the patient is in the prone position. Use of larger tubes is associated with a higher incidence of sore throat than the use of smaller tubes (716–718). Some studies have shown a higher incidence with "difficult" intubation, but others have shown no correlation. Straining on the tube may increase the number of complaints (719). Duration of intubation and age have been found to have little effect (140,141,146,718). Limiting intracuff pressure will decrease the incidence of sore throat (192,714).

Studies looking at the effect of topical lidocaine, steroids, and lubricants on the cuff on sore throat offer conflicting evidence (140,142,146,710,711,720–725). Most studies show that an increase in cuff-to-trachea contact area increases sore throat (109, 143,146,414,718,722,726), although one study showed conflicting results (727). The incidence is quite high with the sponge cuff (109).

Hoarseness

The incidence of hoarseness following intubation for surgical procedures has been reported as being between 4% and 67% (717,720,723,728,729). Its incidence may be decreased by use of tubes with low-pressure cuffs, smaller tubes, and lubrication with lidocaine jelly (717,720,730), and the incidence may be increased with difficult intubation and duration of intubation.

Nerve Injuries

Numbness of the face and tongue on one side of the face has been reported in a patient placed in the prone position (731). It is postulated that the etiology was compression of the buccal and lingual nerves between the tube and the ramus of the jaw. Trigeminal nerve damage has been reported (732).

Laryngeal Edema

Edema may occur anywhere along the path of the tube, including the uvula, epiglottis, aryepiglottic folds, ventricular folds, vocal cords, and the retroarytenoid and subglottic spaces (159,361,733–736). Laryngeal edema is also called postintubation croup, uvular edema postintubation inflammation, acute edematous stenosis, stridor, and subglottic edema.

The edema encroaches on the airway lumen, increasing airway resistance. This is especially so in the young child, in whom there is a disproportionate increase in resistance with a decrease in the lumen. Because the cricoid cartilage completely surrounds the subglottic region, no external expansion of the swollen tissues may occur and subglottic edema not infrequently necessitates emergency reintubation or tracheostomy.

Acute laryngeal edema has a peak incidence between 1 and 4 years of age (737). It is most commonly seen after surgery involving the head and neck and surgery performed with the patient positioned other than supine. It is more common in adult females than adult males (738).

Presentation

Acute edema may manifest itself any time during the first 48 hr after extubation. Usually, the first signs are evident 1 to 2 hr postoperatively. In its mildest form, there is hoarseness or croupy cough. In more severe cases, respiratory obstruction will occur. Decompensation can be rapid.

Etiologies (737)

Inflammation.   Inflammatory conditions include preexisting inflammation of the larynx, bacterial contamination, and chemical irritation.

Mechanical Trauma.   Trauma during intubation may result from inadequate anesthesia or muscle relaxation, roughness, or trying to insert too large a tube. Excessive motion secondary to rotation of the head, bucking, and swallowing will contribute to the mechanical irritation.

Allergy.   An allergic reaction to the tube itself or materials used in lubrication or sterilization has been postulated as a mechanism.

Prevention

Prevention begins with avoiding irritant stimuli, particularly an oversize tracheal tube. If there is an upper respiratory infection, use of a face mask should be strongly considered. Tubes, sprays, and lubricants used on the tubes should be sterile. Intubation should be atraumatic and adequate anesthetic depth and/or good muscle relaxation should be maintained to prevent movement of the tube. Movements of the head should be kept to a minimum. Most studies show that cortiocosteroids are not useful in preventing laryngeal edema (738–740).

Treatment

Aggressive treatment with racemic epinephrine and humidified oxygen are indicated. Use of a helium-oxygen mixture may be of benefit.

Vocal Cord Paralysis

Vocal cord paralysis and paresis have been reported after tracheal intubation in spite of the intubation being atraumatic and the site of the surgery being unrelated to the neck area (332,511,741–755).

It can be unilateral or bilateral. It may originate from pressure exerted by the distended cuff on branches of the recurrent laryngeal nerve (741,743,746,756). The most susceptible area of the nerve is thought to be 6 to 10 mm below the vocal cords (301,744). Placing the cuff at least 1.5 cm below the cords should reduce the incidence (469,756). Nasogastric tubes and esophageal stethoscopes can cause posterior cricoid inflammation with resultant vocal cord paralysis (755,757). It has been reported with both high- and low-pressure cuffs.

Hoarseness and mild aspiration may occur after unilateral paralysis. With bilateral paralysis, signs of airway obstruction may follow immediately after extubation or be delayed for several hours. The usual maneuvers to relieve obstruction (neck extension, insertion of an airway, and jaw lift) will be ineffective (333). Laryngoscopy will reveal motionless vocal cords that remain adducted. Obstruction may be relieved by positive pressure ventilation by mask, but reintubation is the definitive treatment. Most cases of vocal cord dysfunction resolve spontaneously, usually within days or weeks (755).

Ulcerations

Ulcerations (erosions) of the larynx and trachea can occur secondary to intubation trauma or while the tube is in place. They are very common, even when a tube has been in place for only a short time. The incidence and severity increase with the duration of intubation.

Ulcers are commonly found on the posterior parts of the larynx and the anterior and lateral aspects of the trachea at the sites of the cuff and the tube tip (449,758–760). They vary from superficial lesions involving only the mucosa to deep ones in which the underlying cartilage is exposed. The end result will depend on the location and severity as well as other factors, such as infection, that affect the healing process. If the ulcers are superficial, i.e., when the basement membrane is intact, regeneration to normal epithelium occurs relatively quickly (761). When the damage is deeper, the regeneration follows the same pattern as for the superficial damage but is more protracted. If the ulcer is very deep, scar tissue may form. Tracheal ulcers may result in the normal ciliated epithelium being replaced with a stratified squamous epithelium with postextubation arrest of mucus transport. An ulcer may erode into a vessel or through the wall of the trachea. Symptoms of ulceration include pain and hoarseness. Vocal exertion usually aggravates these symptoms.

Use of low-pressure cuffs for long-term intubation will reduce (but not eliminate) the incidence and severity of ulcerations at the cuff level. Use of a flexible tube from the Y piece to the tube will allow free movement of the patient's head and neck and reduce movement between the trachea and the tube.

Granuloma of the Vocal Cord

The incidence of granuloma of the vocal cords (also called postintubation granuloma, contact ulcer granuloma, intubation granuloma, or postanesthesia granuloma) varies from 1 in 800 to 1 in 20,000 intubations. Most cases are in adults, and they are more common in women than men, but occur only rarely in children. The highest incidence is associated with head and neck surgery.

The most common location is on the posterior portions of the cords on or near the vocal processes of the arytenoid cartilages. The lesions are usually unilateral.

The initial lesion is believed to be an ulcer. Granulation tissue forms and develops into a sessile lesion.

Symptoms commonly include persistent hoarseness, intermittent loss of voice, pain or discomfort in the throat, a feeling of fullness or tension in the throat, chronic cough, hemoptysis, and pain extending to the ear. Some cases are symptomless. Occasionally, respiratory obstruction with dyspnea and cyanosis occur. Symptoms may start after in-

tubation or may not develop for as long as several months.

A number of prophylactic measures have been suggested, including use of a proper sized tube and gentle atraumatic intubation as well as avoiding friction between the tube and larynx by a proper depth of anesthesia or use of muscle relaxants. A short period of vocal rest succeeding every intubation has been recommended (762).

Persistent hoarseness after intubation warrants laryngeal examination to exclude the presence of a lesion. If the examination reveals ulceration over the vocal processes, the development of a granuloma may be prevented by strict voice rest to allow healing to take place.

The granuloma may heal spontaneously and removal should be postponed until it is apparent this is not going to take place, unless the granuloma interferes with respiration. Operative removal is most likely to be successful when the lesion has reached the pedunculated stage. Attempts at removal during the sessile stage should be avoided unless there is respiratory embarrassment, as recurrence is likely.

Laryngotracheal Membrane

Formation of a laryngotracheal membrane (subglottic membrane, membranous or pseudomembranous laryngotracheitis, or pseudomembrane) is a relatively uncommon but serious and sometimes fatal complication, as a portion of the membrane may become detached, leading to sudden respiratory obstruction (763–765). Most cases follow an intubation lasting a few hours. In some cases, the intubation was traumatic, but in others, no problems were encountered. Clinically, the picture is one of respiratory obstruction, resembling laryngeal edema with cough, hoarseness, stridor, dyspnea, and suprasternal retractions. The symptoms typically occur later than those associated with edema, usually 24 to 72 hr after extubation (763–765).

If this is not immediately and appropriately treated, it may lead to sudden death. Diagnosis is made by laryngoscopy, followed by bronchoscopy. Unless visualization of the larynx is performed, the condition may be erroneously diagnosed as edema, and an unnecessary tracheostomy may be performed.

Treatment is removal by suction. Removal may not be easy because areas of epithelium still attached to the underlying tissue may be present. If the entire membrane is not removed, it may recur in 24 hr (763).

Glottic and Subglottic Granulation Tissue

Ulcers in the subglottic region may give rise to granulation tissue (18,159,766–770). Their principal importance is that they may cause respiratory obstruction. The onset of symptoms may be immediately after extubation or may be delayed for up to several weeks.

Diagnosis is made by laryngoscopy and/or bronchoscopy. Steroids should be administered. Usually, the granulation tissue will regress and may disappear, but occasionally removal is required. Recurrence is quite common so that repeat bronchoscopies may be necessary.

Nasal Damage

Ulcerations or necrosis of the nasal alae and/or the skin on the bridge of the nose are occasional sequelae of nasotracheal intubation (771,772). This can be prevented by securing the tube so that there is no undue pressure on the nostril (see Fig. 15.24).

Double-Lumen Bronchial Tubes

A double-lumen tube (DLT) is used when it is desired to isolate one lung from the other. Their use has increased greatly with the introduction of disposable plastic tubes and fiberoptic bronchoscopy, which makes location under direct vision possible.

INDICATIONS (723)

Pulmonary Surgical Procedures (774–776)

Intrathoracic surgery performed with the operative lung deflated provides better operating conditions and reduces trauma to the operative lung. The ability to alternate easily and quickly between lung collapse and inflation can help the surgeon to visualize lung morphology and facilitates identification of lobar or intersegmental planes. By improving operative conditions, use of a DLT may shorten surgical time.

Thoracoscopy (777)

Examination of the pleural space (thoracoscopy) is facilitated by deflation of the lung.

Control of Contamination

In situations in which there is contamination in one lung, it may be desirable to isolate that process from the other lung. Placing the patient with the diseased side up for surgery carries the risk that infected material may drain into the dependent lung (775,778,779). Use of a DLT can prevent this.

Control of Hemorrhage (774,775,780)

Hemorrhage can occur in one lung from surgery or trauma, rupture of the pulmonary artery by a Swan-Ganz catheter, or an arteriovenous aneurysm. With a DLT, ventilation can be maintained with the unaffected lung until definitive surgery can be performed.

Bronchopleural or Bronchopleuralcutaneous Fistula or Air Cyst (774,779–783)

A bronchopleural fistula may have such a low resistance to gas flow that most of the tidal volume will flow through the low-resistance pathway and it will be impossible to ventilate the other lung adequately. A unilateral air cyst or bulla may have a valvular opening and can become overinflated when controlled breathing is initiated. A DLT allows isolation of the lung or section of that lung with the fistula or cyst from the ventilatory volume (784).

Tracheobronchial Tree Disruption

Positive pressure ventilation of a lung with a tracheobronchial tree disruption can result in dissection of gas into the pulmonary interstitial spaces or the mediastinum. Use of a DLT allows isolation of the section with the disruption.

Other Indications

Independent (differential) lung ventilation may be useful in the treatment of unilateral pulmonary pathology (785–789). Unilateral bronchopulmonary lavage and selective pulmonary toilet can be performed using a DLT.

CONTRAINDICATIONS (773)

Relative contraindications to the use of DLTs include patients who are at risk of aspiration, patients who have a lesion (airway stricture or endoluminal tumor) somewhere along the pathway of the DLT, small patients in whom a DLT would be too large, patients who will not tolerate being taken off mechanical ventilation even for a short period of time, and those with life-threatening hemorrhage in whom there is insufficient time to insert a DLT.

ANATOMICAL CONSIDERATIONS

The right mainstem bronchus is shorter, straighter, and has a larger diameter than the left. It takes off from the trachea at an angle of 25° in adults. The left mainstem bronchus diverges from the median plane at a 45° angle (773). These angles are slightly larger in children (790).

These anatomic considerations mean that it is easier to intubate the right mainstem bronchus than the left. However, it is difficult to place a tube in the right mainstem bronchus without obstructing the right upper lobe orifice.

DESIGN OF DOUBLE-LUMEN TUBES

Connector (788,791–793)

The connector must allow attachment of the two lumens to the breathing system as well as one-lung ventilation, suctioning of one lung at a time, differential ventilation of each lung, application of PEEP to only one lung (with or without tidal ventilation), differential PEEP to both lungs, and one-lung fiberoptic bronchoscopy. Typical connectors are shown in Figures 15.30, 15.33, 15.36, and 15.38.

Tube

The earliest DLTs were made from red rubber. Then single-use DLTs made from PVC became available. PVC tubes are supplied in sterile packages, which include a special intubation stylet, connectors, suction catheters, and sometimes a device to supply continuous positive airway pressure.

The DLT is essentially two tubes bonded together. The tracheal lumen is designed to terminate above the carina and the bronchial segment to extend into the appropriate mainstem bronchus. The distal portion of the bronchial segment is angled to fit into the bronchus for which it is intended. A double-lumen tube is either right- or left-sided, depending on which bronchus the bronchial segment is designed to fit.

There may be a carinal hook to aid in proper placement and to minimize tube movement after placement. Potential problems with carinal hooks include increased difficulty during intubation, trauma to the airway, malposition of the tube because of the hook, and interference with bronchial closure during pneumonectomy (773,794,795). The carinal hook can break off and become lost in the bronchial tree.

Most manufacturers place radiopaque markers at the bottom of the tracheal cuff or at the end of the tracheal lumens. Other marks may be placed above and below the bronchial cuff.

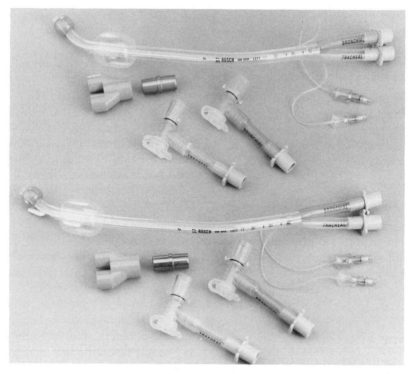

Figure 15.30. Double-lumen tubes with connectors and adaptors for use. *Top,* Robertshaw left DLT. *Bottom,* Carlens DLT. Note the carinal hook. Courtesy of Rusch, Inc.

Cuffs

There are at least two cuffs on each tube. The tracheal cuff is located just above the tracheal orifice and the bronchial cuff just above the termination of the bronchial segment. Some right-sided DLTs have two bronchial cuffs. The bronchial cuff is shorter than the tracheal cuff and causes separation and sealing off of the two lungs from each other. The tracheal cuff has the same function as a cuff on a single-lumen tracheal tube. The bronchial cuff for the right-sided tubes varies in shape, depending on the manufacturer. On some tubes, the cuff has a slot to allow for ventilation of the right upper lobe. Most manufacturers color the bronchial cuff blue. Each cuff has its own inflation system appropriately marked so that it is easy to determine which cuff is being inflated. If the bronchial cuff is blue, there will usually be blue markings on the pilot balloon and/or the inflation device or they may be colored blue.

MARGIN OF SAFETY IN POSITIONING DOUBLE-LUMEN TUBES (796–798)

The length of the tracheobronchial tree between the most distal and proximal acceptable positions for a DLT is called the margin of safety (796,797). It is the length that the tube may be moved without obstructing a conducting airway.

The margin of safety will depend on the length of the lumen into which the cuff is placed and the width of the cuff. If the cuff is narrow or the mainstem bronchus long, the margin of safety will be wider. This does not apply to slotted cuffs in which the margin of safety is related to the length of the slot. The margin of safety will be smaller in females, because the mainstem bronchus is shorter.

Left-Sided Tubes

The outermost acceptable position is when the bronchial cuff is just below the carina. If the tube were pulled farther out, the bronchial cuff could progressively fill the space above the carina and obstruct the trachea and contralateral (right) mainstem bronchus. The most distal acceptable position of a left-sided tube is when the tip of the left lumen is at the proximal edge of the upper lobe bronchial orifice. Further insertion will result in obstruction of the left upper lobe bronchus. The margin of safety is the difference between these outermost and innermost acceptable positions.

Right-Sided Tubes

The margin of safety is defined somewhat differently for right-sided tubes. A right-sided DLT is acceptably positioned if the right upper lobe ventilation slot is aligned with the right upper lobe orifice (773). Thus the margin of safety is the length of the ventilation slot minus the diameter of the right upper lobe orifice. The margin of safety is considerably smaller in right-sided tubes than left-sided ones.

SPECIFIC TUBES

Because of the anatomical differences between the right and left mainstem bronchi, right- and left-sided tubes differ, notably in the degree of angulation of the distal portion of the tube and the design of the bronchial cuff. In addition, the various available tubes have different features and the margin of safety varies with each tube.

Carlens Double-Lumen Tube (775,799,800)

The Carlens double-lumen tube (Fig. 5.31 and also see Fig. 15.30) was the first double-lumen tube used for one-lung ventilation. It was intended for insertion into the left main bronchus. It has a carinal hook.

It was first made of red rubber. Later, a single-use PVC version became available. It is similar in design to the red rubber version, except that the cuffs are low pressure. The margin of safety in positioning a Carlens tube varies from 18 to 23 mm in females and 22 to 27 mm in males (773).

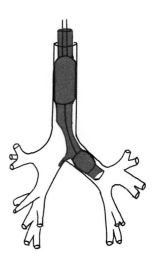

Figure 15.31. Carlens double-lumen tube designed for insertion into the left main bronchus. Note the carinal hook.

White Double-Lumen Tube (801,802)

The White DLT is designed to fit the right mainstem bronchus. It may be made of red rubber (Fig. 15.32) or PVC (Fig. 15.33). There is a carinal hook. On the red rubber version, the bronchial cuff has a slot to correspond to the position of the right upper lobe bronchus. On the PVC version, the cuff for the right mainstem bronchus is circumferential superior to the opening to the right upper lobe bronchus and continues distally behind the opening. This pushes the tube toward the wall of the bronchus.

Robertshaw Left Double-Lumen Tube (774,803,804)

The Robertshaw left DLT was originally made of red rubber (Fig. 15.34). Later single-use tubes made of PVC became available (see Fig. 15.30). It differs from the Carlens tube in that the lumens are larger (while the outside diameter is the same) and D shaped, there is no carinal hook, and it has a more molded curvature to prevent kinking. The angle of the bronchial portion is 40°. Studies have found that the margin of safety varies from 12 to 23 mm in females and from 16 to 27 mm in males (773,799).

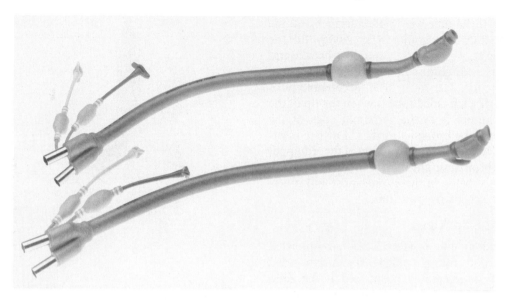

Figure 15.32.   Red rubber double-lumen tubes. *Top,* Robertshaw right DLT. *Bottom,* White DLT. Courtesy of Rusch, Inc.

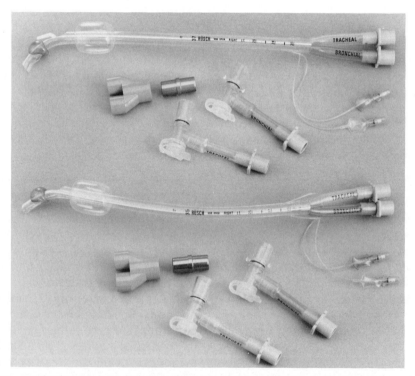

Figure 15.33.   *Top,* PVC White DLT. Note that the cuff is different from that on the red rubber version. *Bottom,* Robertshaw right DLT. Courtesy of Rusch, Inc.

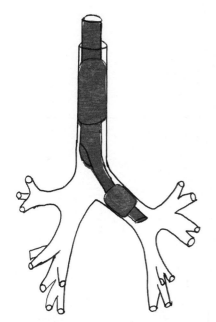

Figure 15.34. Robertshaw left DLT. The angle of the bronchial portion is 40°.

Robertshaw Right Double-Lumen Tube

The Robertshaw right DLT (Fig. 15.35) is available in both red rubber (see Fig. 15.32) and PVC (see Fig. 15.33) and in the same sizes as the left-sided tube. The angle of the bronchial portion is 20°. The bronchial cuff has a slotted opening in the lateral aspect that, when properly positioned, is adjacent to the lumen of the right upper lobe. The right upper lobe slot of the PVC tube is of smaller diameter than that of the red rubber version and, rather than surrounding the slot, the cuff lies proximal to the slot on the lateral surface and extends tangentially toward the medial surface (2,805). The cuff pushes the tube closer to the wall of the bronchus where the upper lobe takes off to effect a more reliable seal. The reported margin of safety in positioning a right-sided Robertshaw tube has been reported to be 11 mm (773,798) or 1 to 4 mm (797).

One study found that when the right-sided red rubber Robertshaw tube was inserted blindly there was a very low incidence of right upper lobe obstruction, and right upper lobe obstruction occurred less frequently

than with right Broncho-Cath tubes (805). Another study found that in more than 90% of cases satisfactory positioning of this tube could be achieved without use of a fiberscope (800).

Broncho-Cath Right-Sided Tube

The Broncho-Cath right-sided tube differs from other right-sided DLTs in the design of the bronchial cuff, which has roughly the shape of an *S*, or a slanted doughnut, with the edge of the cuff nearest the right upper lobe bronchus closer to the trachea than the part of the cuff touching the medial bronchial wall (Figs. 15.37 and 15.38). A slot in the tube just beyond the cuff roughly corresponds to the opening of the right upper lobe bronchus (796).

The margin of safety in positioning was found to be 9 mm in males and 5 mm in females in one study (797) and 1 mm in another (773,798). However, it should be noted that the unique slanted doughnut shape of the right bronchial cuff allows the right upper lobe ventilation slot to ride off the right upper lobe orifice, thereby increasing the margin of

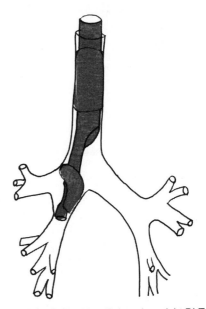

Figure 15.35. Red rubber Robertshaw right DLT. The angle of the portion is 20°. The bronchial cuff has a slot in the lateral aspect.

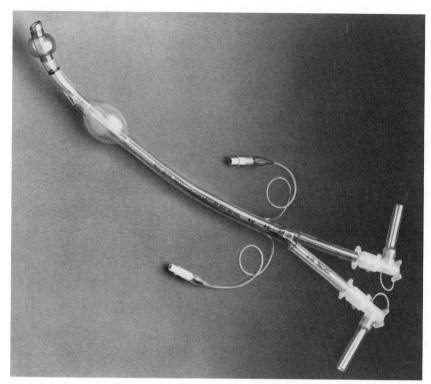

Figure 15.36. Broncho-Cath left DLT. Courtesy of Mallinckrodt Medical, Inc.

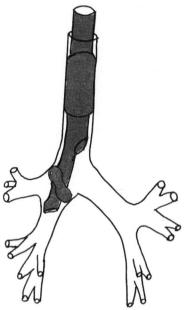

Figure 15.37. Broncho-Cath right DLT. The bronchial cuff has the shape of an *S* or a slanted doughnut, with the edge of the cuff nearest the right upper lobe bron-

safety with this tube (773). One study found that when this tube was inserted blindly, right upper lobe obstruction occurred in 89% of cases (805).

Broncho-Cath Left-Sided Tube (774)

The Broncho-Cath left-sided DLT is similar to the right sided model (see Fig. 15.36). It is available with a carinal hook (806). The bronchial portion of the tube is at an angle of approximately 35° and extends approximately 4.5 cm beyond the tracheal cuff. The margin of safety for placement of this tube has been reported to be approximately 20 mm in males and 15 mm in females in one study (797) and 21 to 25 in females and 25 to 29 in males in two others (773,798).

chus closer to the trachea than the part of the cuff touching the medial bronchial wall. A slot in the tube beyond the cuff corresponds to the opening of the right upper lobe bronchus.

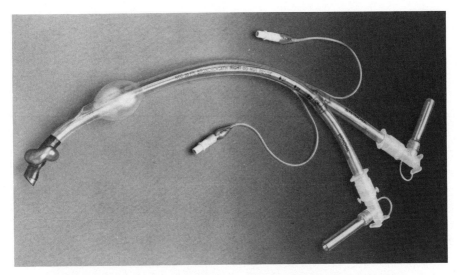

Figure 15.38.   Broncho-Cath right DLT. Courtesy of Mallinckrodt Medical, Inc.

A study comparing this tube with red rubber Carlens and Robertshaw tubes found that there were fewer difficulties with insertion and fewer complications with the Broncho-Cath tube (774).

Sher-i-Bronch Left-Sided Double-Lumen Tube

The Sher-i-Bronch left-sided DLT is similar to other left-sided DLTs (Fig. 15.39*A*). The bronchial segment diverges from the main tube at an angle of 34°. The average margin of safety is reported to be 14 mm in females and 19 mm in males (797).

Sher-i-Bronch Right-Sided Double-Lumen Tube

The Sher-i-Bronch right-sided DLT has two narrow 5-mm cuffs on the bronchial segment, proximal and distal to the right upper lobe ventilation slot, which is 13 to 14 mm long (Fig. 15.40 and see Fig. 15.39). The narrow proximal cuff fits the short right mainstem bronchus (796). In a study comparing the right-sided Sher-i-Bronch with the right-sided Robertshaw and Bronch-Cath tubes, the Sher-i-Bronch was found to provide satisfactory ventilation in the greatest number of cases (807).

TECHNIQUES (809)

Choice of Tube

Right Versus Left

When surgery is performed on the right lung, a left-sided DLT should be used. When surgery is performed on the left lung, either a left- or right-sided DLT may be used.

Because the margin of safety in positioning a right-sided DLT is so small, use of a right-sided DLT for left lung surgery introduces the risk of either blockade of the right upper lobe or the left lung (809). For this reason many people prefer to use a left-sided DLT for left lung surgery (2,797,798,810). During left pneumonectomy, immediately before the time the left mainstem bronchus is clamped, the DLT can be pulled from the bronchus under the surgeon's guidance and can continue to be used for ventilating the remaining right lung. A disadvantage of this technique is the potential risk of decannulation during surgical retraction and manipulation. Because of this some anesthesiologists routinely use right-sided DLTs for left thoracotomies (811).

Other workers believe that avoiding the use of right-sided DLTs is not desirable be-

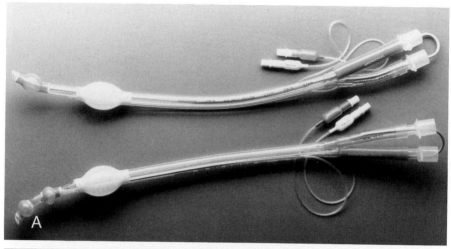

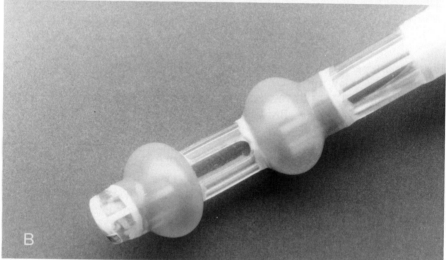

Figure 15.39. Sher-i-Bronch double-lumen tubes. **A,** *Top,* Left-sided tube. *Bottom,* Right-sided tube. **B,** Close-up of right bronchial segment, showing opening to the right upper lobe. Courtesy of Sheridan, Inc.

cause intubation of the nonoperative bronchus ensures surgical access to the entire ipsilateral bronchial tree and eliminates the need for intraoperative tube manipulation should access to the proximal mainstem bronchus be necessary. Moreover, retraction and parenchymal manipulation by the surgeon are unlikely to dislodge or obstruct a tube that lies in the contralateral bronchus.

A right-sided DLT must be used for left lung surgery when there is rupture of the left mainstem bronchus; a lesion in the left mainstem bronchus or the carina; stenosis or compression of the left mainstem bronchus; or distortion of the left mainstem bronchus by either a left lower lobe or left upper lobe tumor, causing the left mainstem bronchus to take off from the trachea at a sharp angle (812).

Size

For adults, both left and right PVC DLTs are available in four sizes: 35 F, 37 F, 39 F,

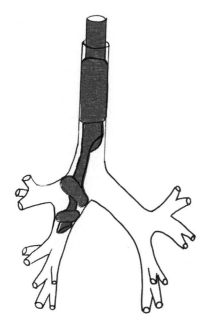

Figure 15.40.   Sher-i-Bronch right DLT. Note the two cuffs proximal and distal to the opening to the right upper lobe.

and 41 F. Most authors recommend using the largest size that can be easily inserted past the glottis. A 35 F tube has been used in children as small as 40 kg without complications (813). A 28 F PVC DLT is available for use in smaller patients.

A large DLT will reduce resistance to flow, facilitate suctioning and passage of a fiberscope, and reduce the chance of advancing the DLT too far down the bronchus. Less air will be needed in the cuffs so there is less chance of pressure damage to the airway. If too small a tube is used, the large endobronchial cuff seal tends to force the entire DLT cephalad, making a functional bronchial seal more difficult.

For adult men, a 41 F DLT is usually used and a 39 F tube for adult women. Rarely is there an indication for a 35 F DLT in adult patients (794). However, inability to introduce a larger tube through the larynx or past the carina or intrinsic or extrinsic obstruction of the mainstem bronchus to be intubated may necessitate use of a smaller tube.

Procedures Before Insertion

The tracheal and bronchial cuffs should be inflated with air and tested for leaks and asymmetrical inflation, making certain that each inflation tube is associated with the proper cuff. The tube and stylet should be lubricated, and the stylet should be placed in the bronchial lumen, making certain that when it is fully inserted it does not extend beyond the tip. If a less-than-optimal view of the larynx is anticipated, the stylet should be left in the lumen. If not, it can be removed and reinserted if needed. The connector should be assembled so that it can be quickly fitted to the tube and the breathing system after intubation.

Insertion

Intubation is performed under direct vision with a rigid laryngoscope. The tube is inserted with the bronchial segment concave anteriorly. This places the tube at a 90° angle from where it will eventually rest. After the tip of the tube has passed the cords, the stylet, if present, should be removed. After the bronchial cuff has passed the cords, the tube is turned 90° so that the bronchial portion points toward the appropriate bronchus. If the tube is to be placed in the left mainstem bronchus, the head and neck should be rotated to the right before rotating and advancing the tube (814,815).

A tube with a carinal hook is inserted with the bronchial segment pointing anteriorly until the bronchial cuff passes the cords. The tube is then rotated 180° so that the hook is anterior. After the hook has passed the vocal cords, the tube is rotated 90° so that the bronchial segment is directed toward the appropriate bronchus (816). The tube is advanced until the hook is engaged by the carina. The hook can be tied closely to the tube with a slip knot to facilitate passage through the larynx, then untied (775).

The tube is advanced until moderate resistance is encountered, or the common two-lumen molding is 1 to 2 cm proximal to the teeth (809). One study found that the average depth of insertion for both male and female patients 170 cm tall was 29 cm and for each 10-cm increase or decrease in height, average placement depth was increased or decreased 1 cm (817).

A DLT can also be placed by inserting a fiberscope into the bronchial lumen and directing it into the appropriate bronchus under direct vision (773,809,818–822). This avoids traumatizing the bronchus or inserting the tube too deeply and ensures that the correct bronchus is intubated on the first attempt. Inserting the fiberscope through a lumen with a self-sealing diaphragm allows ventilation to continue while the fiberscope is in place.

Another technique is to place a well-lubricated, malleable bougie into the correct mainstem bronchus under direct vision using a rigid ventilating bronchoscope (810). The DLT is then inserted over the bougie.

A double-lumen tube can be inserted into a patient with a tracheostomy (823–825). The tracheal cuff may be at the tracheal stoma or lie partly outside the trachea.

Cuff Inflation

Once the tube tip is thought to be in a mainstem bronchus, both cuffs should be inflated. The tracheal cuff should be inflated in a manner similar to that on a tracheal tube.

It is more difficult to inflate the bronchial cuff correctly. Rarely is more than 3 ml required (813). An overinflated bronchial cuff may herniate into the trachea, cause the carina to be pushed toward the opposite side, or result in narrowing of the bronchial segment lumen. One technique is first to inflate the tracheal cuff. The tracheal lumen is then opened to atmosphere. Air is then placed into the bronchial cuff until there is cessation of leak through the open tracheal lumen (773, 836).

A useful technique when the bronchial lumen is in the lung being operated on is to pass a suction catheter through the bronchial lumen when the lung is deflated and leave it

until ready for reinflation (811). This will prevent the bronchial lumen from becoming obstructed by blood or mucus. The catheter must be removed before application of bronchial staples or it may become trapped.

Confirmation of Position

Correct positioning of a double-lumen tube is critical in ensuring that one-lung ventilation proceeds smoothly. If the double-lumen tube is in the correct position, the operative nondependent lung will collapse completely and easily, the surgeon will be able to work efficiently without damaging the operative lung, and the dependent lung will be unobstructed and easy to ventilate (809,827).

When correctly placed, the opening of the tracheal lumen should lie 1 to 2 cm above the carina. The tip of the bronchial lumen should be sufficiently far down the appropriate bronchus that its cuff does not project into the carina, yet not so far down the bronchus as to occlude the upper lobe bronchus on that side.

Whatever method of placement confirmation is used, the entire procedure should be repeated if the position of the head or body is changed, because the tube position can easily change (828,829).

Auscultatory Techniques (800,813,830)

Left-Sided Tubes. With the tracheal cuff inflated and the tracheal lumen connected to the breathing system, both lungs should be auscultated as the reservoir bag is compressed. Auscultation should be performed in the axillary regions and over the upper lung fields to detect differences that might indicate regional hypoventilation. Next, the bronchial cuff should be inflated and both lumens connected to the breathing system. Auscultation should then be repeated.

Next, the tracheal lumen should be occluded with a surgical clamp. Breath sounds should be heard only over the left lung. If breath sounds are heard bilaterally, the tube is too high in the trachea. Both cuffs should be deflated and the tube advanced. If breath sounds are heard only over the right lung, the bronchial lumen is on the right side. If this is the case, both cuffs should deflated, the tube withdrawn until its distal end is above the carina, rotated, then reinserted. The steps outlined above should be repeated.

The bronchial lumen is then clamped, and the patient is ventilated through the tracheal lumen. If the tube is in good position, breath sounds should be heard only over the right lung. If there is marked resistance to ventilation, the tube is either too far into the left bronchus or not deep enough. The tube's position can be determined by deflating the bronchial cuff while continuing to ventilate through the tracheal lumen with the bronchial lumen clamped. If the tip is too deep in the left bronchus, breath sounds will be heard only on the left side. If the tube is not deep enough in the bronchus, breath sounds will be present bilaterally. Depending on where breath sounds are now heard, the tracheal cuff also should be deflated and the tube pulled back or advanced. Both cuffs should be reinflated and the auscultatory sequence repeated.

One of the lumens of the tube should be opened to air and the connector tubing to that side clamped. Breath sounds should be present in the side which is intended to be ventilated. This should be repeated for the opposite side. If after clamping the left bronchial lumen there is difficult ventilation through the tracheal lumen with a marked resistance to air flow, the tube is either too far into the left lumen or not deep enough (830). To determine which, the bronchial lumen should be clamped and ventilation through the tracheal lumen continued. If the tube is too deep in the bronchus, breath sounds will be heard on the left side only. If the tube is not deep enough, breath sounds will be heard bilaterally (830).

Right-Sided Tubes.   Placement of a right double-lumen tube is similar to that of a left-sided one. The important difference is placement in relation to the right upper lobe bron-chus. As has been pointed out, the right upper lobe takes off close to the origin of the right mainstem bronchus. Right double-lumen tubes have certain design features that take into account the anatomical features of the right mainstem bronchus. In spite of the specialized design of right double lumen tubes, the margin of safety is small. After the tube has been placed, auscultation needs to be performed to confirm ventilation of the right upper lobe.

Fiberoptic Techniques

Unfortunately, auscultation maneuvers detect DLT malposition only part of the time because breath sounds can be transmitted from one region of the lung to adjacent areas. Studies have found that DLTs were malpositioned to some extent in as many as 48% of intubations thought to be positioned correctly by auscultation (831,832). A problem with auscultation is that, even if the tube is correctly placed initially, once the patient is prepped and draped the chest is no longer available for auscultation. Another study found that malpositions detected by fiberoptic techniques but not auscultation did not necessarily correlate with poor arterial oxygenation during one-lung anesthesia (833). When positioning of a DLT is checked only by clinical signs, 25% of the time there will be intraoperative problems (804).

Fiberoptic bronchoscopy is the most accurate way to determine DLT position. Many authors believe that fiberoptic confirmation of position of a DLT should be routine (776,831,834). Whenever there is any doubt as to the precise location of the DLT, a fiberscope should be used to check the position (835).

A 4.9-mm-OD fiberscope will not pass down a 35 French tube and is a tight squeeze through a 37 French tube. A pediatric fiberscope (outside diameter less than 4.3 mm) can be passed down the lumens of all adult-size DLTs (773).

Disadvantages of routine fiberscopic evaluation of tube position are that it is time-consuming, requires special equipment and operator experience, and introduces an added source of airway trauma.

Another use for a fiberscope is to act as a light wand to aid in identifying the stump of a disconnected bronchus (776).

Left-Sided Tubes. A small fiberscope is placed in the tracheal lumen (836). The scope may be introduced through the open end of the tube or through a port in the connector specially designed for this purpose.

As the fiberscope is advanced, the carina should come into view. The bronchial portion of the DLT should be seen on the left advancing into the left mainstem bronchus. The top surface of the blue bronchial cuff should be seen just below the carina. However, the bronchial cuff should not herniate over the carina, nor should the carina be pushed over to the right. An unobstructed view of the nonintubated right mainstem bronchus should be obtained.

The fiberscope should then be advanced through the bronchial lumen to check for absence of narrowing of the lumen at the level of the cuff and an unobstructed view of the distal bronchial tree. Failure to check the bronchial lumen may result in problems (837).

Right Sided Tubes. Looking down the left (tracheal) lumen, tube placement needs to be confirmed in the right mainstem bronchus by visualizing the upper surface of the bronchial cuff. The fiberscope is then placed in the right lumen. The right middle-lower lobe bronchial carina distal to the end of the tube should be visualized. The right upper lobe lumen should be located. The endoscopist should be able to look directly into the right upper lobe orifice by flexing the tip of the fiberscope superiorly. There should be no overriding of the right upper lobe ventilation lumen on the bronchial mucosa, and the mucosa should not be covering any part of the lumen.

End-Tidal Carbon Dioxide Techniques

Capnography can be used to check positioning of a double-lumen tube (838). Cap-

nometers attached to each lumen should show synchronous waveforms that are similar in shape and size.

Chext X-Ray

Confirmation of position by chest x-ray may be useful when a fiberscope is not available or for some reason cannot be used. However, it is less precise than the fiberoptic bronchoscopy, is time-consuming, is costly, is awkward to perform, and may dislodge the tube (773).

Stabilization of the Tube

Once the tube has been confirmed to be in the correct position, it should be stabilized at the face. The bronchial cuff should be kept deflated until the lung is isolated or collapsed to minimize pressure damage to the bronchial mucosa.

A determined effort should be made to prevent dislodgement of the tube during turning by holding onto the tube at the level of the incisors and keeping the head immobile or in a neutral or slightly flexed position.

Intraoperative Manipulation (839,840)

It may be possible for the surgeon to assist in correct placement once the chest is open. If it is determined that the tube is in the wrong bronchus, both cuffs are deflated and the tube is withdrawn into the trachea. The surgeon then compresses the bronchus, and the anesthesiologist advances the tube into the correct side under digital surgical guidance. The cuffs are then reinflated. Similar manipulations can be performed if the tube is in the correct bronchus but not in the correct position.

Use of a Left DLT for Left Lung Surgery (774,775,830)

A number of anesthesia personnel prefer to use a left double-lumen tube for left-sided surgery because of the difficulty in placing a right double-lumen tube accurately, provided there is no tumor involving the left mainstem bronchus. Such a tube can be used in procedures below the tip of the tube. If a left pneumonectomy is to be performed, a left DLT can be used until the left mainstem bronchus is to be clamped. At this point, both cuffs are deflated and the tube is pulled back until the tip clears the left bronchus. The tracheal cuff is then reinflated, and the tube is used as a standard tracheal tube.

Replacement of a Double-Lumen Tube with a Single-Lumen Tube

If at the conclusion of a case in which a double-lumen bronchial tube was used it is necessary to have a tube remain in place for continued ventilation, it is usually desirable to replace the DLT with a standard tracheal tube. In most cases, the procedure is as simple as removing one tube and placing another. If the patient was difficult to intubate originally or if circumstances make visualization of the larynx difficult, other techniques should be considered. One would be to advance a flexible jet ventilation catheter (see below) before removal of the DLT, then advance a tracheal tube over the catheter.

Another technique has been described (841). At the conclusion of the case both cuffs are deflated and the double-lumen tube is withdrawn until the bronchial lumen is above the carina. The bronchial cuff is then inflated and the lungs ventilated through the bronchial lumen. The tracheal lumen adaptor is clamped, a 5 × 5 mm opening is created in the wall of the tracheal lumen. A single-lumen tube is then slipped over a fiberscope, and the fiberscope is advanced through the hole in the tracheal lumen and inserted into the trachea. The opening in the DLT is extended, and the DLT is slowly removed. The tracheal tube is then inserted into the trachea over the fiberscope, and the fiberscope is then removed.

HAZARDS ASSOCIATED WITH DOUBLE-LUMEN TUBES

Many of the hazards associated with conventional tracheal tubes can also occur with double-lumen tubes. The type of tube may play a role in the number of complications resulting from the use of DLTs. One study

found that the rate of difficulties or complications was higher with red rubber tubes than PVC ones (774), but another study found no difference (842).

Difficulties with Insertion and Positioning

Insertion of a double-lumen tube is time-consuming. When there is severe tracheobronchial hemorrhage, this can be a major problem. Multiple insertions and repositionings may increase the risk of trauma. PVC tubes may be easier to position than red rubber ones (774,810,843).

Tube Malposition (774,837,844)

In spite of technically correct methods of intubation, difficulty is often experienced (774). Certain physical conditions may make it difficult or impossible for a double-lumen tube to be placed correctly (812,845,846). Even if a correct position is achieved during placement, movement of the head, a change in body positioning, or surgical manipulation may result in tube malposition.

Consequences

Malposition of a DLT can have one or more of the following effects.

Unsatisfactory Lung Deflation (774, 804,831). If the lung cannot be collapsed, operating time will be increased, and in some cases the surgical result may be compromised. Thoracoscopy will be unsatisfactory.

An obstruction in the unventilated lumen will prevent deflation of the unventilated lung (847). Partial withdrawal of the tube or insertion of a bronchial blocker through the bronchial lumen may remedy the situation (848).

Obstruction to Inflation. If the bronchial cuff is too deep, it will obstruct the upper lobe bronchus. This can occur on either the right or left. If the bronchial cuff of a left-sided DLT is not below the carina the cuff may obstruct the trachea and right mainstem bronchus (808). With right-sided tubes, malalignment of the port for the right upper lobe with the upper lobe bronchus can result in bronchial obstruction (805). If the right upper lobe bronchus originates from the trachea above the carina it may be obstructed by the tracheal cuff (849).

Gas Trapping.   Gas trapping, or obstruction to expiration, may be the result of a one-way valvular effect that allows inflation but not deflation. If unrecognized, it can result in cardiorespiratory embarrassment and/or lung parenchymal damage (813).

Failure of Lung Separation.   If the airway to a bronchopleural fistula cannot be isolated from that to the normal lung, tension pneumothorax may develop with positive pressure ventilation or the air leak through the fistula may be so large as to compromise ventilation of the normal lung (844).

With blood or infection in the nondependent lung, an incompletely protected dependent lung may drown in blood or secretions. The need for lung isolation is even greater when a DLT is used to separate the lungs during bronchopulmonary lavage.

Possible Malpositions

Bronchial Portion Inserted into Wrong Mainstem Bronchus.   In some cases the bronchial portion will enter the opposite lung. This should be easy to detect and correct.

Bronchial Portion Inserted Too Far into the Appropriate Bronchus (776,812,830, 832,834,847,849–851). A too-deep insertion may be the result of the use of too small a tube. It will result in obstruction of the upper lobe. In some cases in which the bronchial cuff cannot be visualized looking down the tracheal lumen, no clinical sequelae occur (831).

In a few patients a left-sided DLT placed so that the bronchial cuff is just distal to the carina still may cause left upper lobe obstruction (798,827). One study found that this type of malpositioning is more common with PVC than red rubber Robertshaw tubes (805).

Bronchial Segment Not Advanced Sufficiently Far into Bronchus.   If the tube is not sufficiently advanced into the bronchus, the bronchial cuff may protrude into the trachea. In many cases, no untoward sequelae will occur. Under certain circumstances, however, there may be obstruction of gas flow to the other lung and/or the cuff may produce a valvular obstruction between itself and the tracheal wall, allowing the opposite lung to inflate but not deflate. Another problem is that the endobronchial segment may slip out of its bronchus, especially during positioning of the patient (829).

This type of gas trapping may occur when both lumens are open or may occur only when the bronchial portion is clamped. The trapped gas can be released only by deflating the bronchial cuff.

The need to inject more than 3 ml of air into the bronchial cuff to achieve a seal should alert the user that the tube may be misplaced.

Tip of Bronchial Lumen above the Carina. The tip of the bronchial lumen may be above the carina because of a tracheal lesion that prevents the tube from passing far enough (844). With this malposition there will be unsatisfactory lung deflation and failure of lung separation.

Incorrect Placement with Respect to the Upper Lobe Bronchus.   Malposition with respect to the upper lobe bronchus is particularly a problem with right-sided tubes for which the margin of safety for correct placement is small. The bronchial tip may be in the correct position, but the cuff occludes the lumen to the upper lobe. Even with left-sided tubes, it is possible to obstruct the upper lobe bronchus (831,834,852). The result of such a misplacement is usually hypoxemia and, if the tube is on the operative side, failure of the upper lobe to deflate satisfactorily.

Asymmetrical Bronchial Cuff Inflation. An inflated bronchial can cause the tip of the bronchial lumen to face into the bronchial wall, producing a one-way valvular obstruction (774,853). This allows inflation but not deflation of the lung. It may be more common with red rubber tubes that have been resterilized (774).

Hypoxemia During One-Lung Ventilation

In many instances, hypoxemia during one-lung ventilation is at least partly the result of malpositioning of the DLT. For this reason, whenever hypoxia is a problem, tube position should be reassessed and adjustment made if necessary. Even with correct positioning, hypoxemia can result from blood continuing to flow through the unventilated lung after one-lung ventilation is begun.

An increased FIO_2 will be needed in most cases of one-lung ventilation (774). If hypoxemia continues to be a problem, continuous positive airway pressure (CPAP) between 5 and 10 cm H_2O should be applied to the nonventilated lumen during the deflation phase of a large tidal volume breath (827). More than 10 cm usually distends the lung to the degree that surgical exposure is compromised.

The reader is referred to Chapter 6 for a discussion of devices used to deliver CPAP. Some double-lumen tube manufacturers include a CPAP device with a mechanism for adjusting the level of PEEP with each DLT.

Other measures to improve oxygenation include dependent lung PEEP, occasional ventilation of the nondependent lung (one breath every 5 to 10 min), and clamping of the pulmonary artery before excluding the lung from ventilation.

A change from two-lung to one-lung ventilation does not usually result in a significant increase in P_{CO_2}, provided minute volume is maintained at the same value. However, because the tidal volume is the same, more pressure must be applied during inspiration to overcome the increased resistance to higher flow through the single lumen of the DLT and to compensate for the decreased compliance of the single lung.

Obstruction to Inflation

Many cases of obstruction to inflation are the result of malpositioning of the tube. In addition, overinflation of the bronchial cuff can cause narrowing of the lumen (812,831).

In one reported case, the bronchial cuff was left deflated until one-lung ventilation was to begin (854). Necrotic tumor migrated into the bronchus of the dependent lung, causing airway obstruction when one-lung ventilation was begun.

Trauma

Airway trauma anywhere in the respiratory tract is a possibility whenever intubation with a DLT is performed. Rupture of a mainstem bronchus by the bronchial cuff has been reported (358,855–859). The trachea may be ruptured (348,558). These complications may not be discovered until hours after the initial injury (358,551).

Air leak, subcutaneous or mediastinal emphysema, airway hemorrhage, and cardiovascular instability should alert the user to the possibility of airway damage. The bronchial cuff should be deflated and the integrity of the previously intubated bronchus checked at the time of testing the bronchial stump for leaks.

Measures to reduce airway trauma include removing the stylet after the tip of the tube has passed the vocal cords, avoiding overinflating cuffs, deflating the tracheal and bronchial cuffs when repositioning the patient or the tube, and not advancing the tube when resistance is encountered. Using PVC tubes with high-volume, low-pressure cuffs (860–862) has been recommended to reduce trauma, but proof that high pressures cause increased airway damage during short-term intubation is lacking. It has been recommended that the bronchial cuff be kept deflated until needed to minimize the chance of pressure damage to the bronchial mucosa (859). This may not be prudent if there is endobronchial tumor, as necrotic tumor may migrate into the other lung (854).

Tube Problems

Reported problems with double-lumen tubes include the following:

1. The cuff balloons were mislabeled (863,864).

2. Tubes have been sold with distortion of the main lumen such that a suction catheter would not pass (865).
3. A slit in the septum made it impossible to isolate one bronchus.
4. A defect made the bronchial lumen kink on itself (866).
5. During surgery, the tubing to the bronchial cuff split so that it was impossible to keep the cuff inflated (848).
6. A protuberance on the wall of the tube caused obstruction of the tracheal lumen (867).

Surgical Complications

Clamping of the carinal hook by the surgeon has occurred (801). The bronchial cuff may be punctured.

A case has been reported in which the surgeon placed a suture through the artery and the double lumen tube. On removal, the suture was broken and the patient exanguinated (700).

It is possible that the surgical procedure could result in a tight stenosis, which could entrap the bronchial tube and make extubation difficult (868). These possibilities should be considered when excessive resistance to extubation is encountered; reexploration of the chest may be warranted.

If the bronchial lumen is in the surgical side by mistake and this is not recognized, it is possible that when the bronchus is stapled and divided, the tip of the tube will be likewise stapled and divided.

Circulatory Collapse

A mediastinal mass was compressed and displaced by a DLT in such a way that it compressed the great vessels from the heart (869).

Increased Resistance (870–872)

Increased resistance has not proved to be a significant problem in the operating room, because positive pressure ventilation is almost always used. Resistance could become a problem if a DLT is left in place after surgery and spontaneous ventilation is attempted. Although PVC tubes have thinner walls and more gentle curves than red rubber tubes, studies show little difference in resistance among the various tubes (805,872).

Coaxial Systems for One-Lung Ventilaton

Use of a coaxial system in which a bronchial tube is placed within a large-bore tracheal tube has been described (873–876). The inner tube can be used as a bronchial blocker or as a conduit for suction or for differential ventilation or application of PEEP.

Tracheal and bronchial intubation are performed separately. The bronchial tube can be positioned blindly or by use of a rigid bronchoscope or a fiberscope (873). Bronchial intubation can be attempted many times without haste, while the patient can be ventilated using the tracheal tube.

Advantages of this technique include the ability to remove the bronchial tube at the end of the operation without having to reintubate the patient. Should a problem with the bronchical tube occur, the tracheal tube provides a means of ventilation.

This technique has been used in intensive care patients. The bronchial tube can be positioned and removed many times a day, leaving the main tracheal tube in place.

A disadvantage of this method is the necessity to use a large (at least 9 mm ID) tracheal tube. Another disadvantage is that this technique results in a higher resistance than use of a DLT with a comparable external diameter (872).

Single-Lumen Bronchial Tubes

A single-lumen tube placed in the main bronchus of the nonoperative lung can be used to maintain ventilation while the other lung is blocked and isolated from the ventilated lung.

EQUIPMENT

In the past, there were special tubes for bronchial intubation, including the Gordon-Green, Brompton Pallister, Mackray, and Macintosh-Leatherdale tubes (877). These are no longer available. Today bronchial intubation is usually carried out with a long small-diameter tracheal tube (878,879). A long tube can be created by anastamosing two shorter tubes (880,881) or may be obtained from a veterinary products supplier (882). It is important that the tube have a narrow cuff and beyond this a short length of tube and short bevel.

INDICATIONS

These tubes are used in situations where lung separation is desired and for some reason, a double-lumen tube cannot be used. They have been used most frequently in pediatric patients whose airways are too small for double lumen tubes (779,783,883–893). In patients presenting with massive hemoptysis, endobronchial intubation with a single-lumen tube is often the easiest and quickest method of effectively separating the lungs, especially if the left lung is bleeding (815). Such a tube may also be useful when a double-lumen tube cannot be placed (776). A single-lumen bronchial tube may be used to treat atelectasis (894).

TECHNIQUES

Before insertion, the correct length for the tube can be estimated from a lateral chest X-ray by measuring the distance from the mouth to the carina and adding 1 cm (783).

The tube may be placed before surgery and withdrawn into the trachea for two-lung ventilation when the indication for one-lung ventilation is no longer present (779). It can be placed blindly but is more dependably placed using a fiberscope or rigid bronchoscope (892,895,896). If placed blindly, the tube usually tends to enter the right mainstem bronchus. The chance of intubating the left bronchus will be increased if the tube is

rotated 180° from its usual position before advancing it beyond the carina and the head is turned to the right (814,815,879,897).

Another method is to insert a stylet into the chosen bronchus using a rigid bronchoscope (898). The bronchoscope is then removed and an appropriate single-lumen tube inserted into position over the stylet.

Correct positioning can be confirmed by auscultation, x-rays, and/or fiberoptic bronchoscopy.

DISADVANTAGES (2)

With either right- or left-sided mainstem bronchial intubation, but especially on the right, the upper lobe bronchus is easily obstructed (885). This can result in marked hypoxemia. It may be possible to rotate the tube so that the bevel faces the orifice of the right upper lobe bronchus (878). It is impossible to ventilate both lungs at the beginning of anesthesia and the collapsed lung cannot be suctioned or reexpanded and ventilated until the tube is withdrawn into the trachea. Finally, use of a bronchial tube does not allow application of CPAP to the operative lung.

Bronchial-Blocking Devices

With a bronchial blocker, the bronchus of a diseased lobe or lung is blocked while the balance of the lung is ventilated with a standard tracheal tube or endobronchial intubation of the other lung can be performed.

INDICATIONS

Indications for bronchial blockers are similar to those for a double-lumen tube, with the exception of independent lung ventilation. They are often used in pediatric patients in whom use of a DLT is not possible (887,891,899–901). A bronchial blocker can be used to block a bronchus if a double-lumen tube fails to perform properly (848). Another use is selective reinflation of a lung with lobar atelectasis in patients receiving mechanical ventilation (902). Use of a blocker eliminates the need to change tubes at the conclusion of surgery if artificial ventilation is to be used postoperatively. Blockers are occasionally helpful in controlling pulmonary bleeding (903). They also can be used for short-term control of a major air leak from a bronchopleural fistula.

DEVICES

A blocker typically consists of a central tube surrounded by an inflatable cuff. This allows suctioning, insufflation of oxygen, lavage, and ventilation down the central lumen.

Univent Bronchial-Blocking Tube (809,904–911)

The Univent tube is a single-lumen cuffed PVC tube that has a small lumen along its concave side (Figs. 15.41 and 15.42). The small channel contains a tubular bronchial blocker 2 mm in diameter that has a cuff on

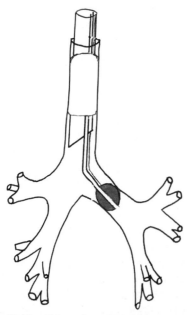

Figure 15.41. Univent bronchial blocker. The cuffed tracheal tube has a small lumen along its concave side, which contains a tubular cuffed bronchial blocker. The blocker can be advanced into a mainstem bronchus or smaller airway.

the end of it. There are radiopaque rings at both ends of the cuff. The blocker can be advanced up to 8 cm beyond the main body of the tube and can block airways smaller than the mainstem bronchus. The Univent tube is available in sizes down to 6.0 mm ID. It has a slightly larger-than-usual external diameter for its internal diameter because of the space taken by the blocker.

All functions possible with a DLT can be performed with a Univent tube, except differential lung ventilation (810). Intermittent reexpansion or suctioning of the lung during operation is easily accomplished without dislodgment of the blocker. One indication for its use may be a patient on anticoagulant therapy because insertion of the Univent tube may cause less trauma than a DLT (912). However, perforation of the tip of the blocker through a bronchus has been reported (913). Use of operative lung CPAP with the Univent tube has been described (904).

The Univent tube may be easier to insert and position correctly than a double-lumen tube (809,905,908,909,914), although one study found that in three of eight cases the Univent failed to occlude the bronchus, requiring replacement with a DLT (912). This contrasts with satisfactory reports from other investigators (908,909). It also offers a larger lumen for ventilation and pulmonary toilet of the unaffected lung.

Embolectomy Catheter

A balloon-tipped embolectomy catheter can be used as a bronchial blocker (899–902,915–917). It comes in a variety of sizes so that it can be used to block a second-order as well as a mainstem bronchus and can be used in both adults and children. It comes with a stylet in place so that it is possible to place a curvature at the distal tip.

Swan-Ganz Catheter

The Swan-Ganz catheter has been used in small pediatric patients (887,902).

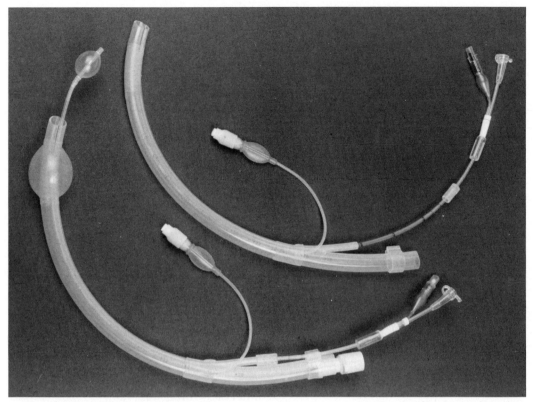

Figure 15.42. Univent bronchial-blocking tubes. *Top,* The bronchial blocker is retracted. *Bottom,* The bronchial blocker is advanced and the cuff is inflated. Courtesy of Vitaid.

Magill Blocker

The Magill bronchial blocker is a fine catheter equipped with an inflatable cuff. It can be used in children.

Foley Catheter

A urinary catheter inserted down one lumen of a DLT has been used when there was a problem with the DLT (848).

TECHNIQUES OF INSERTION (915,916,918)

Univent

Before intubation, both cuffs should be inflated and checked for leaks. After the cuffs have been deflated, the blocker is pushed back and forth to ensure free movement. The blocker is then fully retracted into the main body of the tube.

The Univent is inserted as a unit into the trachea. The cuff on the tracheal tube is inflated, and the patient is ventilated. A fiberscope is inserted into the lumen of the tube while ventilation is maintained around it. The bronchial blocker is located by moving it in and out of its lumen, and the main tube is turned so that the ridge housing the movable blocker is directed toward the side to be blocked. The blocker is then advanced into the desired position under direct vision and secured in place with its balloon deflated. The fiberscope is then withdrawn.

Blind insertion of the bronchial blocker is also possible. The whole tube is turned so that the concavity of the tube faces the side to be blocked. The blocker is advanced into the mainstem bronchus, and the cuff is inflated. This method has not proved very successful in practice (911).

Another method of placing the Univent blocker is to first insert the tube into the trachea. A fiberscope is inserted into the bronchus to be blocked, and the tube is advanced into that bronchus. The blocker is then advanced into the bronchus, and the tube is withdrawn into the trachea, leaving the blocker in the bronchus.

Once the blocker is placed, its position should be checked using a fiberscope (919) or x-rays and auscultation (889,917).

When the bronchus needs to be blocked, the lung is deflated with the blocker open to atmosphere, then suction is applied to the blocker's lumen until complete collapse is achieved. The bronchial blocker cuff should be inflated using the least amount of air that will provide a seal. This can be achieved by attaching a CO_2 analyzer to the proximal end of the blocker and noting when the CO_2 waveform disappears (920). When the need for the blocker is no longer present, the cuff is deflated and the blocker withdrawn into the main tube.

Other Bronchial Blockers

Before use, the cuff on the bronchial blocker should be tested for leaks, and the blocker should be fitted with a stylet. The blocker may be inserted into the trachea either before intubation with the tracheal tube or alongside it after intubation.

The blocker can be inserted using a bronchoscope or blindly (921). Alternately the bronchoscope can be used to place a flexible stylet in the bronchus (922). The blocker is inserted over the stylet, which is then removed.

The blocker also can be inserted beside the tracheal tube. A fiberscope is passed to the end of the single-lumen tube through a self-sealing diaphragm (which permits continued positive pressure ventilation around the fiberscope), and the blocker is visualized. The blocker is rotated until its distal tip is in the desired mainstem bronchus.

Another technique of insertion employs two elbow connectors with self-sealing dia-

phragm ports in series (923). The distal end of the connectors is connected to the patient's single-lumen tracheal tube. The fiberscope is passed through the port, which offers a straight line down the tracheal tube. The blocker is placed through the other port.

DISADVANTAGES (733,814)

With blockers other than the Univent, the blocker and tracheal tube are separated, and there may be difficulty in maintaining or changing the position of the blocker (908). Also, the obstructed lung segment cannot be suctioned or reexpanded until the blocker is removed.

Hazards include the possibility of loss of a portion of the blocker (919). A blocker can slip out of position (912). If it slips into the trachea, separation of the lungs will be lost and life-threatening ventilatory obstruction may occur.

The amount of air needed to inflate the bronchial cuff so that it blocks the bronchus may cause it to exert a high pressure on the wall of the bronchus (924).

Stylets and Bougies

SYTLETS

A stylet (introducer or intubation guide) is designed to fit inside a tracheal tube so that the tube maintains a predetermined, fixed shape. It is most commonly used to facilitate insertion of the tube. It can also be used to check the patency of a tube before intubation. Lighted intubation (flexible lighted) stylets and optical stylets (stylet laryngoscopes) are discussed in Chapter 14.

Description (925)

A variety of stylets are available (Figs. 15.43–15.46). Some have special nonfriction coverings (926–928). A stylet should have enough malleability so that its shape can be changed easily, yet enough rigidity to maintain its shape during insertion. It should be

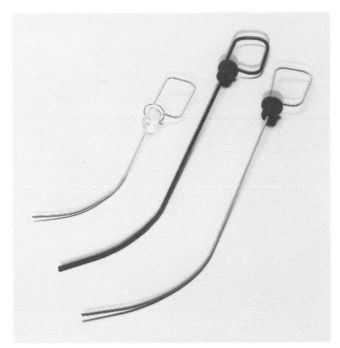

Figure 15.43. Malleable stylets with adjustable stops. The stop fits into the tracheal tube and prevents the stylet from protruding beyond the distal tip of the tube. Courtesy of Polamedco, Inc.

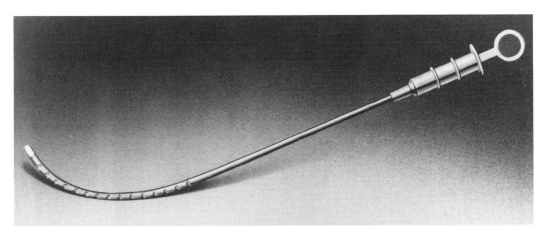

Figure 15.44. Salem/Resce guide. The distal tip can be flexed by means of the proximal grip handle. The guide should be adjusted so that it fits securely into the tracheal tube with the tip extending 2½ to 3 inches beyond the end of the tube. Courtesy of Scientific Sales International, Inc.

resistant to chipping and breaking. The distal end should be smooth to minimize trauma to soft tissues and the tube. It must be at least as long as the tube into which it is introduced.

There should be a means to limit the stylet's advancement into the tube (see Figs. 15.43 and 15.44). If none is present, the stylet should be bent acutely at the proximal end (see Fig. 15.45). The proximal end of the stylet may have an attachment that will fit firmly into the tracheal tube and prevent rotation of the tube on the stylet.

Some stylets allow the user to manipulate the shape of the stylet during insertion (see

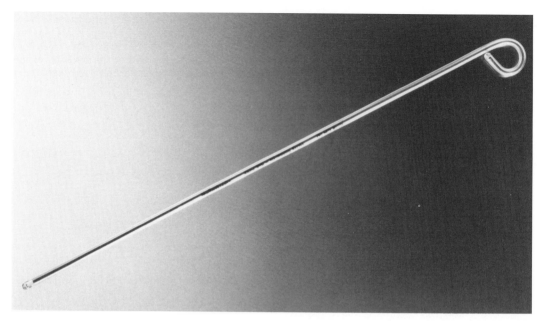

Figure 15.45. Malleable stylet. The proximal end must be bent to prevent it from protruding past the end of the tracheal tube. Courtesy of Mallinckrodt Medical, Inc.

Figure 15.46. Chenoweth stylet. The shape can be altered with the tube in situ. It is designed to intensify breath sounds to assist directing blind placement. The flexible portion should be inserted until its tip is just inside the distal tip of the tracheal tube. Courtesy of Aspen Medical, Inc.

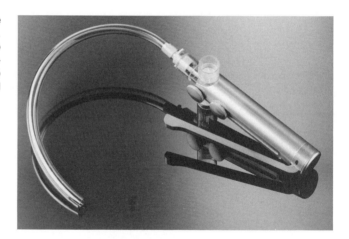

Figs. 15.44 and 15.46). These may be especially useful in patients with cervical spine injuries (929).

Techniques for Use

A stylet should always be available when intubation is being performed. Many anesthesiologists routinely use a stylet, whereas others reserve its use for difficult intubations.

Some tracheal tubes require a stylet to give them sufficient rigidity for insertion. A stylet is often useful when only the arytenoids or epiglottis can be visualized.

Unless the stylet has a nonstick coating, a thin film of lubricant should be spread over its length before insertion. If this is not done, it may be difficult to remove the stylet after the tube is in place. Unless otherwise stated in the manufacturer's directions, the stylet should be inserted into the tube until the distal end is just inside the distal tip of the tracheal tube and should be fixed so that the tip cannot advance. Removing the connector from the tube before inserting the stylet may make it easier to withdraw the stylet and decrease the likelihood of damage to the stylet (926). The tube and stylet should then be bent to the desired shape. For routine intubations, a straight or slightly curved configuration is used. When an anterior larynx is encountered, a *J* or hockey stick configuration, with the distal end of the tube bent anteriorly to an angle of 70° to 80°, is most commonly used. Bending the midpoint of the tube to the right or left at an angle of 70° to 80° to the first bend may result in a better view of the larynx (930). The larynx is exposed in the usual manner, and the tracheal tube is inserted. As soon as the distal part of the tube is believed to have passed the vocal cords, the tube is advanced over the stylet.

A slightly different technique involves inserting the stylet into the tube and angling the distal portion anteriorly (295,931). The stylet is then removed from the tube. The tube is passed into the patient to the vicinity of the larynx, and then the stylet is inserted. This technique may result in decreased trauma.

Problems with Stylets

Use of a stylet may result in trauma with serious consequences (379,380,382). Part of the stylet may be sheared off during removal from the tube (503–505,932–934). The inflation tube can become entangled in the stylet (935). Finally, the stylet may damage the tracheal tube.

BOUGIES (936)

A bougie also is called a guide, intubation or tube guide, guiding catheter, director, stylet catheter, endotracheal tube introducer, introducer, elastic stylet, tracheal tube replacement obturator, and tube changer (Fig. 15.47). It can be used to aid intubation when the operator recognizes some anatomical

landmarks but cannot direct the tip of the tracheal tube into the laryngeal inlet or when movement of the head and/or neck is undesirable (937–940). It is also used for tracheal tube replacement. A bougie can serve as a backup safety measure when changing tracheal tubes (325). Another use is to distinguish esophageal from tracheobronchial intubation (434,396). A bougie can also be used in a patient who is intubated and at the point at which it is thought extubation would be well tolerated but in whom postextubation ventilation and/or reintubation would be difficult (324,325,941–943).

Description

A variety of materials have been used to make bougies, including gum elastic and polyethylene tubing. Other devices such as suction catheters, embolectomy catheters, and nasogastric tubes have been used as bougies (944,947). The tip of the distal end may be angled (948). The proximal end of the bougie may be adapted to allow administration of oxygen or jet ventilation (see Fig. 15.47).

Technique of Use

The bougie is advanced under direct vision to the area where the trachea is thought to be located. If the bougie is solid when it enters the trachea the stepwise advance of the distal end over the tracheal rings will produce a clicking sensation (949). If it is hollow, the proximal end may be attached to a capnograph, which will show regular variations with ventilation (950). Once the bougie is felt to be in the trachea, the tracheal tube is advanced over it using a rotary motion. Sometimes after successful placement of a bougie in the trachea it is difficult or impossible to thread the tracheal tube over it (951). Advancement of the tube may be enhanced by leaving the laryngoscope in the mouth and by rotating the tracheal tube so that the bevel faces posteriorly (952,953). The bougie is then withdrawn.

An alternate technique is to pass the bou-

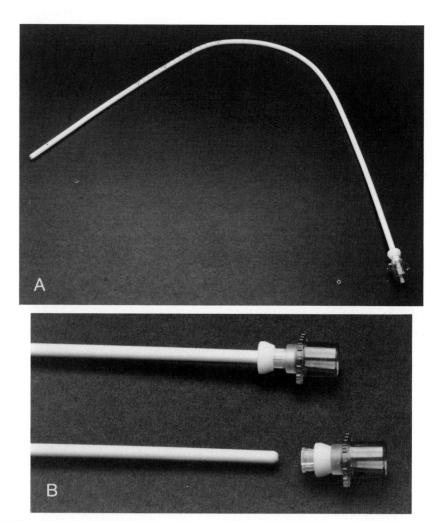

Figure 15.47. **A,** Bougie, which also can be used as an aid in intubation. **B,** Note the marks showing the distance from the tip and the holes near the tip. The proximal connections allow administration of oxygen, jet ventilation, connection to a CO_2 analyzer, or suctioning. Courtesy of Cook Critical Care, a division of Cook, Inc.

gie over a guide inserted translaryngeally and passed retrograde to the oropharynx (933,954).

A bougie can be used as a tube exchanger (changer). Tubes inserted either orally or nasally can be changed using this device (955). A lumen and a 15-mm connection at one end will allow insufflation of oxygen during the changing process. It should have marks to indicate the distance from the tip (see Fig. 15.47*B*). To exchange a tube, the connector on the existing tube is removed (956). The tube changer is inserted into the tube and ad-

vanced to the tracheal tube's full length. Insertion farther than this may result in trauma (383,957). The changer is held steady while the tracheal tube is removed. Care must be taken that the changer is not pulled from the trachea. The replacement tracheal tube is slipped over the changer and passed into the trachea.

In a patient to be extubated in whom reintubation or mask ventilation might be difficult, a bougie can be inserted into the trachea through the extant tracheal tube, which is then removed, leaving the bougie in place.

Patients tolerate a bougie readily, and because it is only a few millimeters in diameter, it represents a negligible obstruction to closure of the vocal cords. It then can serve as a guide if reintubation is necessary. If the bougie is hollow, attachment of an adaptor to the proximal end allows administration of oxygen, suctioning, or aspiration of gases from the distal end (324,950). Jet ventilation through such a catheter can provide a satisfactory minute volume in most cases (957).

Forceps

A forceps can be used to direct a tracheal tube into the larynx or a gastric tube or other device into the esophagus. It also can be used to insert pharyngeal packing and to retrieve foreign objects. Forceps should be readily available whenever an intubation is performed.

DESCRIPTION

A popular type of forceps is Magill's (467). These are designed so that when the grasping ends are in the axis of the tracheal tube, the handle is to the right. Thus the operator can expose the larynx using a laryngoscope held in the left hand and hold the forceps in the right hand, out of the line of sight. Modifications of Magill's forceps and other forceps have been described (958–966) as have other devices to manipulate the tube during intubation (967–970).

PROBLEMS WITH FORCEPS

Cuff damage may occur, especially when forceps are used with high-volume cuffs (921). It is suggested that tubes be picked up at the tip, not the cuff. Another way to avoid cuff damage is to file the teeth from the end of the forceps (959). The forceps may cause damage to the airway mucosa. Another problem is that one arm of the forceps may become lodged in the Murphy eye (29).

REFERENCES

1. Demers RR, Sullivan MJ, Paliotta J. Airflow resistances of endotracheal tubes. JAMA 1977; 237:1362.
2. Bolder PM, Healy TEJ, Bolder AR, Beatty PCW, Kay B. The extra work of breathing through adult endotracheal tubes. Anesth Analg 1986;65:853–859.
3. Brochard L, Rua F, Lorino H, Lemaire F, Harf A. Inspiratory pressure support compensates for the additional work of breathing caused by the endotracheal tube. Anesthesiology 1991;75:739–745.
4. Le Souef PN, England SJ, Bryan AC. Total resistance of the respiratory system in preterm infants with and without an endotracheal tube. J Pediatr 1984;104:108–111.
5. Shapiro M, Wilson RK, Casar G, Bloom K, Teague RB. Work of breathing through different sized endotracheal tubes. Crit Care Med 1986;14:1028–1031.
6. Wall MA. Infant endotracheal tube resistance: effects of changing length, diameter and gas density. Crit Care Med 1980;8:38–40.
7. Bersten AD, Rutten AJ, Vedig AE, Skowronski GA. Additional work of breathing imposed by endotracheal tubes, breathing circuits, and intensive care ventilators. Crit Care Med 1989;17:671–677.
8. Brown ES, Hustead RF. Resistance of pediatric breathing systems. Anesth Analg 1969;48:842–848.
9. Bolder PM, Healy TEJ, Bolder AR, Beattty PCW, Kay B. The extra work of breathing through adult endotracheal tubes. Anesth Analg 1986;65:853–859.
10. Fiastro JF, Habib MP, Quan SF. Pressure support compensation for inspiratory work due to endotracheal tubes and demand continuous positive airway pressure. Chest 1988;93:449–505.
11. Gullahorn GM, Banner MJ, Berman LS. Pressure support ventilation to decrease work of breathing imposed by pediatric endotracheal tubes. Anesthesiology 1991;75:A256.
12. Hendricks HHL. Minimizing work of breathing through endotracheal tubes. Crit Care Med 1987;15:989–990.
13. Boretos JW, Battis CG, Goodman L. Decreased resistance to breathing through a polyurethane pediatric endotracheal tube. Anesth Analg 1972;51:292–296.
14. Blom H, Rytlander M, Wisborg T. Resistance of tracheal tubes 3.0 and 3.5 mm internal diameter. A comparison of four commonly used types. Anaesthesia 1985;40:885–888.
15. Bunnage SM, Bennett MJ. Nd-YAG laser airway surgery. resistance of tracheal tubes partially oc-

cluded by flexible bronchoscope. Anesthesiology 1985;63:A162.

16. Baier H, Begin R, Sackner MA. Effect of airway diameter, suction catheters and the bronchofiberscope on airflow in endotracheal and tracheostomy tubes. Heart Lung 1976;5:235–238.

17. Matthews JG, Ingenito E, Davison B, Barker S, Kacmarek R, Drazen JM. Endotracheal tube resistance. The effects of tube curvature, tube interfaces, gas-liquid interaction and airflow direction. Anesthesiology 1992;77:A280.

18. Badenhorst CH. Changes in tracheal cuff pressure during respiratory support. Crit Care Med 1987;15:300–302.

19. Hatch DJ. Tracheal tubes and connectors used in neonates—dimensions and resistance to breathing. Br J Anaesth 1978;50:959–964.

20. Brown ES. Resistance factors in pediatric endotracheal tubes and connectors. Anesth Analg 1971;50:355–360.

21. Fleming BG, Nott MR. Resistance measurement and connectors. Anaesthesia 1988;43:1057.

22. Steen JA. Impact of tube design and materials on complications of tracheal intubation. Probl Anesth 1988;2:211–224.

23. Carroll RG, Kamen JM, Grenvick A, Safan P, Robison E, Stoner DL, Sheridan DS, McGinnis GE. Recommended performance specifications for cuffed endotracheal and tracheostomy tubes: a joint statement of investigators, inventors, and manufacturers. Crit Care Med 1973;11:155–156.

24. American Society for Testing and Materials. Standard specification for cuffed and uncuffed tracheal tubes (ASTM F1242-89). Philadelphia: ASTM, 1989.

25. Hirshman CA. Anaphylactic reactions to latex-containing medical devices. ASA Newslet 1992;56(8):21–22.

26. Murphy FJ. Two improved intratracheal catheters. Anesth Analg 1941;20:102–105.

27. Baranowski AP. Unusual tracheal tube obstruction leading to an unusual bronchoscopic technique. Anaesthesia 1989;44:359–360.

28. Gregory GA. Pediatric Anesthesia. In: Miller RD, ed. Anesthesia. Vol. 2. San Francisco: Churchill Livingstone, 1981:1214.

29. Harrison JF. A problem with Murphy's eye. Anaesthesia 1986;41:445.

30. MacGillivray RG, Odell JA. Eye to eye with Murphy's law. Anaesthesia 1986;41:334.

31. Nichols KP, Zornow MH. A potential complication of fiberoptic intubation. Anesthesiology 1989;70:562–563.

32. Ovassapian A. Failure to withdraw flexible fiberoptic laryngoscope after nasotracheal intubation. Anesthesisology 1985;63:124–125.

33. Mackenzie CF, McDowell EM, Helrich M. Reduc-

tion of tracheal tube tip damage using a new tube. 1984;Crit Care Med 12:259.

34. Pashayan AG, Gravenstein JS. Helium retards endotracheal tube fires from carbon dioxide lasers. Anesthesiology 1985;62:274–277.

35. Cole F. An endotracheal tube for babies. Anesthesiology 1945;6:627–628.

36. Brandstater B. Dilatation of the larynx with Cole tubes. Anesthesiology 1969;31:378–379.

37. Glauser EM, Cook CK, Bougas TP. Pressure-flow characteristics and dead spaces of endotracheal tubes used in infants. Anesthesiology 1961;22:339–341.

38. Ring WH, Adair JC, Elwyn RA. A new pediatric endotracheal tube. Anesth Analg 1975;54:273–274.

39. Brunsoman JK, Altman VA, Johnson MA, Peterson LJ. A new endotracheal tube for maxillofacial surgery. J Oral Surg 1980;38:847–848.

40. Olson KW, Culling DC. An alternative use for a nasotracheal tube. Can J Anaesth 1989;36:252–253.

41. Barker SWJ, Tremper KK. A new look at pressure loss through endotracheal tubes: RAE and CAT tubes. Anesth Analg 1986;65:S170.

42. Black AE, Mackersie AM. Accidental bronchial intubation with RAE tubes. Anaesthesia 1991;46:42–43.

43. Shanahan EC. A nasotracheal tube for faciomaxillary surgery. Anaesthesia 1983;38:289–290.

44. Mackersie AM. The length of RAE preformed tubes: a reply. Anaesthesia 1991;46:792.

45. Chung RA, Liban JB. Ludwig's angina and tracheal tube obstruction. Anaesthesia 1991;46:228–239.

46. Beckers HL. Use of a stabilized, armored endotracheal tube in maxillofacial surgery. Anesthesiology 1982;56:309–310.

47. Steen JA, Lindhold C, Brdlik GC, Foster CA. Tracheal tube forces on the posterior larynx: index of laryngeal loading. Crit Care Med 1982;10:186–189.

48. Calder I. When the endotracheal tube will not pass over the flexible fiberoptic bronchoscope. Anesthesiology 1992;77:398.

49. Burns THS. Danger from flexometallic endotracheal tubes. Br Med J 1956;1:439–440.

50. Abramowitz MD, McNabb TG. A new complication of flexometallic endotracheal tubes. Br J Anaesth 1976;48:928.

51. Cohen DD, Dillon JB. Hazards of armored endotracheal tubes. Anesth Analg 1972;51:856–858.

52. Catane R, Davidson JT. A hazard of cuffed flexometallic endotracheal tubes. Br J Anaesth 1969;41:1086.

53. Forrester AC. Mishaps in anesthesia. Anaesthesia 1959;14:388–399.

54. Kohli MS, Manku RS. Reinforced endotracheal tube—diversion of air from cuff balloon producing obstruction. Anesthesiology 1966;27:513–514.

55. Lall NG. Airway obstruction with latex armoured endotracheal tube. Indian J Anaesth 1969;17:297.

56. Jacobson J. A hazard of armored endotracheal anesthesia. Anesth Analg 1969;48:37–41.

57. Mirakhur RK. Airway obstruction with cuffed armoured tracheal tubes. Can Anaesth Soc J 1974;21:251–258.

58. Munson ES, Stevens DS, Redfern RE. Endotracheal tube obstruction by nitrous oxide. Anesthesiology 1980;52:275–276.

59. Ng TY, Krimili BI. Hazards in use of anode endotracheal tube: a case report and review. Anesth Analg 1975;54:710–714.

60. Ohn K, Wu W. Another complication of armored endotracheal tubes. Anesth Analg 1980;59:215–216.

61. Robbie DS, Pearce DJ. Some dangers of armoured tubes. Anaesthesa 1959;14:379–385.

62. Ripoli I, Lindhold C, Carroll R, Grenvik A. Spontaneous dislocation of endotracheal tubes: a problem with too soft tube material. Crit Care Med 1978;6:101–102.

63. Rendell–Baker L. A hazard alert: reinforced endotracheal tubes. Anesthesiology 1980;53:268–269.

64. Walton WJ. An invaginated tube. Br J Anaesth 1967;39:520.

65. Wright PJ, Mundy JVB. Tracheal tubes in neuroanesthesia. Nylon reinforced latex rubber tracheal tubes. Anaesthesia 1987;42:1012–1014.

66. Wright PJ, Mundy JVB, Mansfield CJ. Obstruction of armoured tracheal tubes: case report and discussion. Can J Anaesth 1988;35:195–197.

67. Adamson DH. A problem of prolonged oral intubation: case report. Can Anaesth Soc J 1971;18:213–214.

68. Gemma M, Ferrazza M. "Dental trauma" to oral airways. Can J Anaesth 1990;37:951.

69. Hoffmann CO, Swanson GA. Oral reinforced endotracheal tube crushed and perforated from biting. Anesth Analg 1989;69:552–553.

70. McTaggart RA, Shustack A, Noseworthy T, Johnston R. Another cause of obstruction in an armored endotracheal tube. Anesthesiology 1983;59:164.

71. Martens P. Persistent narrowing of an armoured tube. Anaesthesia 1992;47:716–717.

72. Spiess BD, Rothenberg DM, Buckley S. Complete airway obstruction of armoured endotracheal tubes. Anesth Analg 1991;73:95–96.

73. Davies RM. Faulty construction of a reinforced latex endotracheal tube. Br J Anaesth 1963;35:128–129.

74. Hedden M, Smith RBF, Torpey DJ. A complication of metal spiral-imbedded latex endotracheal tubes. Anesth Analg 1972;51:859–862.

75. Malone BT. A complication of Rusch armored endotracheal tubes. Anesth Analg 1975;54:756.

76. Dunn GL. Letter to the editor. Can Anaesth Soc J 1975;22:379–380.

77. Carden E, Crutchfield W. Anaesthesia for microsurgery of the larynx (A new method). Can Anaesth Soc J 1973;20:378–389.

78. Carden E, Ferguson GB, Crutchfield WM. A new silicone elastomer tube for use during microsurgery on the larynx. Ann Otol Rhinol Laryngol 1974;83:360–365.

79. Cooke JE, Hood JB, Thomas JD. A method for inserting the Carden tube. Anesth Analg 1976;55:882–883.

80. El-Naggar M, Keh E, Stemmers A, Copllins VJ. Jet ventilation for microlaryngoscopic procedures: a further simplified technic. Anesth Analg 1974;53:797–804.

81. Edelman JD, Wingard W. Carden-tube insertion. Anesthesiology 1978;49:220–221.

82. Singh A. A safe method of insertion of Carden's tube. Anaesthesia 1982;37:104–105.

83. Carden E. Carden tube. Can Anaesth Soc J 1980;27:512.

84. Soder CM, Haight J, Fredrickson JL, Scott AA. Mechanical ventilation during laryngeal surgery. An evaluation of the Carden tube. Can Anaesth Soc J 1980;27:111–116.

85. Carden E, Vest HR. Further advances in anesthetic technics for microlaryngeal surgery. Anesth Analg 1974;53:584–587.

86. Dawson P, Rosewane F, Wells D. The Montando laryngectomy tube. Can J Anaesth 1989;36:486–487.

87. Fry ENS. Difficult tracheal intubation. Anaesthesia 1985;40:206.

88. Glinsman D, Pavlin EG. Airway obstruction after nasal-tracheal intubation. Anesthesiology 1982;56:229–230.

89. Badgwell JM, McLeod ME, Lerman J, Creighton RE. End-tidal pCO_2 monitoring in infants and children during ventilation with the Air-Shields Ventimeter Ventilator. Anesthesiology 1986;65:A418.

90. Miller BR. Problems associated with endotracheal tubes with monitoring lumens in pediatric patients. Anesthesiology 1987;67:1018–1019.

91. Green JM, Gonzalez RM, Sonbolian N, Rehkopf P. The resistance to carbon dioxide laser ignition of a new endotracheal tube. Xomed Laser-Shield II. J Clin Anesth 1992;4:89–92.

92. Dillon F, Sosis M, Heller S. Evaluation of a new foil wrapped silicone endotracheal tube designed for laser airway surgery. Anesthesiology 1991;75:A392.

93. Sosis M, Pritikin J, Caldarelli D, Ivankovitch AD. Effect of blood on the combustibility of laser resistant tracheal tubes. Anesthesiology 1992; 77:A579.

94. Hawkins DB, Joseph MM. Avoiding a wrapped endotracheal tube in laser laryngeal surgery: experiences with apneic anesthesia and metal laser flex endotracheal tubes. Laryngoscope 1990; 100:1283–1287.

95. Garry B, Hivens HE. Laser safety in the operating room. Cancer Bull 1989;41:219–223.

96. Sosis MB. What is the safest endotracheal tube for Nd-YAG laser surgry?—A comparative study. Anesth Analg 1989;69:802–804.

97. Sosis MB. Which is the safest endotracheal tube for use with the CO_2 laser? A comparative study. J Clin Anaesth 1992;4:217–219.

98. Sosis M, Braverman B, Ivankovich AD. An evaluation of special tracheal tubes with the KTP laser. Anesth Analg 1991;72:S267.

99. Fried MP, Mallampati SR, Liu FC, Kaplin S, Caminear DS, Samonte BS. Laser resistant stainless steel endotracheal tube. Experimental and clinical evaluation. Lasers Surg Med 1991;11:301–306.

100. Anonymous. Laser-resistant endotracheal tubes and wraps. Health Devices 1990;19:109–139.

101. Sosis M, Dillon F. Reflection of CO_2 laser radiation from laser-resistant endotracheal tubes. Anesth Analg 1991;73:338–340.

102. Sprung J, Conley SF, Brown M. Unusual cause of difficult extubation. Anesthesiology 1991; 74:796.

103. Sosis M, Dillon F. Hazards of a new, clear, unmarked polyvinylchloride tracheal tube designed for use with the Nd-YAG laser. J Clin Anesth 1991;3:358–360.

104. Norton ML, Vos P. New endotracheal tube for laser surgery of the larynx. Ann Otol Rhinol Laryngol 1978;87:554–557.

105. Sosis M. Large air leak during laser surgery with a Norton tube. Anesthesiol Rev 1989;16:39–41.

106. Skaredoff MN, Poppers PJ. Beware of sharp edges in metal endotracheal tubes. Anesthesiology 1983;58:595.

107. Sosis MB. Hazards of laser surgery. Semin Anesth 1990;9:90–97.

108. Kamen JM, Wilkinson CJ. A new low-pressure cuff for endotracheal tubes. Anesthesiology 1971;34:482–485.

109. Loeser EA, Machin R, Colley J, Orr D, Bennett GM, Stanley TH. Postoperative sore throat importance of endotracheal tube conformity versus cuff design. Anesthesiology 1978;49:430–432.

110. Bernhard WN, Yost L, Turndorf H, Danziger F. Cuffed tracheal tubes: physical and behavioral characteristics. Anesth Analg 1982;61:36–41.

111. Cohen DD. Note on endotracheal tubes. Anesthesiology 1970;33:463.

112. Bernhard WN, Cottrell JE, Sivakumaran C, Patel K, Yost L, Turndorf H. Adjustment of intra-cuff pressure to prevent aspiration. Anesthesiology 1979;50:363–366.

113. Mehta S, Mickiewicz M. Pressure in large volume, low pressure cuffs. its significance, measurement and regulation. Intensive Care Med 1985;11:267–272.

114. Seegobin RD, Van Hasselt GL. Endotracheal cuff pressure and tracheal mucosal blood flow: endoscopic study of effects of four large volume cuffs. Br Med J 1984;288:965–968.

115. Mehta S. Safe lateral wall cuff pressure to prevent aspiration. Ann R Coll Surg Engl 1984;66:426–427.

116. Bernhard WN, Yost LC, Turndorf H, Cottrell JE, Paegle RD. Physical characteristics of and rates of nitrous oxide diffusion into tracheal tube cuffs. Anesthesiology 1978;48:413–417.

117. Chandler M. Pressure in tracheal tube cuffs. Anaesthesia 1986;41:287–293.

118. Greene SJ, Cane RD, Shapiro BA. A foam cuff endotracheal tube T-piece system for use with nitrous oxide anesthesia. Anesth Analg 1986;65:1359–1360.

119. Mehta S. Effects of nitrous oxide and oxygen on tracheal tube cuff gas volumes. Br J Anaesth 1981;53:1227–1231.

120. Revenas R, Lindholm CE. Pressure and volume changes in tracheal tube cuffs during anaesthesia. Acta Anaesth Scand 1976;20:321–326.

121. Raeder JC, Borchgrevink PC, Sellevold OM. Tracheal tube cuff pressures. The effects of different gas mixtures. Anaesthesia 1985;40:444–447.

122. Stanley TH, Kawamura R, Graves C. Effects of nitrous oxide on volume and pressure of endotracheal tube cuffs. Anesthesiology 1974;41:256–262.

123. Stanley TH. Effects of anesthetic gases on endotracheal tube cuff gas volumes. Anesth Analg 1974;53:480–482.

124. Stanley TH. Nitrous oxide and pressures and volumes of high and low-pressure endotracheal-tube cuffs in intubated patients. Anesthesiology 1975;42:637–640.

125. Latto IP. The cuff. In: Latto IP, Rosen M, eds. Difficulties in tracheal intubation. London: Bailliere Tindall, 1985:48–74.

126. Lineberger CL, Johnson MD. A method for preventing endotracheal tube cuff overdistention caused by nitrous oxide diffusion. Anesth Analg 1991;72:843–844.

127. Morgan P. Prevention of nitrous oxide-induced increases in endotracheal tube cuff pressure. Anesth Analg 1991;73:232.

128. Fischer CG, Cook DR. Endotracheal tube cuff

pressure in the use of nitrous oxide. Anesth Analg 1991;73:99.

129. Brandt L. Nitrous oxide in oxygen and tracheal tube cuff volumes. Br J Anaesth 1982;54:1238–1239.

130. Ikeda D, Schweiss JF. Tracheal tube cuff volume changes during extracorporeal circulation. Can Anaesth Soc J 1980;27:453–457.

131. Partridge BL. Nitrous oxide and endotracheal tube cuff leaks. Anesthesiology 1988;68:167–168.

132. Patel RI, Oh TH, Epstein BS. Effects of nitrous oxide on pressure changes of tracheal tube cuffs following inflation with air and saline. Anaesthesia 1983;38:44–46.

133. Patel RI, Oh TH, Chandra R, Epstein BS. Tracheal tube cuff pressure. Changes during nitrous oxide anaesthesia following inflation of cuffs with air and saline. Anaesthesia 1984;39:862–864.

134. Ballantine RIW. A discontinued endotracheal tube. Anaesthesia 1981;36:74.

135. Kosanin R, Maroff M. Continuous monitoring of endotracheal intracuff pressures in patients receiving general anesthesia utilizing nitrous oxide. Anesthesiol Rev 1981;8:29–32.

136. Carroll R, Hedden M, Safar P. Intratracheal cuffs: performance characteristics. Anesthesiology 1969;31:275–281.

137. Dobrin P, Canfield T. Cuffed endotracheal tubes: mucosal pressures and tracheal wall blood flow. Am J Surg 1977;133:562–568.

138. Wu W, Lim I, Simpson FA, Turndorf H. Pressure dynamics of endotracheal and tracheostomy cuffs. Crit Care Med 1973;1:197–202.

139. Cooper JD, Grillo HC. Analysis of problems related to cuffs on intratracheal tubes. Chest 1972;62:21S–27S.

140. Jensen PJ, Hommelgaard P, Sondergaard P, Eriksen S. Sore throat after operation: influence of tracheal intubation, intracuff pressure and type of cuff. Br J Anaesth 1982;54:453–457.

141. Loeser EA, Orr DL, Bennett GM, Stanley TH. Endotracheal tube cuff design and postoperative sore throat. Anesthesiology 1976;45:684–687.

142. Loeser EA, Stanley TH, Jordan W, Machin R. Postoperative sore throat: influence of tracheal tube lubrication versus cuff design. Can Anaesth Soc J 1980;27:156–158.

143. Crawley BE, Cross DE. Tracheal cuffs. A review and dynamic pressure study. Anaesthesia 1975;30:4–11.

144. Guyton D, Banner MJ, Kirby RR. High-volume, low-pressure cuffs. Are they always low pressure? Chest 1991;100:1076–1081.

145. Lewis FR, Schlobohm RM, Thomas AN. Prevention of complications from prolonged tracheal intubation. Am J Surg 1978;135:452–457.

146. Loeser EA, Bennett GM, Orr DL, Stanley TH.

147. Cross DE. Recent developments in tracheal cuffs. Resuscitation 1973;2:77–81.

148. Bernhard WN, Yost L, Joynes D, Cothalis S, Turndorf H. Intracuff pressures in endotracheal and tracheostomy tubes. Related cuff physical characteristics. Chest 1985;87:720–725.

149. Bunegin L, Albin M. Rauschnuber R, Smith RB. A new method for evaluating the relationship of mucosal contact pressure to endotracheal tube cuff pressure. Anesthesiology 1985;63:A198.

150. Tonnesen AS, Vereen L, Arens JF. Endotracheal tube cuff residual volume and lateral wall pressure in a model trachea. Anesthesiology 1981;55:680–683.

151. Mehta S. Performance of low-pressure cuffs. An experimental evaluation. Ann R Coll Surg Engl 1982;64:54–56.

152. Nordin U. The trachea and cuff-induced tracheal injury. Acta Otolaryngol Suppl (Stockh) 1977;345:1–74.

153. Stauffer JL, Olson DE, Petty TL. Complications and consequences of endotracheal intubation and tracheotomy. A prospective study of 150 critically ill adult patients. Am J Med 1981;70:65–76.

154. Jaeger JM, Wells NC, Blanch PB. Mechanical ventilation of a patient with decreased lung compliance and tracheal dilatation. J Clin Anesth 1992;4:147–152.

155. Loeser EA, Hodges M, Gliedman J, Stanley TH, Johansen RK, Yonetani D. Tracheal pathology following short-term intubation with low- and high-pressure endotracheal tube cuffs. Anesth Analg 1978;57:577–579.

156. Bunegin L, Albin MS, Smith RB. Canine tracheal blood flow after endotracheal tube cuff inflation during normotension and hypotension. Anesth Analg 1993;76:1083–1090.

157. King K, Mandava B, Kamen JM. Tracheal tube cuffs and tracheal dilatation. Chest 1975;67:458–462.

158. Dinnick OP. Tracheal cuffs. Anaesthesia 1975;30:553–554.

159. MacKenzie CF, Shin B, McAslan TC, Blanchard CL, Cowley RA. Severe stridor after prolonged endotracheal intubation using high-volume cuffs. Anesthesiology 1979;50:235–239.

160. Pippin LK, Short DH, Bowes JB. Long-term tracheal intubation practice in the United Kingdom. Anaesthesia 1983;38:791–795.

161. Pavlin EG, VanNimwegan D, Hornbein TF. Failure of a high-compliance low-pressure cuff to prevent aspiration. Anesthesiology 1975;42:216–219.

162. Macrae W, Wallace P. Aspiration around high-

volume, low-pressure endotracheal cuff. Br Med J 1981;283:1220.

163. Routh G, Hanning CD, Ledingham IM. Pressure on the tracheal mucosa from cuffed tubes. Br Med J 1979;1:1425.

164. Seegobin RD, van Hasselt GL. Aspiration beyond endotracheal cuffs. Can Anaesth Soc J 1986;33:273–279.

165. Sweatman AJ, Tomasello PA, Loughhead MO, Orr M, Datta T. Misplacement of nasogastric tubes and oesophageal monitoring devices. Br J Anaesth 1978;50:389–392.

166. Stark P. Inadvertent nasogastric tube insertion into the tracheobronchial tree. A hazard of new high-residual volume cuffs. Radiology 1982;142:239–240.

167. Nakao MA, Killam D, Wilson R. Pneumothorax secondary to inadvertent nasotracheal placement of a nasoenteric tube past a cuffed endotracheal tube. Crit Care Med 1983;11:210–211.

168. Lee T, Schrader MW, Wright BD. Pseudo-failure of mechanical ventilator caused by accidental endobronchial nasogastric tube insertion. Respir Care 1980;25:851–853.

169. Carey TS, Holcombe BJ. Endotracheal intubation as a risk factor for complications of nasoenteric tube insertion. Crit Care Med 1991;19:427–429.

170. Dodd CM, Loken RG, Williams RT. Hazards associated with passage of nasogastric tubes. Can J Anaesth 1988;35:541–542.

171. Elder S, Meguid MM. Pneumothorax following attempted nasogastric intubation for nutritional support. J Parenter Enteral Nutr 1984;8:450–452.

172. Carroll RG, Grenvick A. Proper use of large diameter, large residual volume cuffs. Crit Care Med 1973;1:153–154.

173. Power KJ. Foam cuffed tracheal tubes. Clinical and laboratory assessment. Br J Anaesth 1990;65:433–437.

174. Kamen JM, Wilkinson C. Removal of an inflated endotracheal tube cuff. Anesthesiology 1977;46:308–309.

175. MacKenzie CF, Klose S, Browne DRG. A study of inflatable cuffs on endotracheal tubes. Br J Anaesth 1976;48:105–110.

176. Elliott CJR. Problems of cuff deflation. Anaesthesia 1973;28:535–537.

177. Tavakoli M, Corssen G. An unusual case of difficult extubation. Anesthesiology 1976;45:552–553.

178. Birkhan HJ, Heifetz M. "Uninflatable" inflatable cuffs. Anesthesiology 1965;26:578.

179. Diaz JH. Continuous monitoring of intracuff pressures in endotracheal tubes. Anesthesiology 1988;68:813–814.

180. Morris JV, Latto IP. An electropneumatic instrument for measuring and controlling the pressures in the cuffs of tracheal tubes [The Cardiff cuff controller]. J Med Eng Technol 1985;9:229–230.

181. Scott AA. Pressure monitoring device for low pressure cuffs on tracheostomy tubes. Can Anaesth Soc J 1974;21:120–122.

182. Cox PM, Schatz ME. Pressure measurements in endotracheal cuffs: a common error. Chest 1974;65:84–87.

183. McGinnis GE, Shively JG, Patterson RL, Magovern GJ. An engineering analysis of intratracheal tube cuffs. Anesth Analg 1971;50:557–564.

184. Magovern GJ, Shively JG, Fecht D, Thevoz F. The clinical and experimental evaluation of a controlled-pressure intratracheal cuff. J Thorac Cardiovasc Surg 1972;64:747–756.

185. Leigh JM, Maynard JP. Pressure on the tracheal mucosa from cuffed tubes. Br Med J 1979;1:1173–1174.

186. Carroll RG. Evaluation of tracheal tube cuff designs. Crit Care Med 1973;1:45–46.

187. Brandt L. Pressures on tracheal tube cuffs. Anaesthesia 1981;37:597–598.

188. Burns SM, Shasby DM, Burke PA. Controlled pressure cuffed endotracheal tubes may not be controlled. Chest 1983;83:158–159.

189. Kumar CM, Scott G. Lanz valve—a method of circumventing a leaking valve. Anaesthesia 1986;41:772.

190. Brandt L. Prevention of nitrous oxide-induced increases in endotracheal tube cuff pressure. Anesth Analg 1991;72:262–263.

191. Sosis M, Braverman B, Ivankovich A. Evaluation of a new system to prevent nitrous oxide induced tracheal tube cuff overinflation. Anesthesiology 1992;77:A580.

192. Mandoe H, Nikolajsen L, Lintrup U, Jepsen D, Molgaard J. Sore throat after endotracheal intubation. Anesth Analg 1992;74:897–900.

193. Gravenstein N, Burwick N. Recoil of inflation syringe plunger limits excessive endotracheal tube cuff pressure. Anesthesiology 1988;69:A730.

194. Resnikoff E, Katz JA. A modified epidural syringe as an endotracheal tube cuff pressure-controlling device. Anesth Analg 1990;70:208–211.

195. Stanley TH, Foote JL, Lu WS. A simple pressure-relief valve to prevent increases in endotracheal tube cuff pressure and volume in intubated patients. Anesthesiology 1975;43:478–481.

196. Kay J, Fisher JA. Control of endotracheal tube cuff pressure using a simple device. Anesthesiology 1987;66:253.

197. Kim J. The tracheal tube cuff pressure stabilizer and its clinical evaluation. Anesth Analg 1980;59:291–296.

198. Latto IP, Willis BA, Dyson A. The Cardiff cuff controller. Br J Anaesth 1987;59:651P–652P.

199. Willis BA, Latto IP, Dyson A. Tracheal tube cuff pressure. Clinical use of the Cardiff cuff controller. Anaesthesia 1988;43:312–314.

200. Willis BA, Latto IP. Profile-cuffed tracheal tubes

and the Cardiff cuff controller. Anaesthesia 1989;44:524.

201. Lawler PG, Rayner RR. The limitations of the Shiley pressure relief adaptor. Anaesthesia 1982;37:865.

202. American Society for Testing and Materials. Standard specification for tracheal tube connectors (ASTM F1243-89). Philadelphia: ASTM, 1989.

203. Branson R, Lam AM. Increased resistance to breathing: a potentially lethal hazard across a co-axial circuit-connector coupling. Can J Anaesth 1987;34:S90–S91.

204. Villforth JC. FDA safety alert: breathing systems connectors. Rockville, MD: FDA, September 2, 1983.

205. Shupak RC. A new tracheal tube for head and neck surgery. Anesthesiology 1984;60:621–622.

206. Smith WDA. The effects of external resistance to respiration. Part II. Resistance to respiration due to anaesthetic apparatus. Br J Anaesth 1961;33:610–627.

207. Galloon S. The resistance of endotracheal connectors. Br J Anaesth 1957;29:160–165.

208. Hayes SR, Johnson K, Munson ES. Removal of endotracheal tube connectors. Anesth Analg 1987;66:1059–1060.

209. Scott RPF, Chapman I. A problem with the Argyll tracheal tube. Anaesthesia 1987;42:1123.

210. Sosis M, Dillon F. What is the safest foil tape for endotracheal tube protection during Nd-YAG laser surgery? A comparative study. Anesthesiology 1990;72:553–555.

211. Sosis MB. Anesthesia for laser surgery. Int Anesthesiol Clin 1990;28:119–131.

212. Snow JC, Kripke J, Strong MS, Jako GJ, Meyer MR, Vaughan CW. Anesthesia for carbon dioxide laser surgery on the larynx and trachea. Anesth Analg 1974;53:507–512.

213. Patel V, Stehling LC, Zauder HL. A modified endotracheal tube for laser microsurgery. Anesthesiology 1979;51:571.

214. Patil KF, Hicks JN. Prevention of fire hazard associated with use of carbon dioxide lasers. Anesth Analg 1981;60:885–888.

215. Vourc'h G, Tannieres ML, Freche G. Anaesthesia for microsurgery of the larynx using a carbon dioxide laser. Anaesthesia 1979;34:53–57.

216. Sosis MB. Evaluation of five metallic tapes for protection of endotracheal tubes during CO_2 laser surgery. Anesth Analg 1989;68:392–393.

217. Sosis M, Heller S. A comparison of five metallic tapes for protection of endotracheal tubes during CO_2 laser surgery. Can J Anaesth 1988;35:S63.

218. Sosis MB. In response. Anesth Analg 1991;72:415–416.

219. Willianson R. Why 70 watts to evaluate metal tapes for CO_2 laser surgery? Anesth Analg 1991;72:414–415.

220. Sosis M, Dillon F. Prevention of CO_2 induced laser tracheal tube fires with Laser-Guard protective coating. Can J Anaesth 1989;36:S88–S89.

221. Gonzalez C, Smith M, Reinisch L. Endotracheal tube safety with the erbium:ytrium aluminum garnet laser. Ann Otol Rhinol Laryngol 1990;99:553–555.

222. Burgess GE, LeJeune FE. Endotracheal tube ignition during laser surgery of the larynx. Arch Otolaryngol 1979;105:561–562.

223. Brightwell AP. A complication of the use of the laser in ENT surgery. J Laryngol Otol 1983;97:671–672.

224. Kaeder CS, Hirshman CA. Acute airway obstruction: a complication of aluminum tape wrapping of tracheal tubes in laser surgery. Can Anaesth Soc J 1979;26:138–139.

225. Ngeow YK, Kashima H. More about protection of endotracheal tubes during laser microlaryngeal surgery. Anesthesiology 1981;55:714.

226. Fontenot R, Bailey BJ, Stiernberg CM, Jenicek JA. Endotracheal tube safety during laser surgery. Laryngoscope 1987;97:919–921.

227. Hirshman CA, Leon D. Ignition of an endotracheal tube during laser microsurgery. Anesthesiology 1980;53:177.

228. Hirshman CA, Smith J. Indirect ignition of the endotracheal tube during carbon dioxide laser surgery. Arch Otolaryngol 1980;106:639–641.

229. Kalhan S, Regan AG. A further modification of endotracheal tubes for laser microsurgery. Anesthesiology 1980;53:81.

230. Uejima T. Cuffed endotracheal tubes in pediatric patients. Anesth Analg 1989;68:423.

231. Malmros C, Fletcher R, Jonmarker C, Nordstrom L. Cuffed endotracheal tubes for paediatric cardiac surgery cause a low incidence of post-operative airway problems. Anesthesiology 1991;75:A931.

232. Browning DH, Graves SA. Incidence of aspiration with endotracheal tubes in children. J Pediatr 1983;102:582–584.

233. Stenqvist O, Sonander H, Nilsson K. Small endotracheal tubes. Ventilator and intratracheal pressures during controlled ventilation. Br J Anaesth 1979;51:375–381.

234. Mackenzie CF, Shin B, Whitley N, Helrich M. Human tracheal circumference as an indicator of correct cuff size. Anesthesiology 1980;53:S414.

235. Chandler M, Crawley BE. Rationalization of the selection of tracheal tubes. Br J Anaesth 1986;58:111–116.

236. Mackenzie CF, Shin B, Whitley N, Schellinger D. The relationship of human trachea size to body habitus. Anesthesiology 1979;51:S378.

237. Mackenzie CF, McAslan C, Shin B, Schellinger D, Helrich M. The shape of the human adult trachea. Anesthesiology 1978;49:48–50.

238. Mehta S, Myat HM. The cross-sectional shape and

circumference of the human trachea. Ann R Coll Surg Engl 1984;66:356–358.

239. DiCarlo JV, Sanders AI, Sweeney MF. Airway complications of endotracheal intubation in pediatric patients. Effect of endotracheal tube fit. Anesthesiology 1988;69:A775.

240. Finholt DA, Henry DB, Raphaely RC. Factors affecting leak around tracheal tubes in children. Can Anaesth Soc J 1985;32:326–329.

241. Finholt DA, Audenaert SM, Stirt JA, et al. Endotracheal tube leak pressure and tracheal lumen size in swine. Anesth Analg 1986;65:667–671.

242. Sweeney MF, Egar M, Williams TA, Fuhrman BP. Total respiratory resistance in the intubated pediatric patient. Anesthesiology 1985;63:A477.

243. Lane GA, Pashley RT, Fishman RA. Tracheal and cricoid diameters in the premature infant. Anesthesiology 1980;53:S326.

244. Penlington GN. Endotracheal tube sizes for children. Anaesthesia 1975;24:494–495.

245. Anonymous. Standards for CPR and ECC. JAMA 1986;255:2972.

246. Gregory GA. Respiratory care of the child. Crit Care Med 1980;8:582–587.

247. Fukuoka RH, Kelly JW, Franklin CM. Correlation between ETT size, distal digit diameter and the Penlington formula. Anesth Analg 1991;72:S85.

248. Hinkle AJ, Arnold DE. Pediatric airway device selection with a body length tape measure. Anesthesiology 1991;75:A402.

249. Hinkle AJ. A rapid and reliable method of selecting endotracheal tube size in children. Anesth Analg 1988;67:S92.

250. Zulliger JJ, Garvin JP, Schuller DE, Birck HG, Beach TP, Frank JE. Assessment of intubation in croup and epiglottitis. Ann Otol Rhinol Laryngol 1982;91:403–406.

251. Downes JJ. Pediatric tracheal tube consideration. Paper presented at a workshop on tracheal tubes, Valley Forge, PA. April 30–May 1, 1981.

252. Board J. Endotracheal tube diameter. Anaesth Intensive Care 1982;10:91–92.

253. McCoy E, Barnes S. A defect in a tracheal tube. Anaesthesia 1989;44:525.

254. McLean RF, McLean J, McKee D. Another cause of tracheal tube failure. Can J Anaesth 1989;36:733–734.

255. Smith MB, Watts JD. Splitting tubes. Anaesthesia 1992;47:363.

256. Heusner JE, Viscomi CM. Endotracheal tube cuff failure due to valve damage. Anesth Analg 1991;72:270.

257. Gold ML. Use of petroleum jelly. Anesthesiology 1985;63:339–340.

258. Lee CM. "Training" of pediatric endotracheal tubes. Anesth Analg 1987;66:920.

259. McMillan DD, Rademaker AW, Buchan KA, Reid A, Machin G, Sauve RS. Benefits of orotracheal and nasotracheal intubation in neonates requiring ventilatory assistance. Pediatrics 1986;77:39–44.

260. Fletcher R, Olsson K, Helbo-Hansen S, Nihlson C, Hederstrom P. Oral or nasal intubation after cardiac surgery? A comparison of effects on heart rate, blood pressure and sedation requirements. Anaesthesia 1984;39:376–378.

261. Donn SM, Blane CE. Endotracheal tube movement in the preterm neonate: oral versus nasal intubation. Ann Otol Rhinol Laryngol 1985;94:18–20.

262. Duke PM, Coulson JD, Santos JI, Johnson JD. Cleft palate associated with prolonged orotracheal intubation in infancy. J Pediatr 1976;89:990–991.

263. Erenberg A, Nowak AJ. Palatal groove formation in neonates and infants with orotracheal tubes. Am J Dis Child 1984;138:974–975.

264. Boice JB, Krous HF, Foley JM. Gingival and dental complications of orotracheal intubation. JAMA 1976;236:957–958.

265. Saunders BS, Easa D, Slaughter RJ. Acquired palatal groove in neonates. A report of two cases. J Pediatr 1976;89:988–989.

266. Bach A, Boehrer H, Schmidt H, Geiss HK. Nosocomial sinusitis in ventilated patients. Anaesthesia 1992;47:335–339.

267. Coppolo DP, May JJ. Self-extubations in a 12-month experience. Chest 1990;98:165–169.

268. Berry FA, Blankenbaker WL, Ball CG. A comparison of bacteremia occurring with nasotracheal and orotracheal intubation. Anesth Analg 1979;52:873–876.

269. Dinner M, Tjeuw M, Artusio JF. Bacteremia as a complication of nasotracheal intubation. Anesth Analg 1987;66:460–462.

270. McShane AJ, Hone R. Prevention of bacterial endocarditis: does nasal intubation warrant prophylaxis? Br Med J 1986;292:26–27.

271. Rowse CW. Bacteraemia induced by endotracheal intubation. Br Dent J 1981;151:363.

272. Arens JF, LeJeune FE, Webre DR. Maxillary sinusitis: a complication of nasotracheal intubation. Anesthesiology 1974;40:415–416.

273. Aebert H, Hunefeld G, Regel G. Paranasal sinusitis and sepsis in ICU patients with nasotracheal intubation. Intensive Care Med 1988;15:27–30.

274. Deutschman CS, Wilton PB, Sinow J, Thienprasit P, Konstantinides FN, Cerra FB. Paranasal sinusitis. A common complication of nasotracheal intubation in neurosurgical patients. Neurosurgery 1985;17:296–299.

275. Deutschman CS, Wilton P, Sinow J, Dibbell D, Konstantinides FN, Cerra FB. Paranasal sinusitis associated with nasotracheal intubation. A fre-

quently unrecognized and treatable source of sepsis. Crit Care Med 1986;14:111–114.

276. Fassoulaki A. Nasotracheal intubation, paranasal sinusitis and head injuries. Br J Anaesth 1989;62:236.

277. Fassoulaki A, Pamouktsoglou P. Prolonged nasotracheal intubation and its association with inflammation of paranasal sinuses. Anesth Analg 1989;69:50–52.

278. Hansen M, Poulsen MR, Bendixen DK, Hartman-Andersen F. Incidence of sinusitis in patients with nasotracheal intubation. Br J Anaesth 1988;61:231–232.

279. Halac E, Indiveri DR, Obregon RJ, Begue E, Casanas M. Complication of nasal endotracheal intubation. J Pediatr 1983;103:166.

280. Knodel AR, Beekman JF. Unexplained fevers in patients with nasotracheal intubation. JAMA 1982;248:868–870.

281. Linden BE, Aguilar EA, Allen SJ. Sinusitis in the nasotracheally intubated patient. Arch Otolaryngol Head Neck Surg 1988;114:860–861.

282. O'Reilly MJ, Reddick EJ, Black W, et al. Sepsis from sinusitis in nasotracheally intubated patients. A diagnostic dilemma. Am J Surg 1984;147:601–604.

283. Pope TL, Stelling CB, Leitner YB. Maxillary sinusitis after nasotracheal intubation. South Med J 1981;74:610–612.

284. Pedersen J, Schurizek BA, Melsen NC, Juhl B. The effect of nasotracheal intubation on the paranasal sinuses. A prospective study of 434 intensive care patients. Acta Anaesthesiol Scand 1991;35:11–13.

285. Salord F, Gaussorgues P, Marti-Flich J, et al. Nosocomial maxillary sinusitis during mechanical ventilation: a prospective comparison of orotracheal versus the nasotracheal route for intubation. Intensive Care Med 1990;16:390–393.

286. Willatts SM, Cochrane DF. Paranasal sinusitis. A complication of nasotracheal intubation. Br J Anaesth 1985;57:1026–1028.

287. Grindlinger GA, Niehoff J, Hughes SL, Humphrey MA, Simpson G. Acute paranasal sinusitis related to nasotracheal intubation of head-injured patients. Crit Care Med 1987;15:214–217.

288. Katkov WN, Ault MJ. Endotracheal intubation in massive hemoptysis. Advantages of the orotracheal route. Crit Care Med 1989;17:968.

289. Quintin L, Ghignone M, Odelin P, Trinquier R, Ruvnat L, Du Gres B. Decreasing the incidence of upper airway bleeding when using a large-size nasotracheal tube. Anesthesiology 1985;62:374.

290. Kay J, Bryan R, Hart HB, Minkel DT, Munshi C. Sequential dilatation. A useful adjunct in reducing blood loss from nasotracheal intubation. Anesthesiology 1985;63:A259.

291. Berger JM, Stirt JA. Aid to nasotracheal intubation. Anesthesiology 1983;58:105.

292. Moore DC. Bloodless turbinectomy following blind nasal intubation. Faulty technique. Anesthesiology 1990;73:1057.

293. Tahir AH. A simple manoeuvre to aid the passage of nasotracheal tube into the oropharynx. Br J Anaesth 1970;42:631–632.

294. Dryden GE. Use of a suction catheter to assist blind nasal intubation. Anesthesiology 1976;45:260.

295. Cohen PJ. An endotracheal-tube barb. Anesthesiology 1977;47:77.

296. Berry FA. The use of a stylet in blind nasotracheal intubation. Anesthesiology 1984;61:469–471.

297. Bennett EJ, Grundy EM, Patel KP. Visual signs in blind nasal intubation. A new technique. Anesthesiol Rev 1978;5:18–20.

298. Danzl DF, Thomas DM. Nasotracheal intubations in the emergency department. Crit Care Med 1980;8:677–682.

299. Liew RPC. A technique of naso-tracheal intubation with the soft Portex tube. Anaesthesia 1973;28:567–568.

300. Barriot P, Riou B. Retrograde technique for tracheal intubation in trauma patients. Crit Care Med 1988;16:712–713.

301. Mehta S. Intubation guide marks for correct tube placement. A clinical study. Anaesthesia 1991;46:306–308.

302. Owen RL, Cheney FW. Endobronchial intubation: a preventable complication. Anesthesiology 1987;67:255–257.

303. Yates AP, Harries AJ, Hatch DJ. Estimation of nasotracheal tube length in infants and children. Br J Anaesth 1987;59:524–526.

304. Mamawadu BR, Miller R. Endotracheal cuff inflation. An improved technique. Anesthesiol Rev 1977;4:46–47.

305. Chandler S. Air volume in endotracheal tube cuffs. Anesthesiology 1980;53:437.

306. Mehta S. Aspiration around high-volume low-pressure endotracheal cuff. Br Med J 1982;284:115–116.

307. Wedley JR, Mathias DB. Endotracheal cuffs. Anaesthesia 1976;31:114.

308. Fenje N, Steward DJ. A study of tape adhesive strength on endotracheal tubes. Can J Anaesth 1988;35:198–202.

309. Richards SD. A method for securing pediatric endotracheal tubes. Anesth Analg 1981;60:224–225.

310. Mikawa K, Maekawa N, Goto R, Yaku H, Obara H. Transparent dressing is useful for the secure fixation of the endotracheal tube. Anesthesiology 1991;75:1123–1124.

311. Benumof JL. Conventional (laryngoscopic) orotracheal and nasotracheal intubation (single-

lumen type). In: Benumof JL, ed. Clinical procedures in anesthesia and intensive care. Philadelphia: JB Lippincott, 1992:115–148.

312. Bosman YK, Foster PA. Endotracheal intubation and head posture in infants. S Afr Med J 1977;52:71–73.

313. Dykes ER, Anderson R. Technic for fixation of endotracheal tubes. Anesth Analg 1964;43:238–240.

314. Klein DS. An endotracheal tube fixation device constructed from discarded oxygen tubing and umbilical tape. Anesthesiology 1984;60:76.

315. Steward DJ. Fixation of reinforced silicone tracheal tubes. Anesthesiology 1985;63:334.

316. Boyd GL, Funderburg BJ, Vasconez LO, Guzman G. Long-distance anesthesia. Anesth Analg 1992;74:477.

317. Garcia-Tornel S, Martin JM, Carits J, Toberna L, Garcia ME. Method of fixating tubes in infants and children. Respir Care 1978;22:58.

318. Molho M, Lieberman P. Safe fixation of oro- and nasotracheal tubes for prolonged intubation in neonates, infants and children. Crit Care Med 1975;3:81–82.

319. Stubbing JF, Young JVI. Circumpalatal fixation of an orotracheal tube. Anaesthesia 1985;40:916–917.

320. Jobes DR, Nicolson SC: An alternative method to secure an endotracheal tube in infants with midline facial defects. Anesthesiology 1986;64:643–644.

321. Birmingham PK, Horn B. An infant model to facilitate endotracheal tube fixation in the pediatric ICU patient. Anesthesiology 1989;70:163–164.

322. Gowdar K, Bull MJ, Schreiner RL, Lemons JA, Gresham EL. Nasal deformities in neonates. Their occurrence in those treated with nasal continuous positive airway pressure and nasal endotracheal tubes. Am J Dis Child 1980;134:954–957.

323. Alfery DD. Changing an endotracheal tube. In: JL Benumof, ed. Clinical procedures in anesthesia and intensive care. Philadelphia: JB Lippincott, 1992:177–194.

324. Bedger RC, Chang J. A jet-style endotracheal catheter for difficult airway management. Anesthesiology 1987;66:221–223.

325. Benumof JL. Additional safety measures when changing endotracheal tubes. Anesthesiology 1991;75:921–922.

326. Desai SP Fencl V. A safe technique for changing endotracheal tubes. Anesthesiology 1980;53:267.

327. Garla PGN, Skaredoff M. Tracheal extubation. Anesthesiology 1992;76:1058.

328. Benumof JF. Management of the difficult adult airway. Anesthesiology 1991;75:1087–1110.

329. Benumof JL. Management of the difficult airway. The ASA algorithm (ASA Refresher Course #134). New Orleans: ASA, 1992.

330. Jaffe BF. Postoperative hoarseness. Am J Surg 1972;123:432–437.

331. Kambic V, Radsel Z. Intubation lesions of the larynx. Br J Anaesth 1978;50:587–590.

332. Peppard SB, Dickens JH. Laryngeal injury following short-term intubation. Ann Otol Rhinol Laryngol 1984;92:327–330.

333. Stout DM, Bishop MJ. Perioperative laryngeal and tracheal complications of intubation. Probl Anesth 1988;2:225–234.

334. Prasertwanitch Y, Schwarz JJH, Vandam LD. Arytenoid cartilage dislocation following prolonged endotracheal intubation. Anesthesiology 1974;41:516–517.

335. Nicholls BJ, Packham RN. Arytenoid cartilage dislocation. Anaesth Intensive Care 1986;14:196–198.

336. Gray B, Huggins NJ, Hirsch N. An unusual complication of tracheal intubation. Anaesthesia 1990;45:558–560.

337. Frink EJ, Pattison BD. Posterior arytenoid dislocation following uneventful endotracheal intubation and anesthesia. Anesthesiology 1989;70:358–360.

338. Quick CA, Merwin GE. Arytenoid dislocation. Arch Otolaryngol 1978;104:267–270.

339. Chatterji S, Gupta NR, Mishra TR. Valvular glottic obstruction following extubation. Anaesthesia 1984;39:246–247.

340. Castella X, Gilabert J, Perez C. Arytenoid dislocation after tracheal intubation. An unusual cause of acute respiratory failure? Anesthesiology 1991;74:613–615.

341. Keane WM, Denneny JC, Rowe LD, Atkins JP. Complications of intubation. Ann Otol Rhinol Laryngol 1982;91:584–587.

342. Tintinalli JE, Claffey J. Complications of nasotracheal intubation. Ann Emerg Med 1981;10:142–144.

343. Binning R. A hazard of blind nasal intubation. Anaesthesia 1974;29:366–367.

344. Cooper R. Bloodless turbinectomy following blind nasal intubation. Anesthesiology 1989;71:469.

345. Kawamoto M, Shimidzu Y. A balloon catheter for nasal intubation. Anesthesiology 1983;59:484.

346. Knuth TE, Richards JR. Mainstem bronchial obstruction secondary to nasotracheal intubation. A case report and review of the literature. Anesth Analg 1991;73:487–489.

347. Mayumi T, Miyabe M. Complete endotracheal tube obstruction after nasotracheal intubation. Can Anaesth Soc J 1984;31:344–345.

348. Vitkun SA, Sidhu US, Lagade MRG, Poppers PJ. Intranasal trauma caused by a sharp-edged laser-resistant (silicone) endotracheal tube. Anesthesiology 1985;62:834–835.

349. Kras JF, Marchmont-Robinson H. Pharyngeal

perforation during intubation in a patient with Crohn's disease. Am J Oral Maxillofac Surg 1989;47:405–407.

350. Daly WM. Unusual complication of nasal intubation. Anesthesiology 1953;14:96.

351. Adelman MH. Perforation of the pyriform sinus, a sequela of endotracheal intubation. J Mt Sinai Hosp 1953;19:665–667.

352. Bembridge JL, Bembridge M. Pneumomediastinum during general anaesthesia: case report. Can J Anaesth 1989;36:75–77.

353. Dubost C, Kaswin D, Duranteau A, Jehanno C, Kaswin R. Esophageal perforation during attempted endotracheal intubation. J Thorac Cardiovasc Surg 1979;78:44–51.

354. de Espinosa H, de Paredes CG. Traumatic perforation of the pharynx in a newborn baby. J Ped Surg 1974;9:247–248.

355. Evron S, Beyth Y, Samueloff A, Eimerl D Schenker JG. Pulmonary complications following endotracheal intubation for anesthesia in breech extractions. Intensive Care Med 1985;11:223–225.

356. Eldor J, Ofek B, Abramowitz HB. Perforation of oesophagus by tracheal tube during resuscitaton. Anaesthesia 1990;45:70–71.

357. Finer NN, Stewart AR, Ulan OA. Tracheal perforation in the neonate. Treatment with a cuffed endotracheal tube. J Pediatr 1976;89:510–512.

358. Guernelli N, Bragaglia RB, Briccoli A, Mastrofjrilli M, Vecchi R. Tracheobronchial ruptures due to cuffed Carlens tubes. Ann Thorac Cardiovasc Surg 1979;28:66–68.

359. Hawkins DB, Seltzer DC, Barnett TE, Stoneman GB. Endotracheal tube perforation of the hypopharynx. West J Med 1974;120:282–286.

360. Hirach M, Abramowitz HB, Shapira S, Barki Y. Hypopharyngeal injury as a result of attempted endotracheal intubation. Radiology 1978;128:37–39.

361. Harmer M. Complications of tracheal intubation. In: Latto IP, Rosen M, eds. Difficulties in tracheal intubation. London: Bailliere Tindall, 1985:36–47.

362. Johnson KG, Hood DD. Esophageal perforation associated with endotracheal intubation. Anesthesiology 1986;64:281–283.

363. Kanarek KS, David RF. Traumatic perforation of the esophagus in a newborn. J Fla Med Assoc 1979;66:288–289.

364. Levine PA. Hypopharyngeal perforation. Arch Otolaryngol 1980;106:578–580.

365. Myers EM. Hypopharyngeal perforation: a complication of endotracheal intubation. Laryngoscope 1982;92:583–585.

366. McLeod BJ, Summer E. Neonatal trachea perforation. Anaesthesia 1986;41:67–70.

367. Norman EA, Sosis M. Iatrogenic oesophageal perforation due to tracheal or nasogastric intubation. Can Anaesth Assoc J 1986;33:222–226.

368. Orta DA, Cousar JE, Yergin BM, Olsen GN. Tracheal laceration with massive subcutaneous emphysema: a rare complication of endotracheal intubation. Thorax 1979;34:665–669.

369. O'Neill JE, Giffin JP, Cottrell JE. Pharyngeal and esophageal perforation following endotracheal intubation. Anesthesiology 1984;60:487–488.

370. Stauffer JL, Petty TL. Accidental intubation of the pyriform sinus. A complication of "roadside" resuscitation. JAMA 1977;237:2324–2325.

371. Schild JP, Wuilloud A, Kollberg H, Bossi E. Tracheal perforation as a complication of nasotracheal intubation in a neonate. J Pediatr 1976;88:631–632.

372. Smith BAC, Hopkinson RB. Tracheal rupture during anaesthesia. Anaesthesia 1984;39:894–898.

373. Serlin SP, Daily WJR. Tracheal perforation in the neonate. A complication of endotracheal intubation. J Pediatr 1975;86:596–597.

374. Talbert JL, Rodgers B, Felman AH, Moazam F. Traumatic perforation of the hypopharynx in infants. J Thorac Cardiovasc Surg 1977;74:152–156.

375. Touloukian RJ, Beardsley GP, Ablow RC, Effmann EL. Traumatic perforation of the pharynx in the newborn. Pediatrics 1977;59:1019–1022.

376. Tan CSH, Tashkin DP, Sassoon H. Pneumothorax and subcutaneous emphysema complicating endotracheal intubation. South Med J 1984;77:253–255.

377. Topsis J, Kinas HY, Kandall SR. Esophageal perforation—a complication of neonatal resuscitation. Anesth Analg 1989;69:532–534.

378. Wolff AP, Kuhn FA, Ogura JH. Pharyngeal-esophageal perforations associated with rapid oral endotracheal intubation. Ann Otol 1972;81:258–261.

379. Wengen DFA. Piriform fossa perforation during attempted tracheal intubation. Anaesthesia 1987;42:519–521.

380. Young PN, Robinson JM. Cellulitis as a complication of difficult tracheal intubation. Anaesthesia 1987;42:569.

381. Pembleton WE, Brooks JW. Esophageal perforation of unusual etiology. Anesthesiology 1976;45:680–681.

382. Majumdar B, Stevens RW, Obara LG. Retropharyngeal abscess following tracheal intubation. Anaesthesia 1982;37:67–70.

383. Seitz PA, Gravenstein N. Endobronchial rupture from endotracheal reintubation with an endotracheal tube guide. J Clin Anaesth 1989;1:214–217.

384. Minkel DT, Kay J, Cheng EY, Munshi C. Reducing blood loss from nasotracheal intubation by combining a warmed tube with vasoconstrictors. Anesth Analg 1987;66:S120.

385. Munson ES, Lee R, Kushing LG. A new complication associated with the use of wire-reinforced endotracheal tubes. Anesth Analg 1979;58:152.

386. Basagoitia JN, LaMastro M. Another complication of tracheal intubation. Anesth Analg 1990;70:460–461.

387. Tahir AH, Adriani J. Failure to effect satisfactory seal after hyperinflation of endotracheal cuff. Anesth Analg 1971;50:540–543.

388. Herrema IH. Hazardous tracheal tube pilot balloons. Anaesthesia 1986;46:673.

389. McLintock TTC, Watson E. Failure to inflate the cuff of a tracheal tube. Anaesthesia 1989;44:1016.

390. Redahan CP, Young T. Failure to inflate the cuff of a tracheal tube. Anaesthesia 1989;44:1016.

391. Anonymous. Anesthetic "misintubation" alleged. 1.5 million malpractice suit filed. Biomed Safe Stand 1981;11:67.

392. Anonymous. Anesthesia allegedly incorrect in $520,000 settlement. Biomed Safe Stand 1983;13:79.

393. Anonymous. Anesthesia-related errors alleged in patient deaths & disabilities: suits filed. Biomed Safe Stand 1984;14:65.

394. Adriani J. Unrecognized esophageal placement of endotracheal tubes. South Med J 1986;79:1591–1592.

395. Ballester EE, Torres A, Rodriguez-Roisin, Agusti-Vidal A. Pneumoperitoneum. An unusual manifestation of improper oral intubation. Crit Care Med 1985;13:138–139.

396. Birmingham PK, Cheney FW, Ward RJ. Esophageal intubation. A review of detection techniques. Anesth Analg 1986;65:886–891.

397. Vinen JD, Gaudry PL. Pneumoperitoneum complicating cardiopulmonary resuscitation. Anaesth Intensive Care 1986;14:193–195.

398. Lababidi Z, Bland H, James E. Retrieval of an endotracheal tube from the esophagus. J Pediat Rev 1978;93:1025.

399. Ford RWJ. Confirming tracheal intubation—a simple manoeuvre. Can Anaesth Soc J 1983;30:191–193.

400. Dhamee MS. Signs of endotracheal intubation. Anaesthesia 1981;36:328–329.

401. Howells TH, Riethmuller RJ. Signs of endotracheal intubation. Anaesthesia 1980;35:984–986.

402. Heiselman D, Potacek J, Snyder JV, Grenvik A. Detection of esophageal intubation in patients with intrathoracic stomach. Crit Care Med 1985;13:1069–1070.

403. Linko K, Paloheimo M Tammisto T Capnography for detection of accidental oesophageal intubation. Acta Anaesth Scand 1983;27:199–202.

404. Pollard BJ, Junius F. Accidental intubation of the oesophagus. Anaesth Intensive Care 1980;8:183–186.

405. Sharar SR, Bishop MJ. Complications of tracheal intubation. J Intensive Care Med 1992;7:12–23.

406. Stirt JA. Endotracheal tube misplacement. Anaesth Intensive Care 1982;10:274–276.

407. Peterson AW, Jacker LM. Death following inadvertent esophageal intubation. A case report. Anesth Analg 1973;32:398–401.

408. Baraka A, Tabakian H, Idriss A, Taha S. Breathing bag refilling. Anaesthesia 1989;44:81–82.

409. Andersen KH, Hald A. Assessing the position of the tracheal tube. The reliability of different methods. Anaesthesia 1989;44:984–985.

410. Charters P. Normal chest expansion with oesophageal placement of a tracheal tube. Anaesthesia 1989;44:365.

411. Cundy J. Accidental intubation of oesophagus. Anaesth Intensive Care 1981;9:76.

412. Ogden PN. Endotracheal tube misplacement. Anaesth Intensive Care 1983;11:273–274.

413. Uejima T. Esophageal intubation. Anaesth Analg 1987;66:481–482.

414. Howells TH. Oesophageal misplacement of a tracheal tube. Anaesthesia 1985;40:387.

415. Gillespie JH, Knight RG, Middaugh RE, Menk EJ, Baysinger C. Efficacy of endotracheal tube cuff palpation and humidity in distinguishing endotracheal from esophageal intubation. Anesthesiology 1988;69:A265.

416. Warden JC. Accidental intubation of the oesophagus and preoxygenation. Anaesth Intensive Care 1980;8:377.

417. Sosis MB, Sisamis J. Pulse oximetry in confirmation of correct tracheal tube placement. Anesth Analg 1990;71:309–310.

418. Hirsch NP. Confirmation of tracheal tube placement. Anaesthesia 1988;43:72.

419. Batra AK, Cohn MA. Uneventful prolonged misdiagnosis of esophageal intubation. Crit Care Med 1980;11:760–764.

420. Munro TN. Oesophageal misplacement of a tracheal tube. Anaesthesia 1985;40:919–920.

421. Horton WA, Ralston S. Cuff palpation does not differentiate oesophageal from tracheal placement of tubes. Anaesthesia 1988;43:803–804.

422. Horton WA, Perera S, Charters P. Further developments in tactile tests to confirm laryngeal placement of tracheal tubes. Anaesthesia 1988;43:240–244.

423. Charters P, Wilkinson K. Tactile orotracheal tube placement test. A bimanual tactile examination of the positioned orotracheal tube to confirm laryngeal placement. Anaesthesia 1987;42:801–807.

424. Nunn JF. The oesophageal detector device. Anaesthesia 1988;43:804.

425. Wee MYK. The oesophageal detector device. Assessment of a new method to distinguish oesopha-

geal from tracheal intubation. Anaesthesia 1988;43:27–29.

426. Pollard B. Oesophageal detector device. Anaesthesia 1988;43:713–714.

427. Morton NS, Stuart JC, Thomson MF, Wee MYK. The oesophageal detector device. successful use in children. Anaesthesia 1989;44:523–524.

428. O'Leary JJ, Pollard BJ, Ryan MJ. A method of detecting oesophageal intubation or confirming tracheal intubation. Anaesth Intensive Care 1988;16:299–301.

429. Salem MR, Baraka A, Brennan AM, Czinn EA, Heyman HJ. Efficacy of the self-inflating bulb in detecting esophageal intubation in the presence of a nasogastric tube. Anesthesiology 1992; 77:A1066.

430. Zaleski L, Abello D, Gold MI. Esophageal detector device. comparison with capnogram. Anesthesiology 1992;77:A508.

431. Baraka A, Salem MR, Brennan AM, Mimmagadda U, Heyman HJ. Use of self-inflating bulb in detecting esophageal intubation following "esophageal ventilation." Anesthesiology 1992;77:A294.

432. Thean K, Webster S. Failure of test for tracheal intubation. Anaesth Intensive Care 1989;17:236–237.

433. Lee ST. Partial lung ventilation test for differentiating esophageal and laryngeal intubation. Anesth Analg 1988;67:903–904.

434. Kalpokas M, Russell WJ. A simple technique for diagnosing oesophageal intubation. Anaesth Intensive Care 1989;17:39–43.

435. Birmingham PK, Cheney FW Jr. Incorrect tube placement. Prevention of a fatal complication. In: Bishop MJ, ed. Physiology and consequences of tracheal intubation. Vol. 2. No. 2. Problems in anesthesia. Philadelphia: JB Lippincott, 1988:278–279.

436. Owen RL, Cheney FW. Use of an apena monitor to verify endotracheal intubation. Respir Care 1985;30:974–976.

437. Wee MYK, Walker KY. The oesophageal detector device. Anaesthesia 1991;46:869–871.

438. Zbinden S, Schupfer G. Detection of oesophageal intubation: the cola complication. Anaesthesia 1989;44:81.

439. Abrahams N, Goldacre M, Reynolds EOR. Removal of swallowed neonatal endotracheal tube. Lancet 1970;2:135–136.

440. Bowen A,III, Dominguez R. Swallowed neonatal endotracheal tube. Pediatr Radiol 1981;10:178–179.

441. Dickson JAS, Fraser GC. "Swallowed" endotracheal tube: a new neonatal emergency. Br Med J 1967;1:811–812.

442. Flynn GJ, Lowe AK. Endotracheal tube swallowed by a neonate. Med J Aust 1973;1:62–63.

443. Finucane BT, Shanley V, Ricketts RR. "Disappearing" endotracheal tube following meconium aspiration. A possible solution to the problem. Anesthesiology 1989;71:469–470.

444. Hoffman S, Jedeikin R. Swallowed endotracheal tube in an adult. Anesth Analg 1984;63:457–459.

445. Kennedy S. Swallowed neonatal endotracheal tube. Lancet 1970;2:264.

446. Lee KW, Templeton JJ, Dougal RM. Tracheal tube size and post-intubation croup in children. Anesthesiology 1980;53:S325.

447. Mitchell SA, Shoults DL, Herren AL, Benumof JL. Deglutition of an endotracheal tube: case report. Anesth Analg 1978;57:590–591.

448. Mucklow ES. "Swallowed" endotracheal tube. Br Med J 1967;2:618.

449. Prinn MG. "Swallowed" endotracheal tube. Br Med J 1967;3:176.

450. Storch A, Calderwood GC. Endotracheal tube swallowed by neonate. J Pediatr 1970;77:123.

451. Stool SE, Johnson D, Rosenfeld PA. Unintentional esophageal intubation in the newborn. Pediatrics 1971;48:299–301.

452. Seto K, Goto H, Hacker DC, Arakawa K. Right upper lobe atelectasis after inadvertent right main bronchial intubation. Anesth Analg 1983;62:851–854.

453. Brunel W, Coleman DL, Schwartz DE, Peper E, Cohen NH. Assessment of routine chest roentgenograms and the physical examination to confirm endotracheal tube position. Chest 1989;96:1043–1045.

453a. Dronen S, Chadwick O, Nowak R. Endotracheal tip position in the arrested patient. Ann Emerg Med 1982;108:116–117.

453b. Bednarek FJ, Kuhns LR. Endotracheal tube placement in infants determined by suprasternal palpation: a new technique. Pediatrics 1975;56:224–229.

453c. Kuhns LR Poznanski AK. Endotracheal tube position in the infant. J Pediatr 1971;78:991–996.

453d. Wells AL, Wells TR, Landing BH, Cruz B, Galvis DA. Short trachea, a hazard in tracheal intubation of neonates and infants. Syndromal associations. Anesthesiology 1989;71:367–373.

453e. Blatchley D. Signs of endotracheal intubation. Anaesthesia 1981;36:328.

453f. Conrady PA, Goodman LR, Lainge F, Singer MM. Alteration of endotracheal tube position. Crit Care Med 1976;4:8–12.

453g. Donn SM, Kuhns LR. Mechanism of endotracheal tube movement with change of head position in the neonate. Pediatr Radiol 1980;9:37–40.

453h. Lingenfelter AL, Guskiewicz RA, Munson ES. Displacement of right atrial and endobronchial catheters with neck flexion. Anesth Analg 1978;57:371–373.

453i. Roopchand R, Roopnarinesingh S, Ramsewak S. Instability of the tracheal tube in neonates. Anaesthesia 1989;44:107–109.

453j. Todres ID, deBros F, Kramer SS. Endotracheal tube displacement in the newborn infant. J Pediatr 1976;89:126–127.

453k. Toung TJK, Grayson R, Saklad J, Wang H. Movement of the distal end of the endotracheal tube during flexion and extension. Anesth Analg 1985;64:1030–1032.

454. Heinonen J, Takki S, Tammisto T. Effect of the Trendelenburg tilt and other procedures on the position of endotracheal tubes. Lancet 1969;1:850–853.

455. Birmingham PK, Cheney FW. Incorrect tube placement. Probl Anestheisa 1988;2:278–291.

456. Todres ID, deBros F, Kramer SS. Endotracheal tube displacement in the newborn. Papers presented at the American Society of Anesthesiologists' meeting. 1975:27–28.

457. Goodman LR, Conrardy PA, Laing F, Singer MM. Radiologic evaluation of endotracheal tube position. Am J Roentgenol 1976;127:433–434.

458. Bloch EC, Ossey K, Ginsberg B. Tracheal intubation in children. A new method for assuring correct depth of tube placement. Anesth Analg 1988;67:590–592.

459. Roberts J. Fundamentals of tracheal intubation. New York: Grume & Stratton, 1983.

460. Gorback MS, Ravin CE. Reinforced endotracheal tube placement. Radiographic misdiagnosis. Radiology 1987;162:597.

461. Sosis M. Hazards of a new system for placement of endotracheal tubes. Anesthesiology 1988;68:299.

462. Schellinger RR. The length of the airway to the bifurcation of the trachea. Anesthesiology 1964;25:169–172.

463. Aldrete JA, Wright AJ. Airway assessment systems. Anesthesiol News, July 12, 1992:12.

464. Morgan GAR, Steward DJ. Linear airway dimensions in children. including those with cleft palate. Canad Anaesth Soc J 1982;29:1–8.

465. Tochen ML. Orotracheal intubation in the newborn infant: a method for determining depth of tube insertion. J Pediatr 1979;95:1050–1051.

466. Coldiron JS. Estimation of nasotracheal tube length in neonates. Pediatrics 1968;41:823–828.

467. Mattila MAK, Heikel PE, Suutarinen, Lindfors EL. Estimation of a suitable nasotracheal tube length for infants and children. Acta Anaesth Scand 1971;15:239–246.

468. Russell WJ, Smith JA. Endotracheal tube markings. Anaesth Intensive Care 1985;13:210–211.

469. Mehta S. Endotracheal intubation: friend or foe? Br Med J 1986;292:694.

470. Loew A, Thiebeault DW. A new and safe method to control the depth of endotracheal intubation in neonates. Pediatrics 1974;54:506–508.

471. Wallace CT, Cooke JE. A new method for positioning endotracheal tubes. Anesthesiology 1976;44:272.

472. Dietrich KA, Strauss RH, Cabalka AK, Zimmerman JJ, Scanlan KA. Use of flexible fiberoptic endoscopy for determination of endotracheal tube position in the pediatric patient. Crit Care Med 1988;16:884–887.

473. O'Brian D, Curran J, Conroy J, Bouchier-Hayes D. Fibre-optic assessment of tracheal tube position. A comparison of tracheal tube position as estimated by fibre-optic bronchoscopy and by chest x-ray. Anaesthesia 1985;40:73–76.

474. Vigneswaran R, Whitfield JM. The use of a new ultra-thin fiberoptic bronchoscope to determine endotracheal tube position in the sick newborn infant. Chest 1981;80:174–177.

475. Smith BL. Confirmation of the position of an endotracheal tube. Anaesthesia 1975;30:410.

476. Chander S, Feldman E. Correct placement of endotracheal tubes. NY State J Med 1979;79:1843–1844.

477. Ehrenwerth J, Nagle S, Hirsch N, LaMantia K. Is cuff palpation a useful tool for determining endotracheal tube position? Anesthesiology 1986;65:A137.

478. Cullen DJ, Newbower RS, Gemer M. A new method for positioning endotracheal tubes. Anesthesiology 1975;48:596–599.

479. Triner L. A simple maneuver to verify proper positioning of an endotracheal tube. Anesthesiology 1982;57:548–549.

480. Kopman EA. A simple method for verifying endotracheal tube placement. Anesth Analg 1977;56:121–124.

481. Hauser GJ, Muir E, Kline LM, Scheller T, Holbrook PR. Prospective evaluation of a nonradiographic device for determination of endotracheal tube position in children. Crit Care Med 1990;18:760–763.

482. Zwass MS, Schriener MS, Raphealy RC. Noninvasive determination of tracheal tube position in infants and children. Anesthesiology 1988;69:A178.

483. Cote CJ, Szyfelbein SK, Liu LMP, Firestone S, Goudsouzian NG, Welch J. Intraoperative events diagnosed by expired carbon dioxide monitoring in children. Can Anaesth Soc J 1986;33:315–320.

484. Gandhi SK, Munshi CA, Kampine JP. A sudden warning sign of an accidental endobronchial intubation. A sudden drop or sudden rise in $PaCO_2$? Anesthesiology 1986;65:114–115.

485. Riley RH, Marcy JH. Unsuspected endobronchial intubation—detection by continuous mass spectrometry. Anesthesiology 1985;63:203–204.

486. Riley RH, Finucane KE, Marcey JH. Early warning sign of an accidental endobronchial intubation. A sudden drop or sudden rise in PaCO$_2$? In reply. Anesthesiology 1986;65:115.

487. Stewart RD, LaRosee A, Kaplan RM, Ilkhanipour K. Correct positioning of an endotracheal tube using a flexible lighted stylet. Crit Care Med 1990;18:97–99.

488. Watson CB, Clapham M. Transillumination for correct tube positioning. Use of a new fiberoptic endotracheal tube. Anesthesiology 1984;60:253.

489. Heller RM, Cotton RB. Early experience with illuminated endotracheal tubes in premature and term infants. Pediatrics 1985;75:664–666.

490. Barker SJ, Tremper KK. Detection of endobronchial intubation by noninvasive monitoring. J Clin Monit 1987;3:292–293.

491. Alberti J, Hanafee W, Wilson G, Bethune R. Unsuspected pulmonary collapse during neuroradiologic procedures. Radiology 1967;89:316–320.

492. Bernard SA, Jones BM. Endotracheal tube obstruction in a patient with status asthmaticus. Anaesth Intensive Care 1991;19:121–123.

493. Seifert RD, Starsnic M, Zwillenberg D. Acute obstruction of the left mainstem bronchus following an attempted nasotracheal intubation. An unusual case report. Anesthesiology 1985;62:799–800.

494. Tahir AH. Endotracheal tube lost in the trachea. JAMA 1972;222:1061–1062.

495. Whyte MP. Aspiration of an endotracheal tube. JHEP 1977;6:332.

496. McGrath RB, Einterz RM. Aspiration of a nasotracheal tube. A complication of nasotracheal intubation and mechanism for retrieval. Chest 1987;91:148–149.

497. Milstein J, Rabinovitz J, Goetzman B. A foreign body hazard in the neonate. Anesth Analg 1977;56:726–727.

498. Harrington JF. An unusual cause of endotracheal tube obstruction. Anesthesiology 1984;61:116–117.

499. Chiu T, Meyers EF. Defective disposable endotracheal tube. Anesth Analg 1976;55:437.

500. Doyle LA, Conway CF. A hazard of cuffed endotracheal tubes. Anaesthesia 1967;22:140–141.

501. Loughrey JD. Danger of cuffed endotracheal tube during tracheostomy. Br J Anaesth 1967;39:692.

502. Smotrilla MM, Nagel EL, Moya E. Failure of inflatable cuff resulting in foreign body in the trachea. Anesthesiology 1966;27:512–513.

503. Restall CJ. Plastic-covered wire stylet. Anesth Analg 1976;55:755.

504. Martin P, Campbell AM. Tracheal intubation: a complication. Anaesthesia 1992;47:75.

505. Larson CE, Gonzalez RM. A problem with metal endotracheal tubes and plastic-coated stylets. Anesthesiology 1989;70:883–884.

506. Yeung ML, Lett Z. An uncommon hazard of armoured endotracheal tubes. Anaesthesia 1974;29:186–187.

507. Anonymous. Laser-resistant tracheal tube to be modified following recall. Biomed Safe Stand 1987;17:138.

508. Desmeules H. Defective tracheal tube connector. Can Anaesth Soc J 1982;29:404.

509. Lahay WD. Defective tracheal tube connector. Can Anaesth Soc J 1982;29:80–81.

510. Jackson S, Welch GW. Foreign body from a tube of anesthetic ointment. Anesthesiology 1987;67:154–155.

511. Holley HS, Gildea JE. Vocal cord paralysis after tracheal intubation. JAMA 1971;215:281–284.

512. Kamhol SL, Rothman NI, Underwood PS. Fiberbronchoscopic retrieval of iatrogenically introduced endobronchial foreign body. Crit Care Med 1979;7:346–348.

513. Liew PC. A hazard due to a commercially available topical spray. Anaesthesia 1973;28:346.

514. Debnath SK, Waters DJ. Leaking cuffed endotracheal tubes: two case reports. Br J Anaesth 1968;40:807.

515. Jayasuriya KD, Watson WF. P.V.C. cuffs and lignocaine-base aerosol. Br J Anaesth 1981;53:1368.

516. Reinders M, Gerber HR. Cuff failure of PVC tracheal tubes. Anaesthesia 1989;44:524–525.

517. Walmsley AJ, Burville LM, Davis TP. Cuff failure in polyvinyl chloride tracheal tubes sprayed with lignocaine. Anaesthesia 1988;43:399–401.

518. Wong RM. An unusual source of leakage fron the cuff of an endotracheal tube. Anaesth Intensive Care 1977;5:389.

519. Phillips B. Defect in a cuffed tube. Anaesthesia 1971;26:237.

520. Lacoste L, Thomas D. Unusual complication of tracheal intubation. Anesth Analg 1992;74:474–475.

521. Blitt CD, Wright WA. An unusual complication of percutaneous internal jugular vein cannulation, puncture of an endotracheal tube cuff. Anesthesiology 1974;40:306–307.

522. Brown HI, Burnard RJ, Jensen M, Wightman AE. Puncture of endotracheal-tube cuffs during percutaneous subclavian-vein catheterization. Anesthesiology 1975;43:112–113.

523. Hannington-Kiff JG. Faulty superset plastic catheter mounts. A cautionary tale applicable to other mass-produced disposable products. Anaesthesia 1991;46:671–672.

524. Nixon C. Endotracheal tube connector fracture—an avoidable hazard. Canad Anaesth Soc J 1986;33:251.

525. Oyston J, Holtby H. Fracture of a RAE endotracheal tube connector. Can J Anaesth 1988;35:438–439.

526. Angelillo JC, Kosanin R, Fox WD. Damage to endotracheal tube during maxillofacial surgery. Anesthiol Rev 1986;13:17–20.

527. Bamforth BJ. Complications during endotracheal anesthesia. Anesth Analg 1963;42:727–733.

528. Fagraeus L, Angelillo JC, Dolan EA. A serious anesthetic hazard during orthognathic surgery. Anesth Analg 1980;59:150–152.

529. Job CA, Betcher AM, Pearson WT, Fernandez MA. Intraoperative obstruction of endobronchial tubes. Anesthesiology 1979;51:550–553.

530. Ketzler JT, Landers DF. Management of a severed endotracheal tube during LeFort osteotomy. J Clin Anesth 1992;4:144–146.

531. Levack ID, Scott DHT. Conservative management of intra-operative cuff puncture in a bronchial tube. Anaesthesia 1985;40:1020–1021.

532. Mosby EL, Messer EJ, Nealis MF. Intraoperative damage to nasotracheal tubes during maxillary surgery:report of cases. J Oral Surg 1978;36:963–964.

533. Orr DL. Airway compromise during oral and maxillofacial surgery: case report and review of potential causes. Anesth Prog 1978;25:161–168.

534. Peskin RM, Sachs SA. Intraoperative management of a partially severed endotracheal tube during orthognathic surgery. Anesth Prog 1986;33:247–251.

535. Schwartz LB, Sordill WC, Liebers RM, Schwab W. Difficulty in removal of accidentally cut endotracheal tube. J Oral Maxillofac Surg. 1982;40:518–519.

536. Tseuda K, Carey WJ, Gonty AA, Bosomworth PB. Hazards to anesthetic equipment during maxillary osteotomy: report of cases. J Oral Surg 1977;35:47.

537. Spear RM, Sauder RA, Nichols DG. Endotracheal tube rupture, accidental extubation, and tracheal avulsion. Three airway catastrophes associated with significant decrease in leak pressure. Crit Care Med 1989;17:701–703.

538. McLean R, Houston P, Carmichael F, Bernstein M. Disruption of an armoured endotracheal tube caused by biting. Can Anaesth Soc J 1985;32:313.

539. Fisher MM. Repairing pilot balloon lines. Anaesth Intensive Care 1988;16:500–501.

540. Sills J. An emergency cuff inflation technique. Respir Care 1986;31:199–201.

541. Stimmel S, Gutierrez CJ. Emergency cuff-inflation technique revisited [Letter]. Respir Care 1986;31:538.

542. Watson E, Harris MM. Leaking endotracheal tube. Chest 1989;95:709.

543. Schcubert A, von Kaenel WE, Ilyes L. A comparison of techniques for sealing pinhole endotracheal cuff leaks. Anesthesiology 1989;71:A466.

544. Schubert A, Kaenel WV, Ilyes L. A management

option for leaking endotracheal tube cuffs. Use of lidocaine jelly. J Clin Anesth 1991;3:26–31.

545. Tinkoff G, Bakow ED, Smith RW. A continuous-flow apparatus for temporary inflation of damaged endotracheal tube cuffs. Respir Care 1991;35:423–426.

546. Verborgh C, Camu F. Management of cuff incompetence in an endotracheal tube. Anesthesiology 1987;66:441.

547. Vitkun SA, Lagasse RS, Kyle KT, Poppers PJ. Application of the Grieshaber air system to maintain endotracheal tube cuff pressure. J Clin Anaesth 1990;2:45–47.

548. Wagner DL, Gammage GW, Wong M. Tracheal rupture following the insertion of a disposable double-lumen endotracheal tube. Anesthesiology 1985;63:698–700.

549. Tornvall SS, Jackson KH, Oyanedel T. Tracheal rupture, complication of cuffed endotracheal tube. Chest 1971;59:237–239.

550. Thompson DS, Read RC. Rupture of the trachea following endotracheal intubation. JAMA 1968;204:995–997.

551. Kumar SM, Pandit SK, Cohen PJ. Tracheal laceration associated with endotracheal anesthesia. Anesthesiology 1977;47:298–299.

552. Gaukroger PB, Anderson G. Tracheal rupture in an intubated critically ill patient. Anaesth Intensive Care 1986;14:199–201.

553. de Lange JJ, Booij LHDJ. Tracheal rupture. Anaesthesia 1985;40:211–212.

554. Kubota Y, Toyoda Y, Kubota H. A potential complication associated with a tracheal tube with Murphy eye. Anaesthesia 1989;44:866–867.

555. Cozine K, Rosenbaum LM, Askanazi J, Rosenbaum SH. Laser-induced endotracheal tube fire. Anesthesiology 1981;55:583–585.

556. Fried MP. Complications of CO_2 laser surgery of the larynx. Laryngoscope 1983;93:275–278.

557. Fried MP. A survey of the complications of laser laryngoscopy. Arch Otolaryngol Head Neck Surg 1984;110:31–34.

558. Snow JC, Norton ML, Saluja TS. Fire hazard during CO_2 laser microsurgery on the larynx and trachea. Anesth Analg 1976;55:146–147.

559. Vourcih G, Tannieres M, Freche G. Ignition of a tracheal tube during laryngeal laser surgery. Anaesthesia 1979;34:685.

560. Van Der Spek AFL, Spargo PM, Norton ML. The physics of lasers and implications for their use during airway surgery. Br J Anaesth 1988;60:709–729.

561. Gravenstein JS. Anesthesia for laser surgery (ASA Refresher Course #263). New Orleans: ASA, 1989.

562. Casey KR, Fairfax WB, Smith SJ, Dixon JA. Intratracheal fire ignited by the Nd-YAG laser during

treatment of tracheal stenosis. Chest 1983;84:295–296.

563. Denton RA, Dedhia HV, Abrons HL, Jain PR, Lapp NL, Teba L. Long-term survival after endobronchial fire during treatment of severe malignant airway obstruction with the Nd:YAG laser. Chest 1988;94:1086–1088.

564. Krawtz S, Mehta AC, Wiedemann HP, DeBoer G, Schoepf KD, Tomaszewski MZ. Nd-YAG laser-induced endobronchial burn. Management and long term follow-up. Chest 1989;95:916–918.

565. McLaren ID, Bellman MH, Cooley J. Effects of the argon laser on anaesthetic gases and endotracheal tubes. Br J Anaesth 1983;55:1001–1004.

566. Pashayan AG, Gravenstein JS, Cassisi NJ, McLaughlin G. The helium protocol for laryngotracheal operations with CO₂ laser. A retrospective review of 523 cases. Anesthesiology 1988;68:801–804.

567. Loeb RG, Soriano SG. Helium decreases the flammability of endotracheal tubes. Anesth Analg 1990;70:S246.

568. Goode JG, Murray TR, Murray P, Harbaugh M. The protective effect of helium on silicone endotracheal tube flammability. Anesthesiology 1991;75:A393.

569. Plost J, Campbell SC. The non-elastic work of breathing through endotracheal tubes of various sizes. Am Rev Respir Dis 1984;129:A106.

570. Simpson JI, Schiff GA, Wolf GL. The effect of helium on endotracheal tube flammability. Anesthesiology 1990;73:538–540.

571. Sosis M. Nitrous oxide is contraindicated in endoscopic surgery. Can J Anaesth 1987;34:539.

572. Sosis M. Nitrous oxide should not be used during laser endoscopic surgery. Anesth Analg 1987;66:1054–1055.

573. Shapiro JD, El-Baz NM. N₂O has no place during oropharyngeal and laryngotracheal procedures. Anesthesiology 1987;66:447–448.

574. Byles PH, Kellman RM. The hazard of nitrous oxide during laser endoscopic surgery. Anesthesiology 1983;59:258.

575. Ohashi N, Asai M, Ueda S, Imamura J, Watanabe Y, Mizukoshi K. Hazard to endotracheal tubes by CO₂ laser beam. ORL J Otorhinolaryngol Relat Spec 1985;47:22–25.

576. Sosis MB, Dillon FX. Saline-filled cuffs help prevent laser-induced polyvinylchloride endotracheal tube fires. Anesth Analg 1991;72:187–189.

577. LeJeune FE, Guice C, LeTard F, Marice H. Heat sink protection against lasering endotracheal cuffs. Ann Otol Rhinol Laryngol 1982;92:606–607.

578. Sosis M, Dillon F. Saline filled cuffs help prevent polyvinylchloride laser induced endotracheal tube fires. Can J Anaesth 1989;36:S142–S143.

579. Anonymous. Laser-resistant tracheal tubes. Technol Anesth 1992;12:1–5.

580. Herbert JT, Berlin I, Eberle R. Jet ventilation via a copper endotracheal tube for CO₂ laser surgery of the oropharynx. Laryngoscope 1985;95:1276–1277.

581. Cozine K, Stone JG, Shulman S, Flaster ER. Ventilatory complications of carbon dioxide laser laryngeal surgery. J Clin Anesth 1991;3:20–25.

582. Wegrzynowicz ES, Jensen NF, Pearson KS, Wachel RE, Scamman FL. Airway fire during jet ventilation for laser excision of vocal cord papillomata. Anesthesiology 1992;76:468–469.

583. Brutinel WM, Cortese DA, Edsell ES, McDougall JC, Prakash UBS. Complications of Nd:YAG laser surgery. Chest 1988;94:902–903.

584. Dumon JF, Shapshay S, Boorcereau J, et al:Principles for safety in application of neodymium-YAG laser bronchology. Chest 1984;86:163–168.

585. Anonymous. Airway fires. Reducing the risk during laser surgery. Technol Anesth 1990;11(2):1–4.

586. Elton DR, Berkowitz GP. Endotracheal tube obstruction in neonates. Perinatol Neonatol 1981;5:75–80.

587. Duffy BL. Delayed onset of respiratory obstruction during endotracheal anesthesia. S Afr Med J 1976;50:1551–1552.

588. Johnson JT, Maloney RW, Cummings CW. Tracheostomy tube: cuff obstruction. JAMA 1977;238:211.

589. Jago RH, Millar JM. Airway obstruction—an unusual presentation. Br J Anaesth 1985;57:541–542.

590. Kruczek ME, Hoff BH, Keszler BR, Smith RB. Blood clot resulting in ball-valve obstruction in the airway. Crit Care Med 1982;10:122–123.

591. Flemming DC. Hazards of tracheal intubation. In: Orkin FK, Cooperman LH, eds. Complications in anesthesiology. Philadelphia: JB Lippincott, 1983:165–172.

592. de Soto H, Johnston JF. Pulmonary edema caused by endotracheal tube occlusion. Anesthesiol Rev 1987;14:39–40.

593. Hull JM. Occlusion of armoured tubes. Anaesthesia 1989;44:790.

594. Anonymous. Tracheal tube kinking. Health Devices 1978;7:292–293.

595. Berwick EP, Chadd GD, Cox PN, Loxley CGW, Moskovits PE, Ravalia A. Armoured tracheal tubes for neuroanesthesia. Anaesthesia 1986;41:775–776.

596. Kubota Y, Toyoda Y, Kubota H, Ishida H. Armoured tubes are necessary for neuroanesthesia. Anaesthesia 1986;41:1064–1065.

597. Rao CC, Krishna G, Trueblood S. Stenting of the

endotracheal tube to manage airway obstruction in the prone position. Anesth Analg 1980;59:700–701.

598. Wilks DH, Tullock WC, Klain M. Airway obstruction caused by a kinked Hi-Lo jet endotracheal tube during high frequency jet ventilation. Anesth Analg 1989;69:116–118.

599. Yamashita M, Motokawa K. A simple method for preventing kinking of 2.5-mm ID endotracheal tubes. Anesth Analg 1987;66:803–804.

600. Yamashita M, Motokawa K. Preventing kinking of disposable preformed endotracheal tubes. Can Anaesth Soc J 1987;34:103.

601. Arai T, Kuzume K. Endotracheal tube obstruction possibly due to structural fault. Anesthesiology 1983;59:480–481.

602. Callander CC. Intubation risk with patients with tracheostomy. Anaesthesia 1988;43:1061.

603. Batra AK. Complication following traumatic endotracheal intubation. Crit Care Med 1985;14:80.

604. Carter GL, Holcomb MC. An unusual cause of endotracheal tube obstruction. Anesthesiol Rev 1978;5:51–53.

605. Barat G, Ascorve A, Avello F. Unusual airway obstruction during pneumonectomy. Anaesthesia 1976;31:1290–1291.

606. Henzig D, Rosenblatt R. Thrombotic occlusion of a nasotracheal tube. Anesthesiology 1979;51:484–485.

607. Hitchen JE, Wiener AP. Unexpected obstruction of a nasotracheal tube: report of case. J Oral Surg 1973;31:722–724.

608. Robinson BC, Jarrett WJ. Postoperative complication after blind nasotracheal intubation for reduction of a fractured mandible: report of case. J Oral Surg 1971;29:340–343.

609. Torres LE, Reynolds RC. A complication of use of a microlaryngeal surgery endotracheal tube. Anesthesiology 1980;53:355.

610. Boysen K. An unusual case of nasotracheal tube occlusion. Anaesthesia 1986;40:1024.

611. Butt W. Unusual cause of endotracheal tube obstruction in a neonate. Anaesth Intensive Care 1986;14:95.

612. Scamm FL, Babin RW. An unusual complication of nasotracheal intubation. Anesthesiology 1983;59:352–353.

613. Powell DR. Obstruction to endotracheal tubes. Br J Anaesth 1974;46:252.

614. Stark DCC. Endotracheal tube obstruction. Anesthesiology 1976;45:467–468.

615. Jenkins AV. Unexpected hazard of anaesthesia. Lancet 1959;1:761–762.

616. Haselhuhn DH. Occlusion of endotracheal tube with foreign body. Anesthesiology 1958;19:561–562.

617. Wittman FW. Airway obstruction due to a foreign body. Anaesthesia 1982;37:865–866.

618. Dutton CS. A bizarre cause of obstruction in an Oxford non-kink endotracheal tube. Anaesthesia 1962;17:395–396.

619. Stewart KA. Foreign body in endotracheal tube. Br Med J 1958;2:1226.

620. Rainer EH. Foreign body in endotracheal tube. Br Med J 1958;2:1357.

621. Goudsouzian NG, Ryan JF, Moench B. An unusual cause of endotracheal tube obstruction in a child. Anesthesiol Rev 1980;7:23–24.

622. Galley RL. Foreign body. Anaesth Intensive Care 1987;15:471.

623. Peers B. Another intubation hazard. Anaesthesia 1975;30:827.

624. Uehira A, Tanaka A, Oda M, Sato T. Obstruction of an endotracheal tube by lidocaine jelly. Anesthesiology 1981;55:598–599.

625. McLellan I. Blockage of tracheal connectors with K-Y jelly. Anaesthesia 1975;30:413–416.

626. Blitt CD. Case report: complete obstruction of an armored endotracheal tube. Anesth Analg 1974;58:624–625.

627. Anonymous. Unusual occlusion of small tracheal tubes. Technol Anesth 1989;9(7):1–2.

628. Cook WP, Schultetus RR. Obstruction of an endotracheal tube by the plastic coating sheared from a stylet. Anesthesiology 1985;62:803–804.

629. Zmyslowski WP, Kam D, Simpson GT. An unusual cause of endotracheal tube obstruction. Anesthesiology 1989;70:883.

630. Ehrenpreis MB, Oliverio RM. Endotracheal tube obstruction secondary to oral preoperative medication. Anesth Analg 1984;63:867–868.

631. Singhal M, Gupta M, Singhal CK. Tube in tube. A case of acute airway obstruction. Br J Anaesth 1984;56:1317.

632. Galway JE. Airway obstruction. Anaesthesia 1972;27:102–103.

633. Singh CV. Bizarre airway obstruction. Anaesthesia 1977;32:812–813.

634. Mimpriss TJ. Respiratory obstruction due to a round worm. Br J Anaesth 1972;44:413.

635. Ireland R. Potential hazard of Doughty tongue plate. Anaesth Intensive Care 1986;14:209.

636. Palmieri AM, Scanni E, Spatola R, Cortesano P. Endotracheal tube obstruction. Anaesth Intensive Care 1986;14:209.

637. Populaire C, Robarb S, Souron J. An armoured endotracheal tube obstruction in a child. Can J Anaesth 1989;36:331–332.

638. Bachand R, Fortin G. Airway obstruction with cuffed flexometallic tracheal tubes. Can Anaesth Soc J 1976;23:330–333.

639. Seuffert GW, Urbach KF. An additional hazard of

endotracheal intubation. Can Anaesth Soc J 1968;15:300–301.

640. Pryer DL, Pryer RLR, Williams AF. Fatal respiratory obstruction due to faulty endotracheal tube. Lancet 1960;2:742–743.

641. Harmel MH. Intubation of the trachea does not absolutely insure a patent airway. N Y State J Med 1956;56:2125–2126.

642. Guedj P, Eldor J. Endotracheal cuff herniation. Resuscitation 1991;21:293–294.

642. Forrest F, Millett S. Intermittent obstruction of tracheal tube revealed during pressure-supported ventilation. Anaesthesia 1991;46:799–800.

643. Davidson I, Zimmer S. Cuff herniation. Anaesthesia 1989;44:938–939.

644. Brasch RC, Heldt GP, Hecht ST. Endotracheal tube orifice abutting the tracheal wall: a cause of infant airway obstruction. Radiology 1981;141:387–391.

645. Martin J, Hutchinson B. Tracheal tube obstruction by prominent aortic knuckle. Anaesthesia 1986;41:86–87.

646. Sapsford DJ, Snowdon SL. If in doubt, take it out. Obstruction of tracheal tube by prominent aortic knuckle. Anaesthesia 1985;40:552–554.

647. Stoen R, Smith-Erichsen N. Airway obstruction associated with an endotracheal tube. Intensive Care Med 1987;13:295–296.

648. Sperry K, Smialek JE. The investigation of an unusual asphyxial death in a hospital. JAMA 1986;255:2472–2474.

649. Patterson KW, Keane P. Missed diagnosis of cuff herniation in a modern nasal endotracheal tube. Anesth Analg 1990;71:561–569.

650. Gould AB, Seldon TH. An unusual complication with a cuffed endotracheal tube. Anesth Analg 1968;47:239–240.

651. Feinberg SE, Klein SL. Airway obstruction with the RAE endotracheal tube. J Maxillofac Surg 1983;41:260–262.

652. Bishop MJ. Endotracheal tube lumen compromise from cuff overinflation. Chest 1981;80:100–101.

653. Chan MCY. Collapse of endotracheal tubes. Anaesth Intensive Care 1981;9:289–290.

654. Dunn HC. A defective endotracheal tube. N Z Med J 1988;101:460.

655. Famewo CE. A not so apparant cause of intraluminal tracheal tube obstruction. Anesthesiology 1983;58:593.

656. Hoffman S, Freedman M. Delayed lumen obstruction in endotracheal tubes. Br J Anaesth 1976;48:1025–1028.

657. Hebert RC, DeSessa PC. Compression of an endotracheal tube lumen by its cuff. A case report. Respir Care 1981;26:653–654.

658. Ketover AK, Feingold A. Collapse of a disposable endotracheal tube by its high-pressure cuff. Anesthesiology 1975;48:108–110.

659. Muir J, Davidson-Lamb R. Apparatus failure-cause for concern. Br J Anaesth 1980;52:705–706.

660. Perel A, Katzenelson R, Klein E, Cotev S. Collapse of endotracheal tubes due to overinflation of high-compliance cuffs. Anesth Analg 1977;56:731–733.

661. Patel K, Teviotdale B, Dalal FY. Internal herniation of a Murphy endotracheal tube. Anesthesiol Rev 1978;5:60–61.

662. Roland P, Stovner J. Brain damage following collapse of a "polyvinyl" tube. elasticity and permeability of the cuff. Acta Anaesth Scand 1975;19:303–309.

663. Priem L, Guntupalli K, Sladen A, Faulds J. Inadvertent tracheal tube obstruction. Heart Lung 1982;11:285.

664. Hutchinson M, Himes TM, Davis LE. Preventing multiple body tube mix-ups. Nursing 1987;87:57.

665. Fergusson NV, Fang WB. Unusual problems of nasotracheal intubation. Anesthesiol Rev 1985;12:33–36.

666. Saade E. Unusual cause of endotracheal tube obstruction. Anesth Analg 1991;72:841–842.

667. Chamberlin DA, Tatham PF. Defective adaptor delays resuscitation. Lancet 1970;1:188.

668. McKinley AC. Occlusion of an endotracheal tube connector. Anesthesiology 1977;47:480.

669. Nott MR, Wainwright AC. Imperforate apparatus causing total airway obstruction. Anaesthesia 1977;32:77–78.

670. Osterud A. Dangerous fault in disposable connector for orotracheal tube. Br J Anaesth 1974;46:952.

671. Sansome AJ. Creasing of a paediatric tracheal tube connector. Anaesthesia 1990;45:343.

672. Zebrowski ME. Buckled adaptor. Anesthesiology 1979;51:276–277.

673. Lieman BC, Hall ID, Stanley TH. Extirpation of endotracheal tube secretions with a Fogarty arterial embolectomy catheter. Anesthesiology 1985;62:847.

674. Sizer J, Pierce JMT. Unblocking tracheal tubes. Anaesthesia 1992;47:278–279.

675. Roberts KW. New use for Swan-Ganz introducer wire. Anesth Analg 1981;60:67.

676. Lamb JD. Passage of suction catheter via ETT cited as possibly misleading waste of time. APSF Newslett 1990;5:44.

677. Elpern EH, Jacobs ER, Bone RC. Incidence of aspiration in tracheally intubated adults. Heart Lung 1987;16:527–531.

678. Petring OU, Adelhoj B, Jensen BN, Pedersen NO, Lomholt N. Prevention of silent aspiration due to leaks around cuffs of endotracheal tubes. Anesth Analg 1986;65:777–780.

679. Janson BA, Poulton TJ. Does PEEP reduce the

incidence of aspiration around endotracheal tubes? Can Anaesth Soc J 1986;33:157–161.

680. Healey J. Fine bore feeding tubes. Anaesth Intensive Care 1983;11:81.

681. Adams AL. A complication following guided nasotracheal intubation. Anesthesiology 1983;58:105–106.

682. Gravenstein N, Pashayan AG. More on eliminating CT scan artifact due to endotracheal tubes. Anesthesiology 1988;68:823.

683. Tashiro C, Yagi M, Kinoshita H. Use of an endotracheal tube without radiopaque marker for cervical CT scans. Anesthesiology 1987;67:1022.

684. Black AE, Hatch DJ, Nauth-misir N. Complications of nasotracheal intubation in neonates, infants and children. A review of 4 years' experience in a children's hospital. Br J Anaesth 1990;65:461–467.

685. Dorsey M, Schwider L, Benumof JL. Unintentional endotracheal extubation by orogastric tube removal. Anesthesiol Rev 1988;15:30–33.

686. Allison JM, Gunawardene WMS. Problems with cuffs on tracheal tubes. Anaesthesia 1984;39:191.

687. Bourne TM, Tate K. Failed cuff deflation. Anaesthesia 1990;45:76.

688. Brock-Utne JG, Jaffe RA, Robins B, Ratner E. Difficulty in extubation. A cause for concern. Anaesthesia 1992;47:229–230.

689. Sivaneswaran N, O'Leary J. Failure of endotracheal tube cuff deflation. Anaesth Intensive Care 1984;12:88.

690. Tanski J, James RH. Difficult extubation due to a kinked pilot tube. Anaesthesia 1986;41:1060.

691. Sklar GS, Alfonso AE, King BD. An unusual problem in nasotracheal extubation. Anesth Analg 1976;55:302–303.

692. Fagraeus L. Difficult extubation following nasotracheal intubation. Anesthesiology 1978;49:43–44.

693. Grover VK. Difficulty in extubation. Anaesthesia 1985;40:198–199.

694. Khan RM, Khan TZ, Ali M, Khan MSA. Difficult extubation. Anaesthesia 1988;43:515.

695. Lall NG. Difficult extubation. A fold in the endotracheal cuff. Anaesthesia 1980;35:500–501.

696. Mishra P, Scott DL. Difficulty at extubation of the trachea. Anaesthesia 1983;38:811.

697. Ng TY, Datta TD. Difficult extubation of an endotracheal tube cuff. Anesth Analg 1976;55:876–877.

698. Pavlin EG, Nelson E, Pulliam J. Difficulty in removal of tracheostomy tubes. Anesthesiology 1976;44:69–70.

699. Bhaskar PB, Scheffer RB, Drummond JN. Bilateral fixation of a nasotracheal tube by transfacial Kirschner wires. J Oral Maxillofac Surg 1987;45:805–807.

700. Dryden GE. Circulatory colapse after pneumonec-tomy (an unusual complication from the use of a Carlens catheter): case report. Anesth Analg 1977;56:451–452.

701. Hilley MD, Henderson RB, Giesecke AH. Difficult extubation of the trachea. Anesthesiology 1983;59:149–150.

702. Lee C, Schwartz S, Mok MS. Difficult extubation due to transfixation of a nasotracheal tube by Kirschner wire. Anesthesiology 1977;46:427.

703. Lang S, Johnson DH, Lanigan DT, Ha H. Difficult tracheal extubation. Can J Anaesth 1989;36:340–342.

704. Guntupalli KK, Bouchek CD. Cricothyroid puncture of an undeflatable endotracheal tube cuff. Crit Care Med 1984;12:924.

705. Yau G, Jong W, Oh TE. Failure of endotracheal tube cuff deflation. Anaesth Intensive Care 1990;18:425.

706. Tashayod M, Oskoui B. A case of difficult extubation. Anesthesiology 1973;39:337.

707. Mehta S. The risk of aspiration in presence of cuffed endotracheal tubes. Br J Anaesth 1972;44:601–605.

708. Gard MA, Cruickshank LFG. Factors influencing the incidence of sore throat following endotracheal intubation. Can Med Assoc J 1961;84:662–665.

709. Harding CJ, McVey FK. Interview method affects incidence of postoperative sore throat. Anaesthesia 1987;42:1104–1107.

710. Lund LO, Daos FG. Effects on postoperative sore throats of two analgesic agents and lubricants used with endotracheal tubes. Anesthesiology 1965;26:681–683.

711. Conway CM, Miller JS, Sugden FLH. Sore throat after anesthesia. Br J Anaesth 1960;32:219–223.

712. Alexopoulous C, Lindholm CE. Airway complaints and laryngeal pathology after intubation with an anatomically shaped endotracheal tube. Acta Anaesthesiol Scand 1983;27:339–344.

713. Fink BR. Laryngeal complications of general anesthesia. In: Orkin FK, Cooperman LH, eds. Complications in anesthesiology. Philadelphia: JB Lippincott, 1983:144–151.

714. Saarnivaara L, Grahne B. Clinical study on an endotracheal tube with a high-residual volume, low-pressure cuff. Acta Anaesth Scand 1981;25:89–92.

715. Monroe MC, Gravenstein N, Saga-Rumley S. Postoperative sore throat: effect of oropharyngeal airway in orotracheally intubated patients. Anesth Analg 1990;70:512–516.

716. Stout D, Dwersteg J, Cullen BF, Bishop MJ. Correlation of endotracheal tube size with sore throat and hoarseness. Anesth Analg 1986;65:S155.

717. Stout DM, Bishop MJ, Dwersteg JF, Cullen BF. Correlation of endotracheal tube size with sore throat and hoarseness following general anesthesia. Anesthesiology 1987;67:419–421.

718. Wilson JE, Ozinga DW, Baughaman VL. Sore throat—does endotracheal tube size really matter? Anesthesiology 1989;71:A458.

719. Hartsell CJ, Stephen CR. Incidence of sore throat following endotracheal intubation. Can Anaesth Soc J 1964;11:307–312.

720. Jones MW, Catling S, Evans E, Green DH, Green JR. Hoarseness after tracheal intubation. Anaesthesia 1992;47:213–216.

721. Loeser EA, Kaminsky A, Diaz A, Stanley TH. The influence of endotracheal tube cuff design and lubrication on postoperative sore throat. Anesthesiology 1981;55:A121.

722. Loeser EA, Kaminsky A, Diaz A, Stanley TH, Pace NL. The influence of endotracheal tube cuff design and cuff lubrication on postoperative sore throat. Anesthesiology 1983;58:376–379.

723. Stock MC, Downs JB. Lubrication of tracheal tubes to prevent sore throat from intubation. Anesthesiology 1982;57:418–420.

724. Stride PC. Postoperative sore throat. topical hydrocortisone. Anaesthesia 1990;45:968–971.

725. Winkel E, Knudsen J. Effect on the incidence of postoperative sore throat of 1 percent cinchocaine jelly for endotracheal intubation. Anesth Analg 1971;50:92–94.

726. Stenqvist O, Nilsson K. Postoperative sore throat related to tracheal tube cuff design. Can Anaesth Soc J 1982;29:384–386.

727. Sprague NB, Archer PL. Magill versus Mallinckrodt tracheal tubes. A comparative study of postoperative sore throat. Anaesthesia 1987;42:306–311.

728. Jones GOM, Hale DE, Wasmuth CE, Homi J, Smith ER, Viljoen J. A survey of acute complications associated with endotracheal intubation. Cleve Clin Q 1968;35:23–31.

729 Baron SH, Kohlmoos HW. Laryngeal sequelae of endotracheal anesthesia. Ann Otol Rhinol Laryngol 1951;60:767–792.

730. Ishida T, Yoshiya I, Morita Y, Shirae K. Quantitative analysis of tracheal damage. Crit Care Med 1983;11:283–285.

731. Winter R, Munro M. Lingual and buccal nerve neuropathy in a patient in the prone position. A case report. Anesthesiology 1989;71:452–454.

732. Faithfull NS. Injury to terminal branches of the trigeminal nerve following tracheal intubation. Br J Anaesth 1985;57:535–537.

733. Haselby KA, McNiece WL. Respiratory obstruction from uvular edema in a pediatric patient. Anesth Analg 1983;62:1127–1128.

734. Newman T, Franssen R. Uvular edema in pediatric patients. Anesth Analg 1984;63:701–702.

735. Ravindran R, Priddy S. Uvular edema, a rare complication of endotracheal intubation. Anesthesiology 1978;48:374.

736. Seigne TD, Felske A, DelGiudice PA. Uvular edema. Anesthesiology 1978;49:375–376.

737. Koka BV, Jeon IS, Andre JM, MacKay I, Smith RM. Postintubation croup in children. Anesth Analg 1977;56:501–505.

738. Darmon J, Rauss A, Dreyfuss D, et al. Evaluation of risk factors for laryngeal edema after tracheal extubation in adults and its prevention by dexamethasone. A placebo-controlled double-blind, multicenter study. Anesthesiology 1992;77:245–251.

739. Ferrara TB, Georgieff MK, Ebert J, Fisher JB. Routine use of dexamethasone for the prevention of postextubation respiratory distress. J Perinatol 1989;9:287–290.

740. Tellez DW, Galvis AG, Storgion SA, Amer HN, Hoseyni M, Deakers TW. Dexamethasone in the prevention of postextubation stridor in children. J Pediatr 1991;118:289–294.

741. Brandwein M, Abramson AL, Shikowitz MJ. Bilateral vocal cord paralysis following endotracheal intubation. Arch Otolaryngol Head Neck Surg 1986;112:877–882.

742. Baraka A, Hemady K, Yamut F, Yazigi W, Canalis RF. Postoperative paralysis of phrenic and recurrent laryngeal nerves. Anesthesiology 1981;55:78–80.

743. Cox RH, Welborn SG. Vocal cord paralysis after endotracheal anesthesia. South Med J 1981;74:1258–1259.

744. Cavo JW. True vocal cord paralysis following intubation. Laryngoscope 1985;95:1352–1359.

745. David DS, Shah M. Vocal cord paralysis following intubation. JAMA 1971;216:1645–1646.

746. Ellis PDM, Pallister WK. Recurrent laryngeal nerve palsy and endotracheal intubation. J Laryngol Otol 1975;89:823–826.

747. Gibbin KP, Egginton MJ. Bilateral vocal cord paralysis following endotracheal intubation. Br J Anaesth 1981;53:1091–1092.

748. Komorn RM, Smith CP, Erwin JA. Acute laryngeal injury with short-term endotracheal anesthesia. Laryngoscope 1973;83:683–690.

749. Kennedy RL. Questions and answers. Anesth Analg 1977;56:321–322.

750. Lim EK, Chia KS, Ng BK. Recurrent laryngeal nerve palsy following endotracheal intubation. Anaesth Intensive Care 1987;15:342–345.

751. Mass L. Another post-endotracheal vocal cord paralysis of uncertain etiology. Anesthesiol Rev 1975;2:28–30.

752. Minuck M. Unilateral vocal cord paralysis following endotracheal intubation. Anesthesiology 1976;45:448–449.

753. Nuutinen J, Karja J. Bilateral vocal cord paralysis following general anesthesia. Laryngoscope 1981;91:83–86.

754. Salem MR, Wong AY, Barangan, Canalis RF,

Shaker MH, Lotter AM. Postoperative vocal cord paralysis in paediatric patients. Br J Anaesth 1971;48:696–699.

755. Whited RE. Laryngeal dysfunction following prolonged intubation. Ann Otol 1979;88:474–478.

756. Anonymous. Laryngeal paralysis after endotracheal intubation. Lancet 1986;1:536–537.

757. Friedman M, Toriumi DM. Esophageal stethoscope. Another possible cause of vocal cord paralysis. Surv Anesth 1989;33:243–244.

758. Dubick MN, Wright BD. Comparison of layrngeal pathology following long-term oral and nasal endotracheal intubations. Anesth Analg 1978; 57:663–668.

759. Burns HP, Dayal VS, Scott A, van Nostrand AWP, Bryce DP. Laryngotracheal trauma: observations on its pathogenesis and its prevention following prolonged orotracheal intubation in the adult. Laryngoscope 1979;89:1316–1325.

760. Weymuller EA, Bishop MJ, Fink BR, Hibbard AW, Spelman FA. Quantification of interlaryngeal pressure exerted by endotracheal tubes. Acta Otol Rhinol Laryngol 1983;92:444–447.

761. Nordin U. The regeneration after cuff-induced tracheal injury. Acta Otolaryngol 1982;94:541–555.

762. Bergstrom J. Post-intubation granuloma of the larynx. Acta Otolaryngol 1964;57:113–118.

763. Etsten B, Mahler D. Subglottic membrane. A complication of endotracheal intubation. N Engl J Med 1951;245:957–960.

764. Lewis RN, Swerdlow M. Hazards of endotracheal anaesthesia. Br J Anaesth 1964;36:504–515.

765. Muir AP, Straton J. Membranous laryngo-tracheitis following endotracheal intubation. Anaesthesia 1954;9:105–113.

766. Tonkin JP, Harrison GA. The effect on the larynx of prolonged endotracheal intubation. Med J Aust 1966;2:581–587.

767. Young N, Steward S. Laryngeal lesions following endotracheal anaesthesia: a report of twelve adult cases. Br J Anaesth 1953;25:32–42.

768. Strome M, Ferguson CF. Multiple postintubation complications. Ann Otol 1974;83:432–438.

769. King EG. Aftermath of intubation. Emerg Med 1983;154:201–209.

770. Fine J, Finestone SC. An unusual complication of endotracheal intubation: report of a case. Anesth Analg 1973;52:204–206.

771. Barkin ME, Trieger N. An unusual complication of nasal-tracheal anesthesia. Anesth Prog 1976;23:57–58.

772. Rennie T, Catania AF, Haanaes HR. Ulceration of the nasal ala and dorsum secondary to improper support of the nasoendotracheal tube. J Am Assoc Nurse Anesth 1978;46:282–285.

773. Benumof JL. Anesthesia for thoracic surgery. Philadelphia: WB Saunders, 1987.

774. Burton NA, Watson DC, Brodsky JB, Mark JBD. Advantages of a new polyvinyl chloride double-lumen tube in thoracic surgery. Ann Thorac Surg 1983;36:78–84.

775. Bjork VO, Carlens E, Friberg O. Endobronchial anesthesia. Anesthesiology 1953;14:60–72.

776. MacGillivray RG, Rocke DA, Mahomedy AE. Endobronchial tube placement in repair of ruptured bronchus. Anaesth Intensive Care 1987;15:459–462.

777. Brodsky JB, Welti RS, Mark JBD. Thoracoscopy for retrieval of intrathoracic foreign bodies. Anesthesiology 1981;54:91–92.

778. Bjork VO, Carlens E. The prevention of spread during pulmonary resection by the use of a double-lumen catheter. J Thorac Surg 1950; 20:151–157.

779. Baraka A, Dajani A, Maktabi M. Selective contralateral bronchial intubation in children with pneumothorax or bronchopleural fistula. Br J Anaesth 1983;55:901–904.

780. Carron H, Hill S. Anesthetic management of lobectomy for massive pulmonary hemorrhage. Anesthesiology 1972;37:658–659.

781. Brown CR. Postpneumonectomy empyema and bronchopleural fistula—Use of prolonged endobronchial intubation: a case report. Anesth Analg 1973;52:439–441.

782. Dennison PH, Lester ER. An anaesthetic technique for the repair of bronchopleural fistula. Br J Anaesth 1961;33:655–659.

783. Cullum AR, English ICW, Branthwaite MA. Endobronchial intubation in infancy. Anaesthesia 1973;28:66–70.

784. Ratliff JL, Hill JD, Tucker H, Fallat R. Endobronchial control of bronchopleural fistulae. Chest 1977;71:98–99.

785. Bochenek KJ, Brown M, Skupin A. Use of a double-lumen endotracheal tube with independent lung ventilation for treatment of refractory atelectasis. Anesth Analg 1987;66:1014–1017.

786. Glass DD, Tonnesen AS, Gabel JC, Arens JF. Therapy of unilateral pulmonary insufficiency with a double lumen endotracheal tube. Crit Care Med 1976;4·323–326.

787. Murray JF. Treatment of acute total atelectasis. Anaesthesia 1985;40:158–162.

788. Mullelm M, Baraka A. A simple double lumen adapter for differential lung ventilation. Anaesthesia 1988;43:254–255.

789. Venus B, Pratap KS, Tholt TO. Treatment of unilateral pulmonary insufficiency by selective administration of continuous positive airway pressure through a double-lumen tube. Anesthesiology 1980;53:74–77.

790. Kubota Y, Toyoda Y, Nagata N, Kubota H, Sawada S, Murakawa M, Fujimori M. Tracheobron-

chial angles in infants and children. Anesthesiology 1986;64:374–376.

791. Sibai AN, Baraka A. A new double lumen tube adaptor. Anaesthesia 1986;41:628–630.

792. Tanguturi S, Capan LM, Patel K, Turndorf H. A new double-lumen tube adapter. Anesth Analg 1980;59:507–508.

793. Worsley MH, Hawkins DJ, Scott DHT. Attachments to double lumen bronchial tubes. Anaesthesia 1990;45:1001–1002.

794. Newman RW, Finer GE, Downs JE. Routine use of the Carlens double-lumen endobronchial catheter. J Thorac Cardiovasc Surg 1961;42:327–339.

795. Edwards EM, Hatch DJ. Experiences with double-lumen tubes. Anaesthesia 1965;20:461–467.

796. Benumof JL. Improving the design and function of double-lumen tubes. J Cardiothorac Anesth 1988;2:729–733.

797. Benumof JL, Partridge BL, Salvatierra C, Keating J. Margin of safety in positioning modern double-lumen endotracheal tubes. Anesthesiology 1987;67:729–738.

798. Keating JL, Benumof JL. An analysis of margin of safety in positioning double-lumen tubes. Anesthesiology 1985;63:A563.

799. Bryce-Smith R. A double-lumen endobronchial tube. Br J Anaesth 1959;31:274–275.

800. Butman BB. Experience with the Carlens double-lumen catheter for anesthesia in thoracic surgery. N Y State J Med 1954;54:2463–2466.

801. Clarke AD. The White double lumen tube. A report on its use in fifty cases. Br J Anaesth 1962;34:822–824.

802. White GMJ. A new double lumen tube. Br J Anaesth 1960;32:232–234.

803. Robertshaw FL. Low resistance double-lumen endobronchial tubes. Br J Anaesth 1962;34:576–579.

804. Read RC, Friday CD, Eason CN. Prospective study of the Robertshaw endobronchial catheter in thoracic surgery. Ann Thorac Surg 1977;24:156–161.

805. McKenna MJ, Wilson RS, Botelho RJ. Right upper lobe obstruction with right-sided double-lumen endobronchial tubes. A comparison of two tube types. J Cardiothorac Anesth 1988;2:734–740.

806. Alfery DD. Increasing the margin of safety in positioning left-sided double-lumen endotracheal tubes. Anesthesiology 1988;69:149–150.

807. Slinger P, Triolet W. A clinical comparison of three different designs of right-sided double-lumen endobronchial tubes. Can J Anaesth 1989;36:S59–S60.

808. Benumof J. Anesthesia for thoracic surgery (ASA Refresher Course #175). New Orleans: ASA, 1985.

809. Benumof JL. Anesthesia for pulmonary surgery

810. Rocke DA, MacGillivray RG, Mahomedy AE. Positioning of double lumen tubes. Anaesthesia 1986;41:770–771.

811. Burk WJ. Should a fiberoptic bronchoscope be routinely used to position a double-lumen tube? Anesthesiology 1988;68:826.

812. Watson CB. Problems with endobronchial intubation. Anesthesiol Rev 1986;13:52–55.

813. Brodsky JB. Complications of double-lumen tracheal tubes. Probl Anesth 1988;2:292–306.

814. Neustein SM, Eisenkraft JB. Proper lateralization of left-sided double-lumen tubes. Anesthesiology 1989;71:996.

815. Kubota H, Kubota Y, Toyoda Y, Ishida H, Asada A, Matsuura H. Selective blind endobronchial intubation in children and adults. Anesthesiology 1987;67:587–589.

816. El-Etr AA. Improved technic for insertion of the Carlens catheter. Anesth Analg 1969;48:738–740.

817. Brodsky J, Benumof JL, Ehrenworth J, Ozaki GT. Depth of placement of left double-lumen endobronchial tubes. Anesth Analg 1991;73:570–572.

818. Matthew EB, Hirschmann RA. Placing double-lumen tubes with a fiberoptic bronchoscope. Anesthesiology 1986;65:118–119.

819. Ovassapian A, Braunschweig R, Joshi CW. Endobronchial intubation using flexible fiberoptic bronchoscope. Anesthesiology 1983;59:A501.

820. Ross DG. Fiberoptic intubation and double-lumen tubes. Anaesthesia 1990;45:895.

821. Shulman MS, Brodsky JB, Levesque PR. Fibreoptic bronchoscopy for tracheal and endobronchial intubation with a double-lumen tube. Can J Anaesth 1987;34:172–173.

822. Shinnick JP, Freedman AP. Bronchofiberscopic placement of a double-lumen endotracheal tube. Crit Care Med 1982;10:544–545.

823. Coe VL, Brodsky JB, Mark JBD. Double-lumen endotracheal tubes for patients with tracheostomies. Anesth Analg 1984;63:882.

824. Simpson PM. Tracheal intubation with a Robertshaw tube via a tracheostomy. Br J Anaesth 1976;48:373–375.

825. Seed RF, Wedley JR. Tracheal intubation with a Robertshaw tube via a tracheostomy. Br J Anaesth 1977;49:639.

826. Jenkins AV. An endobronchial cuff indicator for use in thoracic surgery. Br J Anaesth 1979;51:905–906.

827. Benumof JL. Anesthesia for pulmonary surgery (ASA Refresher Course #213). New Orleans: ASA, 1989.

828. Riley RH, Marples FL. Relocation of a double-lumen tube during patient positioning. Anesth Analg 1992;75:1071.

(ASA Refresher Course #225). New Orleans: ASA, 1991.

829. Saito S, Dohi S, Naito H. Alteration of double-lumen endobronchial tube position by flexion and extension of the neck. Anesthesiology 1985;62:696–697.

830. Brodsky JB, Mark JBD. A simple technique for accurate placement of double-lumen endobronchial tubes. Anesthesiol Rev 1983;10:26–30.

831. Smith GB, Hirsch NP, Ehrenwerth J. Placement of double-lumen endobronchial tubes. Br J Anaesth 1986;58:1317–1320.

832. Cohen E, Goldofasky S, Neustein S, Camunas JC, Thys DM. Fiberoptic evaluation of endobronchial tube position: red rubber vs polyvinylchloride. Anesth Analg 1989;68:S54.

833. Cohen E, Neustein S, Camunas JC, Thys DM. Does fiberoptic evaluation of endobronchial tube position improve outcome? Anesth Analg 1990;70:S62.

834. Hirsch NP, Smith GB. Malposition of left-sided double-lumen endobronchial tubes. Anesthesiology 1985;63:563.

835. Benumof JL. Fiberoptic bronchoscopy and double-lumen tube position. Anesthesiology 1986;65:117–118.

836. MacGillivray RG, Rocke DA, Mahomedy AE. Correct placement of bronchial tubes. Anaesthesia 1987;42:570.

837. Asai T. Torsion of a double-lumen tube in the left bronchus. Anesthesiology 1992;76:1064–1065.

838. Shafieha MJ, Sit J, Kartha R, et al. End-tidal CO_2 analyzers in proper positioning of the double-lumen tubes. Anesthesiology 1986;64:844–845.

839. Stevens JJ. Direct (transthoracic) endobronchial intubation. Anesthesiology 1980;53:83–84.

840. Cohen E, Kirschner PA, Goldofsky S. Intraoperative manipulation for positioning of double-lumen tubes. Anesthesiology 1988;68:170.

841. Gatell JA, Barst SM, Desiderio DP, Kolker AC, Scher CS. A new technique for replacing an endobronchial double-lumen tube with an endotracheal single-lumen tube. Anesthesiology 1990;73:340–341.

842. Hurford WE, Alfille PH, Bailin MT, et al. Placement and complications of double-lumen endotracheal tubes. Anesth Analg 1992;74:S141.

843. Clapham MCCC, Vaughan RS. Bronchial intubation. A comparison between polyvinylchloride and red rubber double lumen tubes. Anaesthesia 1985;40:1111–1114.

844. Black AMS, Harrison GA. Difficulties with positioning Robertshaw double lumen tubes. Anaesth Intensive Care 1975;3:299–311.

845. Cohen JA, Denisco RA, Richards TS, Staples ED, Roberts AJ. Hazardous placement of a Robertshaw-type endobronchial tube. Anesth Analg 1986;65:100–101.

846. Saito S, Dohi S, Tajima K. Failure of double-lumen endobronchial tube placement. Congenital tracheal stenosis in an adult. Anesthesiology 1987;66:83–85.

847. Brodsky JB. Malposition of left-sided double-lumen endobronchial tubes. Anesthesiology 1985;62:667–669.

848. Conacher JD. The urinary catheter as a bronchial blocker. Anaesthesia 1983;38:475–477.

849. Brodsky JB, Mark JBD. Bilateral upper lobe obstruction from a single double-lumen tube. Anesthesiology 1991;74:1163–1164.

850. Greene ER, Gutierrez FA. Tip of polyvinyl chloride double-lumen endobronchial tube inadvertently wedged in left lower lobe bronchus. Anesthesiology 1986;64:406.

851. Varma YS. An unusual complication with the Bryce-Smith double-lumen tube. A case report. 1969;41:551–552.

852. Gibbs N, Giles K. Malposition of left-sided double-lumen endobronchial tubes. Anaesth Intensive Care 1986;14:92–93.

853. Desai FM, Rocke DA. Double lumen tube design fault. Anesthesiology 1990;73:575–576.

854. Maguire DP, Spiro AW. Bronchial obstruction and hypoxia during one-lung ventilation. Anesthesiology 1987;66:830–831.

855. Heiser M, Steinberg JJ, MacVaugh H, Klineberg PL. Bronchial rupture, a complication of the use of the Robertshaw double-lumen tube. Anesthesiology 1979;51:88.

856. Hannallah M, Gomes M. Bronchial rupture associated with the use of a double-lumen tube in a small adult. Anesthesiology 1989;71:457–459.

857. Foster JMG, Alimo EB. Ruptured bronchus following endobronchial intubation. Br J Anaesth 1983;55:687–688.

858. Brodsky JB, Shulman MS, Mark JBD. Airway rupture with a disposable double-lumen tube. Anesthesiology 1986;64:415.

859. Burton NA, Fall SM, Lyons T, Graeber GM. Rupture of the left main-stem bronchus with a polyvinylchloride double-lumen tube. Chest 1983;83:928–929.

860. Brodsky JB, Adkins MO, Gaba DM. Bronchial cuff pressures of double-lumen tubes. Anesth Analg 1989;69:608–610.

861. Neto PPR. Bronchial cuff pressure: comparison of Carlens and polyvinylchloride (PVC) double lumen tubes. Anesthesiology 1987;66:255–256.

862. Neto PPR. Bronchial cuff pressure of endobronchial double-lumen tubes. Anesth Analg 1990;71:209.

863. Bickford-Smith P, Evans CS. Error in labelling. Anaesthesia 1987;42:572.

864. Jenkins V. Unusual difficulty with double-lumen endo-bronchial tube. Anaesthesia 1963;18:236–237.

865. Anonymous. Tracheal tube lumens may be distorted. Biomed Safe Stand 1989;19:68.

866. Wyatt R, Garner S. A defect in Robertshaw double lumen endotracheal tubes corrected. Anaesthesia 1981;36:830–831.

867. Campbell C, Viswanathan S, Riopelle JM, Naraghi M. Manufacturing defect in a double-lumen tube. Anesth Analg 1991;73:825–826.

868. Akers JA, Riley RH. Failed extubation due to "sutured" double-lumen tube. Anaesth Intensive Care 1990;18:577.

869. Wells DG, Zelcer J, Podolakin W, Baker TG, Wilson AC, White A. Cardiac arrest from pulmonary outflow tract obstruction due to a double-lumen tube. Anesthesiology 1987;66:422–423.

870. Lack JA. Endobronchial tube resistances. Br J Anaesth 1974;46:461–462.

871. Hammond JE, Wright DJ. Comparison of the resistances of double-lumen endobronchial tubes. Br J Anaesth 1984;56:299–302.

872. Chiaranda M, Rossi A, Manani G, Pinamonti O, Braschi A. Measurement of the flow-resistive properties of double-lumen bronchial tubes in vitro. Anaesthesia 1989;44:335–340.

873. Conacher ID. A coaxial technique for facilitating one-lung ventilation. Anaesthesia 1991;46:400–403.

874. Nazari S, Trazzi R, Moncalvo F, Zonta A. Campani M. Selective bronchial intubation for one-lung anaesthesia in thoracic surgery. Anaesthesia 1986;41:519–526.

875. Nazari S, Trazzi R, Moncalvo F, Carahella F, Bellinzona G, Braschi A, Scaroni M, Mapelli A. A new method for separate lung ventilation. Surv Anesth 1988;32:355–356.

876. Welsh BE. Selective bronchial intubation. Anaesthesia 1987;42:82.

877. White GMJ. Evolution of endotracheal and endobronchial intubation. Br J Anaesth 1960;32:235–245.

878. McLellan I. Endobronchial intubation in children. Anaesthesia 1974;29:757–758.

879. Baraka A, Akel S, Muallem M, et al. Bronchial intubation in children. Does the tube bevel determine the side of intubation. Anesthesiology 1987;67:869–870.

880. Bragg CL, Vukelich GR. Endotracheal tube extension for endobronchial intubation. Anesth Analg 1989;69:548–549.

881. Holzman RS. A tracheal tube extension for emergency tracheal reanastomosis. Anesthesiology 1989;70:170–171.

882. Riebold TW. Source of specialized endotracheal tubes. Anesthesiology 1989;71:322–323.

883. Baskoff JD, Stevenson RL. Endobronchial intubation in children. Anesthesiol Rev 1981;8:29–31.

884. Brooks JG, Bustamante SA, Koops BL, et al. Selective bronchial intubation for the treatment of severe localized pulmonary interstitial emphysema in newborn infants. J Pediatr 1972;91:648–652.

885. Baraka A, Slim M, Dajani A, Lakkis S. One-lung ventilation of children during surgical excision of hydatid cysts of the lung. Br J Anaesth 1982;54:523–528.

886. Dickman GL, Short BL, Krauss DR. Selective bronchial intubation in the mangement of unilateral pulmonary interstitial emphysema. Am J Dis Child 1977;131:365.

887. Dalens B, Labbe A, Haberer J. Selective endobronchial blocking vs selective intubation. Anesthesiology 1982;57:555–556.

888. Fisk GC. Endobronchial anaesthesia in young children. Br J Anaesth 1966;38:157.

889. Hogg CE, Lorhan PH. Pediatric bronchial blocking. Anesthesiology 1970;33:560–562.

890. Mathew OP, Thach BT. Selective bronchial obstruction for treatment of bullous interstitial emphysema. J Ped 1980;96:475–477.

891. Rao CC, Krishna G, Grosfeld JL, Weber TR. One lung pediatric anesthesia. Anesth Analg 1981;60:450–452.

892. Watson CB, Bowe EA, Burk W. One-lung anesthesia for pediatric thoracic surgery. A new use for the fiberoptic bronchoscope. Anesthesiology 1982;56:314–315.

893. Yeh TF, Pildes RS, Salem MR. Treatment of persistent tension pneumothorax in a neonate by selective bronchial intubation. Anesthesiology 1978;49:37–38.

894. Sachdeva SP. Treatment of post-operative pulmonary atelectasis by active inflation of the atelectatic lobe(s) through an endobronchial tube. Acta Anaesth Scand 1974;18:65–70.

895. El-Baz N, Faber LP, Kittle F, Warren W, Ivankovich AD. Bronchoscopic endobronchial intubation with a single lumen tube for one-lung anesthesia. Anesthesiology 1986;65:A480.

896. Aps C, Towey RM. Experiences with fibre-optic bronchoscopic positioning of single-lumen endobronchial tubes. Anaesthesia 1981;36:415–418.

897. Bloch EC. Tracheo-bronchial angles in infants and children. Anesthesiology 1986;65:236–237.

898. Russell GN, Frazer S, Richardson JC. Difficult bronchial intubation. Anaesthesia 1987;42:82.

899. Cant WF, Tinker JH, Tarhan S. Bronchial blockade in a child with a bronchopleural-cutaneous fistula using a balloon-tipped catheter. Anesth Analg 1976;55:874–876.

900. Vale R. Selective bronchial blocking in a small child. Br J Anaesth 1969;41:453–454.

901. Welsh BE. Selective bronchial intubation. Anesthesiology 1987;42:82.

902. Maewal HK, Kirk BW. Balloon catheter re-expan-

sion of atelectatic lung. Crit Care Med 1976;4:301–303.

903. Brodsky JB. Complications of double-lumen tracheal tubes. In: Bishop, MJ ed. Physiology and consequences of tracheal intubation [Special Issue]. Probl Anesth 1988;2(2):292–306.

904. Benumof JL, Gaughan S, Ozaki GT. Operative lung constant positive airway pressure with the Univent bronchial blocker tube. Anesth Analg 1992;74:406–410.

905. Hultgren BL, Krishna PR, Kamaya H. A new tube for one lung ventilation. experience with univent tube. Anesthesiology 1988;65:A481.

906. Inoue H, Shohtsu A, Ogawa J, Kawada S, Koide S. New device for one-lung anesthesia. endotracheal tube with moveable blocker. J Thorac Cardiovasc Med 1982;83:940–941.

907. Inoue H, Shohtsu A, Ogawa J, Koide S, Kawada S. Endotracheal tube with moveable blocker to prevent aspiration of intratracheal bleeding. Ann Thorac Surg 1984;37:497–499.

908. Inoue H. Endotracheal tube with movable blocker (Univent). Jpn J Med Inst 1989;59:241–244.

909. Kamaya H, Krishna PR. New endobronchial tube (Univent tube) for selective blockade of one lung. Anesthesiology 1985;63:342–343.

910. Karwande SV. A new tube for single lung ventilation. Chest 1987;92:761–763.

911. MacGillivray RG. Evaluation of a new tracheal tube with a moveable bronchus blocker. Anaesthesia 1988;43:687–689.

912. Herenstein R, Russo JR, Mooka N, Capan LM. Management of one-lung anesthesia in an anticoagulated patient. Anesth Analg 1988;67:1120–1122.

913. Schwartz DE, Yost CS, Larson MD. Pneumothorax complicating the case of a Univent endotracheal tube. Anesth Analg 1993;76:443–445.

914. Hultgren BL, Krishna PR, Kamaya H. A new tube for one lung ventilation. Experience with Univent tube. Anesthesiology 1986;56:A481.

915. Lines V. Selective bronchial blocking in a small child. Br J Anaesth 1969;41:893.

916. Ginsberg RJ. New technique for one-lung anesthesia using an endobronchial blocker. J Thorac Cardiovasc Surg 1981;82:542–546.

917. Cay DL, Csenderits LE, Lines V, Lomaz JG, Overton JH. Selective bronchial blocking in children. Anaesth Intensive Care 1975;3:127–130.

918. Oxorn D. Use of fiberoptic bronchoscope to assist placement of a Fogarty catheter as a bronchial blocker. Can J Anaesth 1987;34:427–428.

919. Arai T, Hatano Y. Yet another reason to use a fiberoptic bronchoscope to properly site a double lumen tube. Anesthesiology 1987;66:581–582.

920. Essig K, Freeman JA. Alternative bronchial cuff inflation technique for the Univent tube. Anesthesiology 1992;76:478–479.

921. Stark DCC. Anesthesia for thoracic surgery. Anesthesiol Rev 1980;7:14–19.

922. Finucane BT, Kupshik HL. A flexible stilette for replacing damaged tracheal tubes. Can Anaesth Soc J 1978;25:153–154.

923. Larson CE, Gasior TA. A device for endobronchial blocker placement during one-lung anesthesia. Anesth Analg 1990;71:311–312.

924. Hannallah M. The Univent tube. Bronchial cuff inflation. Anesthesiology 1991;75:165.

925. Cobley M, Vaughn RS. Recognition and management of difficult airway problems. Br J Anaesth 1992;68:90–97.

926. Linder GS. A new polyolefin-coated endotracheal tube stylet. Anesth Analg 1974;53:341–342.

927. Linder GS. More on wire stylets. Anesth Analg 1977;56:325.

928. Marshall J. Self-lubricated stylet for endotracheal tubes. Anesthesiology 1968;29:385.

929. Salem MR, Nimmagadda UR, Salazar JL, Heyman HJ. Evaluation of a new intubation guide in patients with cervical spine injuries. Crit Care Med 1990;18:S199.

930. Smith M, Buist RJ, Mansour NY. A simple method to facilitate difficult intubation. Can J Anaesth 1990;36:144–145.

931. Berry FA. Anesthesia for the child with a difficult airway. In: Berry FA, ed. Anesthetic management of difficult and routine pediatric patients. New York: Churchill Livingston, New York, 1990:167–198.

932. Fishman RL. Reuse of a disposable stylet with life-threatening complications. Anesth Analg 1991;72:266–267.

933. Kubota Y, Toyoda Y, Kubota H, Ueda Y. Shaping tracheal tubes. Anaesthesia 1987;42:896.

934. Kubota Y, Toyoda Y, Kubota H. No more complications with stylets. Anaesthesia 1992;47:628.

935. Kataria B, Starnes M. Another problem with a stylet in an endotracheal tube. Anesth Analg 1989;68:422.

936. Macintosh RR. An aid to oral intubation. Br Med J 1949;1:28.

937. Latto IP. Management of difficult intubation. In: Latto IP, Rosen M, eds. Difficulties in tracheal intubation. London: Bailliere Tindall, 1985:99–141.

938. Nolan JP, Wilson ME. An aid to oral intubation in patients with potential cervical spine injuries. Anesth Analg 1992;75:153–154.

939. Benson PF. The gum-elastic bougie: a life saver. Anesth Analg 1992;74:318.

940. Finucane BT, Kipshik HL. A flexible stilette for replacing damaged tracheal tubes. Can Anaesth Soc J 1978;25:153–154.

941. Benumof J. Part I. Management of the difficult airway. fiberoptic and retrograde techniques (ASA Refresher Course #163). New Orleans: ASA, 1990.

942. Cooper RM. Use of an endotracheal ventilation catheter for difficult extubations. Can J Anaesth 1991;39:A107.

943. Gaughan S, Benumof J, Ozaki G. Quantifiation of the jet function of a jet stylet. Anesthesiology 1991;75:A119.

944. Coveler LA. More on management of the difficult airway. Anesthesiology 1987;67:154.

945. Bailey AG, Knopes K, Ciraulo S. Use of the Fogerty embolectomy catheter to change a pediatric endotracheal tube. Anesth Analg 1988;67:1016.

946. Mostafa SM. Complications of difficult intubation. Anaesthesia 1987;42:1241–1242.

947. Gormley MJ, Lee DS. Make a difficult intubation simple. Anesthesiology 1988;68:811–812.

948. McCarroll SM, Lamont BJ, Buckland MR, Yates APB. The gum-elastic bougie: old but still useful. Anesthesiology 1988;68:643–644.

949. Kidd JF, Dyson A, Latto IP. Successful difficult intubation. Use of the gum elastic bougie. Anaesthesia 1988;43:437–438.

950. Artru AA, Schultz AB, Bonneu JJ. Modification of an Eschmann introducer to permit measurement of end-tidal carbon dioxide. Anesth Analg 1989;68:129–131.

951. Boys JE. Failed intubation in obstetric anesthesia. Br J Anaesth 1983;55:187–188.

952. Cossham PS. Difficult intubation. Br J Anaesth 1985;57:239.

953. Dogra S, Falconer R, Latto IP. Successful difficult intubation. Tracheal tube placement over a gum-elastic bougie. Anaesthesia 1990;45:774–776.

954. Freund PR, Rooke A, Schwid H. Retrograde intubation with a modified Eschmann stylet. Anesth Analg 1988;67:605–606.

955. Montgomery G, Dueringer J, Johnson C. Nasal endotracheal tube change with an intubating stylette after fiberoptic intubation. Anesth Analg 1991;72:713.

956. Millen JE, Glauser FL. A rapid simple technic for changing endotracheal tubes. Anesth Analg 1978;57:735–736.

957. Gaughan SD, Benumof JL, Ozaki GT. Quantification of the jet function of a jet stylet. Anesth Analg 1992;74:580–585.

958. Agosti L. Modification of Magill's intubating forceps. Anaesthesia 1976;31:574.

959. Aun NC, Jawan B, Lee JH. A modification of Magill's forceps. Anesthesiology 1988;68:649.

960. Burtles R. A new design of intubation forceps. Br J Anaesth 1987;59:1475–1477.

961. Klaustermeyer WB. An oropharyngeal loop to guide nasotracheal intubation. Am Rev Respir Dis 1970;102:978.

962. Liberman H. A new intubating forceps. Anaesth Intensive Care 1978;6:162–163.

963. Pelimon A, Simunovic Z. Modified Magill forceps for difficult tracheal intubation. Anaesthesia 1987;42:83.

964. Rees DF. A modification of Magill's forceps. Anaesthesia 1976;31:302–303.

965. Vonwiller JB, Liberman H, Maver E. Modified Magill forceps for difficult tracheal intubation. Anaesthesia 1987;42:777.

966. Zuck D. Magill intubating forceps. Br J Anaesth 1982;54:373.

967. Munson ES, Cullen SC. Endotracheal intubation in a patient with ankylosing spondylitis of the cervical spine. Anesthesiology 1965;26:365.

968. Singh A. Blind nasal intubation. Anaesthesia 1966;21:400–402.

969. Chester MH. Tracheal tube guide to facilitate nasotracheal intubation. Anesthesiology 1984;60:522–523.

970. Berman AJ. Device for nasotracheal intubation. Anesthesiology 1962.23:130–131.

Chapter 16

Gas Monitoring

Definitions
Comparison of Nondiverting and
  Diverting Monitors
  Nondiverting
  Diverting
Technology
  Mass Spectrometry

Raman Light Scattering Gas
  Analysis
Infrared Analysis
Paramagnetic Oxygen Analysis
Electrochemical Analysis
Piezoelectric Analysis
Chemical Carbon Dioxide Detection

Gases
  Oxygen
  Carbon Dioxide Analysis
  Volatile Anesthetic Agents
  Nitrous Oxide
  Nitrogen

One study showed that nearly 60% of critical incidents during anesthesia involve either the patient's respiratory system or the gas delivery system (1). Reliable, affordable, and easy-to-use monitors of respiratory and anesthetic gas concentrations are now available. Many monitors use more than one technology to measure different gases. Some combine gas analysis with other types of monitoring such as pulse oximetry and respirometry (Fig. 16.1).

Definitions (2–5)

1. Delay time (transit time, response time, time delay, lag time) is the time from a step change in concentration or partial pressure at the sampling site to achievement of 10% of the step change in reading at the gas monitor.

2. Response (rise) time is the time required to display a rise from 10% to 90% of the change in gas value in volumes percent or partial pressure with a step change at the sampling site. Fast response times are essential to obtaining accurate inspiratory and end-tidal values and waveforms at high respiratory rates. An instrument with a slow response time may display low peak expiratory and high inspiratory readings, because it cannot track the gas concentrations rapidly enough (6).

3. The total system response time is the sum of the delay and rise times.

4. The sensor (measuring head or chamber) is the part of a respiratory gas monitor that is sensitive to the presence of the gas.

5. The sensor area is the part of the sensor at which the gas is detected.

6. A nondiverting (mainstream, direct probe, flow through, in-line, on airway, nonsampling) monitor is one that measures the gas concentration at the sampling site. The sensor is usually connected by a cable to the display module.

7. A diverting (sidestream, withdrawal, sampling, aspirating, sniffer, sampled system) monitor is one that transports a portion of the gas being measured from the sampling site through a sampling tube to the sensor, which is remote from the sampling site.

8. The sampling site is the location at which respiratory gases are diverted for measurement to a remote sensor in a diverting

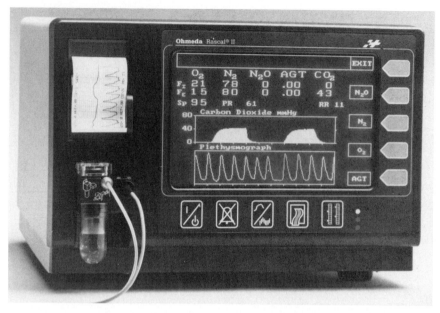

Figure 16.1. Display panel for Raman light scattering gas analyzer. Inspired and expired concentrations for the gases are displayed. Below this is a CO_2 waveform. This particular unit also has a pulse oximeter and plethysmographic waveform. Courtesy of Ohmeda, a division of BOC, Inc.

monitor or the location of the sensor area in a nondiverting monitor.

9. The sampling tube is the conduit for transfer of gases from the sampling site to the sensor in a diverting gas monitor.

10. An alarm is a warning signal that is activated when the concentration(s) of the gas(es) being monitored reaches or exceeds the alarm limit. Alarms for gas monitors fall into three categories: (*i*) high priority, which requires immediate operator response; (*ii*) medium priority, which requires prompt operator response; (*iii*) low priority, which requires operator awareness.

11. An alarm set point is the setting of the adjustment control or display value that indicates the reading at or beyond which the alarm is intended to be activated.

12. An alarm system of a monitor consists of those parts that establish the alarm set point(s) and activate an alarm when the reading is less than or equal to the low alarm set point or is equal to or greater than the high alarm set point.

13. A display is a device that visually indicates quantitative or qualitative information.

14. Shelf life is that period when a gas monitor or any of its components are stored in the original container.

15. Useful life is that period of time during which the performance of an analyzer or any of its components meets the requirements of the applicable standard.

16. Warmup time is the time necessary for the monitor to meet the accuracy specified by the manufacturer.

17. Accuracy is the ability of an instrument to indicate the actual concentration of the gas it is measuring.

18. Resolution is the ability of an instrument to distinguish between two measured values that are different.

19. Span is the output of an analyzer measuring a gas with a concentration equivalent to the mid- or full-scale reading of the instrument or to calibrate the analyzer at a mid- or full-scale reading, using a reference gas.

20. Level is the concentration of a gas in a gaseous mixture. It may be expressed either as volumes percent or partial pressure.

21. The partial pressure of a gas is the pressure that that gas in a gas mixture would exert if it alone occupied the volume of the mixture at the same temperature.

22. The percent (%, V/V, volumes percent, vol %) of a gas is the level of that gas in a mixture, expressed as a percentage volume fraction.

Comparison of Nondiverting and Diverting Monitors (7–9)

NONDIVERTING (10)

In a nondiverting instrument the patient's respiratory gas stream passes through a wide-bore chamber (cuvette) with two windows. The cuvette (Fig. 16.2) is placed between the breathing system and the mask or tracheal

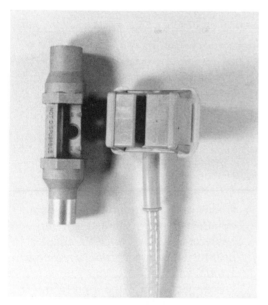

Figure 16.2. Mainstream infrared CO_2 analyzer. At the *left* is the cuvette, which is placed between the breathing system and the patient. At the *right* is the sensor, which houses the light source and detector.

tube, directly in the path of the patient's exhaled gases (Fig. 16.3*A*). The sensor, which houses both the light source and detector, fits over the cuvette (Fig. 16.4). The windows of the cuvette are usually made from sapphire, which is transparent to infrared light. Infrared light shines through the window on one side of the adaptor, and the sensor receives the light on the opposite side. To ensure that water vapor does not condense on the windows and obstruct the optical path, the sensor contains a heater that warms the adaptor to slightly above body temperature. Calibration is performed using sealed reference gas cells.

Advantages

1. Mainstream monitors have good response times because there is no delay time. The gas waveform is not degraded during transport.
2. Because no gas is removed from the breathing system, it is not necessary to scavenge these devices or to increase the fresh gas flow to compensate for gas removed from the breathing system.
3. Water and secretions are seldom a problem with this type of analyzer, although secretions on the windows of the cuvette can cause erroneous readings.
4. Contamination of the sample by fresh gas flow is less likely than with a diverting monitor.
5. A standard gas is not required for calibration.
6. These monitors use fewer disposable items than diverting monitors.
7. This type of monitor can be adapted to act as a diverting monitor so that it can be used to monitor exhaled gases in nonintubated, spontaneously breathing patients (11,12) or to find leaks in carbon dioxide insufflation equipment (13).

Disadvantages

1. To obtain end-tidal values, these analyzers require that the airway adaptor and

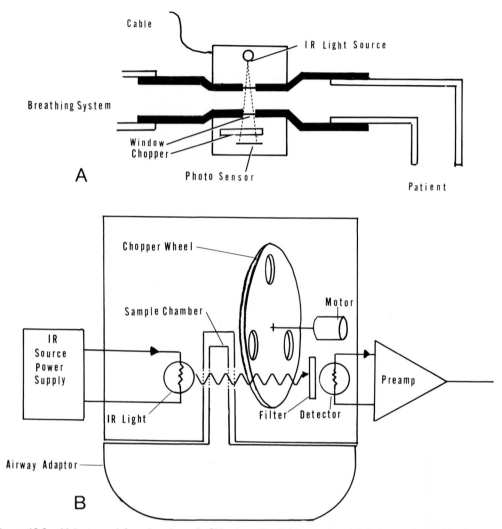

Figure 16.3. Mainstream infrared analyzer **A**, Side view. The light source and detector are housed in the sensor, which fits over the cuvette. The IR light shines through the sapphire windows of the cuvette and is detected by the photosensor. **B**, Cross-sectional view. Gases pass through the airway adaptor (cuvette). The infrared light that is transmitted through the windows is filtered and then detected by the photodetector in the sensor.

analysis module be placed near the patient. The sensor is somewhat heavy and cumbersome enough to cause traction on the tracheal tube. Newer adapters are more lightweight.

2. Use of the airway adapter between the patient and the Y piece will increase dead space, adding from 5 to 17 ml for adult-size adapters and 0.6 to 2 ml for pediatric adapters (14,15). However, studies show that end-tidal CO_2 values obtained using a mainstream infrared analyzer with a pediatric adapter in healthy neonates and infants are close to arterial values (14).

3. Disconnections can be a problem (16–19).

4. Condensed water, secretions, or blood on the windows of the cuvette will interfere with light transmission.

5. The sensor may become dislodged from the cuvette. If it is completely dislodged, no waveform will be seen. If it is slightly dislodged (see Fig. 16.4), the reading may be incorrect although the waveform appears normal (17,20,21).

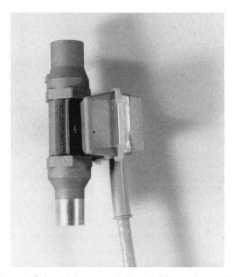

Figure 16.4. Mainstream infrared CO_2 analyzer. The sensor fits over the cuvette as shown. Note that in this picture the sensor does not completely cover the windows of the cuvette; this can result in falsely low CO_2 readings.

6. The sensor is vulnerable to trauma and may be expensive to repair or replace. Newer units are more resistant to mechanical trauma (9).

7. Warmup time is usually longer than with the diverting type.

8. Calibration is usually not automatic.

9. At present, mainstream monitors can only measure carbon dioxide. They do not have the capability of measuring nitrogen, nitrous oxide, and/or anesthetic agents. The user must indicate the presence of nitrous oxide so a correction for this can be used (Fig. 16.5).

10. A mainstream monitor is difficult to use on nonintubated, spontaneously breathing patients.

11. The adapter must be cleaned and disinfected between uses. There is potential for cross-contamination between patients if this is not done properly.

12. Thermal skin burns have been reported with use of a mainstream analyzer despite use of multiple layers of gauze, which kept the sensor from direct contact with the skin (22). To prevent this, it may be necessary to interpose a piece of aluminum foil between two pieces of soft material to reflect the radiant en-

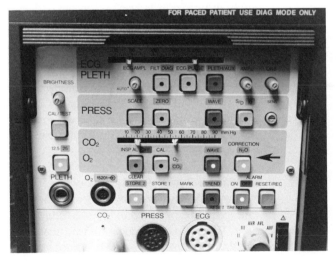

Figure 16.5. Controls for mainstream infrared CO_2 analyzer. Note the *arrow* pointing to N_2O correction button. Because nitrous oxide cannot be measured using a mainstream sensor, the user must indicate the presence of nitrous oxide so a correction can be made by the analyzer.

ergy. Prolonged contact of the sensor assembly with the patient could cause pressure injury.

DIVERTING

In diverting analyzers, gas is continuously drawn from the sampling site through a thin plastic sampling tube into the monitor where the measurement is made. Keeping the sampling tube as short as possible will decrease the delay time and result in a more satisfactory waveform.

The sampling site should be away from the fresh gas port. When a Mapleson breathing system is used, continuous inflow of fresh gas close to the sampling site can result in erroneous readings.

The sensing site can be a T adaptor placed in the breathing system between two components or between the breathing system and the patient (Fig. 16.6). Alternately, a hole that will accept a small tubing can be drilled into a component such as the elbow adaptor or tracheal tube connector (23,24). Disposable breathing systems with built-in sample ports are available.

Face masks have relatively large dead space relative to tidal volume so that it is difficult to obtain end-tidal values if the sampling site is between the mask and breathing system. In this case, the sampling catheter

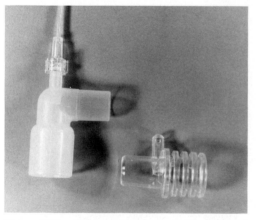

Figure 16.6. Adaptors for sampling with a diverting gas monitor.

can be taped to the upper lip or placed in the patient's nares or the lumen of an oral or nasopharyngeal airway. With a laryngeal mask, the end of the sampling catheter should be placed at the distal end of the LMA (25).

Special tracheal tubes that incorporate a sampling lumen that extends to the middle or distal end of the tube are available. Some are described in Chapter 15. Alternately, a small catheter can be inserted through a modified connector and advanced into the tracheal tube (26–28). This may be associated with increased airway resistance and a greater likelihood that the sampling tube will become obstructed with water or secretions. However, it may result in measurements that more closely approximate alveolar values, especially in small patients with breathing systems in which the fresh gas flow can mix with exhaled gases (29–34).

In spontaneously breathing, unintubated patients, the end of the sampling tube can be placed in front of or inside the patient's nostril (12,35) or a nasopharyngeal airway (36,37). If the patient is a mouth breather, it can be placed in front of the mouth or in the posterior nasopharynx. Methods to attach the tubing to modified nasal cannulae (38–48) and oxygen masks (49–52) have been described. A number of devices for this purpose are now available commercially (Fig. 16.7). Such monitoring is useful for sedated patients during regional or local anesthesia, patients in the postanesthesia care unit, and patients receiving infusions of epidural opioids. Most of these devices are well-tolerated by patients and do not interfere with administration of supplemental oxygen. Intranasal irritation, blocking of the catheter, and mechanical interference by the surgeon can be problems.

On some sidestream monitors the flow rate can be varied. Flow rates between 50 and 500 ml/min have been used. Ideally, the flow rate should be matched to the size of each patient. When tidal volume and dead space are small, the volume removed becomes large in proportion. However, it has been suggested

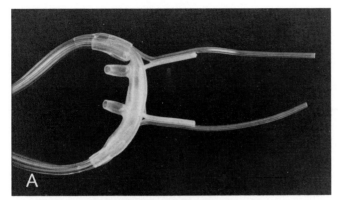

Figure 16.7. Devices to allow simultaneous administration of gas via nasal cannulae and gas sampling. **A,** This device is designed for patients who are predominantly mouth breathers. The oral sampling prongs can be cut and shaped to suit individual patients. Courtesy of Biochem International, Inc. **B,** This device has a septum between the two nasal prongs. One prong is used for administration of oxygen and one for gas sampling.

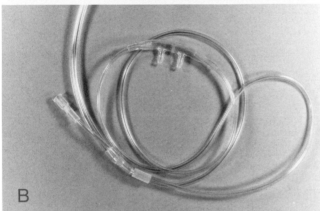

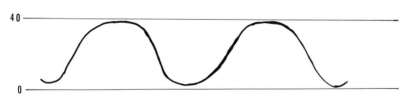

Figure 16.8. Too low a sampling rate with a sidestream capnometer will result in a low peak and, often, elevation of the baseline. Erroneous values for both inspired and end-tidal carbon dioxide will be reported.

that a sampling flow rate less than 150 ml/min not be used, as delay time and rise time are inversely proportional to the sampling flow rate and low sampling flows may result in an elevated baseline, erroneously low peak readings and absence of an end-tidal plateau (53), especially when the respiratory rate is fast and tidal volume is small (Fig. 16.8). A high flow rate will decrease the delay and rise times, but may cause fresh gas to be entrained into the sample line. This will cause incorrect end-tidal readings and a capnogram with a decrease in the CO_2 level at the end of the expiratory plateau (Fig. 16.9) (54).

These analyzers are usually zeroed using room air or automatically using electronics and calibrated against a gas of known composition.

Advantages

1. Sampling from patients who are not intubated is relatively easy.

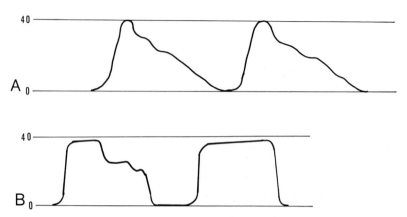

Figure 16.9.   Contamination of expired sample by fresh gas or ambient air may be caused by placing the sampling site too near the fresh gas inlet, a leak, or too high a sampling flow rate. **A,** A large leak is indicated by the progressive decrease in the plateau. **B,** Here, the contamination is of lesser magnitude and a dropoff occurs at the end of the plateau. At the *right,* the leak has been corrected.

2. Warmup is usually faster than with mainstream devices.
3. Calibration and zeroing are usually automatic. Occasional calibration to a standard is necessary but is usually easy to accomplish.
4. The patient interface is lightweight and inexpensive.
5. The added dead space is minimal.
6. The potential for cross-contamination between patients is low if the adaptor and sample tube are changed between patients.
7. With some technologies several gases can be measured simultaneously. This may allow automatic correction for nitrous oxide and/or oxygen.
8. The connection to the sampling site can be used to administer bronchodilators (55).
9. A diverting capnometer can be used to detect leaks in carbon dioxide insufflation equipment (13).
10. These devices allow monitoring of gas levels when the monitor must be remote from the patient, as during magnetic resonance imaging (56–58).

Disadvantages

1. A major problem with sidestream devices is that particulate matter and/or water can cause the sampling tubing to become obstructed (59–61). Manufacturers have addressed this problem with traps (Fig. 16.10) (which must be emptied periodically), filters, or hydrophobic membranes (which must be changed periodically) and nafion tubing (which allows water to rapidly diffuse though its walls), thus lowering the water content of the gas sample. Many water traps are easily overwhelmed so that water enters the measurement system (2). Placing a heat and moisture exchanger between the patient and the sampling site will decrease the amount of water in the aspirated sample. The sampling tube may also be obstructed by kinking or external pressure.
2. Gases flowing to the monitor must be either diverted to the scavenging system or returned to the breathing system. If scavenging is employed, the fresh gas flow may need to be increased to compensate for the gas removed.
3. Some delay time is inevitable.
4. Leaks in the sampling system can cause erroneous readings and/or deformation of the waveforms.
5. Accuracy decreases with increasing respiratory rate, when the I:E ratio changes from 1:1 and with longer sampling lines (62,63). When the I:E ratio is greater than

1, the errors appear first in the end-tidal or expiratory data, and when the ratio is less than 1, the errors appear first in the inspiratory data. Other factors that may affect accuracy are the sample flow rate and the composition of the sampling tube. Fresh gas from the breathing system may dilute exhaled gases.

6. A supply of calibration gas may need to be kept.

7. A number of disposable items (adaptors and catheters) must be used.

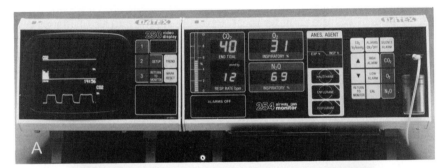

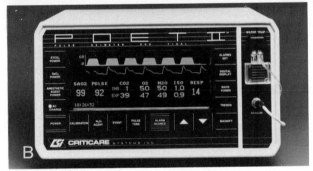

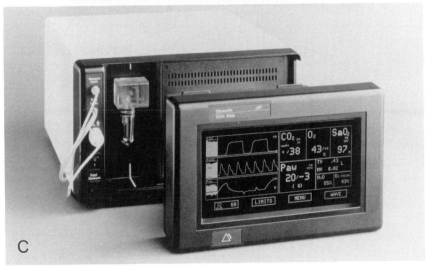

Figure 16.10. Sidestream infrared monitors. CO_2 and anesthetic agents are measured using infrared technology, and another technology is used to measure oxygen levels. Note also the water traps. **A,** Courtesy of Datex, Inc. **B,** Courtesy of Criticare Systems, Inc. **C,** Courtesy of Ohmeda, a division of BOC, Inc.

Technology

MASS SPECTROMETRY (64)

The mass spectrometer can be used to measure inspired and end-tidal concentrations of oxygen, nitrogen, carbon dioxide, nitrous oxide, and the volatile anesthetic agents. Argon and/or helium can be measured on some units.

The mass spectrometer is so named because it spreads components of a gas mixture into a spectrum, according to their mass:charge ratios. By analyzing the spectrum, the composition and relative abundance of each component of a gas sample can be determined. The gas sample cannot be re-

turned to the breathing system and must be vented to a scavenging system.

The mass spectrometer differs from most other measuring devices in that it measures gas levels in volumes percent, not partial pressure. This can cause inaccurate readings if a gas that the mass spectrometer cannot measure is present.

These units are calibrated with cylinders containing mixtures of the gases to be analyzed and with room air.

Two basic types are available: shared (multiplexed) and dedicated (stand alone, single room, mini-mass spectrometer). With a shared system the mass spectrometer is located centrally, usually outside of the anesthetizing sites, but within the operating room suite. There are multiple stations from which

Figure 16.11. Shared mass spectrometer. The mass spectrometer is locally centrally. Long sample tubings pass from each sampling location through specially installed ductwork to the multiplexer, which sequentially directs sample flows to the mass spectrometer. Information derived centrally is relayed to the individual stations and displayed. The central display and printer are optional.

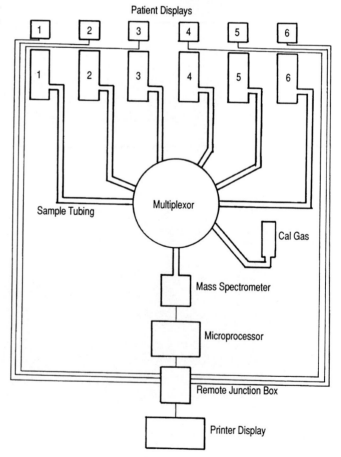

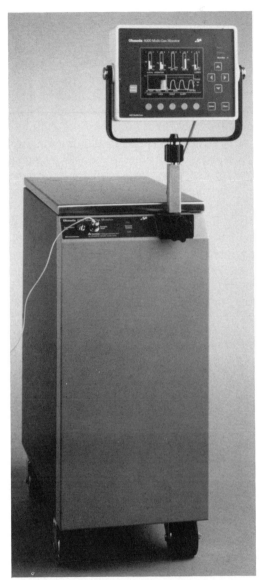

Figure 16.12. Dedicated mass spectrometer. The display monitor can be separated from the rest of the unit. Courtesy of Ohmeda, a division of BOC Health Care, Inc.

gases are sampled and to which data are returned (Fig. 16.11). Long tubings pass from each station through specially installed ductwork to a valve box (multiplexer) at the inlet of the mass spectrometer. The valve box sequentially directs the sample flows to the mass spectrometer, so that one station at a

time is sampled. Information derived centrally is relayed to the individual stations and displayed. It also can be displayed centrally. Such an arrangement permits one central analyzer to function as part of a computerized system, which may serve up to 31 sampling locations on a time-shared basis.

A dedicated mass spectrometer (Fig. 16.12). is used in only one location. It consists of two parts: the analyzer and the display/control unit, which are connected by a cable. A short tubing carries the gas sample from the sampling site to the analyzer. It uses a lower sampling flow rate than a shared mass spectrometer.

Components

Sample Gas Tubing

Gas is transported from the sampling site to the mass spectrometer through a narrow tubing, called the sample gas tubing (inlet line, sample gas transport tube, sample capillary tube, sampling catheter or tube, transport tube, aspirating tube, sample line). With a dedicated mass spectrometer, only a single short tubing is required. With a shared system, a short tubing is used to transport gas from the sampling site to a headwall plate located in the wall or ceiling. This plate has two connectors. One accepts the sampling tube and the other is an electrical connection that transmits information to and from a display unit. From the headwall plate a longer catheter extends to the central mass spectrometer.

The tubing must be made of a material that is resistant to the gases being sampled and will not allow the gases being measured to diffuse out or outside air to be drawn in. Of the various materials tried, nylon has proved most satisfactory (65,66). Nafion, a braided nylon tubing, is permeable to water vapor and will allow most water to diffuse through its walls to atmosphere, is commonly used.

These lines should be as short as possible to ensure a minimum delay time. Long sampling lines will cause smeared inspired and end-tidal peaks with erroneous readings, especially at high respiratory rates and high I:E ratios (62). Signal distortion can be lessened by increasing the sampling flow, but there is a limit to the amount of improvement that can be achieved (67).

Particulate matter and fluids may obstruct the sample gas tube. Adverse consequences may include distorted waveforms, inaccurate measurements and damage to the monitor. For these reasons a filter is commonly used between the breathing system and the sampling tubing. Despite this, fluid may be aspirated into the tube, causing malfunction (68).

Sample Pump

A pump is needed to withdraw the gas from the sampling site at flow rates up to 240 ml/min for shared units and 30 ml/min for dedicated units. A pressure drop from approximately 760 torr at the inlet to less than 50 torr at the mass spectrometer inlet is common (64). The gas profiles from several breaths can be stored in the sampling line without significant loss of information by continuously pulling through the lines going to stations not being monitored but at a slower rate than the mass spectrometer sampling rate. When the line is connected to the mass spectrometer, the flow rate is accelerated.

Multiplexer

The multiplexer (switching mechanism, multiplexing valve) serially samples from each station that has the remote monitor turned on for a specified period of time or for a certain number of breaths, then sends the gas sample on to the mass spectrometer (see Fig. 11). It then switches to a new sample line. The sequence of sampling is controlled by the central station computer. With some units, the sequence can be overridden if a particular station requests an immediate (stat) analysis. This will put that station next in line for sampling.

Some mass spectrometers use a rotary valve for multiplexing. This sequentially directs the gas sample to the mass spectrometer. Others use electronically controlled three-way solenoid valves on each sample gas tubing. Gas is continually sampled from all patient lines. At any moment in time, the solenoid valves direct gas from one sampling line into the mass spectrometer unit for analysis and gas in the other lines to a scavenging system. Gas from the sample line is drawn into the mass spectrometer at twice the original sampling rate. This permits analysis of stored line data in less time. Less time per patient location is required with this method compared with direct sampling. However, if the solenoid valve mechanism malfunctions, the entire system will be out of order. If the rotary valve malfunctions, only one station may be affected.

Vacuum Pump

The creation and manipulation of ions must be carried out in a high vacuum to avoid interference by outside air and to minimize random collisions between the ions and residual gases. The vacuum pump maintains a very low pressure, normally less than 10^{-5} torr within the ionization chamber. Achievement of a suitable vacuum may take up to 15 min.

Sample Inlet System

A very small amount of the gas sampled enters the ionization chamber through the sample inlet (molecular leak inlet system, capillary inlet system, molecular leak, molecular inlet leak), a tiny hole or porous plug. The pressure falls from 20 to 50 torr to approximately 5 to 10^{-5} torr, and its mode of flow changes from viscous to molecular. Viscous flow exists when the density of the gas molecules is high enough to provide consistent interaction (collisions) between the various molecules in a mixture, thereby preventing separation of one gas species from another. Molecular flow occurs when the pressure and density are so low that the molecules rarely collide with one another and are only affected by collisions with the walls of the container (64).

Ion Source

Electrons are emitted by a heated wire filament, focused magnetically or electrically and directed into the ionization chamber. There they pass across the chamber and are collected by a positively charged plate on the opposite side.

Neutral molecules of the sample gas enter the ionization chamber and are bombarded by the electrons. Some molecules are transformed into positively charged ions of the same mass as the molecule from which they were produced. Some molecules are split into fragments, one or more of which are positively charged. The positively charged ions

then travel into the ion focal system, a set of electrodes that establishes an electrostatic field. The ions are accelerated, focused into a beam, and projected into the analyzer section.

Analyzer

The analyzer (ion filter) separates ions according to mass. There are several types, based on the method of separation (64). Two have been used for monitoring gases in anesthesia.

Magnetic Sector (8). The most common type of mass spectrometer is the magnetic sector (magnetic deflector) analyzer, so named because it uses a magnet to separate the ions (Fig. 16.13). Within the ionization chamber is a magnetic field at right angles to the ions' direction of travel. When a charged

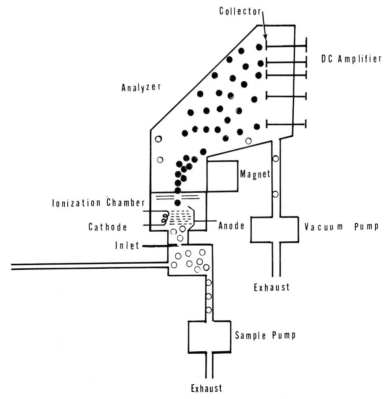

Figure 16.13. Magnetic sector mass spectrometer. The *open circles* represent un-ionized molecules; the *closed circles*, ions. A magnetic field acting on the ions does the same thing as a prism does with a light beam: It separates the different components, in this case according to their mass:charge ratios.

particle moves across a magnetic field, its path is deflected into an arc whose radius of curvature is determined by its mass:charge ratio. The degree of deflection is greater for lighter than for heavier ions, if they have equal charges. Thus a number of separate ion beams will exit the magnetic field.

The ion collectors (cathodes, detectors, detector plates, collector electrodes, ion counters, Faraday cups) are the metal plates that receive the ions. These are placed at locations that correspond to the trajectories of the mass:charge ratios of the ion species for which the mass spectrometer has been programmed. The number of ions impacting on each plate during a fixed time interval is detected and an electric current that is proportional to the concentration of the gas in the original sample is produced.

A disadvantage of this type of analyzer is the need to specify the gases being monitored in advance of purchase (69). Most mass spectrometers use seven collectors. More collectors can sometimes be added.

Quadrupole Mass Filter (70). A quadrupole mass spectrometer works on the principle that a controlled oscillating electric field can prevent all but a narrow range of charged molecules from reaching a target (Fig. 16.14). Four parallel electrically conducting rods are arranged at the corners of a square. Opposite rods are connected together electrically. There is only one collector, which is at the end of the rods.

To the two pairs of rods are applied equal but opposite potentials, each of which has direct current and radiofrequency voltage components. Gas molecules enter the unit and are ionized, and the ions are accelerated along the longitudinal axis of the four rods. To reach the collector the ions must traverse this region without colliding with any of the rods. Radiofrequency and direct current voltage generators are applied to the two pairs of rods so that the quadrupole's electrostatic charge changes in steps. For any given radiofrequency to direct current voltage level, only ions of a specific mass:charge ratio avoid collision with one of the rods and reach the collector at the distal end of the chamber. All other ions collide with one of the rods and, because of the DC voltage, are discharged. The number of hits on the collector for each ion mass:charge ratio is detected and

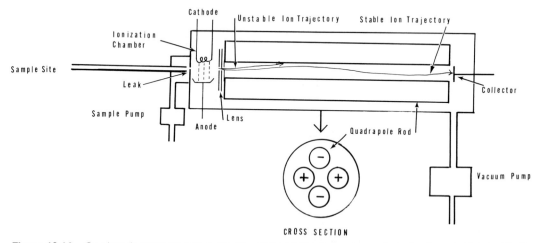

CROSS SECTION

Figure 16.14. Quadrupole mass spectrometer. The name of this device comes from the four parallel electrically conducting rods arranged symmetrically. All electrons, except those of a selected mass:charge ratio, strike the sides of the quadrupole and are discharged. The number of hits on the collector for each mass:charge ratio is detected and is proportional to the partial pressure of the selected gas in the sample.

apportioned to indicate the concentration of the selected gas in the sample. This cycle of filtering out all but one mass:charge ratio of ion and then measuring its abundance is repeated until each component of the mixture of gases has been analyzed. The process occurs so rapidly as to appear almost instantaneous and the response time of this type of analyzer is almost identical to that of a magnetic sector unit.

Compared with the magnetic sector, the quadrupole mass spectrometer is smaller and more lightweight and has a lower sampling rate (64). One advantage of a quadrupole system is that it may be adapted to measure new or additional gases by changes in software.

Processing Circuit

The measured currents from the collector(s) are entered into a computer that converts them into numbers representing the fractional components of the different constituents or partial pressures for each gas. Two special mechanisms are used for dealing with the data: a spectrum overlap erasure and an automatic summing circuit.

Spectrum Overlap Eraser (71,72). A major problem in the use of mass spectrometry during anesthesia is the overlap in the spectra of several gases. Nitrous oxide and carbon dioxide, which both have the same atomic mass, are detected at the same mass:charge ratio. Likewise, isoflurane and enflurane have the same molecular weight and would be indistinguishable by a collector.

Spectrum overlap erasing allows evaluation of individual gases or agents when more than one contribute to the signal at a specific mass:charge ratio. When compounds enter the analyzer, fragmentation (cracking), in which a molecule is split into smaller positively charged ions, occurs. This results in the production of a mass spectrogram (cracking pattern) rather than a discrete peak for each molecule. Fortunately, gas molecules frag-

ment in a fixed proportion. One fragment is detected as the sole output of that gas at a particular mass number. The proportion of the parent substance in the original gas mixture as well as the contribution made by the parent substance to the outputs detected at the mass:charge ratios of the other gases present can then be determined.

Automatic Summing Circuit. Another problem with mass spectrometry is that the amount of charged material arriving at the collectors may vary with time. An automatic summing circuit (automatic stability control, automatic sensitivity control) electronically adds together all the measured concentrations of gases being monitored and adjusts the sensitivity to maintain the sum at 100%. Thus it corrects automatically for alterations in barometric pressure and water vapor and ignores gases for which the mass spectrometer has not been programmed. One problem is that if a gas for which the mass spectrometer is not programmed, e.g., helium, is used the gas will not be detected by the mass spectrometer and the automatic summing circuit will show erroneously high concentrations of the other gases (73).

Computer algorithms have been created to detect maximum and minimum CO_2 levels and, thereby, to identify inspiration and end expiration. Other gases measured at these times are displayed as inspired and end-tidal values. The computer also permits the entry of alarm limits and activation of alarms when these limits are exceeded.

Displays

Data display is a function of software design and can be tailored to the needs of the user. Most units provide a simple menu and controls so that the operator can select the display format and alarm limits (Fig. 16.15). Typically, the screen will display a capnogram and sometimes one other waveform, inspired and expired gas concentrations in numerics or bar graphs, trend data, and

Figure 16.15. Display unit for shared mass spectrometer. Inspired and end-tidal readings for the gases measured are displayed. To the right are trend data, and at the bottom is the CO_2 waveform display. Note the stat control at the bottom. Courtesy of Marquette Electronics.

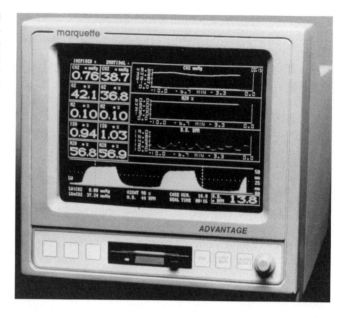

alarm values. With shared systems, units may emit a beep when a new analysis is displayed.

Shared System Versus Stand-Alone Technology

The shared system offers advantages in initial cost and maintenance costs, because there is one instead of many systems to maintain. Disadvantages include the lack of real-time monitoring and increased delay time for each sample. If the system goes down, the entire operating room suite may be without monitoring. Two shared mass spectrometers can be linked to help solve this problem (74). Because CO_2 monitoring is probably of greatest importance, the manufacturers of shared systems offer optional continuous infrared CO_2 detectors, which are placed in series between the patient sampling tube and the headwall adaptor at each sampling location.

Stand-alone units can be moved from location to location, whereas a shared system can only be used in the locations to which it was connected during the installation of the system.

Advantages

Multigas Capability

It can measure nearly every gas of importance to anesthesia.

Multiple Agent Detection

It can detect mixtures of volatile anesthetic agents (75).

Fast Response Time

The response time is fast enough to allow end-tidal measurements of the gases being measured, although accurate values may not be obtained at high respiratory frequencies. Mass spectrometer systems are adequate for respiratory and anesthetic gas monitoring from relatively long lines for the respiratory rates typically encountered in an adult population (62). A time-shared mass spectrometer is suitable for some pediatric patients, if they are not too distant from the analyzer. A stand-alone mass spectrometer can accurately measure expired gas concentrations in subjects requiring tidal volumes as low as 3 to 4 ml and at respiratory rates up to 80 breaths/min (76).

Convenience

Mass spectrometers are fairly easy to use, maintain, and calibrate. With a shared system, minimal space is needed. However, the stand-alone version requires several square feet of floor space.

Reliability

Most mass spectrometer systems function reliably for long periods with little down time.

Low Cost

Despite the large initial equipment and personnel expenses to install and maintain a mass spectrometer, multipatient monitoring with a single, centrally located mass spectrometer results in relatively low cost per patient (77).

Disadvantages

Measurement of Only Preprogrammed Gases

With a mass spectrometer, the reliability of the readings presupposes that no gases other than those for which it is programmed are present in the gas sample. When an unknown, unmeasured gas is introduced into a mass spectrometer, the concentrations of the measured gases will be computed as if they alone were present and the concentrations reported by the analyzer will be erroneously high (78). This can result in significant errors if a gas such as helium is used in significant concentrations (73,79).

In mass spectrometers that are programmed for helium analysis, another problem may arise (80). Some spectrometers cannot evacuate the helium quickly from the high-vacuum chamber of the analyzer. After analyzing a gas mixture containing helium, the shared mass spectrometer will switch to the next station before all the helium has been evacuated from the chamber, and the partial pressures of the sample from the station not using helium will be erroneously low.

Some substances, such as those found in propellants used in bronchodilators, may be erroneously read as anesthetic agents or carbon dioxide (81–83). There may be a decrease or increase in the CO_2 or anesthetic agent reading (84). Fortunately, the effect of propellant gases is transient. If a shared unit is being used, the aerosol should be administered while the spectrometer is sampling other stations. If sampling is continuous, removing the sample port briefly from the circuit during administration of medication will prevent incorrect readings.

Necessity for Scavenging

The gas aspirated must be scavenged. It cannot be returned to the breathing system. The fresh gas flow may need to be increased to compensate for the gas removed.

Turn-Around Time

Shared systems have a small but finite turn-around time when sampling between stations. The delay may be unacceptable for detection of sudden changes such as those seen with air embolism or for verifying placement of a tracheal tube. Some systems can be programmed to sample certain locations more frequently than others to facilitate detection of certain events. Alternately, another type of monitoring than mass spectrometry may be used during such cases.

The frequency of sampling and time from sampling to display of results depends on four factors: (*i*) distance from the mass spectrometer to the sampling location; (*ii*) number of stations on line at a particular time; (*iii*) the number of breaths or time sampled (dwell time); and (*iv*) priority settings. Priority settings enable the user to obtain a stat analysis (see Fig. 16.15). In the stat mode the multiplexer is commanded to sample from the stat location. Frequent use of this mode will delay the updating of information from other sampling locations.

Down Time

Although extremely reliable, any shared system will eventually be out of operation for some time and the entire operating room suite may be without full monitoring. For this reason it is recommended that a time-shared mass spectrometer always be used with other means to measure oxygen and carbon dioxide at each station. As mentioned above, manufacturers of shared systems have made available infrared CO_2 detectors as add-on options. Most anesthesia machines have oxygen analyzers.

To reduce down time, a spare mass spectrometer may be purchased (85). If there is more than one mass spectrometer in close proximity, it may be possible to link them to

provide continuous monitoring during system failure (74,77).

Special Installation Required

With a shared system, the central unit requires a separate room, which may need independent air-conditioning. Special ductwork to each anesthetizing location must be installed.

Difficulties in Monitoring Remote Locations

With a shared system mass spectrometer, there are limits as to how far away from the central mass spectrometer a sampling station can be located.

Movement of a dedicated unit requires a closedown and a startup time of 6 min or

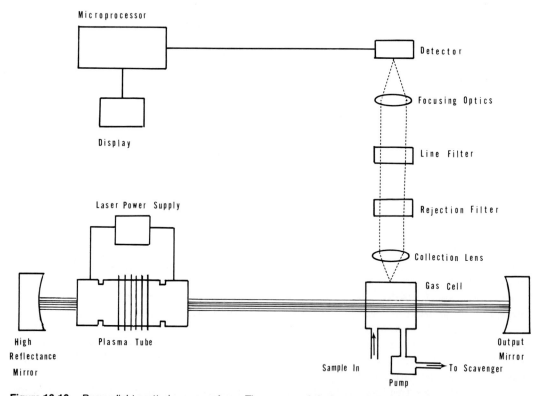

Figure 16.16. Raman light scattering gas analyzer. The gas sample is drawn continuously into the sample (gas) cell. Light traversing this cell is scattered. The scattered light is directed by the collection lens through a series of filters that select particular wavelengths corresponding to the gases being analyzed. The light is then imaged onto the detector and quantified.

more. A special startup and closedown sequence must be followed.

Warmup Time

The dedicated mass spectrometer requires a fairly long warmup time to evacuate the analyzing chamber.

Space

The dedicated mass spectrometer takes up space in the operating room. A special room is needed for a shared system.

RAMAN LIGHT SCATTERING GAS ANALYSIS (86,87)

Technology

In Raman light scattering gas analysis (Raman spectroscopy) an argon laser emits monochromatic light. When this light interacts with gas molecules that have intramolecular bonds, some of its energy is converted into the vibrational and rotational modes within the molecule. A fraction of the energy absorbed is reemitted at new wavelengths in a phenomenon called Raman scattering. The wavelength shift and amount of scattering can be used to determine the constituents of a gas mixture. This technology can be applied to all gases likely to be present in the respiratory gas mixture, including carbon dioxide, oxygen, nitrogen, nitrous oxide, and anesthetic agents (2). Monoatomic gases such as helium, xenon, and argon do not exhibit Raman scattering and cannot be measured using this technology.

A Raman spectrometer is shown in Figure 16.16. The gas mixture to be analyzed is drawn continuously into the instrument. The light source is placed so that the beam traverses the sample cell. Lenses mounted perpendicular to the beam collect the scattered light and direct it through a series of filters that select particular wavelengths corresponding to the gases being analyzed. The scattered light is imaged onto a detector and quantitated by counting photons. Because the shift in frequency is different for each gas, analysis of the frequencies in the scattered light provides identification of the gases present. The intensity of the scattered light at each wavelength is directly proportional to the partial pressure of a particular gas. A computer processes the data, providing a readout on a display screen (see Fig. 16.1).

The Raman spectrometer periodically calibrates itself automatically, using an internal argon cylinder for zero and room air for gain. This takes about 8 sec. The machine needs to be periodically calibrated with test gases.

Advantages (88)

Multiple Gas Capability

The Raman spectrometer can identify and measure inspired and expired partial pressures for nearly every gas of interest in anesthesia, including CO_2, nitrous oxide, oxygen, nitrogen, hydrogen, and the volatile anesthetic agents.

Multiple Agent Detection

Mixtures of volatile agents can be detected.

Fast Response Time

Although the response time is slower than that for mass spectrometry, it is adequate for breath-by-breath end-tidal monitoring in adults (88).

Portability

This monitor can be easily transported to remote locations.

Fast Startup Time

It has a very short startup time. This is especially advantageous if the monitor must be moved. Early models could be turned off between cases. With newer models, it is recommended that they be kept in a standby mode. If the analyzer must be turned off, the startup time is longer.

Convenience

The Raman spectrometer is easy to use and requires relatively little maintenance.

No Need for Scavenging Gases

Because the aspirated gases undergo no physical change during analysis, they can be returned to the breathing system. The gases can also be vented to the scavenging system.

Accuracy

It has a high degree of accuracy (87).

No Artifacts with Propellants

Aerosol propellants that affect the readings of a mass spectrometer do not affect the accuracy of the Raman spectrometer (84). It also gives accurate readings in the presence of unknown or unusual gases such as helium or ethanol.

Disadvantages

Inaccuracy with Pediatric Patients

With small tidal volumes and high respiratory rates, the readings may be inaccurate.

Size

Although the later versions are smaller than the first models, the analyzer is still fairly large.

INFRARED (IR) ANALYSIS (89,90)

Infrared (IR) analyzers are based on the fact that gases that have two or more dissimilar atoms in the molecule (nitrous oxide, carbon dioxide, and the halogenated agents) have specific and unique absorption spectra of IR light. Infrared analyzers use IR wavelengths that are different from the absorption spectra of other compounds present to identify particular gases. The nonpolar molecules of argon, nitrogen, helium, xenon, and oxygen do not absorb IR light and cannot be measured using this technology.

Infrared CO_2 analyzers may be diverting or nondiverting. Infrared analyzers that mea-sure anesthetic agents are diverting. Because the gases are not altered, the sample can be returned to the breathing system.

Most infrared instruments have an accuracy of $\pm 0.2\%$ for CO_2 over the range of 0% to 10% and $\pm 2.0\%$ for N_2O over the range of 0% to 100%. For typical halogenated agents, the accuracy is $\pm 0.4\%$ over a range of 0% to 5% (89). Most investigators believe that these monitors are sufficiently accurate for clinical purposes (91–97), although they tend to underestimate the inspired level and overestimate end-tidal values at high respiratory rates (98). With increasing respiratory rate, accuracy is diminished more for volatile anesthetic values than CO_2 (99).

Advances in electronic circuitry have led to the introduction of infrared volatile anesthetic and CO_2 monitors that are integrated into the anesthesia machine.

Optical (8)

Sidestream. Figure 16.17 shows a sidestream analyzer. IR light is focused continuously on a spinning (chopper) wheel. The wheel has holes with filters specially selected for the gases to be measured. The gas to be measured is pumped continuously through a sample (measuring) chamber. The selectively filtered and pulsed light is passed through the sample chamber and also through a reference chamber with no absorption qualities. The light is then passed on to an IR light detector (photosensor). The amount of light absorbed by the sample gas is proportional to the partial pressures of gases whose IR light absorption patterns correspond to the wavelengths selected by the filters on the chopper wheel. The more light detected, the less gas present, and conversely, the less light detected, the more gas present.

The changing light levels on the photosensor produce changes in the electrical current that runs through it. Electrical signals are sent to an amplifier and processed by rectifiers that generate the actual measuring signal (the difference between the reference chamber and the measuring chamber). The mea-

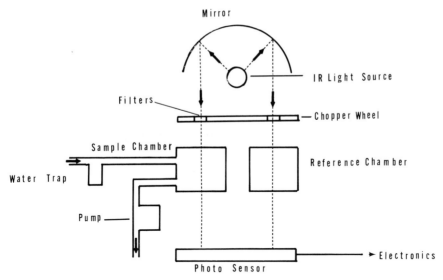

Figure 16.17. Sidestream optical infrared analyzer. A beam of IR light is at one end and a photodetection device is at the other. The chopper wheel contains several filters, which are divided into sections that will allow passage of only the frequencies most readily absorbed by the gases to be measured. The filtered and pulsatile IR light is directed through both the sample chamber and a reference chamber with no absorption qualities. The amount of IR light absorbed at each frequency depends on the levels of gases in the sample chamber.

suring signal is then directed to the display unit.

Rotating the filter wheel thousands of times per minute provides hundreds of readings for each respiratory cycle. For practical purposes, the waveform on the display is continuous.

Early sidestream optical IR analyzers used one wavelength to measure potent inhaled agents and were unable to distinguish between agents or to detect a mixture of agents (100). When such an analyzer is used, the clinician must select which agent is to be monitored (see Fig. 16.10). If an incorrect agent is selected, incorrect values will be reported (101–104). If enflurane is administered and isoflurane is erroneously selected or if isoflurane is administered and enflurane erroneously selected, the error will be minimal. If isoflurane is administered and the dial is set for halothane, the reading will be up to nine times the actual partial pressure. If enflurane is being delivered and the analyzer is programmed to monitor halothane, the reading will be up to five times the correct value. If

halothane is being delivered and the dial on the analyzer is set to enflurane or isoflurane, the reading will be erroneously low by a factor of up to nine. If enflurane or isoflurane is administered and halothane is erroneously selected, the reading on the monitor will be erroneously high. If halothane is administered and enflurane or isoflurane is mistakenly selected, the reading will be erroneously low—a potentially dangerous situation, because the user may increase the delivered concentration. Newer IR analyzers use multiple wavelengths to both identify and quantify the potent inhaled agents (105–108). This eliminates the need for the user to select which anesthetic agent is to be monitored and allows detection of a mixture of agents.

Most sidestream analyzers have fixed sampling rates (usually 150 ml/min), although some permit selection of other rates. The measuring cell is calibrated to zero using gas free of the gases of interest (usually room air) and to a standard level using a calibration gas mixture. Several optical sidestream infrared monitors are shown in Figure 16.10.

Mainstream. A mainstream infrared CO_2 analyzer is shown in Figure 16.3. Infrared light is directed through the sample chamber, which is formed by the airway adaptor. The adaptor has sapphire windows that seal the sample chamber and define the optical depth of the gas in the adapter. After passing through the sample chamber, the light goes through three ports in a rotating wheel, which contains (*i*) a sealed cell with a known high CO_2 concentration, (*ii*) a chamber vented to the sensor's internal atmosphere, and (*iii*) a sealed cell containing only nitrogen. The radiation then passes through a filter that screens the light to the correct wavelength to isolate CO_2 information from interfering gases and onto a photodetector. The signal is amplified and sent to the display module.

Calibration of this device is performed using two sealed cells in a molded plastic unit that attaches to the control unit. It is shaped so that the sensor can clip over either cell. The low calibration cell contains 100% nitrogen whereas the high cell contains a known partial pressure of carbon dioxide. The actual value is printed on the unit and must be programmed into the control unit. Correction factors for nitrous oxide and/or oxygen must be made manually (see Fig. 16.5).

Photoacoustic (8,109,110)

Photoacoustic spectroscopy (PAS) is a method of measuring partial pressures of gases based on the fact that absorption of IR light by molecules causes them to expand and thereby increases the pressure of the gas. If the light is delivered in pulses, the pressure increase will be intermittent. If the frequency of pulsation is in the audible range, the changes in pressure will create a sound wave that can be detected by a microphone. The amplitude of the signal caused by the pressure fluctuation is directly proportional to the partial pressure of gas present.

A photoacoustic gas analyzer is shown in Figure 16.18. Broad-band infrared radiation

is used to produce the increase in pressure, but to differentiate between the signals for each measured gas, it is necessary to divide the emitted beam into three different sections. For this, a chopper disk with three concentric bands of holes is employed. This causes the emitted radiation to be modulated at three different frequencies. The divided light beam then passes through three different optical filters, which form one wall of the measurement chamber. Each of these filters allows only infrared radiation of a specific wavelength to pass through so that the wavelengths of the emitted light are matched to the infrared absorption spectra of the gases to be measured. The filters on the measuring cell are positioned to match the pulses of radiation emerging from the chopper wheel. The frequency at which the light is turned on and off is selected to get the maximum acoustic response.

The PAS system has better long-term stability than traditional IR instruments because it measures IR absorption directly rather than indirectly (109). Accuracy is similar to that of the mass spectrometer (111).

Anesthetic agent identification is not possible with PAS. However, because photoacoustic monitors use a different wavelength for measuring these agents from optical infrared monitors, the errors in the readings when an incorrect agent is selected are less (104,109,112).

Advantages of IR Analysis

Multigas Capability

IR analyzers are capable of measuring carbon dioxide, nitrous oxide, and all of the commonly used potent volatile agents.

Volatile Agent Detection

Although the first IR analyzers were unable to identify anesthetic agents and mixtures of agents, some new models provide agent detection and can detect and quantify mixtures.

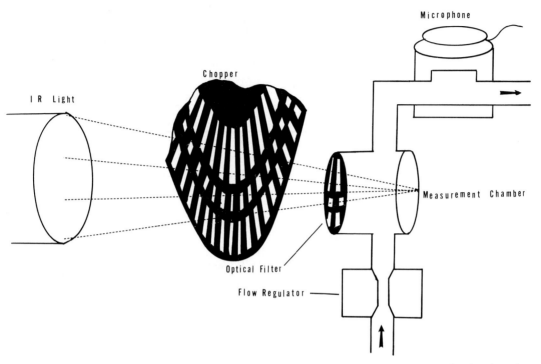

Figure 16.18. Photoacoustic infrared analyzer. The gas sample is drawn into the measurement chamber through a flow regulator. This makes the sample flow rate independent of changes in the patient's airway pressure. Light from an infrared source is aimed toward a window in the measurement chamber. Before the light enters the chamber, it passes through a spinning chopper wheel that causes it to pulsate. To differentiate between the three signals caused by carbon dioxide, nitrous oxide, and anesthetic agents, the chopper has three concentric bands of holes. This causes the light to pulsate at three different frequencies. Each light beam then passes through an optical filter that only allows light of a specific wavelength to pass through. Thus the frequencies and wavelengths of the incident light are matched to the IR absorption spectra of the three gases to be measured. In the measurement chamber, each beam excites one of the gases, causing it to expand and contract at a frequency equal to the pulsation frequency of the appropriate infrared beam. The periodic expansion and contraction of the gas sample produces a fluctuation of audible frequency that can be detected by a microphone.

No Need to Scavenge Gases

After measurement, the gases can be returned to the breathing system if desired or vented to the scavenging system.

Portability

The units are small, compact, and lightweight.

Quick Response Time

The response time for the infrared monitors is fast enough to measure both inspired and exhaled concentrations. Response times for anesthetic agents and nitrous oxide are longer than for CO_2 (89).

Short Warmup Time

The warmup time is short. The instruments do not need to be kept in a standby mode.

Convenience

Although early units required a complicated calibration with test gases with each use, this is no longer necessary. Periodic calibration with a standardized gas mixture is sufficient.

No Artifact with Aerosols

Aerosol propellants do not affect infrared spectrometers (84). However, infrared analyzers that use absorption bands in the far infrared range to identify volatile anesthetic agents might respond to some aerosol propellants (84). Fruit-flavored extract does not affect the accuracy of the photoacoustic infrared analyzer (113).

Disadvantages

Oxygen and Nitrogen Not Measured

Unlike mass spectrometry and Raman spectroscopy, oxygen does not respond to infrared technology. Monitors that also offer oxygen analysis along with infrared analysis must use a different technology for measurement of oxygen.

Interference among Gases

Oxygen is not absorbed by infrared light but causes broadening of the CO_2 absorption spectra, which results in lowered CO_2 readings (2,89). In a typical infrared carbon dioxide analyzer, 95% oxygen causes a 0.5% decline in the measured CO_2 (114). Some units have a user-actuated electronic offset for oxygen (115).

There is some overlap of the carbon dioxide and nitrous oxide infrared absorption peaks so that nitrous oxide can cause falsely high carbon dioxide readings, with an increase of 0.1% to 1.4 torr per 10% nitrous oxide (2). Most infrared analyzers that measure both CO_2 and nitrous oxide automatically correct for nitrous oxide's effect on the CO_2 reading. Some analyzers require the user to indicate when nitrous oxide is present (see Fig. 16.5).

Inaccuracy with Alcohols and Acetone

Ethanol, methanol, isopropanol, or acetone vapor in the sampled gases can cause spurious high readings when volatile agents, especially halothane, are being measured (91,112,113,116–121). Alcohol in a xylo-caine spray may cause abnormal readings (122). The magnitude of the interference varies with the monitor. Newer analyzers may be unaffected (106,110). Nafion tubing allows some alcohol to escape and modify the interference (121).

Interference from Water Vapor (123)

Water vapor absorbs infrared light at many wavelengths and will cause increased CO_2 and volatile agent readings (89). Monitors use nafion tubing, water traps, filters, and/or hydrophobic membranes to minimize this.

PARAMAGNETIC OXYGEN ANALYSIS (110,124,125)

When introduced into a nonhomogeneous magnetic field, some substances locate themselves in the strongest portion of the field. These substances are termed paramagnetic. Of the gases of interest in anesthesia, only oxygen is paramagnetic.

When a gas containing oxygen is passed through a switched magnetic field, the gas will expand and contract, causing a pressure wave proportional to the partial pressure of oxygen present. To obtain a high degree of accuracy it is necessary to compare the pressure in the gas sample to a reference signal obtained using air.

A paramagnetic oxygen analyzer is shown in Figure 16.19. Reference (air) and sample gases are pumped through the analyzer. The two gas paths are joined by a differential pressure or flow sensor. The magnet is switched on and off rapidly. If the streams of sample and reference gas have different oxygen partial pressures, the magnet will cause their pressures to differ. This difference is detected by the pressure transducer and converted into an electrical signal that is displayed as oxygen partial pressure (or converted to volumes percent). The short rise time of this technique allows measurement of inspired and end-tidal oxygen levels at high respiratory rates.

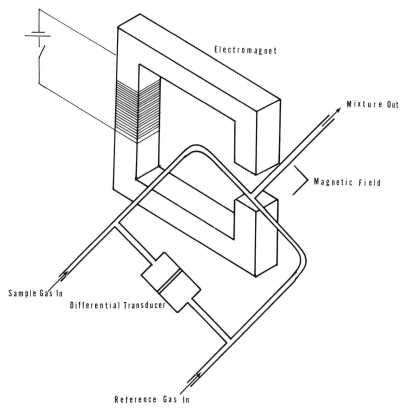

Figure 16.19. Paramagnetic oxygen analyzer. A reference gas of known or no oxygen content and the gas whose oxygen level is to be measured are pumped through the analyzer and converge into a tube at the outlet. The two gas paths are joined at their midpoints by a differential pressure or flow sensor. The magnet is switched on and off at a rapid rate. Because the reference and sample gases have different oxygen levels, the pressures in the paths will differ. The pressure difference is detected by the sensor.

Some monitors combined PAS infrared analysis of CO_2, anesthetic agents, and nitrous oxide with paramagnetic oxygen analysis. Switching the magnet on and off at a certain frequency generates a pressure wave that can be detected in the acoustic spectrum. The frequency at which the magnetic field oscillates is different from the pulsation frequencies used for PAS, so the oxygen signal can be detected using the same microphone as is used for the other gases and vapors.

One problem with these instruments is that if the gas from the analyzer is returned to the breathing system, the room air that is used as a reference gas will dilute the other gases and cause an increase in nitrogen (114).

ELECTROCHEMICAL ANALYSIS

An electrochemical oxygen analyzer consists of a sensor, which is exposed to the gas to be sampled, and the analyzer box, which contains the electric circuitry, display, and alarms (Fig. 16.20).

The sensor contains two electrodes, a cathode and an anode, surrounded by electrolyte gel. An electrode is a material on which a chemical reaction can occur (yielding a voltage) or can be made to occur (by imposing a voltage). The electrolyte is held in

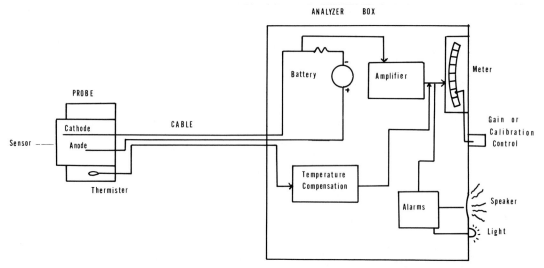

Figure 16.20. Electrochemical oxygen analyzer. The sensor is connected by a cable to the analyzer box, which contains the meter, alarms, and controls. A thermistor compensates for changes in oxygen diffusion caused by temperature. An amplifier is present in the polarographic analyzer. Those monitors with manual calibration require adjustment of a gain control until the correct reading is obtained for a standard oxygen concentration. Those with automatic calibration simply require a button to be pressed in the presence of a gas of standard concentration (usually air). This puts the monitor into calibration mode, and it returns to normal readings automatically when calibration is complete.

place by a membrane that is nonpermeable to ions, proteins, or other such materials, yet permeable to gases such as oxygen. The membrane prevents evaporation of the electrolyte. It should not be touched because dirt and grease reduce its usable area.

Oxygen diffuses through the membrane and electrolyte to the cathode, where it is reduced, causing a current to flow between the electrodes. The rate at which oxygen enters the cell and generates current is proportional to the partial pressure of oxygen in the gas outside the membrane. For convenience, however, the display scale is usually marked in percent oxygen. A gain control allows the analyzer to be calibrated with gas containing a known partial pressure of oxygen.

These analyzers respond slowly to changes in oxygen pressure, so that they cannot be used to measure end-tidal concentrations.

There are two basic types of sensors: galvanic cell and polarographic electrode. The polarographic analyzer has a faster response time than the galvanic (126–128). This is probably not clinically significant but does facilitate calibration.

Technology

Galvanic Cell

A galvanic cell (fuel cell, microfuel cell) sensor is shown in Figure 16.21. It consists of a lead anode and a gold cathode surrounded by a potassium hydroxide electrolyte (129,130). The cathode acts as the sensing electrode and is not consumed. The hydroxyl ions formed there react with the lead anode, forming lead oxide. The lead anode is gradually consumed (worn out).

Cathode: $O_2 + 2H_2O + 4e^- \rightarrow 4OH^-$

Anode: $4OH^- + 2Pb \rightarrow 2PbO$
$$+ 2H_2O + 4e^-$$

Because the current is strong enough to operate the meter, a separate power source is not required to operate the analyzer. A power source (either battery or wall current) is required for alarms.

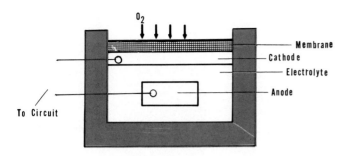

Figure 16.21. Galvanic cell sensor. The membrane is permeable to gases but not to liquids. At the cathode, oxygen molecules are reduced to hydroxide ions. At the anode, hydroxide ions give up electrons. An electron flow between the anode and cathode is generated, which is directly proportional to the partial pressure of oxygen in the sample gas. Redrawn from a drawing furnished by Biomarine Industries, Inc.

The sensor comes packaged in a sealed container from which oxygen has been removed and its limited life begins when the package is opened (129,131). Its useful life is cited in percent hours, which is the product of hours of exposure and oxygen percentage. If it is left in areas of high oxygen concentration, the life expectancy will be decreased. Sensor life can be prolonged by leaving it exposed to air when not in use. Galvanic sensors require no membrane or electrolyte replacement. The entire sensor must be replaced when it becomes exhausted.

Polarographic Electrode

A polarographic (Clark electrode) sensor is shown in Figure 16.22. It consists of a silver anode, a platinum or gold cathode, KCl electrolyte, and a gas-permeable membrane (129,131–133). There is a power source (battery or AC line) for inducing a potential between the anode and the cathode.

Oxygen molecules diffuse through the membrane and the electrolyte. When a polarizing voltage is applied to the cathode, electrons combine with the oxygen molecules and reduce them to hydroxide ions:

Cathode: $O_2 + 2H_2O + 4e^- \rightarrow 4OH^-$

Anode: $4Ag + 4Cl^- \rightarrow 4AgCl + 4e^-$

A current that is proportional to the partial pressure of oxygen in the sample flows between the anode and cathode.

Polarographic sensors may be either preassembled, disposable cartridges or units that can be disassembled and reused by

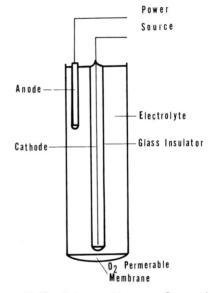

Figure 16.22. Polarographic sensor. Oxygen diffuses through the membrane and electrolyte to the cathode. When a polarizing voltage is applied to the cathode, the oxygen molecules are reduced to hydroxide ions. The current flow between cathode and anode will be proportional to the partial pressure of oxygen. Redrawn from Bageant RA. Oxygen analyzers. Respir Care 1976; 21:415.

changing the membrane and/or electrolyte (126). The sensor remains unconsumed when not turned on, so the analyzer should be kept on standby when not in use.

Use

Calibration

The calibration procedure should be performed daily before use and at least every 8

Figure 16.23. The electrochemical oxygen analyzer is calibrated by exposing the sensor to room air.

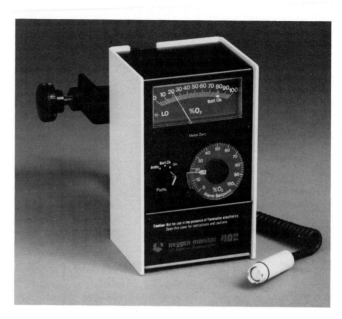

hr after that. Some instruments remind the user when calibration is due and will not give a reading unless calibration is performed. The calibration can be checked quickly by exposing the sensor to room air and verifying that it indicates approximately 21% oxygen (Fig. 16.23). Because the calibration procedure will vary with each analyzer, the manufacturer's instructions should be consulted.

Checking the Alarms

In some polarographic oxygen analyzers, there are three batteries: two for operating the sensor and one for the alarms (134). Checking the battery-test function may not check the battery for the alarms.

The sensor should be put in room air and the low oxygen alarm set above 21%. The visual signal should flash and the audible alarm sound. If the unit has a high oxygen alarm, the setting for that should be moved below 21%. The visual and audible signals should be activated. If the lamp(s) fails to light or the audible alarm is weak, the batteries should be replaced and the alarms rechecked. If this fails to remedy the situation, the unit should

be returned to the manufacturer for servicing or replacement.

Placement in the Breathing System

Sites for placement in breathing systems are discussed in Chapters 6 and 7. The service life of the sensors of some galvanic cell analyzers is reduced by exposure to carbon dioxide, so locating the sensor on the inspiratory side of the system may be preferable.

The junction between the cable and the sensor should not be under strain. The sensor should be upright or tilted slightly to prevent moisture from accumulating on the membrane.

Setting Alarms Limits

Alarms should be set at levels sufficient to sustain a reasonable margin of safety appropriate for the specific clinical situation, without creating false signals or inappropriate distraction.

The low oxygen level alarm should be set a little below the minimum and the high oxygen level alarm a little above the maximum acceptable concentrations. There should be places on the anesthesia record for recording the alarm limits and the oxygen percentages.

Advantages

Ease of Use

Modern oxygen analyzers are dependable, accurate, and user friendly. The warmup time is short.

Cost

These instruments cost far less than other means of oxygen analysis. Compared with the cost of a catastrophic event associated with administration of a hypoxic mixture, the cost of an oxygen analyzer is insignificant.

Automatic Enabling

Oxygen analyzers that are a component part of the anesthesia machine are automatically activated when the machine is turned on. Thus the possibility of the user forgetting to turn it on is eliminated.

Disadvantages

Maintenance

While maintenance on the newer models has been simplified, some instruments need frequent membrane and electrolyte changes.

Calibration

These instruments need to be calibrated before use each day and at least every 8 hr.

User Enabling

Instruments that are not an integral part of anesthesia machines need to be turned on by the user.

Difficulty Using Outside the Breathing System

With spontaneously breathing patients who are not connected to a breathing system and who are receiving oxygen via mask or nasal cannulae, it is difficult to monitor the inspired oxygen concentration using these instruments.

Inaccuracy

A study of oxygen analyzers in a simulated clinical environment found that electrochemical analyzers had a high percentage of errors, most commonly caused by humidity (135).

Slow Response Time

These analyzers cannot be used to measure end-tidal oxygen.

PIEZOELECTRIC ANALYSIS (136,137)

Technology

The levels of potent anesthetic agents can be measured using piezoelectric analysis. The analyzer uses vibrating crystals that are coated with a layer of lipid (Fig. 16.24). When exposed to a volatile anesthetic agent, the vapor is adsorbed into the lipid. The resulting change in the mass of the lipid alters the vibration frequency of the crystal. By use of an electronic system consisting of two oscillating circuits, one of which has an uncoated (reference) crystal and the other a coated (detector) crystal, an electric signal is generated, which is proportional to the vapor level.

The first device using this technology was a mainstream device, which had many problems associated with its use. Newer models are sampling devices (Fig. 16.25) and have a superior performance compared with the earlier model (137).

Advantages

Accuracy

Investigations show an accuracy of better than 0.1% (136–138). Water vapor and nitrous oxide affect the reading, but the worst case interference is less than 0.1%.

The analyzer does not give artifactual re-

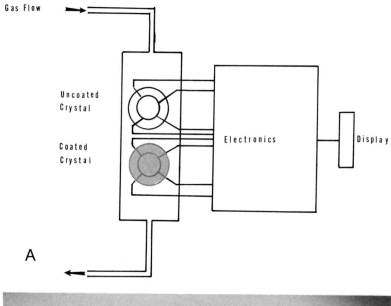

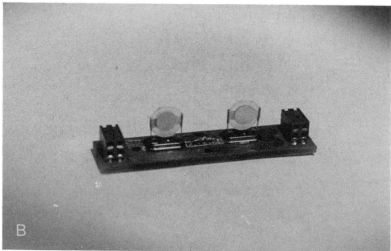

Figure 16.24. **A,** Piezoelectric analyzer. One vibrating crystal is coated with lipid, and the other is uncoated. By comparing the vibration frequencies of the crystals, the level of anesthetic agent in the gas being analyzed can be measured. **B,** Piezoelectric crystals. Courtesy of Biochemical International, Inc.

sults in the presence of aerosol propellants used to administer bronchodilators (84). Although alcohol adheres to the surface of a coated crystal it has a minimal effect on readings (116).

Fast Response Time

Newer models can measure inspired and expired levels of halogenated agents.

No Need for Scavenging

Because the agents are not altered, the gas removed can be returned to the breathing system.

Short Warmup Time

The warmup period is shorter than with an infrared analyzer or mass spectrometer (136).

Compactness

These units are small.

Disadvantages

Only One Gas Measured

This analyzer cannot measure oxygen, carbon dioxide, nitrogen, or nitrous oxide.

No Agent Discrimination

This device cannot discriminate between agents. If the wrong agent is selected the reading can be in error by as much as 118% (136). With a mixture of agents, the reading will be very close to the sum of the delivered percents of the agents (139).

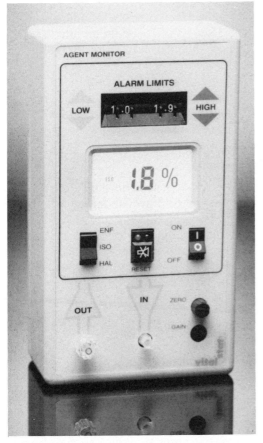

Figure 16.25. Piezoelectric anesthetic agent monitor. The agent to be measured must be selected. Courtesy of Vital Signs, Inc.

CHEMICAL CO$_2$ DETECTION (140–143)

Technology

The colorometric CO$_2$ detector contains hygroscopic filter paper impregnated with a colorless liquid base and an indicator that changes color as a function of the pH. When the detector is exposed to CO$_2$ in expired gas, hydrogen ions are formed from the hydration of CO$_2$, the detector becomes more acidic and the indicator changes color (141). During inspiration of CO$_2$-free gas, the color of the indicator returns to its resting state.

The device is shown in Figure 16.26. The filter paper is visible through a clear window. The color chart on the dome was designed to be read under fluorescent light. An auxiliary color chart included in each package should be consulted if other lighting is encountered. The inlet and outlet ports are standard 15 mm, so the device fits between the tracheal tube and the breathing system or resuscitation bag. With Mapleson systems it may be possible to place the detector elsewhere in the breathing system (144).

The filter paper is normally colored purple in room air. At CO$_2$ concentrations between 0.5% and 2% the color changes to tan and at concentrations over 2%, yellow. The mean minimum concentration of carbon dioxide needed to produce a color change is 0.54% with a range from 0.25% to 0.60% (143). This is important because of the minimum amount of circulation and hence carbon dioxide present during resuscitation.

Use

The device should be left in its gas-impermeable foil package until ready for use. The indicator will permanently change colors if exposed for a prolonged period to low concentrations of CO$_2$ or other acids in the air. The filter paper should be purple before the device is used.

The device is designed to differentiate placement of a tracheal tube in the esophagus from placement in the tracheobronchial tree when a capnometer is unavailable. It may

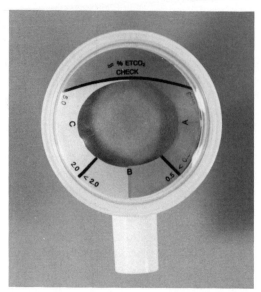

Figure 16.26. Colorometric CO_2 detector. A color code is printed around the outside of the dome to provide a reference. The detector quantifies the level of carbon dioxide measured into three concentrations: less than 0.5%, 0.5% to 2%, and greater than 2%.

have a major application in intubation at remote locations and during transfer of intubated patients where space is limited, as in an ambulance or helicopter.

The manufacturer recommends a minimum of six breaths be given before a determination is made to avoid errors caused by CO_2 forced into the stomach during mask ventilation or caused by prophylactic antacids or cola in the stomach. Usually, the color change is seen long before this.

Reducing the relative humidity of exhaled gases by insertion of a heat and moisture exchanger (HME) to trap moisture before it reaches the device markedly prolongs the operational life of this device (145). Use with a active humidifier will shorten its useful life (146).

Although the speed of the color change diminishes over time, the device should continue for up to 2 hr to change back to purple within seconds if the device is dislodged or emptied of CO_2 (147).

Advantages

1. The device is easy to use and can be left attached for an extended period of time, making it possible to detect late tube dislodgement.
2. Its performance is not affected by nitrous oxide or anesthetic vapors (148).
3. Its small size allows it to be used in locations where access to a carbon dioxide monitor is not possible.
4. The device is portable and requires no power source.
5. Compared with other methods of CO_2 analysis the cost is low.
6. Studies show the device to be very accurate in diagnosing esophageal intubation, even in small children (140–142,144,148,149–153).
7. The device also serves to indicate the effectiveness of resuscitation after the tracheal tube has been correctly positioned (154,155).
8. It offers minimal resistance to flow.
9. The device is always ready for use, does not require sterilization, and limits the risk of transmission of infection.

Disadvantages

1. It may take several breaths before conclusions can be drawn about the location of the tracheal tube. If the tube is in the esophagus, dilation of the stomach with these breaths may increase the risk of aspiration.
2. The 38-ml dead space precludes using this device in spontaneously breathing children.
3. False-negative results may occur. It may not be effective with very low tidal volumes and low end-tidal carbon dioxide concentrations (156,157). However, studies indicate the device should produce a detectable color change in most patients during CPR (143). During CPR, a positive test correctly indicates that the tracheal tube is in the airway, but a negative

result (suggesting esophageal placement) requires an alternate method of confirming tracheal tube position (150). Failure to inflate the tracheal tube cuff may cause equivocal color change (141).

4. Contamination of this device with drugs instilled in the trachea or gastric contents can irreversibly damage it (147,158,159).
5. False-positives can occur if there is CO_2 in the stomach (from ingestion of carbonated beverages, administration of antacids, or mask ventilation). The display may initially turn color, and only slowly revert to its original color (160,161).
6. Difficulty in distinguishing color changes has been reported (161).

Gases

OXYGEN

The need for continuous in-line oxygen monitoring, pointed out many years ago (162), is now routine practice. Problems with oxygenation have accounted for a great number of the serious complications attributable to general anesthesia.

The standards for basic intraoperative monitoring during administration of general anesthesia approved by the American Society of Anesthesiologists include measurement of the level of oxygen in the breathing system. The 1988 anesthesia machine standard requires that the anesthesia machine be equipped with an oxygen analyzer that annunciates high-priority alarm signals when the measured oxygen level is below the user-preset alarm threshold (163).

Standard Requirements

An international standard on oxygen analyzers was published in 1988 (164). A U.S. standard, which slightly modifies the international standard, was published in 1992 (3). The following requirements are in the U.S. standard. Most of the same information is also in the international standard.

1. Oxygen readings shall be within $\pm 3\%$ of the actual oxygen level over a temperature range of 15° to 40°C. This accuracy shall be maintained for at least 8 hr of continuous use. Analyzers must meet the requirement for accuracy following exposure to cyclic positive pressure of 100 cm H_2O and negative pressure of 15 cm H_2O in the breathing system at a rate of 10 cycles/min for 10 min.

2. Humidity up to 100%, concentrations of nitrous oxide up to 80%, carbon dioxide up to 5%, halothane up to 4%, enflurane up to 5%, and isoflurane up to 5% shall not cause the readings to vary from actual level by more than 5%.

3. The instructions for use with each analyzer shall include the stability of measurement accuracy, the response time, the temperature range, the gas diversion rate for sampling-type analyzers, the time from switching on to obtaining specified operating performance, effects of interfering gases or vapors, cycling pressure and barometric pressure, and the expected useful life of the sensors if they are intended to be replaced during the useful lifetime of the analyzer.

4. High-priority signals provided with an oxygen analyzer shall be both visual and auditory. Medium-priority signals shall be visual.

5. If a low alarm limit is provided, it shall not be adjustable or preset below 15%. There must be a visual indication to the user when a low alarm limit is adjusted to below 21%. If a manual control is provided to override the low-oxygen-level alarm, it shall only override the auditory signal and shall automatically cancel after not more than 120 sec following its most recent activation.

Technology

Oxygen levels may be measured using mass spectrometry, Raman scattering, electrochemical analysis, or paramagnetic analysis. Electrochemical analysis can measure mean concentrations in the inspiratory or expiratory pathways. The other three methods have sufficiently rapid response times that both inspired and end-tidal levels can be measured. Electrochemical and paramagnetic analysis measure only oxygen whereas Raman spectroscopy and mass spectrometry measure several other gases.

Cost is a factor in deciding which technology to purchase. The electrochemical analyzer is relatively inexpensive compared with other technologies. Maintenance of a mass spectrometer or Raman analyzer is more involved than that for an electrochemical analyzer.

Space requirements vary among the different technologies. An electrochemical or paramagnetic analyzer takes up very little space. The display unit for a shared mass spectrometer takes up more space. A dedicated mass spectrometer or Raman spectrometer requires more space.

The location where the oxygen analyzer is to be used is important. If anesthesia must be administered in remote locations such as obstetrics or radiology, a shared mass spectrometer system is not useful. An oxygen analyzer, dedicated mass spectrometer, or a Raman analyzer will be needed.

A disadvantage of a shared mass spectrometer system is the time interval between samples, which reduces its effectiveness in early detection of critical events. This is not a problem with the other technologies. In some cases with nonintubated, spontaneously breathing patients it may be desirable to measure the inspired oxygen. This is possible with a diverting device such as the mass spectrometer, Raman spectrometer, or paramagnetic analyzer but not with an electrochemical monitor.

A good case could be made for using more than one device to monitor oxygen, especially if a shared system mass spectrometer is in use. With a shared mass spectrometer, several minutes could elapse before a low oxygen concentration was detected, so an electrochemical analyzer should be used to cover the time between readings. Use of an electro-chemical analyzer as a backup in case of failure of other gas concentration monitors is a good idea.

If use of helium is contemplated, an electrochemical analyzer should be used to supplement the mass spectrometer, which may display erroneously high oxygen readings (73).

Applications of Oxygen Analysis

Detection of Hypoxic or Hyperoxic Mixtures

The importance of a sufficient level of oxygen is obvious. The first line of defense against hypoxemia is avoidance of inhalation of a hypoxic gas mixture. Reported causes of hypoxic mixtures are many and varied, but if oxygen analysis is used, the problem can be detected in time to avert a catastrophe. Low inspiratory and end-tidal oxygen levels provide an earlier warning of inadequate oxygen than pulse oximetry (94).

Use of oxygen analysis will result in safe use of low flow techniques, so that it can pay for itself. Oxygen analysis can also help to prevent problems resulting from hyperoxygenation such as awareness, damage to the lungs and eyes, and airway fires with laser use.

Detection of Disconnections and Leaks

An oxygen monitor can often detect disconnections in the breathing system (94,165–168). However, it cannot be depended on for this purpose (169–171). Whether or not the oxygen level falls at the point being monitored depends on several factors, including the type of breathing system in use, the position of the sensor in the system, the site of disconnection, whether the patient is breathing spontaneously or ventilation is being controlled and the type of ventilator in use (169).

With a sidestream analyzer a decrease in inspired and expired oxygen may result from a leak in the sampling system (172). Disconnection of the tubing to an oxygen mask may be detected using a diverting oxygen analyzer (50).

Other

Knowledge of expired oxygen concentration allows estimates of the patient's metabolic rate, oxygen consumption, and cardiac output and can aid in the diagnosis of malignant hyperthermia. An increased difference between inspiratory and end-tidal oxygen is a sensitive indication of hypoventilation (94,173). The concentration of nitrous oxide can be estimated from the concentration of oxygen.

CARBON DIOXIDE ANALYSIS

The ASA standards for basic intraoperative monitoring includes end-tidal carbon dioxide monitoring for verification of tracheal intubation as of January 1, 1991 (174). A court case has held that a reasonably prudent hospital would supply a carbon dioxide monitor to a patient undergoing general anesthesia (175).

Carbon dioxide analysis provides a means for assessing ventilation and can detect many equipment- and patient-related problems that other monitors may either fail to detect or detect so slowly that patient safety may be compromised (176). A closed claims analysis found the capnography plus pulse oximetry was potentially preventative in 93% of the preventable anesthetic mishaps (177). In one study, 10% of intraoperative problems were initially diagnosed by continuous carbon dioxide monitoring (178).

The respiratory cycle (i.e., inspiration versus expiration) is defined in terms of carbon dioxide measurement so determination of end-tidal values for other gases depends on measurement of CO_2.

Capnometry is the measurement and numerical display of CO_2 level during the respiratory cycle. A capnometer is the device that performs the measurement and displays the readings. Capnography is a graphic rec-

ord with display on a screen or paper of carbon dioxide concentration. A capnograph is the machine that generates the waveform, and the capnogram is the actual waveform.

The Capnometer

Standards Requirements

A U.S. standard on capnometers was published in 1992 (4). It contains the following specifications.

1. The carbon dioxide reading shall be within $\pm 12\%$ of the actual value or ± 4 mm Hg (0.53 kPa), whichever is greater, over the full range of the capnometer.

2. The manufacturer shall provide information on the carbon dioxide measurement range, accuracy of measurements, the stability of measurement accuracy, the rise time and the flow required to meet the disclosed rise time, the carbon dioxide level alarm range and its accuracy, the operating and nonoperating (storage) temperature ranges, and time from switching on to obtaining the specified operating performance.

3. The manufacturer must disclose any adverse interference caused by specified concentrations of oxygen, nitrous oxide, halothane, enflurane, isoflurane, ethanol, acetone, and chlorodifluromethane.

4. Alarms

a. The capnometer shall have a high carbon dioxide reading alarm for both inspired and exhaled carbon dioxide.

b. It should have a low carbon dioxide reading alarm for exhaled carbon dioxide.

c. Alarm set points for both high and (if provided) low carbon dioxide reading alarms shall be operator adjustable.

d. All alarms must be provided with a default setting.

e. When the capnometer is switched on, the high carbon dioxide reading alarm shall be medium priority.

f. If a low carbon dioxide reading alarm is provided it shall be medium priority.

g. If the capnometer has an automatic

change in alarm priority setting, it shall change only to a higher alarm priority and only after activation of the alarm.

h. If the capnometer has an operator-adjustable high carbon dioxide reading alarm priority control, it shall allow the operator to change the alarm priority between medium and high priority only after the capnometer is switched on.

i. The audible components of the alarms should be designed to allow silencing until the capnometer is placed in use (that is, connected to the patient) to reduce nuisance alarms.

j. Temporary silencing of audible alarms, if provided, shall not exceed 2 min. Permanent silencing of audible alarms is allowed. Visual signal(s) shall continue until the alarming condition no longer exists. The audible signal shall reset automatically when the condition causing the alarm is no longer present.

Technology

Methods to measure CO_2 levels include mass spectrometry, Raman scattering gas analysis, infrared analysis, and chemical colorometric analysis. Infrared CO_2 analyzers may be diverting or nondiverting.

A wide variety of display formats are available on CO_2 monitors. These include a meter with a needle, bar graph, strip chart recorder, oscilloscope, and liquid crystal display. The CO_2 level may be reported as either partial pressure or a percentage. The CO_2 level may be displayed continuously or as peak (normally end-tidal) value. The minimum inspired level may also be shown. Many capnometers have more than one speed. Slower speeds are used for trending and faster ones for waveform observation. Most have optional recorders. Other parameters such as respiratory rate and I:E ratio may be displayed.

Many capnometers are part of multipurpose monitors and include parameters such as blood pressure, pulse oximetry, and analysis of other gases. The CO_2 waveform may be one of several waveforms on a video display.

To check the function and calibration of a capnometer, the user may exhale into the device. A normal-appearing waveform and a normal end-tidal CO_2 reading indicate that the device is functioning correctly (90). Likewise, exhaling into the chemical colorometric device should produce a prompt color change.

Water Vapor Considerations (123)

Water vapor dilutes the CO_2 in a gas sample. Because new sampling catheter materials are permeable to water, gas entering the capnometer sample cell will have the water vapor concentration of room air, even though the gas being measured may have a water vapor pressure of up to 47 mm Hg.

If the capnometer does not make an internal correction, it will calculate the partial pressure using the following formula:

$$P_{CO_2} = F_{CO_2} \times Pb$$

where Pb is atmospheric pressure. With 5% CO_2 and an atmospheric pressure of 760

$$P_{CO_2} = 0.05 \times 760$$
$$P_{CO_2} = 38 \text{ mm Hg}$$

To calculate the end-tidal CO_2 level correctly, the formula should be

$$P_{CO_2} = F_{CO_2} \times (Pb - 47)$$

Using the same figures as above,

$$P_{CO_2} = 0.05 \times (760 - 47)$$
$$P_{CO_2} = 35.65 \text{ mm Hg}$$

For mainstream analyzers, the error is far less, although a small decrease from body temperature may result in the analyzer reading slightly less.

Atmospheric Pressure Considerations (2,90,179,180)

Atmospheric pressure can influence the CO_2 reading. Some instruments incorporate a barometer to compensate for changes in atmospheric pressure. Others require the user to enter the correct atmospheric pressure manually and then compensate appropriately. Still others do not correct for atmospheric pressure.

The 1992 capnometer standard (4) states that if automatic compensation for barometric pressure is not provided, the accompanying documents of a capnometer shall contain an explanation that the readings in concentration units are correct only under the pressure at which the capnometer is calibrated.

Mass Spectrometer. A mass spectrometer measures gases in volumes percent. If the reading is converted to partial pressure, the atmospheric pressure must be known to obtain a correct reading. Furthermore, because the mass spectrometer does not measure water vapor, a correction needs to be made for this.

$$P_{CO_2} = F_{CO_2}\ 100 \times (\text{atmospheric pressure} - \text{water vapor pressure})$$

At 760 mm Hg atmospheric pressure and a F_{CO_2} of 5%

$$P_{CO_2} = 0.05 \times (760 - 47)\ \text{mm Hg}$$
$$= 36\ \text{mm Hg}$$

If atmospheric pressure is reduced to 500 mm Hg,

$$P_{CO_2} = 0.05 \times (500 - 47)\ \text{mm Hg}$$
$$= 23\ \text{mm Hg}$$

Sidestream Infrared and Raman Analyzers. The sidestream infrared and Raman analyzers measure partial pressure. Calibration is normally accomplished from a tank whose contents are known in volumes percent. If the atmospheric pressure at calibration time is known, the analyzer can compute the partial pressure of the calibration gas. Its readings will always reflect the partial pressure of the gas being measured, regardless of changes in atmospheric pressure.

When a sidestream infrared or Raman analyzer reports results in volumes percent, the atmospheric pressure at measurement time must be known to compute the value correctly.

$$F_{CO_2}$$
$$= \text{partial pressure (atmospheric pressure} - \text{water vapor pressure}) \times 100$$

At 760 mm Hg atmospheric pressure and a CO_2 level of 38 mm Hg,

$$F_{CO_2} = 38\ (760 - 47) \times 100 = 5\%$$

If the atmospheric pressure is reduced to 500 mm Hg,

$$F_{CO_2} = 38\ (500 - 47) \times 100 = 8\%$$

So if the correction for atmospheric pressure is not made, the capnometer will show erroneously low concentrations at increased altitude (180).

Mainstream Infrared Analyzers. Mainstream infrared instruments are calibrated from sealed gas cells whose partial pressure are known. These instruments will always report measurements in units of partial pressure correctly (2). If this analyzer reports results in volumes percent, the atmospheric pressure at measurement time must be known. Corrections are similar to those for mainstream infrared and Raman analyzers.

Clinical Significance of Capnometry

Carbon dioxide is formed in the body cells as a product of metabolism, transported by the blood, and excreted by the lungs. If the patient is connected to a breathing system, it has to travel through this system before it is eliminated. Therefore, changes in exhaled carbon dioxide may reflect changes in metabolism, circulation, respiration, the airway, or breathing system function. Tables 16.1 to 16.4 list some causes of changes in exhaled carbon dioxide.

Metabolism

Every cell in the body produces carbon dioxide. Monitoring CO_2 elimination gives a measure of metabolic rate. Table 16.1 lists

Table 16.1.   Capnography and Capnometry with Altered Carbon Dioxide Production[a]

	Waveform on Capnograph	End-Tidal CO_2	Inspiratory CO_2	End-Tidal to Arterial Gradient
Absorption of carbon dioxide from peritoneal cavity	Normal	↑	0	Normal
Injection of sodium bicarbonate	Normal	↑	0	Normal
Pain, anxiety, shivering	Normal	↑	0	Normal
Increased muscle tone (as from muscle relaxant reversal)	Normal	↑	0	Normal
Convulsions	Normal	↑	0	Normal
Hyperthermia	Normal	↑	0	Normal
Hypothermia	Normal	↓	0	Normal
Increased depth of anesthesia (in relation to surgical stimulus)	Normal	↓	0	Normal
Use of muscle relaxants	May see curare cleft	↓	0	Normal
Increased transport of carbon dioxide to the lungs (restoration of peripheral circulation after it has been impaired, e.g., after release of a tourniquet)	Normal	↑	0	Normal

[a]Normal end-tidal carbon dioxide is 38 torr (5%). Inspired carbon dioxide is normally 0. The arterial to end-tidal gradient is normally less than 5 torr.

some causes of increased or decreased carbon dioxide production. An increase in end-tidal carbon dioxide is a reliable indicator of increased metabolism only in mechanically ventilated subjects. In spontaneously breathing patients, Pet_{CO_2} may not increase as a result of hyperventilation (181).

Metabolic causes of increases in expired carbon dioxide include increased temperature (182), shivering, convulsions, excessive production of catecholamines, administration of blood or bicarbonate (183), release of an arterial clamp or tourniquet (184–187), glucose in the intravenous fluid (188), parenteral hyperalimentation (189), and carbon dioxide used to inflate the peritoneal cavity during laparoscopy (190) or a joint during arthroscopy (191).

Of great importance is early diagnosis of the syndrome of malignant hyperthermia, which is a hypermetabolic state with a massive increase in carbon dioxide production. This increase occurs early, before the rise in temperature. Early detection of this is one of the most important reasons for routinely monitoring carbon dioxide (178,192–196).

Capnometry can be used to monitor the effectiveness of treatment.

Carbon dioxide production falls with decreased temperature, increased muscle relaxation, and increased depth of anesthesia (197).

Circulation

Carbon dioxide is transported to the lungs by the circulatory system. Table 16.2 lists some of the circulatory causes of changes in exhaled carbon dioxide. A decrease in end-tidal CO_2 is seen with a decrease in cardiac output if ventilation remains constant (198–200). With a sustained reduction in cardiac output, the end-tidal CO_2 will begin to increase as CO_2 levels in the tissues and venous blood rise and CO_2 delivery to the lung moves toward baseline levels.

In addition to reduced cardiac output, reduced blood flow to the lungs can result from surgical manipulations of the heart or thoracic vessels (201,202), wedging of a pulmonary artery catheter, and pulmonary embolism (thrombus, tumor, gas, fat, marrow, or amniotic fluid) (203–207). If the embolized gas is CO_2, the end-tidal CO_2 may increase (208). Although not as sensitive as the Doppler for detecting air embolism, carbon dioxide monitoring is less subjective, is unaffected by electrosurgery apparatus, and can be used in major ENT cases for which the Doppler method is not applicable. Capnography may not be sufficiently sensitive to detect fat and marrow microemboli (209). Although an embolus will cause a drop in end-tidal CO_2 acutely, over time peripheral CO_2 retention may cause the end-tidal CO_2 to return to normal (210).

Exhaled CO_2 is a better guide to the presence of circulation than the ECG, pulse, or blood pressure (211). The effectiveness of resuscitation measures can be gauged by capnometry (154,212–219). The capnograph is not susceptible to the mechanical artifacts associated with chest compression like the ECG, and chest compressions do not have to be interrupted to assess circulation (9). However, if high-dose epinephrine is used, end-tidal carbon dioxide is not a good indicator of resuscitation measures (220). End-tidal carbon dioxide levels may be of use in predicting the outcome of resuscitation (152,213,217–219,221–225).

Respiration

When carbon dioxide reaches the lung it is removed from the body by ventilation of the alveoli. Carbon dioxide monitoring allows continuous, noninvasive assessment of carbon dioxide elimination and also gives information about the rate, frequency, and depth of respiration. For patients breathing spontaneously, exhaled carbon dioxide levels can help to provide an estimate of the depth of anesthesia.

Measurement of end-tidal carbon dioxide allows control of ventilation with fewer blood gas determinations. End-tidal analysis has the advantages of being noninvasive and available on a breath-by-breath basis. Hyperventilation induced by drawing arterial blood samples that results in erroneously low arterial carbon dioxide levels is not a problem with end-tidal analysis.

Table 16.3 lists some respiratory causes of increased and decreased end-tidal carbon dioxide. A capnometer with appropriate alarms can warn of esophageal intubation, a disconnection, apnea, extubation, complete obstruction of a tracheal tube, ventilator malfunction, or complete obstruction of the sampling catheter, all of which will result in no carbon dioxide being detected. A change in compliance, partial obstruction of a tracheal tube, upper airway obstruction, poor mask fit, a leaking tracheal tube cuff, or partial disconnection will result in a drop to a low but nonzero value. Problems such as esophageal intubation and apnea are identified much more quickly by capnometry than by pulse oximetry (226).

A dependable means to determine when a tracheal tube has been positioned in the airway is obviously of great value. In one study of misadventures in anesthesia, placement of the tracheal tube in the esophagus was the leading cause of death or cerebral damage

Table 16.2. Capnographic and Capnometric Alterations as a Result of Circulatory Changes

	Waveform on Capnograph	End-Tidal CO_2	Inspiratory CO_2	End-Tidal to Arterial Gradient
Decreased transport of carbon dioxide to the lungs (impaired peripheral circulation)	Normal	↓	0	Normal
Decreased transport of carbon dioxide through the lungs (pulmonary embolus, either air or thrombus; surgical manipulations)	Normal	↓	0	Elevated
Right to left shunt	Normal	↑	0	Elevated
Increased patient dead space	Normal	↓	0	Elevated

Table 16.3.   Capnometry and Capnography with Respiratory Problems

	Waveform on Capnograph	End-Tidal CO_2	Inspiratory CO_2	End-Tidal to Alveolar Gradient
Disconnection	Absent	0		
Apneic patient, stopped ventilator	Absent	0		
Hyperventilation	Normal	↓	0	Normal
Hypoventilation, mild to moderate	Normal	↑	0	Normal
Upper airway obstruction	Abnormal	↑	0	Elevated
Rebreathing, e.g., (under drapes)	Baseline elevated	↑	↑	Normal
Esophageal intubation	Absent		0	

(227). An extensive discussion of ways to detect inadvertent esophageal placement is found in Chapter 15. CO_2 monitoring is usually considered the best method to verify tracheal tube placement (226,228,229). It can also detect placement of a tube in a false passage (230).

Carbon dioxide detection of tracheal tube placement in the esophagus has some drawbacks and limitations. Bronchospasm, equipment malfunction, or application of PEEP to a loosely fitted uncuffed tracheal tube can result in failure to detect expired CO_2 (231,232). The analyzer may be in a calibration mode when the tube is placed or a shared mass spectrometer system may be sampling another location. During cardiopulmonary resuscitation, if no effective circulation is present, CO_2 may not be present in the lung.

If esophageal intubation has occurred, very small waveforms may be seen transiently on the capnograph caused by CO_2 that has entered the stomach during mask ventilation or by certain beverages or medications (160,161,233–235). If a tracheal tube is placed in the esophagus, this CO_2 could give the impression that the tube is correctly placed in the trachea. However, rapidly diminishing concentrations and abnormal waveforms will usually differentiate esophageal from tracheal intubation (228,233,236,237).

A CO_2 monitor can be used to monitor respiratory rate and exhaled CO_2 in unintubated patients breathing spontaneously (11,12,35,37,41–44,46–49,51,52,238). Apnea and/or airway obstruction can be detected. If ventilation of the breathing space is inadequate, rebreathing will occur and can be detected by a rising inspired carbon dioxide level (43,238). Although some studies have shown a poor correlation between the peak expired and arterial CO_2 using this method of monitoring (36,37,239–241), others have yielded good results (12,39,43,46,242,243). Peak CO_2 values correlate more closely with Pa_{CO_2} values than average end-tidal levels (244). Poor correlation is associated with partial airway obstruction and high respiratory rates (244). Results may be improved by isolating insufflated oxygen from exhaled gases, observing the waveform for normal configuration, and decreasing the oxygen flow rate (46,243,245). In mouth breathers, the cannula may be realigned over the mouth or the mouth may be closed (246).

Capnometry can be used to facilitate blind oral or nasotracheal intubation in the spontaneously breathing patient (247–250). After passage of the tube into the pharynx, observation of CO_2 waveform and/or peak CO_2 is used to guide the tube into place.

Capnometry can be useful in determining the position of a double-lumen endobronchial tube (251,252). CO_2 waveforms from either lung or both lungs can be monitored. Correct placement can be checked by analyzing the waveform from each lung and also during clamping and unclamping of each lumen.

Carbon dioxide monitoring can serve as a

warning of accidental endobronchial intubation. This may result in an acute fall or rise in end-tidal CO_2 (253–255). However, changes in oxygenation will normally be more pronounced (although occurring more slowly) than changes in capnometry.

End-tidal carbon dioxide monitoring can be used to aid in weaning patients from artificial ventilation (256).

Breathing System Function

If there is a problem with the breathing system that results in an inspired carbon dioxide greater than zero, exhaled carbon dioxide will rise. Examples of such problems are listed in Table 16.4 and include a leak (257), faulty or exhausted absorbent, channeling or a bypassed absorber, increased dead space, inadequate fresh gas flow to a Mapleson system, a defect in the inner tube of a Bain system (258), accidental administration of CO_2, and a defective nonrebreathing valve (259–264). With an expiratory valve leak, the inspired CO_2 level is inversely related to inspiratory flow, because as inspiratory flow increases, a smaller portion of each breath passes through the incompetent expiratory valve (259,265,266).

Carbon dioxide monitoring is useful for detecting disconnections and/or extubation (178,267). Continuous monitoring of airway CO_2 will detect a disconnection as rapidly as the time delay setting of the apnea alarm allows, unless the patient begins to breathe spontaneously. However, if a Mapleson D system is being used with a ventilator and there is a disconnection at the patient connection, the ventilator may continue gradually to push gas from the expiratory limb past the sampling site at the patient end of the breathing system (268). This may result in failure to detect a disconnection for a prolonged period of time.

Correlation Between Arterial and End-tidal Carbon Dioxide Levels (269)

Numerous studies have demonstrated that the correlation between arterial and end-tidal carbon dioxide tensions in children and adults without cardiorespiratory dysfunction

Table 16.4. Capnographic and Capnometric Alterations Seen with Equipment Problems

	Waveform on Capnograph	End-Tidal CO_2	Inspiratory CO_2	End-Tidal to Arterial Gradient
Increased apparatus dead space	Baseline Elevated	↑	↑	Normal
Circle system: faulty unidirectional valve, faulty or exhausted absorbent, bypassed absorber (may be masked by high fresh gas flows)	Baseline Elevated	↑	↑	Normal
Inadequate fresh gas flow to a Mapleson system	Baseline Elevated	↑	↑	Normal
Problems with the inner tube of a Bain system	Baseline Elevated	↑	↑	Normal
Malfunctioning nonrebreathing valve with rebreathing	Baseline Elevated	↑	↑	Normal
Obstruction to expiration in the breathing system	Abnormal	↑	0	Elevated
Leakage in breathing system	Abnormal	↓	0	Elevated
Water in sampling cell	Abnormal	↑	↑	Elevated
Water blocking sampling line	Absent			
Leakage in sampling line	Abnormal	↓	0	Elevated
Too low a flow rate with aspiration devices	Abnormal	↓	↑	Elevated
Too high a flow rate with aspiration devices	Abnormal	↓	0	↑
Inadequate seal around endotracheal tube	Abnormal	↓	0	↑

is good enough to warrant routine monitoring (14,270–279). End-tidal CO_2 is usually lower than Pa_{CO_2}, as a result of dilution of gas from well-perfused alveoli by gases from alveoli that are overventilated relative to perfusion and normal physiological shunt. This gradient is normally 2 to 5 torr (269). It may be less is children (14,29,280).

Although it is generally true that there is a linear relationship between peak expired and arterial CO_2 levels, there are limitations to this linearity and erroneous clinical decisions may be made if the two values are assumed to be equal or to change proportionally (281). Tables 16.1 to 16.4 show some conditions with altered arterial-to-alveolar gradients.

Problems with Sampling

Sampling problems are especially difficult when using a sidestream analyzer to monitor patients with small tidal volumes. When a sidestream capnometer is used with a Mapleson system, dilution of exhaled gas during the latter portion of expiration by fresh gas containing no CO_2 can occur if the expiratory flow rate is less than the sampling flow rate of the capnometer. This can cause the measured end-tidal carbon dioxide level to be lower than actual (34,280,282). Measured end-tidal values should be accepted only when the alveolar phase is flat or has a small positive slope. Even then the Pet_{CO_2} values may underestimate the Pa_{CO_2} (280).

To increase the accuracy of measured end-tidal CO_2 values while using these circuits, there should be as much distance as possible between the sampling site and the fresh gas inlet. The magnitude of the difference between proximal and distal sampling will depend on several factors, which include the patient's weight, the type of ventilator and breathing circuit, the fresh gas flow, the sampling rate, the expiratory flow rate, and whether spontaneous or controlled ventilation is used (29,31,32,34,280,283–287) Although sampling from the distal part of the tracheal tube may provide slightly better estimates of Pa_{CO_2}, most studies show that sampling from the proximal part of the tube provides acceptable readings (30,32,286–288). In critically ill neonates, distal sampling may be necessary (33).

Other maneuvers to obtain a Pet_{CO_2} reading that is closer to the Pa_{CO_2} with Mapleson systems include using lower fresh gas flows, extending the time of expiratory flow, adding dead space between the breathing system and gas sampling point, discontinuing fresh gas flow for single breath analysis, and using a circuit that automatically interrupts the fresh gas flow after inspiration or prevents mixing of exhaled and fresh gases (271,280,283,288).

Even with a conventional circle system, dilution of patient gas may occur, especially if the sampling site is far from the patient's airway (34).

Mainstream capnometers, while adding dead space and bulkiness, do not suffer from the problems associated with sampling capnometers and may yield end-tidal CO_2 values more closely approximating Pa_{CO_2} in infants (14,33,289–291).

If the rise time of the analyzer is prolonged, the end-tidal carbon dioxide reading may be falsely low when high respiratory rates are used (6). With sidestream analyzers, rise time will be longer with lower sampling flow rates. For this reason, it has been recommended that a sampling flow rate less than 150 ml/min not be used (53). Kinking of the sampling catheter can cause the sampling flow rate to be decreased.

During high-frequency ventilation Pet_{CO_2} is a poor index of Pa_{CO_2} (292,293). For this reason, it is necessary to measure Pet_{CO_2} by single tidal volume breaths during ventilation lapses (293–296).

Another source of sampling error is a leak at the interface of the patient and the equipment. A poor mask fit, use of an uncuffed tracheal tube or a tube with a defective cuff, or a loose connection or crack in the sampling catheter may cause an erroneously low end-tidal carbon dioxide reading.

Mask ventilation will result in a higher

dead space, especially in children, and may result in low peak expired CO_2 levels if the sampling site is between the mask and the breathing system.

If a patient has not fully exhaled before the next breath, the end-tidal value will be falsely low (15). In this situation, a gentle squeeze of the patient's chest or abdomen will often produce a sample of alveolar gas with a plateau.

Disturbances in the Ventilation:Perfusion Ratio (297)

In the lung, the ideal unit has a normally ventilated alveolus adjacent to a normally perfused capillary. In an inadequately perfused alveolus (high V:Q), there is decreased transfer of carbon dioxide between blood and lung with a resultant increase in the alveolar-to-arterial gradient. Clinical conditions that alter the volume and/or distribution of pulmonary blood flow include pulmonary embolism, stenosis or occlusion of the pulmonary artery, reduced cardiac output, pulmonary hypotension, and various heart lesions (201,269,298–302). Studies suggest there is no significant change in dead space during induced hypotension in young and healthy patients, but older patients are prone to develop an increase (303,304).

Patients undergoing thoracotomy undergo a variety of changes that alter the ventilation:perfusion ratio and make the difference between the arterial and end-tidal CO_2 values unstable (269,305).

The end-tidal to arterial CO_2 gradient increases as venous admixture (right to left shunt) occurs (269). This can be caused by atelectasis, endobronchial intubation, or certain cyanotic congenital heart diseases. The effect is less dramatic than that caused by an increase in dead space, but when the venous admixture is large (as in cyanotic congenital heart disease) its percentage contribution can be considerable (270,299,301).

Changes in body position such as placement in the lateral decubitus position may cause an increase in the Pa/Pet_{CO_2} gradient (306,307).

Patients with airway disease have an uneven distribution of ventilation and, to a lesser extent, of blood flow. This leads to an increased gradient (269,279,302,308,309). However, the difference tends to be stable. Arterial blood gases can be measured to establish the difference between arterial and end-tidal carbon dioxide. Once the difference is established, end-tidal values provide a reliable estimate of arterial carbon dioxide in hemodynamically stable patients (310).

In neonates in intensive care, arterial and end-tidal CO_2 correlate poorly, the relationship being principally determined by the severity of pulmonary disease (125,311).

If airways disease limits full exhalation, the end-tidal volume will be falsely low. In this situation, a gentle squeeze on the patient's chest or abdomen will assist a full exhalation and produce a sample of alveolar gas (312).

Capnometer Inaccuracy (2)

There are a number of factors related to the capnometer that may result in an inaccurate Pet_{CO_2} reading. These include lack of display resolution, instability, changes in atmospheric pressure, temperature dependence, improper calibration, drift, noise, selectivity, pressure effects from the sampling system or patient environment, water vapor, and foreign substances (2).

With some analyzers, the true gas zero reference is obtained from filtered room air. In some monitors CO_2-containing gas may enter the zeroing sample, leading to a shift in the baseline and causing falsely low CO_2 readings with a normal-looking waveform (159).

Other

A significant discrepancy between Pa_{CO_2} and Pet_{CO_2} may occur in patients taking acetazolamide, which delays the conversion of HCO_3^- to CO_2 (313).

End-tidal CO_2 is occasionally higher than arterial CO_2 (12,244,271,280,281,286,314–

316). Causes include errors in the calibration of the capnometer, rebreathing, and inadvertent addition of CO_2 to the inspired gas (123,317–319). Pet_{CO_2} may exceed Pa_{CO_2} if functional residual capacity is reduced, as in pregnant or obese patients or during laparoscopy (274–276,320).

Capnography (15,288,321)

Most carbon dioxide monitors include a waveform. Nearly all older capnometers include an analog output that can be connected to an oscilloscopic display for a low-cost capnograph (322). Most capnograms are calibrated so that values for end-tidal CO_2 can be estimated. Some capnographs have the ability to monitor waveforms and can alert the viewer when the waveform should be checked.

The ability to see and interpret exhaled carbon dioxide waveforms greatly enhances the usefulness of carbon dioxide monitoring. Waveforms can be displayed on an oscilloscope or printed on paper. Slow speeds can be used to show trends. Faster speeds are used for examination of individual waveforms.

Examination of the waveform will often explain readings that appear inaccurate. If the capnometer reads several peaks per breath (as can be seen with certain artifacts) or does not note breaths that do not have a recognizable plateau, the respiratory rate and peak CO_2 readings will be inaccurate.

The waveform should be examined systematically for height, frequency, rhythm, baseline, and shape. Height depends on the end-tidal level of carbon dioxide. Frequency depends on the respiratory rate. Rhythm depends on the state of the respiratory center or ventilator settings. The baseline should be zero (unless carbon dioxide is deliberately added to the inspired gases).

The shape of the normal waveform is illustrated in Figure 16.27. Only one shape is considered normal. Phase I of exhalation begins at A. During this phase the end-tidal CO_2 is zero. The gas being exhaled is dead space gas from the tracheal tube, bronchi, and bronchioles and has the same CO_2 level as the last portion of the previous inhalation.

Phase II of exhalation begins at B and continues to C. As gas from alveoli begins to be exhaled the level of carbon dioxide rises rapidly (BC). Gas exhaled during this time is a combination of dead space and alveolar gas.

Phase III of exhalation begins at C and continues to just before D. As carbon dioxide from the alveoli is exhaled, a plateau, which is never absolutely flat (CD), is seen. The very last portion of exhaled gas, identified by point D, is termed the end-tidal point. The CO_2 level here is at its maximum. In normal individuals this is 5% to 5.5%, or 35 to 40 torr.

It is phase III that is most telling of airway disease. A steep slope is an indication that obstruction to flow is present (269). The end-tidal gas is most reflective of gas levels in the alveoli.

As the patient inhales, the level of carbon dioxide falls abruptly to zero (DE) and remains at zero until the next exhalation.

Examination of the waveform will reveal whether or not an alveolar plateau is present. If it is not, the numerical value obtained may not be equivalent to the end-tidal level and the correlation between arterial and end-tidal CO_2 is not likely to be good.

There are a number of special situations that are demonstrated by waveform analysis. The reader is referred to the excellent atlas of capnography by Smalhout (211). Some common waveforms are shown in Figures 16.8 and 16.9 as well as in Figures 16.28–16.41.

VOLATILE ANESTHETIC AGENTS

The measurement of concentrations of volatile anesthetic gases is becoming common practice. At least one country (Germany) has adopted it as a standard of care (331). Belgium is scheduled to do the same in 1995.

Standard Requirements

A U.S. standard for anesthetic gas monitors is available (5). The following are provisions of that document.

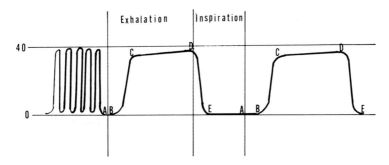

Figure 16.27. Normal CO_2 waveform. A slow recording is shown at the *left*. The curves are long and thin and close together. All the peaks reach the same height. At the *right* are two single waveforms, each representing a single exhalation/inhalation cycle. The capnogram is read from left to right. *AB* is the exhalation of CO_2-free gas contained in dead space at the beginning of expiration. *BC* represents the expiratory upstroke, or the emptying of connecting airways and the beginning of the emptying of alveoli. As exhalation continues, gas from alveoli in regions with relatively short conducting airways appears and mixes with dead space gas from regions with relatively long conducting airways, resulting in an increasing CO_2 level. *CD* shows the expiratory, or alveolar, plateau. Because of uneven emptying of alveoli, the slope continues to rise gently. Point *D* shows the best approximation of alveolar CO_2 (end of expiration, beginning of inspiration). *DE* represents the inspiratory downstroke; as the patient inhales, CO_2-free gas enters the patient's airway and the airway CO_2 level abruptly falls to zero. *EA* shows the completion of inspiratory pause, during which the CO_2 level remains at zero. Characteristics of the normal capnogram include (*i*) rapid increase from *B* to *C*, (*ii*) nearly horizontal plateau between *C* and *D*, (*iii*) rapid decrease from *D* to *E* to zero, and (*iv*) a zero baseline (*EA* + *AB*). A good alveolar plateau greatly increases the changes that the end-tidal reading is a reliable estimate of the alveolar level. Points *B, C, D,* and *E* are sharp but slightly rounded.

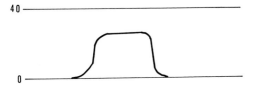

Figure 16.28. Low end-tidal CO_2 with a good alveolar plateau may be the result of hyperventilation or an increase in dead space ventilation. Comparison of Pet_{CO2} with Pa_{CO2} is necessary to distinguish these two conditions.

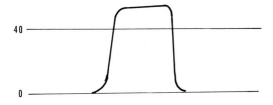

Figure 16.29. Elevated end-tidal CO_2 with good alveolar plateau may be caused by hypoventilation or increased CO_2 delivery to the lungs.

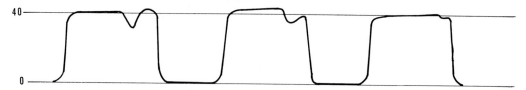

Figure 16.30.   Curare cleft or notch, which is seen during spontaneous ventilation. The capnogram on the *left* shows the notch. As the muscle relaxant is reversed the curve becomes normal in shape. The cleft is in the last third of the plateau and is caused by a lack of synchronous action between the intercostal muscles and the diaphragm most commonly caused by inadequate muscle relaxant reversal. The depth of the cleft is proportional to the degree of muscle paralysis. The notch also is seen in patients with cervical transverse lesions, flail chest, hiccups, and pneumothorax and when a patient tries to breathe during mechanical ventilation.

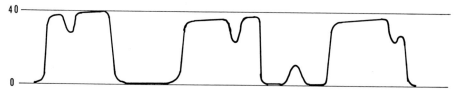

Figure 16.31.   Spontaneous respiratory efforts during mechanical ventilation. The capnogram shows small breaths at various places during expiration and inspiration. Causes include maladjusted ventilator (hypoventilation), inadequate muscle paralysis, severe hypoxia, or the patient waking up. The end-tidal CO_2 may rise slightly because of increasing metabolism of the contracting respiratory muscles. This pattern may also be caused by pressure on the patient's chest or ventilator malfunction (323).

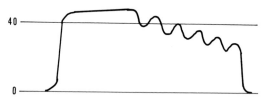

Figure 16.32.   Cardiogenic oscillations appear as small, regular, tooth-like humps at the end of the expiratory phase. They are believed to represent the effects of the contraction and relaxation of the heart and intrathoracic great vessels on the lungs, forcing air in and out. The rate of oscillation matches that of a simultaneously recorded heart rate on the ECG. A number of factors contribute to the appearance of cardiogenic oscillations. These include the presence of negative intrathoracic pressure, a low respiratory rate, diminution in the vital capacity:heart size ratio, a low inspiratory:expiratory ratio, low tidal volumes, and muscular relaxation (324,325). In many cases, adjustment of the ventilator rate, flow, or tidal volume will remove this pattern from the screen. Other times, however, it cannot be corrected. Cardiogenic oscillations are the rule rather than the exception in pediatric patients as a result of the relative size of the infant's heart and stroke volume compared with thoracic size (326). Capnograms from patients suffering severe emphysema tend not to register cardiogenic oscillations. Less sophisticated capnometers may count each oscillation as a breath, displaying a respiratory rate higher than the real one.

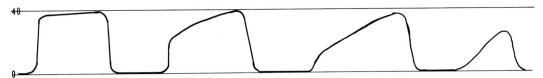

Figure 16.33. Prolonged expiratory upstroke. At the *left* is a normal waveform. The other three curves show progressive slanting and prolongation of the expiratory upstroke. As expiration is progressively prolonged, inspiration may start before expiration is complete so that the end-tidal P_{CO_2} reading is decreased. This is indicative of obstruction to gas flow caused by a partially obstructed tracheal tube or obstruction in the patient's airways (chronic obstructive lung disease, bronchospasm, asthma, or upper-airway obstruction).

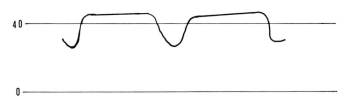

Figure 16.34. The baseline is elevated, and the waveform is normal in shape. This may be caused by an incompetent expiratory valve or exhausted absorbent in the circle system, insufficient fresh gas flow to a Mapleson system, problems with the inner tube of a Bain system, deliberate addition of carbon dioxide to the fresh gas, or in some cases, an incompetent inspiratory valve. It may also be the result of rebreathing under drapes in a spontaneous breathing patient who is not intubated (238,327).

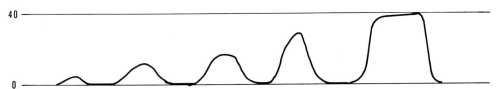

Figure 16.35. On return to spontaneous ventilation, the first breath is typically of small volume. Subsequent breaths show progressively higher peaks with gradual resumption of a normal waveform.

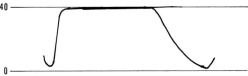

Figure 16.36. Incompetent inspiratory unidirectional valve. The waveform shows a prolonged CO_2 plateau and an inspiratory downstroke that is less steep. The inspiratory phase is shortened, and the baseline may or may not reach zero, depending on the fresh gas flow (264,261,328). A similar pattern may be seen with suction applied to a chest tube (329).

1. For halogenated anesthetic gases, the difference between the mean anesthetic gas reading and the anesthetic gas level shall be within ±(0.15% vol % + 15% of the anesthetic gas level). In addition, 6 standard deviations (SD) of the anesthetic gas readings shall be less than or equal to 0.6 vol %. This means that greater than 68% of all readings occur within 0.1 vol % of the mean reading, over 95% of all readings occur within 0.2 vol % of the mean reading, and more than 99% of all readings occur within 0.3 vol % of the mean reading.

2. High concentration alarms are mandatory. Low concentration alarms are optional. The alarm set point for both high and low concentration alarms must be operator adjustable. The high gas reading alarm(s) shall be medium priority. The visual indication shall be yellow, flashing at 0.4 to 0.8 Hz. If low concentrations alarm(s) are provided, they must be low priority. The visual signal is a constant yellow light.

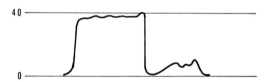

Figure 16.37. Irregular plateau and/or baseline may result from displacement of the tracheal tube into the upper larynx or lower pharynx with intermittent ventilation of the stomach and lungs or from pressure on the chest which causes small volumes of gas to move in and out of the lungs.

3. Temporary silencing of audible alarms shall not exceed 2 min.

Measurement Techniques

The volatile anesthetic agents can be measured using mass spectrometry, Raman scattering gas analysis, infrared analysis, or oscillating crystal technology. Response times for volatile agent monitors vary (332). Factors that decrease the response time include decreasing the length or internal diameter of the sample tube and increasing aspirating flow. The composition of the sample line is important; the partition coefficient of the halogenated agent in the material of a tube correlates with the response time (332).

Usefulness of Anesthetic Agent Monitoring (333)

Vaporizer Function and Contents

A primary advantage of monitoring inspired gases is the ability to assess the accuracy of a vaporizer by sampling from the common gas outlet of the anesthesia machine. Agent-specific analyzers can detect an incorrect agent, and non–agent-specific analyzers will usually show unusual readings when an agent error is made. They also allow determination of the concentration of agent when a setting below the lowest calibration on a vaporizer is dialed or when the vaporizer is used with gas flows outside those for which it is calibrated. Finally, anesthetic agent monitoring will alert the user when a vaporizer has become empty.

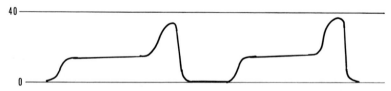

Figure 16.38. A leak in the sampling line during positive pressure ventilation (59,172,330). A plateau of long duration is followed by a peak of brief duration. The height of the plateau is inversely proportional to the size of the leak. The brief peak is caused by the next inspiration when positive pressure transiently pushes undiluted end-tidal gas through the sampling line. If nitrogen is being monitored, an increase will be noted. This pattern is not seen if the patient is breathing spontaneously. A falsely low end-tidal carbon dioxide reading can be obtained owing to air entrainment, but no terminal hump is seen.

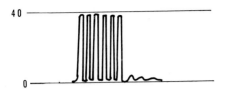

Figure 16.39. A sudden drop of end-tidal CO_2 to zero is usually caused by an acute event relating to the airway, such as extubation, esophageal intubation, complete breathing system disconnection, ventilator malfunction, or a totally obstructed tracheal tube. It may also be the result of a plugged gas sampling tube.

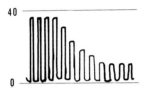

Figure 16.40. The causes of a sudden drop of end-tidal CO_2 to a low but nonzero value include a poorly fitting tracheal tube or mask, a leak or partial disconnection in the breathing system, and a partial obstruction of a tracheal tube.

Inadvertent Administration

Anesthetic agent monitors can detect when a vaporizer is inadvertently left in the on position. They can also detect when a vaporizer not in use is allowing significant amounts of vapor to leak into the fresh gas line.

Information on Uptake and Elimination

Monitoring levels of volatile anesthetic agents provides information on uptake and elimination. The difference between inspired and expired levels provides a measure of patient saturation.

Teaching Low-Flow Anesthesia

Anesthetic agent monitoring can be used to demonstrate the relationship between levels in the fresh gas line and those in the breathing system. This makes them useful in teaching low-flow anesthesia.

Information on Anesthetic Depth

Knowledge of volatile agent concentrations may alter the incidence of hypotension and/or hypertension, provide evidence that the patient who is paralyzed is neither awake nor grossly overdosed, permit more rapid awakening of the patient, and aid in the diagnosis of delayed emergence.

Studies show that volatile anesthetic agents are involved in up to one-third of cardiac arrests in anesthesia (333,334).

End-tidal partial pressure of volatile anesthetic agents can be used as a measure of anesthetic depth. However, caution should be exercised. A study on anesthetized patients found that clinically useful prediction of arterial levels from end-tidal levels was difficult (335). Anesthetic agent monitoring should not be regarded as a replacement for other means of measuring depth, but as an additional source of information. Only by combining knowledge of levels with other variables such as respiration and blood pressure can depth be inferred.

Detection of Contaminants

Contaminants in the nitrous oxide supply were detected with an agent monitor that indicated the presence of a volatile agent when no vaporizer was turned on (336).

NITROUS OXIDE

Standard Requirements

The standard for anesthetic gas monitors (5) requires that the difference between the

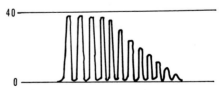

Figure 16.41. Events that cause an exponential decrease in end-tidal CO_2 include sudden hypotension owing to massive blood loss or obstruction of the vena cava, circulatory arrest with continued pulmonary ventilation, and pulmonary embolism (air, clot, thrombus, or marrow).

mean reading and the actual nitrous oxide level be within $\pm(2.0$ vol % $+$ 8% of the nitrous oxide level). In addition, 6 SD of the nitrous oxide reading (for a given level) shall be less than or equal to 10.0 vol %. This means that more than 68% of all readings occur within 1.7 vol % of the mean reading, over 95% of all readings occur within 3.3 vol % of the mean reading, and more than 99% of all readings occur within 5.0 vol % of the mean reading.

Technology

Nitrous oxide can be measured by infrared, mass spectrometry, or Raman scattering technology.

Significance of Nitrous Oxide Levels

Analysis of nitrous oxide will show whether the flowmeters are functioning properly. At the end of a case, the washout of nitrous oxide will avoid diffusion hypoxia. A decrease may be caused by entrainment of room air (172,330).

NITROGEN (333)

Standards

There are currently no standards for monitors that measure nitrogen.

Technology

Nitrogen can be measured only by mass spectrometry or Raman scattering. Intermittent monitoring with a shared mass spectrometer could miss a sudden increase in nitrogen (337).

Significance

Verifying Adequate Denitrogenation

An important use of nitrogen monitoring is to ensure adequate denitrogenation before induction. This is a special concern with pediatric patients, patients with lung disease, and patients who have a reduced functional residual capacity (as may be caused by obesity or pregnancy) as well as during a rapid sequence induction.

Detection of Venous Air Emboli (338)

A rise in exhaled nitrogen indicates that air from some source has entered the breathing system. During certain surgical procedures, this is most likely the result of air entering a venous sinus or open vein, provided that the breathing system is tight enough that no air can be entrained. Used in connection with CO_2 monitoring, nitrogen monitoring provides the necessary information to distinguish between the occurrence of air emboli and other physiological events that cause reduced carbon dioxide elimination.

Monitoring Breathing System Integrity

Normally, during general anesthesia the level of nitrogen in the breathing system drops rapidly at first then more slowly. A slow drop or a rise may be caused by room air entering through a leak, disconnection, poorly fitting mask, or uncuffed tracheal tube (339).

Breathing out of synchrony with a ventilator may cause air to be entrained around a tracheal tube (330).

A leak in the sampling system can cause nitrogen to be detected (59,341). To determine if this is occurring, pure oxygen from the anesthesia machine should be sampled. If the monitor continues to show nitrogen, air is leaking into the sampling line.

Detecting Nitrogen Accumulation

In spite of high initial gas flows, excreted nitrogen can built up in the breathing system during low-flow anesthesia. Nitrogen levels as high as 15% have been reported during closed system anesthesia (342). Such a level can cause a significant decrease in the levels of oxygen, nitrous oxide, and volatile agents.

REFERENCES

1. Cooper JB, Newbower RS, Kitz RJ. An analysis of major errors and equipment failure in anesthesia management. Considerations for prevention and detection. Anesthesiology 1984;60:34–42.
2. Raemer DB, Calalang I. Accuracy of end-tidal car-

bon dioxide tension analyzers. J Clin Monit 1991;7:195–208.

3. American Society for Testing and Materials. Specification for oxygen monitors (F-1462-93). Philadelphia: ASTM, 1993.

4. American Society for Testing and Materials. Specification for capnometers (F-1456-92). Philadelphia: ASTM, 1992.

5. American Society for Testing and Materials. Specification for the minimum performance and safety requirements for components and systems of anesthetic gas monitors (F-1452-92). Philadelphia: ASTM, 1992.

6. Brunner JX, Westinskow DR. How the rise time of carbon dioxide analyzers influences the accuracy of carbon dioxide measurements. Br J Anaesth 1988;61:628–638.

7. Block FE, McDonald JS. Sidestream versus mainstream carbon dioxide analyzers. J Clin Monit 1992;8:139–141.

8. Deluty SH. Capnography: how does it work and what can we learn from it? Prog Anesth 1990;4:273–288.

9. Good ML. Principles and practice of capnography (ASA Refresher Course #234). New Orleans: ASA, 1992.

10. Kinsella SM. Assessment of the Hewlett-Packard HP47210A capnometer. Br J Anaesth 1985;57:919–923.

11. Marks LF. Monitoring of tidal carbon dioxide in spontaneously breathing patients using a mainstream analysing monitor. Anaesthesia 1991;46:154–155.

12. Lenz G, Heipertz W, Epple E. Capnometry for continuous postoperative monitoring of nonintubated, spontaneously breathing patients. J Clin Monit 1991;7:245–248.

13. Pesonen P, Luukonen P. Use of a capnometer to detect leak of carbon dioxide during laparoscopic surgery. Anesthesiology 1992;76:661.

14. Badgwell JM, Heavner JE. End-tidal carbon dioxide pressure in neonates and infants measured by aspiration and flow-through capnography. J Clin Monit 1991;7:285–288.

15. Swedlow DB. Capnometry and capnography. The anesthesia disaster early warning system. Semin Anesth 1986;5:194–205.

16. Seow LT, Davis R. Circuit disconnections. Anaesth Intensive Care 1988;16:242.

17. Quarmby R, Schmitt L. A simple, inexpensive device to prevent airway disconnection when using remote capnometry. Anesth Analg 1989;69:414–415.

18. Lenoir RJ. Hewlett-Packard HP4720A capnometer. Br J Anaesth 1986;58:1204.

19. Anonymous. Hewlett-Packard Model 47210A Capnometers. Technol Anesth 1987;8:4.

20. Hurley MR, Paull JD. A spuriously low end-tidal carbon dioxide. Anaesth Intensive Care 1991;19:615–616.

21. Ornstein E. False-positive abrupt decrease in $EtCO_2$ during craniotomy in the sitting position. Anesthesiology 1985;62:542.

22. Reder RF, Brown EG, DeAsla RA, Jurado RA. Thermal skin burns from a carbon dioxide analyzer in children. Ann Thoracic Surg 1983;35:329–330.

23. Beaumont AC, Diamond JG. CO_2 measurement and the Minilink system. Anaesthesia 1989;44:535.

24. Machin JR, MacNeil A. Gas sampling from a facemask for capnography. Anaesthesia 1986;41:971.

25. Spahr-Schopfer IA, Hartley EJ, Bissonnette B. Pediatric laryngeal masks and capnometry. Anesth Analg 1993;76:S412.

26. Reid MF, Matthews A. A simple arrangement to sample expired gas in small children. Anaesthesia 1988;43:902–903.

27. Levytam S, Kavanagh BP, Cooper RM, Nierenberg H, Roger S, Sandler AN. Distal tracheal capnography following general anesthesia. Anesth Analg 1993;76:S223.

28. Duthie GM. Measurement of end-tidal carbon dioxide tension in adults. Anaesthesia 1984;39:605.

29. Badgwell JM, McLeod ME, Lerman J, Creighton RE. End-tidal P_{CO_2} measurements sampled at the distal and proximal ends of the endotracheal tube in infants and children. Anesth Analg 1987;66:959–964.

30. Hillier SC, Badgwell JM, McLeod E, Creighton RE, Lerman J. Accuracy of end-tidal PCO$_2$ measurements using a sidestream capnometer in infants and children ventilated with the Sechrist infant ventilator. Can J Anaesth 1990;37:318–321.

31. McEvedy BAB, McLeod ME Mulera M, Kirpalani H, Lerman J. End-tidal transcutaneous and arterial PCO$_2$ measurements in critically ill neonates. A comparative study. Anesthesiology 1988;69:112–116.

32. Rich GF, Sullivan MP, Adams JM. Is distal sampling of end-tidal CO_2 necessary in small subjects. Anesthesiology 1990;73:265–268.

33. McEvedy BAB, McLeod ME, Kirpalani H, Volgyesi GA, Lerman J. End-tidal carbon dioxide measurements in critically ill neonates: a comparison of sidestream and mainstream capnometers. Can J Anaesth 1990;37:322–326.

34. Schieber RA, Namnoum A, Sugden A, Saville AL, Orr RA. Accuracy of expiratory carbon dioxide measurements in small subjects. J Clin Monit 1985;1:149–155.

35. Bonsu AK, Tamilarasan A, Bromage PR. A nasal catheter for monitoring tidal carbon dioxide in

spontaneously breathing patients. Anesthesiology 1989;71:318.

36. Dunphy JA. Accuracy of expired carbon dioxide partial pressure sampled from a nasal cannula II. Anesthesiology 1988;68:960–961.

37. Norman EA, Zeig NJ, Ahmad I. Better designs for mass spectrometer monitoring of the awake patient. Anesthesiology 1986;64:664.

38. Ackerman WE, Juneja MM, Reaume D. Measurement of $ETCO_2$ and respiratory rate from a nasal cannula during cesarean section. Anesthesiology 1989;71:A976.

39. Bowe EA, Boysen PG, Broome JA, Klein EF. Accurate determination of end-tidal carbon dioxide during administration of oxygen by nasal cannulae. J Clin Monit 1989;5:105–110.

40. Bowie EA, Hyman WD, Payne DR, Muth DH. Comparison of modified nasal cannulae for sampling end-tidal carbon dioxide during oxygen administration. J Clin Monit 1991;7:107–108.

41. Desmarattes R, Kennedy R, Davis DR. Inexpensive capnography during monitored anesthesia care. Anesth Analg 1990;71:100–101.

42. Goldman JM. A simple, easy, and inexpensive method for monitoring $ETCO_2$ through nasal cannulae. Anesthesiology 1987;67:606.

43. Gallacher BP. The measurement of end tidal carbon dioxide concentrations using modified nasal prongs in ophthalmologic patients under regional anesthesia. Reg Anesth 1991;16:189.

44. Ibarra E, Lees DE. Error in measurement of oxygen uptake due to anesthetic gases when using a mass spectrometer. Anesthesiology 1985;63:572.

45. Keener T, Phillips B. Assessment of airflow in sleep studies by oronasal CO_2 detection. Chest 1989;88:316.

46. Roy J, McNulty SE, Torjman MC. An improved nasal prong apparatus for end-tidal carbon dioxide monitoring in awake sedated patients. J Clin Monit 1991;7:249–252.

47. Turner KE, Sandler AN, Vosu HA. End-tidal CO_2 monitoring in spontaneously breathing adults. Can J Anaesth 1989;36:248–249.

48. Zimmerman D, Loken RG. Modified nasal cannula to monitor $ETCO_2$. Can J Anaesth 1992;39:1119.

49. Huntington CT, King H. A simpler design for mass spectrometer monitoring of the awake patient. Anesthesiology 1986;65:565–566.

50. Hanowell LH, Kanefield J. Case report. The importance of monitoring inspired oxygen concentrations during regional anesthesia. Reg Anesth 1988;13:126–127.

51. Inomata S, Nishikawa T. Early detection of airway obstruction with a capnographic probe attached to an oxygen mask. Can J Anaesth 1992;39:744.

52. Pressman MA. A simple method of measuring $ETCO_2$ during MAC and major regional anesthesia. Anesth Analg 1988;67:905–906.

53. Gravenstein N. Capnometry in infants should not be done at lower sampling flow rates. J Clin Monit 1989;5:63–64.

54. Epstein RA, Reznik AM, Epstein MAF. Determinants of distortions in CO_2 catheter sampling systems. A mathematical model. Respir Physiol 1980;41:127–136.

55. Craen RA, Hickman JA. Use of end-tidal CO_2 sampling connector to administer bronchodilators into the anaesthetic circuit. Anaesth Intensive Care 1991;19:299–300.

56. Patteson SK, Chesney JT. Anesthetic management for magnetic resonance imaging: problems and solutions. Anesth Analg 1992;74:121–128.

57. Peden CJ, Menon DK, Hall AS, Sargentoni J, Whitwam JG. Magnetic resonance for the anaesthetist. Part II. Anaesthesia and monitoring in MR units. Anaesthesia 1992;47:508–517.

58. Shellock FG. Monitoring sedated pediatric patients during MR imaging. Radiology 1990;177:586–587.

59. Skeehan TM, Biebuyck JF. Erroneous mass spectrometer data caused by a faulty patient sampling tube: case report and laboratory study. J Clin Monit 1991;7:313–319.

60. Raynond RN, Tolley PM. Water damage to capnography equipment. Anaesth Intensive Care 1992;20:249.

61. Carlon GC, Miodownik S, Ray C, Kopec IC. An automated mechanism for protection of mass spectrometry sampling tubing. J Clin Monit 1988;4:264–266.

62. Paulsen AW. Factors influencing the relative accuracy of long-line time-shared mass spectrometry. Biomed Instrum Technol 1989;23:476–480.

63. Scamman FL. Accuracy of a central mass spectrometer system at high respiratory frequencies. J Clin Monit 1977;4:227–229.

64. Sodol IE, Clark JS, Swanson GD. Mass spectrometers in medical monitoring. In: Webster, JG, ed. Encyclopedia of medical devices and instrumentation. New York: Wiley, 1988:1848–1859.

65. Scamman FL, Fishbaugh JK. Frequency response of long mass-spectrometer sampling catheters. Anesthesiology 1986;65:422–425.

66. Lerou JGC, van Egmond J, Kolmer HHB. Evaluation of long sampling tubes for remote monitoring by mass spectrometry. J Clin Monit 1990;6:39–52.

67. Cramers CA, Leclercq PA, Lerou JG, Kolmer B. Mass spectrometry in monitoring anaesthetic gas mixtures using long sampling tubes. Band broadening in capillary tubes caused by flow and diffu-

sion. In: Vickers MD, Crul J, eds. Mass spectrometry in anesthesiology. New York: Springer-Verlag, 1981:120–130.

68. Munshi CA, Bardeen-Henschel A. Mass spectrometer failure: an unusual cause. J Clin Monit 1987;3:288–290.

69. Buckingham JD, Holme AE. Mass spectrometry for respiratory gas analysis. Br J Clin Equip 1977;2:142–148.

70. Beatty PCW. The spectralab-M quadrupole medical mass spectrometer. J Med Eng Technol 1988;12:265–272.

71. Beatty PCW. Potential inaccuracies in mass spectrometers with spectrum overlap erasure units used during anaesthesia. Clin Phys Physiol Meas 1984;5:93–104.

72. Davis WOM, Spence AA. A modification of the MGA 200 mass spectrometer to enable measurement of anaesthetic gas mixtures. Br J Anaesth 1979;51:987–988.

73. Williams EL, Benson DM. Helium-induced errors in clinical mass spectrometry. Anesth Analg 1988;67:83–85.

74. Steinbrook RA, Elliott WR, Goldman DB, Philip JH. Linking mass spectrometers to provide continuing monitoring during system failure. J Clin Monit 1991;7:271–273.

75. Munshi C, Dhamee S, Bardeen-Henschel A, Dhruva S. Recognition of mixed anesthetic agents by mass spectrometer during anesthesia. J Clin Monit 1986;2:121–124.

76. Perkins WJ, Marsh BT. Continuous and accurate end-tidal CO_2 and anesthetic concentration measurements at high respiratory frequencies. Anesthesiology 1991;75:A486.

77. Frazier WT, Odom SH. Efficiency and expense of time-shared mass spectrometer systems. Biomed Instrum Technol 1989;23:481–484.

78. McCleary U. Potential effects of an unknown gas on mass spectrometer readings. Anesthesiology 1985;63:724–725.

79. Siegel M, Gravenstein N. Evaluation of helium interference with mass spectrometry. Anesth Analg 1988;67:887–889.

80. Gravenstein JS, Gravenstein N, van der Aa JJ, Paulus DA. Pitfalls with mass spectrometry in clinical anesthesia. Int J Clin Monit Comp 1984;1:27–34.

81. Gravenstein N, Theisen GJ, Knudsen AK. Misleading mass spectrometer reading caused by an aerosol propellant. Anesthesiology 1985;62:70–72.

82. Kharasch ED, Sivarajan M. Aesosol propellant interference with clinical mass spectrometers. J Clin Monit 1991;7:172–174.

83. Theisen GJ, Gravenstein N, Knudsen AL,

Jphnson JV, Yost RA. More on mass spectrometers and aerosol propellants. Anesthesiology 1985;63:568–569.

84. Elliott WR, Raemer DB, Goldman DB, Philip JH. The effects of bronchodilator-inhaler aerosol propellants on respiratory gas monitors. J Clin Monit 1991;7:175–180.

85. Paulsen AW. Spare mass spectrometer vs linking systems in the event of a single system failure. J Clin Monit 1992;8:319–320.

86. Van Wagenen RA, Westinskow DR, Benner RE, Gregonis DE, Coleman DL. Dedicated monitoring of anesthetic and respiratory gases by Raman scattering. J Clin Monit 1986;2:215–222.

87. Westenskow DR, Smith KW, Coleman DL, Gregonis DE, Van Wagenen RA. Clinical evaluation of a Raman scattering multiple gas analyzer for the operating room. Anesthesiology 1989;70:350–355.

88. Westinskow DR, Coleman DL. Can the Raman scattering analyzer compete with mass spectrometers. An affirmative reply. J Clin Monit 1989;5:34–36.

89. Walker SD. Respiratory gas measurements by infrared technology. Biomed Instrum Technol 1989;23:466–469.

90. Mogue LR, Rantala B. Capnometers. J Clin Monit 1988;4:115–121.

91. Colquhoun AD, Gray WM, Asbury AJ:An evaluation of the Datex Normac anaesthetic agent monitor. Anaesthesia 1986;41:198–204.

92. Ilsey AH, Plummer JL, Runciman WB, Cousins MJ. An evaluation of three volatile anaesthetic agent monitors. Anaesth Intensive Care 1986;14:437–442.

93. Jameson LC, Springman SR. Laboratory performance of two commercially available infrared anesthetic monitors and a mass spectrometer. Anesthesiology 1988;69:A301.

94. Luff NP, White DC. Evaluation of the Datex "Normac" anaesthetic agent monitor. Anaesthesia 1985;40:555–559.

95. Schulte GT, Block FE. Infrared-paramagnetic vs. mass spectrometer measurement of anesthetic and respiratory gas values. Anesthesiology 1988;69:A225.

96. Springman SR, Jameson LC. A comparison of two infrared gas monitors and a multiplexed mass spectrometer with a stand-alone mass spectrometer in adult patients. Anesthesiology 1988;69:A302.

97. Zbinden AM, Westenskow D, Thomson DA, Funk B, Maertens J. A laboratory investigation of two new portable gas analyzers. Int J Clin Monit Comp 1986;2:151–161.

98. Synott A, Wren WS. Accuracy of the Datex Nor-

mac anaesthetic vapour analyser. Anaesthesia 1986;41:322.

99. Jameson LC, Popic PM. Adverse effect of respiratory rate on volatile anesthetic reporting in three infrared anesthetic monitors. Anesthesiology 1991;75:A418.

100. McPeak H, Palayiwa E, Madgwick R, Sykes MK. Evaluation of a multigas anaesthetic monitor. The Datex Capnomac. Anaesthesia 1988;43:1035–1041.

101. Bjoraker DG. The Ohmeda 5250 respiratory gas monitor. Anesthesiol Rev 1990;17:44–48.

102. Deriaz H, Baras E, Benmosbah L, Duranteau R, Lienhart A. Misfilled vaporizer: can it be detected with a monochromatic infrared analyzer? Anesthesiology 1989;71:A364.

103. Gravenstein N, Guyton D. Infrared analysis of anesthetic gases: impact of selector switch setting, anesthetic mixtures, and alcohol. J Clin Monit 1989;5:292.

104. Nielsen J, Kann T, Moller JT. Evaluation of two newly developed anesthetic agent monitors: Bruel & Kjaer anesthetic agent monitor 1304 (BK1304) and Datex Capnomac Ultima (Ultima). Anesthesiology 1990;73:A538.

105. Jameson LC. Detection and quantification of mixed volatile anesthetics by Poet II and a mass spectrometer. Anesthesiology 1990;73:A440.

106. Lai NC. Multiple-filter infrared system as an alternative to mass spectrometer. J Clin Monit 1991;7:87–89.

107. Munshi CA, Brennan S. Evaluation of Poet II (Criticare) multigas infrared analyzer. Anesthesiology 1990;73:A478.

108. Sosis MB, Braverman B, Ivankovich AD. Evaluation of a new three wavelength infrared anesthetic agent monitor. Anesth Analg 1993;76:S408.

109. Mollgaard K. Acoustic Gas—measurement. Biomed Inst Technol 1989;23:495–497.

110. McPeak HB, Palayiwa E, Robinson GC, Sykes MK. An evaluation of the Bruel and Kjaer monitor 1304. Anaesthesia 1992;47:41–47.

111. Abenstein JP, Welna JO. Clinical evaluation of a photoacoustic gas analyzer. Anesthesiology 1991;75:A463.

112. Guyton DC, Shomaker TS. Effect of incorrect agent setting or alcohol on a photoacoustic gas monitor. J Clin Monit 1991;7:120.

113. Alphin RS, Guyton DC. Photoacoustic spectroscopy (PAS) effects of anesthetic gas mixtures and of ethanol. Anesthesiology 1991;75:A419.

114. Eisenkraft JB, Raemer DB. Monitoring gases in the anesthesia delivery system. In: Ehrenwerth J, Eisenkraft JB, eds. Anesthesia equipment. Principles and applications. New York: CV Mosby, 1993:201–220.

115. Anonymous. Carbon dioxide monitors. Health Devices 1986;15:255–272.

116. Crawford MW, Volgyesi GA, Carmichael FJ, Creighton R, Lerman J. The effect of ethanol vapor on the detection of inhalational anesthetics using infrared and piezoelectric monitors. Anesthesiology 1990;73:A522.

117. Doyle DJ. Factitious readings from anaesthetic agent monitors. Can J Anaesth 1988;35:667–671.

118. Foley MA, Wood PR, Peel WJ, Jones GM, Lawler PG. The effect of exhaled alcohol on the performance of the Datex Capnomac. Anaesthesia 1990;45:232–234.

119. Guyton D, Gravenstein N. Alcohol interference with infrared anesthetic gas analysis. Anesthesiology 1989;71:A464.

120. Taylor PM, Clarke KW. Performance of the Datex infrared anaesthetic agent monitor. Anaesthesia 1992;47:448.

121. Volgyesi GA, Crawford MW. The effect of alcohols and acetone on the 3.3 nm infrared anesthetic agent monitors. Anesthesiology 1991;75:A488.

122. Yamashita M, Tsuneto S. Alcohol vapour and the Normac analyser. Anaesthesia 1987;42:209.

123. Severinghaus JW. Water vapor calibration errors in some capnometers. Respiratory conventions misunderstood by manufacturers? Anesthesiology 1989;70:996–998.

124. Kocache R. Oxygen analyzers. In: Webster JG, ed. Encyclopedia of medical devices and instrumentation. New York: Wiley, 1988:2154–2161.

125. Merilainen PT. A fast differential paramagnetic O_2-sensor. Int J Clin Monit Comput 1988;5:187–195.

126. Anonymous. Oxygen analyzers for breathing circuits. Health Devices 1983;12:183–197.

127. Erdmann K, Jantzen JAH, Etz C, Dick WF. Evaluation of two oxygen analyzers by computerized data acquisition and processing. J Clin Monit 1986;2:105–113.

128. Ilsey AH, Runciman WB. An evaluation of fourteen oxygen analysers for use in patient breathing circuits. Anaesth Intensive Care 1986;14:431–436.

129. Figallo EM, Smith RB, Pautler S, Reilly KR. Continuous oxygen analyzers in clinical anesthesia. Anesthesiol Rev 1978;5:25–31.

130. Roe PG, Tyler CKG, Tennant R, Barnes PK. Oxygen analysers. An evaluation of five fuel cell models. Anaesthesia 1987;42:175–181.

131. Bageant RA. Oxygen analyzers. Respir Care 1976;21:410–416.

132. Smith AC, Hahn CEW. Electrodes for the measurement of oxygen and carbon dioxide tensions. Br J Anaesth 1969;41:731–741.

133. Wilson RS, Laver MB. Oxygen analysis: advances

in methodology. Anesthesiology 1972;37:112–116.

134. Mazze N, Wald A. Failure of battery-operated alarms. Anesthesiology 1980;53:246–248.

135. Bengtson JP, Sonander H, Stenqvist O. Oxygen analyzers in anaesthesia. performance in a simulated clinical environment. Acta Anaesthesiol Scand 1986;30:656–659.

136. Westenskow DR, Silva FH. Laboratory evaluation of the vital signs (ICOR) piezoelectric anesthetic agent analyzer. J Clin Monit 1991;7:189–194.

137. Humphrey SJE, Luff NP, White DC. Evaluation of the Lamtec anaesthetic agent monitor. Anaesthesia 1991;46:478–481.

138. Westenskow DR, Silva FH. Evaluation of the vital stat (ICOR) anesthetic agent analyzer. Anesthesiology 1989;71:A358.

139. Schulte GT, Block FE. What really happens when the wrong agent is poured into a vaporizer? Anesthesiology 1991;75:S420.

140. Denman WT, Hayes M, Higgins D, Wilkinson DJ. The Fenem CO_2 detector device. Anaesthesia 1990;45:465–467.

141. Goldberg JS, Rawle PR, Zehnder JL, Sladen RN. Colorimetric end-tidal carbon dioxide monitoring for tracheal intubation. Anesth Analg 1990;70:191–194.

142. O'Flaherty D, Adams AP. The end-tidal carbon dioxide detector. Anaesthesia 1990;45:653–655.

143. Jones BR, Dorsey MJ. Sensitivity of a disposable end-tidal carbon dioxide detector. J Clin Monit 1991;7:268–270.

144. Higgins D. Confirmation of tracheal intubation in a neonate using the Fenem CO_2 detector. Anaesthesia 1990;45:591–592.

145. Ponitz AL, Gravenstein N, Banner MJ. Humidity affecting a chemically based monitor of exhaled carbon dioxide. Anesthesiology 1990;73:A515.

146. Feinstein R, White PF, Westerfield SZ III. Intraoperative evaluation of a disposable end-tidal CO_2 monitor. Anesthesiology 1989;71:A460.

147. Anonymous. End-tidal CO_2 detector questions arise. JEMS 1991;16:22–23.

148. Strunin L, Williams T. The FEF end-tidal carbon dioxide detector. Anesthesiology 1989;71:621–622.

149. Bhende MS, Thompson AE, Howland DF. Validity of a disposable end-tidal carbon dioxide detector in verifying endotracheal tube position in piglets. Crit Care Med 1991;19:566–568.

150. Bhende MS, Thompson AE Cook DR, Saville AL. Validity of a disposable end-tidal CO_2 detector in verifying endotracheal tube placement in infants and children. Ann Emerg Med 1992;21:142–145.

151. Kelly JS, Wilhoit RD, Brown RE, Case LD. Validation of a colorimetric end-tidal carbon dioxide detector in children. Anesthesiology 1991;75:A946.

152. Varon AJ, Morrina J, Civetta JM. Clinical utility of a colorimetric end-tidal CO_2 detector in cardiopulmonary resuscitation and emergency intubation. J Clin Monit 1991;7:289–293.

153. Winston RS, Layon AJ, Gravenstein N, Gallagher J. Detection of esophageal intubation with a new chemical monitor of end-tidal carbon dioxide. Crit Care Med 1990;18:S216.

154. Higgins D, Hayes M, Denman W, Wilkinson DJ. Effectiveness of using end tidal carbon dioxide concentration to monitor cardiopulmonary resuscitation. Br Med J 1990;300:581.

155. Varon AJ, Morrina J, Civetta JM. Use of colorimetric end-tidal carbon dioxide monitoring to prognosticate immediate resuscitation from cardiac arrest. Anesthesiology 1990;73:A412.

156. Freid EB, Good ML, Bonett S, Gravenstein N. Disposable end-tidal CO_2 detector. Tidal volume threshold. Anesthesiology 1990;73:A464.

157. Mehta MP, Symreng T, Sum Ping JST. Reliability of FEF end-tidal CO_2 detector during CPR. Anesthesiology 1990;73:A473.

158. Muir JD, Randalls PB, Smith GB. End tidal carbon dioxide detector for monitoring cardiopulmonary resuscitation. Br Med J 1990;301:41–42.

159. Hruby J, Marvulli T. A carbon dioxide calibration error during automatic correction of measurements in the N1000 Nellcor pulse oximeter/capnometer. J Clin Monit 1990;6:339.

160. Petrioanu G, Widjaja B, Bergler WF. Detection of oesophageal intubation: can the "cola complication" be potentially lethal? Anaesthesia 1992.47:70–71.

161. Ping STS, Mehta MP, Symreng T. Accuracy of the FEF CO_2 detector in the assessment of endotracheal tube placement. Anesth Analg 1992;74:415–419.

162. Mazze RI. Therapeutic misadventures with oxygen delivery systems. The need for continuous inline oxygen monitors. Anesth Analg 1972;51:787–792.

163. American Society for Testing and Materials. Standard specification for minimum performance and safety requirements for components and systems of anesthesia gas machines (F-1161-88). Philadelphia: ASTM, 1988.

164. International Organization for Standardization. Oxygen analyzers for monitoring patient breathing mixtures—safety requirements (USO 7767). Geneve, Switzerland: ISO, 1988.

165. Knaack-Steinegger R, Thomson DA. The measurement of expiratory oxygen as disconnection alarm. Anesthesiology 1989;70:343–344.

166. McGarrigle R, White S. Oxygen analyzers can de-

tect disconnections. Anesth Analg 1984;63:464–465.

167. Meyer RM. A case for monitoring oxygen in the expiratory limb of the circle. Anesthesiology 1984;61:347.

168. Ritchie PA. Another use for an oxygen analyser. Anaesthesia 1984;39:1038–1039.

169. Marks MM, Wrigley FRH. Oxygen analysers as disconnection alarm. Can Anaesth Soc J 1981;28:611.

170. Spooner RB. Oxygen analyzers unreliable as disconnection alarms. Anesth Analg 1984;63:962.

171. Spooner RB. The measurement of expired oxygen as disconnection alarm. Anesthesiology 1989;71:994.

172. Zupan J, Martin M, Benumof JL. End-tidal CO_2 excretion waveform and error with gas sampling line leak. Anesth Analg 1988;67:579–581.

173. Linko K, Paloheimo M. Inspired end-tidal oxygen content difference. A sensitive indicator of hypoventilation. Crit Care Med 1989;17:345–348.

174. Cheney FW. ASA closed claims project progress report. The effect of pulse oximetry and end-tidal CO_2 monitoring on adverse respiratory events. ASA Newslett 1992;56(6):6–10.

175. Anonymous. From the literature. Standards of care and capnography. APSF Newslett 1991;6:20–21.

176. Lillie PE, Roberts JG. Carbon dioxide monitoring. Anaesth Intensive Care 1988;16:41–44.

177. Tinker JH, Dull DL, Caplan RA, Ward RJ, Cheney FW. Role of monitoring devices in prevention of anesthetic mishaps. A closed claims analysis. Anesthesiology 1989;71:541–546.

178. Cote CJ, Liu LMP, Szyfelbein SK, et al. Intraoperative events diagnosed by expired carbon dioxide monitoring in children. Can Anaesth Soc J 1986;33:315–320.

179. Hilberman M. Capnometer readings at high altitude. Anesthesiology 1990;73:354–355.

180. James MF, White JF. Anesthetic considerations at moderate altitude. Anesth Analg 1984;63:1097–1105.

181. Alas VD, Geddes LA, Voorhees WD, Bourland JD, Schoenlein WE. End-tidal CO_2, CO_2 production, and O_2 consumption as early indicators of approaching hyperthermia. Biomed Instrum Technol 1990;24:440–444.

182. Donati F, Maille J, Blain R, Boulanger M, Sahab P. End-tidal carbon dioxide tension and temperature changes after coronary artery bypass surgery. Can Anaesth Soc J 1985;32:272–277.

183. Okamoto H, Hoka S, Kawasaki T. Changes in end-tidal CO_2 following sodium bicarbonate administration reflect cardiac output and hemoglobin levels. Anesthesiology 1992;77:A247.

184. Wang LP, Hagerdal M. Reported anesthetic complications during an 11 year period. A retrospective study. Acta Anaesthesiol Scand 1992;36:234–240.

185. Dickson M, White H, Kinney W, Kambam JR. Extremity tourniquet deflation increases end-tidal P_{CO_2}. Anesth Analg 1990;70:457–458.

186. Giuffrida JG. Extremity tourniquet deflation increases end-tidal PCO_2. Anesth Analg 1990;71:568.

187. Patel AJ, Choi C, Giuffrida JG. Changes in end tidal CO_2 and arterial blood gas levels after release of tourniquet. South Med J 1987;80:213–216.

188. Hagerdal M, Caldwell CB, Gross JB. Intraoperative fluid management influences carbon dioxide production and respiratory quotient. Anesthesiology 1983;59:48–50.

189. Salem MR. Hypercapnia, hypocapnia, hypoxemia. Semin Anesth 1987;6:202–215.

190. Khan RM, Maroof M, Bhatti TH, Hamalawy H, Abbas JS. Correlation of end tidal CO_2 and hemodynamic variation following CO_2 insufflation during laparoscopic cholecystectomy. Anesthesiology 1992;77:A464.

191. Goode JG, Gumnit RY, Carel WD, McKenna M. Hypercapnia during laser arthroscopy of the knee. Anesthesiology 1990;73:551–553.

192. Baudendistel L, Goudsouzian N, Cote C, Strafford M. End-tidal CO_2 monitoring. Its use in the diagnosis and management of malignant hyperthermia. Anaesthesia 1984;39:1000–1003.

193. Dunn CM, Maltry DE, Eggers GWN. Value of mass spectrometry in early diagnosis of malignant hyperthermia. Anesthesiology 1985;63:333.

194. Holzman RS. Mass spectrometry for early diagnosis and monitoring of malignant hyperthermia crisis. Anesthesiol Rev 1988;15:31–34.

195. Neubauer KR, Kaufman RD. Another use for mass spectrometry. Detection and monitoring of malignant hyperthermia. Anesth Analg 1985;64:837–839.

196. Triner L, Sherman J. Potential value of expiratory carbon dioxide measurement in patients considered to be susceptible to malignant hyperthermia. Anesthesiology 1981;55:482.

197. Jordan WS, Jordan RB, Westenskow DR, Hayes JK. CO_2 production (VCO_2) related to anesthetic depth. Anesthesiology 1984;51:A173.

198. Isserles SA, Breen PH. Can changes in end-tidal PCO_2 measure changes in cardiac output. Anesth Analg 1991;73:808–814.

199. Shibutani K, Whelan G, Zung N, Ferlazzo P. End-tidal CO_2. A clinical noninvasive cardiac output monitor. Anesth Analg 1991;72:S251.

200. Shibutani K, Komatsu T, Kashiwagi N, Bairamian M, Kumar V. End-tidal PCO_2 reflects changes of cardiac output. Anesthesiology 1990;73:A506.

201. Schuller JL, Bovill JG, Nijveld A. End-tidal carbon

dioxide concentration as an indicator of pulmonary blood flow during closed heart surgery in children. A report of two cases. Br J Anaesth 1985;57:1257–1259.

202. Schuller JL, Bovill JG. Severe reduction in end-tidal PCO_2 following unilateral pulmonary artery occlusion in a child with pulmonary hypertension. Evidence for reflex pulmonary vasoconstriction. Anesth Analg 1989;68:792–794.

203. Symons NLP, Leaver HK. Air embolism during craniotomy in the seated position: a comparison of methods for detection. Can Anaesth Soc J 1985;32:174–177.

204. Hurter D, Sebel PS. Detection of venous air embolism. A clinical report using end-tidal carbon dioxide monitoring during neurosurgery. Anaesthesia 1979;34:578–582.

205. Drummond JC, Prutow RJ, Scheller MS. A comparison of sensitivity of pulmonary artery pressure, end-tidal carbon dioxide, and end-tidal nitrogen in the detection of venous air embolism in the dog. Anesth Analg 1985;64:688–692.

206. Carroll GC. Capnographic trend curve monitoring can detect 1-ml pulmonary emboli in humans. J Clin Monit 1992;8:101–106.

207. Byrick RJ, Forbes D, Waddell JP. A monitored cardiovascular collapse during cemented total knee replacement. Anesthesiology 1986;65:213–216.

208. Shulman D, Aronson HB. Capnography in the early diagnosis of carbon dioxide embolism during laparoscopy. Can Anaesth Soc J 1984;31:455–459.

209. Byrick RJ, Kay JC, Mullen JB. Capnography is not as sensitive as pulmonary artery pressure monitoring in detecting marrow microembolism. Anesth Analg 1989;68:94–100.

210. Mazumdar B, Skinner SC, Thisted R, Breen PH. Does end-tidal PCO_2 detect recovery of CO_2 elimination after pulmonary embolism in the dog. Anesth Analg 1993;76:S252.

211. Smalhout B. Monitoring in the operating room. Adv Med 1982;5(April).

212. Falk JL, Rackow EC, Weil MH. End-tidal carbon dioxide concentration during cardiopulmonary resuscitation. N Engl J Med 1988;318:607–611.

213. Gudipati CV, Weil MH, Bisera J, Deshmukh HG, Rackow EC. Expired carbon dioxide: a noninvasive monitor of cardiopulmonary resuscitation. Circulation 1988;77:234–239.

214. Barton C, Callaham M. Lack of correlation between end-tidal carbon dioxide concentrations and $PaCO_2$ in cardiac arrest. Crit Care Med 1991;19:108–110.

215. Kalenda Z. The capnogram as a guide to the efficacy of cardiac massage. Resuscitation 1976;6:259–263.

216. Lepilin MG, Vasilyev AV, Bildinov OA, Rostovtseva NA. End-tidal carbon dioxide as a noninvasive monitor of circulatory status during cardiopulmonary resuscitation. A preliminary clinical study. Crit Care Med 1987;15:958–959.

217. Sanders AB, Atlas M, Ewy GA, Kern KB, Bragg S. Expired P_{CO2} as an index of coronary perfusion pressure. Am J Emerg Med 1985;3:147–149.

218. Sanders AB, Ewy GA, Bragg S, Atlas M, Kern KB. Expired PCO_2 as a prognostic indicator of successful resuscitation from cardiac arrest. Ann Emerg Med 1985;12:948–952.

219. von Planta M, von Planta I, Weil MH, Bruno S, Bisera J, Rackow EC. End tidal carbon dioxide as an haemodynamic determinant of cardiopulmonary resuscitation in the rat. Cardiovasc Res 1989;23:364–368.

220. Paradis NA, Martin GB, Rivers EP, Goetting MC, Appleton TJ, Nowak RM. End tidal CO_2 and high dose epinephrine during cardiac arrest in humans [Abstract]. Crit Care Med 1990;18:S276.

221. Barton CW, Callaham ML. Successful prediction by capnometry of resuscitation from cardiac arrest. Ann Emerg Med 1988;17:393.

222. Callaham M, Barton C. Prediction of outcome of cardiopulmonary resuscitation from end-tidal carbon dioxide concentration. Crit Care Med 1990;18:358–362.

223. Gazmuri RJ, von Planta M, Weil MH, Rackow EC. Arterial PCO_2 as an indicator of systemic perfusion during cardiopulmonary resuscitation. Crit Care Med 1989;17:237–240.

224. Kern KB, Sanders AB, Voorhees WD, Babbs CF, Tacker WA, Ewy GA. Changes in expired end-tidal carbon dioxide during cardiopulmonary resuscitation in dogs: a prognostic guide for resuscitation efforts. J Am Coll Cardiol 1989;13:1184–1189.

225. Sanders AB, Kern KB, Otto CW, Milander MM, Ewy GA. End-tidal carbon dioxide monitoring during cardiopulmonary resuscitation. JAMA 1989;262:1347–1351.

226. Guggenberger H, Lenz G, Federle R. Early detection of inadvertent oesophageal intubation: pulse oximetry vs. capnography. Acta Anesthesiol Scand 1989;33:112–115.

227. Utting JE, Gray TC, Shelley FC. Human misadventures in anaesthesia. Can Anaesth Soc J 1979;26:472–478.

228. Linko K, Paloheimo M, Tammisto T. Capnography for detection of accidental oesophageal intubation. Acta Anaesthesiol Scand 1983;27:199–202.

229. Vaghadia H, Jenkins LC, Ford RW. Comparison of end-tidal carbon dioxide, oxygen saturation and clinical signs for the detection of oesophageal intubation. Can J Anaesth 1989;36:560–564.

230. Duberman S. Learning from near-misses. ASA Newslett 1985;1:12–13.

231. Dunn SM, Mushlin PS, Lind LJ, Raemer D. Tracheal intubation is not invariably confirmed by capnography. Anesthesiology 1990;73:1285–1287.

232. Markovitz BP, Silverberg M, Godinez RI. Unusual cause of an absent capnogram. Anesthesiology 1989;71:992–993.

233. Garnett AR, Gervin CA, Gervin AS. Capnographic waveforms in esophageal intubation: effect of carbonated beverages. Ann Emerg Med 1989;18:387–390.

234. Ping STS, Mehta MP, Symreng T. Reliability of capnography in identifying esophageal intubation with carbonated beverage or antacid in the stomach. Anesth Analg 1991;73:333–337.

235. Zbinden S, Schupfer G. Detection of oesophageal intubation: the cola complication. Anaesthesia 1989;44:81.

236. Good ML, Modell JH, Rush W. Differentiating esophageal from tracheal capnograms. Anesthesiology 1988;69:A266.

237. Sum Ping ST. Esophageal intubation. Anesth Analg 1987;66:483.

238. Zeitlin GL, Hobin K, Platt J, Woitkoski N. Accumulation of carbon dioxide during eye surgery. J Clin Anesth 1989;1:262–267.

239. Urmey WF. Accuracy of expired carbon dioxide partial pressure sampled from nasal cannula. I. Anesthesiology 1988;68:959–960.

240. Louwsma DL, Silverman DG. Reproducibility of end tidal CO_2 measurements in sedated patients receiving supplemental O_2 by nasal cannula. Anesthesiology 1988;69:A268.

241. Dunphy JA. Accuracy of expired carbon dioxide partial pressure sampled from a nasal cannula. II. Anesthesiology 1988;68:960–961.

242. McNulty SE, Torjman M, Toy J, Seltzer JL. Correlation between arterial carbon dioxide and end tidal carbon dioxide using a nasal sampling port. Anesthesiology 1989;71:A354.

243. Mogue LR, Rantala B. Reply. J Clin Monit 1989;5:63–64.

244. McNulty SE, Roy J, Torjman M, Seltzer JL. Relationship between arterial carbon dioxide and end-tidal carbon dioxide when a nasal sampling port is used. J Clin Monit 1990;6:93–98.

245. Roth JV, Wiener LB, Barth LJ, Profeta JP. A new CO_2 sampling nasal cannula for oxygenation and capnography. Anesthesiology 1991;75:A481.

246. Witkowski TA, McNulty SE, Epstein RH. A comparison of three techniques for monitoring end-tidal CO_2 in awake sedated patients. J Clin Monit 1991;7:92.

247. Schmidt SI, Latham J. Blind oral intubation directed by capnography. J Clin Anesth 1991;3:81.

248. King H-K, Wooten DJ. Blind nasal intubation by monitoring end-tidal CO_2. Anesth Analg 1989;69:412–413.

249. Dohi S, Inomata S, Tanaka M, Ishizawa Y, Matsumiya N. End-tidal carbon dioxide monitoring during awake blind nasotracheal intubation. J Clin Anesth 1990;2:415–419.

250. Dinner M, Steuer M. Capnography as an aid to blind nasal intubation (BNI). Anesthesiology 1992;77:A469.

251. Shafieha MJ, Sit J, Kartha R, et al. End-tidal CO_2 analyzers in proper positioning of the double-lumen tube. Anesthesiology 1986;64:844–845.

252. Shankar KB, Moseley HSL, Kumar AY. Dual end-tidal CO_2 monitoring and double-lumen tubes. Can J Anaesth 1992;39:100.

253. Chang P, Johnson D, Hurst T, Reynolds B, Lang S, Mayers I. Changes in end-tidal CO_2 with bronchial occlusion and one lung canine ventilation. Anesth Analg 1991;72:S34.

254. Gandhi SK, Munshi CA, Kampine JP. Early warning sign of an accidental endobronchial intubation. A sudden drop or sudden rise in PA CO_2. Anesthesiology 1986;65:114–115.

255. Gandhi SK, Munshi CA, Coon R, Bardeen-Henschel A. Capnography for detection of endobronchial migration of an endotracheal tube. J Clin Monit 1991;7:35–38.

256. Thrush DN, Mentis SW, Downs JB. Weaning with end-tidal CO_2 and pulse oximetry. J Clin Anesth 1991;3:456–460.

257. Martin DG. Leak detection with a capnograph. Anaesthesia 1987;42:1025.

258. Lee JJ. Capnography and the Bain coaxial breathing system. Anaesthesia 1991;46:899.

259. Berman LS, Pyles ST. Capnographic detection of anaesthesia circle valve malfunctions. Can J Anaesth 1988;35:473–475.

260. Carlon GC, Ray C, Miodownik S, Kopec I, Groeger JS. Capnography in mechanically ventilated patients. Crit Care Med 1988;16:550–556.

261. Kumar AY, Bhavani-Shankar K, Moseley HS, Delph Y. Inspiratory valve malfunction in a circle system: pitfalls in capnography. Can J Anaesth 1992;39:997–999.

262. Pyles ST, Berman LS, Modell JH. Expiratory valve dysfunction in a semiclosed circle anesthesia circuit—verification by analysis of carbon dioxide waveform. Anesth Analg 1984;63:536–537.

263. Parry TM, Jewkes DA, Smith M. A sticking flutter valve. Anaesthesia 1991;46:229.

264. van Genderingen HR, Gravenstein N, van der Aa JJ, Gravenstein JS. Computer-assisted capnogram analysis. J Clin Monit 1987;3:194–200.

265. Goldman JM. Inspiratory flow rate affects inspired CO_2 concentration in the presence of a circle cir-

cuit expiratory valve leak. J Clin Monit 1992;8:176–177.

266. Anlognini J. Capnograph questioned. APSF Newslett 1990;5:21.

267. Epstein RA. The elusive "disconnect alarm" examined. APSF Newslett 1988;3:39.

268. Levins FA, Francis RI, Burnley SR. Failure to detect disconnexion by capnography. Anaesthesia 1989;44:79.

269. Fletcher R. The arterial-end-tidal CO_2 difference during cardiothoracic surgery. J Cardiothorac Anesth 1990;4:105–107.

270. Lindahl SGE, Yates AP, Hatch DJ. Relationship between invasive and noninvasive measurements of gas exchange in anesthetized infants and children. Anesthesiology 1987;66:168–175.

271. Fletcher R, Jonson B. Deadspace and the single breath test for carbon dioxide during anaesthesia and artificial ventilation. Br J Anaesth 1984;56:109–119.

272. Phan CQ, Tremper KK, Lee SE, Barker SJ. Noninvasive monitoring of carbon dioxide. A comparison of the partial pressure of transcutaneous and end-tidal carbon dioxide with the partial pressure of arterial carbon dioxide. J Clin Monit 1987;3:149–154.

273. Reid CW, Martineau RJ, Miller DR, Hull KA, Baines J, Sullivan PJ. A comparison of transcutaneous, end-tidal and arterial measurements of carbon dioxide during general anesthesia. Can J Anaesth 1992;39:31–36.

274. Shankar KB, Moseley H, Kumar Y, Vemula V. Arterial to end tidal carbon dioxide tension difference during Caesarean section anaesthesia. Anaesthesia 1986;41:698–702.

275. Shankar KB, Moseley H, Vemula V, Ramasamy M, Kumar Y. Arterial to end-tidal carbon dioxide tension difference during anaesthesia in early pregnancy. Can J Anaesth 1989;36:124–127.

276. Shankar KB, Moseley H, Kumar Y, Vemula V, Krishnan A. Arterial to end-tidal carbon dioxide tension difference during anaesthesia for tubal ligation. Anaesthesia 1987;42:482–486.

277. Takki S, Aromaa U, Kauste A. The validity and usefulness of the end-tidal pCO_2 during anaesthesia. Ann Clin Res 1972;4:278–284.

278. Valentin N, Lomholt B, Thorup M. Arterial to end tidal carbon dioxide tension difference in children under halothane anaesthesia. Can Anaesth Soc J 1982;29:12–15.

279. Whitesell R, Asiddao C, Gollman D, Jablonski J. Relationship between arterial and peak expired carbon dioxide pressure during anesthesia and factors influencing the difference. Anesth Analg 1981;60:508–512.

280. Badgwell JM, Heavner JE, May WS, Goldthorm JF, Lerman J. End-tidal PCO_2 monitoring in in-

fants and children ventilated with either a partial-rebreathing or non-rebreathing circuit. Anesthesiology 1987;66:405–410.

281. Raemer DB, Francis D, Philip JH, Gabel RA. Variation in PCO_2 between arterial blood and peak expired gas during anesthesia. Anesth Analg 1983;62:1065–1069.

282. Kaplan RF, Paulus DA. Error in sampling of exhaled gases. Anesth Analg 1983;62:955–956.

283. Bissonnette B, Lerman J. Single breath end-tidal CO_2 estimates of arterial PCO_2 in infants and children. Can J Anaesth 1989;36:110–112.

284. Gravenstein N, Lampotang S, Beneken JEW. Factors influencing capnography in the Bain circuit. J Clin Monit 1985;1:6–10.

285. Rich GF, Sullivan MP, Adams JM. Is distal sampling of end tidal CO_2 necessary in small subjects? Anesthesiology 1989;71:A1005.

286. Rich GF, Sconzo JM. Continuous end-tidal CO_2 sampling within the proximal endotracheal tube estimates arterial CO_2 tension in infants. Can J Anaesth 1991;38:201–203.

287. Halpern L, Bissonnette B. Visualizing the mixing of fresh gas and expired gas in the Mapleson D circuit. A laboratory model. Anesthesiology 1991;75:A421.

288. Halpern L, Bissonnette B. A new endotracheal tube connector for sampling end-tidal CO_2 in infants. Anesthesiology 1991;75:A930.

289. Bissonnette B, Lerman. Single breath end-tidal CO_2 estimates of arterial PCO_2 in infants and children. Can J Anaesth 1989;36:110–112.

290. Pascucci RC, Schena JA, Thompson JE. Comparison of a sidestream and mainstream capnometer in infants. Crit Care Med 1989;17:560–562.

291. From RP, Scamman FL. Ventilatory frequency influences accuracy of end-tidal CO_2 measurements. Anesth Analg 1988;67:884–886.

292. Capan LM, Ramanathan S, Sinha K, Turndorf H. Arterial to end-tidal CO_2 gradients during spontaneous breathing, intermittent positive-pressure ventilation and jet ventilation. Crit Care Med 1985;13:810–813.

293. Mortimer AJ, Cannon DP, Sykes MK. Estimation of arterial pCO_2 during high frequency jet ventilation. Br J Anaesth 1987;59:240–246.

294. Mihm FG, Feeley TW, Rodarte A. Monitoring end-tidal carbon dioxide tensions with high-frequency jet ventilation in dogs with normal lungs. Crit Care Med 1984;12:180–182.

295. Mason CJ. Single breath end-tidal pCO_2 measurement during high frequency jet ventilation in critical care patients. Anaesthesia 1986;41:1251–1254.

296. Algora-Weber A, Rubio JJ, De Villota ED, Cortes JL, Gomez D, Mosquera JM. Simple and accurate monitoring of end-tidal carbon dioxide tensions

during high-frequency jet ventilation. Crit Care Med 1986;14:895–897.

297. Paulus DA. Capnography. Int Anesthesiol Clin 1989;27:167–175.

298. Puri GD, Venkatraman R, Singh H. End-tidal CO_2 monitoring in mitral stenosis patients undergoing closed mitral commissurotomy. Anaesthesia 1991;46:494–496.

299. Burrows FA. Physiologic dead space, venous admixture, and the arterial to end-tidal carbon dioxide difference in infants and children undergoing cardiac surgery. Anesthesiology 1989;70:219–225.

300. Fletcher R. The relationship between the arterial to end-tidal PCO_2 difference and hemoglobin saturation in patients with congenital heart disease. Anesthesiology 1991;75:210–216.

301. Lazzell VA, Burrows FA. Stability of the intraoperative arterial to end-tidal carbon dioxide partial pressure difference in children with congenital heart disease. Can J Anaesth 1991;38:859–865.

302. Hatle L, Rokseth R. The arterial to end-expiratory carbon dioxide tension gradient in acute pulmonary embolism and other cardiopulmonary diseases. Chest 1974;66:352–357.

303. Niall C, Wilton MB. End-tidal pCO_2 monitoring and alveolar dead space with controlled hypotension. Anesthesiology 1984;61:A494.

304. Salem MR, Paulissian R, Joseph NJ, Ruiz J, Klowden AJ. Effect of deliberate hypotension on arterial to peak expired carbon dioxide tension difference. Anesth Analg 1988;67:S194.

305. Heneghan CPH, Scallan MJH, Branthwaite MA. End-tidal carbon dioxide during thoracotomy. Its relation to blood level in adults and children. Anaesthesia 1981;36:1017–1021.

306. Pansard JL, Cholley B, Devilliers C, Clergue F, Viars P. Variation in arterial to end-tidal CO_2 tension differences during anesthesia in the "kidney rest" lateral decubitus position. Anesth Analg 1992;75:506–510.

307. Cholley B, Pansard JL. Clergue F, Devilliers C, Viars P. Differences between $PaCO_2$ induced by the lateral decubitus position during anesthesia. Anesthesiology 1990;73:A490.

308. Fletcher R. Smoking, age and the arterial-end-tidal PCO_2 difference during anaesthesia and controlled ventilation. Acta Anaesthesiol Scand 1987;31:355–356.

309. Yamanaka MK, Sue DY. Comparison of arterial-end-tidal P_{CO2} difference and dead space/tidal volume ratio in respiratory failure. Chest 1987;92:832–835.

310. Perrin F, Perrot D, Holzapfel L, Robert D. Simultaneous variations of $PaCO_2$ in assisted ventilation. Br J Anaesth 1983;55:525–530.

311. Watkins AMC, Weindling AM. Monitoring of end

tidal CO_2 in neonatal intensive care. Arch Dis Child 1987;62:837–839.

312. Swedlow DB. Capnography—a useful clinical monitor for the anesthesiologist (ASA Refresher Course #223). New Orleans, ASA, 1987.

313. Lee TS, Wong YH, Tseng CS. Reliability of $ETCO_2$ to reflect $PACO_2$ in rabbits treated with acetazolamide. Anesthesiology 1986;65:A140.

314. Moorthy SS, Losasso AM, Wilcox J. End-tidal P CO_2 greater than $PaCO_2$. Crit Care Med 1984;12:534–535.

315. Russell GB, Graybeal JM, Strout JC. Stability of arterial to end-tidal carbon dioxide gradients during postoperative cardiorespiratory support. Can J Anaesth 1990;37:560–566.

316. Rampton AJ, Mallaiah S, Garrett CPO. Increased ventilation requirements during obstetric general anaesthesia. Br J Anaesth 1988;61:730–737.

317. Gibbs MN, Braunegg PW, Hensley FA, Larach DR. Hazard associated with CO_2 as the cooling gas during endobronchial Nd:YAG laser therapy. Anesthesiology 1988;68:966–967.

318. Bowie JR, Knox P, Downs JB. Rebreathing reduces arterial to end-tidal CO_2 gradient. Anesthesiology 1992;77:A470.

319. Steinbrook RA, Fencl V, Gabel RA, Leith DE, Weinberger SE. Reversal of arterial-to-expired CO_2 partial pressure differences during rebreathing in goats. J Appl Physiol 1983;55:736–741.

320. Brampton WJ, Watson RJ. Arterial to end-tidal carbon dioxide tension difference during laparoscopy. Anaesthesia 1990;45:210–214.

321. Ward SA. The capnogram: scope and limitations. Semin Anesth 1987;6:216–228.

322. Block FE. A carbon dioxide monitor that does not show the waveform is worthless. J Clin Monit 1988;4:213–214.

323. Hensler T, Dhamee MS. Anesthesia machine malfunction simulating spontaneous respiratory effort. J Clin Monit 1990;6:128–131.

324. Benjamin E, Kaplan JA, Iberti TJ. Expiratory sawtooth pattern or cardiogenic oscillations of the capnogram. Crit Care Med 1986;14:172.

325. Nuzzo PF. Capnography in infants and children. Perinatol Neonatol 1978;2:30, 31, 34–36.

326. Anonymous. Capnograph's role in patient monitoring. Anesth News 1981;7:8–12.

327. Bowe EA, Hyman WD, Klein EF. Carbon dioxide rebreathing during cataract surgery. Anesth Analg 1990;70:S31.

328. Good ML. Capnography. Uses, interpretation and pitfalls (ASA Refresher Course #212). New Orleans: ASA, 1989.

329. Berk AM, Pace N. Use of the capnograph to detect leaks in the anesthesia circuit. Anesthesiology 1992;77:836–837.

330. Martin M, Zupan J. Unusual end-tidal CO_2 waveform. Anesthesiology 1987;66:712–713.
331. Wallen RD. Technology implementation and performance in anesthetic gas analysis. Anesthesiology 1990;73:A518.
332. Frei FJ, Zbinden AM, Wecker H, Thomson D. Parameters influencing the response time of volatile anesthetics monitors. Int J Clin Monit Comput 1989;6:21–30.
333. Jameson LC. Are end-tidal anesthetic concentrations clinically useful? (ASA Refresher Course # 422). New Orleans: ASA, 1988.
334. Keenan RL, Boyan CP. Cardiac arrest due to anesthesia. JAMA 1985;253:2373–2377.
335. Frei FJ, Zbinden AM, Thomson DA, Rieder HU. Is the end-tidal partial pressure of isoflurane a good predictor of its arterial partial pressure? Br J Anaesth 1991;66:331–339.
336. Johnson EB. Detection of contaminated nitrous oxide. Anesthesiology 1987;66:257.
337. Matjasko J, Daffern G, Marquis B, Mackenzie C. End-tidal nitrogen and venous air embolism in dogs breathing N_2O. Anesthesiology 1985;63:A390.
338. Matjasko J, Petrozza P, Mackenzie CF. Sensitivity of end-tidal nitrogen in venous air embolism detection in dogs. Anesthesiology 1985;63:418–423.
339. Lanier WL. Intraoperative air entrainment with Ohio Modulus anesthesia machine. Anesthesiology 1986;64:266–268.
340. Matjasko J, Gunselman J, Delaney J. Mackenzie CF. Sources of nitrogen in the anesthesia circuit. Anesthesiology 1986;65:229.
341. Komatsu T, Nishiwakii K, Shimada Y. A system for automated spectral analysis of arterial blood pressure oscillation. Anesthesiol Rev 1988;15:46–49.
342. Barton F, Nunn JF. Totally closed circuit nitrous oxide/oxygen anesthesia. Br J Anaesth 1975;47:350–357.

Chapter 17

Vigilance Aids and Monitors

Part 1
Peripheral Nerve Stimulators

Muscle relaxants are employed in anesthesia for muscular relaxation and/or abolition of patient movement. Monitoring of the degree of neuromuscular block (NMB) present is accomplished by delivering an electrical stimulus near a peripheral motor nerve, causing it to depolarize. The evoked response of the muscle(s) innervated by that nerve is determined in large part by the degree of NMB present.

Advantages of Routine Use of Nerve Stimulators

Use of nerve (neuromuscular) stimulators allows determination of the state of relaxation on a minute-to-minute basis. Numerous studies have documented enormous variation in patients' responses to fixed doses of muscle relaxants. Disease states and perioperative medications can also modify the responses.

During induction, the stimulator helps to determine the onset of NMB and can be used to diagnose abnormal sensitivity to relaxants. During maintenance, the stimulator can be used as a guide to titrate the relaxant to the needs of the operative procedure so that both underdosage and overdosage of neuromuscular blocking drugs are avoided. Too deep a NMB may result in intraoperative awareness or postoperative respiratory complications and may necessitate artificial support of ventilation in the postoperative period. Underdosage may result in inadequate relaxation or undesirable patient movement. In a study on closed claims against anesthesiologists, eye injuries constituted 3% of claims (1). Patient movement during anesthesia was the mechanism of injury in 30% of those cases. Peripheral nerve stimulators were not used in any of the claims for movement under anesthesia.

At the end of a procedure, use of a stimulator allows the dose of reversal agent, if required, to be adjusted to the patient's needs and aids in assessment of the adequacy of recovery from NMB. Studies have shown that a significant percentage of patients entering the postanesthesia care unit have an unacceptable level of NMB (2–13). Such residual muscle weakness could lead to life-threatening impairment of ventilation. Although one study found that evaluation of NMB during anesthesia did not influence the total dose of relaxant used or the incidence of postoperative residual NMB (11), others have found that use of a nerve stimulator does result in less post-op residual NMB (9,12).

Peripheral nerve stimulators have been used for locating nerves for regional block (14,15). However, the current needed for stimulation of peripheral nerves is far below that needed for monitoring NMB. Stimulators with controls for both functions are available (16).

An unusual use for a stimulator was therapeutic suppression of a ventricular pacemaker (17).

Equipment

The equipment used for estimating NMB is inexpensive, easy to use, noninvasive (unless needle electrodes are used), and permits evaluation of the state of relaxation regardless of the patient's level of consciousness or cooperation.

THE STIMULATOR

The stimulator is an electronic instrument capable of delivering different types of stimuli at varying intensity at varying intervals. Several types of stimulators are shown in Figure 17.1. Desirable features include compactness, lightness, and simplicity. Controls should be large and easy to adjust. The device should be easily secured to an intravenous pole, hose tree, or anesthesia machine. For safety reasons a battery-operated stimulator with a battery check is preferred.

Current

Current, not voltage, is the determining factor in nerve stimulation. Because impedance may change, only those stimulators that maintain a constant current can ensure unchanging stimulation. Although most modern stimulators are claimed by their manufacturers to deliver a constant current, the majority do so only within a certain range of impedances (18).

To evaluate neuromuscular block properly, the current must be of adequate intensity. The force of muscle contraction is proportional to the number of activated muscle fibers. If a motor nerve is stimulated with sufficient intensity, all the muscle fibers supplied by that nerve will contract and the maximum force of contraction will be obtained. Maximal stimulation current is determined by increasing the stimulation intensity stepwise until little or no further increase in response amplitude is observed. In the clinical setting, it is customary to use stimuli of greater than maximal (supramaximal) intensity to ensure reproducible responses. Supramaximal stimulation can be ensured if the current is 2.75 times that which first produces an identifiable response, with a minimum of 20 mA (19).

While it has traditionally been taught that less than supramaximal stimulation may lead to overestimation of the level of NMB present, recent studies have shown that this is not always the case (5,20,21). Use of a submaximal current may be especially useful in patients recovering from anesthesia, because patient discomfort increases with increasing current (20,22).

Constant current stimulators are calibrated in milliamperes and deliver whatever voltage is required to achieve the set current. Currents suitable for stimulating nerves usu-

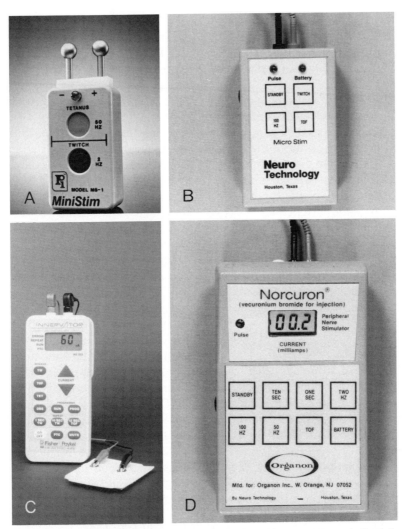

Figure 17.1. Neuromuscular stimulators. **A,** This simple device has only two patterns of stimulation: tetanus and single twitch. The delivered current cannot be varied and is not displayed. Note the metal ball electrodes. Courtesy of Professional Instruments, a subsidiary of Life Tech, Inc. **B,** This unit has three modes of stimulation: single stimulus (twitch), tetanus, and train of four. The current is varied using a rheostat at the side, but there is no display of the current being delivered. **C,** This unit has four patterns of stimulation: single twitch (available at 0.1 and 1 Hz), train of four (which can be repeated automatically every 12 sec), 50-Hz tetanus, and double burst stimulation. It also is capable of delivering the stimulus pattern for obtaining a posttetanic count. The selected current is displayed in the window. Failure to deliver this current will cause a mark to be displayed to the right of the word *error.* Note that the connections for the lead wires are of different colors. The electrodes to the side of the stimulator are specially designed for neuromuscular stimulation. **D,** This unit has three modes of stimulation: single stimulus (which can be delivered at 0.1, 1, or 2 Hz), tetanus (which is available at a frequency of 50 to 100 Hz) and TOF. Stimulus current is varied using a rheostat at the side. The delivered current is displayed in a window, to the left of which is an indicator that lights when a stimulus is being delivered. Battery status can be checked.

ally lie between 20 and 50 mA for surface electrodes and between 5 and 8 mA for needle electrodes (23,24). It is recommended that stimulators be capable of delivering at least 50 to 60 mA and that adult patients be stimulated with at least 20 mA if surface electrodes are used (19).

Display of the current is useful in alerting the user to the possibility of a disconnection, lead wire breakage, weak battery, or poorly conducting electrodes, as the current will then be reduced or absent. Some stimulators have a signal that warns when the selected current is not being delivered.

Investigations of the current output of several nerve stimulators found significant differences among the devices tested (25,26). Some delivered a lower current as impedance increased. This could produce less than supramaximal stimulation and a decreased muscular response, leading to overestimation of NMB.

Frequency

The frequency of stimuli is usually expressed in Hertz (Hz), which is 1 cycle/sec; 0.1 Hz is equal to 1 stimulus every 10 sec; and 10 Hz is 10 stimuli every 1 sec. Commonly used rates of stimulation vary from 0.1 to 100 Hz.

Frequent stimulation promotes fatigue and can lead to an increase in local blood flow, which will result in more rapid delivery of relaxant to the stimulated muscle.

Waveform

Ideally, the stimulus waveform should be rectangular and monophasic. Biphasic waves may produce repetitive stimulation, which can lead to underestimation of the degree of NMB present (27).

Duration

The duration should be as short as possible, less than 0.2 msec (27). If the duration of the pulse is over 0.5 msec, a second action potential may be triggered (28).

Patterns

Single Twitch

Single-twitch stimuli are usually delivered at a frequency of 0.1 or 1 Hz. It should not be applied more frequently than every 10 sec as this is associated with a progressively diminished response and could result in overestimation of NMB (29).

The strength of a (control) response is noted (Fig. 17.2A). The strengths of subsequent responses are then compared with the control and expressed as a percentage of the control (single-pulse or -twitch depression, $T_1\%$, $T_1:T_c$) With both a nondepolarizing and a depolarizing block, there will be progressive depression of the response as the block develops. A decrease in temperature will also cause a reduction in twitch response (30–32).

The single stimulus is useful in establishing a supramaximal stimulus and for identifying when conditions satisfactory for intubation have been achieved. It can be used (in conjunction with a tetanic stimulus) to monitor relatively deep levels of NMB (the posttetanic count, discussed below).

There are several disadvantages associated with its use. There needs to be a prerelaxant control twitch. It cannot distinguish between a depolarizing and nondepolarizing block. Most important, the presence of full-twitch height does not guarantee that full recovery from NMB has occurred (33).

Train of Four (34)

The train of four (TOF, T_4) consists of consecutive single pulses delivered at a frequency of 2 Hz for 2 sec (4 stimuli at 0.5-sec intervals) (see Fig. 17.2B). The train of four should not be repeated more frequently than every 10 to 12 sec (29). Some have recommended an interval of not less than 20 sec. Many modern stimulators do not allow train-of-four stimulation to be repeated more often.

The train-of-four pattern seen with a depolarizing block differs from that of a non-

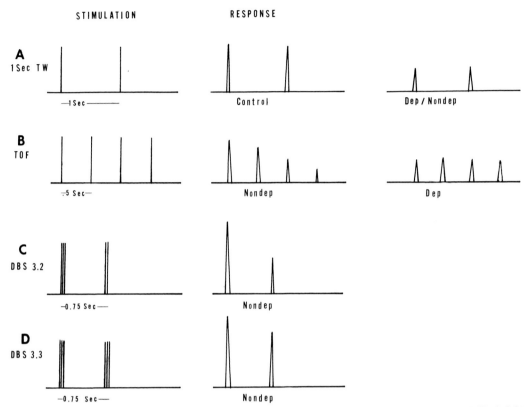

STIMULATION   RESPONSE

Figure 17.2. Patterns of stimulation and response. **A,** Single stimulus stimulation at 1 Hz (1 stimulus/sec). The height of the control twitches are noted. With either a depolarizing or a nondepolarizing block, twitch height is decreased. **B,** Train-of-four stimulation. Four successive single stimuli are delivered with 0.5-sec intervals. With a nondepolarizing block, there will be progressive depression of the response with each stimulus (fade). With a depolarizing block, the responses will be depressed equally. **C and D,** Double-burst stimulation. Three stimuli are delivered at 50 Hz, followed 0.75 sec later by two or three similar stimuli. There will be depression of the response to the second burst with a nondepolarizing block. Note the increased height of the response to the first burst compared with that seen with train-of-four stimulation.

depolarizing block (see Fig. 17.2*B*). With a depolarizing block, there is equal depression of height with all four twitches. With a nondepolarizing block, there is progressive depression of twitch height with each twitch (fade). As the block is deepened, the fourth twitch will be eliminated first, then the third, and so on (Fig. 17.3). Thus counting the number of twitches (train-of-four count or TOFC) permits quantitative assessment of a nondepolarizing block (35). With recovery or reversal of a nondepolarizing block, the TOF count increases, then fade decreases.

The train-of-four ratio (T_r, T_4 ratio, T_4:T_1, $T_r\%$, TOF ratio, TOFR) is the ratio of the magnitude of the fourth response to that of the first in a given train. It may be expressed as a percentage or a fraction. It provides an index of the degree of nondepolarizing neuromuscular block. In the absence of nondepolarizing block, the TOFR is approximately 1.0 (100%). The deeper the block, the lower the TOFR (see Fig. 17.3). A progressive decrease in TOFR is seen below a skin temperature of 32°C (30). Because TOFR requires that four twitches be present, it cannot be used to monitor deep NMB.

Accurate assessment of the TOFR may

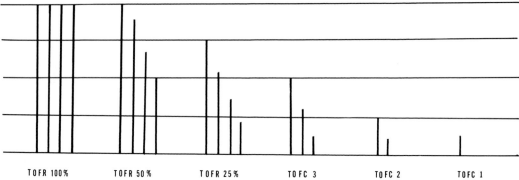

Figure 17.3.   Onset and progressive deepening of nondepolarizing block using train-of-four stimulation. When there is no NMB present, all four responses are equal. With onset of the block, there is progressive depression of twitch height with each twitch (fade). As the block progresses, the last twitch is lost and the train-of-four count is less than four.

not require a supramaximal stimulus (5,20,21). Testing at 10 mA above the lowest current at which four responses can be elicited may provide values that are consistent with those of supramaximal testing (36).

Train of four has several advantages. It is a more sensitive indicator of residual NMB than the single twitch (37). Establishment of a control is not necessary. It can distinguish between a depolarizing and a nondepolarizing block and has proved of value in detecting and following the development of a phase II block following succinylcholine administration.

The main disadvantage of train of four is that it is not possible to detect fade reliably using visual or tactile methods (38–45).

Double-Burst Stimulation (DBS)

Double-burst stimulation (minitetanus) consists of two short tetanic stimuli separated by 750 msec. Although different combinations of stimuli have been used, the two most common are $DBS_{3,3}$ and $DBS_{3,2}$. $DBS_{3,3}$ consists of a burst of three 0.2-msec impulses at 50 Hz, followed 750 msec later by an identical burst (see Fig. 17.2C). $DBS_{3,2}$ is a burst of three impulses followed by two such impulses 750 msec later (see Fig. 17.2D). DBS

may be performed reliably with submaximal stimulation (39). It should not be repeated at intervals of less than 12 sec (41).

The primary use of DBS has been to detect residual NMB. Numerous studies show that it is more sensitive than TOF for identifying fade, using visual or tactile monitoring (39–43,46–50). It also has been used for intraoperative assessment of NMB (51). Studies show a strong correlation between the TOF and $D_2:D_1$ ratios at both supramaximal and submaximal currents (52).

DBS causes more discomfort than train-of-four stimulation, but less than tetanic stimulation (22).

Tetanic Stimulation

Tetanus is a rapidly repeated stimulus. In the absence of NMB, this causes sustained contraction of the stimulated muscles. With a depolarizing block, tetanus will be depressed in amplitude but sustained. With a nondepolarizing block, tetanus is depressed in amplitude and there also is a nonsustained contraction (fade or decrement). With a profound block, there is no response to tetanic stimulation. Fade after tetanic stimulation is a more sensitive index of NMB than the single twitch, but it is not sufficiently sensitive to be used for assessing the adequacy of recovery (53). It may be better to use 100 Hz than 50 Hz when assessing residual NMB (54).

The frequency used most commonly is 50 Hz, because it stresses the neuromuscular junction to the same extent as a maximal voluntary effort. At lower frequencies, fade may not be seen when significant nondepolarizing block is present. As the frequency increases, the block appears to be more pronounced. This can lead to overestimation of the NMB present (55,56).

The duration of the tetanic stimulus is important, because it affects fade. A duration of 5 sec is standard. With a nondepolarizing block, fade is normally seen after only 1 or 2 sec.

Posttetanic facilitation (potentiation, PTF) refers to a transient augmentation of response to stimulation that follows a tetanic stimulus. It is seen with a nondepolarizing, but not a depolarizing, block and is greater with deeper NMB (57). It is maximal in about 3 sec and lasts up to 2 min following a tetanic stimulus of 50 Hz applied for 5 sec (57–60). Tetanic stimulation should not be repeated more often than every 2 min as this could lead to underestimation of the NMB. Some of the newer stimulators limit how frequently tetanic stimulation can be applied.

In situations where NMB is so profound that there is no response to single twitch or train of four, it may be possible to evaluate the block by using the posttetanic count (PTC) (61). This is performed by administering single stimuli at 1 Hz, followed by a tetanic stimulus of 50 Hz for 5 sec. After a 3-sec pause, the single-twitch stimuli at 1 Hz are repeated and the number of posttetanic responses are counted. The number of posttetanic responses increases as the depth of NMB decreases. The time to appearance of the first twitch in pretetanic train of four is inversely related to the number of posttetanic twitches present (61–65). The actual time varies among the different relaxants, being longer with longer-acting drugs.

A significant disadvantage of tetanic stim-

ulation is that it is very painful. Therefore, it should be avoided in the unanesthetized patient.

ELECTRODES

Stimulation is achieved by placing two electrodes along a nerve and passing a current through them. Stimulation can be carried out either transcutaneously using surface electrodes or percutaneously with needle electrodes.

Types

Surface Electrodes

Surface (gel, patch, pad) electrodes are disposable, pregelled electrodes that have adhesive surrounding a gelled foam pad in contact with a metal disc with a knob for attachment to the electrical lead. They are readily available, easily applied, self-adhering, noninvasive, and comfortable. The electrode-skin resistance decreases with a large conducting area, as do skin burns and pain. However, a large conducting area may make it difficult to obtain supramaximal stimulation, so it may be better to use pediatric electrodes.

Electrodes specially designed for peripheral nerve stimulation are available. These have a different thickness than ECG electrodes and chemical buffers to maintain skin surface pH. They are available in a dual-element configuration (see Fig. 17.1C).

Metal Electrodes

Some stimulators are supplied with two metal balls or plates spaced about 1 inch apart, which attach directly to the stimulator (see Fig. 17.1A) These are convenient to use, but they may not make good contact with the patient. Burns have been reported with their use (66).

Needle Electrodes

Special needle electrodes for nerve stimulators are available commercially, but ordinary metal injection needles can be used.

They should be short and thin with metal, not plastic, hubs. The needles should be placed subcutaneously. Inserting them deeper may produce direct muscle excitation and/or cause damage to the nerve. The angle of insertion should be parallel to the nerve to avoid mechanical stimulation and/or injury. There should be a few centimeters between needles. They should be held in place with tape as movement of the tips may influence monitoring.

Use of needle electrodes markedly reduces the impedance so they are useful when supramaximal stimulation cannot be achieved using surface electrodes. This usually occurs when the skin is thickened, cold, or edematous or in obese, hypothyroid, or renal-failure patients (67,68).

Although they give the best contact, they have been associated with complications (broken needles, infection, and intraneural placement). Placement in an awake patient causes discomfort. Too high a current in conjunction with needle electrodes may result in burns.

Polarity (69,70)

Stimulators produce a direct current by using one negative and one positive electrode. Maximal effect is achieved when the negative electrode is placed close to the nerve being stimulated (23,69). If the polarity of the electrodes is unknown, the connections can be reversed to determine which arrangement evokes the greater response. If the electrodes are spaced less than 5 cm apart, the effect of polarity is minimal (69).

Methods of Evaluating Evoked Responses

VISUAL

Visual assessment can be used to count the number of responses present with a train-of-four stimulus, to detect the presence of fade with TOF or DBS or posttetanic facilitation with tetanic stimulation, and to deter-

mine the posttetanic count. However, studies have shown that it is difficult to determine accurately the TOFR or to compare a single-twitch height to its control visually (39,45). Visual recognition of fade with TOF stimulation may be more accurate at lower currents (38, 39).

TACTILE (71)

Tactile monitoring is accomplished by placing the evaluator's fingertips on the muscle to be stimulated so that there is a slight preload and feeling the strength of contraction (Fig. 17.4). It is more sensitive than visual monitoring for assessing NMB using TOF (44). It can be used to determine the presence or absence of responses and/or fade with TOF, DBS, and tetanic stimulation. The posttetanic count can be determined (72). If there is a response to all four stimuli with TOF stimulation, the T_4 ratio can be estimated. However, it is difficult for even trained observers to detect fade unless the TOF ratio is below 40% (38–45). Determination of single-twitch depression also is not accurate using tactile monitoring.

MECHANOMYOGRAM (MMG)

The mechanomyogram uses a force-displacement transducer, such as a strain gauge, attached to a finger or other part of the body

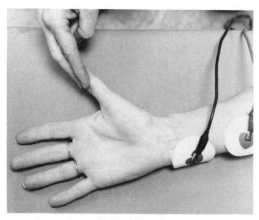

Figure 17.4. For tactile evaluation of thumb adduction, the hand is supine and a slight preload is applied.

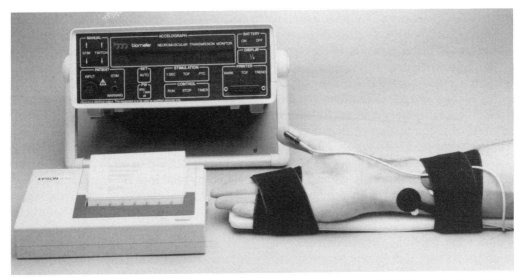

Figure 17.5. Accelerography. The piezoelectric wafer is attached to the moving part, in this case the thumb. When the thumb moves, an electrical signal proportional to the acceleration is produced. The monitor allows determination of single twitch depression, train-of-four count or ratio and/or the posttetanic count. Responses can be displayed using the printer. Courtesy of Biometer International A/S.

that will move when stimulated, to quantitate the response to nerve stimulation. The transducer converts the contractile force into an electrical signal, which is amplified and displayed on a monitor screen or recorded on a chart. Single-twitch height, response to tetanic stimulation, and the T_4 ratio can be accurately measured using a mechanomyogram.

Many mechanical monitoring devices (71,73–87) and feedback systems using mechanical monitoring (88,89) have been described in the literature.

Use of the mechanomyogram entails a number of difficulties. The devices are cumbersome and difficult to set up for stable and accurate measurements. Proper transducer orientation is essential. Small shifts in the angle of applied force can produce significant changes in the transducer output. The technique requires isometric conditions and the application of a constant preload (90).

ACCELEROGRAPHY (91,92)

A relatively new method of monitoring is based on measurement of acceleration. A pi-

ezoelectric ceramic wafer or a small aluminum rod with two electrodes is fixed to the moving part (Fig. 17.5). When the part moves, an electrical signal proportional to the acceleration is produced. This method requires less fixation of the extremity than the mechanomyogram and does not require that a preload be applied, but merely that the muscle on which the measurement is being made can move freely. This method can be used to assess NMB at the hand with the patient's arm tucked at his or her side.

Studies show a close relationship between TOF ratios measured by accelerography and the mechanomyogram (91–99) or electromyography (98,100,101).

ELECTROMYOGRAPHY (EMG) (102,103)

When a motor nerve is stimulated, a biphasic action potential is generated in each of the muscle cells it supplies, unless some degree of NMB exists. The sum of a number of these action potentials can be sensed using electrodes placed over the muscle being stimulated. The two stimulating electrodes are placed along the path of the nerve to be stimulated in the same way as for other methods of evaluating responses. For recording purposes, three electrodes, two receiving (sensing, recording) and one grounding, are used. The best signal is obtained by placing the active receiving electrode over the motor area of the muscle with the indifferent (reference) electrode over the tendon or insertion site. The grounding electrode, whose function is to decrease stimulation artifacts, should be placed between the stimulating and recording electrodes. Better results will be seen when the electrodes have been in contact with the skin for at least 15 min before calibration (cure time). Movement artifact can be minimized by simple limb fixation and applying a constant pretension to the muscle being recorded (103,104).

The evoked EMG signal is filtered, rectified, amplified, and then displayed and/or recorded at a much slower speed. Measurements may be made of the peak amplitude of the major deflection from the isoelectric line,

the sum of the amplitudes of the major positive and negative deflections, or the area under the curve (integrated EMG activity) (105). Changes in latency, duration of the action potential and the power density spectrum have been studied (106,107). The T_4 ratio can be accurately measured using the EMG.

Machines (neuromuscular transmission analyzers) that combine stimulation and evaluation functions are available (Fig. 17.6). They automatically determine the supramaximal stimulus, establish a control response, stimulate at a preselected interval, measure the response, and compare it to the control. Available features include an alarm to warn when the single pulse response exceeds a chosen value and a printer to provide a permanent record. Most have built-in safety features to warn of errors in functioning, loose connections, increased skin resistance, absence of supramaximal stimulation, etc. Most show the EMG waveform and au-

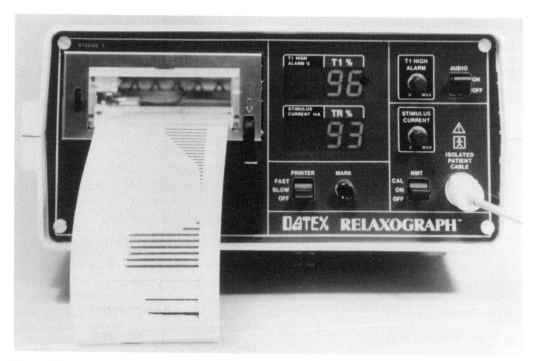

Figure 17.6. EMG monitor. The T_1%, TOF ratio, and TOF count can be measured and are displayed in the boxes to the right of the printer. Responses can be recorded using the printer. A T_1% high alarm is present. Train-of-four stimulation is performed automatically every 20 sec. Courtesy of Datex Medical Instrumentation, Inc.

tomatically adjust the gain so that the waveform occupies the full scale.

With a nondepolarizing NMB, the amplitude of the action potential is decreased and there is fade with successive responses elicited by TOF. Frequently, the amplitude does not return to 100% of control with recovery, although TOF will equal approximately 100%.

Feedback control techniques using EMG have been described (89,108–117).

A number of studies comparing evoked EMG and MMG responses have been published (89,98,110,118–135). With a nondepolarizing block, a correlation is usually seen, although the two techniques do not give identical information. With a depolarizing block, the relationship is more complex and studies show contradictory results (120,125,131,134,135).

Use of the EMG has several advantages over mechanical monitoring. It does not require a bulky apparatus near the muscle being monitored and avoids problems with transducer orientation. The stimulating and receiving electrodes can be applied before the patient enters the operating room. It can be measured from muscles that are not accessible for mechanical recording. It can be performed in small infants. The site of stimulation does not have to be accessible to anesthesia personnel. The EMG can be used to monitor intense NMB when the response to TOF is below the threshold of detection (121).

There are disadvantages to the use of the EMG. It is sensitive to electrical interference. The response may vary according to the muscle used (125). The equipment takes some care and time to set up.

Choice of Monitoring Site (136)

The site of stimulation should be away from the surgical field. If visual or tactile monitoring is to be used, the location must be accessible to the anesthesia personnel. If a muscle in an arm or leg is used, the blood pressure should be measured on a different extremity. If the patient has an upper-motor-neuron lesion, the affected extremities should not be used (137).

ULNAR NERVE

The ulnar nerve is the nerve most commonly used because of its accessibility during most surgical procedures and because of the anatomy of the muscles involved. The ulnar nerve innervates the adductor pollicis, abductor digiti quinti, and the first dorsal interosseous muscles. The force of contraction of the adductor pollicis muscle is most commonly monitored. The response is easily seen, felt, or quantified. Because this muscle is on the side of the arm opposite to the site of stimulation, there is little direct muscle stimulation, which could lead to underestimation of the NMB. For EMG monitoring, another muscle may be preferable.

The nerve can be stimulated at the wrist or elbow. Stimulation at the wrist will produce thumb adduction and flexion of the fingers. Stimulation at the elbow produces hand adduction as well, and finger movements may be falsely interpreted as a nerve-muscle response. If a mechanomyogram or electromyogram is used for measuring the response, the stimulating electrodes should be close to the wrist to limit motion of the hand. Placing the electrodes at the elbow may be preferable in children, to avoid direct muscle stimulation artifact.

At the wrist, the two electrodes are usually placed along the ulnar aspect of the distal forearm, approximately 2 cm proximal to the junction of the hand and wrist (Fig. 17.7*A*). Alternately, the positive electrode may be placed on the dorsal side of the wrist (Fig. 17.8). At the elbow, the electrodes should be placed over the sulcus of the medial epicondyle of the humerus (see Fig. 17.7*B*). Caution must be exercised to ensure that the electrodes do not cause direct ulnar nerve compression.

With other than EMG monitoring, it is important to restrict monitoring of the evoked response to thumb adduction. If the

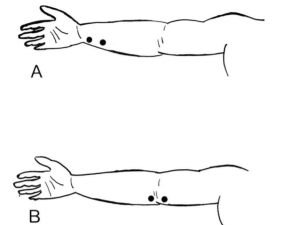

Figure 17.7. Placement of electrodes for ulnar nerve stimulation. **A,** The electrodes are placed along the ulnar aspect of the distal forearm. **B,** The electrodes are placed over the sulcus of the medial epicondyle of the humerus.

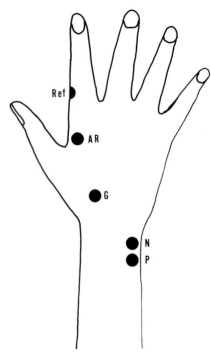

Figure 17.9. Sites for receiving electrodes for EMG monitoring with ulnar nerve stimulation and recording from the dorsal interosseous muscle. The active receiving electrode is placed in the web between the index finger and the thumb and the reference electrode, at the base of the second finger. *Ref,* reference electrode; *AR,* active receiving electrode; *G,* grounding electrode; *N,* negative-stimulating electrode; *P,* positive-stimulating electrode.

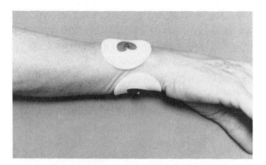

Figure 17.8. Alternate placement of electrodes for ulnar nerve stimulation. The negative electrode is placed along the ulnar aspect of the ventral side of the wrist. The positive electrode is placed on the dorsal side.

other fingers are observed, a pure indirect response cannot be guaranteed, so that the degree of NMB may be underestimated (28,125).

When EMG monitoring is used, the recording electrodes can be placed over the abductor digiti quinti (hypothenar), the adductor pollicis brevis (thenar), or the first dorsal interosseous muscle. The electrical resistance of the palm skin may vary because of the production of sweat and may be increased in manual workers because of keratinization

(138). The dorsum of the hand is less affected than the palm in both respects, so that use of the dorsal interosseous muscle may be preferred (139).

To record the reaction of the dorsal interosseous muscle, the active receiving electrode is placed in the web between the index finger and the thumb, and the other electrode is placed at the base of the second finger (Fig. 17.9). Surface electrodes are simple to fix here, are easy to maintain in position, and are seldom disturbed by hand movements (139).

For the hypothenar EMG, both electrodes are placed on the palmar side over the hypothenar eminence or the active electrode is placed on the hypothenar eminence and the

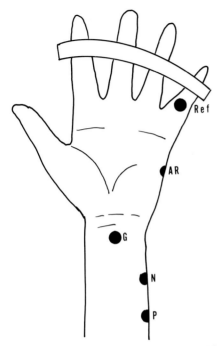

Figure 17.10. Placement of electrodes for EMG monitoring from the hypothenar eminence. The active electrode is placed over the hypothenar eminence. The reference electrode may be placed more distally on the hypothenar eminence, below the second line on the ring finger or at the base of the fifth finger as shown. *Ref,* reference electrode; *AR,* active receiving electrode; *G,* grounding electrode; *N,* negative-stimulating electrode; *P,* positive-stimulating electrode.

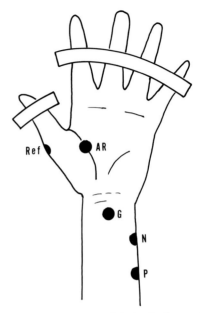

Figure 17.11. Placement of electrodes for monitoring the EMG from the thenar eminence. The active receiving electrode is placed over the thenar eminence. The reference electrode may be placed as shown here or at the proximal phalanx of the middle or index finger. *Ref,* reference electrode; *AR,* active receiving electrode; *G,* grounding electrode; *N,* negative-stimulating electrode; *P,* positive-stimulating electrode.

other below the second line on the ring finger or at the base of the dorsum of the fifth finger (Fig. 17.10) (140). Use of the hypothenar muscles has the advantage that the hand does not need to be rigidly immobilized, because there is little motion artifact (23). The belly of the hypothenar eminence is large and superficial so that the amount of tissue between muscles and recording electrodes is small, reducing the likelihood of measurement artifact (134,141). However, the short latency may produce stimulus artifact (142).

If the thenar muscle EMG is recorded, electrodes are placed on the thenar eminence and the proximal phalanx of the middle or index finger (100) or the lateral side of the base of the thumb (Fig. 17.11). Interference

caused by median nerve stimulation is often a problem. The thenar muscles are less superficial than the hypothenar ones. Abduction of the thumb with a constant pretension will bring the muscles closer to the skin and minimize movement (23,104).

MEDIAN NERVE (70)

The median nerve is larger than the ulnar, but less superficial. It can be stimulated at the wrist, by placing the electrodes medial to where the electrodes would be placed for ulnar nerve stimulation This results in thumb adduction. The EMG signal can be monitored from the thenar muscles.

POSTERIOR TIBIAL NERVE (143–145)

To stimulate the posterior tibial nerve, electrodes are placed behind the medial malleolus of the tibia and anterior to the Achilles

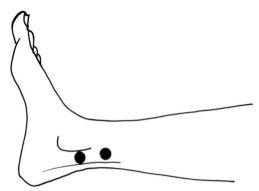

Figure 17.12. Placement of electrodes for stimulating the posterior tibial nerve. The negative electrode is placed behind the medial malleolus, anterior to the Achilles tendon. The positive electrode is placed just proximal to the negative electrode. Stimulation causes plantar flexion of the great toe.

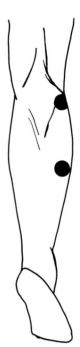

Figure 17.14. Electrode placement for stimulating the peroneal (lateral popliteal) nerve. The electrodes are placed lateral to the neck of the fibula. Stimulation causes dorsiflexion of the foot.

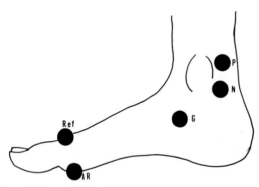

Figure 17.13. EMG monitoring using the posterior tibial nerve. The active receiving electrode is placed over the flexor hallucis brevis and the reference electrode, on the big toe. *Ref*, reference electrode; *AR*, active receiving electrode; *G*, grounding electrode; *N*, negative-stimulating electrode; *P*, positive-stimulating electrode.

tendon (Fig. 17.12). Stimulation causes plantar flexion of the big toe. If EMG monitoring is used, the receiving electrodes are placed on the flexor hallucis brevis on the plantar surface of the foot or on the intermetatarsal muscles with the reference electrode on the big toe (Fig. 17.13).

This site, rarely used, offers many advantages. It is especially useful in children, when it is difficult to find room on the arm because of other monitors or invasive lines, and when the hand is inaccessible or for other reasons

(amputation, burns, or infection) cannot be used. However, patients with peripheral vascular disease, metabolic neuropathies, or foot deformities may have poor evoked responses (146).

PERONEAL NERVE

To stimulate the peroneal (lateral popliteal) nerve, electrodes are placed near the popliteal fossa, lateral to the neck of the fibula (Fig. 17.14). Stimulation causes dorsiflexion of the foot.

FACIAL NERVE

For stimulation of the facial nerve, three configurations of electrodes have been used.

1. The negative electrode is placed just anterior to the inferior part of the ear lobe, and the other electrode is placed just posterior or inferior to the lobe (Fig. 17.15). Stimulation at this site will make it likely that muscle con-

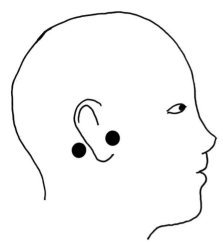

Figure 17.15. Electrode placement for stimulating the facial nerve. The negative electrode is placed anterior to the earlobe. The positive electrode is placed posterior or inferior to the earlobe.

tractions are the result of stimulation of the nerve rather than direct muscle stimulation.

2. The negative electrode is placed just anterior to the earlobe, and the positive electrode is placed over the lateral margin of the contralateral eyebrow (147). This results in direct muscle stimulation on the contralateral side and indirect stimulation on the ipsilateral side.

3. One electrode is placed lateral to and below the lateral canthus of the eye, and the other electrode is placed anterior to the earlobe (148,149) or 2 cm lateral to and above the lateral canthus (150). This placement may result in direct muscle stimulation.

The frontalis, orbicularis oculi, and corrugator muscles are observed for twitch. If the EMG is to be used, sensing electrodes are placed over the frontalis muscle. However, electromyographic activity of the frontalis muscle is affected by the level of anesthesia and may be increased with certain stimuli, making it less than ideal for monitoring. Accelerography can be used to monitor the response to stimulation of the facial nerve (151).

The facial nerve may be useful for monitoring NMB when the arms and legs are not accessible. However, the facial muscles, like the diaphragm, are relatively resistant to neuromuscular blocking drugs (148,149,151, 152). Therefore, managing NMB by stimulation of the facial nerve will result in relaxation greater than that from stimulating a limb nerve if equivalent responses are used. Great caution should be used when using facial nerve stimulation to assess recovery from NMB. The responses may show complete recovery while significant NMB is still present (8,148,153,154).

Stimulating the facial nerve is useful in detecting the onset of relaxation in the muscles of the jaw, larynx, and diaphragm.

MANDIBULAR NERVE (155)

The mandibular nerve, a branch of the trigeminal, supplies the masseter muscle. It can be stimulated by placing the negative electrode anterior and inferior to the zygomatic arch and by placing the positive electrode on the forehead. Stimulation causes closure of the jaw. The onset of NMB in this muscle is faster than in hand muscles (155–157). In adults, this muscle is more sensitive to both depolarizing and nondepolarizing drugs than the muscles of the hand (156,158). In children, the sensitivity may be equal (157).

Use

BEFORE INDUCTION

Before induction of anesthesia, the stimulator unit should be connected to surface electrodes positioned over the nerve selected. If EMG monitoring is to be used, the receiving electrodes must be placed at least 15 min before induction.

The electrode sites should be dry and free of excessive hair. An electrode should not be placed over scar tissue or any other type of lesion or an area of erythema. Proper preparation of the skin will decrease resistance. Even the best electrodes cannot stimulate well if the skin is covered by a layer of insu-

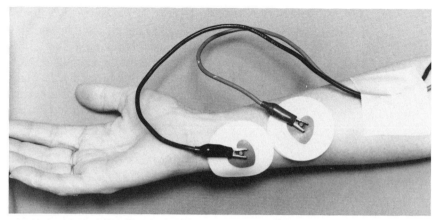

Figure 17.16. Electrodes in place. Creating loops and securing the wires with tape will decrease the likelihood that the wires will be pulled off the electrodes.

lating dead cells and oil. The skin should be wiped with a solvent (alcohol, acetone, or ether), then dried and rubbed briskly with a dry gauze pad till a slight redress is visible (159).

The electrodes should be checked to verify that the gel is moist. It is important to avoid spreading of the gel or overlap of adhesive while placing the electrodes on the skin. A gel bridge between the electrodes can short circuit them and lead to poor stimulation (23). It is a good practice when placing an electrode to press the adhesive onto the skin while avoiding pressure at the center. After the disc is secured, the center should be depressed to ensure good contact between the gel and the skin. After the wire is attached to the snap of the electrode, a piece of tape should be placed over the wire to prevent movement. It is also good practice to create a loop of the wires with tape to prevent displacement (Fig. 17.16).

INDUCTION

After induction and before administering any muscle relaxants, the stimulator should be switched on, and the clinician should feel or observe the response, as a final check on the functional integrity of the system. The stimulator should be adjusted to provide supramaximal stimulation by applying single-twitch stimuli at 0.1 Hz, and the output of the stimulator should be increased until the response shows no increase with an increase in current. Starting stimulation earlier or applying it more frequently will make it appear as if the time of onset of NMB were shorter (160–162). The same effect will result from use of train-of-four stimulation.

If a maximal stimulation is not achieved with a current of 50 to 70 mA, the electrodes should be checked for proper placement, polarity, and drying. The wire connections should be checked. If maximal stimulation still cannot be achieved, needle electrodes should be used. After maximal stimulation is achieved, the output should then be increased another 10% to 20%.

Correct EMG electrode placement should be verified by observing the quality of the evoked waveform, which should approximate a sine wave. The gain control should be adjusted so that the waveform occupies the full scale (163).

INTUBATION

The onset of NMB will occur sooner in the diaphragm and the facial, laryngeal, and jaw muscles than the hand (155,156,164,165) The diaphragm and muscles of the vocal cords and face are more resistant to neuromuscular blocking drugs than limb muscles.

On the other hand, the masseter muscle is more sensitive to relaxants than hand muscles (158,166).

Monitoring the response of the facial muscle will reflect the time of onset and the level of NMB at the airway musculature more closely than monitoring of peripheral muscles (148,149,151), which will underestimate the rate of onset of NMB in the airway musculature and may overestimate the degree of block so that a dose of relaxant sufficient to abolish response in a limb muscle may not completely block the response of the vocal cords or diaphragm (96,165,167–170). Whatever nerve it used, it is recommended that single twitch at 0.1 Hz be used and that the clinician wait until the twitch is barely perceptible before attempting laryngoscopy and intubation.

It should be kept in mind that the response to intubation is a function of both muscular block and the level of anesthesia. It is possible to intubate a patient with less-than-complete muscular paralysis if a sufficient depth of anesthesia is present.

The response to stimulation will usually disappear for a variable period of time, then appear and increase progressively to full recovery. Additional relaxants should not be given until there is evidence of some recovery to make sure the patient does not have an abnormal response. However, it is not necessary to wait for complete recovery.

MAINTENANCE

During a surgical procedure the aim of monitoring is to produce optimal paralysis and optimal recovery following anesthesia. The degree of NMB required depends on many factors, including the type of surgery, the anesthetic technique, and the level of anesthesia. It is important that the patient be kept warm, especially the peripheral areas where neuromuscular response is being monitored to avoid impairment of nerve conduction or increased skin resistance.

It is important to compare the reaction to nerve stimulation with the clinical condition of the patient, as there may be a discrepancy between the degree of relaxation of the peripheral muscles and that of the abdominal wall muscles. If the surgeon feels that relaxation is inadequate, the anesthesiologist should confirm that the depth of anesthesia is sufficient and that the nerve stimulator is working properly. With some stimulators, it may be necessary to place electrodes on the user's arm and stimulate with a low current.

Train of four is usually considered the most useful pattern for monitoring NMB during maintenance of anesthesia. With a nondepolarizing agent, fade is observed. As the block becomes deeper, the fourth twitch disappears, then progressively the third, second, and first.

With tactile or visual monitoring, the goal for most cases in which abdominal muscle relaxation is required should be to maintain at least one response to train-of-four stimulation in a peripheral nerve (171). If no response is present, further administration of relaxants is not indicated. If two responses are present, abdominal relaxation should be adequate, using balanced anesthesia (172). Presence of three twitches is usually associated with adequate relaxation if a volatile agent is used. Deeper levels of NMB may be required for upper abdominal or chest surgery or if diaphragmatic paralysis is needed. If the facial muscles are used, at least one twitch should be added to the above.

The EMG waveform decreases in both amplitude and latency during the first few minutes of anesthesia in the absence of neuromuscular blocking drugs (23,173,174). This is true of narcotic-based balanced anesthesia techniques as well as those employing volatile anesthetics. Consequently, monitoring of single twitch depression may give misleading results.

Muscle relaxants are sometimes administered in cases that do not require paralysis, such as eye surgery or laser surgery of the vocal cords, to guarantee that movement does not occur. To ensure total diaphragmatic paralysis, the NMB should be so intense that there is no response to posttetanic stimulation (175). One approach is to give a bolus of a short-acting muscle relaxant when a response appears following tetanic stimulation (176).

RECOVERY AND REVERSAL (177)

When relaxation is no longer required, administration of neuromuscular blocking drugs should be discontinued. As recovery progresses, the responses to TOF will progressively appear. As recovery progresses further, fade will disappear.

If there is residual NMB on completion of surgery, it should be reversed by the administration of an anticholinesterase, unless there are indications for the patient to remain paralyzed postoperatively. The ease of reversal of a nondepolarizing NMB is inversely related to the degree of block at the time of reversal. If at least one twitch is present, reversal will usually be successful. At deep levels of NMB (i.e., absence of response to TOF), complete antagonism may be difficult to achieve, irrespective of the dose of the reversal drug.

A considerable body of evidence exists to show that a TOFR of 70% or greater in a limb muscle on mechanomyogram indicates adequate recovery from NMB (37,73,178–181). Absence of heaviness of the eyelids, blurred vision, and difficulty in swallowing may require a higher TOFR. Unfortunately, using visual or tactile monitoring, fade with TOF stimulation can only be reliably determined up to a TOFR of about 40% (44,45). Double-burst stimulation is more reliable for detecting fade and should be used if available. However, failure to detect fade with DBS does not guarantee that the TOFR is greater than 70%. One study showed that a sustained response to tetanus at 100 Hz for 5 sec measured by MMG is correlated with a TOFR over 75% (54).

The response to single-twitch stimulation should not be used to assess recovery, because return to 100% of control can be achieved when other tests show residual NMB. Absence of fade with 50-Hz tetanic stimulation is similarly unsatisfactory (53). The facial muscles should not be used to determine the adequacy of recovery, because a satisfactory response in these muscles can be present while the TOFR in a limb muscle is significantly less and at a level at which respiratory impairment may exist (182).

If EMG monitoring is being used, residual anesthetic effects usually prevent the return of $T_1\%$ to preanesthetic reference levels (174). However, the T_4 ratio should exceed 90% (126).

If visual or tactile methods of evaluation are being used, when all four responses to train of four appear equal, it is appropriate to apply a 50-Hz tetanic stimulus (71). A sustained response and absence of posttetanic potentiation provide additional indications of the absence of significant residual NMB. However, at present, no pattern of nerve stimulation that allows visual or tactile evaluation of the response to reliably exclude residual NMB is available (174).

Irrespective of the method used to assess the adequacy of recovery from NMB, the clinician should use as many criteria as practical to ascertain the return of muscle strength to a level strong enough to provide protection of the upper airway and provide adequate ventilation (183). The criteria depend on whether the patient is awake and responds to command or asleep. Clinical criteria in an awake patient include the ability to (i) open the eyes widely on command, (ii) sustain protrusion of the tongue, (iii) sustain head lift for at least 5 sec, (iv) sustain hand grip, and (v) cough effectively. Clinical criteria in an asleep patient include an adequate tidal volume and an inspiratory force of at least 25 cm H_2O negative pressure.

POSTOPERATIVE PERIOD

Even if a nerve stimulator has not been used during an operation, it can be of diagnostic value postoperatively. A TOFR less than 70% and/or fade or posttetanic potentiation with tetanic stimulation suggest residual paralysis.

If the patient is not anesthetized, it is preferable to use less than supramaximal stimulation (20,36,52). This decreases the discomfort associated with stimulation and may improve the accuracy of visual assessment (39).

Hazards

BURNS

Burns have been reported using a stimulator with metal ball electrodes, tetanic stimulation, and the stimulator set to deliver maximal stimulation (66,184). No burns have been reported with surface electrodes, although erythema at the electrode sites may be seen (159,185). Electrodes should not overlap, as gel could diffuse between them and this could result in burns. A high current for stimulation in association with use of needle electrodes may result in burns.

PARESTHESIAS

Thumb paresthesias were reported in nine patients whose muscular function was monitored mechanically (186). Care must be taken to avoid pressure on nerves.

COMPLICATIONS ASSOCIATED WITH INVASIVE TECHNIQUES

When needle electrodes are used, possible complications include penetration of the nerve by the needle, infection, bleeding, pain, and damage to arteries or other tissues.

PAIN

Patient discomfort will be reduced by using lower currents and avoiding tetanic stimulation when the patient is awake.

REFERENCES

1. Gild WM, Posner KL, Caplan RA, Cheney FW. Eye injuries associated with anesthesia. Anesthesiology 1992;76:204–208.
2. Andersen BN, Madsen JV, Schurizek BA, Juhl B. Residual curarisation. A comparative study of atracurium and pancuronium. Acta Anaesthesiol Scand 1988;32:79–81.
3. Bevan DR, Smith CE, Donati F. Postoperative

neuromuscular blockage. A comparison between atracurium, vecuronium, and pancuronium. Anesthesiology 1988;69:272–276.
4. Beemer GH, Rozental P. Postoperative neuromuscular function. Anaesth Intensive Care 1986;14:41–45.
5. Brull SJ, Ehrenwerth J, Connelly NR, Silverman DG. Assessment of residual curarization using low-current stimulation. Can J Anaesth 1991;38:164–168.
6. Howardy-Hansen P, Rasmussen JA, Jensen BN. Residual curarization in the recovery room: atracurium versus gallamine. Acta Anaesthesiol Scand 1989;33:167–169.
7. Jensen E, Werner M, Viby-Mogensen J. Bilateral measurement (BM) of neuromuscular blockade using mechanomyography. Anesthesiology 1989;71:A822.
8. Jones KA, Lennon RL, Black S. Methods of intraoperative monitoring of neuromuscular function and residual blockade in the recovery room. Anesthesiology 1989;71:A946.
9. Hartmannsgruber M, Gravenstein N. Routine use of nerve stimulator reduces incidence of postoperative muscle weakness. J Clin Monit 1992;8:185–186.
10. Lennmarken C, Lofstrom JB. Partial curarization in the postoperative period. Acta Anaesthesiol Scand 1991;28:260–262.
11. Pedersen T, Viby-Mogensen J, Bang U, Olsen NV, Jensen E, Engboek J. Does perioperative tactile evaluation of the train-of-four response influence the frequency of postoperative residual neuromuscular blockade? Anesthesiology 1990;73:835–839.
12. Shorten GD, Ali H, Merk H. Perioperative neuromuscular monitoring and residual curarization. Br J Anaesth 1992;68:438P–439P.
13. Viby-Mogensen J, Jorgensen BC, Ording H. Residual curarization in the recovery room. Anesthesiology 1979;50:539–541.
14. Nielsen CH, Arnold DE. Performance of peripheral nerve stimulators for regional anesthesia. Anesthesiology 1989;71:A464.
15. Raj PP, Rosenblatt R, Montgomery SJ. Use of the nerve stimulator for peripheral blocks. Regional Anesth 1980;5:14–21.
16. Sansome AJ, de Courcy JG. A new dual function nerve stimulator. Anaesthesia 1989;44:494–497.
17. Ducey JP, Fincher CW, Baysinger CL. Therapeutic suppression of a permanent ventricular pacemaker using a peripheral nerve stimulator. Anesthesiology 1991;75:533–536.
18. Mylrea KC, Hameroff SR, Calkins JM, Blitt CD, Humphrey LL. Evaluation of peripheral nerve stimulators and relationship to possible errors in assessing neuromuscular blockade. Anesthesiology 1984;60:464–466.
19. Kopman AF, Lawson D. Milliamperage require-

ments for supramaximal stimulation of the ulnar nerve with surface electrodes. Anesthesiology 1984;61:83–85.

20. Brull SJ, Ehrenwerth J, Silverman DG. Stimulation with submaximal current for train-of-four monitoring. Anesthesiology 1990;72:629–632.

21. Brull SJ, Connelly NR, O'Connor TZ, Silverman DG. Consistency of accelographic train-of-four ratios at varying currents. Anesthesiology 1990;73:A867.

22. Connelly NR, Silverman DG, O,Conner TZ, Brull SJ. Subjective responses to train-of-four and double burst stimulation in awake patients. Anesth Analg 1990;70:650–653.

23. Edmonds HL Jr, Paloheimo M, Wauquier A. Computerized EMG monitoring in anesthesia and intensive care. Schoutlaan, The Netherlands: Instrumentarium Science Foundation, 1988.

24. Mehta MP, Choi WW. Monitoring of neuromuscular blockade. In: Webster JA, ed. Encyclopedia of medical devices and instrumentation. New York: Wiley, 1988:2034–2041.

25. Brull SJ, Elwood J, Ehrenwerth J, Silverman DG. Train of four assessment at various monitor currents. Anesthesiology 1988;69:A468.

26. Mylrea KC, Hameroff SR, Calkins JM, Blitt CD, Humphrey LL. Evaluation of peripheral nerve stimulators and relationship to possible errors in assessing neuromuscular blockade. Anesthesiology 1984;60:464–466.

27. Epstein RA, Wyte SR, Jackson SH, Sitter S. The electromechanical response to stimulation by the block-aid monitor. Anesthesiology 1969;30:43–47.

28. Ali HH, Miller RD. Monitoring of neuromuscular function. In: Miller RD, ed. Anesthesia. 2nd ed. New York: Churchill Livingston, 1986:871–887

29. Ali HH, Savarese JJ. Stimulus frequency and dose-response curve to *d*-tubocurarine in man. Anesthesiology 1980;52:36–39.

30. Eriksson LI, Jensen E, Viby-Mogensen, Lennmarken C. Train-of-four (TOF) response following prolonged neuromuscular monitoring. Influence of peripheral temperature. Anesthesiology 1989;71:A826.

31. Heier T, Caldwell JE, Sessler KL, Kitts JB, Miller RD. The relationship between adductor pollicis twitch tension and core, skin and muscle temperature during nitrous oxide-isoflurane anesthesia in humans. Anesthesiology 1989;71:381–384.

32. Heier T, Caldwell JE, Sessler DI, Miller RD. The effect of local surface and central cooling on adductor pollicis twitch tension using nitrous oxide/isoflurane and nitrous oxide/fentanyl anesthesia in humans. Anesthesiology 1990;72:807–811.

33. Donati F, Bevam JC, Bevan DR. Neuromuscular

blocking drugs in anaesthesia. Can Anaesth Soc J 1984;31:324–335.

34. Ali HH, Utting JE, Gray C. Stimulus frequency in the detection of neuromuscular block in humans. Br J Anaesth 1970;42:967–978.

35. Lee CM. Quantitation of competitive neuromuscular block. Anesth Analg 1975;54:649–653.

36. Silverman DG, Connelly NR, O'Connor TZ, Garcia R, Brull SJ. Accelographic train-of-four at near-threshold currents. Anesthesiology 1992;76:34–38.

37. Ali HH, Savarese JJ, Lebowitz PW, Ramsey FM. Twitch, tetanus and train-of-four as indices of recovery from nondepolarizing neuromuscular blockade. Anesthesiology 1981;54:294–297.

38. Brull SJ, Connelly NR, Sutherland D, Silverman DG. Visual assessment of fade with low intensity stimulating current. Anesthesiology 1990;73:A863.

39. Brull SJ, Silverman DG. Visual assessment of train-of-four and double burst induced fade at submaximal stimulating currents. Anesth Analg 1991;73:627–632.

40. Drenck NE, Ueda N, Olsen V, et al. Manual evaluation of residual curarization using double burst stimulation. A comparison with train-of-four. Anesthesiology 1989;70:578–581.

41. Gill SS, Donati F, Bevan DR. Clinical evaluation of double-burst stimulation. Its relationship to train-of-four stimulation. Anaesthesia 1990;45:543–548.

42. Jones KA, Lennon RL, Stensrud PE, Weber JG, Joyner MJ. Double burst stimulation assessment of nondepolarizing neuromuscular blockade. Anesthesiology 1990;73:A879.

43. Saddler JM, Bevan JC, Donati F, Bevan DR, Pinto SR. Comparison of double-burst and train-of-four stimulation to assess neuromuscular blockade in children. Anesthesiology 1990;73:401–403.

44. Tammisto I, Wirtavouri K, Linko K. Assessment of neuromuscular block: comparison of three clinical methods and evoked electromyography. Eur J Anaes 1988;5:1–8.

45. Viby-Mogensen J, Jensen NH, Engbaek J, Ording H, Skovgaard LT, Chraemmer-Jorgensen B. Tactile and visual evaluation of the response to train-of-four nerve stimulation. Anesthesiology 1985;63:440–443.

46. Ueda N, Viby-Mogensen J, Viby-Olsen N, Drenck W, Tsuda H, Muteki L. The best choice of double burst stimulation pattern for manual evaluation of neuromuscular transmission. J Anesth 1989;3:94–99.

47. Engbaek J, Ostergaard D, Viby-Mogensen J. Double burst stimulation (DBS). A new pattern of nerve stimulation to identify residual neuromuscular block. Br J Anaesth 1989;62:274–278.

48. Ddrenck NE, Ueda N, Olsen V, et al. Manual evaluation of residual curarization using double burst stimulation. A comparison with train of four. Anesthesiology 1989;71:578–581.

49. Crawford NW, Bissonnette B. Double burst characteristics of muscle relaxants in children. Anesthesiology 1991;75:A811.

50. Braude N, Vyvyan HAL, Jordan MJ. Intraoperative assessment of atracurium-induced neuromuscular block using double burst stimulation. Br J Anaesth 1991;66:403P.

51. Braude N, Vyvyan HAL, Jordan MJ. Intraoperative assessment of atracurium-induced neuromuscular block using double burst stimulation. Br J Anaesth 1991;67:574–578.

52. Brull SJ, Connelly NR, Silverman DG. Correlation of train-of-four and double burst stimulation ratios at varying amperages. Anesth Analg 1990;71:489–492.

53. Dupuis Y, Tessonnier JM. Clinical assessment of the muscular response to tetanic nerve stimulation. Can J Anaesth 1990;37:397–400.

54. Causton PR, Lennon RL, Jones KA. Assessment of residual blockade by 50 Hz and 100 Hz tetany. A comparison with train-of-four ratio. Anesth Analg 1992;74:S40.

55. Kopman AF, Epstein RH, Flashburg MH. L Use of 100-Hertz tetanus as an index of recovery from pancuronium-induced non-depolarizing neuromuscular blockade. Anesth Analg 1982;61:439–441.

56. Staanec A, Heyduk J, Stanec G, Orkin LR. Tetanic fade and post-tetanic tension in the absence of neuromuscular blocking agents in anesthetized man. Anesth Analg 1978;57:102–107.

57. Brull SJ, Connelly NR, O'Connor TZ, Silverman DG. Effect of tetanus on subsequent neuromuscular monitoring in patients receiving vecuronium. Anesthesiology 1991;74:64–70.

58. Brull SJ, Connelly NR, Halevy J, O'Connor, Ehrenwerth J, Silverman DG. Effect of tetanus on train-of-four: potentiation and time to recovery. Anesth Analg 1990;70:S38.

59. Brull SJ, Connelly NR, O'Connor TZ, Silverman DG. Effect of tetanus on subsequent double burst stimulation responses. Anesth Analg 1990;70:S40.

60. Silverman DG, Garcia RM, Grosso LM, Brull SJ. Consistency of response to tetanic stimulations at two and five-minute intervals. Anesthesiology 1992;77:A958.

61. Viby-Mogensen J, Howardy-Hansen P, Chraemmer-Jorgensen B, Ording H, Engbaek J, Nielsen A. Posttetanic count (PTC). A new method of evaluating intense nondepolarizing neuromuscular blockade. Anesthesiology 1981;55:458–461.

62. Viby-Mogensen J, Bonsu AK, Muchhal FK, Tamilarasan A, Lambourne A. Monitoring of intense neuromuscular blockade caused by atracurium. Br J Anaesth 1986;58:68S.

63. Gwinnutt CL, Meakin G. Use of the post-tetanic count to monitor recovery from intense neuromuscular blockade in children. Br J Anaesth 1988;61:547–550.

64. Eriksson LI, Lennmarken C, Staun P, Viby-Mogensen J. Use of post-tetanic count in assessment of a repetitive vecuronium-induced neuromuscular block. Br J Anaesth 1990;65:487–493.

65. Bonsu AK, Viby-Mogensen J, Fernando PUE, Muchhal K, Tamilarasan A, Lambourne A. Relationship of post-tetanic count and train-of-four response during intense neuromuscular blockade caused by atracurium. Br J Anaesth 1987;59:1089–1092.

66. Lippmann M, Feilds WA. Burns of the skin caused by a peripheral-nerve stimulator. Anesthesiology 1974;40:82–84.

67. Hunter JM, Kelly JM, Jones RS. Difficulties with neuromuscular monitoring. Anaesthesia 1985;40:916.

68. Miller LR, Benumof JL, Alexander L, Miller CA, Stein D. Completely absent response to peripheral nerve stimulation in an acutely hypothermic patient. Anesthesiology 1989;71:779–781.

69. Berger JJ, Gravenstein JS, Munson ES. Electrode polarity and peripheral nerve stimulation. Anesthesiology 1982;56:402–404.

70. Rosenberg H, Greenhow DE. Peripheral nerve stimulator performance. The influence of output polarity and electrode placement. Can Anaesth Soc J 1978;25:424–426.

71. Viby-Mogensen J. Clinical assessment of neuromuscular transmission. Br J Anaesth 1982;54:209–223.

72. Howardy-Hansen P, Viby-Mogensen J. Gottschau A, Skovgaard LT, Chraemmer-Jorgensen B, Engbaek J. Tactile evaluation of the posttetanic count (PTC). Anesthesiology 1984;60:372–374.

73. Ali H, Kitz RJ. Evaluation of recovery from nondepolarizing neuromusuclar block, using a digital neuromusuclar transmission analyzer. Preliminary report. Anesth Analg 1973;52:740–745.

74. Ali HH. A new device for monitoring force of thumb adduction. Br J Anaesth 1970;42:83–85.

75. Baraka A. Monitoring of neuromuscular transmission in anesthetized man by a bulb-transducer assembly. Anesthesiology 1973;56:402–404.

76. Brunner EA, Badola RP. A simple muscle-twitch monitor. Anesthesiology 1969;31:466–467.

77. Dundas CR, Levack ID, Brockway MS. Monitoring neuromuscular blockade. Anaesthesia 1987;42:1092–1095.

78. Karis JP, Burton LW, Karis JH. A quantitative neuromuscular blockade monitor. Anesth Analg 1980;59:308–310.

79. Nemazie AS, Kitz RJ. A quantitative technique for the evaluation of peripheral neuromuscular blockade in man. Anesthesiology 1967;28:215–217.

80. Nagle J, Perkins H, Ravin M. A simple method for monitoring twitch height. Anesthesiology 1974;41:523–524.

81. Nagashima H, Nguyen HD, Conforti M, Duncalf D, Goldiner PL, Foldes FF. A simple method for monitoring muscular relaxation during continuous infusion of vecuronium. Can J Anaesth 1988;35:134–138.

82. Pearce AC, Williams JP, Jones RM. Vecuronium for short surgical procedures in day patients. Br J Anaesth 1984;56:973–976.

83. Stanec A, Stanec G. The adductor pollicis monitor—apparatus and method for the quantitative measurement of the isometric contraction of the adductor pollicis muscle. Anesth Analg 1983;62:602–605.

84. Tahir AH. A Simple aid to monitoring muscular relaxation. Anesth Analg 1971;50:842–843.

85. Tyrell MF. The measurement of the force of thumb adduction. Anaesthesia 1969;24:626–629.

86. Walts LF. The "boomerang"—a method of recording adductor pollicis tension. Can Anaesth Soc J 1973;20:706–708.

87. Walts LF, Lebowitz M, Dillon JB. A means of recording force of thumb adduction. Anesthesiology 1968;29:1054–1055.

88. Bradlow HS, Rametti LB, Uys PC, Coetzee WP. Microcomputer-based muscle relaxation monitor and controller for clinical use. Med Biol Eng Comput 1985;23:547–555.

89. Ebert J, Carroll SK, Bradley EL. Quantitative comparison of thenar electromyographic and force displacement signals during automated vecuronium infusion. Anesthesiology 1987;67:A343.

90. Donlon JV, Savarese JJ, Ali HH. Cumulative dose-response curves for gallamine: effect of altered resting thumb tension and mode of stimulation. Anesth Analg 1979;58:377–381.

91. Jensen E, Viby-Mogensen, Bang U. The accelograph: a new neuromuscular transmission monitor. Acta Anaesth Scand 1988;32:49–52.

92. Viby-Mogensen, Jensen E, Werner M, Nielsen HK. Measurement of acceleration; a new method of monitoring neuromuscular function. Acta Anaesth Scand 1988;32:45–48.

93. Ueda N, Muteki T, Poulsen A, L-Espensen J. Clinical assessment of a new neuromuscular transmission monitoring system (Accelerograph). Jpn J Anesth 1989;3:90–93.

94. Werner MU, Jensen E, Nielsen HK, Viby-Mogensen J. Assessment of the evoked acceleration response during recovery from vecuronium and atracurium induced block. Anesthesiology 1987;67:A344.

95. Werner MU. Monitoring of neuromuscular transmission in infants and children. A comparison between an acceleration responsive transducer and a force displacement transducer. Anesthesiology 1988;69:A474.

96. Werner MU, Nielsen HK, May O, Djernes M. Assessment of neuromuscular transmission by the evoked acceleration response. Acta Anaesthesiol Scand 1988;32:395–400.

97. May O, Nielsen HK, Werner MU. The acceleration transducer—an assessment of its precision in comparison with a force displacement transducer. Acta Anaesthesiol Scand 1988;32:239–243.

98. Meretoja OA, Brown WA, Cass NM. Simultaneous monitoring of force, acceleration and electromyogram during computer-controlled infusion of atracurium in sheep. Anaesth Intensive Care 1990;18:486–489.

99. Itagaki T, Tai K, Katsumata N, Suzuki H. Comparison between a new acceleration transducer and a conventional force transducer in the evaluation of twitch responses. Acta Anaesthesiol Scand 1988;32:347–349.

100. Meretoja OA, Werner MU, Wirtavuori K, Luosto T. Comparison of thumb acceleration and thenar EMG responses in the pharmacodynamic evaluation of neuromuscular blockade. Anesthesiology 1988;69:A270.

101. Meretoja OA, Werner MU, Wirtavuori K, Luosto T. Comparison of thumb acceleration and thenar EMG in a pharmacodynamic study of alcuronium. Acta Anaesthesiol Scand 1989;33:545–548.

102. Calvey TN. Assessment of neuromuscular blockade by electromyography: a review. J R Soc Med 1984;77:56–59.

103. Sakabe T, Nakashima K. The Datex relaxograph NMT-100. Anesthesiol Rev 1990;17:45–51.

104. Paloheimo M, Edmonds HL Jr. Minimizing movement-induced changes in twitch response during integrated electromyography. In reply. Anesthesiology 1988;69:143.

105. Pugh ND, Kay B, Healy TEJ. Electromyography in anaesthesia. A comparison between two methods. Anaesthesia 1984;39:574–577.

106. Pugh ND, Harper NJN, Healy TEJ, Petts HV. Effects of atracurium and vecuronium on the latency and the duration of the negative deflection of the evoked compound action potential of the adductor pollicis. Br J Anaesth 1987;59:195–199.

107. Harper NJN, Pugh ND, Healy TEJ Petts. Changes in the power spectrum of the evoked compound action potential of the adductor pollicis with the onset of neuromuscular blockade. Br J Anaesth 1987;59:200–205.

108. Asbury AJ, Linkens DA. Clinical automatic control of neuromuscular blockade. Anaesthesia 1986;41:316–320.

109. Clutton-Brock TH, Black AMS, Huitton P. Simplified feed-back control of neuromuscular block. Br J Anaesth 1987;59:135P–136P.

110. DeVries JW, Ros HH, Booij HDJ. Infusion of vecuronium controlled by a closed-loop system. Br J Anaesth 1986;58:1100–1103.

111. Ebert J, Carroll SK, Bradley EL. Closed-loop feedback control of muscle relaxation with vecuronium in surgical patients. Anesth Analg 1986;65:S44.

112. Jaklitsch RR, Westenskow DR. Closed-loop control of neuromuscular blockade during anesthesia. J Clin Monit 1987;3:301.

113. Lampard DG, Brown WA, Cass NM, Ng KC. Computer-controlled muscle paralysis with atracurium in the sheep. Anaesth Intensive Care 1986;14:7–11.

114. Quill TJ, Reves JG, Jacobs JR, Glass PS. Automatic computer control of neuromuscular blockade. Anesthesiology 1987;67:A641.

115. Ritchie G, Ebert JP, Jannett TC, Kissin I, Sheppard LC. A microcomputer based controller for neuromusuclar block during surgery. Ann Biomed Eng 1985;13:3–15.

116. Wait CM, Goat VA, Blogg CE. Feedback control of neuromuscular blockade. A simple system for infusion of atracurium. Anaesthesia 1987;42:1212–1217.

117. Webster NR, Cohen AT. Closed-loop administration of atracurium. Anaesthesia 1987;42:1085–1091.

118. Astley BA, Katz RL, Payne JP. Electrical and mechanical responses after neuromuscular blockade with vecuronium, and subsequent antagonism with neostigmine or edrophonium. Br J Anaesth 1987;59:983–988.

119. Carter JA, Arnold R, Yate PM, Flynn PJ. Assessment of the Datex relaxograph during anaesthesia and atracurium-induced neuromuscular blockade. Br J Anaesth 1986;58:1447–1452.

120. Donati F, Bevan DR. Muscle electromechanical correlations during succinylcholine infusion. Anesth Analg 1984;63:891–894.

121. Eisenkraft JB, Pirak L, Thys DM. Monitoring neuromuscular blockade. EMG vs twitch tension. Anesth Analg 1986;65:S47.

122. Epstein RA, Epstein RM. The electromyogram and the mechanical response to indirectly stimulated muscle in anesthetized man following curarization. Anesthesiology 1973;38:212–223.

123. Eon B, Blache JL, Aknin PH, Francois G. Quantitative comparison of evoked electromyographic and mechanical responses of the adductor pollicis muscle during a regional neuromusuclar blockade technique with vecuronium. Anesthesiology 1988;69:A469.

124. Engboek J, Ostergaard D, Viby-Mogensen J, Skovgaard LT. Clinical recovery and train-of-four ratio measured mechanically and electromyographically following atracurium. Anesthesiology 1989;71:391–395.

125. Katz RL. Electromyographic and mechanical effects of suxamethonium and tubocurarine on twitch, tetanic and post-tetanic responses. Br J Anaesth 1973;45:849–859.

126. Kopman AF. The relationship of evoked electromyographic and mechanical responses following atracurium in humans. Anesthesiology 1985;63:208–211.

127. Kopman AF. The effect of resting muscle tension on the dose-effect relationship of *d*-tubocurarine; does preload influence the evoked EMG? Anesthesiology 1988;69:1003–1005.

128. Kopman AF. The relationship of evoked electromyographic and mechanical responses following atracurium in humans. Anesthesiology 1985;63:208–211.

129. Kopman AF. The dose-effect relationship of metocurine. The integrated electromyogram of the first dorsal interosseous muscle and the mechanomyogram of the adductor pollicis compared. Anesthesiology 1988;68:604–607.

130. Harper NJN, Bradshaw EG, Healy TEJ. Evoked electromyographic and mechanical responses of the adductor pollicis compared during the onset of neuromuscular blockade by atracurium or alcuronium, and during antagonism by neostigmine. Br J Anaesth 1986;58:1278–1284.

131. Shanks CA, Jarvis JE. Electromyographic and mechanical twitch responses following suxamethonium administration. Anaesth Intensive Care 1980;8:341–344.

132. Windsor JPW, Sebel PS, Flynn PJ. The neuromuscular transmission monitor. A clinical assessment and comparison with a force transducer. Anaesthesia 1985;40:146–151.

133. Weber S, Muravchick S. Does electromyography provide valid measurement of train-of-four? Anesthesiology 1985;63:A186.

134. Weber S, Muravchick S. Electrical and mechanical train-of-four responses during depolarizing and nondepolarizing neuromuscular blockade. Anesth Analg 1986;65:771–776.

135. Weber S, Muravchick S. Monitoring technique affects measurement of recovery from succinylcholine. J Clin Monit 1987;3:1–5.

136. Hudes E, Lee KC. Clinical use of peripheral nerve stimulators in anaesthesia. Can J Anaesth 1987;34:525–534.

137. Graham DH. Monitoring neuromuscular block may be unreliable in patients with upper-motor-neuron lesions. Anesthesiology 1980;52:74–75.

138. Harper NJN. Comparison of the adductor pollicis and the first dorsal interosseous muscles during

atracurium and vecuronium blockade: an electro-myographic study. Br J Anaesth 1988;61:477–478.

139. Kalli I. Effect of surface electrode position on the compound action potential evoked by ulnar nerve stimulation during isoflurane anaesthesia. Br J Anaesth 1990;65:494–499.

140. Paloheimo MPJ, Wilson RCW, Edmonds HL, Lucas LF, Triantafillou AN. Comparison of neuromuscular blockade in upper facial and hypothenar muscles. J Clin Monit 1988;4:256–260.

141. Kopman AF. Monitoring neuromuscular function. Anesthesiology 1986;64:532–533.

142. Kalli I. Effect of surface electrode positioning on the compound action potential evoked by ulnar nerve stimulation in anaesthetized infants and children. Br J Anaesth 1989;62:188–193.

143. Frank LP. But where will I put my twitch monitor? Anesth Analg 1986;65:419–425.

144. Sopher MJ, Sears DH, Walts LF. Neuromuscular function monitoring comparing the flexor hallucis brevis and adductor pollicis muscles. Anesthesiology 1988;69:129–131.

145. Theroux MC, Brandom BW, Cook DR. Neuromuscular monitoring of the flexor hallucis brevis compared with the adductor pollicis in anesthetized children. Anesth Analg 1990;70:S408.

146. Henthorn RW, Cajee RA. A neuromuscular block monitor using the toe flexors. Anesth Analg 1992;74:774.

147. Kempen PM. Clinical use of peripheral nerve stimulators. Can J Anaesth 1988;35:542.

148. Caffrey RR, Warren ML, Becker KE. Neuromuscular blockade monitoring comparing the orbicularis oculi and adductor pollicis muscles. Anesthesiology 1986;65:95–97.

149. Stiffel P, Hameroff SR, Blitt CD, Cork RC. Variability in assessment of neuromuscular blockade. Anesthesiology 1980;52:436–437.

150. Gray JA. Nerve stimulators. Anesthesiology 1975;42:231–232.

151. Ho LC, Crosby G, Sundaram P, Ronner SF, Ojemann RG. Ulnar train-of-four stimulation in predicting face movement during intracranial facial nerve stimultion. Anesth Analg 1989;69:242–244.

152. Pathak D, Sokoll MD, Barcellos W, Kumar V. A comparison of the response of hand and facial muscles to non-depolarising relaxants. Anaesthesia 1988;43:747–748.

153. Sharpe MD, Moote CA, Lam AM, Manninen PH. Comparison of integrated evoked EMG between the hypothenar and facial muscle groups following atracurium and vecuronium administration. Can J Anaesth 1991;38:318–323.

154. Sharpe MD, Moote CA, Manninen PH. Facial nerve TOF stimulation may not indicate adequate recovery of neuromuscular function. Anesth Analg 1990;70:S364.

155. Curran MJ, Ali HH, Savarese JJ, Shash AM. Comparative evoked thumb and jaw force measurement using accelerometry. Anesthesiology 1988;69:A472.

156. Plumley MH, Bevan JC, Saddler JM, Donati F, Bevan DR. Dose-related effects of succinylcholine on the adductor policis and masseter muscles in children. Can J Anaesth 1990;37:15–20.

157. Saddler JM, Bevan JC, Plumley MH, Donati F, Bevan DR. Potency of atracurium on masseter and aductor policis muscles in children. Can J Anaesth 1990;37:26–30.

158. Smith CE, Donati F, Bevan DR. Differential effects of pancuronium on masseter and adductor pollicis muscles in humans. Anesthesiology 1989;71:57–61.

159. Kopman AF. A safe surface electrode for peripheral-nerve stimulation. Anesthesiology 1976;44:343–345.

160. Brull SJ, Connelly NR, Silverman DG. Succinylcholine-induced fasciculations: correlation to loss of twitch response at different stimulation frequencies. Anesthesiology 1990;73:A868.

161. Curran MJ, Donati F, Bevin DR. Onset and recovery of atracurium and suxamethonium-induced neuromuscular blockade with simultaneous train-of-four and single twitch stimulation. Br J Anaesth 1987;59:989–994.

162. Viby-Mogensen J. Monitoring of neuromuscular blockade: technology and clinical methods. In: Agoston S, Bowman WC, eds. Muscle relaxants. 2nd ed. New York: Elsevier, 1990:141–162.

163. Zorab JSM, Bettles ND, Lynn PA, Harris D. A computerized neuromuscular blockade monitor with visual-display unit. A preliminary report. Eur J Anaesth 1984;1:85–92.

164. Smith CE, Donati F, Bevan DR. Effects of succinylcholine at the masseter and adductor pollicis muscles in adults. Anesth Analg 1989;69:158–162.

165. Donati F, Meistelman C, Plaud B. Vecuronium neuromuscular blockade at the adductor muscles of the larynx and adductor pollicis. Anesthesiology 1991;74:833–837.

166. Smith CE, Donati F, Bevan DR. Differential effects of pancuronium on masseter and adductor pollicis muscles in humans. Can J Anaesth 1988;35:S214.

167. Donati F, Antzaka C, Bevan DR. Potency of pancuronium at the diaphragm and the adductor pollicis muscle in humans. Anesthesiology 1986;65:1–5.

168. Donati F, Meistelman C, Plaud B. Vecuronium neuromuscular blockade at the diaphragm, the orbicularis oculi, and adductor pollicis muscles. Anesthesiology 1990;73:870–875.

169. Meistelman C, Plaud B, Donati F. Rocuronium (ORG 9426) neuromuscular blockade at the ad-

ductor muscles of the larynx and adductor pollicis in humans. Can J Anaesth 1992;39:665–669.

170. Waund BE, Waund DR. The margin of safey of neuromuscular transmission in the muscle of the diaphragm. Anesthesiology 1972;37:417–422.

171. Haraldsted VY, Nielsen JW, Joensen F, Dilling-Hansen B, Hasselstrom L. Infusion of vecuronium assessed by tactile evaluation of evoked thumb twitch. Br J Anaesth 1988;61:479–481.

172. Gibson FM, Mirakhur RK, Clarke RSJ, Brady MM. Quantification of train-of-four responses during recovery of block from non-depolarizing muscle relaxants. Acta Anaesth Scand 1987;31:655–657.

173. Meretoja OA, Brown TCK. Drift of the evoked thenar EMG signal. Anesthesiology 1989; 71:A825.

174. Viby-Mogensen J. Clinical measurement of neuromuscular function: an update. Clin Anesthesiol 1985;3(2):467–482.

175. Fernando PUE, Viby-Mogensen J, Bonsu AK, Tamilarasan A, Muchhal KK, Lamabourne A. Relationship between posttetanic count and response to carinal stimulation during vecuronium-induced neuromuscular blockade. Acta Anaesthesiol Scand 1987;31:593–596.

176. Salathe M, Johr M. Use of post-tetanic train-of-four for evaluation of intense neuromuscular blockade with atracurium. Br J Anaesth 1988;61:123.

177. Bevan DR, Donati F, Kopman AF. Reversal of neuromuscular blockade. Anesthesiology 1992;77:785–805.

178. Ali HH, Wilson RS, Savarese JJ, Kitz RJ. The effect of tubocurarine on indirectly elicited train-of-four muscle response and respiratory measurements in humans. Br J Anaesth 1975;47:570–574.

179. Ali HH, Savarese JJ. Monitoring of neuromuscular function. Anesthesiology 1976;45:216–245.

180. Brand JB, Cullen DJ, Wilson NE, Ali HH. Spontaneous recovery from nondepolarizing neuromuscular block correlation between clinical and evoked responses. Anesth Analg 1977;56:55–58.

181. Sharpe MD, Lam AM, Nicholas FJ, Chung DC, Merchant R, Alyafi W, Beauchamp RJ. Correlation between integrated evoked EMG and respiratory function following atracurium administration. Anesthesiology 1987;67:A608.

182. Sharpe MD, Lam AM, Merchant R, Manninen PH. Monitoring of neuromuscular function from the facial muscle and hypothenar muscle—an electromyographical evaluation. Can J Anaesth 1988;35:S119–S120.

183. Ali HH. Monitoring neuromuscular function. Semin Anesth 1989;8:158–168.

184. Myyra R, Dalpra M, Globerson J. Electrical erythema? Anesthesiology 1988;69:440.

185. Pue AF. Disposable EKG pads for peripheral nerve stimulation. Anesthesiology 1976;45:107–108.

186. Sia RL, Straatman NJA. Thumb paresthesia after neuromuscular twitch monitoring. Anaesthesia 1985;40:167–169.

Part 2
Temperature Monitoring

Under general anesthesia a patient loses his or her usual mechanisms for regulating body temperature. Numerous studies have shown that significant temperature changes routinely occur in anesthetized patients

Indications (1–3)

The monitoring guidelines of the American Society of Anesthesiologists state that there shall be a readily available means to measure continuously the patient's temperature. When changes in body temperature are intended, anticipated, or suspected, the temperature shall be measured (4,5).

Monitoring of temperature during all general anesthetics has been advocated by many to facilitate detection of malignant hyperthermia and quantify hyperthermia and hypothermia (2). It should be performed whenever large volumes of cold blood and/or intravenous fluids are administered, when the patient is deliberately cooled and/or warmed, for pediatric surgery of substantial duration, and in hypothermic or pyrexial patients or those with a suspected or known temperature regulatory problem such as malignant hyperthermia. Major surgical procedures, especially those involving body cavities, should be considered a strong indication for temperature monitoring.

Because malignant hyperthermia and severe thermal disturbances are rare during regional or monitored anesthesia, temperature monitoring is usually unnecessary during these procedures (2).

Instruments

A temperature-measuring device functions by using matter with a property (electrical resistance or potential, light direction) that varies with temperature.

Many thermometers simply display the temperature. These are less than optimal, because if a high or low temperature is displayed, it may go unnoticed for some time. Devices with adjustable audible and visual alarms for both high and low temperatures are more satisfactory. Those that are battery powered should have a means to indicate when battery power is low. Trend indicators are available on some instruments.

THERMISTOR

A thermistor is a semiconductive substance whose electrical resistance varies with temperature. In addition to the thermistor, there must be a source of current and a device to measure the current so that the resistance can be converted into a temperature.

Advantages of thermistors include small size of sensors, rapid response, continuous readings, capability of remote readings, and sensitivity to small changes in temperature. They are fairly inexpensive. Probes can be made interchangeable and disposable. Most clinical thermistors have an accuracy of 0.1° to 0.3°C (6–8).

There are disadvantages, however. The resistance gradually increases with age and will change if it is subjected to rapid or large changes of temperature so that recalibration is required. The resistance of a batch of thermistors tends to vary.

THERMOCOUPLE

A thermocouple is the juxtaposition of dissimilar metals. A small difference in electrical potential exists across this junction. This difference varies directly with the temperature. The junctions are united by soldering or welding. There needs to be a source of current and a means to measure the current.

Advantages of thermocouples include accuracy, small size, rapid response, continuous readings, stability, capability of remote reading, and interchangeability of probes. Most clinical thermocouples have an accuracy of approximately 0.1°C (6,8). The materials are inexpensive so that sensor probes can be made disposable.

PLATINUM WIRE (9)

The electrical resistance of platinum wire varies almost linearly with temperature. By employing wire of an extremely small diameter, rapid thermal equilibration occurs. The resistance is measured in a manner similar to a thermistor.

These thermometers are accurate and give continuous readings. Newer models have been made small enough for clinical use. Probes can be made interchangeable.

If a probe with a thermocouple, thermistor, or platinum wire is to be used inside the body, it must be ensheathed in an insulating material so it does not get wet. The end of the probe designed to be inserted into the patient is sealed, and the electrical connection is

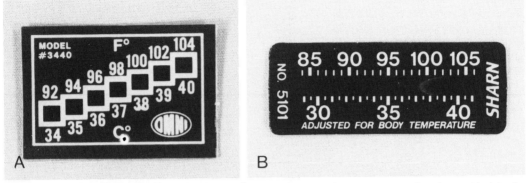

Figure 17.17. The flexible adhesive-backed strips of these liquid-crystal temperature monitors have a black background. To use, the covering over the adhesive is removed, and the monitor is placed on the skin.

made at the other end. The connections need to be kept dry. If one becomes wet, spurious readings can result (7,10,11).

LIQUID CRYSTAL (12,13)

Certain organic compounds in the thermal transformation from solid to liquid state, pass through an intermediate phase that exhibits anisotropic (optically active) properties. The term *liquid crystal state* was coined to describe this phenomenon. When light is shown on such material, crystals at a certain temperature scatter some of the light, producing iridescent colors. The remaining portion of the incident light is transmitted by the crystals. By encapsulating the liquid crystals, the colors form letters and numbers. An absorptive black background prevents reflection of the transmitted light and enhances the resolution of the colors.

Liquid crystal temperature monitors are shown in Figure 17.17. Each consists of a flexible adhesive-backed strip or disc with plastic-encased liquid crystals on a black background. To use, the covering over the adhesive is removed and the disc or strip is placed on the skin. Temperature displayed on these is lower than internal temperature. To compensate for this, some of these devices have a built-in measurement offset (see Fig. 17.17*B*) so that the temperature displayed approximates the temperature at an-

other site in the body. Others have another scale to indicate that temperature (14).

Liquid crystal thermometers have a number of advantages. They are convenient, atraumatic, easy to apply and read, noninvasive, unbreakable, disposable, comfortable for the patient, and inexpensive. They also give fast, continuous readings and involve no electronics, wire, or monitor box. They can be applied before induction and are easily transferred to the recovery area with the patient.

Disadvantages include the need for subjective observer interpretation and the inability to interface with a recording system; they are less accurate than other devices. Extremes of ambient temperature, humidity, and air movement can introduce inaccuracy. They are capable of measuring temperature only on the skin. If left in the sun for an extended period, an error indicating hyperthermia can be induced. Freezing the device causes destruction so that all numbers are visible at once (15). Infrared heating lamps may heat the liquid crystal device directly and cause erroneously elevated readings (13).

INFRARED THERMOMETER (16,17)

The infrared thermometer is a noninvasive device that senses the infrared radiation emitted by a warm object such as the tympanic membrane or ear canal. The measure-

Figure 17.18. The infrared thermometer's probe is inserted into the external ear canal.

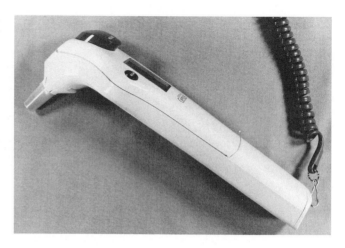

ment is based on the difference between the thermometer's temperature and the temperature of the target. The instrument has an otoscope-like probe (Fig. 17.18). Disposable plastic probe covers are used to preserve hygiene and prevent cerumen buildup on the probe.

Temperatures between 15.5° and 43.3°C can be measured (18). One study showed this device had an accuracy of 0.1°C between 34.0° and 39.5°C (19). Other studies have shown slightly less accuracy (20). It provides a reading in a few seconds.

Because the device does not contact any surface, there should be no trauma associated with its use. These devices are well-tolerated by sleeping or drowsy patients (17). They may offer a more comfortable and less stressful method of temperature monitoring for both patients and healthcare workers, especially compared with rectal temperature probes. A study of two models found that they were stable over a wide range of both patient and ambient temperatures (17).

Disadvantages include the fact that temperature measurement is intermittent. The viewing angle includes both the tympanic membrane and the walls of the ear canal. Poor penetration, improper aiming, and obstructions such as curvatures of the ear canal will result in significantly lower temperatures. Many infrared ear thermometers have

offsets to correct for these factors (16,20). By adding different constants to the temperature measured, the device displays the temperature as if it had been measured simultaneously from a different site in the body.

Sites

There are a number of body sites at which temperature can be monitored. Temperature can vary considerably in different parts of the body at any time as a result of changes in the amount of heat generated or lost. Sites differ in the precision with which they reflect core temperature. The core or deep body thermal compartment is composed of well-perfused tissues in which the temperature is uniform, is relatively resistant to external influences, and reflects the mean temperature of the body's vital organs, e.g., brain, heart, lungs, and viscera. Many believe that true core temperature should be regarded as that of the hypothalamus, because the control center for temperature regulation is located there (2). The accuracy with which a site reflects core temperature may depend on the rate of temperature change. A site that reflects core temperature accurately when temperature change is slow, may fail to reflect rapid changes, such as are seen with cardiac surgery.

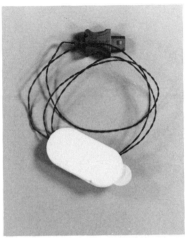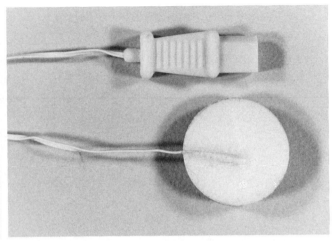

Figure 17.19. These disposable probes for measuring skin temperature stick onto the skin. Note the thermocouple near the surface of the probe to the *right* and the backing that insulates the sensor from ambient conditions.

The site chosen for temperature monitoring should depend on the surgical procedure planned and the reason for temperature monitoring. The site should be convenient and have a fairly consistent temperature gradient between it and a core site. The correlation between temperatures measured at the site and core temperature becomes more important if rapid warming or cooling is anticipated.

SKIN

Skin temperature can be measured by liquid crystal devices or flat metal discs containing thermocouples or thermistors (Fig. 17.19). Some skin probes have a special backing to insulate the sensor from ambient conditions and may have a coating to reflect radiant heat and light. Use of an opaque dressing and/or tape over the sensor may decrease the effect of environmental factors on the reading.

Skin temperature is most commonly measured at the forehead, because this site has a fairly good blood flow and there is not much underlying fat. The back, chest, anterior abdominal wall, fingers, toes, and the inside of the elbow have also been used.

Skin temperature is useful in evaluating the quality of a sympathetic block. A rise in

temperature is an indication that the block is successful. Another use is in microsurgery. An increase in skin temperature may indicate that flow to that area has been successfully reestablished.

Many investigations have confirmed that skin temperature does not accurately reflect core temperature and the difference between skin and core temperatures may vary unpredictably during anesthesia (6,12,21–27). Readings are affected by room temperature and the adequacy of skin perfusion. When these factors are constant, skin temperature correlates modestly with core temperature, and it may be useful as a trend indicator.

Although it has been recommended as a screening device for malignant hyperthermia (28), its usefulness for this purpose has been questioned, as cutaneous vasoconstriction may occur with this syndrome (24,29).

Monitoring skin temperature carries few risks, and the site is easily accessible. It may be useful in situations in which other means of obtaining a temperature cannot be used.

AXILLA

To measure axillary temperature, the probe should be positioned carefully over the axillary artery (6). The arm should be adducted. Equilibration may take 10 to 15 min

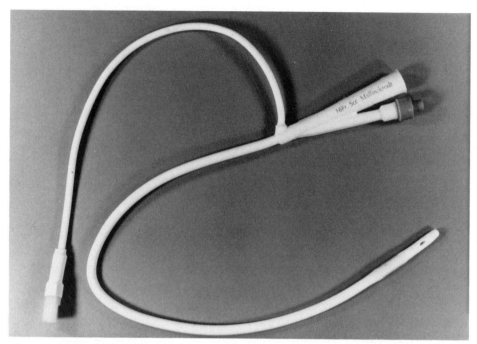

Figure 17.20. Urinary catheter with temperature sensor near the patient end.

(29). It should not be used on the same side as a blood pressure cuff on the upper arm.

Axillary temperature is convenient, noninvasive, and carries little risk. It is most frequently used on infants, especially neonates, because the patient's small size makes other methods difficult to use and the greater surface vasculature of these patients makes them relatively uniform in temperature (16). This site has been rated by nurses as more acceptable to toddlers than other sites (30).

Axillary temperature readings are influenced by contact with the probe, skin perfusion, and proximity of the probe to the axillary artery. Studies differ on how well temperatures measured at this site relate to core temperatures with some showing good (6,25) and some poor (27,31–35) correlation.

NASOPHARYNX

Temperature measurement in the nasopharynx is made with the sensor in contact with the posterior nasopharyngeal wall. This position should put it close to the hypothalamus. Readings taken with a probe in this position are normally not affected by the temperature of the inspired gases (36) but may be if there is leakage of gases around the tracheal tube (37). Although some studies show that the correlation with core temperature is good (23,27,32), another showed readings taken at this site were not reliable (37).

This site cannot be used in unintubated patients. Epistaxis may follow insertion of the probe.

URINARY BLADDER

Urinary catheters with a temperature sensor near the patient end are available (Fig. 17.20). This method of measurement is useful in patients who will need a urinary catheter during the postoperative period.

The temperature of the urinary bladder usually correlates well with temperatures measured by tympanic membrane, pulmonary artery, and esophageal sensors, but it may lag behind during rapid warming or cooling (20,23,25–27,38–42). The correlation will be increased with a high rate of urine flow (40).

This site cannot be used during genitouri-

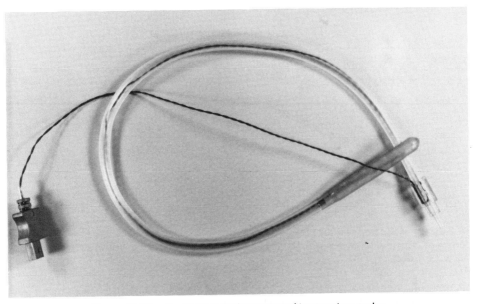

Figure 17.21. Esophageal stethoscope and temperature probe.

nary procedures. Manipulation of the bladder during pelvic surgery may affect the reading (41).

ESOPHAGUS

Measurement of esophageal temperature can be accomplished either with a simple probe, with a esophageal stethoscope that has a temperature sensor (Fig 17.21), or with a gastric tube with the tip of the probe incorporated some distance from the end of the tube (43).

Esophageal temperature should be measured with the sensor located in the lower third or fourth of the esophagus (retrocardiac esophagus) (44). At this depth, the esophagus lies between the heart and the descending aorta. Placement in this position will minimize (but not completely eliminate) the effect of the temperature of inspired gases (6). If the probe is placed higher in the esophagus, the reading may be affected by inspired gases and will be lower than readings obtained when the probe is correctly positioned (37,44–48). If the probe is placed in the stomach, it may record temperatures several degrees higher than core temperature, reflecting liver metabolism; also, response time to

changes in thermal balance is slow with the probe in this position.

The probe is most accurately placed by using an electrocardiographic lead built into the probe (49). The positive lead is attached to the esophageal probe and the negative lead to the right shoulder. A biphasic P wave indicates that the probe tip is at the midatrial level.

In adults, the ideal position is approximately 38 to 46 cm below the central incisors (48), 24 cm below the larynx (44,45), and 45 cm from the nostril (50). In children, the ideal distance in centimeters below the corniculate cartilages is approximated by the following formula (46):

$$10 + (2 \times \text{age in years})/3 \text{ cm}$$

No formula for calculating the distance of insertion of esophageal probes can be expected to give a constant level in every case, so it is advisable to record temperatures up to 2 cm above and below the estimated level before fixing it in place.

When the sensor is part of an esophageal stethoscope, one method of placement is to locate the point of maximum breath and heart sounds. However, studies have shown

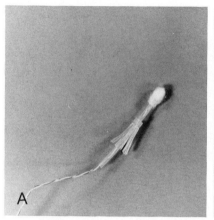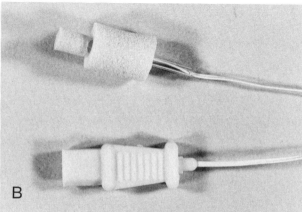

Figure 17.22. Tympanic membrane temperature probes. The sensor is encased in soft foam. **A,** The feather holds the probe in place; it can be moved along the probe. **B,** A piece of soft foam that can be moved along the probe helps to hold the probe in place.

that this method does not place the probe in the correct position (48,51). Measurements of esophageal temperature most closely resembled core temperature when the probe is placed 12 to 16 cm beyond the site of best sounds.

Esophageal temperature has been determined to follow quantitatively and quickly (lag time 80 sec) temperature changes in the pulmonary artery (52). The esophagus is easily accessible during most general anesthesia.

Contraindications to use of an esophageal probe include procedures on the face, oral cavity, nose, airway, or esophagus. It can be used only in intubated patients. It is uncomfortable and poorly tolerated by awake patients, making it useful only in patients under general anesthesia. Correct placement may be difficult and probes may become displaced during intubation, extubation, or intrathoracic or abdominal surgery (53). Esophageal temperatures are unreliable during rapid transfusion of cold blood or fluids and during thoracic and upper abdominal surgery.

When an esophageal probe is used with the patient in the sitting or prone position, oral secretions can track down the leads of the probe to the connection between the probe and monitor cable. This can lead to falsely elevated readings (7).

TYMPANIC MEMBRANE

Research has shown that the central thermoregulatory center is in the hypothalamus. Its main blood supply is the internal carotid artery. The anatomical position of the tympanic membrane deep within the skull and separated from the internal carotid by only the narrow air-filled cleft of the middle ear and a thin shell of bone and its ready accessibility during most surgical procedures make it an attractive site for temperature measurements (54,50).

Contact Type

The temperature of the tympanic membrane can be measured by inserting a thermistor probe into the external auditory canal until it contacts the tympanic membrane. If the probe does not touch the membrane, the reading will not be accurate (55).

Tympanic membrane temperature probes are shown in Fig. 17.22. The sensor is enclosed in soft foam. It usually has a widened segment, piece of foam, or a feather or barb to hold it in place after insertion. The proper placement technique is to pull down the ear lobe and gently insert the probe with a twisting motion until the resistance of the tympanic membrane is encountered (56). The meter reading should stabilize quickly. If it does not, the probe should be slowly advanced until the reading stabilizes.

Numerous studies have shown a close correlation with temperature measured at the esophagus or pulmonary artery (6,27,50, 53,57–59). However, during passive hyperthermia, tympanic temperature may be lower than pulmonary artery and esophageal temperatures (52). Fanning the face will reduce the tympanic temperature but not the temperature in the brain (60). Readings can be rendered inaccurate by cerumen (61).

Advantages include cleanliness and convenience. The site is readily accessible in most cases. Probe placement is simple. It is tolerated by conscious patients, making it useful for postoperative monitoring.

Complications have been reported. Oozing from the ear was noted in two patients in whom large probes were used (58). Trauma to the external auditory canal with subsequent otitis externa has been reported (50). Perforation of the membrane has been reported (56,62). Methods to avoid trauma include otoscopic inspection of the canal and drum before insertion, stopping insertion as soon as resistance is felt, and placement in awake patients. Extra care should be taken to make sure the probe is not pushed into the canal when the head is moved.

Contraindications include any abnormality of the ear that would prevent correct placement, a skull fracture that passes through the osseous meatus, and perforation of the membrane (54).

Infrared

Infrared temperature measurement is performed by inserting an otoscope-like probe into the external ear canal. A reading can be obtained in only a few seconds.

Studies comparing temperatures measured by this method with those from other sites show contradictory results (17–20,30,63–70). Acute otitis media did not influence the reading in three studies (67,68,71) but did in another (72). Interference by cerumen should not affect readings,

because ear wax is reported to be essentially transparent to infrared energy (71).

Infrared ear probes do not contact the tympanic membrane so trauma is not a problem. They allow rapid measurement of temperature with minimal disturbance.

PULMONARY ARTERY

Pulmonary artery temperatures can be recorded in patients who have a pulmonary artery catheter in place. This gives an accurate measure of the temperature of mixed venous blood. For this reason, many consider this the gold standard among sites to monitor temperature. Pulmonary artery temperature correlates well with brain temperature even with rapid cooling and rewarming (32). Unfortunately, it is available only in those patients for whom a Swan-Ganz catheter is required as part of their care.

ORAL CAVITY

Oral temperature is measured by placing a probe in one of the sublingual pockets on either side of the frenulum of the tongue. Probe placement is critical; the temperature of the sublingual pockets can vary significantly from tissues just a few centimeters away (16). Studies have found that oral temperatures were 0.02° to 1.1°C less than those measured in the pulmonary artery (25,73).

RECTUM

In the past, measurement of rectal temperature was commonly performed during anesthesia. However, this is a peripheral site and often poorly reflects core temperature.

Rectal temperature is commonly higher than core temperature, probably because of heating by fecal microorganisms (19,27,32,53,74). It is affected by blood returning from the lower limbs. Changes in temperature at this site tend to lag behind those at other sites because of the areas low blood flow and the presence of rectal contents that form a thermal reservoir (23,32,40,52,58). Although a few studies have found this site reflected core temperature (6,25,27), most investigations have found otherwise (23,35,40,53,75).

This method is not applicable in surgery involving the rectum and most surgery involving the lower pelvic region. Furthermore, it is generally disliked by patients as uncomfortable, hospital personnel as cumbersome, and both as aesthetically objectionable. The probes are prone to extrusion during recovery.

Contraindications include obstetric, gynecologic, and urologic procedures. The readings will be affected by peritoneal lavage and cystoscopy. Bowel perforation is a risk. A pararectal abscess has been reported associated with its use (76).

Use

Reusable probes must be thoroughly cleaned and disinfected between uses. They are subject to wear and tear and must be checked before use.

If the thermometer has a range that includes normal operating room temperature, an attached probe reading air temperature allows a one-point calibration check. When unexpected and extreme temperature readings are made, the accuracy should be verified by another means.

It is important that the connection between the probe and the cable be kept dry to avoid incorrect readings (7,10). Use of waterproof tape is recommended.

Hazards of Thermometry

DAMAGE TO THE MONITORING SITE

There are reports of tympanic membrane perforation and trauma to the external auditory canal following use (50,56,58,62). The rectum and esophagus can also be damaged (76). Epistaxis may occur with a nasopharyngeal probe. Temperature-sensing thermo-

couple wires may protrude from the tip of the probe (77).

BURNS (78–80)

Burns can occur at the site of a temperature probe when the probe acts as a ground for the electrosurgical apparatus. Although the probes are insulated, no insulation can completely block radiofrequency currents, and if there is no other satisfactory return path, the current can burn through insulation (81). Electrosurgical apparatus should have proper safeguards to ensure proper return of current. Temperature probes should be examined before use to detect damage to the insulation. A technique to avoid esophageal burns is to insert the probe into the esophagus via a small tracheal tube (82). The probe may be pulled back into the tube during periods of maximal electrical activity.

A burn associated with temperature monitoring during magnetic resonance imaging has been reported (83). This occurred with a probe designed for use during MRI.

FALSE INFORMATION

A faulty probe can cause an incorrect temperature to be displayed (84,85). Secretions or fluids in the connection between the temperature probe and the reading instrument can result in falsely elevated readings (7,10).

REFERENCES

1. Holloway AM. Monitoring and controlling temperature. Anaesth Intensive Care 1988;16:44–47.
2. Sessler DI. Temperature monitoring should be routine during general anesthesia. Anesthesiol Rev 1992;19:40–43.
3. Kaplan RF. Temperature monitoring need not be done routinely during general anesthesia. Anesthesiol Rev 1992;19:43–46.
4. Anonymous. Standards for basic intra-operative monitoring. APSF Newslett 1987;2:3.
5. Eichorn JH, Cooper JB, Cullen DJ, Maier WR, Philip JH, Seeman RG. Standards for patient monitoring during anesthesia at Harvard Medical School. JAMA 1986;256:1017–1020.
6. Bissonnette B, Sessler KI, LaFlamme P. Intraoperative temperature monitoring sites in infants and

children and the effect of inspired gas warming on esophageal temperature. Anesth Analg 1989;69:192–196.

7. Berman MF. The susceptibility of thermistor-based esophageal temperature probes to errors caused by electrically conductive fluids ("artificial saliva"). J Clin Monit 1992;8:107–110.

8. Imrie MM, Hall GM. Body temperature and anaesthesia. Br J Anaesth 1990;64:346–354.

9. Cliffe P. The measurement of temperature. Anaesthesia 1962;17:215–237.

10. Berman MF. An unusual cause of misleading temperature readings. Anesthesiology 1990;72:208.

11. Wiegert PE. An unusual cause of misleading temperature readings. Anesthesiology 1990;72:208.

12. Burgess GE, Cooper JR, Marino RJ, Peuler MJ. Continuous monitoring of skin temperature using a liquid-crystal thermometer during anesthesia. South Med J 1978;71:516–518.

13. Bjoraker DG. Liquid crystal temperature indicators. Anesthesiol Rev 1990;17:50–56.

14. Shomaker TS, Bjoraker DG. Measurement offset with liquid crystal temperature indicators. Anesthesiology 1990;73:A425.

15. Enright CF. Colorful thermometers. ASTM Stand News, March 1986.

16. Anonymous. Infrared thermometers. An earful of innovation. Technol Anesth 1992;12:1–7.

17. Weiss ME, Pue AF, Smith J III. Laboratory and hospital testing of new infrared tympanic thermometers. J Clin Eng 1991;16:137–144.

18. Ward L, Kaplan RM, Paris PM. A comparison of tympanic and rectal temperatures in the emergency department. Ann Emerg Med 1988;17:198.

19. Shinozaki T, Deane R, Perkins FW. Infrared tympanic thermometer. Evaluation of a new clinical thermometer. Crit Care Med 1988;16:148–150.

20. Nierman DM. Core temperature measurement in the intensive care unit. Crit Care Med 1991;19:818–823.

21. Lacoumenta S, Hall GM. Liquid crystal thermometry during anaesthesia. Anaesthesia 1984;39:54–56.

22. Leon JE, Bissonnette B, Lerman J. Liquid crystalline temperature monitoring: does it estimate core temperature in anaesthetized paediatric patients? Can J Anaesth 1990;37:S98.

23. Moorthy SS, Winn BA, Jallard MS, Edwards K, Smith ND. Monitoring urinary bladder temperature. Heart Lung 1985;14:90–93.

24. Vaughan MS, Cork RC, Vaughan RW. Inaccuracy of liquid crystal thermometry to identify core temperature trends in postoperative adults. Anesth Analg 1982;61:284–287.

25. Ilsley AH, Rutten AJ, Runciman WB. An evaluation of body temperature measurement. Anaesth Intensive Care 1983;11:31–39.

26. Earp JK, Finlayson DC. Urinary bladder/pulmonary artery temperature ratio of less than 1 and shivering in cardiac surgical patients. Am J Crit Care 1992;1:43–52,

27. Cork RC, Vaughan RW, Humphrey LS. Precision and accuracy of intraoperative temperature monitoring. Anesth Analg 1983;62:211–214.

28. Lees DE, Schuette W, Bull JM, Whang-Peng J, Atkinson ER, Macnamara TE. An evaluation of liquid-crystal thermometry as a screening device for intraoperative hyperthermia. Anesth Analg 1978;57:669–674.

29. Sladen RM. Temperature regulation and anesthesia (ASA Refresher Course #243). New Orleans: ASA, 1990.

30. Rogers J, LeBlanc G, Curley M, et al. Evaluation of tympanic membrane thermometer for use with pediatric patients. Pediatr Nurs 1992;17:376–378.

31. Stewart SM, Luhan E, Ruff CL. Incidence of adult hypothermia in the post anesthesia care unit. Perioper Nurs Q 1987;3:57–62.

32. Stone JG, Young WL, Smith CR, Solomon RA, Ostapkovich N, Wang A. Do temperatures recorded at standard monitoring sites reflect actual brain temperature during deep hypothermia. Anesthesiology 1991;75:A483.

33. Kamal GD, Hasell RH, Pyle SM, Carnes RS. Inconsistent relationship between axillary and tympanic temperature following general anesthesia. Anesth Analg 1992;74:S155.

34. Casey WF, Broadman LM, Rice LJ, Dailey M. Comparison of liquid crystal skin temperature probe and axillary thermistor probe in measuring core temperature trends during anaesthesia in paediatric patients. Can J Anaesth 1989;36:S62–S63.

35. Allen GC, Horrow JC, Rosenberg H. Does forehead liquid crystal temperature accurately reflect "core" temperature? Can J Anaesth 1990;37:659–662.

36. Siegal MN, Gravenstein N. Use of a heat and moisture exchanger partially improves the correlation between esophageal and core temperature. Anesthesiology 1988;69:A284.

37. Whitby JD, Dunkin LJ. Cerebral oesophageal and nasopharyngeal temperatures. Br J Anaesth 1971;43:673–676.

38. Mravinac CM, Dracup K, Clochesy JM. Urinary bladder and rectal temperature monitoring during clinical hypothermia. Nurs Res 1989;38:73–76.

39. Lilly JK, Boland JP, Zekan S. Urinary bladder temperature monitoring. A new index of body core temperature. Crit Care Med 1980;742–744.

40. Horrow JC, Rosenberg H. Does urinary catheter temperature reflect core temperature during cardiac surgery? Anesthesiology 1988;69:986–989.

41. Glosten B, Sessler DI, Faure E, Karl L. Bladder vs tympanic core temperature measurement during cesarean section. Anesthesiology 1990;73:A960.

42. Bone ME, Feneck RO. Bladder temperature as an estimate of body temperature during cardiopulmonary bypass. Anaesthesia 1988;43:181–185.

43. Koyama K, Takahashi J, Ochiai R, Takeda J, Nagano M. Evaluation of esophageal temperature measured by gastric tube with thermister. Can J Anaesth 1990;37:S111.

44. Whitby JD, Dunkin LJ. Temperature differences in the oesophagus. Br J Anaesth 1968;40:991–995.

45. Whitby JD, Dunkin LJ. Temperature differences in the oesophagus. Br J Anaesth 1969;41:615–618.

46. Whitby JD, Dunkin LJ. Oesophageal temperature differences in children. Br J Anaesth 1970;42:1013–1015.

47. Siegel MN, Gravenstein N. Passive warming of airway gases (artificial nose) improves accuracy of esophageal temperature monitoring. J Clin Monit 1990;6:89–92.

48. Kaufman RD. Relationship between esophageal temperature gradient and heart and lung sounds heard by esophageal stethoscope. Anesth Analg 1987;66:1046–1048.

49. Brengelmann GL, Johnson JM, Hong PA. Electrocardiographic verification of esophageal temperature probe position. J Appl Physiol 1979;47:638–642.

50. Webb GE. Comparison of esophageal and tympanic temperature monitoring during cardiopulmonary bypass. Anesth Analg 1973;52:729–733.

51. Freund PR, Brengelmann GL. Placement of esophageal stethoscope by acoustic criteria does not consistently yield an optimal location for the monitoring of core temperature. J Clin Monit 1990;6:266–270.

52. Shiraki K, Konda N, Sagawa S. Espophageal and tympanic temperature responses to core blood temperature changes during hyperthermia. J Appl Physiol 1986;61:98–102.

53. Benzinger M. Tympanic thermometry in surgery and anesthesia. JAMA 1969;209:1207–1211.

54. Anonymous. Tympanic thermometry during anesthesia. Arch Otolaryngol 1969;90:28.

55. Sharkey A, Elliott P, Giesecke AH, Lipton JM. Relations between temperature of the external auditory meatus and the esophagus during anesthesia. Anesthesiology 1986;65:A530.

56. Tabor MW, Blaho DM, Schriver WR. Tympanic membrane perforation. Complication of tympanic thermometry during general anesthesia. Oral Surg 1981;51:581–583.

57. Benzinger M, Benzinger TH. Tympanic clinical temperature. Paper presented at fifth symposium on temperature. Washington DC, June 21–24, 1971.

58. Dickey WT, Ahlgren EW, Stephen CR. Body temperature monitoring via the tympanic membrane. Surgery 1970;67:981–984.

59. Ferrara-Love R. A comparison of tympanic and pulmonary artery measures of core temperatures. J Post Anesth Nurs 1991;6:161–164.

60. Shiraki K, Sagawa S, Tajioma F, Yokota A, Hashimoto M, Brengelmann L. Independence of brain and tympanic temperatures in an unanesthetized human. J Appl Physiol 1988;65:428–486.

61. Morley-Forster PK. Unintentional hypothermia in the operating room. Can Anaesth Soc J 1986;33:516–527.

62. Wallace CT, Marks WE, Adkins WY, Mahaffey JE. Perforation of the tympanic membrane. A complication of tympanic thermometry during anesthesia. Anesthesiology 1974;41:290–291.

63. Green MM, Danzl DF, Praszkier H. Infrared tympanic thermography in the emergency department. J Emerg Med 1989;7:437–440.

64. Johnson KJ, Bhatia P, Bell EF. Infrared thermometry of newborn infants. Pediatrics 1991;87:34–38.

65. Nypaver M, Zieserl E, Nachtsheim B, Davis AT. Tympanic membrane thermometers. Caveat emptor. Am J Dis Child 1991;145:403.

66. Ros SP. Evaluation of a tympanic membrane thermometer in an outpatient clinical setting. Ann Emerg Med 1989;18:1004–1006.

67. Terndup TE, Wong A. Influence of otitis media on the correlation between rectal and auditory canal temperatures. Am J Dis Child 1991;145:75–78.

68. Treloar D, Muma B. Comparison of axillary, tympanic membrane, and rectal temperatures in young children. Ann Emerg Med 1988;17:198.

69. Terndrup TE, Allegra JR, Kealy JA. A comparison of oral, rectal, and tympanic membrane temperature changes after ingestion of liquids and smoking. Am J Emerg Med 1989;7:150–154.

70. Rhodes FA, Grandner J. Assessment of an aural infrared sensor for body temperature measurement in children. Clin Pediatr 1990;29:112–115.

71. Kenney RD, Fortenberry JD, Surratt SS, Ribbeck BM, Thomas WJ. Evaluation of an infrared tympanic membrane thermometer in pediatric patients. Pediatrics 1990;85:854–858.

72. Vinci R, Garabedian C, Bauchner H. Accuracy of tympanic thermometry in a pediatric emergency department. Am J Dis Child 1990;144:429.

73. Audiss D, Brengelmann G, Bond E. Variations in the temperature differences between pulmonary artery and sublingual temperatures. Heart Lung 1989;18:294–295.

74. Nilsson K. Maintenance and monitoring of body temperature in infants and children. Pediatr Anaesth 1991;1:13–20.

75. Benzinger TH. Clinical temperature. JAMA 1969;209:1200–1206.

76. Di Paola I, Macneil P. Rectal thermometer complication. Anaesth Intensive Care 1985;13:441.

77. Anonymous. "Tissue agitation" cited in temperature probe recall. Biomed Safe Stand 1989;19:67–68.
78. Parker EO. Electrosurgical burn at the site of an esophageal temperature probe. Anesthesiology 1984;61:93–95.
79. Schneider AJL, Apple HP, Braun RT. Electrosurgical burns at skin temperature probes. Anesthesiology 1977;47:72–74.
80. Wald AS, Mazzia VDB, Spencer FC. Accidental burns. JAMA 1971;217:916–921.
81. Anderson GD. Electrosurgery units, not temperature probes, must be corrected to prevent burns. Anesthesiology 1985;62:834.
82. Weis FR, Kaiser RE. Technique of avoiding esophageal burns. Anesthesiology 1985;62:370.
83. Hall SC, Stevenson GW, Suresh S. Burn associated with temperature monitoring during magnetic resonance imaging. Anesthesiology 1992;76:152.
84. Chapin JW, Moravec M. Faulty temperature probe. Anesthesiology 1980;52:187.
85. Davies AO. Malignant temperature probe. Can Anaesth Soc J 1980;27:179–180.

Part 3
Airway Pressure Monitors

Equipment
Pressure Conditions
  Low Pressure
  Sustained Elevated Pressure
  High Pressure
  Subambient Pressure
  Other
Location of Pressure Monitor in Breathing System

Airway pressure monitors are also known as ventilator or respiratory monitors or alarms; pressure alarms; pressure alarm systems; anesthesia, patient, or breathing circuit monitors; ventilator monitoring alarms; breathing gas interruption monitors; disconnect monitors; and breathing pressure monitors.

When ventilation is manually controlled, the feel of the bag provides a means of continuously monitoring the breathing system pressure. When a ventilator is used this advantage is lost and abnormal pressures may not be detected rapidly. Excessive or inadequate pressure in the breathing system has been a major cause of anesthesia mortality and morbidity (1–5). For these reasons, use of a device that responds to pressure changes within the breathing system and provides warning of a problem with the patient or breathing system during mechanical ventilation is strongly recommended (6). Other parameters such as exhaled carbon dioxide and exhaled volumes may remain relatively normal in the presence of dangerously abnormal pressures. Monitoring of breath sounds with a precordial or esophageal stethoscope and observation of chest wall movements and the breathing system manometer are valuable, but frequently must be intermittent.

Use of these devices should not lead to less use of other devices. A combination of monitoring devices and techniques will increase the likelihood of detecting hazardous conditions.

Equipment

Airway pressure monitors may be freestanding or incorporated into a ventilator and/or anesthesia machine. Most anesthesia ventilators have at least a low-pressure alarm as standard equipment. Add-on alarms are available for many older ventilators.

To be effective, an alarm should be automatically ready to perform its functions when needed. Many freestanding pressure alarms can be interfaced with the on-off switch of a ventilator so that the alarm is activated when the ventilator is turned on. However, such an interface is not compatible with all ventilators and failure of the high-pressure gas source when the interface is operational may result in failure of the low-pressure alarm (6).

A freestanding device may not be activated or may be deactivated, because the alarm is annoying, and not be reactivated again. Simply educating staff not to turn off

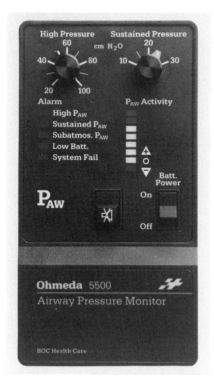

Figure 17.23. Airway pressure monitor. The high and sustained elevated pressure alarm limits are user adjustable. This monitor can be run on main power (with the batteries for back up) or on batteries. Note the low battery indicator and the mute button. Courtesy of Ohmeda, a division of BOC Health Care, Inc.

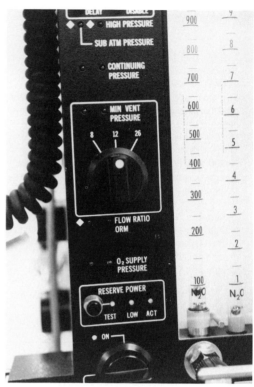

Figure 17.24. Airway pressure monitor. The user has a choice of three low pressures: 8, 12 and 26 cm H_2O. The sustained elevated (continuing), subambient, and high-pressure alarm levels are not adjustable. The delay button is at the top.

an alarm does not eliminate the problem, because even knowledgeable, conscientious, and experienced personnel occasionally forget to turn an alarm on.

Most of these devices are relatively inexpensive, easy to use, reliable, and require little maintenance. They should be either powered from the main electrical system or powered with battery backup or battery powered with battery test capability (Fig. 17.23).

Most pressure alarms have a delay (reset, mute, silencing) control that when activated will delay the audible signal for some or all of the functions (Fig. 17.24; see also Fig. 17.23). It should not be possible to silence an alarm permanently. Such muting should not prevent the visual indicator from functioning. Other desirable features include automatic

activation when a pressure pulse is detected, and protection against accidental inactivation, power failure or impending battery failure (6,7). Some airway pressure monitors have the ability continuously to display pressure waveforms. This is useful for detecting variations from the normal waveform.

Pressure Conditions

The airway pressure monitor alarm may be activated by one or more of the following conditions.

LOW PRESSURE

The basic intraoperative monitoring standards adopted by the American Society of

Anesthesiologists state that when ventilation is controlled by a mechanical ventilator, there shall be in continuous use a device that is capable of detecting disconnection of components of the breathing system (ventilation failure alarm, cycling alarm, pressure failure alarm, disconnect alarm, minimum ventilatory or ventilation pressure alarm, threshold pressure alarm). The device must give an audible signal when its alarm threshold is exceeded (8). Such an alarm has been recommended by several other responsible bodies around the world (9).

These devices are designed to alarm if the pressure in the breathing system fails to exceed a certain level within a fixed time. Devices that allow the user to select the alarm threshold may have distinct values (see Fig. 17.23) or allow continuous variation. The time span should be long enough that the peak pressure must fall below the alarm point for several successive breaths before the alarm will sound. This will avoid false alarms due to short-term disturbances.

Conditions that can be detected by a low-pressure alarm include a disconnection or major leak in the breathing system, failure of the fresh gas flow, a leaking tracheal tube cuff, failure of the ventilator to cycle, an unconnected ventilator, incorrect ventilator settings, failure of the gas supply to the ventilator, increased lung compliance and reduced resistance.

The low-pressure alarm threshold should be set just below the peak pressure reached during inspiration (6,10–12). This pressure will vary not only from patient to patient but even during a given case if tidal volume, inspiratory flow, compliance, or resistance changes. When a choice of low pressures is available, the highest pressure that is below the peak pressure should be selected.

Often the alarm threshold is set at its lowest limit in a misguided attempt to prevent false alarms. If the threshold value is too low, the alarm may be fooled (12–16). It has been suggested that a pressure threshold of less than 8 to 10 cm H_2O is unacceptable (17).

On some of the newer anesthesia machines that have a variable threshold pressure, an advisory will be activated if the threshold is set too far below the peak pressure. Some machines have automatic threshold adjustment.

Problems with low-pressure alarms have been reported. Those operating on batteries will not alarm if the batteries fail (18,19). The alarm can be fooled during use of a PEEP valve if the end expiratory pressure does not fall below the selected low pressure (20,21). Other conditions that may produce a pressure large enough to exceed the threshold when a disconnection occurs include the breathing system connector becoming obstructed by a pillow or surgical drapes; high resistance components such as a heat and moisture exchanger (HME), capnometer cuvette, or humidifier; entrainment of air into the breathing system; partial extubation; and a Mapleson breathing system with a high flow resistance (12,22–26). Oscillation of a water "plug" can falsely silence an alarm; conversely, droplets in the tube can attenuate the detected airway pressure, leading to a false alarm (27–29). It has been suggested that the alarm unit should be positioned higher than the breathing system to prevent water from plugging the line (10). Failure to turn on the ventilator will foil this type of alarm. For these reasons, it is essential that the alarm be checked before use by making a disconnection at the patient connector while the ventilator is cycling.

These monitors are of little or no use during spontaneous breathing when the pressure in the system does not rise and fall appreciably (11).

SUSTAINED ELEVATED PRESSURE

A sustained elevated pressure (continuous or continuing pressure) device compares airway pressure with a certain level to ensure that part of the waveform falls below that level. If it does not, an alarm sounds. Some alarms incorporate a valve that opens after a certain time (30). The selected pressure may be fixed or user adjustable (see Figs. 17.23 and 17.24).

A sustained elevated pressure may lead to decreased patient ventilation or even lung barotrauma in extreme cases (31). Such a pressure can result from several mechanisms: accidental activation of the oxygen flush valve; occlusion or obstruction of the expiratory limb; an improperly adjusted APL valve; occlusion of the scavenging system; a malfunctioning ventilator; or malfunction of a ventilator spill valve (6,7,31–33).

Continuous pressure alarms require lower threshold values and shorter time delays than are required for low-pressure alarms (6).

HIGH PRESSURE

An alarm that responds to a high pressure is important because high pressures may arise and cause serious patient morbidity very rapidly (2). However, some believe that this alarm is not essential, because most ventilators have a safety-relief valve (7). Such an alarm may have a fixed or adjustable pressure threshold (34,35) (see Figs. 17.23 and 17.24). Such an alarm is usually set at a value considered to be the maximum safe airway pressure.

A high pressure generally occurs only when the pressure is not buffered by a bag or ventilator bellows. Situations in which this might occur are airway obstruction, reduced lung compliance, increased airway resistance, a kinked or occluded tracheal tube, a punctured ventilator bellows, occlusion or obstruction of the expiratory limb of the breathing system, or a patient coughing or straining against the tracheal tube (6).

The following factors in various combinations may cause the high-pressure alarm to fail: high respiratory rate; low I:E ratio; low tidal volume; high tubing compliance; low inspiratory flow rate; and low fresh gas inflow from the anesthesia machine (34).

SUBAMBIENT PRESSURE

Subambient pressure alarms respond to pressures that fall below atmospheric pres-

sure by a predetermined amount. Pressures less than atmospheric can be generated by a patient attempting to inhale against an empty reservoir bag, a blocked inspiratory limb, a malfunction of an active scavenging system, a nasogastric tube placed in the trachea, or the refilling of a ventilator with a hanging bellows (6,32,36–38).

OTHER

Some airway pressure monitors have an alarm that sounds if the pressure falls below the selected positive end expiratory pressure (28). Some generate an alarm when a high positive end expiratory pressure is sensed.

Location of Pressure Monitor in the Breathing System

The closer the monitoring site is to the connection with the patient, the closer the pressure monitored is to that of the patient's airway. Placement between the patient and the breathing system may be ideal from this standpoint but presents problems in terms of dead space, disconnections, and contamination and water buildup in the pilot line. The need to connect the pilot line for every case may be unacceptable to many users.

A frequently used site is in the expiratory limb just upstream of the expiratory unidirectional valve (Fig. 17.25). The expiratory limb is preferable to the inspiratory limb, because if there is obstruction to flow in the inspiratory limb and the sensor is upstream of the obstruction, the low-pressure alarm may be fooled (26,39,40).

In the past, the sensor was sometimes located in the ventilator. Under certain circumstances, back pressure sufficient to generate a pressure high enough to inhibit the low-pressure alarm may be generated at the bellows even when there is a disconnection (28,31,41). Also siting the sensing point in the ventilator may result in failure to detect ventilator noncycling or an incorrectly set bag/ventilator selector valve (42, 43).

A pressure-monitoring device can be lo-

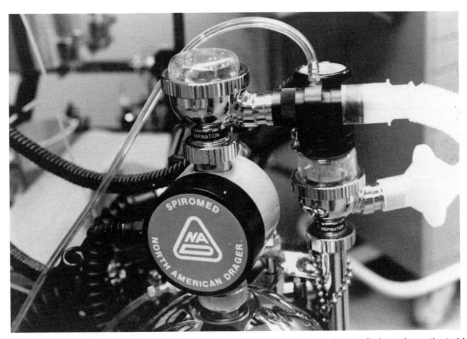

Figure 17.25. The sampling site for the airway pressure monitor is in the expiratory limb on the patient side of the unidirectional valve. Note the sensor for the Spiromed respiratory volume monitor below the expiratory unidirectional valve.

cated on the machine side of the unidirectional valves. With such an arrangement, the sensing line can be kept in place at all times, and its routine is less inconvenient (43). However, although this location may be acceptable for revealing disconnections, it may not be acceptable for revealing high, low, or continuous pressure conditions.

REFERENCES

1. Cooper JB, Newbower RS, Long CD, McPeek B. Preventable anesthesia mishaps. A study of human factors. Anesthesiology 1978;49:399–406.
2. Newton NI, Adams AP. Excessive airway pressure during anaesthesia. Anaesthesia 1979;33:689–699.
3. Holland R. Anesthesia-related mortality in Australia. In: Pierce EC, Cooper JB, eds. Analysis of anesthetic mishaps [Special issue]. Int Anesth Clin 1984;22:61–71.
4. Cooper JB, Newbower RS, Kitz RJ. An analysis of major errors and equipment failures in anesthesia management. Considerations for prevention and detection. Anesthesiology 1984;60:34–42.
5. Keenan RL, Boyan P. Cardiac arrest due to anesthesia. A study of incidence and causes. JAMA 1985;253:2373–2377.
6. Myerson KR, Ilsley AH, Runciman WB. An evaluation of ventilator monitoring alarms. Anaesth Intensive Care 1986;14:174–185.
7. Mimpriss T, Spivey A. A simple disconnect alarm. J Med Eng Technol 1989;13:222–224.
8. Anonymous. Standards for basic intra-operative monitoring. Am Soc Anesth Newslett 1986;50:12–13.
9. Winter A, Spence AA. An international consensus on monitoring [Editorial]. Br J Anaesth 1990;64:263–266.
10. Anonymous. Low-pressure alarms for sensing ventilator disconnects. Health Devices 1983;12:260–261.
11. Epstein RA. The elusive "disconnect alarm" examined. APSF Newslett 1988;3:39.
12. Pryn SJ. Crosse MM. Ventilator disconnexion alarm failures. Anaesthesia 1989;44:978–981.
13. Picard UM, Hancock DE, Pinchak AC. Pressure transients in anesthesia ventilators—failure of disconnect alarm system. Anesthesiology 1987;67:A189.
14. Reynolds AC. Disconnect alarm failure. Anesthesiology 1983;58:488.
15. Schreiber PJ. Corrections concerning alleged disconnect alarm failure. Anesthesiology 1983;59:601.

16. Bourke AE, Snowdon SL, Ryan TDR. Failure of a ventilator alarm to detect patient disconnection. J Med Eng Technol 1987;11:65–67.

17. Lawrence JC. Breathing system gas pressure monitoring and venting, ventilator monitors and alarms. Anaesth Intens Care 1988;16:38–40.

18. Mazza N, Wald A. Failure of battery-operated alarms. Anesthesiology 1980;53:246–248.

19. Anonymous. Pressure alarms, airway. Technol Anesth 1991;11:13.

20. Anonymous. Alert. Breathing circuit alarms. Health Devices 1980;4(22):1.

21. Anonymous. Canadian government issues alert on Monagahan/Hospital 703 ventilator alarm. Biomed Safe Stand 1980;10:135.

22. Ghanooni S, Wilks DH, Finestone C. A case report of an unusual disconnection. Anesth Analg 1983;62:696–697.

23. Murphy PJ, Rabey PG. The Humphrey ADE breathing system and ventilator alarms. Anaesthesia 1991;46:1000.

24. Milligan KA. Disablement of a ventilator disconnect alarm by a heat and moisture exchanger. Anaesthesia 1992;47:279.

25. McEwen JA, Jenkins LC. Complications of and improvements to breathing circuit monitors for anesthesia ventilators. Med Instrum 1983;17:70–74.

26. Slee TA, Pavlin EG. Failure of low pressure alarm associated with the use of a humidifier. Anesthesiology 1988;69:791–793.

27. Anonymous. Airway pressure monitor. Biomed Safe Stand 1982;12:123.

28. Anonymous. Evaluation of ventilator alarms. J Med Eng Technol 1984;8:270–276.

29. Hommelgaard P, Nissen T. A water-insensitive ventilator alarm. Anaesthesia 1979;34:1048–1051.

30. Seed RF. Alarms for lung ventilators. Br J Clin Equip 1978;4:114–121.

31. McEwen JA, Small CF, Jenkins LC. Detection of interruptions in the breathing gas of ventilated anaesthetized patients. Can J Anaesth 1988;35:549–561.

32. Anonymous. Ventilation alarms. Health Devices 1981;10:204–220.

33. Rendell-Baker L, Meyer JA. Accidental disconnection and pulmonary barotrauma. Anesthesiology 1983;58:286.

34. Bashein G, MacEvoy B. Anesthesia ventilators should have adjustable high-pressure alarms. Anesthesiology 1985;63:231–232.

35. Schreiber PJ. Anesthesia ventilators should have adjustable high-pressure alarms: a reply. Anesthesiology 1985;63:232–233.

36. Spielman FJ, Sprague DH. Another benefit of the subatmospheric alarm. Anesthesiology 1981;54:526–527.

37. Stirt JA, Lewenstein LN. Circle system failure induced by gastric suction. Anaesth Intensive Care 1981;9:161–162.

38. Hodgson CA, Mostafa SM. Riddle of the persistent leak. Anaesthesia 1991;46:799.

39. Shribman AJ. Failure of a ventilator alarm. Anaesthesia 1982;37:1044.

40. Mecklenburgh JS, Latto IP, Jones PL, Saunders RL. Failure of Penlon IDP ventilator alarm. Anaesthesia 1983;38:703–704.

41. Sinclair A, VanBergen J. Flow resistance of coaxial breathing systems: investigation of a circuit disconnect. Can J Anaesth 1992;39:90–94.

42. Sarnquist FH, Demas K. The silent ventilator. Anesth Analg 1982;61:713–714.

43. Schreiber P. Safety guidelines for anesthesia systems. Boston: Merchants, 1984.

Part 4
Respirometers

Equipment
  Wright Respirometer
  Drager Volumeter and Minute Volumeter
  Spiromed
  Ohmeda Model 5420 Volumeter
Placement in the Breathing System
Cross-Infection from Respirometers

A respirometer (spirometer, ventilation or respiratory meter or monitor, ventilometer, volume measuring device, flow monitor, respiratory flowmeter) is a device that measures and displays volumetric measurements such as tidal and minute volumes and, sometimes, respiratory rate. Newer models may display continuous flow-volume or pressure-volume loops.

A respirometer is useful to check the actual tidal or minute volume against that set on the ventilator. When equipped with an alarm and placed in the breathing system, a respirometer can aid in detecting occlusions in the breathing system, disconnections, apnea, leaks, and ventilator failure. Some can detect reversed flow. Although there are other ways of detecting these problems—including observation of chest wall movements, monitoring breath sounds using a stethoscope, capnometry, and airway pressure monitoring—use of a respirometer pro-

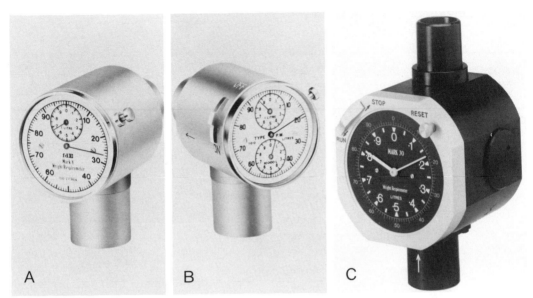

Figure 17.26. Wright respirometers. **A,** This is a small instrument that can be hand held to make selective respiratory measurements or can be inserted into the breathing system. It has two dials: a large peripheral one and a smaller one on the upper part of the main dial. The small dial indicates volumes up to 1 liter and the large dial, up to 100 liters. Note the reset button on the side. **B,** This instrument has three dials. The top small dial reads up to 1 liter, the large dial indicates volumes up to 100 liters, and the bottom small dial reads up to 10,000 liters. Note the on-off control and the directional flow arrow. **C,** This is a larger version of the respirometer, designed to be mounted into a breathing system. The long hand indicates volumes up to 1 liter on the inner scale and the small hand indicates volumes up to 100 liters on the concentric outer scale. Note the directional arrow at the bottom, the reset button, and the on-off control. Courtesy of Ferraris Medical, Inc.

vides additional protection by using a different and unrelated technology. One study found that a respirometer was a better monitor for detecting and classifying breathing system faults than an airway pressure or CO_2 monitor (1). In conjunction with a pressure gauge, a respirometer allows a rough estimate of compliance and resistance.

A major advantage of these devices is that they can be used to detect problems in spontaneously breathing patients as well as those ventilated mechanically. A major disadvantage is that with a ventilator with a hanging bellows even a total disconnection may not be detected.

Equipment

Respirometers suitable for use with anesthetized patients may be strictly mechanical

devices or the flow may be translated into an electronic signal that is processed. Most mechanical devices are not equipped with alarms and do not display respiratory rate. Electronic processing permits display of respiratory frequency and reverse flow as well as low-volume and -frequency alarms.

WRIGHT RESPIROMETER (2–4)

Description

Typical Wright respirometers are shown in Figure 17.26. They are supplied with adaptors to facilitate connection to a mask, tracheal tube, or breathing system. There is an on-off control in the form of a sliding stud and a spring-loaded reset button to set the hands of the scales to zero.

An infant version that can measure volumes down to 15 ml is available (5) (Fig. 17.27). Its dead space is 15 ml.

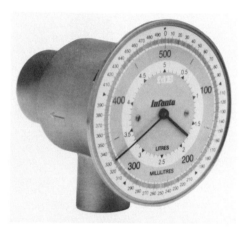

Figure 17.27. Infant version of Wright respirometer. The outer scale goes up to 500 ml and the inner scale goes up to 5 liters. Courtesy of Ferraris Medical, Inc.

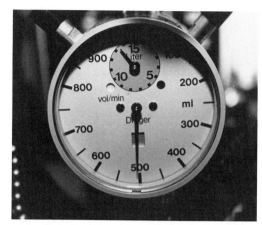

Figure 17.29. Drager volumeter (see text for details).

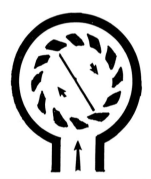

Figure 17.28. Internal construction of Wright respirometer. Gas entering the casing is directed through a series of tangential slots and strikes the rotor vane in the center, causing it to rotate.

The internal construction is shown in Figure 17.28. Gas entering through the outer casing is directed through a series of tangential slots enclosed in a cylindrical housing and strikes a rotor vane, causing it to rotate. The movement of the vane is transferred to the hands on the dial by a gear system.

Evaluation

Most studies have found that the Wright respirometer overreads at high flows and underreads with low flows (2–8), although one investigator found it consistently underread

(9). It will give slightly higher readings with mixtures of nitrous oxide and oxygen than for air (3).

Its advantages include small size and light weight, which makes it very portable. But this may be a significant cause of inaccuracy caused by lint and other pocket dirt and a high incidence of damage from dropping. Guards designed to reduce damage induced by dropping and abuse are available. Another advantage is its low dead space, which makes it suitable for use between the patient and the breathing system.

The main disadvantage is that it has no alarms. Also, it is somewhat difficult to read and does not give respiratory rate. Determination of minute volume requires a watch.

Maintenance can be expensive. Many instruments in use suffer inaccuracy because of poor mechanical condition (8).

DRAGER VOLUMETER AND MINUTE VOLUMETER

Description

The Drager minute volumeter is a large instrument, which is usually permanently mounted on the anesthesia machine and incorporated into the circle system. It is also sold as a separate component.

The instrument is shown in Figure 17.29. Gas flow is from top to bottom. There are two control buttons at the top. When the left button is depressed, a black dot appears on the left side of the face and a timer begins to run. After one minute, the hands stop and a black disc fills the space under the pointer. The minute volume is then displayed. When the right button is depressed, a black dot appears in the right-hand window and the tidal volume is measured. To stop the pointer, the right-hand button is depressed halfway; fully depressing it starts it again.

The internal construction is shown in Figure 17.30. Two hourglass-shaped rotors, which mesh as they rotate, are within the measuring chamber. Gas flow along the sides of the case actuates the rotors. The rotation is transmitted by means of a cog-wheel mechanism to the pointer on the gauge. It responds to flow in both directions.

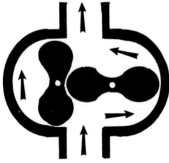

Figure 17.30. Internal construction of Drager minute volumeter. Gas flow along the sides of the case causes the rotors to rotate.

Evaluation

The volumeter tends to give erroneously low readings at low flows and high readings with high flows (4,9). Both instruments are easy to read, but are rather cumbersome and have large dead spaces, making them unsuitable for use between the patient and the breathing system.

SPIROMED

Description

The Spiromed is an electronic respirometer designed for use with North American Drager breathing systems. It employs a displacement rotating-lobe impeller that generates electronic pulses in response to the patient's expiratory flow. The sensor in the breathing system is shown in Figure 17.25 and the display is shown in Figure 17.31. The tidal volume, minute volume, and respiratory rate are continuously displayed in digital form. A self-diagnostic indicator located on the left side of the panel will flash red and green if the electronic system fails. If the system is operating properly it will be green.

Various alarms are built into the device. If no exhaled volume is detected for 15 sec, *LO* is displayed on the breaths-per-minute display accompanied by an intermittent repeating tone. If apnea persists for 30 sec, the *LO* on the breaths-per-minute display is augmented by a repeating tone, and both tidal-

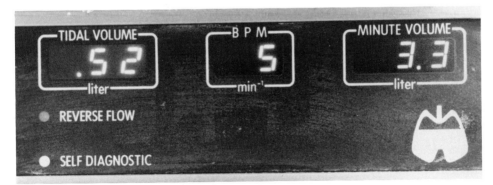

Figure 17.31. Drager Spiromed.

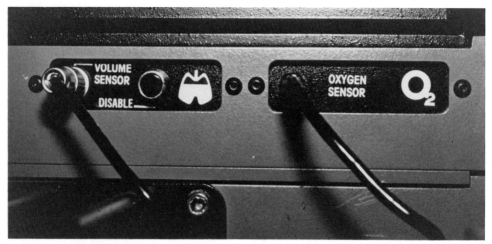

Figure 17.32. Alarm silence button on the side of an anesthesia machine.

and minute-volume displays are blanked. If the minute volume falls below 1 liter/min, *LO* is displayed on the minute-volume display and an intermittently repeating tone is generated. If the measured respiratory rate exceeds 60 breaths/min, *HI* is shown on the breaths-per-minute display. If reversed flow during inspiration is detected, a reversed flow indicator appears on the left side of the front panel, accompanied by a brief audible tone.

A alarm silence button for the Spiromed is located on the side of the anesthesia machine (Fig. 17.32).

Evaluation

This instrument is programmed to measure tidal volumes equal to or greater than 0.15 liter. If the tidal volume is less than 0.15 liter the instrument will automatically add two or more consecutive tidal volumes and reduce the frequency accordingly. The minute-volume display remains correct.

The accuracy of the tidal volume measurement is reported as ±0.04 liter, minute volume as ±10% of reading or 0.1 liter, and respiratory rate as ±8% of reading or 1 breath/min.

OHMEDA 5420 VOLUME MONITOR

Description

The Ohmeda 5420 volume monitor is available in two configurations. It may be an integral part of an anesthesia machine. In this configuration the monitor obtains power from the anesthesia machine and has an internal rechargeable back-up battery pack. The other configuration is a stand-alone unit that can operate off either a remote charger or a battery pack. When the monitor is operating from the battery pack, the heater in the sensor is turned off to conserve power. The instrument can operate for up to 8 hr on battery power.

The monitor consists of a sensor that fits into the breathing system, a display unit that can be mounted on the anesthesia machine, and a coiled electrical cord connecting the two.

The sensor portion (Fig. 17.33) consists of two parts: a cartridge, which is placed in the breathing system, and a clip-on optical coupler, which fits over the cartridge. The clip is marked with arrows to indicate the correct direction of flow through it. It has a dead space of 6 to 10 ml.

As gas passes through the cartridge, it strikes a vane, causing it to spin. The clip contains two light beam sources and an optical sensor. As the vane spins it interrupts the light beams shining through the cartridge. The optical sensor generates a voltage pulse each time one of the light beams is blocked. The number of pulses is proportional to gas flow through the sensor. A com-

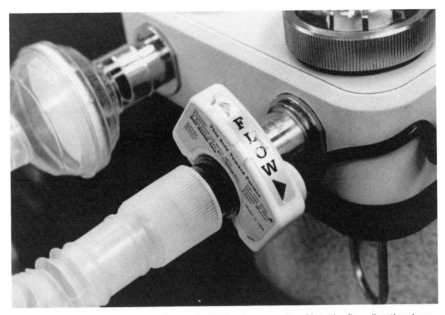

Figure 17.33. Flow sensor for the Ohmeda 5420 volume monitor. Note the flow directional arrow.

puter in the monitor counts these pulses and then calculates tidal volume, minute volume, and respiratory rate. The computer can detect reverse flow by determining the order in which the light beams are blocked. The clip contains a small heater to help prevent condensation. If the light beams are blocked by condensate or other contaminants, the sensor may not work and must be replaced.

Calculations for respiratory rate and minute volume are performed at the end of each detected breath or at 10-sec intervals and averaged over the last six breaths. Averaging helps eliminate artifacts such as coughing.

Values are shown on the liquid crystal display along with any alarm conditions. The display unit is shown in Figure 17.34. An on-off switch is located at the lower right. A switch on the left allows the user to select either tidal volume or minute volume. An alarm silence switch, which will silence all audible tones for 30 sec, is located between these two switches. An alarm light is located just above the alarm silence switch. It will be illuminated during alarm conditions, whether the alarm silence switch is activated or not. At the top are thumb-wheel switches, which allow the operator to select the alarm

levels for low and high minute volumes. The upper minute volume alarm limits can be adjusted to between 1 and 99 liters and the low, between 0.0 and 9.9 liters. Each is disarmed when set to 0.0.

The unit will display respiratory rate and either tidal or minute volume. The respiratory rate is shown by two small digits to the left of the larger volume display. Tidal volume may be displayed in milliliters or liters. Minute volume is displayed in liters. A 15-segment bar graft shows the tidal volume with each breath. Each bar segment represents approximately 50 ml. If the volume exceeds 750 ml, an arrow will display the overflow condition.

Inside a door below the display and switches are two switches. One is for changing the source of power (line or battery). The transition to battery is not automatic on built-in units. When the line power source fails, the monitor is turned off. It is important to switch back to line power when it is restored to avoid running down the batteries. The other switch is to activate the reverse flow detector. A *REV OFF* message appears on the display when the switch is in the off position. When the switch is in the on posi-

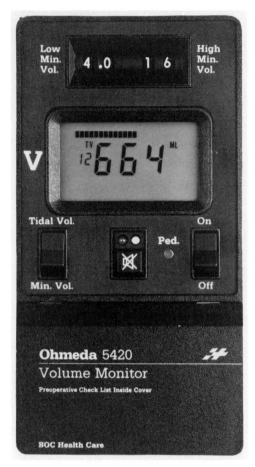

Figure 17.34. Display unit for the Ohmeda 5420 volume monitor. Courtesy of Ohmeda, a division of BOC Health Care, Inc.

tion, reverse flow volumes greater than 50 ml are indicated by an audio tone. This should not be used when the sensor is located where gas flow will be bidirectional.

An alarm will be triggered if the monitor itself malfunctions or the batteries are low. This is indicated by a continuous high tone with a blank display, and the alarm light is continuously on. The apnea alarm will be triggered if a 150-ml breath is not sensed within 30 sec. An apnea message will appear on the screen and the light will flash. There will be a single tone after 30 sec, two tones after 60 sec, three tones after 90 sec, and a continuous tone after 120 sec, if the condition persists. Low- and high-minute-volume

alarms are activated if the exhaled volume falls below or rises above the selected limits. A low- or high-minute-volume message will appear on the screen. An intermittent low tone signifies a low minute volume and an intermittent high tone a high minute volume. If the reverse flow detection switch is in the on position, a reverse flow volume greater than 50 ml will be indicated by a *REV FLOW* message and an audible alarm with a continuous low tone.

The unit is intended for use only on patients over 20 kg. It is not intended for use on patients with shallow and rapid breathing or with a tidal volume less than 150 ml.

Evaluation

The manufacturer specifies an accuracy of either $\pm 8\%$ or ± 40 ml, whichever is greater. Respiratory rate is stated to be accurate to within 1 breath/min.

Placement in the Breathing System

From the standpoint of accuracy, the most desirable location of this device is between the breathing system and the patient, so that the volume of gas measured is that actually exhaled. In this location, fresh gas flow and breathing system compliance do not affect the readings. However, the flow of gas is bidirectional, which affects some instruments. Placing the sensor at this site will increase the dead space. Condensation of water may be a significant problem. Some respirometers are too bulky to place in this position. Use in this position may result in increased damage to the instrument.

A common practice is to locate the respirometer in the exhalation side of the circle just upstream of the expiratory unidirectional valve. An advantage of this position is that if the respirometer can detect reverse flow, a malfunctioning exhalation check valve will be spotted. A respirometer in this location will read accurately during spontaneous respiration. During controlled respiration, it will overread because of the expansion of breathing system components and gas compression (10). The error will be increased by addition of components such as a humidifier to the breathing system, heating the circuit, and decreased lung compliance (11). If the fresh gas inlet in a circle system is downstream of the inspiratory unidirectional valve the spirometer will read inaccurately (10,12–14). If a ventilator with a hanging bellows is used, a respirometer in this position may still indicate flow when a disconnection occurs (15).

The respirometer should not be located downstream of the absorber, because the absorption of carbon dioxide will decrease the volume of gas measured.

Another possible location is on the inspiratory side of the circle system. In this location, the respirometer will display erroneously high readings because of expansion of the tubings and compression of the gases and leaks between the respirometer and the patient. During controlled ventilation, a disconnection may not be detected.

The use of respirometers in Mapleson systems is problematic. Respirometers with turbines, which recognize flow in only one direction, can be inserted between the patient and the breathing system, but this location is generally unsatisfactory because of the bulk of the sensor, increased dead space, and increased likelihood of a disconnection (16).

Cross-Infection from Respirometers

Respirometers have been implicated in the transfer of infection between patients (17). Because of their potential exposure to bacterial contamination, they should not be used in sequential patients until they are disinfected.

REFERENCES

1. Orr JA, Westenskow DR, Farrell RM. Information content of three breathing circuit monitors: a neural network analysis. Anesthesiology 1992;77:A517.

2. Wright BM. A respiratory anemometer. J Physiol 1955;127:25.

3. Nunn JF, Ezi-Ashi TI. The accuracy of the respirometer and ventigrator. Br J Anaesth 1962;34:442–432.

4. Byles PH. Observations on some continuously-acting spirometers. Br J Anaesth 1960;32:470–475.

5. Meeke R, Wren W, Davenport J, O'Griofa P. The measurement of tidal volumes in spontaneously breathing children during general anaesthesia using a Haloscale infant Wright respirometer. Acta Anaesth Scand 1984;28:696–699.

6. Bushman JA. Effect of different flow patterns on the Wright respirometer. Br J Anaesth 1979;51:895–898.

7. Hall KD, Reeser FH. Calibration of Wright spirometer. Anesthesiology 1962;23:126–129.

8. Lunn JN, Hillard EK. The effect of repairs on the performance of the Wright respirometer. Br J Anaesth 1970;42:1127–1130.

9. Kittredge P. Accuracy of clinical ventilation meters. Respir Care 1972;17:181–187.

10. Purnell RJ. The position of the Wright anemometer in the circle absorber system. Br J Anaesth 1968;40:917–918.

11. Feldman JM, Muller J. Tidal volume measurement errors—the impact of lung compliance and a circuit humidifier. Anesthesiology 1990;73:A468.

12. Briere C, Patoine J-G, Audet R. Inaccurate ventimetry by fresh gas inlet position. Can Anaesth Soc J 1974;21:117–119.

13. Campbell DI. Change of gas inflow siting on Boyle Mk3 absorbers. Anaesthesia 1971;26:104.

14. Campbell DI. Volumeter attachment on Boyle circle absorber. Br J Anaesth 1971;43:206–207.

15. Thorpe CM. Ventilators, circle systems and respirometers. Anaesthesia 1992;47:913.

16. Schreiber P. Safety guidelines for anesthesia systems. Boston: Merchants, 1984.

17. Irwin RS, Demers RR, Pratter MR, et al. An outbreak of Actinobacter infection associated with the use of a ventilator spirometer. Respir Care 1980;25:232–237.

Part 5
Pulse Oximetry

Bilirubinemia
Anemia
Equipment
Sensors
Cable
Console
Oximeter Standards
Use
Sites
Fixation
Stabilization
Inspection of Sites
Applications
Monitoring Oxygenation
Controlling Oxygen Administration
Monitoring Circulation
Determining Systolic Blood Pressure
Locating Vessels
Preventing Retinopathy of Prematurity
Monitoring Vascular Volume
Other Uses
Advantages
Accuracy
Independence from Gases and Vapors
Dependability
Fast Response Time
Noninvasiveness
Continuous Measurement
Continuous Pulse Rate
Provision of Separate Respiratory and Circulatory
    Variables
Monitoring of Peripheral Blood Flow
Easy Sensor Application
Convenience
Minimal Site Preparation
Fast Start Time
Verification of Proper Operation
Tone Modulation
User Friendliness
Light weight and Compactness
Rugged Sensors
Variety of Sensor Configurations
No Heating Required
Battery Operated
Economical
Limitations and Disadvantages
Insensitivity to Low Blood Pressure, Low Pulse
    Pressure, and Vasoconstriction
Inaccuracy with Increased Venous Pressure
Interference from Exogenous Dyes
Optical Interference
Nail Polish and Skin Color Interference
Loss of Accuracy at Low Values
Erratic Performance with Irregular Rhythms
Sensitive to Electrical Interference
Saturation Data Not Helpful with High Oxygen Partial
    Pressure

Delayed Detection of Hypoxic Events
False Alarms
Falsely High SpO_2 Readings
Failure to Detect Absence of Circulation
Expensive Sensor
Discrepency in Readings from Different Monitors
Pulse Overload
Patient Injury

Introduction

Pulse oximetry is a noninvasive method of measuring oxygen saturation (SpO_2 or SaO_2) from a light signal transmitted through tissue, taking into account the pulsatile nature of volume changes with blood flow.

A reliable, continuous noninvasive method of measuring oxygen delivery was a goal of researchers for many years. Until the 1980s, noninvasive oximeters, known as ear oximeters, were large, expensive, and cumbersome. They required "arterialization" by heat or chemical treatment, and their utility was limited by technical difficulties in differentiating light absorbance of arterial blood from that of venous blood and tissues.

Technical advances, such as light-emitting diodes (LEDs) miniaturized photodetectors, and microprocessors, allowed the creation of a new generation of oximeters, which are smaller, less expensive, and easier to use than the earlier models. These differentiate the absorption of incident light by the pulsatile arterial component from the static components. Hence they are called pulse oximeters. Many pulse oximeters are combined with other monitors, such as capnometers, into one instrument and may be incorporated into an anesthesia machine.

The American Society of Anesthesiologists made pulse oximetry a standard for intraoperative monitoring on January 1, 1990, and a standard for postanesthesia care unit monitoring on January 1, 1992. International standards for safe practice endorsed by the World Federation of Societies of Anesthesiologists highly recommend continuous use of a quantitative monitor of oxygenation such as pulse oximetry (1). In some states, its use is mandatory. A study of closed claims of anesthetic-related malpractice cases determined that a combination of pulse oximetry and capnography could have prevented 93% of avoidable mishaps (2).

Principles of Operation (3–7)

The pulse oximeter estimates SaO$_2$ by measuring pulsatile signals across perfused tissue at two discrete wavelengths, using the constant component of absorption (that caused by everything except arterial blood) at each wavelength to normalize the signals (8). It then computes the ratio between these two normalized signals and relates this ratio to the arterial oxygen saturation, using an empirical algorithm. Most pulse oximeters currently in use base their calculations on calibration curves derived from studies in healthy volunteers (5).

The two wavelengths allow differentiation of reduced hemoglobin and oxyhemoglobin. Reduced hemoglobin absorbs more light in the red band than does oxyhemoglobin. Oxyhemoglobin absorbs more light in the infrared band.

Fractional oxygen saturation (% HbO$_2$) is the ratio of oxyhemoglobin to the sum of all hemoglobin species present, whether available for reversible binding to oxygen or not (9). Functional oxygen saturation (SaO$_2$) is defined as ratio of oxyhemoglobin to all functional hemoglobins. These must be determined using an in vitro oximeter. For patients with low dyshemoglobin levels, the difference between fractional and functional saturation is very small. However, when the dyshemoglobin levels are elevated, the two values can vary greatly and the pulse oximeter readings are unlikely to agree with either the true fractional or functional saturation values (8).

The principal barrier to the clinical use of oximetry was the difficulty in separating the absorption of light by arterial blood from that of venous blood and tissues. Modern pulse oximeters discriminate between arterial blood and other tissue components by considering only the change in the transmitted light caused by the inflow of arterial blood. The transmitted light signal during diastole serves as a reference. The oximeter pulses the red and infrared LEDs on and off several hundred times per second. The rapid sampling rate allows precise recognition of the times of the peak and trough of each pulse wave. Absorbance data from both peak and trough are saved and used in calculations. At the trough, the vascular bed contains arterial, capillary, and venous blood as well as intervening tissue. At the peak, it contains all this plus a quantity of arterial blood. The presence of this additional arterial blood changes the amount of transmitted light in both red and infrared bands. Most oximeters have a phase of both LEDs off to allow detection and compensation for extraneous light. Light readings during the off period are automatically subtracted from the next sequence. Data from several sequences are used to calculate the oxygen saturation.

A microcomputer in the pulse oximeter monitors and controls signal levels, coordinates the functional elements, performs the calculations, implements signal validity schemes, activates alarms and messages, and monitors its own circuitry to warn of malfunctions.

Physiology

Efficient oxygen transport relies on the ability of hemoglobin reversibly to load and unload oxygen at physiological tensions. The relationship between oxygen tension and oxygen binding is exemplified in the well-known hemoglobin dissociation curve, which plots the oxygen saturation of hemoglobin against the oxygen tension. The sigmoid shape is essential for physiological transport. As oxygen is taken up in the lungs, the blood is nearly fully saturated over a large range of tensions. During passage through the systemic capillaries a large amount of oxygen is released with a relatively small drop in tension. This allows oxygen to be released at sufficiently high concentrations to provide an adequate gradient for diffusion into the cells.

The shape of the oxygen dissociation curve limits the degree of desaturation that can be tolerated. Between 90% and 100% saturation the Pa_{O_2} will be 60 torr or above. Below 90% saturation, the curve becomes steeper and small drops in saturation correspond to large drops in the partial pressure. Thus there is a narrow range of oxygen saturation that can be considered the safety zone and if a problem develops there may not be a great deal of warning before the oxygen level reaches dangerous levels.

Normal arterial oxygen saturation breathing air at sea level is approximately 95%. At an altitude of 5000 feet this drops to 92%, and at 10,000 feet, approximately 88% (10).

Effects of Different Hemoglobin Conditions

Whole blood contains not only reduced hemoglobin and oxyhemoglobin but, frequently, other moieties such as carboxyhemoglobin and methemoglobin. In vitro cooximetry can measure the percentages of other moieties by using more than two wavelengths.

METHEMOGLOBIN (11)

Normally less than 1% of the total hemoglobin, methemoglobin (metHb) is an oxidation product of hemoglobin that forms a reversible complex with oxygen and impairs the unloading of oxygen to tissues.

Acquired methemoglobinemia is unusual. Among the causes are nitrobenzene (12), benzocaine (13,14), prilocaine (15,16), and dapsone (17,18). If methemoglobinemia is suspected, the diagnosis should be con-

firmed by multiwavelength cooximetry, because standard blood gas analysis is not capable of detecting and measuring metHb (19).

Methemoglobin has approximately the same absorption coefficient in the red and infrared bands. When compared with functional saturation, pulse oximeters give falsely low readings for saturations above 85% and falsely high values for saturations below 85%. As methemoglobin increases, SpO_2 seeks the 80% to 85% range and stays there once methemoglobin is above 40% (11,20–24). The discrepancy between SpO_2 and functional saturation increases as the level of metHb increases (11). With treatment of the methemoglobinemia, the SpO_2 readings become more accurate (15,16,18,23).

All two-wavelength pulse oximeters will overread compared with fractional saturation when metHb is present (8).

CARBOXYHEMOGLOBIN

Carboxyhemoglobin (HbCO) exists in varying degrees as a consequence of smoking and urban pollution, but may occur in concentration as high as 45% as a result of smoke inhalation (8).

Carboxyhemoglobin has an absorption spectrum similar to oxyhemoglobin so most pulse oximeters will overread by the percentage of carboxyhemoglobin present (25–27). This must be considered in smokers, victims of fires, and during laser resection of the trachea (28–30).

Pulse oximeters that differentiate between oxyhemoglobin and carboxyhemoglobin are available.

FETAL HEMOGLOBIN

The presence of fetal hemoglobin (Hb F) does not appear to affect the accuracy of pulse oximetry to a clinically important degree (5,31–38), although very high levels will cause some inaccuracy (39). Therefore, pulse oximetry can be used to monitor oxygenation in preterm neonates with predominantly fetal hemoglobin.

HEMOGLOBIN S

The presence of hemoglobin S does not appear to affect the accuracy of pulse oximetry to an important degree.

BILIRUBINEMIA

Severe hyperbilirubinemia can cause an artifactual elevation of methemoglobin and carboxyhemoglobin using in vitro oximetry, but it does not affect pulse oximetry readings (31,33,38,40–43).

ANEMIA

The pulse oximeter is less accurate at low saturations in patients with anemia than those with normal hemoglobin levels (44). The level at which a pulse oximeter finds the sample too dilute is not precisely defined, but is generally accepted to be a hematocrit of less than 10% (45).

Equipment

SENSORS

The sensor (probe) is the part intended to come in direct contact with the patient. It contains two or more LEDs that emit light at specific wavelengths and are 180° opposed to a photodetector (photocell). These are mounted in a receptacle that supports them and maintains them in contact with the pulsatile tissue.

The LEDs provide monochromatic light. This means they emit a constant wavelength throughout their life, so that once calibrated they never need recalibration. The exact wavelengths used vary somewhat with different pulse oximeters. LEDs cause little heating. Thus the sensor can be left in place for long periods of time without thermal injury. LEDs are so inexpensive that they may be used in a disposable sensor.

The light, partially absorbed and modulated as it passes through the tissue sample, is converted into an electronic signal by the photodetector, which passes it on to the console.

Sensors may be reusable or disposable. Disposable sensors are adhesive. Reusable sensors either clip on to the patient like a clothes pin or are attached with adhesive. Disposable sensors are easier to use, but reusable sensors are more economical (46,47). Various methods of preserving disposable probes have been described (48,49). With repeated use, a disposable sensor may give inaccurate readings (50). Disposable sensors may be preferred when cross-contamination is a concern. Tape-on probes are less susceptible to motion artifact and less likely to come off if the patient moves. However, they are usually not as well-shielded from ambient light as slide-on probes. Probes lined with soft material may be associated with fewer motion artifacts (51).

Making it difficult to separate a reusable sensor from the cable will reduce loss of reusable sensors (47). Use of Velcro to hold the reusable probe to the oximeter case when not in use will reduce damage to the probe and make it easy to find (52).

Figures 17.35. through 17.40 show several types of probes that are available. A circumferential design may preclude use in people with extremely large fingers. A metal nose clip from a disposable face mask may be useful in fitting a nasal or flexible probe. Probes may be available in different sizes. If a probe used is too large for the patient, some of the output of the LED can reach the sensor without passing through the tissue and falsely high SpO_2 readings will be produced (53).

CABLE

The probe is connected to the oximeter by a simple, sturdy, electrical cable. The cable should be long enough to connect to various vascular beds while the console is situated in the user's sight. Cables from one manufac-

Figure 17.35. **A,** This disposable probe is most commonly used on the finger, as shown in **B.** Other sites where it has been used include the ear, cheek, tongue, toe, penis, hypothenar or thenar eminence, palm, forefoot, and wrist. Courtesy of Nellcor, Inc.

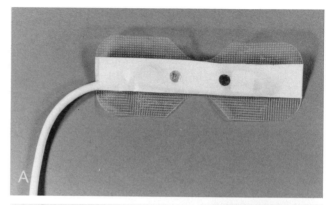

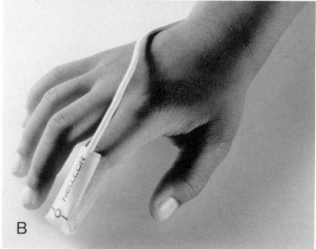

turer should not be used for others even though the cables seem to be interchangeable.

CONSOLE

Many different consoles are available. Most are line operated but can be operated on batteries, making them suitable for use during patient transport. Most units have a bright display, allowing them to be seen easily in a darkened room.

The front panel usually displays percent saturation, pulse rate, and alarm limits. The displayed values for SpO_2 and pulse rate are usually weighted averages. This provides a more acceptable result with lower sensitivity to motion and other "noise."

Some oximeters allow the averaging period to be adjusted. A mode that averages over a longer period of time is better if there is much probe motion, because there will be fewer artifactual readings (54). However, changes in pulse rate or saturation will be reflected more rapidly in a mode that averages over a shorter period of time.

A variety of messages may be provided by the oximeter to inform the operator of its functional status (6). A means of assessing signal strength may be present. Pulse amplitude may be represented using a vertical post with the lighted height of the post rising with an increase in pulse amplitude, by a bar graph on a dot matrix display, or as a plethysmographic waveform.

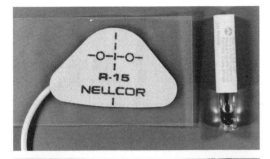

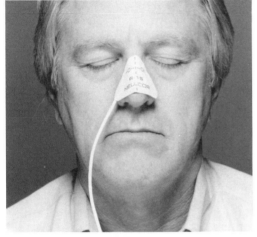

Figure 17.36. A, Disposable probe designed for use on the nose. It may come with a container for degreating the skin. **B,** The disposable nasal probe in place. Courtesy of Nellcor, Inc.

Most instruments provide an audible tone with each pulse and the pitch changes with the saturation. In this way, the operator can be made aware of changes in SpO$_2$ without looking at the oximeter. There may be a means to control volume of the beep.

An increasing number of pulse oximeters offer trend data storage (55). On some units trend data are available even when the unit is turned off. Interfaces for hard copy recording and computer communication are sometimes available.

Alarms are commonly provided for low and high heart rates and low and high saturation. Most units have default alarm limits. Most units generate an alarm when the sensor is not properly applied to the patient or when for some other reason a signal is inadequate.

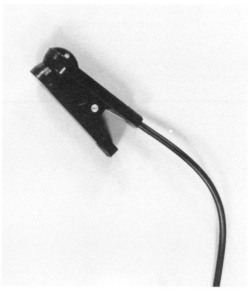

Figure 17.37. Reusable probe designed for use on the ear. This may also be used on various other locations, including the cheek.

Oximeter Standards

A U.S. standard (56) and an international standard (57) were published in 1992. Among the provisions are the following:

1. Manufacturers must disclose the accuracy and range of hemoglobin saturation over which the accuracy is claimed and whether the calibration was to functional or fractional saturation. If provided, the manufacturer must disclose the accuracy and range for the pulse rate and the range over which this accuracy is claimed.
2. If intended for continuous monitoring, the pulse oximeter shall have a low SpO$_2$ alarm.
3. The default limit on a low SpO$_2$ alarm shall be 80% SpO$_2$ or greater.
4. The audible components of alarms should be designed to allow silencing until the pulse oximeter is placed in use.
5. Temporary silencing of audible alarms, if provided, shall not exceed 2 min.

Figure 17.38. Reusable probes for use on fingers or toes in adults and children. In infants, this type of probe can be placed on part of the hand, including some fingers, or part of the foot, including some toes. These probes offer better shielding from ambient light than some other probes.

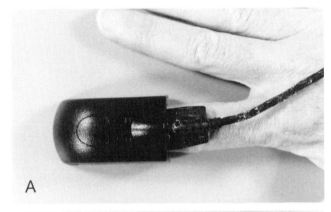

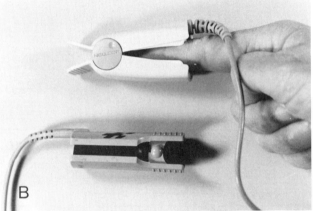

6. Visual indication of signal adequacy should be provided.
7. If a normalized pulse waveform display is provided, a visual display of pulse strength shall also be provided.
8. If a variable pitch audible annunciation is provided for the pulse signal, a pitch or amplitude change in the sound should be provided parallel to the reading. For example, as the SpO_2 reading lowers the sound, pitch should also be lowered.
9. If the pulse oximeter is provided with user-adjustable controls to compensate for dysfunctional hemoglobin, there shall be a clear indication that these controls have been adjusted.
10. If intended for continuous monitoring, a probe fault alarm shall be provided.

Use

SITES

The sensor is attached to a pulsatile vascular bed. Such a bed may include the fingertip; hypothenar or thenar eminence; cheek; penis; toe; earlobe; nose; or in infants, the palm, forefoot, or wrist. It is essential that an assortment of probes be available. If pulsatile flow is inadequate, the sensor site should be changed.

Finger or Toe

The probe is most commonly attached over the fingertip (see Figs. 17.35*B* and 17.38), The failure rate is less when the probe

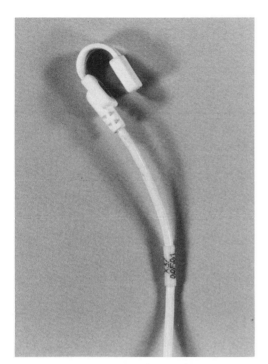

Figure 15.39. Reusable probe for use on finger or toe of pediatric patient. It may also be used on the thenar or hypothenar eminence, the wings of the nostrils, or the nasal septum. The probe should be taped in place.

is placed on the finger than on the earlobe (58,59).

Under conditions of poor perfusion caused by cold, finger probes perform better than ear probes (60). If there is poor circulation, a finger block may restore circulation and oximeter detection (61,62).

A disadvantage of probes placed on an extremity is that desaturation is detected less rapidly than when probes are placed more centrally (63–69). Response time may be quicker when the sensor is placed on the thumb (69).

The finger with the strongest pulsatile signal can be located using the pulse signal strength. Motion artifacts are less frequent when the sensor is placed on one of the larger fingers (51).

In general, the arm opposite from that on which the blood pressure cuff is applied or in which an arterial catheter has been inserted should be used. Insertion of a radial artery catheter is commonly followed by a transient decrease in blood flow and loss of an adequate signal for a pulse oximeter whose probe in placed on a finger of that hand (70). With some monitors, the pulse oximeter is integrated with the noninvasive blood pressure monitor so that the pulse oximeter will not alarm during the inflation cycle.

When one limb is above the other the pulse amplitude and SaO_2 will be greater in the upper than the dependent hand (71). Occasionally, poor function may occur with probe attachment to the same extremity as the intravenous infusion, due to local hypothermia and vasoconstriction.

If there is dark fingernail polish or synthetic fingernails, the probe should be oriented so that it transmits light from one side of the finger to the other side (72).

Nose

The bridge of the nose (see Fig. 17.36*B*), the wings of the nostrils, and the nasal septum have been used (73). The nose clip from a disposable oxygen face mask can be attached to the outer surface of a flexible sensor to make it fit closely (74).

The nose is a convenient location. This site has been recommended as useful under conditions such as hypothermia, hypotension, and infusion of vasoconstrictor drugs (75). The evidence on this is conflicting. One study found that nasal probes often give grossly erroneous results and had a higher failure rate than other probes under conditions of poor perfusion (60). However, a study found that in hypothermic patients the nasal septum was a more reliable site than the finger. Another study found that nasal probes were associated with a higher failure rate than finger probes (76).

Nasal pulse oximeter SpO_2 readings are higher than those with finger probes (73,77) and may be more accurate when compared with blood gas controls (73).

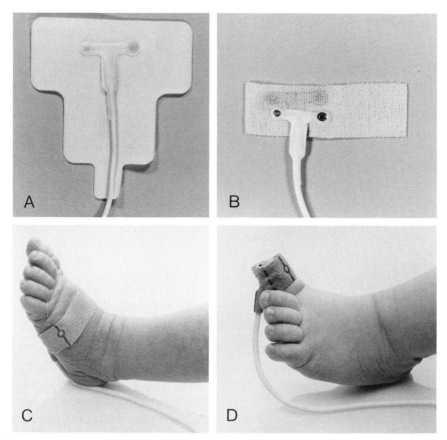

Figure 17.40.   Reusable flexible probes. **A,** This probe is attached to the patient using a disposable adhesive backing. **B,** This probe is attached to an elastic bandage for attachment to the patient. **C** and **D,** The probe is wrapped around the finger, palm, foot, or toe in a manner similar to a common bandage. These probes offer some shielding from ambient light.

Nasal probes respond more rapidly to desaturation than probes placed on extremities.

Ear

The ear probe is useful when the hand is not accessible to the operator, or when significant finger motion is expected. It may be held in place by a thin plastic semicircle hung around the ear. Stabilizing devices such as headbands or around-the-ear loops can be useful when patients are moving. The nose clip from a disposable oxygen face mask can be attached to hold the sensor in place (74).

The earlobe should be massaged for 30 to 45 sec with alcohol or vasodilator cream to increase perfusion and improve oximeter performance.

Response time is faster with an ear probe than with a finger probe (65,66,69,78), but ear probes are associated with a higher failure rate (76). Under conditions of poor perfusion, some ear probes perform well compared with finger probes (60). Ear probes may give more erroneous readings than finger probes in patients with tricuspid incompetence (79).

Tongue

A tongue probe can be made by placing a malleable aluminum strip behind the sensor to allow it to bend around the tongue (80,81).

A disposable probe wrapped around the tip of the tongue in the sagittal plane may also be used (82). The mouth should be closed. It is somewhat difficult to maintain in place during emergence but is reported to be more resistant to signal interference from electrocautery than peripheral sites (80,81). Glossal pulse oximetry has been shown to be accurate (82).

This site may be especially useful in patients with burns over a large percentage of their body surface (81,82).

Cheek

A probe with a metal strip backing can be used at the cheek to perform buccal oximetry (83). An ear probe can also be used (84,85). Buccal pulse oximetry is reported to be more accurate than finger pulse oximetry (86,87).

Other

In infants, flexible probes may work through the palm, foot, penis, or even arm (88) (see Fig. 17.40C). The ankle or lower calf may also be used. Adhesive tape, a Velcro strap, or a nonadhesive wrap such as Coban can be used to attach a flexible probe to the vascular bed. The probe should be snug against the skin but not so tight as to cause vasoconstriction. Circulation distal to the sensor location should be checked frequently. Clip-on reusable probes can be used in infants by placing the probe on part of the infant's hand, including some fingers, or part of the foot, including some toes (89). An ear probe has been used successfully on the palm of neonates. The shaft of the penis has been used (90).

FIXATION

Proper probe placement is critical to good performance. A malpositioned probe can result in false-positive or false-negative alarms (91). The penumbra effect occurs when the probe becomes partially dislodged from the measuring site (92,93). This generally causes a low reading before failure.

Probes can be totally or partially dislodged without being noticed. This may be difficult to determine if the probe is under drapes.

Adhesive probes often stay on better than clip-on probes. It may be beneficial to tape oximeter probes in place when they will be inaccessible during surgery, but it is important to avoid compression of the finger or other part. Wrapping the limb with gauze may serve to fix the probe in position.

STABILIZATION

The pulse search process that occurs when a probe is initially applied (or dislodged) includes sequential trials of various intensities of light in an effort to find one strong enough to transmit through the tissue but not so strong that the device's detection/amplification system is saturated (5). Once a pulse is found, there is generally a delay of a few more seconds while SpO_2 values for several pulses are averaged.

Appearance of a satisfactory waveform is a good indication that the readings are reliable. Comparison of the pulse rate shown by the oximeter and that indicated by an ECG monitor is a good method of ensuring reliability of saturation readings (32). A discrepancy between the rates is frequently an indication of malposition or malfunction of the probe.

Pulse oximetry has been used successfully during magnetic resonance imaging (94–96). Aluminum foil may be used to shield the probe (97). Pulse oximeters specially designed for use in these units are available (98,99).

INSPECTION OF SITES

During prolonged procedures, it is recommended that the site of probe application be inspected for evidence of injury.

Applications

MONITORING OXYGENATION

Hypoxemia is one of the most feared problems associated with anesthesia. Assessment of arterial oxygenation is an essential part of the monitoring of anesthetized patients. Its purpose is to provide warning of hypoxemia, the final common pathway for many life-threatening events so that treatment can be initiated before the hypoxia becomes severe enough to cause irreversible changes. Unlike carbon dioxide, body stores of oxygen are small. Thus changes in oxygenation occur rapidly. The magnitude and speed of a decrease in SpO_2 will depend on the initial SpO_2 and the cause of the decrease. Saturation will fall more quickly with obstructive than central apnea (100).

Anesthetizing Areas

Oxygen desaturation can occur anytime during anesthesia, regardless of the skill and experience of the anesthesiologist. Studies have shown that desaturation greater than 10% occurs in 10% to 53% of anesthetized patients (101–104). Pediatric patients are especially at risk (88,105–109). Most severe desaturations occur during induction or emergence. During maintenance, desaturations are milder but more frequent (110). Studies have shown that a reduction in the number of hypoxemic events occurred when pulse oximetry was used (106,111).

A period of increased risk is during the placement of catheters when the emphasis is on the establishment of monitoring with less attention directed toward the patient (112).

A number of problems can be manifested by desaturation, including pulmonary embolism (113) fat embolism (114), amniotic fluid embolism (115), pulmonary edema (116), pneumothorax (117,118), and malignant hyperthermia (119).

Pulse oximetry may help to detect unsuspected endobronchial intubation (120). This should be considered whenever there is a fall in oxygen saturation. However, it may not always detect endobronchial intubation, especially with elevated FI_{O_2} (5,121,122) and the absence of desaturation does not rule out bronchial intubation (123).

Oximetry is especially useful in managing one-lung anesthesia. Pulse oximetry can also help to assess the effectiveness of measures taken to increase the oxygen saturation (124,125).

Pulse oximetry can be used to assess oxygenation during newborn resuscitation (126).

Oximetry offers great usefulness for patients undergoing conduction anesthesia (127). Often the signs of hypoxia are confused with restlessness from an inadequate block and instead of supplying oxygen and assisting respiration, additional sedation is provided, which compounds the problem. With oximetry, the patient's oxygenation status can be assessed and adjustments made to provide the best SpO_2.

Much surgery, especially ophthalmological operations, is performed with local anesthesia supplemented with sedation. These patients are frequently older and in poor health, so a small amount of sedation may be excessive. Pulse oximetry is a very useful method of monitoring these patients.

Pulse oximetry may be helpful in confirmation of correct tracheal tube placement when a capnograph is not available or nonfunctional (128).

Postanesthesia Care Unit

The recovery room is another situation in which desaturation is common (129–140). Before leaving the recovery room, a trial of room air while observing oxygen saturation may provide an indication of the need for continuing supplemental oxygen.

Transport

Unrecognized oxygen desaturation may occur during transportation between the operating room and the postanesthesia care unit and between this unit and the critical care area or the wards (141–152). Battery-operated pulse oximeters should be used. Pulse oximetry is included on many transport monitors.

Postoperative Period

Patients frequently experience hypoxic episodes in the postoperative period (153–

155). Pulse oximetry can detect these and aid in deciding when supplemental oxygen therapy should be discontinued.

Out-of-Hospital Transport

Pulse oximetry may be useful during transport of patients by helicopter or ambulance (156–161).

CONTROLLING OXYGEN ADMINISTRATION

Oxygen is a drug and should be administered in a dose just sufficient to avoid hypoxemia without side effects. Pulse oximetry allows administration of the lowest concentration of inspired oxygen compatible with safe levels of arterial oxygenation (162).

Oximetry is useful in situations in which as low an oxygen concentration as possible is desired. These include laser procedures in the airway, during which keeping the oxygen concentration low will help diminish the potential for a fire (163).

MONITORING CIRCULATION

Pulse oximetry can be used to detect positions that compromise circulation (164,165). If an arm is positioned in a way that the pulse oximeter is unable to detect a pulse, this is an indication that the position should be altered.

Monitoring oxygen saturation during shoulder arthroscopy has been recommended as a test for brachial artery compression (166). However, an adequate pulse signal may be present with brachial plexus compression (167).

Pulse oximeters may be used to evaluate sympathetic block as indicated by an increase in peripheral blood flow (168,169).

Pulse oximetry has been used as a monitor for reimplanted or revascularized digits (170,171). Continuous saturation monitoring can provide warning of decreased perfusion and allow therapeutic interventions to occur before serious tissue damage results. However, oxygen saturation readings cannot be relied on to exclude vascular compromise in a limb (172).

The pulse oximeter has been used to monitor the effectiveness of CPR measures (173). However, because of artifacts and lag times, it may produce erroneous data (174).

Pulse oximetry can be used to measure palmar collateral circulation (175–182). However, its efficacy has been disputed (183–185). A similar examination of the dorsalis pedis and posterior tibial collateral arteries may be performed (176).

DETERMINING SYSTOLIC BLOOD PRESSURE

A pulse oximeter can be used to determine the systolic blood pressure (186–191). The blood pressure cuff is first applied to the same arm as the pulse oximeter. The cuff is inflated slowly and the pressure at the point at which the waveform is lost is noted. It also can be determined by inflating the cuff well past the systolic pressure and looking for the onset of a signal as the cuff is deflated. This leads to underestimation of the systolic pressure. One study found that the best agreement with Korotokoff sounds and noninvasive blood pressure equipment occurred when the average of blood pressures estimates at the disappearance and reappearance of the waveforms was taken as the systolic pressure (186).

Pulse oximetry may be used in patients with pulseless diseases of the extremities to monitor saturation and systolic blood pressure (192).

LOCATING VESSELS

When performing an axillary nerve block, it is important to locate the axillary artery. In cases where it cannot be palpated, it may be compressed by the searching finger. When this occurs, there should be lack of oxygen saturation in the fingers of that hand (193).

The dorsalis pedis artery can be localized by placing the oximeter probe on the second toe and occluding the posterior tibial artery behind the medial malleolus. As the artery is occluded, the pulse on the oximeter goes away (194).

Pulse oximetry has been used to locate the

femoral artery for cannulation when obesity prevented palpation of a pulse (195).

PREVENTING RETINOPATHY OF PREMATURITY

In premature neonates, administration of oxygen is sometimes associated with retrolental fibroplasia. Pulse oximetry can aid in titrating inspired oxygen by detecting hypoxemia. However, it is generally agreed that pulse oximetry is not adequate for evaluating hyperoxia in this setting (182).

MONITORING VASCULAR VOLUME

If the pulse oximeter begins skipping beats or performing intermittently, the cause could be hypovolemia (196). A correlation has been seen between pulse waveform amplitude variation during positive pressure ventilation and hypovolemia (197).

The diagnosis may sometimes be confirmed by interruption of ventilation for 15 sec. If this causes the pulse oximeter to return to normal or more constant function, a trial of fluid therapy may be warranted.

OTHER USES

Other situations in which oximetry may be useful include weaning from respiratory support (198), during high-frequency jet ventilation (199), and determining the effectiveness of therapeutic bronchoscopy. It can be combined with measurement of mixed venous oxyhemoglobin saturation to estimate oxygen use (200,201).

Pulse oximetry can be used to gauge pulmonary blood flow in infants and children with cyanotic congenital heart lesions and decreased pulmonary blood flow (202).

Advantages

ACCURACY

The instrument is accurate, and accuracy does not change with time. Numerous studies have shown that the difference between saturation determined by pulse oximetry and

by arterial blood gas analysis to be clinically insignificant above an SaO_2 of 70% (6,32,33,38,64,67,75,88,125,203–231). Most manufacturers claim that errors are less than $\pm 3\%$ at saturations above 70% (182). This accuracy should be sufficiently precise for most clinical purposes, except possibly for neonatal hyperoxia.

Pulse oximeters may be less accurate at lower saturations (65,204,214,226,232–235).

INDEPENDENCE FROM GASES AND VAPORS

Pulse oximetry readings are not affected by anesthetic gases or vapors.

DEPENDABILITY

The instruments are dependable. Studies have found that the failure rate, to be less than 2% (236–238). Performance is unaffected if pulse oximeter readings are made on the arm in which an arterial cannula is present (239). The failure rate is increased with ear and nose sensors (76).

FAST RESPONSE TIME

Pulse oximetry has a fast response time, especially compared with transcutaneous measurements (125). This allows rapid determination of changes so that anesthesia personnel can respond in a timely fashion.

NONINVASIVENESS

It is noninvasive, which allows it to be used as a routine monitor. It is readily accepted by awake patients, so it can be applied before induction. The temporary elevation of the Pa_{O_2} induced by pain and apprehension associated with invasive procedures is avoided. The bleeding, arterial insufficiency, embolization, and infection sometimes seen after arterial puncture are avoided.

CONTINUOUS MEASUREMENT

Monitoring is continuous. Developing trends can be detected and remedial action taken before severe hypoxia ensues.

CONTINUOUS PULSE RATE

Pulse oximetry provides a continuous pulse rate.

PROVISION OF SEPARATE RESPIRATORY AND CIRCULATORY VARIABLES (240)

Perfusion is indicated by the pulse strength signal and oxygenation by saturation. Unlike transcutaneous monitoring, the values displayed do not require interpretation. Most oximeters will signal if the flow is not adequate to provide a saturation value. This is helpful in determining a truly low saturation value as opposed to one from low flow.

MONITORING OF PERIPHERAL BLOOD FLOW

There is continuous beat-to-beat monitoring of the quality of the peripheral pulse. This may be helpful in determining whether a hypotensive patient has good cardiac output or is in shock. If blood pressure is low and pulse signal strength is high, the patient is probably vasodilated but perfusing adequately. If, however, both blood pressure and pulse strength are low, perfusion may be inadequate. If a vasoconstrictor agent is administered under these conditions, blood pressure may improve, but pulse strength will usually decline further.

EASY SENSOR APPLICATION

Application of the sensor is simple and fast. No skill is required.

CONVENIENCE

No calibration or changing of electrolyte or membrane is required.

MINIMAL SITE PREPARATION

Site preparation is minimal. "Arterialization" of the skin is not necessary, except when the earlobe is the monitoring site.

FAST START TIME

There is minimal delay in starting. Readout occurs within a few heartbeats after ap-

plication of the sensor. This is a distinct advantage over transcutaneous monitoring, which requires a prolonged warmup time.

VERIFICATION OF PROPER OPERATION

By providing an arterial pulse wave, it gives immediate verification of proper sensor operation.

TONE MODULATION

Changes in pulse tone with varying saturation allow the user to be continuously updated on pulse and SpO_2 without ever taking his or her eyes off the patient.

USER FRIENDLINESS

Most instruments are user friendly. Minimal training is required to learn to operate the instrument.

LIGHT WEIGHT AND COMPACTNESS

The console can be made compact and lightweight. This facilitates use in transport.

RUGGED SENSORS

The sensors are rugged. Although the sensor will take a lot of punishment, reusable sensors are costly to replace.

VARIETY OF SENSOR CONFIGURATIONS

The wide variety of sensor configurations confers broad clinical applicability to all types of patients, including preterm infants (32). The ability to use various vascular beds offers advantages from the standpoint of access during surgery and avoidance of the surgical field.

NO HEATING REQUIRED

No heating of the skin is required. The sensor can be left in place for extended periods without great risk of thermal injury.

BATTERY OPERATED

Most stand-alone units and those associated with a transport monitor are battery operated to facilitate transport.

ECONOMICAL

Estimates of the per-case cost of pulse oximetry range from $1.35 to $2.40 (101,110). Use of pulse oximetry can save money by allowing oxygen administration only when needed and decreasing the number of blood gas analyses (241–243).

Limitations and Disadvantages

INSENSITIVITY TO LOW BLOOD PRESSURE, LOW PULSE PRESSURE, AND VASOCONSTRICTION

Pulse oximeters require adequate plethysmographic pulsations to allow them to distinguish arterial blood light absorption from background venous blood and tissue light absorption (244). Readings may be unreliable or unavailable if there is a loss or diminution of the peripheral pulse (proximal blood pressure cuff inflation, leaning on an extremity, improper positioning, hypotension, hypothermia, cardiopulmonary bypass, low cardiac output, hypovolemia, peripheral vascular disease, or infusion of vasoconstrictor drugs) (60,75,189,244–248). With vasoconstriction, there may false saturation readings without eliminating the pulsatile signal (248,249).

Under these conditions, some pulse oximeters blank the display or give a message such as *Low Quality Signal* or *Inadequate Signal*. Others freeze the display when they are unable to detect a consistent pulse wave. The presence of a functioning pulse oximeter should not be construed as evidence of adequate tissue oxygenation or oxygen delivery to vital organs (182,189,250).

Application of vasodilating cream widens the physiologic limits within which reliable measurements can be obtained (251). Digital nerve blocks may restore oximeter signal detection (61,62,252).

Various methods have been devised for warming cool extremities (253,254). This may increase the pulse amplitude, provided the cardiac output is not depressed. If the patient is in shock, warming the extremity will probably not restore peripheral perfusion.

Although it has been recommended that under these circumstances a nasal or ear probe be used, studies indicate the finger probe perform best under conditions of poor perfusion (60). Placing a probe on the cheek or tongue may work (81).

INACCURACY WITH INCREASED VENOUS PRESSURE

The assumption that all pulsatile flow is arterial allows calculation of SpO_2. Prominent venous pulsations may lead to underestimation of the SaO_2 (255–257). The error may be worse when ear probes are used (79). Venous congestion increases the detection time for hypoxemia (246,248).

Venous pulses in the fingers are increased when the finger is in a dependent position (71). The effect on accuracy may be less when the probe is placed at the distal part of the finger (258).

High airway pressures during artificial ventilation may cause phasic venous congestion, which may be recognized by the oximeter as a pulse wave (259). In some cases, it may be necessary to turn off the ventilator to obtain a correct reading (259).

INTERFERENCE FROM EXOGENOUS DYES

Certain intravenous dyes including methylene blue, indocyanine green, indigo carmine, and fluorescein can interfere with readings and introduce errors (260–263). If methylene blue is injected into the uterine cavity, it will cause a lowering of the pulse oximetry readings (264,265). The magnitude of the change is dose dependent. Fortunately, the effect is usually minimal within a minute of administration (266,267). In vitro oximetry is also affected by methylene blue (17,268).

OPTICAL INTERFERENCE

Stray light or light flickering at frequencies similar to the frequencies of the light-emitting diode pulse rate, including sunlight, operating room lights, infrared heating lamps, light sources for various scopes, xenon lamps, and bilirubin lights, can enter the photodetector, resulting in inaccurate or erratic readings (7,269–278). Partial dislodgement of the probe may result in inaccurate readings (71,93). Oximeters vary significantly in their susceptibility to optical interference (247).

This should be suspected if the pulse rate displayed on the pulse oximeter does not correspond to that on other monitors. Although excessive ambient light usually prevents the oximeter from tracking the pulse, in some instances it can result in apparently normal but inaccurate measurements.

There are a number of ways of minimizing the effects of external optical interference. These include selection of the correct sensor for the patient and use, correct application of the sensor so the detector is across from the LEDs, making certain the sensor remains properly positioned, and shielding the sensor from bright light and other nearby sensors. It is usually sufficient to cover the probe with an opaque material such as a surgical towel, gauze, finger cot, blanket, alcohol wire pack, or other foil shield (49,279,280). Infrared light may not be shielded adequately by a blanket or towel (269). For infants, the foot can be wrapped in gauze, which cuts out extraneous light and reduces movement (281).

NAIL POLISH AND SKIN COLOR INTERFERENCE

Nail polish may or may not have an effect on readings (282,283). Some shades of black, blue, and green (but not red or purple) nail polishes may significantly lower saturation readings (284,285). Up to a 6% error in saturation has been reported.

Long fingernails can cause inaccurate readings (286). Synthetic nails may interfere with pulse oximetry (240). One way to avoid this (besides removing the polish or the fingernail) is to orient the finger probe so it transmits light from one side of the finger to the other side (72).

Fingerprinting ink will cause a low satu-ration reading (287). Henna, a stain used by some Middle Eastern women on the fingers and toes, can cause a low saturation reading (288). Children who have been finger painting with blue paints may exhibit low oxygen saturation readings (289).

The presence of onychomycosis, a yellowish gray color caused by fungus, can cause falsely low SpO_2 readings (290).

Oximeter readings may be erroneously high in patients with dark skin color (209,291–295). There is also a higher incidence of failure to detect a signal in such individuals.

Although there is one report of dried blood on a finger causing erroneous low saturation readings (295), other authors have found that dried blood does not affect the accuracy of the pulse oximeter (296,297).

LOSS OF ACCURACY AT LOW VALUES

Measurement of SpO_2 is less accurate at low values (33,64–66,68,208,210,214,215, 221,226,231,233–235,298–300).

ERRATIC PERFORMANCE WITH IRREGULAR RHYTHMS

Irregular heart rhythms can cause erratic performance. If the SpO_2 is stable, the signal strength is adequate, and at least three consecutive pulsatile plethysmograms are noted, there should not be a difference in saturation from that which would be found if normal sinus rhythm were present. Pulse oximetry is accurate in patients with dysrhythmias, provided the SpO_2 is stable and the plethysmogram is noise free and has reasonable amplitude (301). The SpO_2 may be correct even if the pulse rate is not.

SENSITIVE TO ELECTRICAL INTERFERENCE

Electrosurgical interference can cause the oximeter to give an incorrect pulse count (usually by counting extra beats) or falsely to detect a decrease in oxygen saturation (302). This problem may be increased in patients with weak pulse signals (6). False alarms caused by this can be frequent and annoying.

However, the effect is transient, limited to the duration of the cauterization. Manufacturers have made significant progress in reducing their instruments' sensitivity to electrical interference (6,182,247). Some monitors display a notice when significant interference is present.

There are a number of steps that will reduce electrical interference (302). These include locating the electrosurgery grounding plate as close to, and the oximeter sensor as far from, the surgical field as possible; routing the cable from the sensor to the oximeter away from the electrosurgery apparatus; keeping the pulse oximeter sensor and console as far as possible from the surgical site and the electrosurgery grounding plate and table; raising the high pulse rate alarm; and operating the unit in a rapid response mode. The electrosurgical apparatus and pulse oximeter should not be plugged into the same power source.

SATURATION DATA NOT HELPFUL AT HIGH OXYGEN PARTIAL PRESSURE

At high saturations, small changes in saturation are associated with relatively large changes in Pa_{O_2}. Thus it has limited ability to distinguish high but safe levels of arterial oxygen from excessively elevated levels (303).

DELAYED DETECTION OF HYPOXIC EVENTS

While the response time of the pulse oximeter is generally regarded as fast, there may be a significant delay between a change in alveolar oxygen tension and a change in the oximeter reading. It is possible for arterial oxygen to reach dangerous levels before the pulse oximeter alarm is activated (304).

Delay in pulse oximeter response is related to sensor location (69,78,305). Desaturation is detected earlier when the sensor is placed more centrally. Lag time will be decreased if blood flow to the site is increased (306) and increased with poor perfusion (189). Venous obstruction, peripheral vasoconstriction, cold, and motion artifacts will

cause increases in detection time for hypoxemia (51,246,248). Increasing the time over which the pulse signals are averaged increases the delay time.

FALSE ALARMS

A high percentage of pulse oximetry alarms are spurious (307,308–312). False alarms are most commonly caused by motion artifact but also are associated with poor signal quality, sensor displacement, and electrocautery interference. Motion artifact is usually not a problem during general anesthesia, but if the patient is shivering or moving about, as in the recovery room, it can be significant.

Delaying the time between detection of low SpO_2 and alarm activation and lowering the low SpO_2 alarm limit can reduce the number of false alarms (311,313).

Some false alarms can be avoided by simple measures such as putting the probe on a different arm from the automated blood pressure cuff or in a location where it will not be affected by pressure (308). On some pulse oximeters, turning off the low pulse rate alarm prevents them from alarming when a blood pressure cuff is inflated for a certain period of time (6). If the pulse oximeter is on the same hand as the nerve stimulator, artifact can occur with stimulation (314). Evoked potential monitoring can also produce a motion artifact.

The susceptibility of a pulse oximeter to motion artifact is influenced by the duration of time over which the pulsing signals are averaged to give a final reading, which may be changed by the user with some units (315). Longer averaging times reduce motion interference.

Artifacts caused by motion can be decreased by careful sensor positioning. Ear, cheek, and nose probes may be more useful than finger probes in restless patients. Flexible probes that are taped in place tend to be less susceptible to motion artifacts than clip-on probes (6). Probes lined with soft material may be associated with fewer motion artifacts (51). Smaller fingers are more susceptible to motion artifact (51).

Some pulse oximeters have sophisticated methods to reject noise and motion artifacts. Frequent running averages of saturation throughout a pulse pressure wave are carefully weighted to avoid showing sudden changes, and many factors are taken into account to determine when to indicate no reading if the signal quality is poor (316). Use of neural networks may reduce false alarms (317).

Synchronizing the pulse oximeter with the ECG monitor is another way of minimizing motion artifacts (51,54). Those components of the signal that are coupled to the ECG pass unchanged, whereas those that are random with respect to the ECG (e.g., motion artifact or other noise) are attenuated. However, the oximeter may synchronize with ECG artifacts generated by motion or shivering, resulting in erroneous readings (6). Furthermore, with this system, the pulse rate displayed by the oximeter is necessarily equal to the pulse rate show by the ECG monitor; therefore, when using this system, equality of the pulse rates indicated by the ECG and oximeter should not be used as an indication that the displayed saturation data are valid.

Pulse oximeters that display the arterial plethysmographic waveform have an advantage over those that display only the amplitude of the signal, because this allows the operator to assess the quality of the signal from which the saturation is derived and to observe any noise such as motion artifacts that may alter its accuracy (318).

Following a pulse oximeter alarm, one should first look to the message display for a *probe off* message and to the plethysmographic waveform for evidence of motion or electrocautery interference. Many oximeters give an artifact message with motion.

FALSELY HIGH SpO$_2$ READINGS

The pulse oximeter may overestimate SpO$_2$ if the sensor is malpositioned (91). Optical interference can result in falsely elevated readings (272,276), as may use of too large a probe (53). Cases of unexplained falsely elevated oximeter readings have been reported (319).

FAILURE TO DETECT ABSENCE OF CIRCULATION

Some pulse oximeters show pulses despite inadequate tissue perfusion (189,248) or even when no pulse is present (174,278, 320,321). Ambient light may produce a false signal (277).

EXPENSIVE SENSOR

Use of disposable sensors can be costly. Although intended for single use, many clinicians reuse disposable sensors for a number of patients. Methods for prolonging the life of disposable probes have been described (49,322,323). Some disposable sensors can be returned to the manufacturer for recycling (46).

DISCREPANCIES IN READINGS FROM DIFFERENT MONITORS

A discrepancy in readings between two different brands of oximeter on the same patient at the same time is not uncommon (9,324). One reason for the difference is the way pulse oximeters are calibrated (325). A monitor calibrated to fractional saturation will not correlate with one calibrated to functional saturation.

PULSE OVERLOAD

In the presence of very large pulses, some pulse oximeters can become overloaded and read zero (326).

PATIENT INJURY

Burns can result if probes of different manufacturers are used with oximeters other than that for which they were designed (327–330) or if a damaged probe is used (331–334). Mild burns are relatively common (335,336).

Ischemic injuries associated with reuseable finger probes have been reported (337–340). The risk may be increased by prolonged probe application, compromised perfusion of the extremity, or tight application of tape.

Injuries ranging from burns and mild skin necrosis to tanned areas under the probe have been reported in children when probes were left in place for long periods of time (341–343).

First-, second-, and third-degree burns associated with pulse oximetry during MRI as a result of induced skin current beneath looped cables acting as antennae have been reported (344–346).

To avoid these injuries, frequent inspection of probe sites and site rotation are recommended. When a probe is placed on a finger or toe, it is recommended that the light source should be placed on the nail rather than the pulp of the digit (343). Gloves can be placed on the hand to protect from thermal burns without affecting the accuracy of the instrument (347). Any freezing of the pulse oximeter display should be investigated to aid in detection of short circuits.

During MRI, the danger of burns can be reduced by the following measures:

1. All potential conductors should be checked before use to ensure the absence of frayed insulation, exposed wires, and other hazards.
2. All unnecessary conductive materials such as unused surface coils should be removed from the bore of the MR system before initiation of patient monitoring.
3. The sensor should be placed as far from the imaging site as possible.
4. All cables or wires from monitoring devices that come into contact with the patient should be positioned so that no loops are formed.
5. If possible, no potential conductors should touch the patient at more than one location.
6. A thick layer of thermal insulation should be placed between any wires or cables and the patient's skin.
7. Monitoring devices that do not appear to

be operating properly during imaging should be removed from the patient immediately.

Despite these limitations, pulse oximetry is a practical method for monitoring oxygenation and its use has become the standard of care for all anesthetized patients. It is likely that its routine use could reduce the number of anesthetic mishaps and malpractice claims.

REFRENCES

1. Gravenstein JS. International standards for safe practice endorsed by WFSA. APSF Newslett 1992;7:29–31.
2. Tinker JH, Dull DL, Caplan RA, Ward RJ, Cheney FW. Role of monitoring devices in prevention of anesthetic mishaps. A closed claims analysis. Anesthesiology 1989;71:541–546.
3. Tremper KK, Barker SJ. Pulse oximetry. Anesthesiology 1989;70:98–108.
4. Wukitsch MW, Petterson MT, Tobler DR, Pologe JA. Pulse oximetry. Analysis of theory, technology, and practice. J Clin Monit 1988;4:290–300.
5. Kelleher JF. Pulse oximetry. J Clin Monit 1989;5:37–62.
6. Alexander CM, Teller LE, Gross JB. Principles of pulse oximetry. Theoretical and practical considerations. Anesth Analg 1989;68:368–376.
7. Anonymous. Pulse Oximeters. Health Devices 1989;18:185–230.
8. Reynolds KJ, Palayiwa E, Moyle JTB, Sykes MK, Hahn CEW. The effect of dyshemoglobins on pulse oximetry. Part I: theoretical approach. Part II: experimental results using an in vitro test system. J Clin Monit 1993;9:81–90.
9. Pologe JA. Functional saturation versus fractional saturation. what does pulse oximetry read. J Clin Monit 1989;5:298–299.
10. Petty TL. Clinical pulse oximetry. Boulder, CO: Ohmeda, 1986,
11. Barker SJ, Tremper KK, Hyatt J. Effects of methemoglobinemia on pulse oximetry and mixed venous oximetry. Anesthesiology 1989;70:112–117.
12. Kumar A, Chawla R, Ahuja S, Girdhar KK, Bhattacharya A. Nitrobenzene poisoning and spurious pulse oximetry. Anaesthesia 1990;45:949–951.
13. Severinghaus JW, Xu Fa-Di, Spellman MJ. Benzocaine and methemoglobin. Recommended actions. Anesthesiology 1991;74:385–386.
14. Anderson ST, Hajduczek J, Barker SJ. Benzocaine-induced methomoglobinemia in an adult:

accuracy of pulse oximetry with methemoglobinemia. Anesth Analg 1988;67:1099–1101.

15. Marks LF, Desgrand D. Prilocaine associated methaemoglobinaemia and the pulse oximeter. Anaesthesia 1991;46:703.

16. Bardoczky GI, Wathieu M, D'Hollander A. Prilocaine-induced methemoglobinemia evidenced by pulse oximetry. Acta Anaesthesiol Scand 1990;34:162–164.

17. Eisenkraft JB. Pulse oximeter desaturation due to methemoglobinemia. Anesthesiology 1988; 68:278–282.

18. Trillo PA, Aukburg S. Dapsone-induced methemoglobinemia and pulse oximetry. Anesthesiology 1992;77:594–596.

19. Varpm AK. Methemoglobinemia and pulse oximetry. Crit Care Med 1992;20:1363–1364.

20. Delwood L, O'Flaherty D, Prejean EJ, Popat M, Giesecke AH. Methaemoglobinaemia and pulse oximetry. Anaesthesia 1992;47:80.

21. Delwood L, O'Flaherty D, Prejean EJ, Giesecke AH. Methemoglobinemia and its effect on pulse oximetry. Crit Care Med 1991;19:988.

22. Rieder HU, Frei FJ, Zbinden AM. Thomson DA. Pulse oximetry in methaemoglobinaemia. Anaesthesia 1989;44:326–327.

23. Schweitzer SA. Spurious pulse oximeter desaturation due to methaemoglobinaemia. Anesth Intensive Care 1991;19:269–271.

24. Watcha MF, Connor MT, Hing AV. Pulse oximetry in methemoglobinemia. Am J Dis Child 1989;143:845–847.

25. Vegfors M, Lennmarken C. Carboxyhemoglobinaemia and pulse oximetry. Br J Anaesth 1991;66:625–626.

26. Gonzalez A, Gomez-Arnay J, Pensado A. Carboxyhemoglobin and pulse oximetery. Anesthesiology 1990;73:573.

27. Barker SJ, Tremper KT. The effect of carbon monoxide inhalation on pulse oximetry and transcutaneous pO$_2$. Anesthesiology 1987;66:677–679.

28. Goldhill DR, Hill AJ, Whitburn RH, Feneck RO, George PJM, Keeling P. Carboxyhaemoglobin concentrations, pulse oximetry, and arterial blood-gas tensions during jet ventilation for Nd-YAG laser bronchoscopy. Br J Anaesth 1990;65:749–753.

29. Hodges MR, Preece LP, Downs JB. Clinical experience with pulse oximetry in the presence of elevated carboxyhemoglobin. Anesthesiology 1989; 71:A369.

30. Tashiro C, Koo YH, Fukumitsu K, Tomi K, Mashimo T, Yoshiya I. Effects of carboxyhemoglobin on pulse oximetry in humans. J Anesth 1988;2:36–40.

31. Anderson JV. The accuracy of pulse oximetry in neonates: effects of fetal hemoglobin and bilirubin. J Perinatol 1987;7:323.

32. Deckardt R, Steward DJ. Noninvasive arterial hemoglobin oxygen saturation versus transcutaneous oxygen tension monitoring in the preterm infant. Crit Care Med 1984;12:935–939.

33. Fanconi S, Doherty P, Edmonds JF, Barker GA, Bohn DJ. Pulse oximetry in pediatric intensive care. Comparison with measured saturations and transcutaneous oxygen tension. J Pediatr 1985;107:362–366.

34. Harris AP, Sendak MJ, Donham RT, Thomas M, Duncan D. Absorption characteristics of human fetal hemoglobin at wavelengths used in pulse oximetry. J Clin Monit 1988;4:175–177.

35. Pologe JA, Raley DM. Effects of fetal hemoglobin on pulse oximetry. J Perinatol 1987;7:324–326.

36. Praud J-P, Carofilis A, Bridey F, Lacaille F, Dehan M, Gaultier CL. Accuracy of two wavelength pulse oximetry in neonates and infants. Pediatr Pulminol 1989;6:180–182.

37. House JT, Schultetus RR, Gravenstein N. Continuous neonatal evaluation in the delivery room by pulse oximetry. J Clin Monit 1987;3:96–100.

38. Ramanathan R, Durand M, Larrazabal C. Pulse oximetry in very low birth weight infants with acute and chronic lung disease. Pediatrics 1989;79:612–617.

39. Jennis MS, Peabody JL. Pulse oximetry. An alternative method for the assessment of oxygenation in newborn infants. Pediatrics 1988;79:524–528.

40. Beall SN, Moorthy SS. Jaundice, oximetry, and spurious hemoglobin desaturation. Anesth Analg 1989;68:806–807.

41. Chelluri L, Snyder JV, Bird JR. Accuracy of pulse oximetry in patients with hyperbilirubinemia. Respir Care 1991;36:1383–1386.

42. Veyckemans F, Baele P, Guillaume JE, Willems E, Robert A, Clerbaux T. Hyperbilirubinemia does not interfere with hemoglobin saturation measured by pulse oximetry. Anesthesiology 1989;70:118–122.

43. Veyckemans F, Baele PL. More about jaundice and oximetry. Anesth Analg 1990;70:335–336.

44. Severinghaus JW, Koh SO. Effect of anemia on pulse oximeter accuracy at low saturation. J Clin Monit 1990;6:85–88.

45. Lee S, Tremper KK, Barker SJ. Effects of anemia on pulse oximetry and continuous mixed venous hemoglobin saturation monitoring in dogs. Anesthesiology 1991;75:118–122.

46. Anonymous. Hospitals look for savings in pulse oximetry sensors. Technol Anesth 1992;13(5):1–2.

47. Maruschak GF, Johnson RM. Pulse oximeter cost per use—securing savings. Anesthesiology 1989;71:167–168.

48. Foltz BD. Another technique for extending the life

of oximetry monitoring probes. Anesth Analg 1987;66:367–374.

49. Alpert CC, Cooke JE. Extending the life of oximetry monitoring probes. Anesth Analg 1986;65:826–827.

50. Racys V, Nahrwold ML. Reusing the Nellcor pulse oximeter probe. Is it worth the savings? Anesthesiology 1987;66:713.

51. Langton JA, Hanning CD. Effect of motion artefact on pulse oximeters. Evaluation of four instruments and finger probes. Br J Anaesth 1990;65:564–570.

52. Yoder RD. Preservation of pulse oximetery sensors. Anesthesiology 1988;68:308.

53. Zahka KG, Dean MJ. Failure of pulse oximetry to detect severe hypoxia: importance of sensor selection. Clin Pediatr 1988;27:403–404.

54. Barrington KJ, Finer NN, Ryan CA. Evaluation of pulse oximetry as a continuous monitoring technique in the neonatal intensive care unit. Crit Care Med 1988;16:1147–1153.

55. Pasterkamp H, Daien D. The use of a personal computer for trend data analysis with the Ohmeda 3700 pulse oximeter. J Clin Monit 1988;4:215–222.

56. American Society for Testing and Materials. Specification for pulse oximeters (F1415–92). Philadelphia: ASTM, 1992.

57. International Organization for Standardization. Pulse oximeters for medical use—requirements (ISO 9919–1992). Geneve: ISO, 1992.

58. Barker SJ, Le N, Hyatt J. Failure rates of transmission and reflectance pulse oximetry for various sensor sites. J Clin Monit 1991;7:102–103.

59. Swedlow DB, Running V, Feaster SJ. Ambient light affects pulse oximeters: a reply. Anesthesiology 1987;67:865.

60. Clayton DG, Webb RK, Ralston AC, Duthie D, Runciman WB. Pulse oximetry probes. A comparison between finger, nose, ear and forehead under conditions of poor perfusion. Anaesthesia 1991;46:260–265.

61. Grayson RF, Bourke DL. Digital block for pulse oximetry failure. Anesthesiology 1991;75:A407.

62. Bourke DL, Grayson RF. Digital nerve blocks can restore pulse oximeter signal detection. Anesth Analg 1991;73:815–817.

63. Berko RS, Kagle DM, Alexander CM, Giuffre M, Gross JB. Evaluation of the Ohmeda Biox 3700 pulse oximeter during rapid changes in arterial oxygen saturation. Anesthesiology 1986;65:A130.

64. Kagle DM, Alexander CM, Berko RS, Giuffre M, Gross JB. Evaluation of the Ohmeda 3700 pulse oximeter: steady-state and transient response characteristics. Anesthesiology 1987;66:376–380.

65. Severinghaus JW, Naifeh KH. Accuracy of response of six pulse oximeters to profound hypoxia. Anesthesiology 1987;67:551–558.

66. Severinghaus JW, Naifeh KH, Koh SO. Errors in 14 pulse oximeters during profound hypoxia. J Clin Monit 1989;5:72–81.

67. Warley ARH, Mitchell JH, Stradling JR. Evaluation of the Ohmeda 3700 pulse oximeter. Thorax 1988;42:892–896.

68. Webb RK, Ralston AC, Runciman WB. Potential errors in pulse oximetry. Part II. Effects of changes in saturation and signal quality. Anaesthesia 1991;46:207–212.

69. Young D, Jewkes C, Spittal M, Blogg C, Weissman J, Gradwell D. Response time of pulse oximeters assessed using acute decompression. Anesth Analg 1992;74:189–195.

70. Kurki TS, Sanford TJ, Smity NT, Dec-Silver H, Head N. Effects of radial artery cannulation on the function of finger blood pressure and pulse oximeter monitors. Anesthesiology 1988;69:778–782.

71. Kim J-M, Arakawa K, Benson KT, Fox DK. Pulse oximetry and circulatory kinetics associated with pulse volume amplitude measured by photoelectric plethysmography. Anesth Analg 1986;65:1333–1339.

72. White PF, Boyle WA. Nail polish and oximetry. Anesth Analg 1989;68:546–547.

73. Ezri T, Lurie S, Konichezky S, Soroker D. Pulse oximetry from the nasal septum. J Clin Anesth 1991;3:447–450.

74. Segstro R. Nasal sensor attachment. Can J Anaesth 1989;36:365–366.

75. Yelderman M, New W. Evaluation of pulse oximetry. Anesthesiology 1983;59:349–352.

76. Barker SJ, Hyatt J, Rumack WA. Pulse oximeter failure rates. Effects of manufacturer sensor site and patient. Anesth Analg 1992;74:S15.

77. Rosenberg J, Pedersen MH. Nasal pulse oximetry overestimates oxygen saturation. Anaesthesia 1990;45:1070–1072.

78. Broome IJ, Harris RW, Reilly CS. The response times during anaesthesia of pulse oximeters measuring oxygen saturations during hypoxaemic events. Anaesthesia 1992;47:17–19.

79. Skacel M, O'Hare E, Harrison D. Invalid information from the ear probe of a pulse oximeter in tricuspid incompetence. Anaesth Intensive Care 1990;18:270.

80. Jobes DR, Nicolson SC. Monitoring of arterial hemoglobin oxygen saturation using a tongue sensor. Anesth Analg 1988;67:186–188.

81. Cote CJ, Daniels AL, Connolly M, Szyfelbein SK, Wickens CD. Tongue oximetry in children with extensive thermal injury. Comparison with peripheral oximetry. Can J Anaesth 1992;39:454–457.

82. Hickerson W, Morrell M, Cicala RS. Glossal pulse oximetry. Anesth Analg 1989;69:73–74.

83. Gunter JB. A buccal sensor for measuring arterial oxygen saturation. Anesth Analg 1989;69:417–418.

84. Sosis MB, Coleman N. Use of an Ohmeda ear oximetry probe for "buccal" oximetry. Can J Anaesth 1990;37:489–490.

85. Lema GE. Oral pulse oximetry in small children. Anesth Analg 1991;72:414.

86. O'Leary RJ, Landon M, Benumof JL. Buccal pulse oximeter is more accurate than finger pulse oximeter in measuring oxygen saturation. Anesth Analg 1992;75:495–498.

87. Landon M, Benumof JL, O'Leary RJ. Buccal pulse oximetry: an accurate alternative to the finger probe. Anesthesiology 1992;77:A526.

88. Miyasaka K, Katayama M, Kusakawa I, Ohata J, Kawano T, Honma Y. Use of pulse oximetry in neonatal anesthesia. J Perinatol 1987;7:343–345,

89. Mikawa K, Maekawa N. A simple alternate technique for the application of the pulse oximeter probe to infants. Anaesthesia 1992;77:400.

90. Robertson RE, Kaplan RF. Another site for the pulse oximeter probe. Anesthesiology 1991;74:198.

91. Barker SJ, Hyatt J, Shah NK. The accuracy of malpositioned pulse oximeters during hypoxemia. Anesthesiology 1992;77:A496.

92. Kelleher JF, Ruff RH. The pneumbra effect. Vasomotion-dependent pulse oximeter artifact due to probe malposition. Anesthesiology 1989;71:787–791.

93. Serpell MG. Children's fingers and spurious pulse oximetry. Anaesthesia 1991;46:702–703.

94. Peden CJ, Menon DK, Hall AS, Sargentoni J, Whitwam JG. Magnetic resonance for the anaesthetist. Part II. Anaesthesia and monitoring in MR units. Anaesthesia 1992;47:508–517.

95. Glaser R, Fisher DM. Respiratory monitoring for children undergoing radiation therapy. Anesthesiology 1985;63:123–124.

96. Karlik SJ, Heatherley T, Pavan F, et al. Patient anesthesia and monitoring at a 1.5-T MRI Installation. Magn Reson Med 1988;7:210–221.

97. Wagle WA. Technique for RF isolation of a pulse oximeter in a 1.5-T MR unit. Am J Neuroradiol 1989;10:208.

98. Salvo I, Colombo S, Capocasa T, Torri G. Pulse oximetry in MRI units. J Clin Anesth 1990;2:65–66.

99. Shellock FG, Kimble K. Monitoring heart rate and oxygen saturation during MRI with a fiber-optic pulse oximeter. Abstract of paper presented to the Society of Magnetic Resonance in Medicine. San Francisco, August 10–16, 1991.

100. Hanning CD. Oximetry and anaesthetic practice. (Preoperative, intraoperative, postoperative and critical care). Leicester, UK: BOC Healthcare Group, 1985.

101. Raemer DB, Warren DL, Morris R, Philip BK, Philip JH. Hypoxemia during ambulatory gynecologic surgery as evaluated by the pulse oximeter. J Clin Monit 1987;3:244–248.

102. Moller JT, Joannessen NW, Berg H, Espersen K, Larsen LE. Hypoxaemia during anaesthesia. An observer study. Br J Anaesth 1991;66:437–444.

103. Whitcher C, New W, Bacon BA. Perianesthetic oxygen saturation vs skill of the anesthetist. Anesthesiology 1982;57:A172.

104. Walsh JF. Training for day-case dental anaesthesia. Oxygen saturation during general anaesthesia administered by dental undergraduates. Anaesthesia 1984;39:1124–1127.

105. Bone ME, Galler D, Flynn PJ. Arterial oxygen saturation during general anesthesia for paediatric dental extraction. Anaesthesia 1987;42:879–882.

106. Cote CJ, Goldstein EA, Cote MA, Hoaglin DC, Ryan JF. A single-blind study of pulse oximetry in children. Anesthesiology 1988;68:184–188.

107. Cote CJ, Rolf N, Liu LMP, et al. A single-blind study of combined pulse oximetry and capnography in children. Anesthesiology 1991;74:980–987.

108. Laycock GJA, McNicol LR. Hypoxaemia during induction of anaesthesia—an audit of children who underwent general anaesthesia for routine elective surgery. Anaesthesia 1988;43:981–984.

109. Moorthy SS, Dierdorf SF, Krishna G. Transient hypoxemia during emergence from anesthesia in children. Anesthesiol Rev 1988;15:20–23.

110. McKay WPS, Noble WH. Critical incidents detected by pulse oximeter during anaesthesia. Can J Anaesth 1988;35:265–269.

111. Moller JT, Jensen PF, Johannessen NW, Espersen K. Hypoxaemia is reduced by pulse oximetry monitoring in the operating theatre and in the recovery room. Br J Anaesth 1992;68:146–150.

112. Hensley FA, Dodson DL, Martin DE, Stauffer RA, Larach DR. Oxygen saturation during preinduction placement of monitoring catheters in the cardiac surgical patient. Anesthesiology 1987;66:834–836.

113. Michael S, Fraser RB, Reilly CS. Intra-operative pulmonary embolism. Detection by pulse oximetry. Anaesthesia 1990;45:225–226.

114. Byrick RJ, Forbes D, Waddell JP. A monitored cardiovascular collapse during cemented total knee replacement. Anesthesiology 1986;65:213–216.

115. Quance D. Amniotic fluid embolism: detection by pulse oximetry. Anesthesiology 1988;68:951–952.

116. Mason RA. The pulse oximeter—an early warning device? Anaesthesia 1987;42:784–785.

117. Allberry RAW, Westbrook D. Pulse oximetry. Anaesth Intensive Care 1991;19:130.

118. Laishley RS, Aps C. Tension pneumothorax and pulse oximetry. Br J Anaesth 1991;66:250–252.

119. Bacon AK. Pulse oximetry in malignant hyperthermia. Anaesth Intensive Care 1989;17:208–210.

120. Riley R. Detection of unsuspected endobronchial intubation by pulse oximetery. Anaesth Intensive Care 1989;17:381–382.

121. Barker SJ, Tremper KK, Hyatt J, Zaccari J, Thaure TB. Pulse oximetry may not detect endobronchial intubation. Anesthesiology 1987;67:A170.

122. Barker SJ, Tremper KK, Hyatt J, Heitzmann H. Comparison of three oxygen monitors in detecting endobronchial intubation. J Clin Monit 1988;1:240–243.

123. Barker JS, Tremper KK. Detection of endobronchial intubation by noninvasive monitoring. J Clin Monit 1987;3:292–293.

124. Brodsky JB, Shulman MS, Swan M, Mark JBD. Pulse oximetry during one-lung ventilation. Anesthesiology 1985;63:212–214.

125. Viitanen A, Salmenpera M, Heinonen J. Noninvasive monitoring of oxygenation during one-lung ventilation: a comparison of transcutaneous oxygen tension measurement and pulse oximetry. J Clin Monit 1987;3:90–95.

126. Sendak MJ, Harris AP, Donham RT. Use of pulse oximetry to assess arterial oxygen saturation during newborn resuscitation. Crit Care Med 1986;14:739–740.

127. Davies MJ, Scott DA, Cook PT. Continuous monitoring of arterial oxygen saturation with pulse oximetry during spinal anesthesia. Reg Anesth 1987;12:63–70.

128. Sosis MB, Sisamis J. Pulse oximetry in confirmation of correct tracheal tube placement. Anesth Analg 1991;71:309–310.

129. Moller JT, Wittrup M, Johansen SH. Hypoxemia in the postanesthesia care unit. An observer study. Anesthesiology 1990;73:890–895.

130. Canet J, Ricos M, Vidal F, Early postoperative arterial desaturation. Determining factors and response to oxygen therapy. Anesth Analg 1989;69:207–212.

131. Smith DC, Canning JJ, Crul JF. Pulse oximetry in the recovery room. Anaesthesia 1989;44:345–348.

132. Tomkins DP, Gaukroger P. Oxygen saturation in children following general anaesthesia. Anaesth Intensive Care 1987;15:111.

133. Bach A. Pulse oximetry in the recovery room. Anaesthesia 1989;44:1007.

134. Brown LT, Purcell GJ, Traugott FM. Hypoxaemia during postoperative recovery using continuous pulse oximetry. Anaesth Intensive Care 1990;18:509–516.

135. Glazener C, Motoyama K. Hypoxemia in children following general anesthesia. Anesthesiology 1984;61:A416.

136. Motoyama EK, Glazener CH. Hypoxemia after general anesthesia in children. Anesth Analg 1986;65:267–272.

137. Mertzlufft FO, Jansen U, Dick W. Continuous monitoring of arterial oxygenation in the recovery room using pulse oximetry. Eur J Anaesth 1987;4:64–65.

138. McDonald J, Keneally J. Oxygen saturation in children during transit from operating theatre to recovery. Anaesth Intensive Care 1987;15:360–361.

139. Morris RW, Bushman A, Warren DL, Philip JH, Raemer DB. The prevalence of hypoxemia detected by pulse oximetry during recovery from anesthesia. J Clin Monit 1988;4:16–20.

140. Nakatsuka M, Bolling D. Incidence of postoperative hypoxemia in the recovery room detected by the pulse oximeter. Anesth Analg 1989;68:S209.

141. Blair I, Holland R, Lau W, McCarthy N, Chiah TS, Ledwidge D. Oxygen saturation during transfer from operating room to recovery after anaesthesia. Anaesth Intensive Care 1987;15:147–150.

142. Chripko D, Bevan JC, Archer DP, Bherer N. Decreases in arterial oxygen saturation in paediatric outpatients during transfer to the postanaesthetic recovery room. Can J Anaesth 1989;36:128–132.

143. Katarina BK, Harnik EV, Mitchard R, Kim Y, Admed S. Postoperative arterial oxygen saturation in the pediatric population during transportation. Anesth Analg 1988;67:280–282.

144. Meiklejohn BH, Smith G, Elling AE, Hindocha N. Arterial oxygen desaturation during postoperative transportation: the influence of operation site. Anaesthesia 1987;42:1313–1315.

145. Pullerits J, Burrows RA, Roy WL. Arterial desaturation in healthy children during transfer to the recovery room. Can J Anaesth 1987;34:470–473.

146. Patel R, Norden J, Hannallah RS. Oxygen administration prevents hypoxia during post-anesthetic transport in children. Anesthesiology 1988;69:616–618.

147. Riley RH, Davis NJ, Finucane KE, Christmas P. Arterial oxygen saturation in anaesthetised patients during transfer from induction room to operating room. Anaesth Intensive Care 1988;16:182–186.

148. Smith DC, Crul JF. Early postoperative hypoxia during transport. Br J Anaesth 1988;61:625–627.

149. Tyler IL, Tantisira B, Winter PM, Motoyama EK.

Continuous monitoring of arterial oxygen saturation with pulse oximetry during transfer to the recovery room. Anesth Analg 1985;64:1108–1112.

150. Tompkins DP, Gaukroger PB, Bentley MW. Hypoxia in children following general anesthesia. Anaesth Intensive Care 1988;16:177–181.

151. Tait AR, Kyff JV, Crider B, Santibhavank V, Learned D. Post-operative arterial oxygen saturation—up in a puff of smoke. Anesth Analg 1989;68:S284.

152. Tait AR, Kyff JV, Crider B, Santibhavank V, Learned D, Finch JS. Changes in arterial oxygen saturation in cigarette smokers following general anesthesia. Can J Anaesth 1990;37:423–428.

153. Lampe GH, Wauk LZ, Whitendale P, Way WL, Kozmary SV, Donegan JH, Eger EI. Postoperative hypoxemia after nonabdominal surgery. A frequent event not caused by nitrous oxide. Anesth Analg 1990;71:597–601.

154. Choi HJ, Little MS, Garber SZ, Tremper KK. Pulse oximetry for monitoring during ward analgesia. Epidural morphine versus parenteral narcotics. J Clin Monit 1989;5:87–89.

155. McKenzie AJ. Perioperative hypoxaemia detected by intermittent pulse oximetry. Anaesth Intensive Care 1989;17:412–417.

156. Aughey K, Hess D, Eitel D, et al. An evaluation of pulse oximetry in prehospital care. Ann Emerg Med 1991;20:887–891.

157. Short L, Hecker RB, Middaugh RE, Menk EJ. A comparison of pulse oximeters during helicopter flight. J Emerg Med 1989;7:639–643.

158. Hankins CT. The use of pulse oximetry during infant transport from outside facilities. J Perinatol 1987;7:346.

159. Puttick NP, Lawler PGP. Pulse oximetry in mountain rescue and helicopter evacuation. Anaesthesia 1989;44:867.

160. Runcie CJ, Reeve W. Pulse oximetry during transport of the critically ill. J Clin Monit 1991;7:348–349.

161. Talke P, Nichols RJ, Traber DL. Monitoring patients during helicopter flight. J Clin Monit 1990;6:139–140.

162. Brodsky JB, Shulman MS. Oxygen monitoring of bleomycin-treated patients. Can Anaesth Soc J 1984;31:488.

163. Lennon RL, Hosking MP, Warner MA, et al. Monitoring and analysis of oxygenation and ventilation during rigid bronchoscopic neodymium-YAG laser resection of airway tumors. Surv Anesth 1988;32:100.

164. Skeehan TM, Hensley FA Jr. Axillary artery compression and the prone position. Anesth Analg 1986;65:518–519.

165. Hovagim AR, Backus WW, Manecke G, Lagasse R, Sidhu U, Poppers PJ. Pulse oximetry and patient positioning. A report of eight cases. Anesthesiology 1989;71:454–456.

166. Herschman ZJ, Frost EAM, Goldiner PL. Pulse oximetry during shoulder arthroscopy. Anesthesiology 1986;65:565.

167. Gibbs N, Handal J, Nentwig MK. Pulse oximetry during shoulder arthroscopy. Anesthesiology 1987;67:150–151.

168. Vegfors M, Tryggvason B, Sjoberg F, Lennmarken C. Assessment of peripheral blood flow using a pulse oximeter. J Clin Monit 1990;6:1–4.

169. Ngeow J, Shay P, Neudachin L. Plethysmographic pulse oximetry. A teaching tool in lumbar sympathetic blockade. Anesthesiology 1990;73:A1086.

170. Graham B, Paulus DA, Caffee HH. Pulse oximetry for vascular monitoring in upper extremity replantation surgery. J Hand Surg 1986;11:687–692.

171. Skeen JT, Bacus WW, Hovagim AR, Poppers PJ. Intraoperative pulse oximetry in peripheral revascularization in an infant. J Clin Monit 1988;4:272–273.

172. Clay NR, Dent CM. Limitations of pulse oximetry to assess limb vascularity. J Bone Joint Surg 1991;73:344.

173. Narang VPS. Utility of the pulse oximeter during cardiopulmonary resuscitation. Anesthesiology 1986;65:239–240.

174. Moorthy SS, Dierdorf SF, Schmidt SI. Erroneous pulse oximetry data during CPR. Anesth Analg 1990;70:339.

175. Matsuki A. A modified Allen's test using a pulse oximeter. Anaesth Intensive Care 1988;16:126–127.

176. Nowak GS, Moorthy SS, McNiece WL. Use of pulse oximetry for assessment of collateral arterial flow. Anesthesiology 1986;64:527.

177. Cheng EY, Lauer, KK, Stommel KA, Guenther NR. Evaluation of the palmar circulation by pulse oximetry. J Clin Monit 1989;5:1–3.

178. Pillow K, Herrick IA. Pulse oximetry compared with Doppler ultrasound for assessment of collateral blood flow to the hand. Anaesthesia 1991;46:388–390.

179. Persson E. The pulse oximeter and Allen's test. Anaesthesia 1992;47:451.

180. Raju R. The pulse oximeter and the collateral circulation. Anaesthesia 1986;41:783–784.

181. Rozenberg B, Rosenberg M, Birkhan J. Allen's test performed by pulse oximetry. Anaesthesia 1988;43:515–516.

182. Severinghaus JW, Kelleher JF. Recent developments in pulse oximetry. Anesthesiology 1992;76:1018–1038.

183. Glavin RJ. Pulse oximeter and Allen's test. Anaesthesia 1992;47:917.

184. Lovinsohn DG, Gordon L, sessler DI. The Allen's test. Analysis of four methods. J Hand Surg 1991;16A:279–282.

185. Glavin RJ, Jones HM. Assessing collateral circulation in the hand. Four methods compared. Anaesthesia 1989;44:594–595.

186. Chawla R, Kumarvel V, Girdhar KK, Sethi AK, Indrayan A, Bhattacharya A. Can pulse oximetry be used to measure systolic blood pressure? Anesth Analg 1992;74:196–200.

187. Greenblott GB, Gerschultz S, Tremper KK. Blood flow limits and signal detection comparing five different models of pulse oximeters. Anesthesiology 1989;70:367–368.

188. Korbon GA, Wills MH, D'Lauro F, Lawson D. Systolic blood pressure measurement. Doppler vs pulse oximeter. Anesthesiology 1987;67:A188.

189. Severinghaus JW, Spellman MJ. Pulse oximeter thresholds in hypotention and vasoconstriction. Anesthesiology 1990;73:532–537.

190. Talke P, Nichols RJ, Traber DL. Does measurement of systolic blood pressure with a pulse oximeter correlate with conventional methods? J Clin Monit 1990;6:5–9.

191. Wallace CT, Baker JD, Alpert CC, Tankersley SJ, Conroy JM, Kerns R. Comparison of blood pressure measurement by doppler and by pulse oximetry techniques. Anesth Analg 1987;66:1018–1019.

192. Chawla R, Kumarvel V, Girdhar KK, Sethi AK, Bhattacharya A. Oximetry in pulseless disease. Anaesthesia 1990;45:992–993.

193. Sullivan MJ, Cooke JE, Baker JD III, Conroy JM, Bailey MK. Axillary block utilizing the pulse oximeter. Anesthesiology 1989;71:166–167.

194. Katz Y, Lee ME. Pulse oximetry for localization of the dorsalis pedis artery. Anaesth Intensive Care 1989;17:114.

195. Introna RPS, Silverstein PI. A new use for the pulse oximeter. Anesthesiology 1986;65:342.

196. James DJ, Brown RE. Vascular volume monitoring with pulse oximetry during paediatric anaesthesia. Can J Anaesth 1990;37:266–267.

197. Partridge BL. Use of pulse oximetry as a noninvasive indicator of intravascular volume status. J Clin Monit 1987;3:263–268.

198. Withington DE, Ramsay JG, Saoud AT, Bilodeay J. Weaning from ventilation after cardiopulmonary bypass. Evaluation of a non-invasive technique. Can J Anaesth 1991;38:15–19.

199. Carlson CA, Gravenstein JS, Banner MJ, Boyson PG. Monitoring techniques during anesthesia and HFJV for extracorporeal shock-wave lithotripsy. Anesthesiology 1985;63:A178.

200. Rasanen J, Downs JB, Hodges MR. Continuous monitoring of gas exchange and oxygen use with dual oximetry. J Clin Anesth 1988;1:3–8.

201. Rasanen J, Downs JB, Malec DJ, Oates K. Oxygen tensions and oxyhemoglobin saturations in the assessment of pulmonary gas exchange. Crit Care Med 1987;15:1058–1061.

202. Stemp LI. Another use for pulse oximetry. Anesthesiology 1992;77:1236.

203. Anonymous. Pulse oximeters. Health Devices 1989;18:185–230.

204. Boxer RA, Gottesfeld I, Singh S, LaCorte MA, Parnell VA, Walker P. Noninvasive pulse oximetry in chldren with cyanotic congenital heart disease. Crit Care Med 1987;15:1062–1064.

205. Chapman KR, D'Urzo A, Rebuck AS. The accuracy and response characteristics of a simplified ear oximeter. Chest 1983;83:860–864.

206. Cecil WT, Petterson MT, Lamoonpun S, Rudolph CD. Clinical evaluation of the Biox IIA ear oximeter in the critical care environment. Respir Care 1985;30:179–183.

207, Cecil WT, Morrison LS, Lampoonpun S. Clinical evaluation of the Ohmeda Biox III pulse oximeter. A comparison of finger and ear cuvettes. Respir Care 1985;30:840–845.

208. Chapman KR, Liu FLW, Watson RM, Rebuck AS. Range of accuracy of two-wavelength oximetry. Chest 1986;89:540–542.

209. Cecil WT, Thorpe KJ, Fibuch EE, Tuohy GF. A clinical evaluation of the accuracy of the Nellcor N-100 and Ohmeda 3700 pulse oximeters. J Clin Monit 1988;4:31–36.

210. Chapman KR, Liu FLW, Watson RM, Rebuck AS. Range of accuracy of two wavelength oximetry. Chest 1986;89:540–542.

211. Fait CD, Wetzel RC, Dean JM, Schleien CL, Gioia FR. Pulse oximetry in critically ill children. J Clin Monit 1985;1:232–235.

212. Hess D, Kochansky M, Hassett L, Frick R, Rexrode WO. An evaluation of the Nellcor N-10 portable pulse oximeter. Respir Care 1986;31:796–802.

213. Gabrielczyk MR, Buist RJ. Pulse oximetry and postoperative hypothermia. Anaesthesia 1988; 43:402–404.

214. Knill RL, Clement JL, Kieraszewicz HT, Dodgson BG. Assessment of two noninvasive monitors of arterial oxygenation in anesthetized man. Anesth Analg 1982;61:582–586.

215, Lynn AM, Bosenberg A. Pulse oximetry during cardiac catherization in children with congenital heart disease. J Clin Monit 1986;2:230–233.

216. Kim SK, Baidwan BS, Petty TL. Clinical evaluation of a new finger oximeter. Crit Care Med 1984;12:910–912.

217. Mihm FG, Halperin BD. Noninvasive detection of profound arterial desaturations using a pulse oximetry device. Anesthesiology 1985;62:85–87.

218. Mackenzie N. Comparison of a pulse oximeter

with an ear oximeter and an in-vitro oximeter. J Clin Monit 1985;1:156–160.

219. Mendelson Y, Kent JC, Shahnarian A, Welch GW, Giasi RM. Evaluation of the Datascope Accusat pulse oximeter in healthy adults. J Clin Monit 1988;4:59–63.

220. Macnab AJ, Baker-Brown G, Anderson EE. Oximetry in children recovering from deep hypothermia for cardiac surgery. Crit Care Med 1990;18:1066–1069.

221. Nickerson BG, Sarkisian C, Tremper K. Bias and precision of pulse oximeters and arterial oximeters. Chest 1988;93:515–517.

222. Russell RIR, Helms PJ. Comparative accuracy of pulse oximetry and transcutaneous oxygen in assessing arterial saturation in pediatric intensive care. Crit Care Med 1990;18:725–727.

223. Rebuck AS, Chapman KR, D'Urzo A. The accuracy and response characteristics of a simplified ear oximeter. Chest 1983;83:860–864.

224. Ries AL, Farrow JT, Clausen JL. Accuracy of two ear oximeters at rest and during exercise in pulmonary patients. Am Rev Respir Dis 1985;132:685–689.

225. Shippy MB, Petterson MT, Whitman RA, Shivers CR. A clinical evaluation of the BTI Biox II ear oximeter. Respir Care 1984;29:730–735.

226. Sidi A, Rush W, Gravenstein N, Ruiz B, Paulus DA, Davis RF. Pulse oximetry fails to accurately detect low levels of arterial hemoglobin oxygen saturation in dogs. J Clin Monit 1987;3:257–262.

227. Southall DP, Bingall S, Stebbens VA, Alexander JR, Rivers RPA, Lissauer T. Pulse oximeter and transcutaneous arterial oxygen measurements in neonatal and paediatric intensive care. Arch Dis Child 1987;62:882–888.

228. Tytler JA, Seeley HF. The Nellcor N-100 pulse oximeter. A clinical evaluation in anaesthesia and intensive care. Anaesthesia 1986;41:302–305.

229. Tweeddale PM, Douglas NJ. Evaluation of Biox IIA ear oximeter. Thorax 1985;40:825–827.

230. Taylor MB, Whitwam JG. The accuracy of pulse oximeters. Anaesthesia 1988;43:229–232.

231. Sendak MJ, Harris AP, Donham RT. Accuracy of pulse oximetry during oxyhemoglobin desaturation in dogs. Anesthesiology 1988;68:111–114.

232. Thrush D, Hodges M. The accuracy of pulse oximetry during hypoxemia. Anesthesiology 1992;77:A537.

233. Ridley SA. A comparison of two pulse oximeters. Anaesthesia 1988;43:136–140.

234. Reynolds KJ, Moyle JTB, Sykes MK, Hahn CEW. Response of 10 pulse oximeters to an in vitro test system. Br J Anaesth 1992;68:365–369.

235. Fanconi S. Reliability of pulse oximetry in hypoxic infants. J Pediatr 1988;112:424–427.

236. Freund PR, Overand PT, Cooper J, et al. A pro-

spective study of intraoperative pulse oximetry failure. J Clin Monit 1991;7:253–258.

237. Gillies BSA, Overand PT, Bosse S, et al. Failure rate of pulse oximetry in the post anesthesia care unit. Anesthesiology 1990;73:A1009.

238. Overand PT, Freund PR, Cooper JO, et al. Failure rate of pulse oximetry in clinical practice. Anesth Analg 1990;70:S289.

239. Morris RW, Nairn M, Beaudoin M. Does the radial arterial line degrade the performance of a pulse oximeter? Anaesth Intensive Care 1990;18:107–109.

240. New WJ. Pulse oximetry. J Clin Monit 1985;1:126–129.

241. DiBenedetto RJ, Graves SA, Grevenstein N, Melio FA, Konecek CL. O_2 as needed based on pulse oximetry in the postanesthesia care unit. A way to save. Anesthesiology 1992;77:A1127.

242. King T, Simon RH. Pulse oximetry for tapering supplemental oxygen in hospitalized patients. Chest 1987;92:713–716.

243. Roisen MF, Schreider B, Austin W. Pulse oximetry. Reducing cost and improving the quality of care with smart technology. Anesthesiology 1990;73:A536.

244. Clayton DG, Webb RK, Ralston AC, Duthie D, Runciman WB. A comparison of the performance of twenty pulse oximeters under conditions of poor perfusion. Anaesthesia 1991;46:260–265.

245. Falconer RJ, Robinson BJ. Comparison of pulse oximeters: accuracy at low arterial pressure in volunteers. Br J Anaesth 1990;65:552–557.

246. Langton JA, Lassey D, Hanning CD. Comparison of four pulse oximeters. Effects of venous occlusion and cold-induced peripheral vasoconstriction. Br J Anaesth 1990;65:245–247.

247. Morris RW, Nairn M, Torda TA. A comparison of fifteen pulse oximeters. Part I: a clinical comparison. Part II: a test of performance under conditions of poor perfusion. Anaesth Intensive Care 1989;17:62–73.

248. Wilkins CJ, Moores M, Hanning CD. Comparison of pulse oximeters. Effects of vasoconstriction and venous engorgement. Br J Anaesth 1989;62:439–444.

249. Severinghaus JW. Pulse oximetry uses and limitations (ASA Refresher Course #211). New Orleans: ASA, 1989.

250. Lawson D, Norley I, Korbon G, Loeb R, Ellis J. Blood flow limits and pulse oximeter signal detection. Anesthesiology 1987;67:599–603.

251. Palve H, Vuori A. Pulse oximetry during low cardiac output and hypothermia states immediately after open heart surgery. Crit Care Med 1989;17:66–69.

252. Freund PR, Bowdle TA, Neuenfeldt T, Posner K.

Reversal of intraoperative pulse oximetry failure by digital nerve block. Anesth Analg 1991;72:S81.

253. Gupta A. Vegfors M. A simple solution. Anaesthesia 1992;47:822.

254. Paulus DA, Monroe MC. Cool fingers and pulse oximetry. Anesthesiology 1989;71:168–169.

255. Mark JB. Systolic venous waves cause spurious signs of arterial hemoglobin desaturation. Anesthesiology 1989;71:158–160.

256. Sami HM, Kleinman BS, Lonchyna VA. Central venous pulsations associated with a falsely low oxygen saturation measured by pulse oximeter. J Clin Monit 1991;7:309–312.

257. Stewart KG, Rowbottom SJ. Inaccuracy of pulse oximetry in patients with severe tricuspid regurgitation. Anaesthesia 1991;46:668–670.

258. Kao YJ, Norton RG. A quantitative study of venous congestion on pulse oximetry. Can J Anaesth 1991;38:A154.

259. Scheller J, Loeb R. Respiratory artifact during pulse oximetry in critically ill patients. Anesthesiology 1988;69:602–603.

260. Scheller MS, Unger RJ, Kelner MJ. Effects of intravenously administered dyes on pulse oximetry readings. Anesthesiology 1986;65:550–552.

261. Sidi A, Paulus DA, Rush W, Gravenstein N, Davis RF. Methylene blue and indocyanine green artifactually lower pulse oximetry readings of oxygen saturation. Studies in dogs. J Clin Monit 1987;3:249–256.

262. Kessler MR, Eide T, Humayun B, Poppers PJ. Spurious pulse oximeter desaturation with methylene blue injection. Anesthesiology 1986;65:435–436.

263. Gorman ES, Shnider MR. Effect of methylene blue on the absorbance of solutions of haemoglobin. Br J Anaesth 1988;60:439–444.

264. Robinson DN, McFadzean WA. Pulse oximetry and methylene blue. Anaesthesia 1990;45:884–885.

265. Scott DM, Cooper MG. Spurious pulse oximetry with intrauterine methylene blue injection. Anaesth Intensive Care 1991;19:267–284.

266. Unger R, Scheller MS. More on dyes and pulse oximeters. Anesthesiology 1987;67:148–149.

267. Eide TR, Humayun-Scott B, Poppers PJ. More on dyes and pulse oximeters. In reply. Anesthesiology 1987;67:149.

268. Eisenkraft JB. Methylene blue and pulse oximetry readings: spuriouser and spuriouser! Anesthesiology 1988;68:171.

269. Anonymous. Ambient light interference with pulse oximeters. Technol Anesth 1988;8:3.

270. Amar D, Neidzwski J, Wald A, Finck AD. Fluorescent light interferes with pulse oximetry. J Clin Monit 1989;5:135–136.

271. Anonymous. Pulse oximeter inteference from surgical lighting. Health Devices 1987;16:50–51.

272. Anonymous. Pulse oximeter interference from surgical lighting. Technol Anesth 1987;7:8–9.

273. Anonymous. Ambient light interference with pulse oximeters. Health Devices 1987;16:346–347.

274. Brooks TD, Paulus DA, Winkle WE. Infrared heat lamps interfere with pulse oximeters. Anesthesiology 1984;61:630.

275. Block FE. Interference in a pulse oximeter from a fiberoptic light source. J Clin Monit 1987;3:210–211.

276. Costarino AT, Davis DA, Keon TP. Falsely normal saturation reading with the pulse oximeter. Anesthesiology 1987;67:830–831.

277. Hanowell L, Eisele JH, Downs D. Ambient light affects pulse oximeters. Anesthesiology 1987;67:864–865.

278. Munley AJ, Sik MJ. An unpredictable and possibly dangerous artefact affecting a pulse oximeter. Anaesthesia 1988;43:334.

279. Siegel MN, Gravenstein N. Preventing ambient light from affecting pulse oximetry. Anesthesiology 1987;67:280.

280. Zablocki AD, Rasch DK. A simple method to prevent interference with pulse oximetry by infrared heating lamps. Anesth Analg 1987;66:915.

281. Samuels SI, Shochat SJ. A new technique for stabilizing the oxygen saturation monitor probe in infants and children. Anesth Analg 1986;65:213.

282. Kataria BK, Lampkins R. Nail polish does not affect pulse oximeter saturation. Anesth Analg 1986;65:824.

283. Kataria BK, Lampkins R. Nail polish does not affect pulse oximeter saturation. Anesth Analg 1986;65:824.

284. Cote CJ, Goldstein EA, Fuchsman WH, Hoaglin DC. The effect of nail polish on pulse oximetry. Anesth Analg 1988;67:683–686.

285. Rubin AS. Nail polish color can affect pulse oximeter saturation. Anesthesiology 1988;68:825.

286. Tweedie IE. Pulse oximeters and fingernails. Anaesthesia 1989;44:268.

287. Battito MF. The effect of fingerprinting ink on pulse oximetry. Anesth Analg 1989;69:256.

288. Goucke R. Hazards of henna. Anesth Analg 1989;69:416–417.

289. Sneyd JR. "Finger-painting" and the pulse oximeter. Anaesthesia 1991;46:420–421.

290. Ezri T, Szmuk P. Pulse oximeters and onychomycosis. Anesthesiology 1992;76:153.

291. Cahan C, Decker MJ, Hoekje PL, Strohl KP. Agreement between noninvasive oximetric values for oxygen saturation. Chest 1989;97:814–819.

292. Emery JR. Skin pigmentation as an influence on

the accuracy of pulse oximetry. J Perinatol 1987;7:329–330.

293. Ries AL, Prewitt LM, Johnson JJ. Skin color and ear oximetry. Chest 1989;96:287–290.

294. Volgyesi GA, Spahr-Schopfer I, Bissonnette B. The effect of skin pigmentation on the accuracy of pulse oximetry: an in vitro study. Can J Anaesth 1991;38:A155.

295. Hopkins PM. An erroneous pulse oximeter reading. Anaesthesia 1987;44:868.

296. Rosewarne FA, Reynolds KJ. Dried blood does not affect pulse oximetry. Anaesthesia 1991;46:886–887.

297. Oyston J, Ordman A. Erroneous explanation for an erroneous pulse oximeter reading. Anaesthesia 1990;45:258.

298. Mendelson Y, Kent JC, Shahnarian A, Welch GW, Giasi RM. Simultaneous comparison of three noninvasive oximeters in healthy volunteers. Medical Instrum 1987;21:183–188.

299. Sendak MJ, Harris AP, Donham RT. Accuracy of pulse oximetry during severe arterial oxygen desaturation. Anesthesiology 1986;65:A133.

300. Sarnquist FH, Todd C, Whitcher C. Accuracy of a new non-invasive oxygen saturation monitor. Anesthesiology 1980;53:S163.

301. Wong DH, Tremper KK, Davidson J, et al. Pulse oximetry is accurate in patients with dysrhythmias and a pulse deficit. Anesthesiology 1989;70:1024–1025.

302. Block FE, Detko GJ. Minimizing interference and false alarms from electrocautery in the Nellcor N-100 pulse oximeter. J Clin Monit 1986;12:203–205.

303. Barker SJ, Tremper KK, Gamel DM. A clinical comparison of transcutaneous P_{O_2} and pulse oximetry in the operating room. Anesth Analg 1986;65:805–808.

304. Verhoeff F, Sykes MK. Delayed detection of hypoxic events by pulse oximeters. Computer simulations. Anaesthesia 1990;45:103–109.

305. Reynolds LM, Jobes DR, Nicholson SC, Escobar A, McGonigle ME. Changes in oxygen saturation in children are detected earlier by centrally placed pulse oximeter sensors. Anesthesiology 1992; 77:A1178.

306. Ding Z, Shibata K, Yamamoto K, Kobayashi T, Murakami S. Decreased circulation time in the upper limb reduces the lag time of the finger pulse oximeter response. Can J Anesth 1992;39:87–89.

307. Wilson S. Conscious sedation and pulse oximetry. False alarms? Pediatr Dent 1990;12:228–232.

308. Rolf N, Cote CJ. Incidence of real and false positive capnography and pulse oximetry alarms during pediatric anesthesia. Anesthesiology 1991; 75:A476.

309. Wiklund L, Hok B, Jordeby-Jonsson A, Stahl K. Postanesthesia monitoring. More than 75% of pulse oximeter alarms are trivial. Anesthesiology 1992;77:A582.

310. Anonymous. Delay circuit may reduce pulse oximetry false alarms. Biomed Safe Stand 1992;22:162–163.

311. Pan PH, James CF. Effects of default alarm limit settings on alarm distribution in telemetric pulse oximetry network in ward setting. Anesthesiology 1991;75:A405.

312. Jones RDM, Lawson AD, Gunawardene WMS, Roulson CJ, Brown AG, Smith ID. An evaluation of prolonged oximetric data acquisition. Anesth Intensive Care 1992;20:303–307.

313. Pan PH. False alarms distribution in intraoperative pulse oximetry. Anesthesiology 1992; 77:A494.

314. Marks LF, Heath PJ. An unusual pulse oximeter artifact. Anaesthesia 1990;45:501.

315. Ralston AC, Webb RK, Runciman WB. Potential errors in pulse oximetry. Anaesthesia 1991;46:291–295.

316. Ralston AC, Webb RK, Runciman WB. Potential errors in pulse oximetry. Part I. Pulse oximeter evaluation. Anaesthesia 1991;46:202–206.

317. Egbert TP, Westenskow DR. Detection of artifact in pulse oximetry signals using a neural network. Anesthesiology 1992;77:A521.

318. Taylor MB. Erroneous actuation of the pulse oximeter. A reply. Anaesthesia 1987;42:1116.

319. Norman GV, Cheney FW. Falsely elevated oximeter reading dangerous on one lung. APSF Newslett 1989;4:23.

320. Norley I. Erroneous actuation of the pulse oximeter. Anesthesiology 1987;42:1116.

321. Dawalibi L, Rozario C, van den Bergh AA. Pulse oximetry in pulseless patients. Anaesthesia 1991;46:990–991.

322. Shlamowitz M, Miguel R. Prolonging the lifespan of disposable Nellcor pulse oxisensors. J Clin Monit 1990;6:160.

323. Tharp AJ. A cost-saving method of modifying the Nellcor pulse oximeter finger probe. Anesthesiology 1986;65:446–447.

324. Strohl KP, House PM, Holic JF, Fouke JM, Cheung PW. Comparison of three transmittance oximeters. Med Instrum 1986;20:143–149.

325. Choe H, Tashiro C, Fukumitsu K, Yagi M, Yoshiya I. Comparison of recorded values from six pulse oximeters. Crit Care Med 1989;17:678–681.

326. Armstrong N, Perrin LS. Pulse oximeter overload. Anesthesiology 1992;76:148.

327. Anonymous. Safety alert. Pulse oximeter sensors can cause burns at skin-contact site. Biomed Safe Stand 1990;20:91–92.

328. Anonymous. Different manufacturers' patient probes and pulse oximeters. Technol Anesth 1990;11:2–3.

329. Willingham MC. A warning in the use of pulse oximeters: I. Anesthesiology 1990;73:358.

330. Murphy KG, Secunda JA, Rockoff MA. Severe burns from a pulse oximeter. Anesthesiology 1990;73:350–352.

331. Sloan TB. Finger injury by an oxygen saturation monitor probe. Anesthesiology 1988;68:936–938.

332. Mills GH, Ralph SJ. Burns due to pulse oximetry. Anaesthesia 1992;47:276–277.

333. Anonymous. Potential burn hazard from pulse oximeter adapter cables. Biomed Safe Stand 1992;22:28.

334. Anonymous. Oximeters, ear. Technol Anesth 1985;6:10.

335. Polar SM. Cutaneous injuries associated with pulse oximeters. J Clin Monit 1992;8:185.

336. Alexander R, Levison A. Burns from a pulse oximeter [Letter]. Clin Intens Care 1991;2:188.

337. Rubin MM, Ford HC, Sadoff RS. Digital injury from a pulse oximeter probe. J Oral Maxillofac Surg 1991;49:301–302.

338. Berge KH, Lanier WL, Scanlon PD. Ischemic digital skin necrosis. A complication of the reusable Nellcor pulse oximeter probe. Anesth Analg 1988;67:712–713.

339. Bannister J, Scott DHT. Thermal injury associated with pulse oximetry. Anaesthesia 1988;43:424–425.

340. Chemello PD, Nelson SR, Wolford LM. Finger injury resulting from pulse oximeter probe during orthognathic surgery. Oral Surg Oral Med Oral Pathol 1990;69:161–163.

341. Bethune DW, Baliga N. Skin injury with a pulse oximeter. Br J Anaesth 1992;69:665.

342. Miyasaka K, Ohata J. Burn, erosion, and "sun" tan with the use of pulse oximetry in infants. Anesthesiology 1987;67:1008–1009.

343. Pettersen B, Kongsgaard U, Aune H. Skin injury in an infant with pulse oximetry. Br J Anaesth 1992;69:204–205.

344. Bashein G, Syrovy G. Burns associated with pulse oximetry during magnetic resonance imaging. Anesthesiology 1991;75:382–383.

345. Shellock FG, Slimp GL. Severe burn of the finger caused by using a pulse oximeter during MR imaging. AJR Am J Roentgenol 1989;153:1105.

346. Kanal E, Shellock FG. Burns associated with clinical MR examinations. Radiology 1990;175:585.

347. Ackerman WE, Juneja MM, Baumann RC, Kaczorowski DM. The use of a vinyl glove does not affect pulse oximeter monitoring. Anesthesiology 1989;70:558–559.

Part 6
Alarms

Audible Signal
Alarm Signal Identification
Visual Signal
Alarm Prioritization
Organization of Alarms
Alarm Set Points
False Alarms
   False-Positive Alarms
   False-Negative Alarms
Alarm Silencing
Smart Alarms

Alarms are warning signals automatically generated by equipment to indicate abnormal or unusual conditions. The purposes of an alarm are to get attention, transfer information, enhance vigilance, and warn of an existing or developing adverse condition (1–3). Another purpose may be to transfer responsibility from the device's manufacturer to the user (4).

The number of alarms in the anesthetizing areas has increased greatly for several reasons. First, the number and variety of monitors has increased. Second, because of an increased emphasis on patient safety and the realization that anesthesia personnel are human (and, therefore, fallible), manufacturers have been putting more alarms on each piece of equipment. To add further confusion, alarms may originate from devices such as electrosurgical apparatus, lasers, warming blankets, and infusion pumps. The result is that anesthesia personnel are faced with a variety of disturbing signals, often just when the patient needs their undivided attention.

Audible Signals

It is essential that there be means of alerting personnel to a change in the anesthesia machine, breathing system or patient, for there will always be occasions when his or her vigilance will be reduced or attention lowered by the need to perform other tasks (5). An audible signal is a potent attention getter, attracting attention faster and more reliably than a visual signal (6).

Ideally an auditory signal should attract attention without startling anybody. Unfortunately, the qualities that make sounds attention getting also tend to make them annoying. Some are so unpleasant that the principal response may be to want to make the offensive noise go away rather than address the condition that generated the alarm. Manufacturers may deliberately make alarm sounds intrusive and loud to ensure that their equipment will not be faulted for failing to alert the clinician to a deteriorating situation.

Many alarms are steady pure-tone signals that are easily masked by louder and more complex equipment noises that may contain tones of the same frequency (7). As a result, in a noisy environment and especially if many monitors are alarming simultaneously, an alarm sound may not be noticed.

There are a number of options available in alarm sound technology, including variations in pattern, pitch, tone, frequency, and loudness (8). In 1993, a standard for electronically generated alarm signals for use in anesthesia and respiratory care was published (9). Some of its specifications are shown in Table 17.1.

The standard requires that alarm sounds have a fundamental frequency between 150 and 1000 Hz based on standard musical pitches. There must be at least four frequency components ranging from 300 to 4000 Hz and these must be related so that they form a distinct sound. Adjustable alarms must have an intensity between 45 and 85 db. Those with fixed intensity must be between 70 and 85 db.

An approach favored in Europe are the Patterson sounds (10). These tones, originally developed for aviation, were modified

for medical equipment. There are three general alarm sounds for advisory, caution, and warning and six categories for ventilation, oxygenation, cardiovascular, artificial perfusion, drug administration, and temperature. Concerns about using these sounds have been raised, stemming from questions about their applicability to the operating room setting in view of advances that have been made in monitoring devices and technology, and concern that their use will worsen noise and stress in the operating room (8,10).

Alarm Signal Identification

Once an alarm is activated, the next step is to identify its origin. It is important that the clinician be able quickly to identify any alarm, because many monitors are not in his or her immediate field of view and the clinician cannot always turn around. Inability to identify an alarm will delay or prevent the appropriate remedial action (2,5). An audible signal that cannot be identified is distracting, and this may exacerbate a difficult situation (8).

Many alarms are high-pitched, continuous tones that are difficult to differentiate from one another and may be difficult to locate because the sound seems to come from all directions. Many anesthesiologists have trouble identifying audible alarms (11–15).

Visual Signal

While sounds draw attention to a problem, visual signals give more specific information. Their principal drawback is that in a situation in which the individual responsible for reacting to an alarm is required to use his or her vision for other tasks, a visual message may go unnoticed (12). Another problem is that it may not be possible for the individual to turn around and look at the alarm (e.g., during laryngoscopy).

Table 17.1.   Alarm Signals

Alarm Category	Operator Response	Audible Indicators	Indicator Color	Flashing Frequency
High priority	Immediate	Not medium or low priority	Red	1.4 to 2.8 Hz
Medium priority	Prompt	Not high or low priority	Yellow	0.4 to 0.8 Hz
Low priority	Awareness	Not high or medium priority	Yellow	Constant

From American Society for Testing and Materials. Specification for alarm signals in medical equipment used in anesthesia and respiratory care. (F1463-93) Philadelphia: ASTM, 1993.

Alarm lights can be coded by color, brightness, size, location, and flashing frequency (8). Flashing lights are more noticeable and have traditionally been used for more crucial information.

The alarm standard requirements for visual signals are shown in Table 17.1. Alphanumeric or computer-generated graphic displays of alarm messages, including centralized alarm displays, are exempt from the color and flashing frequency requirements shown in the table. Visual signals must be clearly legible at a distance of 1 m. High- and medium-priority signals must be distinguishable at 4 m.

Alarm Prioritization

All alarms are not equally important. The information that an alarm conveys may represent an emergency, the potential for an emergency, or just an unusual condition. Frequently, there is no correlation between an alarm sound and the urgency of the condition it annunciates (16).

The alarm standard divides alarms into three priorities: high, medium, and low. A high-priority alarm indicates a condition that requires immediate action. Medium priority implies a potentially dangerous situation that requires a prompt response. A low-priority alarm indicates that only operator awareness is required. It may or may not have an audible indicator. Audible and vi-

sual indicators should reset automatically after the alarm condition ceases to exist.

The object of prioritization is to minimize interference from less important alarm conditions during an emergency. It will not reduce the number of alarms, but may make them more tolerable. It has been suggested that only the alarm sound corresponding to the most urgent of the prevailing alarm conditions should be annunciated; all other sounds should be temporarily suppressed (2). Once the most urgent alarm condition is resolved, the sound corresponding to the next highest priority condition would then be initiated. This priority interlock should be limited to audible annunciation; lower-priority alarm visual indications need not be suppressed, because they are unobtrusive.

Organization of Alarms

In a typical monitoring environment, alarm messages arrive in an unorganized pattern. Visual indicators intended to specify the exact nature of the alarm are randomly dispersed, resulting in delay in identifying the problem.

A recent development designed to aid alarm identification is the single integrated display (2). Typical ones are shown in Figures 17.41 and 17.42. The display is connected to various monitors. When an alarm condition is present, it can be identified in this area. Thus anesthesia personnel need

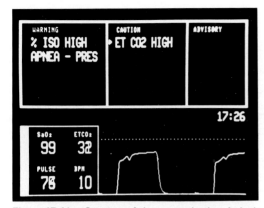

Figure 17.41. One type of alarm organization. A single integrated display connects to various monitors. When an alarm condition is present. it can be identified in this area. Various data from monitors are displayed below, with a CO_2 waveform on the right. Courtesy of North American Drager.

look in only one place to identify the problem. A disadvantage of this is that a crowded display may be difficult to read in a crisis. Also, it may not be possible to integrate all monitors into a single display.

Alarm Set Points

The criteria that determine when a particular alarm is activated are called the alarm set points (threshold values, limits, thresholds, settings). Set points should be displayed continuously or be capable of being displayed at the user's discretion.

Limits can be set by either the manufacturer or the user. Those set by the manufacturer may be default values (those that the monitor automatically assumes when it is turned on) or the monitor may analyze data collected for a certain period of time after monitoring has commenced and set the limits based on measured values (5).

Set points may be user variable, allowing the user to change them according to his or her preferences. In most cases, the monitor returns to the default values after it is turned off.

To ensure that an alarm sounds before a dangerous condition has occurred without creating frequent spurious signals requires intelligence on the part of both the alarm and the user (8,17). Many operators set limits to extremes unlikely to be encountered clinically. Others simply use the limits set by the last person who used the device. Others keep the thresholds close to the safe limits, changing the thresholds often to prevent the occurrence of false alarms. Unfortunately, this may lead the user to disable the alarm (8,18).

Setting unrealistic set points can result in an increase in either false-positive or false-negative alarms (5,19). The farther thresholds are from normal values, the greater the probability that a dangerous condition will occur without activating the alarm. On the other hand, the closer the thresholds are to normal values, the more likely it is that false alarms will be produced.

Thresholds for detection of significant change are not the same for all patients. If one attempts to find limits that include the safety zone for all patients, the result will be too many false alarms. However, if the limits are set at their extremes the alarms are of no value with normal patients. A reasonable alternative is for the manufacturer to set default limits for average patients and allow the user to adjust the limits for each patient.

It is good practice to record alarm set points on the anesthesia record. This provides evidence that the alarms were activated. It may also increase the operator's awareness of the alarms and/or make it more likely that appropriate limits will be set.

False Alarms (19)

If an alarm fails to generate a signal when it should (false negative), the patient's well-being will be threatened. If it is activated

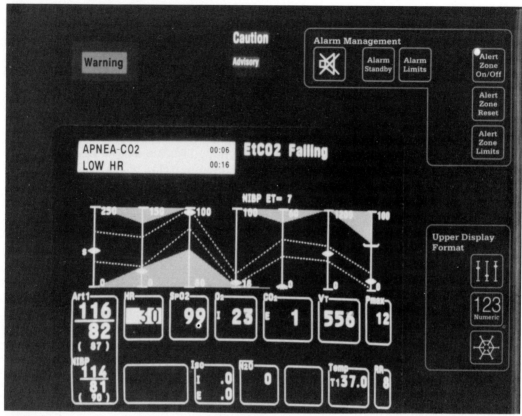

Figure 17.42. Another type of alarm organization. Warnings, advisories, and cautions are displayed on the top of the screen. Data from various monitors are displayed both numerically and pictorially. Numerical data are at the bottom. Above, measured data are displayed relative to the alarm limits. This particular display also has "alert zones," indicated by the dashed lines. When activated, these cause the system to monitor the relationship of the measured parameters to the alert zone. If a reading is outside this alert zone, the system will sound a caution. A alarm silence button is at the top, just right of the middle. Pressing it will cause any alarm that is sounding to be silenced. When an alarm is sounding, either the warning or caution indicator will flash. Pressing the alarm silence button will cause the alarm to stop flashing, but the message will still be displayed. Courtesy of Ohmeda, a division of BOC Health Care, Inc.

without proper cause (false positive), it is annoying and this may lead to its being ignored, silenced, or turned off.

FALSE-POSITIVE ALARMS

Many alarms are spurious and only a small number indicate patient risk (20–25). A false alarm requires time and effort to check the actual conditions. This will result in less attention to other tasks and may lead to an inappropriate action. False alarms are a source of irritation and a threat to patient care, because the operator becomes increasingly likely to ignore the signals, disable the entire alarm system, silence the alarm without looking for the cause, or set the alarm limits at extreme values. Disabling of alarms is common (26–28).

There are a number of possible reasons for false alarms, including alarm malfunction, artifacts, inappropriate settings or default values, and extraneous sounds being mistaken for an alarm signal.

Setting wide alarm limits will result in

fewer alarms (22). The manufacturer may incorporate narrow default limits to protect itself. If they are not reset, there will be a high incidence of unnecessary alarms. False alarms may be reduced by changing alarm limits at certain times, because clinical ranges vary during different phases of anesthesia (29).

An artifact can cause the monitor to sense a value outside the alarm limits. Examples of this include interference with the ECG from other electrical devices, movement of an oximeter probe and pressure on a blood pressure cuff during cycling (30). Artifacts can be reduced by careful placement of sensors (31). On some monitors, delaying the time between detection of a condition and alarm activation will reduce the number of false alarms (18,32). On some pulse oximeters, the time over which signals are averaged can be varied. Increasing the averaging time will decrease the number of false alarms.

Some false alarms can be reduced by integration of monitors. An example is synchronizing the pulse oximeter and noninvasive blood pressure monitors. If the oximeter probe is on the same arm as the blood pressure cuff, no alarm will sound if no pulse is detected when the cuff is inflated. Another example is the pulse oximeter and electrocardiogram. SpO$_2$ values are rejected unless the pulse rate measured on the oximeter matches that on the ECG.

FALSE-NEGATIVE ALARMS

A false-negative alarm may occur if an alarm limit is set so that a condition that can cause harm does not trigger the alarm. A false-negative alarm can also be created by turning the alarm volume so low that the audible signal cannot be heard.

Alarm Silencing

Once an audible alarm signal has succeeded in capturing the operator's attention, it is no longer required and becomes a hindrance (2). It needs to be silenced (muted, reset, paused, disabled, delayed) to provide time to correct the situation.

Most manufacturers provide a means to at least temporarily silence the auditory signal. The silencing time varies with the instrument and is sometimes variable. Some monitors indicate the elapsed time. The alarm standard requires that there be a visual indication that a high- or medium-priority alarm signal has been silenced.

Smart Alarms (19,22,33–43)

The latest development in alarm technology is the smart (intelligent) alarm. When an alarm condition is sensed, the smart alarm will identify the source of the alarm, analyze the data, provide the operator with a list of possible conditions that could have triggered the alarm, and may present information that will aid in determining the correct way to deal with the condition that triggered the alarm.

It is anticipated that this advanced data analysis will reduce false alarms by weighing the signal strength and looking at other parameters. It should also improve anesthesia safety by decreasing the time required to correct problems (37).

REFERENCES

1. Beneken JEW, van der Aa JJ. Alarms and their limits in monitoring. J Clin Monit 1989;5:205–210.
2. Schreiber PJ, Schreiber J. Structured alarm systems for the operating room. J Clin Monit 1989;5:201–204.
3. Quinn ML. Semipractical alarms. A parable. J Clin Monit 1989;5:196–200.
4. Hayman WA, Drinker PA. Design of medical device alarm systems. Med Instrum 1983;17:103–106.
5. Sykes MK. Panel on practical alarms. J Clin Monit 1989;5:192–193.
6. Morgan CT, Cook JS III, Chapanis A, Lund MW. Eds. Human engineering guide to equipment design. New York: McGraw-Hill, 1963.
7. Stanford LM, McIntyre JWR, Hogan JT. Audible alarm signals for anaesthesia monitoring equipment. Int J Clin Monit Comp 1985;1:251–256.

8. Weinger MB, Smith NT. Vigilance, alarms, and integrated monitoring systems. In: Ehrenwerth J, Eisenkraft JB, Eds. Anesthesia equipment, principles and applications. St. Louis: CV Mosby, 1993:350–384.

9. American Society for Testing and Materials. Specification for alarm signals in medical equipment used in anesthesia and respiratory care (F1463–93). Philadelphia: ASTM, 1993.

10. Weinger MB. Proposed new alarm standards may make a bad situation worse. Anesthesiology 1991;74:791–792.

11. Finley GA, Cohen AJ. Perceived urgency and the anaesthetist: responses to common operating room monitor alarms. Can J Anaesth 1991;38:958–964.

12. Griffith RL, Raciot BM. A survey of practicing anesthesiologists on auditory alarms in the operating room. In: Hedley-Whyte, J, Ed. Operating room and intensive care alarms and information transfer (STP 1152). Philadelphia: American Society for Testing and Materials, 1992:10–18.

13. Loeb RG, Jones BR, Leonard RA, Behrman K. Recognition accuracy of current operating room alarms. Anesth Analg 1992;75:499–505.

14. Samuels SI. An alarming problem. Anesthesiology 1986;64:128–129.

15. Schmidt SI, Baysinger CL. Alarms: help or hindrance? Anesthesiology 1986;64:654–655.

16. Beinlich IA, Gaba DM. The ALARM monitoring system—intelligent decision making under uncertainty. Anesthesiology 1989;71:A337.

17. Kerr JH. Alarms and excursions [Editorial]. Anaesthesia 1986;41:807–808.

18. Anonymous. Delay circuit may reduce pulse oximetry false alarms. Biomed Safe Stand 1992;22:162–163.

19. Kerr JH. Warning devices. Br J Anaesth 1985;57:696–708.

20. Koski EMJ, Makivirta A, Sukuvaara T, et al. Frequency and reliability of alarms in the monitoring of cardiac postoperative patients. Int J Clin Monit Comput 1990;7:129–133.

21. Wiklund L, Hok B, Jordeby-Jonsson A, Stahl K. Postanesthesia monitoring. More than 75% of pulse oximeter alarms are trivial. Anesthesiology 1992;77:A582.

22. Watt RC, Miller KE, Navabi MJ, Hameroff SR, Mylrea KC. An approach to "smart alarms" in anesthesia monitoring. Anesthesiology 1988;69:A241.

23. Schaaf C, Block FE. Evaluation of alarm sounds in the operating room. J Clin Monit 1989;5:300–301.

24. O'Carroll TM. Survey of alarms in an intensive therapy unit. Anaesthesia 1986;41:742–744.

25. Kestin IG, Miller BR, Lockhart CH. Auditory alarms during anesthesia monitoring. Anesthesiology 1988;69:106–109.

26. McIntyre JWR. Ergonomics. Anaesthetists' use of auditory alarms in the operating room. Int J Clin Monit Comput 1985;2:47–55.

27. Anonymous. Critical alarms: patients at risk. Technol Anesth 1987;7(10):1–6.

28. Sury MRJ, Hinds CJ, Boustred M. Accidental disconnexion following inactivation of Servoventilator alarm. Anaesthesia 1986;41:91.

29. van Oostrom JH, Gravenstein C, Beneken JEW, Gravenstein JS. Improving alarm systems: how to define acceptable vital signs during general anesthesia. J Clin Monit 1992;8:159–160.

30. Spraker TE. Alarm strategies for anesthesia: where we've been; where we are now; where we're going. J Clin Monit 1989;5:301.

31. Barker SJ, Hyatt J, Shah NK. The accuracy of malpositioned pulse oximeters during hypoxemia. Anesthesiology 1992;77:A496.

32. Pan PH, James CF. Effects of default alarm limit settings on alarm distribution in telemetric pulse oximetry network in ward setting. Anesthesiology 1991;75:A405.

33. Anonymous. Alarms in the operating room. Can J Anaesth 1991;38:951.

34. Egbert TP, Westenskow DR. Detection of artifact in pulse oximetry signals using a neural network. Anesthesiology 1992;77:A521.

35. Fukui Y, Masuzawa T. Knowlege-based approach to intelligent alarms. J Clin Monit 1989;5:211–216.

36. Orr JA, Westenskow DR. A breathing circuit alarm system based on neural networks. Anesthesiology 1989;71:A338.

37. Orr JA, Simon FH, Bender H-J, Westenskow DR. Response time with smart alarms. Anesthesiology 1990;73:A447.

38. Orr JA, Westenskow DR. Evaluation of a breathing circuit alarm system based on neural networks. Anesthesiology 1990;73:A445.

39. Orr JA, Kuck K, Farrell RM, Westenskow DR. Neural network breathing circuit alarms in an anesthesia workstation. Anesthesiology 1991; 75:A1005.

40. Pan PH. False alarms distribution in intraoperative pulse oximetry. Anesthesiology 1992;77:A494.

41. van Oostrom JH, van der Aa JJ, Beneken JEW, Gravenstein JS. Intelligent alarms in the anesthesia circle breathing system. Anesthesiology 1989; 71:A336.

42. Westenskow DR, Loeb RG, Brunner JX, Pace NL. Expert alarms and autopilot in an anesthesia workstation. Anesthesiology 1988;69:A731.

43. Watt RC, Navabi MJ, Mylrea KC, Hameroff SR. Integrated monitoring "smart alarms" can detect critical events and reduce false alarms. Anesthesiology 1989;71:A338.

Chapter 18

Equipment Checkout, Management, and Legal Issues

Introduction

The idea of a routine checkout procedure analogous to the preflight check for airline pilots to determine whether the equipment is functioning properly and ready for use has become popular (1–3). An electronic checklist may offer advantages a handwritten one does not (4).

Studies have shown that failure to check equipment properly was a factor in up to 33% of critical incidents (4–7). Introduction of a checklist may be a potent factor in reducing the frequency of critical incidents (8).

Failure to perform a proper equipment check before use is common (9,10), and many anesthesia personnel are unable to identify intentionally created faults (11–13). Defects may be found even just after preventive maintenance is performed (14).

The 1988 anesthesia machine standard (15) requires that an outline of operational checks to be carried out before use be provided by the manufacturer, and be located on the machine. User manuals provided by manufacturers for newer machines have fairly complete and detailed directions for checking. These should be read carefully, and the suggested procedures followed.

The Food and Drug Administration, working with representatives of the anesthesia community and industry, compiled a set of apparatus checkout recommendations, which were published in 1986 (16). Unfortunately, this list was too complicated for most users. Also, a study showed that the introduction of this checklist did not improve the ability to detect machine faults (13). An attempt to make the checking procedure more practical and thus more likely to be used resulted in a simplified version, which

Table 18.1.   Simplified Checking Procedure

Emergency Ventilation Equipment
1. Verify backup ventilation equipment is available and functioning[a]
High-Pressure System
2. Check oxygen cylinder supply[a]
   a. Open O_2 cylinder and verify that it is at least half full (about 1000 psi)
   b. Close cylinder
3. Check central pipeline supplies[a]
   a. Check that hoses are connected and that the pipeline gauges read 45 to 55 psi
Low-Pressure System
4. Check initial status of low-pressure system[a]
   a. Close flow control valves and turn vaporizers off
   b. Check fill level and tighten vaporizers' filler caps
   c. Remove O_2 monitor sensor from circuit
5. Perform leak check of machine's low-pressure system[a]
   a. Verify that the machine's master switch and flow control valves are off
   b. Attach "suction bulb" to common (fresh) gas outlet
   c. Squeeze bulb repeatedly until fully collapsed
   d. Verify bulb stays fully collapsed for at least 10 sec
   e. Open one vaporizer at a time and repeat steps c and d, above
   f. Remove sunction bulb and reconnect fresh gas hose
6. Turn on machine's master switch and all other necessary electrical equipment[a]
7. Test flowmeters[a]
   a. Adjust flow of all gases through their full range, checking for smooth operation of floats and undamaged flowtubes
   b. Attempt to create a hypoxic O_2/N^2O mixture and verify correct changes in flow and/or alarm
Breathing System
8. Calibrate O_2 monitor[a]
   a. Calibrate to read 21% in room air
   b. Reinstall sensor in circuit and flush breathing system with O_2
   c. Verify that monitor now reads greater than 90%
9. Check initial status of breathing system
   a. Set selector switch in bag mode
   b. Check that breathing circuit is complete, undamaged, and unobstructed
   c. Verify that CO_2 absorbent is adequate
   d. Install breathing system accessory equipment to be used during the case
10. Perform leak check of the breathing system
    a. Set all gas flows to zero (or minimum)
    b. Close APL valve and occlude Y piece
    c. Pressurize breathing system to 30 cm H_2O with O_2 flush
    d. Ensure that pressure remains at 30 cm for at least 10 sec
Scavenging System
11. Check APL valve and scavenging system
    a. Pressurize breathing system to 50 cm H_2O and ensure its integrity
    b. Open APL valve and ensure that pressure decreases
    c. Ensure proper scavenging connections and waste gas vacuum
    d. Fully open APL valve and occlude Y piece
    e. Ensure absorber pressure gauge reads zero when:
       i. Minimum O_2 is flowing
       ii. O_2 flush is activated
Manual and Automatic Ventilation Systems
12. Test ventilation systems and unidirectional valves
    a. Place a second reservoir bag on the Y piece
    b. Set appropriate ventilator parameters for next patient
    c. Set O_2 flowmeter to 250 ml/min, other gas flows to zero
    d. Switch to automatic ventilation (ventilator) mode
    e. Turn ventilator on and fill bellows and breathing bag with O_2 flush
    f. Verify that during inspiration bellows delivers correct tidal volume and that during expiration bellows fills completely
    g. Check that volume monitor is consistent with ventilator parameters
    h. Check for proper action of unidirectional valves
    i. Exercise breathing circuit accessories to ensure proper function

Table 18.1. *continued*

j. Turn ventilator off and switch to manual ventilation (bag/APL) mode
k. Ventilate manually and ensure inflation and deflation of artificial lungs and appropriate feel of system resistance and compliance
l. Remove second reservoir bag from the Y piece

Monitors

13. Check, calibrate, and/or set alarm limits of all monitors
    a. Capnometer
    b. Pulse oximeter
    c. Oxygen analyzer
    d. Respiratory volume meter (spirometer)
    e. Pressure monitor with high and low airway pressure alarms

Final Position

14. Check final status of machine
    a. Vaporizers off
    b. APL valve open
    c. Selector switch to bag
    d. All flowmeters at zero (or minimum)
    e. Patient suction level adequate
    f. Breathing system ready to use

[a]If the anesthesia person uses the same machine in successive cases, these steps need not be repeated or may be abbreviated after the initial checkout.

was published in 1992 in draft form. This is shown in Table 18.1. A final version of this list is expected to be published in 1993. An attempt has been made to retain or add checks of components that fail more frequently than others and that quickly injure the patient when they do fail (17). Checks of components that fail infrequently or whose isolated failure will not put the patient in immediate danger were removed from the list.

The FDA checkout recommendations are intended for an anesthesia gas delivery system that includes a circle system, a ventilator with an ascending (standing) bellows and a capnograph, pulse oximeter, oxygen analyzer, respiratory volume meter and airway pressure monitor with high and low pressure alarms. Clinicians using equipment that do not conform to this configuration must look for failures that might go unrecognized and adapt the checkout procedure as indicated. For example, if a Mapleson system is to be used, the checking procedure should include this. The manufacturer's user's manual should be consulted for special procedures. Modifications of the checklist should have appropriate peer review.

A copy of the checkout procedure should be kept in the drawer of the anesthesia machine or cart or attached to one of these. A record that the checklist was used should be made and kept for several years. A general rule says, "If it isn't written down, it wasn't done" (18).

Daily Checks before Beginning Anesthesia

The FDA checkout recommendations should be regarded as the minimum basic procedures that should be performed before using an anesthesia machine. Other tests suggested by various parties are given here so that the practitioner can select those which he or she regards as most important. In some cases, the reader may prefer to do a different test to check for proper function of a component. When an alternate test is given, an attempt will be made to point out the advantages and deficiencies of the various tests. The user should read the manufacturer's suggested checking procedures and make alterations or additions to the list as necessary.

It is recognized that it may not be possible to carry out a full check in an emergency situation.

BACKUP VENTILATION EQUIPMENT

Manual Resuscitator

There should be a self-inflating resuscitation bag (described in Chapter 8) in every anesthetizing location. Though rare, certain malfunctions (such as contaminated oxygen supply, loss of oxygen pressure and obstruction of the breathing system) can render the anesthesia machine inoperative (17). Sometimes a problem occurs that cannot be diagnosed quickly. In these cases, a manual resuscitator will allow the user to generate a positive pressure and ventilate the patient while the problem is corrected or the machine replaced.

The resuscitation bag should be inspected for signs of wear such as cracks or tears. Next,

the patient port should be occluded and the bag squeezed (Fig. 18.1). Pressure should build up rapidly to a point at which the bag can no longer be compressed. If there is a pressure-limiting device, it can be checked by connecting a pressure manometer between the patient port and the bag, using a T fitting. If there is an override mechanism on the pressure-limiting device, this should be checked.

To check the bag refill valve, the bag should be squeezed, then the patient port occluded, then the bag released. The bag should reexpand rapidly.

If the resuscitator has a closed reservoir, its function can be checked by performing several compression-release cycles with no oxygen flow into the reservoir. The reservoir should deflate, but the resuscitation bag should continued to expand.

A reservoir bag should be placed over the patient port (Fig. 18.2). Squeezing the resuscitation bag should cause the reservoir bag to inflate. After the resuscitation bag is released,

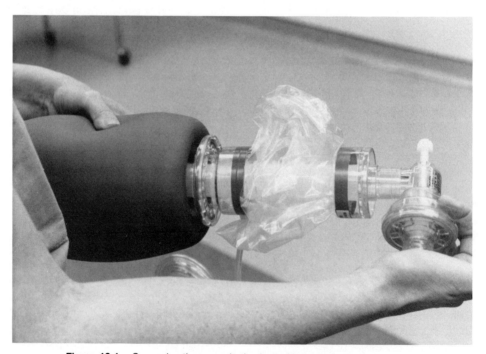

Figure 18.1.   Squeezing the resuscitation bag with the patient port occluded.

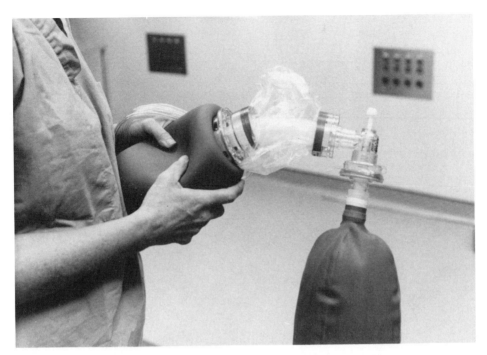

Figure 18.2. The resuscitation bag is checked by placing a reservoir bag over the patient port. Squeezing the resuscitation bag should cause the reservoir bag to inflate. The reservoir bag should then deflate easily when it is squeezed.

patency of the exhalation path should be confirmed by squeezing the reservoir bag. It should deflate easily.

A Mapleson system (see Chapter 6) with a separate oxygen cylinder may also be used for emergency ventilation.

Equipment for the Difficult Airway

There should be immediately available a means to deal with the desperate cannot ventilate/intubate situation (19). Three alternate ventilation methods that can be instituted blindly and quickly and that appear to have a low risk:benefit ratio have been described: the Combitube (discussed in Chapter 15); the laryngeal mask airway (discussed in Chapter 13); and transtracheal ventilation.

Transtracheal ventilation is performed by inserting a large intravenous catheter through the cricothyroid membrane and connecting it to a source of oxygen under pressure (20). There are three systems that

work reliably and can be easily and inexpensive assembled. The first is a jet injector (blow gun) powered by regulated or unregulated central wall oxygen pressure (Fig. 18.3). The second is a jet injector powered by an oxygen tank regulator. The third system uses the anesthesia machine flush valve as the jet injector. The fresh gas outlet of the anesthesia machine is connected to noncompliant oxygen supply tubing by a standard 15-mm tracheal tube connector. The other end of the tubing is connected to the IV catheter. This can be accomplished in several ways. One is shown in Figure 18.4. **NOTE:** Using the anesthesia breathing system or a self-inflating resuscitation bag as a means of a ventilation with a transtracheal catheter *will not* produce effective ventilation (20).

HIGH-PRESSURE SYSTEM

Some authors recommend that before any checking of the anesthesia machine is done

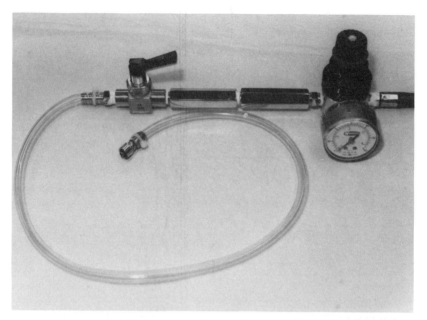

Figure 18.3. This system is designed to deliver oxygen at high flow through a small tubing. The regulator at the right is attached to a 50-psig oxygen source such as the pipeline system. The pressure delivered can be adjusted by turning the knob over the pressure gauge. The flow is controlled by the toggle switch downstream of the regulator. The tubing is attached to a large-bore needle or other device placed percutaneously through the cricothyroid membrane.

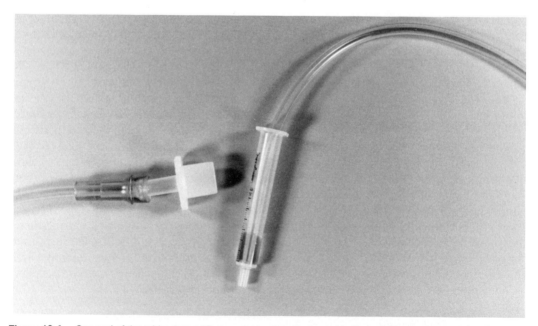

Figure 18.4. One end of the tubing has a 15-mm adaptor for attachment to the machine fresh gas outlet. The other end is firmly glued into the barrel of a 3-ml syringe. This end attaches to a large-bore intravenous catheter inserted percutaneously through the cricothyroid membrane.

that the user smell the gas from the fresh gas outlet to see if vapor has been leaking from a vaporizer.

Cylinder Gas Supply

Before gas supplies are checked, all flow control valves should be closed by turning them completely clockwise. Excessive torque should be avoided. Opening a cylinder or connecting a pipeline hose when a flow control valve is open may cause the indicator to shoot up to the top of the tube and perhaps be damaged, stuck at the top, or not noticed (21–23).

Cylinder gauges should be checked to make certain that they read zero. Yokes should be scanned to make certain any not containing a cylinder are fitted with a yoke plug. All cylinders should be checked to determine that their tags indicate *full* or *in use.*

The pressure in an oxygen cylinder is checked by turning the cylinder valve slowly counterclockwise while observing the related pressure gauge. If a hissing sound occurs when the valve is opened, the cylinder should be tightened in the yoke. If the machine is equipped with a dual cylinder yoke, the pressure in the second cylinder should be checked. The valve on the first cylinder should be closed and the oxygen flush used to release the pressure from the first cylinder. The second cylinder is then opened and its pressure checked.

The cylinder(s) should contain sufficient gas so that in the event of a problem with the pipeline supply, life support can be maintained until the pipeline problem can be corrected or more cylinders obtained. Whether a less-than-full cylinder is acceptable will depend on the particular circumstances. A full E cylinder will indicate about 2200 psi. This is equivalent to about 625 liters. Therefore, one full cylinder will last less than 4 hr at a flow of 3 liters/min. How low a pressure is acceptable will depend on whether additional cylinders are readily available and how low a fresh gas flow the user is willing to use. Hand ventilation as opposed to automatic ventila-

tion will conserve gas. The FDA checklist recommends that the cylinder be at least half full (about 1000 psig). If there are two cylinders and one is completely full, a low pressure in the second cylinder may be acceptable.

Empty or near-empty cylinders should be labeled as empty and replaced with full ones.

The 1992 FDA recommendations do not mention checking the pressures of cylinders containing gas other than oxygen, because these are not essential for life support. If it is planned to use one of these gases, it is reassuring to know that reserve supplies are available on the machine. As discussed in Chapter 1, the contents of a nitrous oxide cylinder may not be reflected by the pressure. The pressure gauge will continue to read 745 psi until all of the liquid has been consumed.

After the pressures are checked, all cylinder valves should be closed. If this is not done, leaks may cause loss of the entire supply. During use, there will be pressure fluctuations in the machine and the pipeline hoses. This is especially true of oxygen when a ventilator is in use. As the ventilator cycles, there will be a transient lowering of pressure in the machine. If the pressure falls below that at the regulator outlet while the cylinder valve is open, gas will be drawn from the cylinder until the pressure increases. Eventually the cylinder will empty and there may be no emergency supply available in the event of pipeline failure.

When piped gases are not going to be used, there should be one full cylinder of each gas to be used and the valve on this should be closed after the pressure has been checked. The other cylinders of these gases should be checked to make certain they have adequate contents for the intended procedure and the valves on these cylinders should be left fully opened.

Pipeline Gas Supply

Many institutions disconnect the hoses from the machine at night to prevent leakage from the hoses or the connections and to allow the machine to be moved for cleaning. If this is the case, the hoses need to be connected to the pipeline system. Fittings should hold firmly, no leaks should be heard and the hoses should be arranged to prevent occlusion. The pipeline gauges should read 45 to 55 psi.

As discussed in Chapter 3, a pipeline pressure gauge will register only pipeline pressure if it is positioned upstream of the check valve at the pipeline inlet, as required by the 1988 ASTM machine standard (15). If it is located downstream of the check valve, as it is on some older machines, the pressure registered will reflect the pressure in the machine (24).

LOW-PRESSURE SYSTEM

Initial Status Check

The check of the low-pressure system is begun by determining that the vaporizers and flow control valves are turned off. The liquid level in each vaporizer, as indicated by the sight glass, should be checked, adding more liquid if needed. Filler caps and drain valves should be checked for tightness.

The oxygen analyzer battery condition (if so equipped) should be checked. Removal of the oxygen sensor from the breathing system and exposing it to room air (see Fig. 16.23) at this point will expedite its calibration later.

Leak Checks of Machine Low-Pressure System

Testing for leaks by pressurizing the breathing system will often not detect leaks in the machine. Many machines are equipped with unidirectional check valves, either near the common outlet or in a vaporizer, to prevent pressures in the breathing system from affecting the accuracy of the flowmeters or vaporizers. Testing the breathing system for leaks by pressurization will reveal only leaks downstream of these check valves. Important leaks, such as those associated with flowmeters, may go undetected.

Negative Pressure Test (25)

The FDA checkout recommends using a suction bulb to create a negative pressure in the machine. The suction bulb is attached to a hose with a 15-mm adaptor, which will fit the anesthesia machine common gas outlet (Fig. 18.5). This device can be constructed by taking a sphygmomanometer bulb and reversing the valve in the end. When reversed, the valve will pull air from the machine side of the bulb instead of adding air. All flowmeters on the machine are turned off. A machine with a minimum mandatory flow must be turned off at the master switch. Squeezing the bulb until it is collapsed will create a negative pressure in the machine. If the bulb remains fully collapsed for 10 sec, there is no significant leak present. If there is a leak in the machine air from atmosphere will be drawn in and the bulb will expand. This test is repeated with each vaporizer turned on to detect leaks in individual vaporizers. The suction bulb should then be removed and the fresh gas hose reconnected.

This negative pressure leak test will work for all makes and models of machines, whether there is a check valve or not, and can be performed on machines that have a high minimum flow rate. It is sensitive enough to detect small leaks (100 ml/min) (17). However, it is possible that the negative pressure could close some leaks and give a false-negative result.

Positive Pressure Tests

There are other ways of testing for leaks in the machine using a positive pressure. When performing a positive pressure test, care must be taken that the pressures do not increase beyond the prescribed limits. There is little room for compression in the machine tubing and no bag to buffer pressure increases. It is conceivable that the pressure could increase to a point at which a flowmeter or other part of the machine could be damaged.

Pressure Gauge Test. A pressure gauge (the gauge from a standard sphygmomanom-

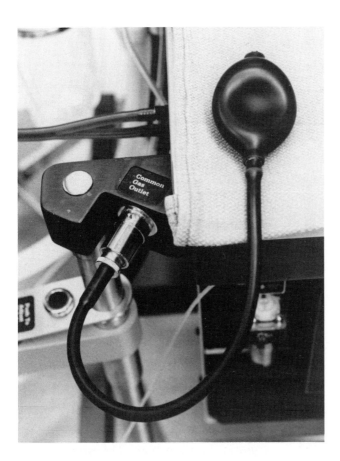

Figure 18.5. The suction bulb is attached to the common gas outlet and squeezed until it is collapsed. It should remain collapsed for at least 10 sec.

eter will do) is attached to the common gas outlet (Fig. 18.6), and the flow control valve is slowly opened until the pressure on the gauge reaches 30 cm H_2O (22 mm Hg). If the machine has a measured-flow vaporizer, the flowmeter associated with that vaporizer should be used. If there is no measured-flow vaporizer, the oxygen flowmeter can be used. The flow is then lowered until a steady pressure reading is achieved. The flow rate on the flowmeter is then equal to the leak rate in the machine. It should be less than 50 ml/min. This check should be repeated with each vaporizer turned on.

Gas Line Occlusion Test. A variation of the above test is to set a flow of 50 ml/min on the oxygen flowmeter and kink the fresh gas line. The indicator in the flowmeter should move downward.

Elapsed Time Pressure Test. If the machine does not have a flowmeter that reads as low as 50 ml/min, the following test may be used. A pressure gauge is attached to the machine outlet. The oxygen flowmeter is slowly turned on until a pressure of 30 cm H_2O is registered on the gauge. The flow is then turned off and the time it takes for the pressure to drop to 20 cm H_2O is observed. The time should be at least 10 sec. A shorter time implies an unacceptably high leak rate. This test should also be repeated with each vaporizer turned on.

Combination Breathing System and Machine Leak Tests. The following two tests can be used to check for leaks in the breathing system and the parts of the machine downstream of the check valves. To perform them, the oxygen sensor must be remounted

Figure 18.6. A pressure gauge from a blood pressure cuff is attached to the delivery hose from the machine. Sufficient flow is established on a flowmeter to maintain a pressure of 22 mm Hg on the pressure gauge. The flow required to maintain that pressure should be less than 50 ml/min.

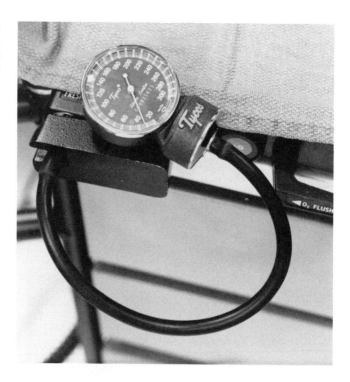

in the breathing system or replaced by a plug.

1. The APL valve is closed and the patient port occluded. The master control switch needs to be turned on. A vaporizer is turned on. The oxygen flush or a high flow on the flowmeter is used to fill the reservoir bag. As the bag begins to distend, the pressure on the manometer begins to rise. As the pressure starts to rise, the flowmeter flow is decreased until the pressure remains at 30 cm H_2O. If this pressure is overshot, the APL valve should be opened briefly. The flow should be no greater than 350 ml/min.

The advantages of this test are that it can be performed quickly without accessory equipment and that it checks the breathing system as well as the low-pressure parts of the machine in those models that do not have a check valve (26). It also allows checking of the continuous positive pressure airway alarm. A disadvantage is that it is relatively insensitive to small leaks.

2. With the machine power switch, flow control valves, and vaporizers off, the ports of the inspiratory and expiratory valves are connected with a hose. The manual/automatic selector is set to "bag," and the APL valve is closed. A test terminal and sphygmomanometer squeeze bulb are connected to the breathing bag mount, and the bulb is squeezed repeatedly until the breathing system pressure gauge reads at least 50 cm H_2O. The pressure drop on the breathing system pressure gauge is observed. If a drop from 50 to 30 cm H_2O takes 30 sec or longer the leak rate is acceptable. After the test is performed, the hose, squeeze bulb, and test terminal are removed. This test may miss leaks in the machine upstream of the check valve.

During use, a leak in the machine or breathing system can be tested for by lowering the fresh gas flow to 300 ml/min (27). The ventilator bellows or reservoir bag should continue to fill.

When the leak test of the machine is complete, residual vapors should be flushed out of the machine by turning on oxygen flow at

1 liter/min for 1 min with all vaporizers off (26). Use of the oxygen flush control will not flush vapors out of the machine, because its flow enters the fresh gas flow downstream of the vaporizers. There should be no noticeable odor in the gas coming from the common gas outlet.

Turn on the Machine's Master Switch

To continue the machine checkout, the on-off switch on the machine needs to be turned on to enable the pneumatics as well as the electronics of the machine.

Tests of Flowmeters

Flowmeters should be examined with no gas flow to make certain that the indicator is at the zero position (or at minimum flow if so equipped). Each flow control valve should be slowly opened and closed while observing the indicator as it rises and falls within the tube. It should move smoothly and respond to small adjustments of the flow control valve. If the indicator is a rotameter or ball it should rotate freely. An indicator with erratic movement or that fails to return to zero may be displaying erroneous flow rates and the machine should be taken out of service until the problem is corrected.

An attempt should be made to create a hypoxic mixture by adjusting the nitrous oxide flow up or the oxygen flow down while the nitrous oxide is flowing. This is not a test of the flowmeters but of the proportioning system. Turning the nitrous oxide flow up should cause the oxygen flow to increase so that a concentration of at least 25% oxygen is maintained. Similar results should occur if a high flow on nitrous oxide is present and the oxygen flow is adjusted downward. If the machine has a ratio alarm, it should be activated.

BREATHING SYSTEM

Calibration of the Oxygen Monitor

If the oxygen monitor sensor was exposed to room air during the check of the low-pres-

sure system it should have had enough time to adjust. It should be calibrated to 21%, and the low oxygen alarm should be checked by setting the alarm limit above 21%. The sensor should then be placed securely in its mount in the breathing system. Flushing with oxygen should result in a reading over 90%. The oxygen monitor should not be recalibrated at a high oxygen concentration, because greater accuracy is needed at low concentrations (17). Some checklists recommend that gas flows be set for 50% oxygen and the reading checked. This also checks the flowmeters.

Initial Status

The breathing system should be inspected to determine that no parts are damaged or missing. The bag-ventilator selector switch should be in the bag position. The pressure gauge should be observed to determine that it reads zero. If there is an absorber bypass, it should be in the nonbypass position.

The absorbent should be noted. If color change extends into the second chamber, the upstream canister should be replaced by the partially charged canister; the exhausted absorbent should be discarded and replaced by fresh absorbent. Accumulated absorbent dust and water should be removed from the absorber dust cup, taking care not to spill either because they are caustic.

At this point, accessory equipment such as a humidifier, circulator, or PEEP valve should be added to the breathing system. Often these are added just before or after the start of the case. This means they will not be included in the checkout procedure and faults or improper installation will not be discovered until a problem has surfaced.

Breathing System Leak Check

To initiate the breathing system check outlined in the FDA protocol, all gas flows should be zero or the minimum possible. The APL valve should be closed and the patient port occluded. The breathing system should be pressurized to 30 cm H_2O by using the oxygen flush (Fig. 18.7). If there is no leak, the pressure will remain at this level for at least 10 sec.

To quantitate the leak, the flow through the oxygen flowmeter needed to maintain the pressure is determined. This will equal the leak present. The breathing system standard (28) requires that this not exceed 300 ml/min.

This test has two advantages (29). First, it does not require accessory test devices. Second, it can be performed quickly. A disadvantage is that it does not test for leaks in the ventilator.

Mapleson Breathing Systems

Mapleson breathing systems need to be connected to the fresh gas source. The APL valve is closed. The patient port is occluded, and the system is pressurized using the oxygen flush. The pressure should be retained at this level for 10 sec. The pressure should be released by opening the APL valve.

Special Test of the Bain System

Potential dangers with the Bain system include the inner tube having a hole, becoming detached at its proximal end, or not extending to the patient end of the outer tubing. If problems with the inner tube are present, the dead space is greatly increased. These problems can be detected by the following test (30–33).

1. A 2 liter/min flow is set on one of the flowmeters.
2. The plunger from a small syringe or a finger is inserted into the distal (patient) end of the outer tube, occluding the inner tube (Fig. 18.8). The flowmeter indicator should fall. The machine relief valve, if present, should open. **NOTE:** If the system has side holes at the patient end of the inner tubing, this test *will not* work (34).

The alternate test is as follows (35):

1. The reservoir bag is filled.
2. The patient port remains open to atmosphere

3. The oxygen flush valve on the machine is activated while observing the reservoir bag. The high flow of gas through the inner tube will produce a Venturi effect, which lowers the pressure in the larger outer tube. If there are no problems with the inner tube, the bag should deflate slightly. If the bag does not deflate or inflates slightly, the inner tube should be checked.

Note: The authors prefer the first test, because the second test may fail to detect major faults (31,36,37).

Special Test of the Lack System (38,39)

To test the integrity of the inner limb of this system, a suitably sized tracheal tube should be inserted well into the inner tubing at the patient end of the system. Blowing down the tracheal tube with the APL valve closed will produce movement of the bag if there is leakage between the inner and outer limbs.

An alternative method is to occlude both the inner and outer limbs with the APL valve open. There should be no gas escape on applying pressure to the reservoir bag. If the inner limb is defective, the bag will collapse and gas will escape through the APL valve.

SCAVENGING SYSTEM AND APL VALVE

The scavenging system should be checked to make sure the APL valve and ventilator are connected to the interface. If an active disposal system is being used, the flow should be adjusted to an acceptable rate. The manufacturer's instructions should be consulted.

Function of the scavenging system and APL valve are checked by closing the APL valve, occluding the patient port, and filling the system using the oxygen flush so that the breathing system pressure gauge reads 50 cm H_2O. The APL valve is then opened. There should be a gradual loss of pressure from the system. This establishes proper function of the APL valve and patency of the transfer tubing. If the scavenging system has a reservoir bag at the interface, it should increase in

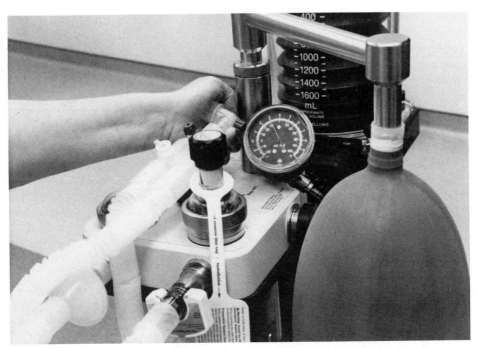

Figure 18.7.   Test for leaks in the breathing system. With all gas flows set to zero or minimum, the APL valve is closed and the patient port occluded. The reservoir bag is filled using the oxygen flush until a pressure of 30 cm H_2O is shown on the gauge. With no additional gas flow, the pressure should remain at this level for at least 10 sec.

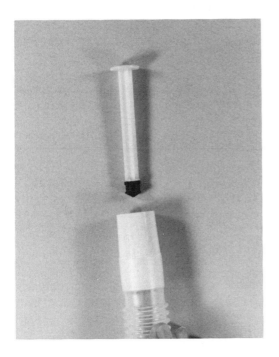

Figure 18.8.   Test of the Bain system. The plunger from a small syringe is inserted into the patient end of the system over the end of the inner fresh gas delivery tubing. The flowmeter indicator should drop.

size when the APL valve is opened and then decrease in size (40).

If the pressure is released by removing the occlusion at the patient port the APL valve and scavenging system patency will not be checked. In addition, this may cause a cloud of absorbent dust to fly into the breathing tubes (41,42).

With the APL valve fully open and the patient port occluded, the negative and positive pressure reliefs on the scavenging interface should be checked. With minimum flow from the machine, there should be negligible negative pressure in the breathing system after the bag in the scavenging system (if present) and the reservoir bag in the breathing system are collapsed. To test the positive relief, the oxygen flush is activated. The breathing system pressure gauge should show minimal positive pressure.

MANUAL AND AUTOMATIC VENTILATION SYSTEMS

Functional Test of Ventilator and Unidirectional Valves (43)

A reservoir bag is placed on the patient port (Fig. 18.9). Ventilator parameters appropriate for the intended patient are set. The oxygen flowmeter should be set at 300 ml/min. The bag-ventilator selector switch should be set in the ventilator mode. The bellows and reservoir bag are filled using the oxygen flush, and the ventilator is turned on. The bellows should move freely and fill completely as the ventilator cycles. If the bellows does not fill, a leak in the ventilator or hose should be suspected. The tidal volume actually delivered as measured with a respiratory volume meter should be compared with that set on the ventilator. A discrepancy suggests a leak. Each ventilator control should be varied and the effects noted. Functions such as manual sigh should be checked.

While the ventilator is cycling, the unidirectional valves should be inspected. The disc in the inspiratory valve should rise during inspiration, and the disc in the exhalation valve should rise during exhalation.

To check the spill valve on the ventilator an oxygen flow of 500 ml/min should be set, and the bellows should be allowed to rise to the top of the housing. The pressure gauge in the breathing system should indicate less than 2.5 cm H_2O, and the bellows should remain at the top of the housing.

The bag should be removed from the patient port and the ventilator allowed to continue cycling. The low airway pressure alarm (and volume monitor alarm if present) should sound after an appropriate delay.

If the ventilator has batteries for back-up power or powering alarms, these should be checked.

To check manual ventilation, the ventilator is turned off and a reservoir bag is placed on the patient port (Fig. 18.10). Another reservior bag is placed on the bag mount. The bag-ventilator selector switch is turned to the bag position. As the reservoir bag on the bag mount in the breathing system is squeezed, inflation and deflation of the bag on the patient port should occur.

In some departments, it is common practice to let the patient breathe through the breathing system while still conscious using a mask. This can also be done by anesthesia personnel (wearing a mask of course) (Fig. 18.11). This will check for obstructions (44). Negative pressure will reveal an obstruction in the inspiratory limb; positive pressure will reveal an obstruction in the expiratory limb (45). While this is being done, the capnograph should be checked to make certain a waveform appears.

Check for Leaks in Ventilator with Hanging Bellows

To check for a leak in a ventilator with a hanging bellows (Fig. 18.12), all flowmeters should be turned off or to the minimum flow. The APL valve is closed and the ventilator turned on. When the bellows is fully contracted against the head of the bellows assem-

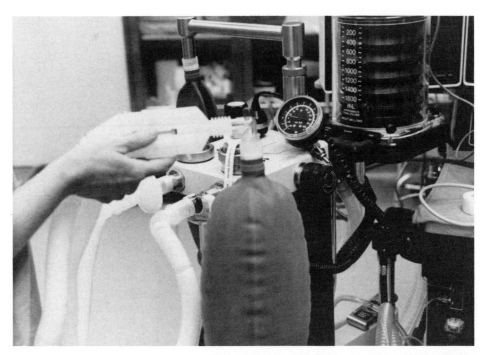

Figure 18.9. Test of ventilator and unidirectional valves. A reservoir bag is placed on the patient port. The oxygen flowmeter is set for a flow of 300 ml/min. Ventilator parameters appropriate for the intended patient are set. The bag-ventilator selector switch should be in the ventilator position. The bellows and reservoir bag are filled, and the ventilator is turned on. The bellows should move freely and fill completely as the ventilator cycles. The unidirectional valves should be observed to make certain the discs move properly.

bly, the patient port is occluded (or the bag-ventilator selector switch is put in the bag position) and the ventilator switched off. The bellows should remain at the top of the housing for at least 10 sec. If it expands downward, a leak is present. Another way of performing this test is to occlude the patient port (or put the bag-ventilator selector switch in the bag position) with the ventilator turned off and move the bellows stop to a larger tidal volume setting. Again, the bellows should not expand downward.

Check of Ventilator Safety-Relief Valve

While the patient port is occluded, the ventilator is turned on. The breathing system pressure should rise no higher than the safety-relief pressure of the ventilator, normally 60 to 75 cm H_2O.

Tests for Incompetent Unidirectional Valves (46,47)

Incompetent unidirectional valves can be detected with a capnograph (see Chapter 16). Reverse flow will be noted if the respirometer is able to detect this condition. If these are not available, one of the following tests can be used.

Breathing Method

The inspiratory limb of the breathing system is detached from the absorber and occluded. Wearing a mask, the tester tries to breath through the Y piece (Fig. 18.13*A*). It should be possible to exhale freely but not inhale. Next the exhalation tube is detached and occluded. The tester should be able to inhale from the Y piece but not exhale (see Fig. 18.13*B*).

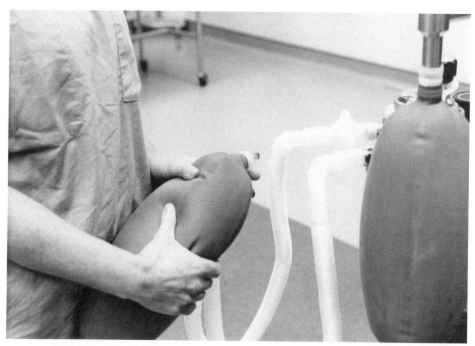

Figure 18.10.   Test for manual ventilation system. A reservoir bag is placed on the patient port. The bag-ventilator switch is turned to the bag position. As the reservoir bag in the breathing system is squeezed the bag on the port should inflate. Squeezing the bag on the patient port should cause the reservoir bag in the breathing system to inflate.

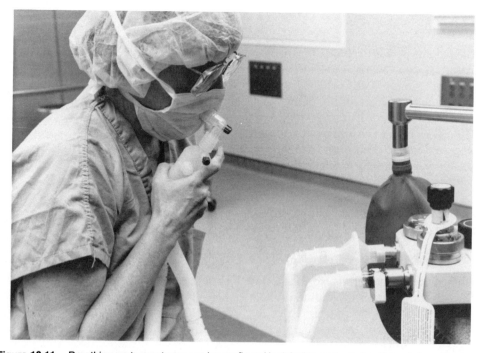

Figure 18.11.   Breathing system patency can be confirmed by inhaling and exhaling through the patient port.

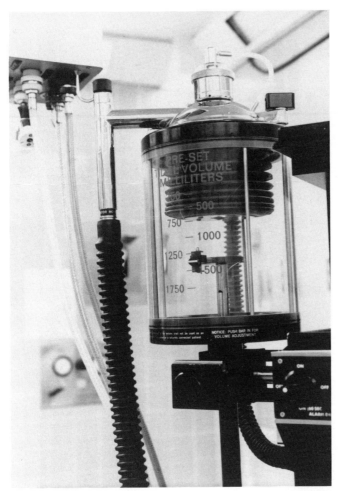

Figure 18.12.   Test for leak in ventilator with hanging bellows. The flowmeters should be turned off or at minimum flow. The APL valve is closed and the ventilator turned on. When the bellows is fully contracted against the head of the bellows assembly, the patient port is occluded (or the bag-ventilator selector switch is put in the bag position) and the ventilator is turned off. The bellows should remain at the top of the housing for at least 10 sec.

Pressure Method

The inhalational valve is checked by connecting a reservoir bag at the usual bag connector site and a corrugated tube to the inhalation outlet. While the exhalation inlet is covered, positive pressure is applied to the corrugated tube. No gas should flow into the tube and the reservoir bag should not fill.

To check the exhalation valve, a reservoir bag is connected to the expiratory limb connection and a corrugated tube to the reservoir bag connection. While the inhalation outlet is covered, positive pressure is applied to the corrugated tube. No gas should flow into the tube and the reservoir bag should not fill.

MONITORS

All monitors should be turned on and calibrated if needed; alarms should be tested and the alarm limits set. The instructions for each particular instrument will need to be followed. The alarm limits should not be so high or low that the alarms sound needlessly or so broad that potentially harmful situations are missed. The sampling tube of a diverting gas monitor should be checked for integrity and connected to the breathing

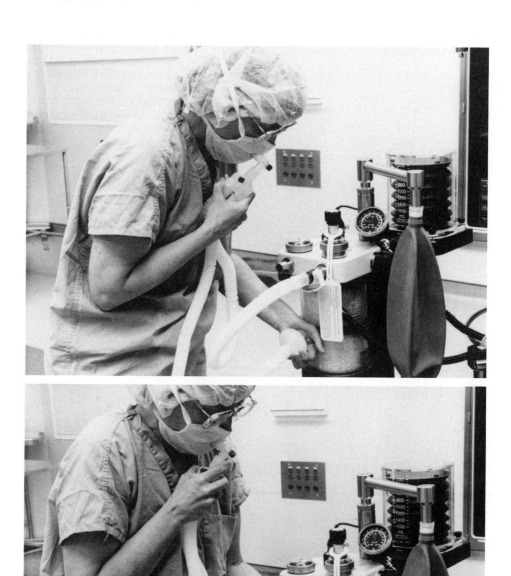

Figure 18.13.   Checks for incompetent unidirectional valves. **Top,** The inspiratory limb is detached and occluded. The tester tries to breathe through the Y piece. It should be possible to exhale freely but not inhale. **Bottom,** The exhalation tubing is detached and occluded. The tester should be able to inhale from the Y piece but not exhale.

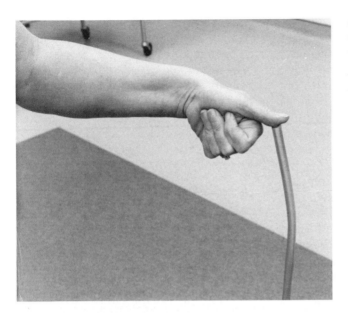

Figure 18.14. Suction check. The strength of the vacuum is tested by determining that the weight of the suction tubing can be supported at waist height by the seal between the tubing and the underside of a finger. If the vacuum is unsatisfactory, the tubing will not remain in contact with the finger.

system near the patient. If there is a water trap it should be emptied.

FINAL MACHINE STATUS

The final status of all controls needs to be checked before the machine is put in use. This includes having all flow control valves closed, all vaporizers in the off position, the bag-ventilator selector switch set to bag, and the APL valve closed.

An inflexible suction catheter should be present. The adequacy of suction can be checked by placing the end of the suction tubing on the underside of the finger (Fig. 18.14). The tubing should stay without support.

Other Machine and Breathing System Checks

While the FDA checkout recommendations are adequate for daily use, other parts may need to be checked, especially after the machine has been altered or serviced.

OXYGEN PRESSURE FAILURE ALARM

Most machines are now equipped with an oxygen pressure failure alarm, which is acti-

vated if there is no or low oxygen pressure in the machine while the master on-off switch is turned on. To test this alarm, the oxygen pipeline hose is disconnected and cylinder closed. Any pressure remaining in the machine should be bled off using the oxygen flush. The alarm should sound. This step was not included in the 1992 FDA checkout recommendations because isolated failure of this component will not injure a patient (17).

LEAKAGE AT THE YOKE

If a cylinder is not properly tightened in a yoke there will be leakage of gas when the cylinder is turned on. If there is a large leak, it will be quite apparent. If the leak is small, it will not be heard but could cause significant loss of gas. To check for leakage at the yoke, after the cylinder pressures have been checked and the valves closed, the cylinder pressure gauges are observed for 2 to 5 min, with no flow on the flowmeters. A drop of more than 50 psig indicates significant leakage.

OXYGEN FAILURE SAFETY VALVE

The oxygen failure safety valve was included as a routine test in the first edition of the FDA checkout but was not made part of the newest version because failures of this device are rare and there are many other methods of detecting the problem (17). This test can be performed using either the pipelines or cylinders as the gas source. A cylinder of each gas on the machine is turned on, leaving the pipeline hoses disconnected. Flows of 2 liters/min are established on the flowmeters for each gas. The oxygen cylinder is then turned off. As the pressure of the oxygen falls, the flows of all other gases except possibly air, as indicated by their flowmeters, should decrease in proportion to the decrease in oxygen flow and eventually shut off. Restoring the oxygen pressure should cause the indicators to return to their previous positions.

To perform the test using pipeline gases, all cylinder valves should be closed and the flow control valves opened until the cylinder pressure gauges register zero. The pipeline hoses are then connected and flows established on all flowmeters. The oxygen hose is disconnected. The indicators of the anesthetic gases should fall with the oxygen indicator.

SPARE COMPONENTS

Extra components of the breathing system should be immediately available. These include an additional disposable system or individual components of reusable systems (Y piece, tubings, and bag).

Checking Other Components

TRACHEAL TUBES

A tracheal tube of the size appropriate for the age and sex of the patient should be ready for use. One larger and one smaller tube should be readily available.

Patency of the lumen should be checked. With clear tubes, simple observation will suffice. With other tubes, it is necessary to look in both ends or, better, insert a stylet. If the anticipated procedure will involve movement of the head or neck, the tube should be tested for kinking. It should be possible to approximate the two ends of the tube without a kink forming.

The cuff should be held inflated for at least 1 min to verify that there are no leaks. It should inflate evenly and not stick to the wall of the tube or decrease the size of the lumen.

Studies show that a tracheal tube whose package has been opened to test the cuff remains sterile for up to 7 days (48).

LARYNGOSCOPES

Laryngoscope malfunction is a frequent problem. At least two handles should be present, each fitted with the type of blade the user anticipates will be best for the patient. The lights should be checked for adequate intensity. Blades of other sizes and shapes should be immediately available and checked for proper function.

ACCESSORY INTUBATION EQUIPMENT

A stylet should be immediately available. If a rapid sequence intubation is planned, the stylet should be fitted to the tube, if not actually in it. An intubating forceps should be immediately available. If a difficult intubation is anticipated, specialized equipment for difficult intubation described in Chapters 14 and 15 should be assembled.

MASKS AND AIRWAYS

An assortment of masks and airways in a variety of sizes should be readily available.

OTHER EQUIPMENT

Special equipment required for particular cases such as extension pipeline hoses, a hot air warming system, etc. should be present and checked before use.

Subsequent Checks on the Same Machine on the Same Day

If a thorough check is performed before the first case of the day, a less complete procedure can be followed before subsequent cases. Those steps are indicated in Table 18.1.

Procedure at the End of the Case

At the conclusion of a case, flowmeters, vaporizers, and suction should be turned off. Monitors that would need recalibration should be left on or put in a standby mode. The absorbent should be checked for signs of exhaustion and changed if indicated (see Chapter 8).

Care at the End of the Day

Following the last case, the pipeline hoses should be disconnected at the wall or ceiling (not at the back of the machine) and coiled over the machine. During the nonuse hours, the external surfaces of the machine should be cleaned. If the pipeline hoses are disconnected, it is more likely the machine will be moved and the floor under it cleaned. If the hoses are disconnected at the back of the machine, they will continue to be pressurized and gas may be lost into the room through leaks. Cylinder valves should be closed. Each flow control valve should be opened until the cylinder and pipeline pressure gauges read zero, then closed. Closing the flow control valve will not conserve any gas, but if they are left open, restoration of the gas supply may forcibly raise the indicator to the top of the flowmeter, causing damage.

Vaporizers should be filled at the conclusion of the day after most operating room personnel have left the room. This will decrease exposure to trace amounts of anesthetic agents.

Liquid should be drained from the base of the absorber. Care must be exercised as the liquid is caustic and should not come in contact with skin.

Checking New or Modified Equipment

Each new anesthesia machine, ventilator, or other complex piece of equipment should be checked for proper functioning before being put to use. Assembly and testing for correct function is best performed by a manufacturer's representative. Often this person will give in-service instructions. A document certifying that the equipment has been checked for proper assembly and function should be obtained and kept.

A manual that contains assembly and installation instructions, maintenance requirements, daily checking procedures, and instructions for use should be supplied with each piece of equipment. This should be read carefully and reviewed periodically. A copy should be kept in the central equipment files and with the equipment itself.

The following series of tests designed to check for crossovers between gas supplies should be performed on all new machines and any time repairs or adjustments are made to a machine. In many states performance of these procedures is a legal requirement (49).

1. All hoses are detached and all cylinder valves closed.
2. The oxygen pipeline hose is connected, and the reading on the pipeline gauge is checked to confirm that it reads between 45 and 55 psig.
3. The oxygen flush is actuated, and flow from the common outlet is confirmed.
4. The ventilator power outlet (if present) is actuated, and presence of flow confirmed.
5. The oxygen flow control valve is opened and flow on the oxygen flowmeter is verified. Flow control valves for other gases are opened to make certain no flow occurs.
6. The flow control valves on measured

flow vaporizer(s) are opened, and flow on the flowmeter(s) is verified.

7. The nitrous oxide pipeline hose is connected, and it is verified that the reading on the pressure gauge is between 45 and 55 psig.
8. The oxygen hose is disconnected.
9. Steps 3, 4, 5, and 6 are repeated. There should be no flow from any flowmeters, the flush valve, or the power outlet.
10. The oxygen pipeline hose is reconnected and a suitably calibrated oxygen analyzer connected to the common outlet. The oxygen flow control knob is turned off.
11. The oxygen flush valve is actuated. More than 90% oxygen should be indicated on the oxygen analyzer.
12. The oxygen flow control valve is opened so that a flow of 5 liters/min is indicated on the flowmeter. More than 95% oxygen should be indicated. The nitrous oxide flow control valve is opened until a 5 liters/min flow is established. A reading of 50% oxygen should be indicated on the oxygen analyzer.
13. All flow control valves are closed.
14. The pipeline hoses are disconnected and steps 2 through 13 repeated, except that the oxygen and nitrous oxide cylinders are used instead of the pipeline hoses. The results should be the same except for the pipeline pressure gauge readings.

After these tests are performed, a complete preuse checking procedure needs to be performed. In addition, there may be special testing procedures recommended by the manufacturer.

Preventive Maintenance

Preventive maintenance includes inspection, testing, cleaning, lubrication, and adjustment of components. Worn or damaged parts are fixed or replaced. Preventive main-tenance has been shown to be effective in preventing equipment failure (50). Many items in an anesthesia machine and ventilator deteriorate with time and use. Preventive maintenance is designed to anticipate predictable failures and replace weakened components before they fail. In some cases an improved part has become available and can be substituted for one likely to fail. Lack of a preventive maintenance program may lead to an unacceptably high rate of breakdowns, premature replacement of major equipment, and unnecessary accidents and hazards (51).

The question of who should perform preventive maintenance has been widely debated. Contracted service is most efficient when anesthesia equipment inventories are minimal or in-house resources are limited.

EQUIPMENT MANUFACTURER UNDER SERVICE CONTRACT

With a service contract, a service representative employed by the manufacturer or the manufacturer's agent comes to the healthcare facility. Sometimes different levels of service can be selected. The intensity of the service will determine the cost.

INDEPENDENT SERVICE COMPANY

There are many independent companies not associated with a particular manufacturer who will service certain equipment on a contractual basis. These contracts vary but are similar to those offered by the manufacturer.

One problem is that it may not always be possible for an independent company to procure manufacturer-approved parts. It is important for the user to determine the extent of the service company's liability coverage.

Laws recently enacted in at least one state require that the credentials of each servicing person be approved by the machine manufacturer or determined by the physician director of the anesthesia department to be equivalent to the credentials of the manufacturer's service person.

IN-HOUSE BIOMEDICAL SERVICES

Use of in-house biomedical services may be an option for much anesthesia equipment. Usually, only larger facilities have the volume of equipment that makes this approach cost effective. In some cases, the intensity of service from outside sources can be reduced. Biomedical technicians can sometimes attend special schools to learn how to service specific equipment.

There are advantages to in-house biomedical maintenance of anesthesia machines, one of which is minimal response time to trouble calls (52). It is optimal to have a biomedical service facility located within the operating room suite. This allows immediate reaction to calls and observation of problems while the equipment is in use. An in-house service located elsewhere in the hospital can be effective if good communication with the operating room is established.

There are a number of potential problems with an in-house maintenance program.

Obtaining Factory-Authorized Parts

Maintenance performed in the facility must use the proper parts. Often these can be ordered from the company, but some companies will not sell parts to uncertified maintenance personnel. Nonstandard parts can affect the ability of the instrument to function properly.

Understanding of the Equipment

To perform proper maintenance, it is necessary to understand how the equipment is constructed and what would happen if it were not assembled correctly. If personnel have been trained and certified by the equipment manufacturer, this should not be a problem.

Modifications

Personnel may be tempted to make changes when doing maintenance. These changes may affect the function of the equipment. Each modification should be carefully and exhaustively evaluated before clinical use to ensure that new modes of failure are not introduced (52). Modifying a piece of equipment puts the modifying party in the category of a manufacturer with all the attendant responsibilities.

Delays in Performing Maintenance

Routine maintenance may not seem important and may not be performed because everything is working well or because other equipment receives higher priority.

Documentation

Documentation of maintenance work must be complete. Outside service contractors usually leave a checklist and a purchase order that shows that the servicing has been performed, what repairs were made, and what parts were replaced.

Laws recently enacted in at least one state stipulate that records must be kept of each machine, including the name of the service person, work performed, and date the work was performed.

Legal Responsibility

The question of liability exposure must be addressed when considering in-house service (52). If a problem occurs as a result of the actions of a service person from outside the hospital, his or her liability insurance should cover the cost. If hospital personnel cause a problem, the hospital will have to shoulder the liability.

Record Keeping

Record keeping on equipment has frequently been neglected in the past. Often it is assumed that the manufacturer's service representative who does periodic preventive maintenance will take care of this task. Common experience does not support this. Record keeping is important for several reasons.

1. It provides proof that an effort has been made to keep the equipment in proper working order. This could have medicolegal significance.
2. It provides a means of communication with the service representative. Representatives frequently come in the late afternoon or evening when anesthesia personnel have left. If there is no written record of problems that have occurred with the equipment, the service representative may not perform the indicated repair(s).
3. It provides a complete, up-to-date record for each piece of equipment. If one piece of equipment malfunctions more frequently than others, consideration should be given to replacing it.
4. It provides a written record that maintenance by a service representative was performed and shows what was done. Service representatives may present only a bill for service and parts and no record of what was actually done.
5. It provides a check on the service rendered by the representative. After equipment is serviced, it should perform well. If a machine develops a problem soon after servicing or if there is an increased frequency of repairs that can be traced to a change in service representatives, one may wish to question that representative's effectiveness.
6. With pieces of equipment such as vaporizers that need to be sent to the manufacturer periodically for servicing, or oxygen analyzers that need to have certain components replaced at intervals, it serves to remind the user when the equipment needs to be serviced or a component replaced. After a vaporizer is serviced, it may be held in reserve before being put into use. This would extend the time before servicing would be due. This can be noted on the form by recording the time when a vaporizer is received from the

manufacturer and when it is actually put into service on a machine.

A record should be kept for each piece of complex equipment such as an anesthesia machine, ventilator, vaporizer, or monitor. This should include identification information; date of purchase; instructions for servicing; and the name, address, and telephone number of the service representative. If a problem with the equipment arises, the date, problem, and corrective action should be recorded. When routine servicing is performed, this should be noted, along with any problems or parts replaced. Each entry should be signed by the person making it.

Should a serious accident that may involve equipment occur, a systematic approach to accident investigation should be made. These steps are discussed in detail in Chapter 12.

Safe Medical Devices Act (53–55)

The Safe Medical Devices Act of 1990 (Public Law 101–629) was designed to make sure that devices entering the market are safe and effective and that if there are serious problems the FDA learns about them quickly so that the devices can be removed from the market quickly. Healthcare facilities are required to report within 10 working days all incidents that reasonably suggest that there is a probability that a medical device caused or contributed to the death, serious illness, or serious injury of a patient. The report should include the reporting facility, product name, model, serial number, name of the manufacturer, and a description of the event. Deaths must be reported to both the manufacturer and the FDA. Other events must be reported to the manufacturer if he is not known to the FDA.

A reporting system needs to be developed within each facility. This should include three components. First is a program that educates all staff members about their responsibilities. Second, there needs to be a procedure that ensures that reports from individuals are forwarded to a review group for analysis and decision making. Finally, a documentation and record-keeping system needs to be in place for the storage and retrieval of all data that may be submitted to the FDA and/or reported to manufacturers.

REFERENCES

1. Charlton JE. Checklists and patient safety [Editorial]. Anaesthesia 1990;45:425–426.
2. Cundy J, Baldock GJ. Safety check procedures to eliminate faults in anaesthetic machines. Anaesthesia 1982;37:161–169.
3. Chopra V, Bovill JG, Spierdijk J. Checklists. Aviation shows the way to safer anaesthesia. APSF Newslett 1991;6:26,29.
4. Feldman JM, Blike G, Cheung KH. New electronic checklists aim at decreasing anesthetist errors. APSF Newslett 1992;7:1–2.
4. Cooper JB, Newbower RS, Kitz RJ. An analysis of major errors and equipment failures in anesthesia management: considerations for prevention and detection. Anesthesiology 1984;60:34–42.
5. Craig J, Wilson ME. A survey of anaesthetic misadventures. Anaesthesia 1981;36:933–936.
6. Cobcroft MD. More misconnected Boyle circuit tubings. Anaesth Intensive Care 1978;6:170–171.
7. Chopra V, Bovill JG, Spierdijk J, Koornneef F. Reported significant observations during anaesthesia: a prospective analysis over an 18 month period. Br J Anaesth 1992;68:13–17.
8. Kumar V, Barcellos WA, Mehta MP, Carter JG. Analysis of critical incidents in a teaching department for quality assurance. A survey of mishaps during anaesthesia. Anaesthesia 1988;43:879–883.
9. Mayor AH, Eaton JM. Anaesthetic machine checking practices. Anaesthesia 1992;47:866–868.
10. Anonymous. FDA re-examines anesthesia safety & equipment check procedures. Biomed Safe Stand 1991;21:17–19.
11. Withiam-Wilson. FDA preuse equipment checklist spurred by accidents, studies. APSF Newslett 1991;6:27.
12. Buffington CW, Ramanathan S, Turndorf H. Detection of anesthesia machine faults. Anesth Analg 1984;63:79–82.
13. March MG, Crowley JJ. An evaluation of anesthesiologists' present checkout methods and the validity of the FDA checklist. Anesthesiology 1991;75:724–729.
14. Drews JH. Hazardous anesthesia machine malfunc-

tion occurring after routine preventive maintenance inspection. Anesth Analg 1983;62:701.
15. American Society for Testing and Materials. Standard specification for minimum prformance and safety requirements for components and systems of anesthesia gas machines (F1161–88). Philadelphia: ASTM, 1988.
16. Carstensen P. FDA issues pre-use checkout. APSF Newslett 1986;1:13–20.
17. Good ML. Comments sought on new FDA pre-anesthesia checklist. APSF Newslett 1992;7:47–51.
18. American Society of Anesthesiologists. Professional liability and the anesthesiologist. Park Ridge, IL: ASA, 1987.
19. Benumof JL. Management of the difficult adult airway. Anesthesiology 1991;75:1089–1110.
20. Benumof JL, Scheller MS. The importance of transtracheal jet ventilation in the management of the difficult airway. Anesthesiology 1989;71:769–778.
21. Dinnick OP. Accidental severe hypercapnia during anaesthesia. Br J Anaesth 1968;40:36, 45.
22. Lomanto C, Leeming M. A safety signal for detection of excessive anesthetic gas flows. Anesthesiology 1970;33:663–664.
23. Prys-Roberts C, Smith WDA, Nunn JF. Accidental severe hypercapnia during anaesthesia. Br J Anaesth 1967;39:257–267.
24. Wilson AM. The pressure gauges on the Boyle international anaesthetic machine. Anaesthesia 1982;37:218–219.
25. Berner MS. Profound hypercapnia due to disconnection within an anaesthetic machine. Can J Anaesth 1987;34:622–626.
26. Eisenkraft JB. The anesthesia delivery system. Part II: Progress in Anesthesiology 1989;3:1–12.
27. Ghani GA. Test for a leak in the anesthesia circle. Anesth Analg 1983;62:855–856.
28. American Society for Testing and Materials. Standard specification for minimum performance and safety requirements for anesthesia breathing systems (F1208–89). Philadelphia: ASTM, 1989.
29. Andrews JJ. The anatomy of modern anesthesia machines (ASA Refresher Course #274). New Orleans. ASA, 1989.
30. Foex P, Crampton-Smith A. A test for co-axial circuits. Anaesthesia 1977;32:294.
31. Heath PJ, Marks LF. Modified occlusion tests for the Bain breathing system. Anaesthesia 1991;46:213–216.
32. Ghani GA. Safety check for the Bain circuit. Can Anaesth Soc J 1984;31:487–488.
33. Jackson IJB. Tests for co-axial systems. Anaesthesia 1988;43:1060–1061.
34. Robinson S, Fisher DM. Safety check for the CPRAM circuit. Anesthesiology 1983;59:488–489.
35. Pethick SL. Correspondence. Can Anaesth Soc J 1975;22:115.

36. Petersen WC. Bain circuit. Can Anaesth Soc J 1978;25:532.
37. Beauprie IG, Clark AG, Keith IC, Spence D, Eng P. Pre-use testing of coaxial circuits: the perils of Pethick. Can J Anaesth 1990;37:S103.
38. Furst B, Laffey DA. An alternate test for the Lack system. Anaesthesia 1984;39:834.
39. Martin LVH, McKeown DW. An alternative test for the Lack system. Anaesthesia 1985;40:80–92.
40. Eisenkraft JB, Sommer RM. Flapper valve malfunction. Anesth Analg 1988;67:1132.
41. Debban DG, Bedford RF. Overdistention of the rebreathing bag, a hazardous test for circle-system integrity. Anesthesiology 1975;42:365–366.
31. Ribak B. Reducing the soda-lime hazard. Anesthesiology 1975;43:277.
43. Grogono AW. Anesthesia ventilators: function, limitations, hazards (ASA refresher Course #275). New Orleans: ASA, 1989.
44. Olympio MA, Stoner J. Tight mask fit could have prevented "airway" obstruction. Anesthesiology 1992;77:822–825.
45. Grundy EM, Bennett EJ, Brennan T. Obstructed anesthetic circuits. Anesthesiol Rev 1976;3:35–36.
46. Kim J, Kovac AL, Mathewson HS. A method for detection of incompetent unidirectional dome valves. A prevalent malfunction. Anesth Analg 1985;64:745–747.
47. Dzwonczyk D, Dahl MR, Steinhauser R. A defective unidirectional dome valve was not discovered during normal testing. J Clin Eng 1991;16:485–490.
48. Moore MW, Bowe EA, Turner JF, Baysinger CL. Opened endotracheal tubes can be saved. Anesthesiology 1992;77:A1059.
49. Compressed Gas Association. Handbook of compressed gases. New York: Van Nostrand Reinhold, 1981:469–470.
50. Holley HS, Carroll JS. Anesthesia equipment malfunction. Anaesthesia 1985;40:62–65.
51. Tamse JG. Preventive maintenance of medical and dental equipment. Paper presented at the AAMI 13th annual meeting, Washington, DC, March 28–April 1, 1978.
52. Welch JP. Clinical engineering in anesthesia. Med Instrum 1985;3:109–112.
53. Emergency Care Research Institute. A Guide for Healthcare Facilities. Plymouth Meeting PA: ECRI, 1991.
54. Anonymous. The Safe Medical Devices Act of 1990—a look at the implications. Biomed Instrum Technol 1991;25:347–360.
55. Anonymous. Highlights of the Safe Medical Devices Act of 1990 (Public Law 101–629). Washington, DC: U.S. Department of Health and Human Services, Public Health Service, Food and Drug Administration Center for Devices and Radiological Health, 1991.

Chapter 19

Cleaning and Sterilization

Most anesthesia equipment is exposed to potentially infectious material during ordinary use, but the role played by anesthesia equipment in the transmission of infections remains controversial.

Definitions

Antiseptic: Any substance that has antimicrobial activity and that can be safely applied to living tissue.

Bacteria: Minute unicellular plant-like organisms. This term is usually applied to the vegetative (growing) forms.

Bacteriostat: An agent that will prevent bacterial growth but does not necessarily kill the bacteria.

Bioburden (Bioload, Microbial Load): The number and types of viable organisms with which an object is contaminated.

Biological Indicator: A sterilization-process monitoring device consisting of a standardized, viable population of microorganisms (usually bacterial spores) of high resistance to the mode of sterilization being monitored. Subsequent growth or failure of the microorganisms to grow under suitable conditions indicates whether or not conditions were adequate to achieve sterilization.

Chemical Indicator: A device, usually with a sensitive chemical or dye, employed to monitor one or more process parameters of a sterilization cycle.

Chemosterilizer (Chemical Sterilant): A chemical used for the purpose of destroying all forms of microbiological life, including bacterial spores.

Cleaning: Removal of all foreign material from objects.

Contamination: The state of actually or potentially having been in contact with microorganisms.

Decontamination: This term has a number of definitions.

1. The process by which contaminated items are rendered safe for personnel who are not wearing protective attire to han-

dle, that is, reasonably free of the probability of transmitting infection (1–5). In
some cases, the decontamination process
is also sufficient to render the items safe
for reuse in patient care.
2. The reduction of microbial contamination to some acceptable level (6,7).
3. Any process that eliminates harmful substances (8).

Decontamination includes thorough cleaning and, whenever necessary for personnel
or patient safety, appropriate application
of a microbicidal process (disinfection or
sterilization).
Disinfectant: A chemical germicide that is
formulated to be used solely on inanimate
objects.
Disinfection: The destruction of many, but
not all, microorganisms on inanimate objects. Formerly, this term was used to designate destruction of only pathogenic organisms but the terms *pathogen* and
nonpathogen are no longer relevant (9). All
microorganisms should be considered potentially pathogenic. The Centers for Disease Control and Prevention (CDC) has
adopted a classification that distinguishes
three levels of chemical disinfection (1) as
shown in Table 19.1.

1. *High-Level Disinfection.* A procedure
that kills all organisms with the exception
of bacterial spores and certain viruses,
such as the Creutzfeldt-Jakob virus (2).
High-level disinfectants are registered
with the Environmental Protection
Agency (EPA) as sterilant/disinfectants,
sporicidal hospital disinfectants, or sterilants (3). Most high-level disinfectants can
produce sterilization with sufficient contact time.
2. *Intermediate-Level Disinfection.* A procedure that kills bacteria, including *Mycobacterium tuberculosis,* some fungi,
and most viruses but not bacterial spores.
Chemical germicides that cause intermediate-level disinfection correspond to

EPA approved "hospital disinfectants"
that are also "tuberculocidal."
3. *Low-Level Disinfection.* A procedure that
kills most bacteria but not *M. tuberculosis,* some fungi, and some viruses. It does
not kill bacterial spores. These chemical
germicides are approved by the EPA as
"sanitizer hospital disinfectants."

Disposable: A device intended for single use
or single-patient use.
Fungicide: An agent that kills fungi.
Germicide: An agent that destroys microorganisms, particularly pathogenic organisms (9).
Mechanical Control (Physical) Monitors:
Sterilizer components that gauge and record time, temperature, humidity, or pressure during a sterilization cycle.
Microbicidal Process: A process designed to
provide an appropriate level of microbial
lethality (kill). Depending on the level of
decontamination needed, this process may
be sanitization, disinfection, or sterilization (1).
Microbiocide: An agent that kills all organisms.
Nosocomial: Pertaining to a hospital.
Reusable: A device intended for multiple
uses.
Sanitization: The process of reducing the
number of microbial contaminants to a
safe or relatively safe level. The term is
generally used in connection with cleaning.
Spore: The normal resting stage in the life
cycle of certain bacteria.
Sporicide: An agent that kills spores.
Sterile/sterility: The state of being free from
all living microorganisms. In practice, sterility is usually described as a probability
function (10,11).
Sterility Assurance Level: The probability of
survival of microorganisms after a terminal sterilization process and a predictor of
the efficacy of the process. For example, a
sterility assurance level of 00.0000%

Table 19.1. Levels of Disinfection[a,b]

	Bacteria				Lipid and Medium Size	Nonlipid and Small Size
Levels	Vegetative	Tubercle	Spores	Fungi		
High	+	+	+[c]	+	+	+
Intermediate	+	+	±[d]	+	+	±[e]
Low	+	−	−	±[f]	+	−

[a]From American National Standards Institute. Good hospital practice: handling and biological decontamination of reusable medical devices (ST35-1991). Arlington, VA: Association for the Advancement of Medical Instrumentation, 1991.
[b]+, a killing effect can be expected when the normal-use concentrations of chemical disinfectants or pasteurization are properly employed; −, little or no killing effect.
[c]Only with extended exposure times are high-level disinfectant chemicals capable of actual sterilization.
[d]Certain intermediate-level disinfectants can be expected to exhibit some sporicidal action.
[e]Some intermediate-level disinfectants may have limited virucidal activity.
[f]Some low-level disinfectants may have limited fungicidal activity.

means that the possibility of a nonsterile items exists, but is only 1×10^{-6} or 1 in 1,000,000.

Sterilization: Destruction of all viable forms of microorganisms. Sterilization is intended to convey an absolute, not a relative meaning (9).

Terminal Sterilization: A sterilization process that is carried out after an item has been placed in its final packaging (1).

Virucide: An agent that kills viruses. The label on a product should indicate which viruses an agent will inactivate.

Viruses: Submicroscopic, noncellular parasitic particles composed of a protein shell and a nucleic acid core.

Role of the Federal Government in Disinfection and Sterilization (5)

The primary U.S. federal government agency involved with disinfection and sterilization procedures and devices is the EPA. Chemical germicides that are formulated as sterilants and disinfectants are registered and regulated by EPA. The EPA requires manufacturers to test formulations for microbicidal efficacy, stability, and toxicity to humans. This agency also approves sterilizers. Certain chemical disinfectants are regulated by the Food and Drug Administration (FDA); occupational exposure to chemical disinfectants and sterilizers is regulated by the Occupational Safety and Health Adminstration (OSHA).

The CDC does not approve, regulate, or test chemical germicides or sterilizers. Rather, it recommends broad strategies to prevent transmission of infections in the healthcare environment (12)

Resistance of Microorganisms to Disinfection and Sterilization

Microorganisms show great variation in their resistance to sterilants and disinfectants. Bacterial spores are the most resistant. *M. tuberculosis,* nontuberculosis mycobacteria, and Gram-negative water bacteria such as *Pseudomonas aeruginosa* and *P. ccpacia* are relatively resistant (5).

Some types of viruses are more resistant than others. Viruses are separated into two classes based on their chemical structure. Lipophilic viruses have a lipid (fat) envelope surrounding the protein coat. Viruses that do not have the lipid envelope are termed naked, or hydrophilic; hydrophilic viruses are generally more resistant to inactivation. To be classified as a high-level disinfectant, a product must be tested against both lipo-philic and hydrophilic viruses and claims may be made only for the particular viruses tested.

Cleaning of Equipment

For all reusable medical devices, the first and most important step in decontamination is thorough cleaning. Cleaning means the removal of foreign matter without any special effort to kill microorganisms. It will usually reduce the bioburden but will not disinfect or sterilize.

Unless an article is clean, there may be insufficient contact between it and the decontaminating agent and sterilization will not be accomplished. Organic material (e.g., blood and protein) inactivates many germicides. Even if the material is rendered sterile, a patient may have a reaction to the residue.

The device manufacturer's instructions should be consulted to determine the appropriate cleaning agents. Presoaking with a specialized product (e.g, a protein-dissolving solution) is sometimes recommended.

Rinsing or wiping articles as soon as possible after use may prevent drying of organic material.

Cleaning procedures should be performed in a designated location that is divided into dirty and clean areas (6). Personnel should wear protective attire and be very cautious not to injure themselves with contaminated instruments.

Equipment should be disassembled and examined for worn or defective parts. The idea is to take each device apart as much as practical to expose the maximum surface area. Tape should be removed. Adhesive residue should be removed with a special solvent.

The parts should then be placed in a basin filled with water and soap or detergent and allowed to soak. This will allow water to penetrate, soften, and loosen soil. The detergent should be chosen for its surface-wetting ac-

tion rather than disinfection activity. It should be noncorrosive to rubber and plastics.

After the equipment has soaked long enough for the detergent to penetrate and loosen organic matter, it should be scrubbed thoroughly inside and out to remove all debris. Particular attention should be paid to corners and grooves in which debris may be hidden.

Cleaning may be accomplished manually, mechanically, or by a combination of manual and mechanical methods. Immersible devices should be cleaned under water to prevent aerosolization of microorganisms. Much equipment is still cleaned manually and requires the use of a stiff brush. An ordinary scrub brush used in surgery is adequate for most cleaning. Test-tube brushes can be used for the lumens of tubes and airways. Special brushes may be supplied for the lumens of instruments such as fiberscopes. Brushes and other cleaning implements should be disinfected or sterilized daily.

Use of lukewarm water/detergent solutions will prevent coagulation and assist in removal of soil. Detergents reduce the forces at the interface between water and oil. They have some bactericidal effect. They are most effective against Gram-positive bacteria. They are not effective against tubercle bacilli and many viruses. Commercial products (e.g., blends of quaternary ammonium compounds with other additives) that provide the double action of cleaning and preliminary disinfection, thereby reducing health hazards during decontamination, are available.

Items that do not lend themselves to cleaning by immersion often may be cleaned by a cloth soaked in detergent and water.

As an alternative to washing by hand, automatic machines for washing equipment are available (13–15). These go through several cycles of washing and rinsing. They may have a final drying cycle. Some also disinfect the equipment by pasteurization or a chemical germicide. The hot water or chemical disinfectant is held in a side tank and is automatically pumped into the holding tub. After the disinfection cycle, the liquid may be pumped back into the side tank for reuse. Contamination of fiberoptic bronchoscopes associated with automated cleaning and disinfecting machines has been reported (16,17).

Equipment that has joints, crevices, lumens, and other areas that are difficult to clean by other methods can be treated in an ultrasonic cleaner after gross soil has been removed. In an ultrasonic cleaner, high-frequency electrical energy is converted into mechanical energy in the form of sound waves. The waves, passing through a solvent, produce submicroscopic bubbles. These bubbles collapse on themselves, generating tiny shock waves that knock debris off surfaces. Ultrasonic cleaning is sometimes superior to scrubbing by hand, because it can remove soil in hard-to-reach areas. When grossly soiled items are placed in the ultrasonic cleaner, the water will become dirty and must be changed.

Rinsing is important to remove soil and residual detergent and keep it from resettling on the equipment. Any organic material and/or residual cleaning agents remaining on an item may inactivate chemical disinfectants or sterilants as well as protect microorganisms from destruction. Some items should be rinsed with distilled or demineralized water to remove minerals from tap water. After rinsing, each item should be inspected to ensure freedom from foreign matter.

Unless steam sterilization, pasteurization, or the Steris system is to be used, the cleaned item should be thoroughly dried. Even if an item is to undergo no further disinfection, drying is important because a humid environment may encourage the growth of Gram-negative organisms (6). If a liquid chemical agent is used to disinfect or sterilize, any water on the equipment will dilute it and make it less effective. If water droplets are left on equipment that is to be gas sterilized, ethylene oxide will dissolve in the water

and form ethylene glycol, which is both toxic and difficult to remove.

Most items may be towel dried or air dried. Air-drying cabinets and hot-air ovens are available. If an item is to undergo ethylene oxide sterilization, only unheated air should be used.

Methods of Disinfection and Sterilization

PASTEURIZATION

With pasteurization, the equipment is immersed in water at an elevated temperature (but below 100°C) for a given time period. The time and temperature recommended vary. Contact time is inversely related to temperature, i.e., for equivalent microbial kill, substantially longer exposure times may be required when the temperature is reduced. A commonly used combination is 77°C for 33 min (18).

This method is a disinfecting process but cannot be depended on for sterilization. CDC guidelines refer to pasteurization as a high-level disinfection process, although this is inconsistent with its classification system because of the inability of the procedure to reliably kill spores and viruses (6).

Pasteurization has been used for breathing tubes, reservoir bags, tracheal and endobronchial tubes, face masks, oral airways, laryngoscope blades, and ventilator bellows (4). It may produce tubing and face masks as clean as an equivalent disposable breathing system, which is not sterile either (4).

The biggest advantage of this method is that the lower temperature is less damaging to equipment than the higher temperatures employed in autoclaving. There are no toxic residues. It is simple, inexpensive, and reliable. The main disadvantage is that the treated equipment is wet and must still be dried and packaged, during which it may become recontaminated. Some materials may deform because of the heat.

AUTOCLAVING

Autoclaving (steam sterilization), which uses moist heat in the form of saturated steam under pressure, is the oldest and most commonly used method for sterilizing equipment in healthcare facilities.

Equipment to be sterilized is first cleaned and then packaged in muslin, linen, or paper. The steam easily penetrates these materials. After sterilization, the packaging material prevents recontamination during subsequent handling and storage.

The chamber is the portion of the sterilizer in which materials are processed and that is sealed off when the door is closed (19). The jacket is the portion surrounding and affixed to the chamber through which steam is circulated and that functions to maintain temperature in the chamber.

The items are placed on a shelf in the chamber, and the door is closed and secured. Before the sterilization cycle is begun, air is evacuated from the chamber. If this is not done, the quantity of steam entering the autoclave is reduced and, with this, the temperature achieved. As steam enters the chamber, it enters the load to be sterilized and gives up its latent heat. Once the intended temperature is reached, the duration of sterilization is set. At the end of this period the steam is exhausted from the autoclave to avoid condensation of water on the load when cool air is admitted.

Variables in Steam Sterilization

Steam sterilization is extremely effective because saturated steam transfers heat energy to materials very rapidly on contact and can destroy even highly resistant bacterial spores in a relatively short time. Microbial destruction will occur most effectively at locations where saturated steam can contact the microorganisms. At locations inaccessible to steam penetration (as might occur with complex medical devices, improperly packaged items or incorrect load configurations), some microbial destruction may occur as a result of dry heat, but dry heat is not as efficient at sterilizing as saturated steam.

Temperature

At sea level, water boils at 100°C. When it is boiled within a closed vessel at increased pressure, the temperature at which it boils and that of the steam it forms will exceed 100°C; the increase depends on the pressure within the chamber. This is the basic principle of the autoclave. Pressure per se has little or no sterilizing effect. It is the moist heat at a suitable temperature, as regulated by the pressure in the chamber, that brings about sterilization.

Time

The higher the temperature, the more rapidly sterilization can be accomplished. The minimum time for sterilization by steam at 121°C is 15 min (20). If the temperature is 126°C, the time is reduced to 10 min. It is 3 min at 134°C and only a few seconds at 150°C (21).

Flash sterilization refers to steam sterilization of unwrapped products. It is recommended only when time does not permit use of a wrapped product. The recommended exposure time and temperature for nonporous loads such as those containing only metal instruments is 3 min at or above 132°C (270°F) (22).

Characteristics of the Steam (11)

Less-than-optimum steam characteristics reduce the efficiency of heat transfer and jeopardize the attainment of sterility. Steam should contain no air, liquid water, or solid particles. A filter that removes liquids and solid particles should be installed in the steam line, just upstream of the autoclave.

Problems with Steam Sterilization (11)

Steam Quality

Steam quality or saturation refers to the level of moisture in steam. Liquid water may be present in the form of "fog" or water droplets. "Wet" steam may condense onto cool surfaces and impede the transfer of heat to items being sterilized. Current standards call for a steam quality greater than 97% (less than 3% liquid water). Low-quality ("wet") steam is one cause of wet packs. It may result from problems in the steam supply itself, or it may occur locally within the chamber when steam contacts a cold load.

Steam Saturation

Steam is said to be saturated when it has the proper balance of pressure and temperature. If the pressure is too great, the steam will change to rain, causing packs to become wet; if the pressure is too low, the steam will be superheated. Superheated steam is less able than saturated steam to transfer its heat energy to the cooler items being sterilized and will interfere with attainment of a uniform temperature in the chamber. Superheating may be caused by the materials being processed. Packs that are overly dry, because they have been accidentally processed twice, or that are reprocessed without laundering or other means of humidification may cause superheating by removing moisture from the steam.

Steam Supply

Variations in steam pressure may affect the temperature come-up time and temperature uniformity within the chamber. Pressure variations may come about because of clogged filters, poorly engineered piping or excessive demands on the steam supply. It is not unusual for problems to occur at the start of winter in cold climates; these problems can often be traced to a marginal steam supply that is overloaded when it is called on to supply building heat.

Air in the Autoclave Chamber (11)

The presence of air in the chamber will impair sterilization. Air is a poor conductor of heat and retards the penetration of steam (23). Temperature fluctuations within the chamber and cold spots in the load are usu-

ally signs that air has not been adequately removed. The modern autoclave evacuates much of the air before steam enters the chamber either by gravity displacement by the steam or a vacuum system. Air can leak back into the chamber through inadequately sealed valves, fittings, and door gaskets.

Equipment Malfunction (11)

Examples of equipment malfunction include out-of-calibration temperature or pressure gauges and controllers, incorrect steam supply pressure, faulty or maladjusted control valves, leaks, clogged vent lines or drain screens, faulty vacuum pumps, defective steam traps, and malfunctioning cycle sequence controllers.

Personnel Errors

Personnel errors include inadequate cleaning of equipment, incorrect pack preparation and packaging methods, and poor loading techniques. There is also the possibility that an entire load is inadvertently not processed.

Steam Sterilization Process Monitoring

There is no monitor or indicator that is able to give assurance that each item in a load is sterile. There are various devices that will give a high level of assurance. These should be used in concert to give the greatest possible confidence that individual items are sterile.

Mechanical Monitors

Mechanical monitors are devices or gauges that indicate the time, temperature, and pressure. They will detect major equipment malfunctions while the cycle is in progress. Most autoclaves provide a permanent record by means of chart recordings or computer-driven printouts.

Biological Indicators (11,24,25)

Biological indicators are standardized preparations of microorganisms resistant to a particular sterilization process. Usually for in-hospital steam sterilization, paper strips impregnated with spores or ampules of spores are used. The strips or ampules are placed in the sterilization chamber, within a special test pack or within packaged items. They are then exposed to the sterilization cycle, retrieved, incubated, and examined for microbial growth. Biological indicators are designed to equal or exceed the resistance of highly resistant, naturally occurring microorganisms on clean medical items.

The CDC recommends use of biological monitors at least once a week (12,22).

The main problem with biological indicators is that time is needed to incubate the bacteria to determine the kill rate.

Chemical Indicators (11)

A chemical indicator (chemical monitor, sterilizer control, chemical control device) is a sterilization-process monitoring device designed to respond with characteristic chemical or physical changes to one or more of the physical conditions (temperature, time, or pressure) within the sterilization chamber.

Chemical indicators are a more practical means of detecting local conditions at multiple points within the load than biological indicators. They can reveal potential problems immediately (or at least before an item is used), whereas biological indicator results are usually not available for several days.

The CDC and all major U.S. organizations that issue sterilization-related standards or guidelines advocate that a chemical indicator be attached to every package that goes through a sterilization cycle (12).

Advantages and Disadvantages

Autoclaving kills all bacteria, spores, and viruses. It allows the interior of a wrapped package to be sterilized. Advantages include speed, good penetration, economy, ease of use, absence of toxic products or residues, and reliability. The material can be prepackaged and kept sterile until used. A great advantage is that the autoclave is available in every modern operating theater. It is the least

expensive means of sterilizing items and provides the quickest turnaround time.

The principal disadvantage of autoclaving is that many pieces of equipment made from heat-sensitive materials are damaged if subjected to steam. Autoclaving can cause blunting of cutting edges, corrosion of metal surfaces, and shortening of the life of electronic components.

LIQUID CHEMICAL AGENTS

Liquid chemical agents (cold sterilization or disinfection) are especially useful for heat-sensitive equipment. Cold sterilization is usually performed by soaking an item in a basin of solution. It can also be accomplished by automated equipment called washer/disinfectors or washer/sterilizers, which typically provide a cycle of cleaning, rinsing, disinfection, rinsing, and sometimes drying. Other automated instruments, such as the Steris system, provide automatic sterilization after an object has been cleaned.

Regulation of Chemical Germicides (5)

The formulations of chemical germicides and their labeling are regulated by the EPA. By law, the labeling for chemical disinfectants must provide information relating to safe and effective use, including the required contact time, the use temperature, the reuse pattern, and the shelf life.

The EPA requires the label of a hospital disinfectant to show clearly the ability of the chemical agent to destroy *M. tuberculosis* and the time and temperature required. If the product is effective against this organism, the label will say "tuberculocidal." Similarly, if a disinfectant product is capable of destroying *P. aeruginosa,* the label will state that it is pseudomonacidal. If the product is effective against the human immunodeficiency virus (HIV), the label must so state.

Safety Considerations in Chemical Disinfection

OSHA has established limits on occupational exposure to glutaraldehyde, formaldehyde, and other chemical disinfectants and sterilants, as shown in Table 19.2. The user should consult the safety data supplied by the disinfectant manufacturer and observe recommended safety precautions. The following general measures should be considered:

1. Adequate ventilation and, if necessary, a vented hood in the disinfection area to evacuate the chemical vapors from glutaraldehyde and other products.
2. Use of lidded containers for the disinfectant solution when appropriate.
3. Appropriate protective clothing and devices for the user, such as gloves, eye protection, and masks.
4. Thorough rinsing of devices with water after disinfection.

Factors Influencing Liquid Chemical Disinfection

Concentration of the Chemical

Generally, the rate of kill of a bacterial population varies directly with the concentration of the disinfectant (26). An exception is the alcohols. Concentration will also influence the ability of a chemical agent to kill or inactivate certain microorganisms. A chemical in very low concentration may inactivate certain organisms, whereas a much higher concentration is required to inactivate others.

Although it is usually true that the stronger the solution, the more effective will be its disinfectant action, a strong solution may be more irritating to tissues and/or injurious to the item being disinfected. In such cases, weaker solutions must be used.

Water left on equipment will dilute the liquid agent and render it less effective. For this reason, most equipment should be dried after it is cleaned. Dilution can become very significant with long-term use and reuse and can potentially reduce the concentration of the chemical agent to a level too low to be effective in killing a sufficient number of certain microorganisms in the recommended exposure time.

Table 19.2. Occupational Exposure Limits for Some Chemical Sterilants and Disinfectants[a,b]

Chemical Agent	OSHA Requirements[c]
Alcohols	Varying PEL
Chlorine dioxide	0.1 ppm 8-hr TWA/0.3 ppm STEL
Ethylene oxide	1.0 ppm 8-hr/TWA 5 ppm STEL
Formaldehyde	1.0 ppm 8-hr TWA/2 ppm STEL
Glutaraldehyde	0.2 ppm 8-hr TWA
Hydrogen peroxide	1.0 ppm 8-hr TWA
Peracetic acid	No limits established
Phenol	5.0 ppm 8-hr TWA

[a]From American National Standards Institute. Good hospital practice: handling and biological decontamination of reusable medical devices (ST35-1991). Arlington, VA: Association for the Advancement of Medical Instrumentation, 1991.
[b]Standard ST35-1991 has been in effect since 1989, but until the end of 1993, compliance methods such as work practices and protective personal equipment will suffice. After this, administrative and engineering controls must have been implemented whenever feasible. A ceiling limit is the highest concentration an employee may be exposed to during any part of the workday.
[c]PEL, permissible exposure limit; *TWA,* time-weighted average; *STEL,* short-term excursion limit (TWA for 15 min).

Temperature

Although these agents are designed to be used at room temperature, increasing the temperature usually increases their effectiveness (27). The product label will usually tell what temperature should be used. If the temperature of the solution is at any time lower than the temperature indicated on the product label, then complete disinfection may not be achieved during the prescribed time period. On the other hand, the temperature should not be high enough that the active ingredients evaporate appreciably.

Evaporation and Light Deactivation

If the solution is in an uncovered container, evaporation can occur. Generally, evaporation is not as critical as dilution. However, if the chemical agent is more volatile than the diluent, then loss of the agent by evaporation can be very important. Chlorine products are especially susceptible to

Table 19.3. Capabilities of Disinfecting Agents[a,b]

Disinfectant	Gram-Positive Bacteria	Gram-Negative Bacteria	Tubercle Bacillus	Spores	Viruses	Fungi
Quats	+	±	0	0	±	±
Alcohols	+	+	+	0	±	±
Glutaraldehydes	+	+	+	±	+	+
Hydrogen peroxide–based compounds	+	+	+	±	+	+
Formaldehyde need other agents	+	+	+	−	+	+
Phenolic compounds	+	+	±	0	±	±
Chlorine	+	+	+	−	+	+

[a]From Chatburn RL. Decontamination of respiratory care equipment: what can be done, what should be done. Respir Care 1989;34:98; and Berry AJ. Infection control in anesthesia. Anesth Clin North Am 1989;7:967–981.
[b]+, good; ±, fair; 0, litte or none.

evaporation. Exposure to light may adversely affect chlorine disinfectants.

pH

Disinfectants may be formulated over a range of pH values, depending on the chemical agent used. Some agents are more effective in killing microorganisms under alkaline conditions while others work best with acidic conditions. The presence of detergents in the disinfectant solution, which may occur if the device is inadequately rinsed after cleaning, can alter the pH of the solution and reduce its effectiveness.

Bioburden

The success of the disinfectant depends on the cleanliness of the items to be processed. Soiled equipment will require longer exposure and/or a stronger concentration for adequate disinfection to be achieved.

Liquid agents vary widely in their effectiveness against various types of microorganisms. Table 19.3 shows the capabilities of some commonly used disinfectant agents.

Characteristics of the Item to Be Disinfected

A disinfectant solution is only effective if it can contact all surfaces of the item to be disinfected. Uneven or porous surfaces resist chemical disinfection. Deeply situated resident flora are not affected by disinfectants applied to the surface (26). Air entrapment prevents contact between the liquid and bubble-covered regions.

Use Pattern and Use Life

The product label must be examined for information on the use pattern, use life, and storage life of the product. It is important to distinguish between the use life of a disinfectant and its use pattern. The use life commonly applies, but is not limited, to disinfectant products that require the mixing of two ingredients for activation. Once a disinfectant solution is mixed, there may be a limited period of time during which the activated solution may be used. That time is its use life. The use pattern refers to how many times the solution can be used. It is event related, not time related. The storage life is the time period after which the unused and/or unactivated product is no longer deemed effective.

Time

The time required for the different chemical agents to function effectively varies from seconds to hours and will depend on the factors just mentioned. Some microorganisms are killed faster than others. It is essential that the minimum time of exposure to a specific chemical solution be observed.

Sterilization Monitors

Test methods are available to determine the efficacy of sterilizing chemical agents. These tests employ standardized carriers onto which the test organism is deposited. The innoculated carrier is then exposed to the sterilizing agent under the conditions recommended for its routine use (exposure time, concentration, temperature, etc.).

Following exposure, the carrier is placed in a growth media and incubated. Growth in the media indicates that the sterilization process failed to destroy the test organisms. No growth indicates that the sterilization process was effective.

Agents (2)

Formaldehyde

Formaldehyde is used as a disinfectant principally in a water-based solution called formalin, which is 37% formaldehyde by weight. The aqueous solution is a bacteriocide, tuberculocide, fungacide, virucide, and sporicide. It is noncorrosive and is not inactivated by organic matter (28).

Although formaldehyde-alcohol is a chemosterilizer and formaldehyde is a high-level disinfectant, its hospital uses are limited by its pungent odor and fumes, which irritate the skin, eyes, and respiratory tract at very low levels (less than 1 ppm) (9). The National Institute for Occupational Safety and Health (NIOSH) has indicated that formaldehyde should be handled as a potential carcinogen and has set an 8-hr time-weighted average employee exposure limit of 1 ppm.

Quaternary Ammonium Compounds (2,6)

Quaternary ammonium compounds, or quats, are a special class of synthetic detergents that possess the useful property of lowering the surface tension of the solution.

Quaternary ammonium compounds are considered low-level disinfectants (28). They are bactericidal, fungal, and viricidal at room temperature within 10 min, but have not demonstrated sporicidal effects. If a spore is coated with a quaternary ammonium compound, it will not develop into a vegetative cell as long as the coating of the germicide remains, but if the coating is removed, the cell can germinate (29,30). These compounds are more effective against Gram-positive than Gram-negative bacteria. They are only marginally effective against *P. aeruginosa*. Quats inactivate HIV but not the hepatitis virus (2).

Quaternary ammonium compounds have enjoyed wide usage as disinfectants and until recently as antiseptics. Since they were introduced in 1935 they have undergone several changes in formulation (2). Early generation quats were affected by factors such as hard water, soap, and anionic residues and proteinaceous soils and were inactivated by organic materials (e.g. cork, cotton, and gauze pads). There were reports of nosocomial infections associated with contaminated quaternary ammonium compounds. The newest generation quaternary ammonium surfactant mixed with a noninionic emulsifier and readily available hydroxyl groups combine to produce synergistic antimicrobial and detergency activities greater than that of the individual components while maintaining the hard water, protein, and anionic tolerance necessary in environmental disinfectants (2,6).

The quats are recommended for use in ordinary environmental sanitization of noncritical surfaces such as floors, furniture, and walls (2). Because they are quick acting, relatively nontoxic and noncaustic, and do not produce noxious fumes, they are useful for initial cleaning procedures (6).

In 1985, the CDC modified its recommendation for cleaning blood or body fluid spills to include cleaning with a detergent followed by decontamination with the use of an EPA-approved hospital disinfectant that is tuberculocidal, which excludes most quaternary ammonium compounds.

Reported problems include an allergic reaction of the tracheal mucosa after use of a quaternary ammonium compound to clean a tracheostomy tube (31) and contact dermatitis (32).

Phenolic Compounds (2,6)

Phenolic compounds (phenols) are a group of compounds derived from carbolic acid (phenol), one of the oldest germicides. They are good bactericides and are active against fungi. They are sometimes viricidal but are not sporicidal except at or above 100°C. They are active in the presence of organic matter and soap (33). They are sometimes combined with detergents to form detergent germicides. Phenolic compounds are very stable. Application of moisture to a surface previously treated with a phenolic compound can redissolve the chemical so that it again becomes bactericidal.

Most phenolic compounds have a bad odor and are irritating to skin (29,34). They are absorbed by rubber and may damage skin or mucous membranes they contact. Phenolics are assimilated by porous materials and the residual disinfectant may cause tissue irritation (2).

Phenolics are considered low-level disinfectants (29) They are not recommended for semicritical items because of the lack of published efficacy data for many of the available formulations and because the residual disinfectant on porous materials may cause tissue irritation even after thorough rinsing (2). They are used mainly on floors and furniture (29) but may be useful on anesthesia equipment such as machines, monitors, carts, and cylinders that do not contact the patient. They have been used for reservoir bags but are absorbed by rubber and may irritate the anesthesiologist's hand. Facial burns may result from their use on masks (35). Depigmentation has been reported (36).

Alcohol (Ethyl or Isopropyl)

Ethyl and isopropyl alcohol are relatively inexpensive disinfectants that are sometimes combined with another agent to enhance the action of the other agent. This is known as a tincture.

Ethyl alcohol is bactericidal in 60% to 90% concentrations (70% is best) and isopropyl alcohol in 60% or greater concentration (90% is best). Both kill most bacteria, including *M. tuberculosis* during an exposure of 1 to 5 min (33,37). They do not kill spores. Their action against viruses is variable, with ethyl alcohol superior to isopropyl alcohol (9). The CDC recommends exposure to 70% ethanol for 15 min to inactivate the hepatitis virus, but 1 min should be adequate for HIV (38). Neither alcohol will inactivate the Creutzfeldt-Jakob virus (39).

Isopropyl and ethyl alcohol have been excluded as high-level disinfectants because of their inability to inactivate bacterial spores and some viruses. They evaporate rapidly, thus making extended contact time difficult to achieve unless the items are immersed.

Alcohols have a cleansing action. They are inactivated by protein, but not by soap (2,28). They are quite volatile. It is not necessary to rinse items soaked in alcohol because it evaporates rapidly.

Alcohols have been used to disinfect fiberoptic endoscopes (40,41) and reusable pressure transducer heads (42,43). However, infections associated with this equipment in an intensive care environment has been reported (44). They are sometimes used to disinfect external surfaces of equipment (e.g., stethoscopes and ventilators) (2). They may be substituted for water as a final rinse when water contamination is a problem (16).

Alcohols can damage the shellac mounting of lensed instruments and tend to swell and harden rubber and certain plastics after prolonged and repeated use (9,45).

Alcohols are flammable so care must be taken not to use them in the presence of open flame or electrical sparks that could ignite the vapor.

Iodophors

An iodophor is a combination of iodine and a solubilizing agent or carrier with the resulting complex providing a sustained-release reservoir of iodine and releasing a small amount of free iodine in aqueous solution. They are bactericidal, virucidal, and tuberculocidal but may require prolonged contact time to kill certain fungi and bacterial spores.

Iodophors are used principally as antiseptics but are capable of intermediate-level and low-level disinfection (9). Iodophors formulated as antiseptics contain significantly less free iodine than those formulated as disinfectants (46).

Peracetic (Peroxyacetic) Acid

Peracetic acid is acetic acid plus an extra oxygen atom. It is bactericidal, sporicidal, fungicidal, and virucidal (47). It remains effective in the presence of organic material.

One problem is that it is corrosive and irritating to skin in a concentrated solution.

Peracetic acid is the active ingredient in the Steris sterilant. This is a single-use concentrate of 35% peracetic acid plus corrosion and degradation inhibitors, which are contained in a sealed single-use container. The concentrate is automatically diluted with sterile water to a final concentration of 0.2% peracetic acid with a pH of about 6.4 before exposure to the instruments to be processed. The concentrate should be used only in the Steris processing system. It is not intended for manual open-pan techniques.

The Steris system is shown in Figure 19.1. Equipment to be sterilized, which must be clean but need not be dry, is placed in a spe-

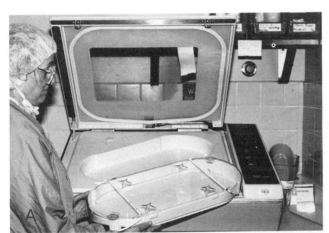

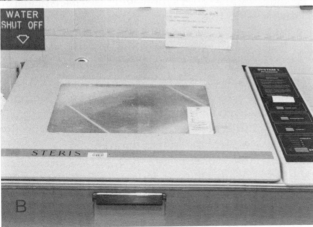

Figure 19.1. The Steris system **A,** Items to be sterilized are cleaned, then placed in a tray. The tray is then placed in the sterilizer. **B,** After the lid is closed and the processing cycle started, the processor automatically opens the sterilant concentrate and mixes it with filtered water. The use dilution of the sterilant enters the tray, covering the instruments, and is circulated for 12 min. It is then drained from the chamber, and the chamber and tray are rinsed four times with sterile water. Next, sterile air is pumped into the chamber to displace the rinse water. A printout confirming that the sterilization parameters were met is provided.

cial tray, which is then placed in the automated tabletop processor.

Each tray has holes in the bottom for fluid entry and drainage. Two different types of trays are available: a flexible one for endoscopes and a lidded (general-purpose) one for items requiring protection from environmental contamination during transportation to the sterile field following processing. The trays are designed to enable the operator to fix instruments so that there is a continuous flow of sterilant on exposed surfaces. Endoscopes with internal channels are connected so that the sterilant flows through the channels.

After the tray is positioned in the sterilizer, a package of sterilant concentrate is placed in the sterilizer. The lid is closed, and the processing cycle is started. During the cycle, the lid is sealed so that there is no exposure of personnel to the sterilant. The processor automatically opens the sterilant concentrate and mixes it with a controlled volume of filtered sterile water heated to 50° to 55°C (122° to 132°F). The use dilution of the sterilant enters the tray, covering the instruments, and is circulated for 12 min. It is then drained from the chamber and the chamber and tray are filled with sterile water. The instruments and chamber are rinsed four times with sterile water, then sterile air is pumped into the chamber to displace the rinse water. The cycle may take from 20 to 30 min, depending on the initial temperature of the water and how extensively the local water supply must be filtered. After the cycle is complete, the unit flushes the diluted sterilant and rinse water directly into a drain.

The processor is an automated microcomputer-controlled device that monitors and maintains the parameters necessary to ensure sterile processing. It will stop the cycle if a process error is detected. At the end of each cycle, a printout confirming that the sterilization parameters were met is provided for quality assurance records.

This system provides a quick method for sterilizing a wide variety of heat-sensitive immersible instruments, including some fiberscopes. It is less damaging to delicate instruments than steam sterilization and is compatible with a wide variety of materials—including plastics, rubber, and most heat-sensitive items.

It is useful for items requiring a quick turnaround time. It is faster than sterilization with ethylene oxide or glutaraldehyde and can be used on wet or dry items. No dilution of the sterilant by personnel is necessary, and the rinse is automatic so personnel are not exposed to any toxic chemicals.

This system does have some disadvantages. Only items that can be totally immersed can be sterilized. Only one scope or a small number of instruments can be processed in a cycle. The use of instruments sterilized in this system should be consistent with "just-in-time" processing and delivery. The processor and trays cannot be used as extended storage devices.

Chlorine and Chlorine Products

Hypochlorites are the most widely used of the chloride disinfectants. They are available in a liquid (e.g., sodium hypochlorite) or solid (e.g., calcium hypochlorite) form. They are inexpensive and fast acting. Alternative compounds that release chlorine and are used in the hospital setting include demand-release chlorine dioxide and chloramine-T (2). These compounds retain chlorine longer and so exert a more prolonged bactericidal effect than the hypochlorites.

These agents are active against all bacteria and viruses but not bacterial spores. Their disinfecting efficacy decreases with an increase in pH.

Household bleach contains 5.25% sodium hypochlorite or 52,500 ppm available chlorine. A 1:100 to 1:1000 dilution is effective against the human immunodeficiency virus (48,49). A 1:5 to 1:10 dilution is an excellent disinfectant for destroying the hepatitis virus (4) and will inactivate the virus of Creutzfeldt-Jakob disease with an exposure time of 1 hr (39,50,51).

Hypochlorite solutions in tap water at pH greater than 8.0 are stable for a period of 1 month when stored at room temperature in closed plastic containers (52,53), but the free available chlorine levels are reduced to 40% to 50% of the original concentration (2).

Inorganic chlorine solutions are useful for spot disinfection of countertops and floors. A 1:10 dilution of 5.25% sodium hypochlorite has been recommended by the CDC for cleaning blood spills (9).

Their use in hospitals is limited by their corrosiveness, inactivation by organic matter and relative instability (2,28). They may leave a residue and are irritating to skin, eyes, and the respiratory tract. A potential hazard is the production of the carcinogen bis-chloromethyl ether when hypochlorite solutions come into contact with formaldehyde and the production of the carcinogen trihalomethane during the hyperchlorination of hot water. A mixture of sodium hypochlorite with acid will affect a rapid evolution of toxic chlorine gas (9).

Hydrogen Peroxide (2,6)

Hydrogen peroxide is an effective bacteriocide, fungicide, virucide, and sporicide (54–57). Synergistic sporicidal effects have been observed with a combination of hydrogen peroxide and peracetic acid (58).

It is commercially available in a 3% solution but can be used in up to a 25% concentration (2,28). It is noncorrosive and is not inactivated by organic matter but is an irritant to the skin and eyes (28). It is said to be safe for use with rubber, plastic, and stainless steel.

Glutaraldehyde (Pentanedial)

Glutaraldehyde is a saturated dialdehyde that is available in alkaline, acid, and neutral formulations. Neutral or alkaline glutaraldehydes possess superior microbiocidal and anticorrosion properties compared with acid glutaraldehydes (9). Novel glutaraldehyde formulations (e.g., glutaraldehyde-phenate, potentiated acid glutaraldehyde, and stabilized alkaline glutaraldehyde) that overcome the problem of rapid loss of stability while generally maintaining excellent microbiocidal activity have been produced (2,9,59,60).

The use of glutaraldehyde-based solutions in hospitals is widespread because of their advantages, which include excellent biocidal properties; activity in the presence of organic matter; noncorrosive action to endoscopic equipment, rubber, or plastic equipment; and noncoagulation of proteinaceous material.

Dilution of glutaraldehyde commonly occurs during use, and it is important to ensure that semicritical equipment is disinfected with an acceptable concentration: 1.0% glutaraldehyde is the minimum effective concentration when used as a high-level disinfectant (61,62). Thorough rinsing of all exposed materials is mandatory, because residual glutaraldehyde is irritating to tissues.

Healthcare workers can be exposed to elevated levels of glutaraldehyde vapor when equipment is processed in poorly ventilated rooms, when spills occur, or when there are open immersion baths. OSHA has established a ceiling limit of 0.2 ppm time-weighted average for an 8-hr workday (63). After January 1, 1994, OSHA plans to toughen its requirements for meeting this limit. It may be difficult to keep the glutaraldehyde exposure below the legal limit in some departments.

Alkaline (Activated) Glutaraldehyde (2,6). Alkaline glutaraldehyde is marketed as a mildly acidic solution that is activated with a bicarbonate buffer, yielding a solution with a pH of 7.5 to 8.5. It may contain a rust inhibitor (64).

It is fungicidal and viricidal in 10 min and deals effectively with most bacteria (except tubercle bacilli) in less than 2 min (2,6,33,65–76). At least 20 min are required to inactivate tubercle bacilli (2,38,77). A minimum of 10 hr may be required to kill spores.

It is noncorrosive to metal with short exposure times, is not harmful to rubber or plastics, and can be used on rigid and flexible endoscopes (6). It is not inactivated by organic matter (28) Alkaline glutaraldehyde should not be heated.

Disinfection can be carried out in a special automatic machine, which is a device with several cycles that perform both cleansing with a detergent and cold disinfection with glutaraldehyde (13,14,78). The glutaraldehyde is held in a side tank and is automatically pumped into the tub. Upon completion of the disinfection cycle, the solution is returned to the side tank for reuse during later cycles.

Thorough rinsing of equipment is mandatory to prevent irritation to tissues. Glutaraldehyde solution causes corrosion of rubber and etching of plastic (79). Pseudomembranous laryngitis has been linked to disinfection of tracheal tubes with glutaraldehyde (80). Sticking of APL valves may occur (81).

Alkaline glutaraldehyde is irritating to the eyes and nasal passages (9). Contact dermatitis has also been reported (83). Gloves, eye protection, and a fume hood are recommended to protect sensitive individuals or to prevent sensitization.

Stick indicators are available to determine the concentration and dilution of glutaraldehyde solutions. The pad of the indicator is immersed in the solution and immediately withdrawn. After 3 min, the color is observed. Bright yellow indicates maximum potency. Faint yellow indicates minimum effectiveness. No color change indicates that the solution should be discarded.

Acid Glutaraldehyde (2,6,83). Acid glutaraldehyde is used as a 2% solution and a pH of 2.7 to 3.7. At room temperature it will kill most bacteria (except tubercle bacilli), viruses, and fungi in 10 min. It is not sporicidal at this temperature. Its microbiocidal activity is increased at higher temperatures, up to 100°C. At 60°C (140°F) it is bactericidal, virucidal, and fungicidal in 5 min; tuberculocidal in 20 min; and sporicidal in 60 min (6).

Acid glutaraldehyde has wetting and penetrating properties. It does not coagulate blood. Although it will not harm rubber, plastic, steel, or lensed instruments, it is not recommended for plated metal instruments.

It can be used in open containers, automatic washing/disinfecting machines, and ultrasonic cleaners. If processing is carried out at elevated temperatures, a closed container should be employed to reduce evaporation.

It does not stain or irritate the hands or irritate the eyes or nostrils. It is not necessary to wear gloves when using it.

Neutral Glutaraldehyde. Neutral glutaraldehyde solution has a pH from 7.0 to 7.5. It is used in a 2% solution but is effective down to 0.2%. It requires activation and has a useful life of 28 days. It kills bacteria (including tubercle bacilli), fungi, and some viruses within 10 min and spores in 10 hr.

A surfactant may be added to lower surface tension and give slight detergency. Special corrosion inhibitors to make it safe for steel and delicate lensed instruments may be added. It can be used on rigid and flexible endoscopes. Gloves should be worn when using it.

Advantages and Disadvantages

Advantages of liquid chemical disinfection include economy, speed, and simplicity. It cannot be used for all types of equipment. Many devices cannot be soaked because their design prevents solution contact or because the aqueous solution would damage electrical circuitry and/or corrode metal components. Prepackaging is not possible and the equipment will be wet. Thus there is an opportunity for recontamination during subsequent rinsing, drying, or wrapping. With most agents, sterility cannot be guaranteed. Finally, some solutions are irritating to tissues and have unpleasant odors.

GAS STERILIZATION

Ethylene oxide (EtO or EO) is a colorless, poisonous gas with a sweet odor that is widely used to sterilize equipment. It is especially useful for heat- and moisture-sensitive materials such as rubber and plastic. As a gas, EO penetrates into crevices and through permeable bags. Items can be packaged before sterilization and stored sterile for extended periods of time.

Ethylene oxide kills bacteria, spores, fungi, and viruses. Because EO sterilization is a more complex and expensive process than steam sterilization, it is usually restricted to objects that might be damaged by heat or excessive moisture.

Ethylene oxide is available commercially in high-pressure tanks and unit-dose ampules and cartridges. It is flammable and explosive in concentrations of 3% or greater in air. Manufacturers have dealt with the fire and explosion hazard in two ways. Some dilute the EO with carbon dioxide or a fluorocarbon. Mixtures containing up to 12% EO in these inert diluents are nonflammable, but retain their sterilizing capacity. Ready-made mixtures are available commercially as compressed gases in cylinders. Other manufacturers use 100% EO, but design equipment specially for gas containment and to minimize the risk of explosion.

Limitations on the use of chlorofluorocarbons may impact ethylene oxide use (84). Fluorocarbons have been implicated in the depletion of the earth's ozone layer. A ban on these substances will impact the use of ethylene oxide. It is anticipated that a new, more environmentally acceptable fluorocarbon mixture will be available to allow continued use of ethylene oxide and fluorocarbon mixtures (4).

A number of standards have been approved for the use of EO sterilization for use in healthcare facilities (85–90).

Preparation for Ethylene Oxide Sterilization

It is important to verify that the product is suitable for sterilization by EO. The manufacturer's instructions for each device should be consulted. Some devices may need to be sterilized at a lower temperature.

Before packaging, items must be disassembled, cleaned, and dried. Disassembly is important because all barriers to the gas's free movement must be removed to allow it to penetrate throughout the whole product. Caps, plugs, valves, and/or stylets must be removed. Hollow-bore products such as needles and tubes must be open at both ends and inspected to ensure an unobstructed lumen.

Items for gas sterilization must be free of water droplets. They should be allowed to dry in ambient air or towel dried. The use of heated forced air should be avoided, because ethylene oxide sterilization depends on the presence of adequate (but not excessive) moisture. The small amount of humidity will not produce significant amounts of ethylene glycol (91). It is advisable to maintain a relative humidity range of 35% to 70% and a temperature range of 18° to 22°C (64° to 72°F) throughout the processing and storage facility (85,88).

Items to be sterilized are placed in wire baskets, metal sterilizer carts, or other carriers that do not absorb EO. The sterilizer manufacturer's instructions for loading should be carefully followed. Items should be loaded loosely to allow penetration of gas throughout the load. Items should be loaded in such a fashion that packages will not contact the operator's hands when the baskets are transferred from the sterilizer to the aerator.

Sterilization

Factors Affecting Ethylene Oxide Sterilization

Concentration of the Gas (92). The solubility of ethylene oxide in the product and the gas diffusion rate through the product will influence the sterilant concentration. The operating pressure of the EO cycle will greatly influence the gas diffusion rate. Packaging can also be a crucial influence.

Temperature. Exposure time can be decreased by increasing the temperature. Operating temperatures in automatic sterilizers are usually preset during manufacturing. Some sterilizer models provide a selection of temperatures, generally 120° to 145°F (49° to 63°C) for a warm cycle and 85° to 100°F (29° to 38°C) for a cold cycle. Some conduct sterilization at room temperature. This is equally efficacious if other factors (exposure time and concentration) are adjusted.

Humidity. Moisture hydrates microbes, making them more susceptible to destruction by EO. Articles and wrappings should be protected from excessive drying before sterilization by storage in an atmosphere of at least 35% relative humidity.

In most automatic sterilizers, humidity is injected into the sterilizer before the ethylene oxide is admitted, or a wet gauze or sponge may be placed in the sterilizer.

Protective Barriers. Blood and other proteinaceous materials can act as barriers to ethylene oxide. Therefore, equipment must be thoroughly cleansed and rinsed before sterilization.

Packaging. The type of wrapping used is very important. It must be permeable to ethylene oxide gas and water vapor and allow for proper aeration. In sterilizers that have a vacuum cycle, the material must allow the air inside the packages to escape. Lists of packagings that are appropriate for EO sterilization are available. (88)

Exposure Time. The time needed for sterilization will depend on the factors mentioned above. In automatic sterilizers, the time generally ranges from 1.5 to 6 hr. Up to 12 hr may be required.

Sterilizers (85)

EO sterilizers are of two types (87): general purpose and special purpose. A general-purpose sterilizer is defined as a chamber-type sterilization system that injects water vapor for humidity adjustment during the cycle and generally uses excursions in pressure from atmospheric levels. A special-purpose EO sterilizer is one that requires prehumidification of items to be sterilized, does not inject water vapor during the cycle, generally

operates at atmospheric pressure, and may or may not have limitations placed by the manufacturers on the items that can be processed.

Manufacturers of general-purpose ethylene oxide sterilizers have developed sophisticated units to ensure that the process is reliable and safe. After the sterilizer chamber is tightly sealed and the controls set, a typical sterilization cycle includes the following phases: (*i*) warming the chamber; (*ii*) evacuating air; (*iii*) introducing moisture and maintenance for a "dwell" period to ensure that the water vapor penetrates the wrappings and materials to be sterilized; (*iv*) introducing the ethylene oxide; (*v*) raising the chamber pressure (in some sterilizers); (*vi*) raising the temperature (if required); (*vii*) exposing for the time required; (*viii*) releasing the pressure in the chamber; and (*ix*) removing the ethylene oxide mixture under vacuum. This is called a purge cycle or phase; some sterilizers are provided with several successive purge phases. Sterilizers without purge cycles can release a cloud of EO gas when the sterilizer door is opened. This necessitates an extraction hood above the sterilizer door with a dedicated exhaust system and potentially exposes the operator to EO gas (4) The last phase is (*x*) reestablishing atmospheric pressure by introduction of filtered air into the chamber.

In most automatic sterilizers, a source of EO gas is provided (by attachment of a cylinder of an EO mixture or insertion of a unit dose cartridge of 100% EO) and then a sterilization cycle is selected and begun. At this point, the sterilizer proceeds to completion, following the above phases, without further operator attention, unless one of its safety features indicates a malfunction or error.

Units that carry out sterilization at room temperature and ambient humidity are available (93). Some have a dedicated exhaust system. Special ventilation cabinets are available for exhausting the EO from these units to atmosphere (94). One type of special-purpose sterilizer provides a single-use ampule of ethylene oxide sealed inside a small gas-release bag. When the ampule is broken, the liquid vaporizes and diffuses out of the gas-release bag into a larger bag into which the materials to be sterilized have been placed. These two bags act as a diffusing chamber and allow the gas to remain long enough for sterilization to be accomplished. A rigid container acts as an open flame and spark shield.

Another type of EO sterilizer that carries out sterilization at room temperature and ambient humidity uses a hermetically sealed plastic pouch that acts both as a protective package and as a gas diffusion membrane. The sterilizer evacuates air from each pouch before the introduction of EO, and injects precisely the amount of gas necessary to sterilize the items. The machine then applies a heat seal, sealing the sterilant within and preventing air from reentering the package (93).

Indicators (95)

Because of the many variables that affect ethylene oxide sterilization, it advisable to have evidence that sterilization is being achieved. Three types of indicators (monitors) are available. For maximum value, they should be used in combination.

Physical Monitors

Physical (mechanical control) monitors include all sterilizer components that measure exposure time, temperature, humidity, and/or pressure during each cycle. They should be examined for proper functioning at the beginning, middle, and end of each cycle.

Chemical Indicators (12)

Chemical indicators change color when certain conditions necessary for sterilization have been met. Color change varies with the product. They are available as tapes, strips, cards, and sheets. They may be implanted or attached to packaging material or enclosed in packages. There are two types of chemical indicators currently available: those that mon-

itor the combination of gas plus moisture and those that monitor heat plus moisture.

Chemical indicators are not sterility indicators and should not replace biological monitors. They only indicate that the package has been subjected to some parameters of the sterilization cycle. Chemical indicators may change color under conditions inadequate for sterilization.

It is recommended that a chemical indicator be used with each package that undergoes ethylene oxide sterilization to prevent sterilized packages from being mixed with nonsterilized items and to detect some failures of sterilization. The user of an ethylene oxide-sterilized item should always check the chemical indicator for color change before the equipment is used.

Biological Indicators (87)

A biological indicator is a calibration of microorganisms (of high resistance to the mode of sterilization being monitored) on or in a carrier, put up in a package that maintains the integrity of the inoculated carrier (which is convenient to the ultimate user), and serves to demonstrate whether sterilization conditions were met (87).

The CDC recommends their use at least once a week (12). They should always be used after installation of a sterilizer and after any repairs or modifications to the sterilizer. They should also be used any time there are changes in packaging procedures or materials and any time major changes are made in the composition of the load (87).

To achieve a high degree of certainty that a sterilizer is functioning properly, and to detect problems in techniques, biological indicators should be placed in the most inaccessible location in the sterilized load (87). They provide assurance that each package has been subjected to proper sterilizing conditions. It should be noted that if the articles to be sterilized have not been properly cleaned before packaging, a biological indicator will not be a valid tool for determining sterility.

At least one biological indicator from the

lot used for testing should be left unexposed to the sterilant, incubated, and treated as a positive control (87).

Aeration

Ethylene oxide not only comes in contact with all surfaces of articles being sterilized but also penetrates some items, which then retain varying amounts. These items need special treatment called aeration (degassing, desorption) to remove enough residual ethylene oxide that a level safe for both personnel and patient use is achieved. Aeration may be done passively in air (ambient aeration) or actively in a mechanical aerator.

Ambient Aeration

Ambient aeration is highly variable because of the lack of control of temperature and air flow. It results in a slower reduction of residual ethylene oxide than mechanical aeration. It is possible that some of the toxicity problems encountered in the early hospital use of ethylene oxide resulted from failure to recognize this.

Items that require 8 to 12 hr of mechanical aeration may require 7 days of ambient aeration (96,97). Some items take 5 to 6 weeks. Thus the hospital must maintain a large and often costly inventory of items. The temperature in the aeration area should be at least 18°C (88).

Ambient aeration may also result in hazardous exposure of workers to ethylene oxide. If ambient aeration is unavoidable (for heat-sensitive items that cannot withstand the elevated temperatures of conventional aerator cabinets or when a closed vented cabinet especially designed for that purpose is not available), measures to minimize traffic in the aeration area and to ensure that personnel who must enter the area are not exposed to ethylene oxide at hazardous concentrations should be taken.

Mechanical Aeration

In mechanical aerators, a stream of filtered air is directed over the sterilized items. This reduces the necessary aeration time.

Factors Affecting Aeration

Composition, Thickness, Configuration, and Weight of the Device and Its Wrapping Material. The amount of residual EO and the length of time needed for it to dissipate depend on the type of material being sterilized. Unwrapped nonporous metal and glass items do not absorb ethylene oxide and require little or no aeration. Plastics, rubber, cloth, paper, and muslin may absorb significant quantities. Items that consist of a combination of absorbent and nonabsorbent materials (e.g., a metal item with rubber parts) must be treated as though they were made entirely of absorbent material. Metal and glass items that are wrapped in EO-absorbent material must be aerated.

The most common material retaining large amounts of EO is polyvinyl chloride. The type and amount of plasticizer in the polyvinyl chloride will strongly influence the amount absorbed. Rubber absorbs less, and polyethylene and nylon still less. Teflon absorbs very little ethylene oxide. When the composition of a device is in doubt, it should be treated as if it were polyvinyl chloride.

Thicker objects require longer aeration time than thin ones because they have a smaller ratio of surface area to volume, which reduces the rate of gas diffusion.

Size and Arrangement of Packages in the Aerator (91). Arranging items loosely in the aerator will allow easier diffusion.

Diluent. Gas mixtures with a fluorocarbon require a longer aeration time than those diluted with carbon dioxide.

Wrappings. The packaging material should allow the easy transfer of gas. Most wrappings freely allow the transfer of ethylene oxide and thus do not present any problem of gas retention.

Temperature at Which Aeration Occurs. Increasing the temperature greatly accelerates the removal of ethylene oxide from items. The usual aeration temperature is 50° or 60°C. If these temperatures would be damaging to a device aeration can be carried out at room temperature in a closed ventilated cabinet especially designed for that purpose or ambient aeration can be used.

Air Flow. Aeration is affected by the rate of air exchange and the air flow pattern.

Characteristics of Sterilization System Used. Use of sterilizers that subject materials to hot gases under elevated pressure can result in higher levels of ethylene oxide in the items sterilized (98).

Intended Use of the Device. Whether the item is to be external to the body, within a body cavity, intravascular, or implanted will affect the acceptable level of residual ethylene oxide.

Time. Because of the many aeration process variables, it is not practical to recommend specific minimum aeration times. Many device manufacturers provide specific aeration recommendations for their devices.

The minimum recommended times for devices that are difficult to aerate are 8 hr at 60°C (140°F), 12 hr at 50°C (120°F), and 7 days at room temperature (21°C) (70°F) (90). When in doubt about aeration requirements for a particular device, these recommendations may be followed as a general rule. It should be noted, however, that some items may require even longer periods.

Complications of Ethylene Oxide Sterilization

Patient Complications

Complications of ethylene oxide sterilization stemming from failure to eliminate residual gas from sterilized items include skin reactions and laryngotracheal inflammation (99–102). When blood is exposed to ethylene oxide–treated materials, destruction of the red cells can occur (103–105). Sensitization and anaphylaxis from exposure to products sterilized with ethylene oxide have been reported (106). The risk of patients developing cancer or suffering other adverse health effects from exposure to ethylene oxide residue left on EO-sterilized medical equipment is negligible (107).

These problems are caused by excessive levels of ethylene oxide or its byproducts, ethylene glycol, and ethylene chlorhydrin, which are left after sterilization. Ethylene glycol is formed by the reaction of ethylene oxide and water. Because even dry materials contain some moisture, some glycol formation is unavoidable. Traces of glycols are generally regarded as relatively harmless and permissible for human exposure (108). Removing all visible water droplets from equipment before sterilization should prevent formation of excessive glycol.

Ethylene chlorhydrin is formed when ethylene oxide comes into contact with chloride ions such as may be present in previously γ-irradiated PVC items. The American National Standards Institute at one time recommended that PVC items that have been γ-irradiated never be resterilized with ethylene oxide (97). Doubt has been cast on this, however, by some workers who have found very low levels of byproducts in γ-irradiated products treated with ethylene oxide (109–111). In the light of this information, resterilization of γ-irradiated PVC tubes is acceptable if strict attention is paid to aeration.

Alterations in Equipment

Repeated exposure of some plastics to ethylene oxide and heat may leach out plasticizers and weaken the structural integrity (112). Rubber and some plastic tracheal tubes may soften and kink more easily (64) or become sticky. Blisters between layers in the walls of latex tracheal tubes with embedded spiral wires can occur, resulting in narrowing of the lumen (64). It is recommended that these tubes not be sterilized by this method (113). Detachment of the balloon of a disposable esophageal stethoscope sterilized with ethylene oxide has been reported (112).

Personnel Complications

Possible Hazards of Exposure to Ethylene Oxide (88). Scientific studies suggest that acute and chronic exposure to ethylene oxide carries increased risks to the health of exposed personnel.

Exposure to liquid EO can cause burns or severe irritation of the skin (114,115). Frost-bite-like symptoms can occur if contact is prolonged.

Acute exposure to significant levels of ethylene oxide gas commonly provokes an irritant response (116,117). Upper respiratory complaints, eye irritation, headache, blunting of taste or smell, and coughing are reported by the majority of people exposed. A peculiar metallic taste is often reported. With higher concentrations, nausea, vomiting, diarrhea, increased fatigability, memory loss, drowsiness, weakness, dizziness, incoordination, chest discomfort, shortness of breath, difficulty swallowing, cramps, and convulsions have been reported (118,119). There are a few reports of the development of pulmonary edema and electrocardiographic changes associated with acute exposure.

The majority of reports on chronic exposure depict effects on the eye (increased corneal thickness, cataract formation, and epithelial keratitis), nervous system (sensory-motor polyneuropathy) and skin (irritant and allergic reactions) (116,119–121). Respiratory infections, anemia, and altered behavior may be found (108). In addition there are concerns that EO may be mutagenic or carcinogenic and that it may adversely affect the reproductive system. An increase in the frequency of chromosome aberrations has been seen in workers accidentally exposed to high concentrations of EO (122). Ethylene oxide induces sister chromatid exchanges, a marker for chormosomal damage in humans (123). Studies have shown a link between exposure to ethylene oxide and leukemia and stomach cancer (124,125). A large-scale study of medical device industry workers exposed to EO before 1978 found that cancer rates were comparable with those in the general population (94). However, statistically significant increases in hematopoietic cancers were observed among men. A potentially significant observation was that a higher incidence of disease was evident for sterilizer operators and others who worked in the sterilizer area.

Chronic exposure in animals causes declines in the rates of body weight gain, increases in the incidence of some types of neoplasms, adverse male reproductive effects, and increases in sister chromatid exchanges in lymphocytes.

Exposure to chlorofluorocarbons used to dilute ethylene oxide can also be dangerous to personnel. These substances can induce respiratory depression, bronchoconstriction, and death in exposed workers (126).

In 1984, OSHA promulgated a standard for occupational exposure to EO. It limited worker exposure to an 8-hr time-weighted average (TWA) of 1 ppm and averaged over a 15-min period (127). An action level of 0.5 ppm as a TWA was also established. A short-term excursion limit (STEL) of 5 ppm was added in 1988.

The OSHA standard requires performance of initial (baseline) monitoring (128). If the 8-hr time-weighted airborne concentration of EO is at or exceeds the action level, employers must begin periodic exposure monitoring and medical surveillance. Below 0.5 ppm no action is required except whenever there has been a change in production-process control equipment, personnel or work practices. If the TWA exceeds 1 ppm, quarterly monitoring must be instituted in conjunction with exposure reduction measures. If the TWA is between 0.5 and 1 ppm, semiannual monitoring is required.

The presence of gaseous EO in very high concentrations is easily detected, because it is irritating to the eyes and mucous membranes, but this should not be depended on. About 600 ppm is the odor threshold, so it is possible to be in a room with dangerously high ethylene oxide concentrations without being aware of it (129).

Sources of EO Exposure. There are eight principal sources of ethylene oxide exposure: the area in front of the sterilizer when the door is opened upon completion of the sterilization cycle; the freshly sterilized goods themselves; the aeration cabinet; the sterilizer; the floor drain; the procedure for changing the tank and/or cartridge; the safety valve; and the supply tanks and cartridges.

Recommendations to Reduce Exposure (77,88,93,130–132) 1. Unnecessary use of EO should be avoided. It should be reserved for those products that must be sterilized and cannot withstand other methods of sterilization.

2. There should be strict adherence to manufacturers' installation and operating instructions for sterilizers and aerators. Each sterilizer and aerator should have regular preventive maintenance to ensure that malfunctions, especially leaks, are minimized and that any malfunctions that occur are detected and corrected. Repairs should be made only by adequately trained personnel. Records should be kept on all malfunctions and repairs.

3. Cylinders of ethylene oxide should be stored in a designated area that meets building codes and OSHA regulations, conforms to the temperature specifications of the gas supplier/manufacturer and is out of the way of traffic. Tanks should not stand free but should be chained upright to a solid structure and the protection cap should be in place when the tank is not in use. The storage room should have some ventilation to prevent the buildup of a significant environmental EO concentration in the event that a container has a leak.

4. EO tanks should be transported on equipment designed to keep them secure during transit.

5. Caution should be exercised not to expose the technician to ethylene oxide when changing tanks and filters. Protective attire (e.g., goggles or a face shield, heavy-duty gloves, full-body suits) should be worn. If monitoring or air sampling results indicate that excessive EO exposures can occur without the use of respirators, personnel must wear a respirator approved for EO use by NIOSH (88,133).

There should be check or shutoff valves in the EO lines close to the connection point to limit the release of EO into the atmosphere during cylinder changes.

A local exhaust hood should be installed as near as possible to the EO cylinder connection area to capture EO released to the air during changeover and leakage around line connections. The exhaust system should be designed so that air movement draws the EO away from personnel. It should exhaust the EO to the outside atmosphere or to an emission control system.

6. Sterilizers and aerators should be located in well-ventilated areas with limited access, away from work stations and storage areas. Personnel traffic patterns should be routed away from the gas sterilization area. Selecting an appropriate location should be a joint decision made by the hospital engineer and the department manager, with advice from the manufacturer's representative.

The room(s) in which the sterilizer and aerator are located should be large enough to ensure adequate EO dilution and to accommodate the loading, unloading, and maintenance of the equipment. The ventilation system should allow at least 10 air changes per hour and be designed to allow air to flow over the sterilizer door opening and ultimately to an exhaust fan or blower system that carries the room air and any ethylene oxide to the outside or an emission control system. Ventilation rates should be monitored and documented at least every 3 months.

7. Entrances to areas where EO is used should be posted with signs warning that high levels of EO are possible. No supplies or unnecessary equipment should be stored in the vicinity of sterilization/aeration equipment, and a minimum number of personnel should be permitted in those areas.

8. All EO sterilizers and sterilizer relief valves must be vented out of the workplace to the outside atmosphere, an emission control system, or a sanitary floor drain. Sterilizers venting to atmosphere should be vented through a dedicated vent line that does not terminate within 25 feet of any building air intake source. Running chamber vent lines in ways that would either release EO within the building or allow the reentry of EO-contaminated air into the building and releasing EO near pedestrian traffic inside or outside the facility must be prohibited.

9. The aerator should also be vented to provide proper exhaust ventilation. Even though residual EO concentrations measured at the vent opening of an aerator are typically less than those measured at the sterilizer discharge point or around the sterilizer door at the end of the sterilization cycle, a poor exhaust ventilation system in combination with an unvented aerator can contribute significantly to background exposure levels.

10. EO sterilizers should meet the following requirements (92). (*i*) The sterilizer should be constructed so that the cycle cannot be initiated or allowed to continue unless all doors are closed and secured. In addition, it should not be possible to open the door when the chamber is under pressure or before the postevacuation cycle is completed. (*ii*) The sterilizer should have purge (air flush) cycles to reduce the amount of residual ethylene oxide on goods that will be removed from the sterilizer. Depending on the volume of EO involved, safe evacuation may be achieved by a nonrecirculating general ventilation system, by a dedicated exhaust system, via evacuation through ducts to the outside atmosphere or emission control system, to a dedicated floor drain after mixing the EO with water, or by a combination of these methods. (*iii*). The sterilizer should be equipped with a means of detecting leaks.

11. Local exhaust ventilation systems should be installed to capture ethylene oxide before it can escape into the general work environment. The ethylene oxide can be collected in a hood of suitable design located as close to the source of EO as possible and exhausted to the outside atmosphere via a fan and duct system. The following are the most common areas where high EO concentrations may occur and where local exhaust systems are recommended: (*i*) as close as possible to the sterilizer, preferably 1 to 2 inches from the top of the door, so as to capture the hot, rising EO vapors as they leave the chamber at the end of the sterilization cycle; (*ii*) the area near the sterilizer pressure relief valve; (*iii*) for sterilizers that discharge to a sanitary system, the area immediately above the line that drains into the sanitary sewer; and (*iv*) the EO cylinder connection points.

12. Employees operating sterilizers or aerators should be properly instructed in the hazards of ethylene oxide and appropriate safety procedures. A continuing education program should be established, and all personnel working around EO should be required to participate in the program. When feasible, workers should be isolated from direct contact with the work environment by the use of automated equipment operated by personnel observing from a closed control booth or room.

13. A combination sterilizer/aerator will reduce EO exposure associated with opening the sterilizer door and removal of items from the sterilizer. However, it may be difficult to justify tying up an expensive sterilizer when a less expensive aerator could be used.

14. Occupational exposure to EO can be avoided by using a loading cart and/or wire baskets (93). These can be moved into and from the sterilizer, then directly into and from the aerator. Items should be loaded in such a manner that they will not touch the operator's hands when the cart or basket is transferred from the sterilizer to the aerator.

15. The single greatest source of EO exposure occurs when the sterilizer door is opened after completion of a sterilization cycle (134–136). Exposure control at this point is essential. Employees should avoid being close to a sterilizer that has just finished a cycle, except as necessary to operate the unit.

Materials should not be left in a closed sterilizer after the cycle is complete, as this will allow high concentrations of EO to build up in the sterilizer and be released into the room when the door is first opened.

The chamber door should be opened 6 inches immediately following a cycle (136). A door-opening device on some large sterilizers allows the operator to push a button, then walk away, while the sterilizer door slowly opens (108). The operator should leave the immediate sterilizer area for a minimum of 15 min after opening the door (88,137). This time allows ethylene oxide to dissipate from the chamber and be removed by the general ventilation system.

The purge characteristics of some newer sterilizers will prevent the buildup of ethylene oxide inside the chamber (88). These sterilizers should be unloaded immediately upon opening the door, because it is at this time that the EO concentration within the chamber is lowest. When in doubt, the manufacturer's instructions should be consulted.

16. Sterilized items should be transferred rapidly to the aerator. Goods should never be handled directly. Transfer carts should be used to remove items from large sterilizers and gloves and forceps for items in small sterilizers. Carts should be pulled, rather than pushed, to the aerator so that personnel are not upwind of the degassing goods. Items should be placed in the aerator without delay. Unaerated items should never be left outside the aerator where they might contaminate the environment or be used inadvertently.

17. Special-purpose sterilizers should be used only in a well-ventilated room. If a sterilizer does not have a venting mechanism other than the door or lid the healthcare facility must determine that the system effectively minimizes employee exposure to EO gas. Possible options include using local exhaust ventilation (such as a laboratory hood) and adding a chemical neutralization system or EO sorbent to the sterilizer. Ventilation cabinets designed for special-purpose EO sterilizers are available (138).

18. All ethylene oxide-sterilized items should be aerated before handling. A mechanical aerator is best. If ambient aeration is unavoidable, the aeration area should be segregated from general work areas and have limited access. It should have good general ventilation and be at a negative pressure with respect to adjoining areas. Storage of supplies in the area must be prohibited.

19. Personnel and environmental monitoring similar to that discussed in Chapter 11 must be practiced to ensure that recommended levels are not exceeded (88,139–151). Leak checks must be performed regularly. The frequency of monitoring required by OSHA depends on the levels found in the work environment (88).

20. A system to detect ventilation system failures and to alert personnel with audible and/or visual alarms should be installed. Alarms for local exhaust ventilation system failures should be installed.

21. Because ethylene oxide can escape from equipment into the work area through faulty or poorly maintained gaskets, valves, and fittings, the gasket seals or sterilizer and aerator doors should be inspected for cracks, tears, debris, and other foreign substances before each load. Sterilizer and aerator valves and fittings should be inspected at least every 2 weeks and replaced as necessary. Intake air filters for the restricted access area should be inspected and cleaned regularly as part of scheduled preventative maintenance.

22. Sterilizers and aerators should be tested for leaks at least every 2 weeks. Also leakage at the EO gas line entrance port within the sterilizer should be checked for at least every 2 weeks (88).

23. Only 1 day's supply of EO cartridges should be stored in the immediate area of the sterilizer (88).

24. Each facility in which EO is used should have a written emergency plan for dealing with ethylene oxide leaks and spills (88,152,153). Development of precautionary measures should be a joint effort of the hospital's sterilization department, its safety department, the local fire department, and perhaps others such as the physician responsible for employee health and a hospital engineer familiar with ventilation systems, air exchange rates, and so forth. The hospital should form an action team responsible for the development and exercise of the written procedures to handle EO leaks and spills (88).

Environmental Problems

Once ethylene oxide is emitted, it remains in the air without breaking down for long periods of time. People who live near facilities with sterilizers or aerators may, therefore, be exposed to airborne ethylene oxide from these sources. Catalytic convertors are now available that break EO down into carbon dioxide and water. Other systems are available that absorb the EO and react it with water, producing ethylene glycol (154). This chemical is then sold, completing the recycle mode.

Advantages and Disadvantages

Ethylene oxide sterilization has many advantages. It is effective against all organisms. It is very reliable, because the gas penetrates into crevices and regions blocked to liquids. It can be used on a wide variety of items, including those that would be damaged by heat or high concentrations of moisture. Indeed, it is the only reliable and practical means for sterilizing many devices in common use today. Damage to most equipment is minimal. Items can be prepackaged and the package sealed. This eliminates the danger of recontamination that can occur during rinsing and packaging following "cold sterilization" and allows the items to remain sterile during long-term storage.

Ethylene oxide has a number of disadvantages. Fires and explosions involving sterilizers have been reported (155,156). Flammable mixtures require special handling. Even with the diluted ethylene oxide mixtures, care must be exercised, because there is a possibility that the gas mixture may become stratified and create a fire or explosion hazard (64).

A major disadvantage is that it may require a long turnaround time because of the need for aeration to eliminate residual EO. This may necessitate having to keep a large stock of equipment.

It is more costly than most other types of disinfection. Installation of the necessary equipment is expensive and if large items are

to be sterilized the equipment will take a great deal of space. Personnel need to be highly trained and supervised to ensure proper sterilization and prevent complications. Frequent biological monitoring is required.

Equipment to be sterilized needs to be dry, which can be difficult to achieve with items such as corrugated tubings. Some materials deteriorate after repeated sterilization, especially at elevated temperatures. It cannot be used to sterilize any medical devices that have petroleum-based lubricants in or on them, because ethylene oxide cannot permeate these (157).

RADIATION STERILIZATION (158)

Radiation sterilization is the dominant process for sterilizing disposable products from the manufacturer. Gamma-radiation (γ-rays) is an electromagnetic wave produced during the disintegration of certain radioactive elements. If the dosage applied to a product is large enough, all microorganisms, including bacterial spores and viruses, will be killed (6).

There are many advantages to γ-radiation (8). The product can be prepackaged in a wide variety of impermeable containers before treatment. The package will not interfere with the sterilization process. The treated items remain sterile indefinitely until the packaging seal is broken. As there is virtually no temperature rise during treatment, thermolabile materials can be sterilized and thermolabile packaging can be used. Equipment may be used immediately after γ-radiation treatment with no risk from retained radioactivity.

Gamma radiation is not practical for everyday use in hospitals. It requires expensive equipment and is used only by large manufacturers to sterilize disposable equipment (159). The importance of γ-radiation is that it does cause changes in some plastics, especially polyvinyl chloride (PVC). When PVC is sterilized by γ-radiation, chloride ions are liberated. It was once thought that a γ-radiated tracheal or tracheostomy tube should not be resterilized with ethylene oxide (160). Evidence now confirms that previously γ-radiated tubes can be resterilized with ethylene oxide (110,111). As always, aeration times must be strictly enforced.

A Program for Anesthesia Equipment

THE STERILIZATION DILEMMA (101,161–163)

Those concerned with anesthesia equipment find themselves faced with a dilemma as to how much time, effort, and money should be expended to try to prevent transmission of infection to patients. Those who argue that more vigorous approaches are not needed and feel that many of the measures being advocated are unreasonable advance the following arguments.

1. Documented cases of cross-infection by contaminated anesthesia equipment are rare. Studies have cast doubt on the likelihood of the breathing system causing postoperative respiratory infections (164,165).
2. Decontamination is difficult, costly, and entails certain dangers to patients and hospital personnel. It entails a heavy capital outlay for equipment, increased work for personnel, and increased space. Considerable training of staff is necessary.
3. The nature of maneuvers required in anesthesia makes sterility impractical.
4. Many forms of sterilization can damage equipment. Liquid and gas chemical sterilization may leave residues that can subsequently harm a patient. Mistakes may be made during reassembly.

Proponents for more vigorous attempts at sterilization argue as follows:

1. Cases of cross-contamination caused by anesthesia equipment have been reported (166,167).

2. The risk of cross-contamination may be greater than is commonly believed because it is frequently difficult to pinpoint the exact cause of a postoperative infection. Patients undergoing anesthesia and surgery are more likely to develop respiratory infections than the normal population. Anesthesia interferes with ciliary and mucus activity and surgery can impair the patient's ability to cough and breathe deeply. Anesthesiologists are caring for immunocompromised patients more often and this group may be unable to protect itself against what formerly were thought to be harmless environmental organisms or insignificant innoculums (7).
3. Although there is general agreement that sterilization of equipment is essential after use in a patient with a respiratory infection or a particularly virulent organism, it is frequently impossible to identify these patients. Any organism is a potential cause of infection. Therefore, all equipment is suspect.
4. Even if the incidence of postoperative respiratory infections resulting from anesthesia apparatus is low, the cost of a single such infection in terms of mortality, morbidity, and economics is high (168).

CDC RATIONALE FOR CLEANING, DISINFECTION, AND STERILIZATION

The CDC has published guidelines on how to prevent or control specific nosocomial infection problems. As shown in Table 19.4, they have divided items into three categories, based on the potential risk of infection involved in their use.

Critical Items

Critical items are those that are introduced into the bloodstream or other normally sterile areas of the body by penetrating skin or mucous membranes. These items must be sterile at the time of use. If an item's sterility is in doubt, it should not be used. This equipment includes vascular needles

Table 19.4. Classification of Devices, Processes, and Germicidal Products

Critical	Sterilization: sporicidal chemical, prolonged contact	Sterilant/disinfectant
Semicritical	High-level disinfection: sporicidal chemical, short contact	Sterilant/disinfectant
Noncritical	Intermediate-level disinfection	Hospital disinfectant with tuberculocidal activity
	Low-level disinfection	Hospital disinfectant without tuberculocidal activity

and catheters, regional block needles and catheters, the interior of associated tubing and connectors, syringes, and urinary catheters.

Semicritical Items

These are devices that come in contact with intact mucous membranes, but do not ordinarily penetrate body surfaces. Sterilization is desirable for these items, but if not easily possible, a high level of decontamination is acceptable (2,12). Intact mucous membranes are generally resistant to infection by common bacterial spores (9). In most cases, meticulous cleaning followed by high-level disinfection gives the user a reasonable degree of assurance that the items are free of pathogens. Evidence that sterilization reduces the risk of infection is lacking (2). Equipment that falls into this category includes endoscopes; laryngoscope blades; esophageal, nasopharyngeal, and rectal temperature probes; face masks; oral and nasal airways; resuscitation bags; breathing circuits and connectors; esophageal stethoscopes; and tracheal and double-lumen tubes (3).

Noncritical Items

Noncritical items are those that do not ordinarily touch the patient or only touch intact skin. In general, intact skin acts as an effective barrier to most microorganisms; thus items that touch only intact skin need only intermediate- or low-level disinfection. Items in this category include stethoscopes (not esophageal); blood pressure cuffs and tubing; pulse oximeter probes and cables; ECG ca-

bles; reusable skin temperature probes, temperature monitor cables; head straps; blood warmers; and the exteriors of the anesthesia machine, monitors, and equipment carts.

ORGANIZATION (1)

Each anesthesia department should have an infection control plan that documents procedures and policies to prevent transmission of infectious agents to patients during their anesthetic care and to minimize exposure of anesthesia personnel to occupational infectious hazards (28).

Considerations before Anesthesia

Use of Bacterial Filters

Bacterial filters have been used on patients requiring respiratory isolation at the time of surgery or to protect patients at increased risk of developing an infection. A variety are available (see Chapter 5).

Use of filters is controversial. Some studies indicate that routine use of filters does not prevent postoperative pulmonary infections (165,169–171). Certain hazards, especially obstruction, are associated with their use.

Choice of Equipment

Reusable Versus Disposable Equipment (172,173). Most departments have struck a balance between disposable and reusable items. The balance, however, needs to be continually reassessed in light of rapidly changing technologies, cost comparisons, universal precautions, and waste management dilemmas. Most departments keep at least some disposable items available for use with known infected cases.

The advantages of disposable equipment include ease of use, convenience, lower unit costs, and a quicker response to innovations in the marketplace. Disposables ensure that the patient will always receive a sterile or clean item, and there is no need for decontamination before use. If labor costs are high, this may be an important consideration. Among the disadvantages of disposables are the costs of keeping sufficient inventory. Storage space can be a problem. The ecological problems of getting rid of disposable items after use and uncertain availability of petroleum products must be considered (8).

Reusable products offer the advantage of reduced storage space as well as consistency of product. Reusables cut down on the waste generated by a facility. However, a reusable device often requires disassembly, cleaning, drying, reassembly, repackaging, and disinfection or sterilization before reuse (173). While equipment is being cleaned it cannot be used. This necessitates a larger inventory. The increased handling increases the risks for injury to the handler. It must be remembered that there is a given life span for reusable equipment.

Reuse of Disposable Equipment. Reuse of disposable items is controversial. Surveys show that up to 65% of hospitals regularly reuse disposable devices (173,174). Although this practice may be advantageous economically, there are many ramifications that need to be considered. Reuse of disposable devices shifts the product liability from the manufacturer to the individual (28).

The CDC believes that there is a lack of evidence indicating increased risk of nosocomial infections associated with the reuse of all single-use items and, therefore, does not recommend against all types of reuse (12). The guidelines indicate that items that cannot be cleaned and sterilized or disinfected without altering their physical integrity and function should not be reprocessed. In addition, reprocessing procedures that result in residual toxicity or compromise the overall safety or effectiveness of the items should be avoided. It recommends that hospitals consider the safety and efficacy of the reprocessing procedure of each item or device separately and the likelihood that the device will function as intended after reprocessing.

FDA guidelines state that if a hospital reuses a disposable item, it must be able to demonstrate (*i*) that the device can be adequately cleaned and sterilized, (*ii*) that the physical characteristics or quality of the device will not be adversely affected, and (*iii*) that the device remains safe and effective for its intended use. Furthermore, (*iv*) they must accept full responsibility for the device's safety and effectiveness (4). It is recommended that an interdisciplinary committee within each healthcare facility be developed to assess all requests to resterilize and reuse any device labeled single-use or disposable by the manufacturer.

Intraoperative Considerations

Care of Equipment

Anesthesia personnel should always work from a clean surface. At the start of a case only those articles that are to be used on that patient should be placed there. During the administration of anesthesia it is important to establish a routine whereby an article not used on a patient is kept separate from those that have been and to be able to identify and isolate all articles that may have been contaminated.

All used articles should be placed in a special receptacle that is physically separated from the clean area. It may contain water with detergent to prevent drying of secretions. At the end of the operation, this receptacle should be taken to the dirty wash-up area. Disposable items should be discarded in suitable containers in the operating room.

Additional isolation of dirty items of equipment such as laryngoscope blades can be achieved by wrapping them in a glove or packaging from a tracheal tube (175).

Decontaminating Spills of Blood and Body Fluids

Spills of blood or body fluids on equipment or environmental surfaces should be cleaned and decontaminated as soon as practical. Visible material should be removed with water and detergent followed by decontamination using a EPA-approved hospital disinfectant that is classified as tuberculocidal (28). A 1:10 to 1:100 dilution of 5.25% sodium hypochlorite has been recommended by the CDC for cleaning blood spills (176,177).

Decontamination of Reusable Equipment

A decontamination program that meets the needs of a given hospital usually results from tailoring several techniques to that hospital's needs. Factors to be considered include cost, types of equipment employed, available facilities, and the importance attributed to sterilization in that hospital. A hospital that has many patients with reduced immunity must be more careful than a surgical center that handles only healthy outpatients. Whatever decontamination plan is devised, it is important that alternate methods be available in the event the primary system fails. Whatever system is devised, certain factors are essential for a successful program.

Physical Arrangements (2)

Ideally, the decontamination area should be physically separate from all other areas of the processing department. However, spatial separation may be adequate, provided that work practices prevent splashing and contamination of clean items and work surfaces. Sinks should be large enough to contain large instruments and there should be enough sinks to accommodate concurrent soaking, washing, and rinsing. Sinks should have attached counters or adjacent work surfaces on which to place soiled and clean items separately. Signs showing where dirty equipment should be placed should be prominently displayed.

Airborne microbial and particulate contamination is likely to be high in the decontamination area because of the presence of grossly soiled items, manual cleaning that produces aerosols, and in some facilities, trash and linen handling. Therefore, it is recommended that the ventilation system for the decontaminated area be designed to maintain negative air pressure relative to surrounding spaces and to remove toxic vapors. Air from the decontamination area should be exhausted to the outdoors without recirculation.

Good traffic control in the decontamination area will protect personnel and visitors from airborne contaminants and from microorganisms present on contaminated items. The area should be restricted to authorized personnel to avoid spreading contamination.

Hand washing facilities should be conveniently located in or near the decontamination area. They should be separate from sinks used in cleaning or rinsing items to be decontaminated.

There should be at least daily cleaning and disinfection of horizontal work surfaces. Floors should be cleaned daily and, when necessary, disinfected. Other surfaces such as walls and storage shelves, should be cleaned on a regular basis and as needed for spot cleaning of soiled areas. Special attention should be paid to the sequence of cleaning to avoid transferring contaminants from dirty to clean areas and surfaces.

Personnel (1)

The responsibility for decontamination of anesthesia equipment should be vested in one individual who devises and administers a comprehensive program. This person should be a member of the infection control committee of the hospital.

It is imperative that cleaning and disinfection or sterilizing of anesthesia equipment be delegated to conscientious, well-trained individuals who understand the principles of containment of contamination and the disinfecting or sterilizing process (1,178).

Most nurses are well-indoctrinated in the principles of aseptic technique. Frequently, however, technicians caring for equipment are without a clinical hospital background. Such people need considerable indoctrination before they can be relied on in practice.

Appropriate attire will minimize the transfer of microorganisms from contaminated items to personnel. Heavy-duty. fluid-resistant protective gloves, a long-sleeved fluid-resistant covering, a face mask and eye protection (goggles or safety glasses) should be worn. Gloves do not offer absolute protection because they may develop small leaks caused by the stresses of the cleaning process. Therefore, it is important that hand washing be performed immediately after cleaning to prevent any further contamination of the worker or environment.

Surveillance

The third factor necessary for a successful decontamination program is surveillance to check the efficiency of decontaminating techniques. CDC guidelines do not recommend monitoring by routine cultures (12). Cultures need only be taken if a problem becomes evident. This policy should result in considerable cost savings (179).

CONSIDERATION OF INDIVIDUAL ITEMS

The level of decontamination required for a particular device depends on the potential hazard arising from its most recent and its intended subsequent use. In general it is best to follow specific manufacturers' instructions for acceptable germicides and decontamination procedures.

Anesthesia Carts

Anesthesia carts are used in many operating rooms as a repository for equipment and drugs. Some attention should be given to the placement of equipment in the drawers.

For instance, a blood pressure cuff that is used on several patients with no attempt to decontaminate it between cases should not be placed in the same drawer as airways or masks that are not kept in sterile containers, but it may be placed in a drawer containing items such as suction catheters and syringes that are kept in disposable wrappers. Equipment such as airways and masks that are not kept in sterile containers should be placed in drawers that are less frequently opened, i.e., not in the same drawer as frequently used drugs. Containers used to hold drugs, syringes, needles, etc. should be made of metal or plastic rather than cardboard to facilitate cleaning.

Horizontal surfaces should be wiped between cases and at the conclusion of the workday with a cloth soaked with a detergent germicide (28). Blood or secretions should be wiped off promptly (7). A clean covering should be placed on the top at the start of each case. Vertical surfaces should be cleaned at the end of the workday or more often if there is an obvious contamination with blood or body fluids.

At least once a week, and following use on a patient with a known communicable disease, the entire cart should be cleaned. All equipment should be removed and the drawers washed with detergent and water and then wiped or sprayed with a germicide. Containers used in the drawers should be washed.

Gas Cylinders

Gas cylinders are transported to the hospital in open trucks and are frequently stored outside. They should be considered dirty when received in the operating room area. Some are furnished in plastic or paper wrappers. Before taking a cylinder into an operating room, the wrapper, if present, should be removed.

The cylinder should be washed with water and detergent and wiped with a cloth soaked in germicide or sprayed with a germicidal spray. After placing the cylinder on the anesthesia machine, it may be considered part of the machine and treated accordingly.

Anesthesia Machines

Anesthesia machines usually remain in the operating room and are not transported to other areas. They are often used to store drugs and equipment and may provide the "clean" and/or "dirty" areas for equipment. The same principles for storage of equipment and separation of clean and dirty areas apply to machines as to carts. The top of an anesthesia machine is a convenient area for keeping equipment. Many machines have a shelf several feet above the table. This can be used for placing a tray holding "clean" equipment or a receptacle for the "dirty" equipment. Items placed there will be separate from the rest of the equipment but readily available.

The machine's countertop should be covered with a fresh, clean towel for each patient. The horizontal surfaces should be wiped between cases and at the end of the workday. At least once a week equipment should be removed from the drawers and the drawers cleaned. The final application should be with a cloth containing a disinfectant solution or a germicidal spray may be used.

Absorber, Unidirectional Valves, and APL Valve

Absorbent has a potent cidal effect on microorganisms and only a low number of resistant spores pass through the absorber (180). Studies strongly suggest that regardless of prior upper airway colonization and duration of anesthesia, patients rarely contaminate these parts with significant levels of bacteria (164,181). Disposable absorbers are available, but offer no more protection against contamination of breathing systems than reusable ones (182).

The manufacturer's instructions should be consulted with respect to disassembling, cleaning, and disinfecting. CO_2 absorbent chambers should be cleaned and disinfected during routine changing of absorbent. The screens should receive particular attention as they are susceptible to the gumming film produced by absorbents. The absorber frame should be cleaned by wiping with a cloth soaked in a detergent germicide. Unidirectional valves are usually easily disassembled and cleaned by wiping the disc, the inside of the plastic dome, and the valve seat with alcohol or a detergent. APL valves can be cleaned by wiping with a detergent. Some canisters will withstand autoclaving once the pressure gauge and valve assemblies have been removed. Some can be sterilized using ethylene oxide.

Some canisters can be disinfected by immersion in a liquid such as glutaraldehyde, as can most APL valves. However, use of glutaraldehyde on APL valves has been reported to cause stickiness and increase the opening pressure (81). Some APL valves may be autoclaved (18,183).

The Reservoir Bag

Disposable rubber and plastic reservoir bags are most commonly used. Most come with disposable tubing or as parts of a completely disposable system. Bags can be cleaned manually or in an automatic washing machine.

Ethylene oxide is probably the most satisfactory means of sterilizing the bag. Aeration times should be carefully observed and the bag filled and emptied a few times before use on a patient.

Bags can be sterilized by autoclaving, provided an adequate wick is placed inside to ensure steam contact with all surfaces (184). Autoclaving will cause rubber bags to deteriorate and will usually melt plastic bags. Some bags may be pasteurized but this also will result in gradual deterioration (183).

Chemical disinfection can be used. The bag must be filled with liquid to remove pockets of air (185). Of the various agents used, glutaraldehyde is probably the most satisfactory, provided adequate rinsing is performed.

Breathing Tubings

The corrugated tubing of the circle system presents a difficult problem. Studies have shown that this tubing is contaminated after use. The closer to the patient, the heavier the contamination (186). Water commonly condenses in the expiratory tubing. If the tubings are lifted up, this water may run down into the mask or tracheal tube. Airborne contamination of anesthetic gases by anesthetic tubing is uncommon (187).

Disposable tubings are usually used today. This may present a storage problem if frequent changes are made. One study showed that use of sterile tubings did not prevent postoperative pulmonary infections (165).

Because of their bulk and construction, tubings are difficult to clean and disinfect. Reusable tubings should be rinsed out under a running tap soon after use to prevent drying. They may then be soaked in a large container containing water and detergent.

The long length and ridges preclude a brush being effective in cleaning. Ultrasonic cleaning has been used to remove debris from corrugated tubing in respiratory therapy (188). A washing machine may be used (189). Another method is to pour detergent and water into one end of the tube and agitating in a seesaw manner (190). After washing, the tubings should be thoroughly dried unless they are to undergo pasteurization. Special tube dryers are available.

Pasteurization has been used for corrugated tubings (186,191). The Y piece should be removed beforehand. Otherwise, a loose fit may result.

Chemical disinfection can be carried out using an automatic washing machine or by immersion in a liquid agent (191). It is important that the tube be inserted vertically, making sure it is filled on the inside and there are no air pockets. One study found that machine-assisted chemical disinfection with glutaraldehyde was superior to machine-assisted pasteurization for respirator tubing (189).

The Y Piece

Y pieces are contaminated in a high percentage of cases. Fortunately, they are relatively easy to clean and sterilize. Disposable Y pieces attached to disposable tubings are usually used today.

After use, the Y piece should be removed from the corrugated tubings and rinsed out under running tap water. They should then be placed in a solution of water and detergent to soak. They can be scrubbed manually or placed in a washing machine. If chemical or ethylene oxide sterilization is to be used, the Y piece should be thoroughly dried. Y pieces may be pasteurized, immersed in liquid agents, or sterilized with ethylene oxide.

Mapleson Systems

One study of Bain circuits found a contamination rate of 8% following single patient use (192). After use, the systems should be disassembled and the components cleaned. The components may be disinfected or sterilized by one of the methods discussed. Metal components can undergo autoclaving. Rubber and plastic parts can undergo gas sterilization or disinfection using a liquid chemical agent.

Adaptors

Adaptors used near the patient are contaminated in a high percentage of cases. Fortunately, they are usually not difficult to clean or sterilize. After use, adaptors should be rinsed under a running tap, then placed in a solution of detergent and water and soaked. They may be washed manually or in a washing machine. Rubber and plastic adaptors may be sterilized with ethylene oxide or in a liquid such as glutaraldehyde. Metal adaptors may be autoclaved or pasteurized.

Anesthesia Ventilators

Ventilators can be protected from contamination by use of a filter in the ventilator hose. This will also protect the patient from a contaminated ventilator.

Anesthesia ventilator tubing and bellows should be cleaned and disinfected at regular intervals (3). Anesthesia ventilators are thought to represent a low risk for infection transmission and need not undergo cleaning and disinfection following each use.

Some ventilators have metal poles to which the hose is attached. These poles can be autoclaved. The manufacturer's instructions should be consulted for treatment of other parts. Parts of the ventilator breathing circuit may be autoclavable. Most ventilator bellows and tubings can be sterilized using ethylene oxide.

Scavenging Equipment

A satisfactory method of treating scavenging equipment is to wash the device in a detergent solution monthly and to change the plastic hoses that connect the device to the breathing system and ventilator at the same time (18).

Face Masks

Face masks are among the most frequently and heavily contaminated pieces of equipment, being subject to microorganisms both from the mouth and airway and from the patient's skin. Frequently, mucus or vomitus gets onto them. Because of their proximity to the patient, transmittal of infection to the patient is a definite possibility. For obviously contaminated cases, disposable masks are available.

Asepsis should be practiced in the use of the face mask. They should not be allowed to drop onto the floor or be exposed to obvious contamination. After use, the mask should be kept near the patient's head or with the dirty equipment.

Immediately after use, the connector should be removed and the mask rinsed in cool tap water. Then it should be soaked and scrubbed. It may be cleaned automatically in a washing machine. Masks should always be thoroughly rinsed and carefully dried, especially if ethylene oxide is to be used for sterilization. Masks should receive high-level disinfection.

Ethylene oxide offers the advantage that the mask can be maintained sterile for long periods of time. Aeration must be adequate or facial burns may result (99). Most automatic ethylene oxide sterilizers employ a vacuum at least once during the sterilization cycle. This vacuum may cause the pneumatic cushion of the mask to balloon and the mask may lose its cushion (101). This can be prevented by removing the plug that seals the pneumatic cushion or by using a sterilizer not employing a vacuum phase.

Autoclaving is sometimes used for face masks. Steam will shorten the life of masks made of conductive rubber. Conductive neoprene face masks are available that will withstand steam sterilization (184). Autoclaving also involves a vacuum phase that will damage the inflated cushion, so before autoclaving, the plug should be removed. Pasteurization also has been used for face masks (193,194).

Liquid chemical agents are widely used for face masks. Thorough rinsing is necessary to remove residual detergent. Facial injury can be caused by a mask improperly sterilized with liquid agents. Phenolic compounds should not be used because they are absorbed by the rubber. Any cracks in the cushion of the mask can let liquid agent into the airspace. When placed on a patient's face, the liquid can be squeezed out, possibly into the eyes.

Head Straps

Head straps should be subjected to periodic cleaning with a detergent, then soaked in a disinfectant solution or sterilized with ethylene oxide.

Airways

Before use, airways should be treated as clean objects and not allowed to drop on the floor. Because they are inserted into a relatively dirty portion of the patient, sterility at the time of use is probably unnecessary.

After removal, they should be treated as dirty equipment. As soon as possible after use, the airway should be rinsed with cold water, then placed in a solution of water and detergent. They should be washed manually using a brush, making sure any channels are cleaned, or washed in a machine (13,14,195). They should be thoroughly rinsed to remove residual detergent.

Pasteurization, liquid chemical disinfection, and ethylene oxide sterilization can be used for airways. Rubber airways may be autoclaved, but this will shorten their useful life.

Laryngoscope Blades, Stylets, and Intubating Forceps (183)

Laryngoscope blades, stylets, and forceps should be stored under clean conditions. Many people believe stylets should be kept sterile, because they are placed inside an tracheal tube. For known contaminated cases disposable laryngoscope blades are available.

All these items will be contaminated after use and should be treated as dirty and not placed on the clean surfaces of the anesthesia machine or anesthesia cart. One suggestion is to invert the glove the operator is wearing over the blade after intubation (196).

The laryngoscope handle should be separated from the blade after use and kept in a clean location. It can be wiped with isopropyl alcohol.

Although it has been reported that simply wiping the blade thoroughly with 70% isopropyl alcohol after use killed most bacteria (197), most authors favor more mechanical cleansing. As soon as possible after use, the blade, stylet, or forceps should be rinsed under a running tap or immersed in a pan of water and detergent. It should be washed mechanically with particular attention given to the area around the light bulb.

Blades, stylets, and forceps may be autoclaved, gas sterilized, or treated with liquid chemicals. Of the liquid chemical agents, alcohol and glutaraldehyde are the most frequently used. If ethylene oxide is used for sterilization, no aeration time is required.

Fiberoptic Scopes

There have been several reports of contamination of endoscopes attributed to either inadequate cleaning, improper selection of a disinfecting agent, insufficient exposure time, or failure to expose a portion of the equipment to the disinfectant (4). Transmission of *M. tuberculosis* by contaminated bronchoscopes has been documented in at least 16 cases (17). Pseudoepidemics—clusters of false infections—of bronchoscopy-related mycobacterial disease have been reported (17). This can lead to unnecessary diagnostic and therapeutic interventions. Reported causes of pseudoepidemics include a damaged suction channel, contaminated tap water, contaminated dye added to the local anesthetic, and contaminated antimicrobial solution in the microbiology laboratory (17). Two pseudoepidemics associated with contaminated bronchoscope cleaning machines have been reported (16,17).

The manufacturer's instructions must be consulted as to cleaning procedures. In most cases, immediately after a scope is removed from the patient the air-water channel should be flushed with water and the scope's surfaces wiped with 70% alcohol The scope's channels should be flushed with a detergent solution, then the scope soaked in the detergent to begin breaking down any organic soil. Special cleaning brushes should be inserted into the channels to remove debris loosened by the detergent. The fiberscope and all of its channels should be thoroughly rinsed with water to remove detergent residue. Excess water should then be removed from the channels to reduce the chance that the disinfectant will be diluted. The exterior of the scope should be dried with a soft cloth to remove excess water.

Following cleaning, fiberoptic scopes should be sterilized or receive high-level disinfection before use (2). Endoscopic instruments are particularly difficult to disinfect and easy to damage because of their intricate design and delicate materials.

The manufacturer's recommendations need to be followed in regard to disinfection and sterilization. One important point to be noted is the head. In some cases it is immersible, whereas in others it is not.

Chemical disinfectants used for endoscopes include alcohol, iodophores, glutaraldehydes, a hydrogen peroxide–based formulation, and a quaternary ammonium compound followed by alcohol (8,40,41,198). The Steris system uses peracetic acid. All lumens and/or channels must be filled with—and the device then immersed in—the disinfectant. All parts of the device must come in contact with the chemical for at least 20 min. After disinfection, the device must be thoroughly rinsed with sterile water to remove all traces of disinfectant and protect patients from the toxic chemicals. If sterile water is not available, the scope can be rinsed first with tap water, then with 70% alcohol.

Ethylene oxide at low temperatures may be used on some instruments (28). It is effective but requires at least 12 hr and is frequently impractical. If a fiberoptic scope is to be gas autoclaved, it may be necessary to install the venting cap before it is sent for gas autoclaving. This allows the gas that permeates the endoscope to escape without rupturing the outer skin (4). The cap is then removed before the endoscope is returned to service or immersed in liquids.

Tracheal and Double-Lumen Tubes and Connectors

The tracheal tube is placed into an area of the body that is normally sterile. The Sub-

committee on Infection Control Policy of the American Society of Anesthesiologists has recommended that tracheal and bronchial tubes be kept sterile until the time of use (3). However, high-level disinfection should be sufficient, because infection caused by spore-bearing organisms is unlikely.

Disposable sterile tubes are available at relatively low cost. These are used routinely in most institutions. The tube should be kept in its package until just before use and the patient end of the tube should not be touched. Sterile lubricant should be used. If possible, the tube should not touch any part of the mouth or pharynx during insertion. One study showed that sterility is maintained up to 5 days after opening the package and confirming cuff integrity (199).

After use, the tube should be treated as a dirty piece of equipment. If the tube is to be disinfected, it is important that secretions be prevented from drying by rinsing in cold running water and soaking in a detergent and water solution. Before immersion, the inflating tube should be plugged to prevent water from entering the tube and cuff. The connector should be removed and tape, etc., taken off. The tube should then be washed inside and out. While washing the tube, one should be careful not to catch the cuff on any sharp object. Tracheal tubes may also be cleaned in a washing machine.

The tube should be rinsed thoroughly, making sure to flush the lumen. Thorough drying is important before chemical disinfection or gas sterilization. Unless the tube is to be autoclaved or pasteurized, the connector should be reinserted after cleaning.

Use of ethylene oxide is a popular method for sterilizing tracheal tubes. The tube and connector must be free of water droplets. The end of the inflating tube should be open. With repeated ethylene oxide sterilization, rubber and some plastic tracheal tubes become softened and kink more easily (64,200). Spiral latex tracheal tubes should not be gas sterilized or steam sterilized with a vacuum applied in the sterilizing cycle, as the latex layers can separate. During anesthesia, anesthetic gases, especially nitrous oxide, may penetrate into the layers, resulting in partial or total occlusion of the inner lumen of the tube (113).

Autoclaving has been used in the past for sterilizing tracheal tubes. However, repeated autoclaving makes tracheal tubes more likely to kink and causes a decrease in the elasticity of the rubber composing the cuffs. Spiral embedded tubes are especially susceptible to damage from autoclaving. Most of the newer tracheal tubes made of plastic will not withstand the high temperatures involved in autoclaving.

When packaging tracheal tubes for autoclaving, the connector should be removed. Otherwise, a loose fit will result. The inflating tube end should be left open. Otherwise, the heat will cause the air in the cuff to expand and may cause the tube to narrow under the cuff. Pasteurization also has been used for tracheal tubes (186).

Liquid chemical disinfection of tracheal tubes has been used. The inflating tube should be closed during immersion to prevent the solution from entering the cuff. The tube will frequently float and needs to be held down with an object that does not distort it or prevent the solution from reaching all surfaces. Thorough rinsing is necessary after all agents except alcohol. Otherwise, tracheitis may result (201,202).

Resuscitation Bags

Resuscitation bags have been implicated as the source of epidemics (203–205). Disposable resuscitation bags are available. The primary source of contamination is the valve. This should be disassembled and cleaned, and if possible, disinfected or sterilized after each use or on a regular basis if dedicated to a single patient. The manufacturer's instructions should be followed.

Blood Pressure Cuffs and Stethoscopes

Blood pressure apparatus can be a reservoir of bacteria (206,207). They should be cleaned with a detergent or disinfectant at the end of the day and when visibly contaminated (3). Periodic sterilization is advisable.

Most cuffs can be soaked in disinfectant solution. After rinsing, the bladder can be reinserted, air pumped into it, and the cuff dried. After drying, the cuff may be subjected to ethylene oxide sterilization if desired.

Stethoscopes can be washed with soap and water and wiped with alcohol. Ear plugs can be cleaned with an alcohol-saturated applicator.

Pressure Transducers

Nosocomial infections associated with contaminated reusable pressure transducers have been reported (208,209). Most anesthesia departments prefer to use sterile disposable transducers.

If reusable transducers are used they should be cleaned and then disinfected with a high-level disinfectant, disinfected with 70% isopropyl alcohol wipes, or sterilized with ethylene oxide (2). They should be stored in a manner to prevent recontamination before use.

AIDS, Hepatitis, TB and Creutzfeldt-Jakob Disease

The question has been raised regarding the need for disinfection or sterilization of medical devices contaminated with blood from patients infected with HIV or hepatitis B virus (HBV) or with respiratory secretions from a patient with pulmonary TB. The CDC has determined that standard disinfection and sterilization procedures are adequate for devices with these organisms. No changes in procedures for cleaning, disinfecting, or sterilizing need be made. Contaminated noncritical environmental surfaces should be cleaned with an EPA-registered disinfectant-detergent. Individuals cleaning spills should wear disposable gloves.

Table 19.5 shows inactivation of HIV and

Table 19.5. Inactivation of Hepatitis B Virus and Human Immunodeficiency Virus by Disinfectants[a]

Disinfectant	Concentration Inactivating HBV (10 min, 20°C)	Concentration Inactivating HIV (10 min, 25°C)
Chlorine dioxide	ND[b]	1:200 dilution
Ethyl alcohol	Not effective	50%
Formaldehyde	10%	1% formalin
Glutaraldehyde	2%	2%
Hydrogen peroxide	ND	0.3%
Iodophor	80 ppm	0.25%
Isopropyl alcohol	70%	35%
Phenolic	Not effective	0.5%
Quaternary ammonium	Not effective	0.08%
Sodium hypochlorite	500 ppm (0.1% to 1%)	50 ppm

[a]From Berry AJ. Infection control in anesthesia. Anesth Clin North Am 1989;7:967–981; and du Moulin GC, Hedley-Whyte J. Hospital-associated viral infection and the anesthesiologist. Anesthesiology 1983;59:51–65.
[b]No data.

HBV by chemical agents. Disinfectants that are classified as tuberculocidal are adequate for inactivation of HBV (28). HIV is inactivated by a wide range of chemical germicides, even those that are classified as low level.

An infectious agent that may require unique decontamination procedures is the virus of Creutzfeldt-Jakob disease (9,39). This virus is extremely resistant to most methods of disinfection and sterilization. After cleaning, steam sterilization for 1 hr at a temperature of 132°C is recommended for contaminated critical and semicritical equipment. When steam sterilization cannot be used, items should be immersed in 1 N sodium hydroxide for 1 hr at room temperature. Noncritical patient care items or surfaces may be disinfected with either bleach (undiluted, or up to 1:10 dilution) or 1 N sodium hydroxide at room temperature for 15 min (9).

Prevention of Occupational Transmission of Infection to Anesthesia Personnel (3)

USE OF BARRIERS

Appropriate barrier precautions such as gloves, fluid-resistant mask, face shield, and gown must be routinely used with all patients to prevent skin and mucous-membrane ex-posure when any contact with blood or body fluids is possible. The choice of barrier should be commensurate with the expected extent of exposure. It has been demonstrated that 98% of anesthesiologists' contacts with patient blood could be prevented by routine use of gloves (210).

HAND WASHING

Hands should be washed as soon as possible after removing gloves or if contaminated by blood or body fluids.

PREVENTION OF NEEDLESTICKS

Contaminated needles should never be recapped, bent or broken by hand for disposable. If absolutely necessary to recap contaminated needles, a single-handed technique (one in which the needle is never directed toward an unprotected hand) or a mechanical protective device should be used. Use of needleless systems should be encouraged. Puncture-resistant containers for needle disposable must be available in all work locations.

EMERGENCY VENTILATION DEVICES

When emergency mouth-to-mouth resuscitation is indicated, mouthpieces, resuscitation bags, or other ventilation devices should be available.

PERSONNEL WITH CUTANEOUS LESIONS

Healthcare workers with breaks in the skin or exudative/weeping lesions should refrain from direct patient contact unless the open area can be protected.

REFERENCES

1. American National Standards Institute. Guideline for the use of ethylene oxide and steam biological indicators in industrial sterilization processes (ST34–1991). Arlington, VA: Association for the Advancement of Medical Instrumentation, 1991.
2. Rutala WA. Draft guideline for selection and use of disinfectants. Am J Infect Control 1989;17:24A–38A.
3. Arnold WP, Hug CC. Recommendations for infection control for the practice of anesthesiology. Park Ridge, IL: American Society of Anesthesiologists, 1991.
4. Rendell-Baker L. Maintenance, cleaning, and sterilization of anesthesia equipment. In: Ehrenwerth J, Eisenkraft JB, eds. Anesthesia equipment, principles and applications. St. Louis: CV Mosby, 1992:492–511.
5. Favero MS. Principles of sterilization and disinfection. Anesth Clin North Am 1989;7:941–949.
6. Chatburn RL. Decontamination of respiratory care equipment. What can be done, what should be done. Respir Care 1989;34:98.
7. Rosenquist RW, Stock MC. Decontaminating anesthesia and respiratory therapy equipment. Anesth Clin North Am 1989;7:951–966.
8. Wasse L, Curtis M. Sterilization versus disinfection of anesthesia breathing circuits. Safety and economic considerations. J Am Assoc Nurse Anesth 1982;50:161–165.
9. Rutala WA. APIC guidelines for infection control practice. Am J Infect Control 1990;18:99–117.
10. Association for the Advancement of Medical Instrumentation. Selection and use of chemical indicators for steam sterilization monitoring in health care facilities (TIR #3). Arlington, VA: AAMI, 1988.
11. American National Standards Institute. Good hospital practice. Handling and biological decontamination of reusable medical devices (ST35–1991). Arlington, VA: Association for the Advancement of Medical Instrumentation, 1991.
12. Garner JS, Favero MS. CDC guidelines for the prevention and control of nosocomial infections. Am J Infect Control 1986;14:110–129.
13. Wilson RD, Traber DL, Allen CR, Priano LL, Bass J. An evaluation of the Cidematic decontamination system for anesthesia equipment. Anesth Analg 1972;51:658–661.
14. Borick PM, Dondershine FH, Hollis RA. A new automated unit for cleaning and disinfecting anesthesia equipment and other medical instruments. Dev Ind Microbiol 1971;12:266–272.
15. Bennett PJ, Cope DHP, Thompson REM. Decontamination of anaesthetic equipment. Anaesthesia 1968;23:670–675.
16. Fraser VJ, Jones M, Murray PR, Medoff G, Zhang Y, Wallace RJ. Contamination of flexible fiberoptic bronchoscopes with mycobacterium chelonae linked to an automated bronchoscope disinfection machine. Am Rev Respir Dis 1992;145:853–855.
17. Gubler JGH, Salfinger M, von Graevenitz A. Pseudoepidemic of nontuberculous mycobacteria due to a contaminated bronchoscope cleaning machine. Report of an outbreak and review of the literature. Chest 1992;101:1245–1249.
18. Browne RA. Infectious diseases and the anaesthetist. Can J Anaesth 1988;35:655–665.
19. Association for the Advancement of Medical Instrumentation. American national standard for hospital steam sterilizers (ST8–1092). Arlington, VA: American National Standards Institute, 1982.
20. Medical Research Council. Sterilization by steam under increased pressure. Lancet 1959;1:425–435.
21. Rendell-Baker L, Roberts RB. Gas versus steam sterilization: when to use which. Med Surg Rev 1969;5:10–14.
22. Association for the Advancement of Medical Instrumentation. Good hospital practice. Steam sterilization using the unwrapped method (flash sterilization) (SSUM-9/85). Arlington, VA: AAMI, 1985.
23. Hoyt A, Chaney AL, Cavell K. Studies on steam sterilization and the effects of air in the autoclave. J Bacteriol 1938;36:639–652.
24. Association for the Advancement of Medical Instrumentation. Biological indicators for saturated steam sterilization processes in health care facilities (ST19–1985). Arlington, VA: American National Standards Institute, 1985.
25. Anonymous. Biological sterilization indicators for steam, EtO & radiation developed by NAmSA. Biomed Safe Stand 1984;14(3):31.
26. Rice HM. Testing of air-filters for hospital sterilizers. Lancet 1958;2:1275–1277.
27. Ascenzi JM, Wendt TM, McDowell JW. Important information concerning the reuse of glutaraldehyde-based disinfectants and their tuberculocidal activity. Arlington, TX: Surgikos Inc, Research Division, October 1984.
28. Berry AJ. Infection control in anesthesia. Anesth Clin North Am 1989;7:967–981.

29. U.S. Department of Health, Education and Welfare. Selection and use of disinfectants in health facilities (HEW Publication #HSM 72–4008). Washington, DC: U.S. Government Printing Office, 1967.

30. Hope T. Prepackaging and sterilization of anesthetic equipment. Nurs Times 1964;60:251–252.

31. Padnos E, Horwitz I, Wunder G. Contact dermititis complicating tracheostomy. Am J Dis Child 1965;109:90–91.

32. Wahlberg JE. Two cases of hypersensitivity to quaternary ammonium compounds. Acta Derm Venereol (Stockh) 1964;42:230–234.

33. Spaulding EH. Chemical disinfection and antisepsis in the hospital. J Hosp Res 1972;9:7–31.

34. Stark DC. Sterilization by chemical agents in infections and sterilization problems. Int Anesth Clin 1972;10:49–65.

35. Herwick RP, Treweek ON. Burns from anesthesia mask sterilized in compound solution of cresol. JAMA 1933;100:407–408.

36. Kahn G. Depigmentation caused by phenolic detergent germicides. Arch Dermatol 1970;102:177–187.

37. Spaulding EH. Principles and application of chemical disinfection. AORN J 1963;1:36–46.

38. Ayliffe GAJ. Hospital disinfection and antibiotic policies. Chemotherapy 1987;6:228–233.

39. du Moulin GC, Hedley-Whyte J. Hospital-associated viral infection and the anesthesiologist. Anesthesiology 1983;59:51–65.

40. Babb JR, Bradley CR, Deverill CEA, Ayliffe GAJ, Melikian V. Recent advances in the cleaning and disinfection of fiberoscopes. J Hosp Infect 1981;2:329–340.

41. Garcia de Cabo A, Larriba PLM, Pinilla JC, Sanz FG. A new method of disinfection of the flexible fiberbronchoscope. Thorax 1978;33:270–272.

42. Talbot GH, Skros M, Provencher M. 70% alcohol disinfection of transducer heads: experimental trials. Infect Control 1985;6:237–239.

43. Platt R, Lehr JL, Marino S, Munoz A, Nash B, Raemer DB. Safe and cost-effective cleaning of pressure monitoring transducers. Infect Control Hosp Epidemiol 1988;9:409–416.

44. Beck–Sague CM, Jarvis WR. Epidemic bloodstream infections associated with pressure transducers: a persistent problem. Infect Control Hosp Epidemiol 1989;10:54–59.

45. Spaulding EWH. Alcohol as a surgical disinfectant. AORN J 1964;2:67–71.

46. Favero MS. Sterilization, disinfection, and antisepsis in the hospital. In: Lennette EH, Balows A, Hausler WJ, Shadomy HJ eds. Manual of clinical microbiology. Washington, DC: American Society for Microbiology, 1985:129–137.

47. Kralovic RC, Badertscher DC. Bactericidal and sporicidal efficacy of a peracetic acid based liquid chemical sterilant [Abstract Q114.302]. Paper presented at the annual meeting of the American Society of Microbiologists, 1988.

48. Martin LS, McDougal JS, Loskoski SL. Disinfection and inactivation of the human T lymphotrophic virus type III/lymphadenopathy-associated virus. J Infect Dis 1985;152:400–403.

49. Spire B, Barre-sinoussi F, Montagnier L, Shermann JC. Inactivation of lymphadenopathy-associated virus by chemical disinfectants. Lancet 1984;2:899–901.

50. Brown P, Gibbs CJ, Amyx HL, et al. Chemical disinfection of Creutzfeld-Jakob disease virus. N Engl J Med 1982;306:1279–1282.

51. Gajdusek DC, Gibbs CJ, Asher DM, et al. Precautions in medical care of and in handling materials from patients with transmissible virus dementia (Creutzfeld-Jakob disease). N Engl J Med 1977;297:1253–1258.

52. Hoffman PN, Death JE, Coates D. The stability of sodium hypochlorite solutions. In: Collins CH, Allwood MC, Bloomfeld SF, Fox A eds. Disinfectants: their use and evaluation of effectiveness. London: Academic Press, 1981.

53. Rutala WA, Cole EC, Thomann CA. Stability and bactericidal activity of chlorine solutions [Abstract 1150]. Paper presented at the twenty-seventh Interscience Conference on Antimicrobal Agents and Chemotherapy, 1987.

54. Schaeffer AJ, Jones JM, Amundsen SK. Bactericidal effect of hydrogen peroxide on urinary tract pathogens. Appl Environ Microbiol 1980;40:337–340.

55. Mentel R, Schmidt J, Investigations on rhinovirus inactivation by hydrogen peroxide. Acta Virol (Praha) 1973;17:451–354.

56. Wardle MD, Renninger GM. Bactericidal effect of hydrogen peroxide on spacecraft isolates. Appl Microbiol 1975;30:710–711.

57. Turner FJ. Hydrogen peroxide and other oxidant disinfectants. In: Block SS, ed. Disinfection, sterilization and preservation. 3rd ed. Philadelphia: Lea & Febiger, 1983:240–250.

58. Leaper S. Influence of temperature on the synergistic sporicidal effect of peracetic acid plus hydrogen peroxide in Bacillus subtitis SA22(NCA 72–52). Food Microbiol 1984;1:199–203.

59. Leach ED. A new synergized glutaraldehyde-phenate sterilizing solution and concentrated disinfectant. Infect Control 1981;2:26–30.

60. Townsend TR, Wee S-B, Koblin B. An efficacy evaluation of a synergized glutaraldehyde-phenate solution in disinfecting respiratory therapy equipment contaminated during patient use. Infect Control 1982;3:240–243.

61. Masferrer R, Marquez R. Comparison of two ac-

tivated glutaraldehyde solutions. Cidex solution and sonacide. Respir Care 1977;22:257–262.

62. Collins FM, Montalbine V. Mycobactericidal activity of glutaraldehyde solutions. J Clin Microbiol 1976;4:408–412.

63. American Conference of Government Industrial Hygenists. Documentation of threshold limit values. 4th ed. p. 204.

64. Anonymous. Ethylene oxide sterilization. Health Devices 1975;5:27–50.

65. Stonehill AA, Krop S, Borick PM. Buffered glutaraldehyde—a new chemical sterilizing solution. Am J Hosp Pharm 1963;20:458–465.

66. Borick PM, Dondershine FH, Chandler VL. Alkalinized glutaraldehyde, a new antimicrobial agent. J Pharm Sci 1964;53:1273–1275.

67. Borick PM. Chemical sterilizers (chemosterilizers). Adv Appl Microbiol 1968;10:291–312.

68. Borick PM. Antimicrobial agents as liquid chemosterilizers. Biotechnol Bioeng 1965;7:435–443.

69. Kelsey JC, Mackinnon IH, Maurer IM. Sporicidal aspects of hospital disinfectants. J Clin Pathol 1974;27:632–638.

70. Haselhuhn DH, Brason FW, Borick PM. "In use" study of buffered glutaraldehyde for cold sterilization of anesthesia equipment. Anesth Analg 1967;46:468–474.

71. Pepper RE, Chandler VL. Sporicidal activity of alkaline alcoholic saturated dialdehyde solutions. J Appl Microbiol 1968;11:384–388.

72. Roberts RB. The anaesthetist, cross-infection and sterilization techniques—a review. Anaesth Intensive Care 1973;1:400–406.

73. Richards M, Levitsky S. Outbreak of Serratia marcescens infections in a cardiothoracic surgical intensive care unit. Ann Thorac Cardiovasc Surg 1975;19:503–513.

74. Snyder RW. Cheatle EL. Alkaline glutaraldehyde as effective disinfectant. Am J Hosp Pharm 1965;22:321–327.

75. Miner NA, McDowell JW, Willcockson GW, Bruckner NI, Stark RL, Whitmore EJ. Antimicrobial and other properties of a new stabilized alkaline glutaraldehyde disinfectant/sterilizer. Am J Hosp Pharm 1977;34:376–382.

76. Saitanu K, Lund E. Inactivation of enterovirus by gluteraldehyde. Appl Soc Microbiol 1975;29:571–574.

77. American Hospital Association. Ethylene oxide sterilization (Guideline Report #8, AHA Technology Series). Chicago: AHA, Division of Management and Technology, 1982.

78. Iddenden FR. New decontamination procedure cuts costs—reduces staff time. Can Hosp 1972;49:26–28.

79. Becker KO. Inhalation therapy department chooses ETO. Hospitals 1971;45:108–111.

80. Belani KG, Priedkalns J. An epidemic of pseudomembranous laryngotracheitis. Anesthesiology 1977;47:530–531.

81. Mostafa SM. Adverse effects of buffered glutaraldehyde on the Heidbrink expiratory valve. Br J Anaesth 1980;52:223–227.

82. Fisher AA. Reactions to glutaraldehyde with particular reference to radiologists and x-ray technicians. Cutis 1981;28:113, 114, 119.

83. Lin KS, Park MK, Baker HA, Sidorowicz A. Disinfection of anesthesia and respiratory therapy equipment with acid glutaraldehyde solution. Respir Care 1979;24:321–327.

84. Anonymous. EPA chlorofluorocarbon restrictions. Price increases certain & medical uses may be banned. Biomed Safe Stand 1988;18:125–126.

85. Automatic, general-purpose ethylene oxide sterilizers and ethylene oxide sterilant sources intended for use in health care facilities (ST24–1987). Arlington, VA: AAMI, 1987.

86. Association for the Advancement of Medical Instrumentation. Selecting airborne ethylene oxide monitoring equipment or services for an EO gas sterilization facility (TIR #1). Arlington, VA: AAMI, 1984.

87. Association for the Advancement of Medical Instrumentation. Good hospital practice: performance evaluation of ethylene oxide sterilizers—ethylene oxide test packs. Arlington, VA: AAMI, 1985.

88. Association for the Advancement of Medical Instrumentation. Good hospital practice: ethylene oxide gas ventilation recommendations and safe use. Arlington, VA: AAMI, 1981.

89. Association for the Advancement of Medical Instrumentation. Automatic, general-purpose ethylene oxide sterilizers and ethylene oxide sterilant sources intended for use in health care facilities. Arlington, VA: AAMI, 1987.

90. Canadian Standards Association. Ethylene oxide sterilizers for hospitals (CSA Standard Z314.1-M1977). Rexdale, Ont. Canada: CSA, 1977.

91. Anonymous. Ethylene oxide sterilization. Hospitals 1971;45:99–100.

92. Fitzpatrick BG, Reich RR. ETO sterilization monitoring: a performance study. J Health Care Mater Manag 1986;4:32–35.

93. Andersen SR, Halleck F, Kaye S, Scheide EM, Schneier ML. Technological innovations in sterilizer design. In: Association for the Advancement of Medical Instrumentation, ed. Inhospital ethylene oxide sterilization. Current issues in EO toxicity and occupational exposure (TAR #8-84). Arlington, VA: AAMI, 1984:21–22.

94. Steenland K, Stayner L, Greife A, et al. Mortality among workers exposed to ethylene oxide. New Eng J Med 1991;324:1402–1407.

95. American National Standards Institute. Biological indicators for ethylene oxide sterilization processes in health care facilities (ST21–1986). Arlington, VA: Association for the Advancement of Medical Instrumentation, 1986.

96. Rendell-Baker L. Ethylene oxide. II. Aeration. Int Anesthesiol Clin 1972;10(2):101–122.

97. American National Standards Institute Sectional Committee Z-79 and ASA Subcommittee on Standardization. Ethylene oxide sterilization of anesthesia apparatus. Anesthesiology 1970;33:120.

98. Andersen SR. Ethylene oxide residues in medical materials. Bull Parenteral Drug Assoc 1973;27:49–57.

99. Anonymous. The physician and the law. Anesth Analg 1970;49:889.

100. Lipton B, Gutierrez R, Blaugrund S, Litwak RS, Rendell-Baker L. Irradiated PVC plastic and gas sterilization in the production of tracheal stenosis following tracheostomy. Anesth Analg 1971;50:578–586.

101. Russell JP. The sterilization dilemma. Where will it end—laboratory aspects. Anesth Analg 1968;47:653–656.

102. Anonymous. Aeration of anesthesia equipment. Hosp Top 1966;44:115.

103. O'Leary RK, Guess WL. The toxiogenic potential of medical plastics sterilized with ethylene oxide vapors. J Biomed Mater Res 1968;2:297–311.

104. Clarke CP, Davidson WL, Johnston JB. Haemolysis of blood following exposure to an Australian manufactured plastic tubing sterilized by means of ethylene oxide gas. Aust N Z J Surg 1966;36:53–56.

105. Hirose T, Goldstein R, Bailey CP. Hemolysis of blood due to exposure to different types of plastic tubing and the influence of ethylene oxide sterilization. J Thorac Cardiovasc Surg 1963;45:245–251.

106. Poothullil J, Shimizu A, Day RP, Dolovich J. Anaphylaxis from the product(s) of ethylene oxide gas. Ann Intern Med 1975;82:58–60.

107. Anonymous. Health risk due to EtO residue on sterilized devices is negligible—HIMA. Biomed Safe Stand 1988;18:138–139.

108. Glaser ZR. Special occupation hazard review with control recommendations for the use of ethylene oxide as a sterilant in medical facilities (Publication No. 77-200). Washington, DC: U.S. Department of Health, Education, and Welfare (NIOSH), 1977.

109. Roberts RB. Gamma Rays + PVC + EO = OK. Respir Care 1976;21:223–224.

110. Stetson JB, Whitbourne JE, Eastman C. Ethylene oxide degassing of rubber and plastic materials. Anesthesiology 1976;44:174–180.

111. Bogdansky S, Lehn PJ. Effects of gamma-irradia-tion on 2-chloro-ethanol formation in ethylene oxide-sterilized polyvinyl chloride. J Pharm Sci 1964;63:802–803.

112. Bryson TK, Saidman LJ, Nelson W. A potential hazard connected with the resterilization and reuse of disposable equipment. Anesthesiology 1979;50:370.

113. Rendell-Baker L. A hazard alert—reinforced endotracheal tubes. Anesthesiology 1980;53:268–269.

114. Anderson SR. Ethylene oxide toxicity. J Lab Clin Med 1971;77:346–355.

115. Andersen SR. Experimentally produced skin reactions to ethylene oxide. In: Association for the Advancement of Medical Instrumentation, ed. Inhospital ethylene oxide sterilization. Current issues in EO toxicity and occupational exposure (TAR # 8–84). Arlington, VA: AAMI, 1984:21–22.

116. Garry VF. Some thoughts on medical surveillance for ethylene oxide exposure. In: Association for the Advancement of Medical Instrumentation, ed. Inhospital ethylene oxide sterilization. Current issues in EO toxicity and occupational exposure (TAR # 8–84). Arlington, VA: AAMI, 1984:1–3.

117. Marshall C, Dolovitch J. Potential effects on humans of short-term high-dose exposure: allergic reactions to ethylene oxide-clinical data and symptoms. In: Association for the Advancement of Medical Instrumentation, ed. Inhospital ethylene oxide sterilization. Current issues in EO toxicity and occupational exposure (TAR #8–84). Arlington, VA: AAMI, 1984:26–27.

118. Anonymous. Hospital employees treated after ethylene oxide leak. Biomed Safe Stand 1992;22:145, 147.

119. Gross JA, Haas ML, Swift TR. Ethylene oxide neurotoxicity. report of four cases and review of the literature. Neurology 1979;29:978–983.

120. Morgan TF. Potential effects on humans of short-term high dose exposure. Effects on the nervous system—clinical data and symptoms. In: Association for the Advancement of Medical Instrumentation, ed. Inhospital ethylene oxide sterilization. Current issues in EO toxicity and occupational exposure (TAR #8–84). Arlington, VA: AAMI, 1984:23–25.

121. Royce A, Moore WKS. Occupational dermatitis caused by ethylene oxide. Br J Ind Med 1955;12:169–171.

122. Lynch DW, Lewis TR, Moorman WJ, et al. Effects on monkeys and rats of long-term inhalation exposure to ethylene oxide. Major findings of the NIOSH Study. In: Association for the Advancement of Medical Instrumentation, ed. Inhospital ethylene oxide sterilization. Current issues in EO toxicity and occupational exposure (TAR #8–84). Arlington, VA: AAMI, 1984:7–10.

123. Garry VF. Sister chromatid exchange in human lymphocytes following exposure to ethylene oxide. In: Association for the Advancement of Medical Instrumentation, ed. Inhospital ethylene oxide sterilization. Current issues in EO toxicity and occupational exposure (TAR #8–84). Arlington, VA: AAMI, 1984:28–30.

124. Hogstedt C, Aringer L, Gukstavsson A. Epidemiologic support for ethylene oxide as a cancer-causing agent. JAMA 1986;255:1575–1578.

125. Hogstedt C, Malmqvist N, Wadman G. Leukemia in workers exposed to ethylene oxide. JAMA 1979;241:1132–1133.

126. Anonymous. Deaths from CFC-113 exposure subject of NIOSH alert. Biomed Safe Stand 1990;20(16):121–122.

127. Anonymous. Ethylene oxide exposure. 15-minute "excursion limit" established by OSHA. Biomed Safe Stand 1988;18:70.

128. Gschwandtner G, Kruger D, Harman P. Compliance with the EtO standard in the United States. J Health Care Mater Manag 1986;4:38–41.

129. Manheimer A. Ethylene oxide: the silent hazard. Respir Ther 1978;8:19–22, 74.

130. Anonymous. Revised guidelines for EO sterilization. AORN J 1976;24:1086–1088.

131. Daley WJ, Morse WA, Ridgway MG. Ethylene oxide control in hospitals. Chicago: American Society of Hospital Central Service Personnel and American Society for Hospital Engineering of the American Hospital Association, 1979.

132. Morford SD. Facility design and engineering controls. In: Association for the Advancement of Medical Instrumentation, ed. Inhospital ethylene oxide sterilization. Current issues in EO toxicity and occupational exposure (TAR #8–84). Arlington, VA: AAMI, 1984:49–51.

133. Grunberg RD. Personal respiratory protection for sterilization processing personnel. In: Association for the Advancement of Medical Instrumentation, ed. Inhospital ethylene oxide sterilization. Current issues in EO toxicity and occupational exposure (TAR #8–84). Arlington, VA: AAMI, 1984:66–67.

134. Samuels TM. Personnel exposures to ethylene oxide in a central service assembly and sterilization area. Hosp Top 1978;56:27–33.

135. Anonymous. Field evaluation of EtO exposure levels. Health Devices 1982;11:249–252.

136. Meeker MH. Inhospital control of EO residue levels through good aeration practices. In: Association for the Advancement of Medical Instrumentation, ed. Inhospital ethylene oxide sterilization. Current issues in EO toxicity and occupational exposure (TAR #8–84). Arlington, VA: AAMI, 1984:85–87.

137. Gunther DA, Barron WR, Durnick TJ, Young JH.

Sources of environmental ethylene oxide gas contamination in a simulated sterilization facility. Paper presented at the 16th annual meeting of the Association for the Advancement of Medical Instrumentation, Washington, DC, May 11, 1981.

138. Anonymous. Safe use of EtO sterilizer aided by new ventilation cabinet. Biomed Safe Stand 1983;13:44.

139. Ridgeway M. Environmental and employee monitoring. Current techniques. In: Association for the Advancement of Medical Instrumentation, ed. Inhospital ethylene oxide sterilization. Current issues in EO toxicity and occupational exposure (TAR #8–84). Arlington, VA: AAMI, 1984:95–97.

140. Denny FJ, Jr. Cost-effective EO Monitoring. the experience of the US Veterans Administration. In: Association for the Advancement of Medical Instrumentation, ed. Inhospital ethylene oxide sterilization. Current issues in EO toxicity and occupational exposure (TAR #8–84). Arlington, VA: AAMI, 1984:98–101.

141. Reichert M. Cost-effective EO monitoring in a health care facility: the experience of Robinson Memorial Hospital. In: Association for the Advancement of Medical Instrumentation, ed. Inhospital ethylene oxide sterilization. Current issues in EO toxicity and occupational exposure (TAR #8–84). Arlington, VA: AAMI, 1984:102–104.

142. Loving TJ, Wooter LL. Cost-effective ethylene oxide monitoring: a case study. In: Association for the Advancement of Medical Instrumentation, ed. Inhospital ethylene oxide sterilization. Current issues in EO toxicity and occupational exposure (TAR #8–84). Arlington, VA: AAMI, 1984:105–107.

143. Anonymous. New passive dosimeter designed for personal and area monitoring for EO gas vapors. Biomed Safe Stand 1986;16:21.

144. Anonymous. EtO & formaldehyde exposure measured by personal monitoring badges. Biomed Safe Stand 1988;18:110.

145. Anonymous. Passive diffusion monitor detects ethylene oxide. Biomed Safe Stand 1988;18:101.

146. Anonymous. Personal chemical exposure monitor badges developed. Biomed Safe Stand 1989;19:29.

147. Anonymous. EtO monitoring analyzer based on crystal growth. Biomed Safe Stand 1990;20:126.

148. Reichert MC. Ethylene oxide environmental monitoring in a health care facility. Med Instrum 1983;17:113–115.

149. Qazi A, Ketcham NH. A new method for monitoring personal exposure to ethylene oxide in the occupational environment. Am Ind Hyg Assoc J 1977;38:635–647.

150. McCullough CE. Microcomputer-based system for real-time computation of time-weighted aver-

age levels of ethylene oxide and other gases. Med Instrum 1985;19:136–140.

151. Anonymous. ETO. 16 commonly asked questions . . . and their answers. J Health Care Mater Manag 1986;4:42.

152. Loving TJ, Wooter LL. Cost-effective ethylene oxide exposure control: a case study. In: Association for the Advancement of Medical Instrumentation, ed. Inhospital ethylene oxide sterilization. Current issues in EO toxicity and occupational exposure (TAR #8–84). Arlington, VA: AAMI, 1984:69–73.

153. Reichart M. Reducing occupational exposure in a health care facility: the experience of Robinson Memorial Hospital. In: Association for the Advancement of Medical Instrumentation, ed. Inhospital ethylene oxide sterilization. Current issues in EO toxicity and occupational exposure (TAR #8–84). Arlington, VA: AAMI, 1984:74–77.

154. Anonymous. New pollution control system designed for hospital EtO sterilizers. Biomed Safe Stands 1986;16:126.

155. Anonymous. Hazard. Amdek Boekel sterilizer. Health Devices 1975;5:50–51.

156. Anonymous. Hazard. 3M models 100 and 200 sterilizers. Health Devices 1975;5:51.

157. Halleck FE. Hazards of EO sterilization in hospitals. Hosp Top 1975;53:45–52.

158. Association for the Advancement of Medical Instrumentation. Process control guidelines for gamma radiation sterilization of medical devices (RS-3/84). Arlington, VA: AAMI, 1984.

159. Olander JW. New facilities and equipment for radiation sterilization. Bull Parenteral Drug Assoc 1963;17:14–21.

160. Artandi C. Sterilization by ionizing radiation. Int Anesthesiol Clin 1972;10(2):123–130.

161. Thomas ET. The sterilization dilemma. Where will it end? Clinical aspects. Anesth Analg 1968;47:657–662.

162. Hamilton WK, Feeley TW. A need for aseptic inhalation anesthesia equipment for each case is unproven. In: Eckenhoff JE, ed. Controversy in anesthesiology. Philadelphia: WB Saunders, 1979:84.

163. Dryden GE. Inhalation anesthesia equipment should be aseptic for each use. In Eckenhoff JE, ed. Controversy in anesthesiology. Philadelphia: WB Saunders, 1979:73–83.

164. Du Moulin GC, Saubermann AJ. The anesthesia machine and circle system are not likely to be sources of bacterial contamination. Anesthesiology 1977;47:353–358.

165. Feeley TW, Hamilton WK, Xavier B, Moyers J, Eger EI. Sterile anesthesia breathing circuits do not prevent postoperative pulmonary infection. Anesthesiology 1982;54:369–372.

166. Olds JW, Kisch AL, Eberle BJ, Wilson JN. Pseudomonas aeruginosa respiratory tract infection acquired from a contaminated anesthesia machine. Am Rev Respir Dis 1972;105:628–632.

167. Joseph JM. Disease transmission by inefficiently sanitized anesthetizing apparatus. JAMA 1952;149:1196–1198.

168. Spengler RF, Greenlough WB III. Hospital costs and mortality attributed to nosocomial bacteremias. JAMA 1978;240:2455–2458.

169. Ping FC, Oulton JL, Smith JA, Skidmore AG, Jenkins LC. Bacterial filters—are they necessary on anaesthetic machines. Can Anaesth Soc J 1979;26:415–419.

170. Garibaldi RA, Britt MR, Webster C, Pace NL. Failure of bacterial filters to reduce the incidence of pneumonia after inhalation anesthesia. Anesthesiology 1981;54:364–368.

171. Luney SR, Milligan KR, Armstrong MB, Alexander JP. The role of bacterial airway filters in the prevention of nosocomial pneumonia in the intensive care unit. Anesth Analg 1993;76:S230.

172. Lees DE. To reuse or not to reuse, that is the question. ASA Newslett 1992;56:13–15.

173. Walton JR. A new controversy in respiratory equipment management. Reusables versus disposed disposables versus reused disposables. Respir Care 1986;31:213–217.

174. Campbell BA, Wells GA, Palmer WN, Martin DL. Reuse of disposable medical devices in Canadian Hospitals. Am J Infect Control 1987;15:196–200.

175. Gadalla F, Fong J. Improved infection control in the operating room. Anesthesiology 1990;73:1295.

176. Garner JS, Simmons BP. Guidelines for isolation precautions in hospitals. Infect Control 1983;4:245–325.

177. Centers for Disease Control. Acquired immune deficiency syndrome (AIDS): precautions for clinical and laboratory staffs. MMWR 1982;31:577–580.

178. Anonymous. Standards for cleaning and processing anesthesia equipment. AORN J 1977;25:1268–1274.

179. Boyce JM, White RL, Spruill EY, Wall M. Cost-effective application of the Centers for Disease Control guideline for prevention of nosocomial pneumonia. Am J Infect Control 1985;13:228–232.

180. Murphy PM, Fitzgeorge RB, Barrett RF. Viability and distribution of bacteria after passage through a circle anaesthetic system. Br J Anaesth 1991;66:300–304.

181. du Moulin GC, Hedley-Whyte J. Bacterial interactions between anesthesiologists, their patients, and equipment. Anesthesiology 1982;57:37–41.

182. Chrusciel C, Mayhall CG, Embrey J, Weir S, Russell M. A comparative study of bacterial contami-

nation of reusable and disposable soda lime absorbers. Anesth Analg 1988;67:S31.

183. Brown RA, Bell R, Pine W, Bosnjak T. Sterilization of anaesthetic equipment. Can J Anaesth 1989;36:359–361.

184. Gibbons CP. Care of anesthesia equipment. Hosp Top 1964;44:109–115.

185. George RH. A critical look at chemical disinfection of anaesthetic apparatus. Br J Anaesth 1975;47:719–722.

186. Clark R. Sterilization of anaesthetic apparatus. In: Proceedings of the third Asian and Australian congress of anesthesia, 1970. London: Butterworth, 1971.

187. Ibrahim JJ, Perceval AK. Contamination of anaesthetic tubing—a real hazard? Anaesth Intensive Care. 1992;20:317–321.

188. Baker R. Sonic energy cleaning in inhalation therapy. Inhal Ther 1968;13:56.

189. Gurevich I, Tafuro P, Ristuccia P, Herrmann J, Young AR, Cunha BA. Disinfection of respirator tubing: a comparison of chemical versus hot water machine-assisted processing. J Hosp Infect 1983;4:199–208.

190. Maltais EA, Webber IM. Disinfection of anesthesia equipment-why not? J Am Assoc Nurse Anesth 1970;38:217–218.

191. Barry AE, Noble MA, Marrie TJ, Paterson IJ. Cleaning of anaesthesia breathing circuits and tubings: a Canadian survey. Can Anaesth Soc J 1984;31:572–575.

192. Enright AC, Moore RL, Parney FL. Contamination and resterilization of the Bain circuit. Can Anaesth Soc J 1976;23:545–549.

193. Schnierson SS. Sterilization by heat. Int Anesthesiol Clin 1972;10(2):67–83.

194. MacCallum FO, Noble WC. Disinfection of anaesthetic face masks. Anaesthesia 1960;15:307–309.

195. Beeuwkes H, Vijver AED. Disinfection in anaesthesia. Br J Anaesth 1959;31:363–366.

196. Barnette RE, Pietrzak WT, BianRosa JJ. On preventing transmission of viral infections. Anesthesiology 1985;62:845.

197. Roberts RB. Cleaning the laryngoscope blade. Can Anaesth Soc J 1973;20:241–244.

198. de Cabo AG, Larriba PLM, Pinila JC, Sanz FG. A new method of disinfection of the flexible fibrebronchoscope. Thorax 1978;33:270–272.

199. Moore MW, Bowe EA, Turner JF, Baysinger CL. Opened endotracheal tubes can be saved. Anesthesiology 1992;77:A1059.

200. Bosomworth PP, Hamelberg W. Effect of sterilization techniques on safety and durability of endotracheal tubes. Anesth Analg 1965;44:576–584.

201. Bamforth BJ. Questions & answers. Anesth Analg 1963;42:658.

202. Keenleyside HB. Reaction to improperly cleaned endotracheal catheter. Anesthesiology 1957;18:505–506.

203. Fierer J, Taylor PM, Gezon HM. Pseudomonas aeruginosa epidemic traced to delivery-room resuscitators. N Eng J Med 1967;276:991–996.

204. Thompson AC, Wilder BJ, Powner DJ. Bedside resuscitation bags. A source of bacterial contamination. Infect Control 1985;6:231–232.

205. Cartwright RY, Hargrove PRJ. Hazard of self-inflating resuscitation bags. Br Med J 1969;4:302.

206. Beard MA, McIntyre A, Rountree PM. Sphygmomanometers as a reservoir of pathogenic bacteria. Med J Aust 1969;2:758–760.

207. Sternlicht AL, VanPoznak A. Significant bacterial colonization occurs on the surface of non-disposable sphygmomanometer cuffs and re-used disposable cuffs. Anesth Analg 1990;70:S450.

208. Centers for Disease Control. Epidmiologic notes and reports: Nosocomial *Pseudomonas cepacia* bacteremia caused by contaminated pressure transducers. MMWR 1974;23(49):423.

209. Centers for Disease Control. Sterilization and disinfection of hospital supplies. MMWR 1977;26:266.

210. Kristensen M, Sloth E, Jensen TK. Relationship between anesthetic procedure and contact of anesthesia personnel with patient body fluids. Anesthesiology 1990;73:619–624.

Index

Page numbers followed by a "t" denote tables; those followed by "f" denote figures.